Vyas's Comprehensive Textbook of Surgery

2nd Edition

Vyas's Comprehensive Textbook of Surgery

2nd Edition

Editors in Chief

Vijay K. Mittal,
MD, FAIS, FICS, FICA, FACS
Former Program Director Surgery
Associate Director of Medical Education
Ascension Providence Hospital, Southfield
Professor of Surgery
Wayne State University
School of Medicine, Detroit, Michigan
Michigan State University
College of Human Medicine, Lansing, Michigan

Dinesh Vyas
MD, FACS
Associate Professor of Surgery
Chair Department of Surgery
College of Medicine
California Northstate University
CMO (Quality) Adventist Dameron, California
Former Program Director Surgery
Former Associate Dean, Research [Surgery]

Editors

Mayur Narayan,
MD, MPH, MBA, FACS
Divion Head of Trauma and Acute Care Surgery
Rutgers University, New Jersey

Rajiv Vohra,
MBBS, MS, FRCSEd, PhD
Consultant Vascular Surgery
University of Birmingham, UK

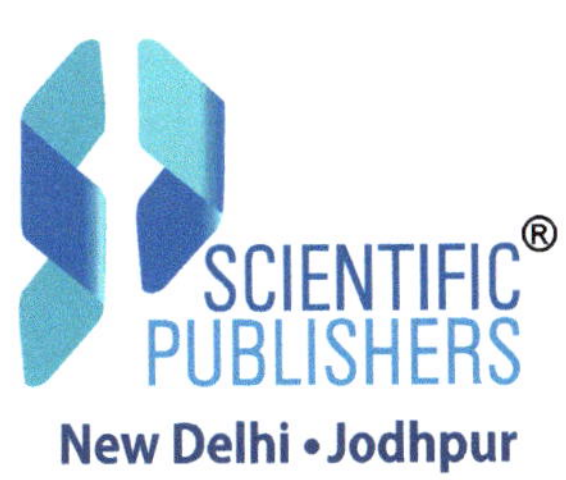

New Delhi • Jodhpur

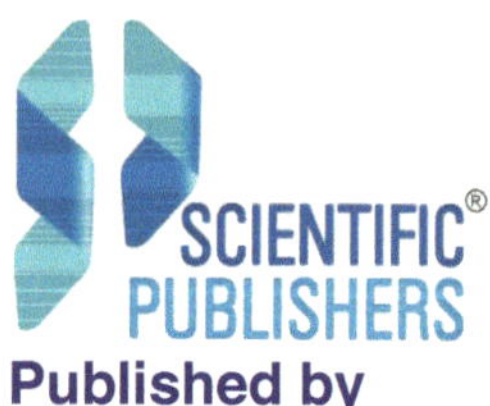

Published by

Jodhpur
5 A, New Pali Road, P.O. Box 91
Jodhpur - 342 001 Rajasthan (India)
E-mail: info@scientificpub.com
Website: www.scientificpubonline.com

New Delhi
4806/24, Ansari Road, Daryaganj,
New Delhi - 110 002 (India)

ISBN: 978-93-94645-59-2 H/B

eISBN: 978-93-94645-60-8 E/B

Printed in India

Dedication:

This textbook is dedicated to:

Dr. Vijay Mittal's late wife, Suresh Lata Mittal, whose constant support and endless sacrifices created a legacy and provided Dr. Mittal the strength to impact the lives of many as a transplant surgeon and program director.

Dr. Dinesh Vyas' brother Mahesh Vyas, an Orthopedic Surgeon (1966-1997) and father Purshottam Das Vyas, a Scientist, Educationist, and Social Worker (1933-2000). Both influenced Dr. Vyas to pursue medicine for those who need it the most.

Preface

This is the second edition of the *Vyas's Comprehensive Textbook of Surgery*, a collaborative effort by distinguished surgical educators. Throughout the development process, the editors and authors remained mindful of the practical limitations and variations involved in treating most general surgical conditions. The result is a comprehensive clinical review that contains numerous practical insights and thousands of illustrations and figures. While the main focus of this book is on the medical and operative management of conditions in the field of general surgery and subspecialties, it also provides extensive coverage of medical management and non-operative treatment of various surgical conditions. The book is written in simple, easy-to-understand language, making it accessible to a wide range of readers, including medical and nursing students, surgery residents, practicing and academic surgeons, and others interested in surgery.

The primary purpose of this book is to provide practical advice on current best practices in surgery. It serves as an easily accessible resource for surgeons seeking information on basic and new surgical diseases, including options for diagnosing diseases and treatment options. The authors provide a rationale for why certain treatments are preferred over others, as well as guidance on managing complications. In addition to providing an overview of general surgery and subspecialties, this textbook also includes discussions of the history of surgery from seven thousand BC, evolution and limitation of TNM staging, simulation, education, clinical research, rural surgery, interventional radiology, and new surgical approaches (such as laparoscopic, endoscopic, and robotic surgery).

Overall, this textbook is a valuable resource for anyone interested in surgery, and is sure to be a go-to reference for surgeons seeking practical advice on the latest techniques and best practices in the field.

Editor's note

Writing a textbook is a fulfilling endeavor and an opportunity to disseminate the art and science of surgery from the editor's perspective. Surgeons and trainees learn different aspects of surgery from different authors; therefore, this textbook will add value to the existing surgical literature. The second edition of *Comprehensive Textbook of Surgery* has been in the works for the past decade, bringing together bright minds from across the world and from some of the best institutions to create a concise resource of knowledge, equivalent to at least 2000 years of experience. Particularly unique to this textbook is the historical, innovative, and global perspective of surgery that could only come from the work of the over one-hundred contributors.

As editors-in-chief, we wholeheartedly appreciate the work of the editors, editorial assistants from California Northstate University, Tanay Sharma and his team at Scientific Publishers, cover page illustrator Wenjia Wang, and all contributors who aided in accomplishing this massive feat. This project could not have happened without our editors Dr. Mayur Narayan from Rutgers University and Dr. Rajiv Vohra from University of Birmingham who provided relentless support, inspiration, and guidance in authoring and editing major portions of this textbook. Next, we must recognize executive editorial assistant Kayla Umemoto, whose initiative and diligence played an essential role in the execution of this textbook. She swiftly managed, executed, and oversaw fulfillment of the material. Professor K Kant from S.N. Medical College in India who supported the global aspect of surgical care and innovation.

We would also like to thank the patients who trusted us with their lives so that we could work with and learn from them. Lastly, I would like to acknowledge the everlasting strength, support, patience, and vision of my wife Arpita, my mother Shyama, my daughter Anoushka, and my son Advitiya which enabled me to complete this vision.

This textbook is a continuation of the previous hard work that resulted in the first edition of *Comprehensive Textbook of Surgery* and this momentum will carry us through future endeavors. Thank you for your time, we hope you enjoy this textbook.

Sincerely,

Dinesh Vyas, MD, FACS
Associate Professor of Surgery, Chair Department of Surgery
California Northstate University
CMO (Quality) Adventist Dameron Hospital
Stockton, California

Vijay Mittal, MD, FAIS (Hon.), FICS, FICA, FACS
Former Program Director, Surgery Residency
Associate Director of Medical Education
Ascension Providence Hospital
Southfield, Michigan
Professor of Surgery

Introduction

Vyas's Comprehensive Textbook of Surgery has been written as a book containing much information that will be encountered by the general surgeon. The target audience of this book includes medical students, nursing students, surgery residents, and surgeons; therefore, it is written in a simple and easy to understand language. The purpose of this book is to be an easily accessible resource for surgeons that provides practical advice on the current best practice available. A group of seven distinguished and accomplished editors, along with over a hundred contributors have provided much information on basic and new surgical diseases, incorporating options for diagnosing diseases, treatment options and explaining why certain treatments should be used over others, and the management of complications. In addition to providing a basic overview of general surgery, we incorporated different ways of practicing surgery including the practice of clinical research, rural surgery, interventional radiology, new surgical approaches (i.e., laparoscopic, endoscopic, and robotic surgery), and surgical education. We hope this book can act as an invaluable resource.

Notice

Medicine is and has been one of the most rapidly evolving areas of science. Advances in research and technology have been instrumental in changing our practice. The experience and exchange of information has enabled better medical care. There are changes that are incorporated into practice at different paces, in different parts of the globe, and that is understandable due to our different resources. There are treatments that have been withdrawn after their introduction, and hence the need for judicious treatment.

Surgeons rely on experience and knowledge when treating their patients and offering them relief from their diseases. Physicians should also be mindful of their own safety, as well as the safety of their team members. There is always a need to constantly check the current literature and the literature provided by the industry.

Publisher, authors, contributors, and editors are not liable for any injury, damage to person, property, product liability, and negligence for any procedure, operation, idea, or instruction in this text. All physicians and caregivers have a responsibility to take the utmost care to keep themselves updated with the current literature. Please ensure that any procedure described in this text should be mastered under proper guidance before practicing.

There is tremendous opportunity to learn every day.

Contributors

Authors

Yavar Abgin, BA
California Northstate University
Elk Grove, California

Arpit Aggarwal, DO
Fellow Colorectal Surgery
Ascension Providence Hospital
Southfield, Michigan

Silvy Celine Akrawe, MD
General Surgery Chief Resident
Ascension Providence Hospital
Michigan State University College of Human Medicine
Southfield, Michigan

Anas Al-Janadi, MD
Vice President of Medical Affairs for Oncology
Spectrum Health Hospital
Grand Rapids, Michigan

Shahini Ananth, BA
California Northstate University
Elk Grove, California

Melissa Arief, MD
Orthopedic, Hand Surgeon
Baylor St. Luke's Medical Center
Houston, Texas

Richard Berri, MD, FACS
Chief of Surgical Oncology and Peritoneal Malignances Program
Program Director, Jerome F. Williams Gastric Cancer Program
General Surgery and Surgical Oncology
Ascension St. John Hospital
Grosse Pointe, Michigan

AmanPreet Bhullar, MD, DGO
Academic Hospitalist and Faculty
Henry Ford Allegiance Hospital
Jackson, Michigan

Jasneet Singh Bhullar, MD, MS, FACS, FASCRS
Colorectal Surgery
Department of Surgery
University of Pittsburgh Medical Center
Williamsport, Pennsylvania

Sreeja Biswas-Roy, MBBS, MD
Instructor in Medicine
Fellow Physician, Pulmonary and Critical Care Medicine
Mayo Clinic
Phoenix, Arizona

Marine Bolliet, MD
General Surgery Resident
Ascension Providence Hospital
Southfield, Michigan

Claire de la Calle, MD
Instructor of Urology
Johns Hopkins University
Baltimore, Maryland

Lawrence Chen, BA
California Northstate University
Elk Grove, California

Laurence Cheung, MD, FACS
Chairman, Department of Surgery, Ascension Providence Hospital
Professor of Surgery
Michigan State University
Lansing, Michigan

Sanjeev Chhangani, MD (Late)
Surgical Critical Care and Anesthesia and Trauma
Harvard Medical School
Boston, Massachusetts

Patrick Collier, MD, PhD
Cardiologist
Cleveland Clinic
Cleveland, Ohio

Pankaj Dangle, MD
Associate Professor of Urology
Indiana University
Indianapolis, Indiana

Ananya Das, MD
Professor of Gastroenterology
Banner Health
Phoenix, Arizona

Martin Duddy, MS
Vascular Surgeon
University Hospital of Birmingham
Birmingham, United Kingdom

Elango Edhayan, MD, FACS
Program Director of General Surgery
Ascension St. John Hospital
Grosse Pointe, Michigan

Jonathan Egle, MD, FACS
General Surgery
Spectrum Health
Niles, Michigan

Richard Englehardt, MD, FACS
General and Bariatric Surgery
Fellowship Program Director for Bariatric and Minimally Invasive Surgery
Clinical Assistant Professor of Surgery
Methodist Hospital
San Antonio, Texas

Puja Van Epps, MD
Assistant Professor of Infectious Disease
Louis Stokes Cleveland Hospital, Case Western Reserve University
Cleveland, Ohio

Sanjay Gandhi, MD
Professor of Cardiology
Wake Forest School of Medicine
Winston-Salem, North Carolina

Nirupa Gopinath, MD
Director of Simulation and Education Center
St. Joseph Mercy Oakland Simulation Center
Pontiac, Michigan

Rakhi Goswami, BS
California State University, East Bay
Hayward, California

Nav Yash Gupta, MD, FACS
Professor of Vascular Surgery
Cedar Sinai Hospital
Los Angeles, California

Sachinder Singh Hans, MD, FACS, FRCS(C)
Director Vascular and Endovascular Services
Henry Ford Macomb Hospital, Clinton Township
Senior Vascular Surgeon, Henry Ford Medical Group
Clinical Assistant Professor of Surgery
Wayne State University School of Medicine
Detroit, Michigan

Sarah D. Hans, MD
Surgery Resident
Ascension St. John Hospital
Grosse Pointe, Michigan

Jimmy Haouilou, MD, FACS, RPVI
Chief of Vascular Surgery
Ascension St. John Hospital
Grosse Pointe, Michigan

Manjunath Haridas, MD, FACS
Surgeon
Manipal Hospital
Bangalore, India

Abdelkader Hawasli, MD
General and Endocrine and Minimally Invasive Surgery
Ascension St. John Hospital
Assistant Professor of Surgery
Wayne State University School of Medicine
Detroit, Michigan

Barry Herschman, MD
Former Chairman of Pathology
Ascension Providence Hospital
Southfield, Michigan

Michael Jacobs, MD, FACS, FICS
Program Director-Hepatobiliary and Pancreas Fellowship Program
Department of Surgery
Ascension Providence Hospital
Clinical Professor of Surgery
Michigan State University College of Human Medicine
Lansing, Michigan

Apram Jyot, MD
General Surgery Chief Resident
Ascension Providence Hospital
Michigan State University College of Human Medicine
Southfield, Michigan

Rahul Kalla, MD, PhD
Assistant Professor of Gastroenterology
University of Edinburgh
Edinburgh, United Kingdom

Armin Kamyab, MD, FACS
Director of Surgical Services, General Surgery and Minimal Invasive Surgery
Cox Monett Hospital
Cox Monett, Missouri

Preet Singh Kang, MD
Assistant Professor of Radiology
Louis Stokes Cleveland Hospital, Case Western Reserve University
Cleveland, Ohio

Kamal Kant, MD, FACS
Professor of Surgery and Former Dean
Dr SN Medical College
Jodhpur, India

Ravi Kapadia, MD, FACS
General and Vascular Surgery
Assistant Professor of Medicine
Marshall University Joan C. Edwards School of Medicine
Huntington, West Virginia

Binit Katuwal, MD
General Surgery Chief Resident
Ascension Providence Hospital
Southfield, Michigan

Manu Kaushik, MD
Department of Surgery
University of Alabama
Birmingham, Alabama

Srinivas Kavuturu, MD, FACS
Assistant Professor
Hepatobiliary Surgeon
Michigan State University
East Lansing, Michigan

Mark Kay, MS
Consultant Vascular Surgeon
Leicester Royal Infirmary
Leicester, United Kingdom

Ashir Kumar, MD
Emeritus Professor of Pediatrics
Michigan State University
East Lansing, Michigan

Tarun Kumar, MD
Professor of Pediatric Surgery
Desmond University
Des Moines, Iowa

Peter Kurniali, MD
Assistant Professor, Medical Oncologist
University of North Dakota
Grand Forks, North Dakota

Gary Lambert, MD, FRCS, MRCS
Consultant Vascular Surgeon
Worcester, England

Austin Lee, BS
California Northstate University
Elk Grove, California

Anthony Ma, BS
California Northstate University
Elk Grove, California

Francisco Igor Macedo, MD
Associate Professor
Department of Surgery and Surgical Oncology, North Florida Surgical Oncology
University of Central Florida School of Medicine Orlando
Gainsville, Florida

David Machado-Aranda, MD, FACS
Assistant Professor, Department of Surgery and Acute Care Surgery
University of Michigan
Ann Arbor, Michigan

Alasdair MacKendrick, MD, FACS
Former Chief of Colorectal Surgery
Emeritus Professor of Surgery
Ascension Providence Hospital
Southfield, Michigan

Sheila Mallenahalli, BS
University of Alabama at Birmingham
Birmingham, Alabama

Manjunath Markandaya, MD
Vascular Neurologist
Prismal Health
Greenville, North Carolina

Scott Marshall, MD
Vascular Neurologist
Intermountain Medical Hospital
Salt Lake City, Utah

Michael Martin, MD, FACS
General Surgery
McLaren Northern Michigan Hospital
Petoskey, Michigan

Morgan McMonagle, FACS
Vascular and Trauma Surgeon
St. Mary's Hospital
London, United Kingdom

Pooja Mittal Green, MD
Maternal Fetal Medicine
St. Joseph Mercy Hospital Medical Center
Ann Arbor, Michigan

Vijay Mittal, MD, FAIS (hon), FICS, FICA, FACS
Former Program Director, Surgery Residency
Associate Director of Medical Education
Ascension Providence Hospital Southfield,
Professor of Surgery
Wayne State University School of Medicine
Michigan State University College of Human Medicine
Michigan

Y.S. Mohan, MD
Neurosurgery and General Surgery
Henry Ford Health System
Detroit, Michigan

Khanjan Nagarsheth, MD
Vascular Surgeon
University of Maryland School of Medicine
Baltimore, Maryland

Edsa Negussie, MD
Chairman, Department of Radiology
Ascension Providence Hospital
Southfield, Michigan

Megan Nelson, MD, FACS
Department of Surgery
Mayo Clinic Health System
Tucson, Arizona

Mayur Narayan, MD, MPH, FACS
Division Head of Trauma and Acute Care Surgery
Robert Wood Johnson Medical School, Rutgers University
New Brunswick, New Jersey

Mukund Patel, MD
Orthopedic Hand Surgeon
New York-Presbyterian Lower Manhattan Hospital
Brooklyn, New York

Yogendra Patel, MD
Acute Care General Surgeon
New York, New York

Sachin V. Patil M.D, FACS
Associate Program Director HPB Fellowship
Ascension Providence Hospital
Southfield, Michigan
Assistant Professor, Michigan State University, College of Human Medicine
Lansing, Michigan

Nitin Puri, MD, FCCP
Co-Director of Center for Critical Care
Division Head Critical Care
Medical Director, Mechanical Circulatory Support
Associate Professor of Medicine
Cooper Medical School of Rowan University
Camden, New Jersey

Vinod Puri, MD, FACS
Former Director of Surgical Critical Care
Ascension Providence Hospital
Associate Professor of Surgery
Wayne State University School of Medicine
Detroit, Michigan

Saurabh Rai, MS
Vascular Surgeon
University Hospital of Birmingham
Birmingham, United Kingdom
Mazumadar Shaw Medical Center
Bangalore, India

Indreesh Ramachandra, MD
Cardiologist
University Hospital of Cleveland, Case Western Reserve University
Cleveland, Ohio

Dinesh Ranjan, MD, FACS
Transplantation, Trauma Surgery, and Surgical Critical Care
Chief of Surgery
Oscar G Johnson Veteran Affairs Medical Center
Iron Mountain, Michigan

Chandramani N. Rao, MD
Family Medicine and Surgery
Kumar Surgical Center
Rochester Hills, Michigan

Pasala Ravichandran, MD, FRCSC, FRCS
Chief of Cardiovascular Surgery
Oregon Health Sciences University and VA Medical Center
Portland, Oregon

Madan Mohan Reddy Paluru, MD
Senior Resident in Surgery
Ascension Providence Hospital
Southfield, Michigan

Neelima Rehil, MD, FCCP
Department of Medicine
Amita Health
Oak Park, Illinois

Reza F. Saidi, MD, FACS
General, Transplant and Hepatobiliary and Pancreatic Surgery
Chief of Transplantation
Associate Professor of Surgery
Upstate Medical University
Syracuse, New York

Asha Shah, MD, FACS
Department of Surgery and Surgical Critical Care
Mid-Michigan Health
University of Michigan Health System
Kalamazoo, Michigan

Simranjit Singh, MD
Department of Clinical Medicine
Indiana University School of Medicine
Indianapolis, Indiana

Ajay Singla, MD, FACS, FRCS
Residency Program Director
Department of Urology
Center for Pelvic Floor Disorders
Massachusetts General Hospital, Harvard Medical School
Boston, Massachusetts

Nirmish Singla, MD, MSc
Assistant Professor
Director, Translational Research in GU Oncology
Department of Urology and Oncology
James Buchanan Brady Urological Institute
Johns Hopkins University School of Medicine
Baltimore, Maryland

Lauren Smithson, MD, FACS
General Surgery
Labrador-Grenfell Health
Happy Valley-Goose Bay, Canada

Magda Stawikowska, MD
Chief Resident of Surgery
Ascension Providence Hospital
Southfield, Michigan

Gokulakkrishna Subhas, MD, FACS, FASCRS
General and Colorectal Surgery
St Luke's Hospital
Sioux City, Iowa

Abhishek Swami, MD
Assistant Professor of Nephrology
Oakland University School of Medicine
Detroit, Michigan

Ethan Tabaie, BS
California Northstate University
Elk Grove, California

Deepa Taggarshe, MD, FACS, FASCRS, MRCS(Edin)
General Surgery and Colorectal Surgery
Ascension Providence Hospital
Clinical Assistant Professor of Surgery
Michigan State University College of Human Medicine
Lansing, Michigan

Alok Tiwari, MS
Consultant Vascular Surgeon
Leicester Royal Infirmary
Leicester, United Kingdom

Kayla Umemoto, BA
California Northstate University
Elk Grove, California

Neha Varshney, MD
Assistant Professor of Pathology
University of Mississippi
Jackson, Mississippi

Wickii T. Vigneswaran, MD, FACS, FCCP
Professor of Surgery
Associate Chief of Cardiac and Thoracic Surgery
Director of Lung and Heart-lung Transplant
University of Chicago
Chicago, Illinois

Sumeet Virmani, MD
Assistant Professor, Department of Radiology and Nuclear Medicine
Rush University Medical Center
Chicago, Illinois

Rajiv Vohra, MBBS, MS, FRCSEd, PhD
Consultant Vascular Surgery
University of Birmingham
Birmingham, United Kingdom

Arpita Vyas, MD
Professor of Pediatric Endocrinology
Washington University School of Medicine
St. Louis, Missouri

Dinesh Vyas, MD, FACS
Associate Professor of Surgery,
Chair Department of Surgery,
California Northstate University,
Chief Medical Quality Officer
Adventist Dameron Hospital,
California

Melissa Wong, MD
General Surgery
Mount Sinai School of Medicine
New York City, New York

Gopala K. Yadavalli, MD
Professor of Infectious Disease
Program Director of Internal Medicine
Boston University
Boston, Massachusetts

William Yoon, MD, FACS
Assistant Professor, General and Vascular Surgery
Clinical Director, Aortic Program, Northshore University Health System
University of Chicago Medical Center
Chicago, Illinois

Gazi Zabari, MD, FACS
Hepatobiliary Surgery, Pancreas, Transplantation, Minimally Invasive Surgery
Director, John C McDonald Regional Transplant Center
Professor of Surgery and Malcolm Fiest Chair
Louisiana State University School of Medicine
Shreveport, Louisiana

Editors in Chief

Dinesh Vyas, MD, FACS
Associate Professor of Surgery,
Chair Department of Surgery,
California Northstate University,
Chief Medical Quality Officer
Adventist Dameron Hospital,
California

Vijay Mittal, MD, FAIS (hon), FICS, FICA, FACS
Former Program Director, Surgery Residency
Associate Director of Medical Education
Ascension Providence Hospital Southfield,
Professor of Surgery
Wayne State University School of Medicine
Michigan State University College of Human Medicine
Michigan

Editors

Mayur Narayan, MD, MPH, FACS
Division Head of Trauma and Acute Care Surgery
Robert Wood Johnson Medical School, Rutgers University
New Brunswick, New Jersey

Rajiv Vohra, MBBS, MS, FRCSEd, PhD
Consultant Vascular Surgery
University of Birmingham
Birmingham, United Kingdom

Executive Editorial Assistant

Kayla Umemoto, BA
California Northstate University
Elk Grove, CA

Editorial Assistants

Shahini Ananth, BA
California Northstate University
Elk Grove, CA

Anthony Ma, BS
California Northstate University
Elk Grove, California

Lawrence Chen, BA
California Northstate University
Elk Grove, CA

Content

SECTION 7: CARDIOTHORACIC AND TRANSPLANT 759—826

SECTION 8: MISCELLANEOUS 827—966

SECTION 1: GENERAL

1. Fluid and Electrolyte
2. Perioperative Cardiac Risk Stratification
3. Surgical Genetics
4. Geriatic Surgical Care
5. Clinical Research
6. Rural Surgery
7. Respiratory Failure and Ventilator Management
8. End of Life Care
9. Interventional Radiology
10. Surgical Infections
11. Treatment of Surgical Infections
12. Acute Kidney Injury
13. Laparoscopic, Endoscopic, and Robotic Techniques
14. Animal and Human Bites
15. Coagulation and Anticoagulation
16. Quality Improvement and patient Safety
17. Simulation in Surgery
18. Surgical Education
19. Global History of Surgery

1

CHAPTER

Fluid and Electrolyte

Arpita Vyas, MD
Rahul Kalla, MD

1.1 INTRODUCTION

Understanding body water and electrolyte distribution is paramount in managing surgical patients with electrolyte derangements. These changes can occur preoperatively, intraoperatively, and postoperatively, and the management is governed by adequate knowledge of the underlying mechanism and appropriate fluid therapy if indicated.

In a normal individual who has not undergone a surgical procedure, there are insensible physiological fluid and electrolyte losses, some of which are outlined in Table 1. A normal individual consumes around 2-3 L of water each day and consumes 3-5 g of salt each day, both of which are regulated by the kidneys.

Normal Body Water and Electrolyte Distribution

Total body water (TBW) contributes to 40-60% of our total body weight, varying with a person's age and sex. At birth, 80% of our body weight comprises the TBW and this contribution rapidly decreases with age. It is also known that the percentage of TBW in lean individuals is 10-20% higher than elderly or obese individuals. Young adult females also tend to have a lower percentage TBW at 50%, compared to age-matched males.

The TBW is compartmentalized in the body with two-thirds being intracellular and one-third being extracellular. An example of the TBW distribution in a 60 kg female is given in Table 2. The chemical composition of fluid compartments is summarized in Table 3.

The composition of electrolytes within each compartment is governed primarily by the potassium, sodium, chloride, and protein content. This is regulated by the ATP driven, Na-K pump located within the cell membrane. Therefore, ion and protein movement are restricted, however, water is freely distributed across the compartments. As a result, if excess water is ingested, it will be equally distributed amongst the compartments. On the other hand, if sodium containing fluids are given, this will expand the intravascular and interstitial volumes. Although there is free movement of water, the direction of flow into the respective compartments is dependent on the osmotic pressure within the compartment. The ultimate goal of water movement is to attain osmotic equilibrium. Osmotic pressure is measured in osmoles (Osm) or milliosmoles (mOsm). To calculate osmolality the following equation is used:

$$\text{Serum osmolality} = \frac{2\text{Na} + \text{glucose}}{18 + \left(\frac{\text{BUN}}{2.8}\right)}$$

Table 1: Fluid and electrolyte losses in normal individual

Fluid Type	Volume Loss (ml)	Potassium Loss (mmol)	Sodium loss (mmol)
Feces	300	10	80
Urine	2000	60	–
Other Losses	700	–	–
Endogenous	–300	–	–
Total	2700	70	80

Table 2: TBW distribution

Intracellular Fluid Volume	Extracellular Fluid Volume (ECV) Total 10L	
2/3rd of total volume 30L	Interstitial Fluid volume is 3/4th of ECV	Plasma volume is 1/4th of ECV
Total = 20L	Total = 7.5L	Total = 2.5L

Table 3: Chemical composition of fluid compartments

Intracellular Fluid Volume	Extracellular Fluid Volume (mEq)	
	Interstitial composition	Plasma composition
Na: 10	Na: 144	Na: 142
K: 150	K: 4	K: 4
Mg: 40	Ca: 3	Ca: 5
HCO_3: 10	Mg: 2	Mg: 3
Mg: 3	Cl: 114 Organic acids: 5 Protein: 1	Cl: 103 HCO_3: 27 Organic acids: 15 Protein: 16

The body tries to maintain the osmolality of the ECF and ICF at 290-310 mOsm. Any change in the compartments will trigger the movement of water across the semi-permeable membrane to equalize the osmolalities. The usual travel of water is from a compartment with a low osmolality to a compartment with a relatively higher osmolality. As the calculation above implies, sodium is a major determinant of osmolality to a degree where one can say that the net movement of water will usually be governed by changes in the concentration of sodium. This theory can be applied clinically when advising patients with hypertension (high intravascular volume) to reduce their salt intake.

ELECTROLYTE DISTURBANCES

Hyponatremia

A low sodium level is usually caused by either the depletion of extracellular sodium or excessive dilution.[1] The extracellular volume status is helpful in identifying the cause. In post-operative patients, hyponatremia is commonly a result of the over-administration of fluid therapy, or a physiological production of ADH as a result of intravascular volume depletion. Figure 1 summarizes the causes of a low sodium level.

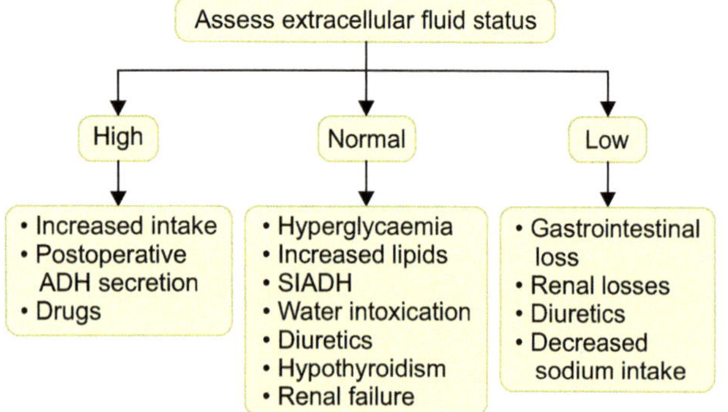

Figure 1: SIADH – Syndrome of inappropriate anti-diuretic hormone secretion

The symptoms of hyponatremia include headache, confusion, seizures, weakness, fatigue, lethargy, vomiting, diarrhea, and salivation. The initial assessment must include fluid status as it will help with the differential diagnoses as mentioned above. The fluid status is assessed by checking blood pressure, peripheral edema, and jugular venous pressure. If the patient is hypovolemic due to extrarenal losses, then a slow correction of sodium with isotonic fluids is indicated. It is pertinent that sodium levels are corrected slowly as rapid correction may result in the permanent demyelination syndrome.

Over administration of sodium free fluids to post-operative patients is a common cause for hyponatremia; therefore, it is pertinent to review the amount and type of fluid input. Normal saline should be used in these situations. Hypertonic saline is rarely used as it can cause circulatory overload.

It is crucial to omit any drugs that may cause a temporary low sodium such as diuretics, proton pump inhibitors, and ACE inhibitors. If the patient is euvolemic, SIADH should be considered. Note that an increase in ADH secretion postoperatively can be a normal physiological response and is a common cause for hyponatremia in these patients. However, SIADH should be considered.

The management of hyponatremia includes diagnosis via urinary sodium, paired osmolalities of urine and serum, and fluid restriction. It is also important to investigate and treat the underlying cause of SIADH.

Hypernatremia

As in hyponatremia, a high sodium level can be subdivided by the extracellular volume status. Commonly a high sodium level is a result of dehydration and low extracellular volume.

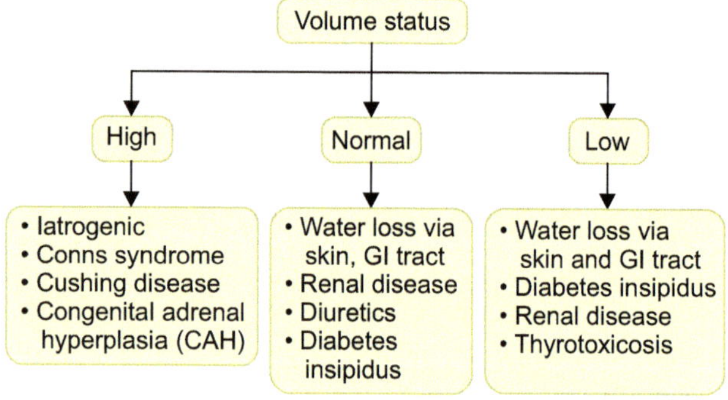

Figure 2: Causes of hypernatremia

Symptoms of hypernatremia include lethargy, thirst, weakness, restlessness, fever, and in severe cases altered conscious level. Note that symptoms rare unless sodium levels are more than 160 mEq/L.

Signs of hypernatremia include evidence of dry mucous membranes and dehydration, oliguria or increased urine output, fever, and tachycardia. Additionally, it can be due to Cushing's disease which has signs such as buffalo hump, centripetal obesity, moon face. If a patient has CAH, the patient may have ambiguous genitalia.

The management of hypernatremia include the following:

- Assess fluid volume status as mentioned previously
- Monitor the fluid input/output chart with daily weights
- If hypovolemic, the most likely cause is dehydration due to extrarenal losses, especially in post-operative patients. Management involves fluid replacement with isotonic solutions and the slow correction of sodium to avoid cerebral edema.
- Certain medications can cause hypernatremia such as antacids with sodium bicarbonate, antibiotics such as ticarcillin, salt tablets, and intravenous hypertonic saline. Such medications should be discontinued.
- If the patient is alert, consider restricting dietary sodium intake temporarily.
- If the above measures fail to correct the Na level, consider other rare causes of hypernatremia such as Cushing's disease, diabetes insipidus, and underlying renal disorders.

Hyperkalemia

High potassium level is defined as a value >5 mEq/L. Severe hyperkalemia is defined as any level >7 mEq/L. The causes are summarized in Figure 3, but usually involve a physiological change of increased absorption, impaired excretion, or excessive release from cells.[2] A high potassium level with ECG changes is a medical emergency and should be treated promptly.

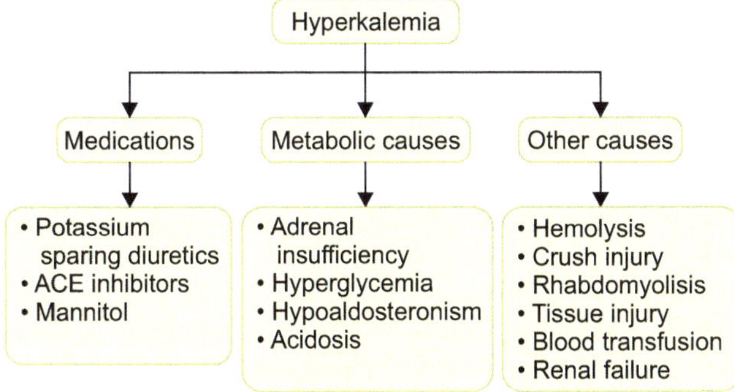

Figure 3: Causes of hyperkalemia

Symptoms of hyperkalemia include mild symptoms include diarrhea, lethargy, nausea, and vomiting. Then weakness and paralysis may ensue. Patients with severe life-threatening hyperkalemia may have symptoms such as chest pain, palpitations, and altered conscious level. ECG will show flattened P waves, a prolonged PR interval, peaked tented T waves, widened QRS complexes, sine wave formation, and arrhythmias such as ventricular fibrillation.

High potassium can be life threatening, but easily correctable and, at a cellular level, the main goal is to drive the extracellular potassium within the cells to protect cardiac conduction cells from the effects of a raised potassium level. Management of hyperkalemia include the following:

- If the patient has ECG changes or is has acute severe hyperkalemia, then the administration of calcium gluconate 10 mL (10%) is required. While administering this drug, cardiac monitoring is needed, and the drug should be discontinued if bradycardia develops.
- The administration of the insulin sliding scale with dextrose will drive the potassium into cells temporarily, approximately 4 hours.
- In acute situations, nebulized salbutamol can also assist in shifting potassium.
- Calcium resins are used to reduce the gastrointestinal absorption of potassium. This is usually given at a 15 g dose orally three times a day, but preparations and route vary.
- Treat the underlying cause to prevent recurrent hyperkalemia.
- Bicarbonate can be used in resistant cases with associated metabolic acidosis. Bicarbonate is useful because metabolic acidosis may be due to high hydrogen ions which can cause a shift of potassium into the extracellular compartments.
- Renal dialysis is usually considered when all medical therapies have been exhausted.
- Once the patient is stabilized, assess the medication history and discontinue drugs that may precipitate hyperkalemia. These include potassium sparing diuretics, oral potassium tablets, ACE inhibitors, and any other drugs that would precipitate renal failure.
- Ensure that a low potassium diet is encouraged until the potassium is in a normal range.

Hypokalemia

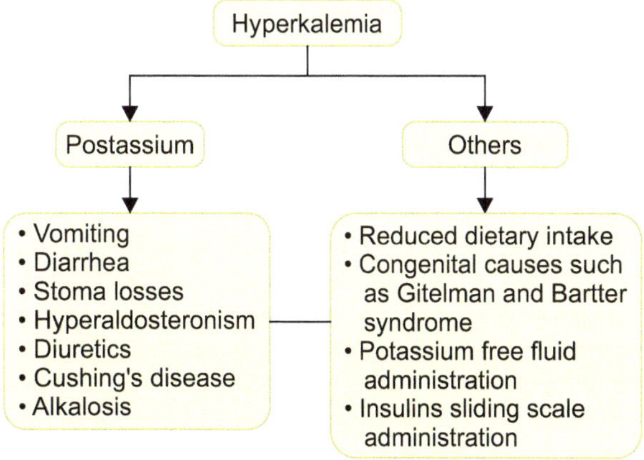

Figure 4: Causes of hypokalemia

Signs and symptoms of hypokalemia include fatigue, lethargy, anorexia, leg cramps, constipation, weakness, hyporeflexia, paresthesia, and ileus. ECG findings include U waves, flattened T waves, ST segment changes, arrhythmias, and eventually cardiac arrest.

The management of hypokalemia is as follows.

- If the potassium level is <3 mEq/L, potassium replacement should be administered at 20-30 mEq/L with ECG monitoring in severe hypokalemia.
- Potassium levels 3 to 3.5 mEq/L can be replaced orally or intravenously.
- Some patients may be resistant to potassium replacement, and in these patients, magnesium levels must be checked as they often co-exist. It will be difficult to correct low potassium if the magnesium level is not corrected first.
- It is also pertinent to omit any drugs that may aid the depletion of potassium temporarily.
- In postsurgical patients, fluid administration must include potassium especially in those who are kept nil by mouth, on an insulin sliding scale, and in stoma patients.

Hypermagnesemia

High magnesium levels are rarely seen in surgical patients unless they are known to have renal disease. In these patients, magnesium levels should be monitored closely. Any medications that may increase serum levels such as magnesium containing antacids and laxatives should be avoided.

Symptoms and ECG changes of hypermagnesemia resemble those in hyperkalemia. Symptoms and signs ensue at a level >6 mEq/L, and levels >10 mEq/L can be fatal.

Management includes fluid replacement with isotonic saline administration to enhance renal excretion. This management may be ineffective in patients with severe renal failure who would require dialysis.

Hypomagnesemia

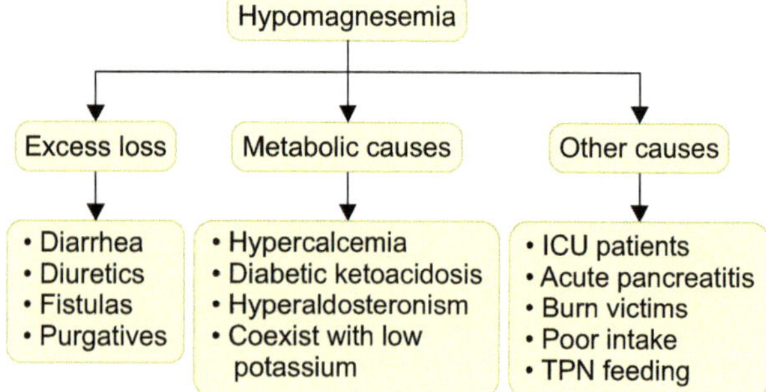

Figure 5: Causes of hypomagnesemia

The signs and symptoms of hypomagnesemia include tremors, delirium or confusion, seizures, hyperactive tendon reflexes, and a positive Chvostek sign. ECG findings include prolonged QT and PR intervals, ST segment depression, flattening or inversion of P waves, torsade's de pointes, and arrhythmias.

Magnesium depletion is a common problem amongst in-patients and those in the critical care units.[5] Management of hypomagnesemia includes magnesium replacements which usually come in two preparations, sulphates and chlorides. If the patient has moderately low magnesium levels, these levels can be replaced by oral therapy. In more severe deficits, parenteral replacement is appropriate and should be done cautiously to avoid over-replacement especially in patients with renal failure. It is useful to know that hypomagnesemia can occur along with low potassium and calcium levels, and therefore these electrolytes should be corrected.

Calcium Homeostasis

Calcium plays an important role in neuromuscular function and at a cellular level. The majority of calcium is stored in the skeletal system, with only 1% in the extracellular fluid. Calcium is distributed as three forms: ionized (40%), albumin-bound (50%) and anion-bound (10%). The serum calcium concentration (4.2–5.2 mEq/L) is regulated by three hormones: chiefly vitamin D, parathyroid hormone, and calcitonin. These hormones have direct and indirect effects on three major organ systems as shown in Figure 6. The acid-base balance also alters the calcium concentration. Acidosis increases the serum calcium concentration as it reduces the protein binding, whereas low serum calcium is seen in alkalosis. The ionized calcium concentration is important in the postoperative surgical patient, especially post-parathyroidectomy patients. The disturbance, although transient, can cause clinical signs and symptoms that would require correction. Figure 7 lists some of the important causes of calcium abnormalities.

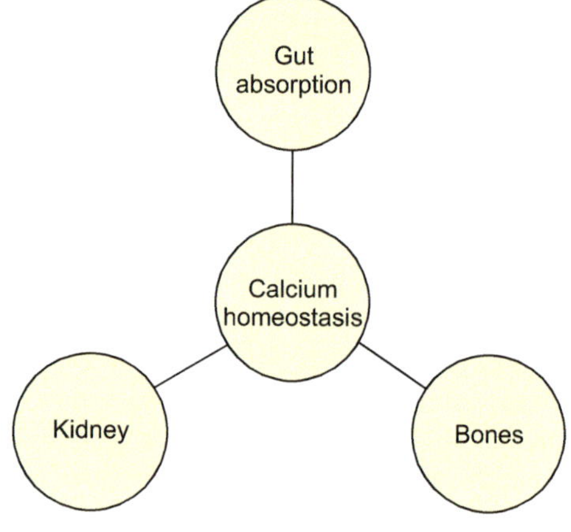

Figure 6: Calcium homeostasis

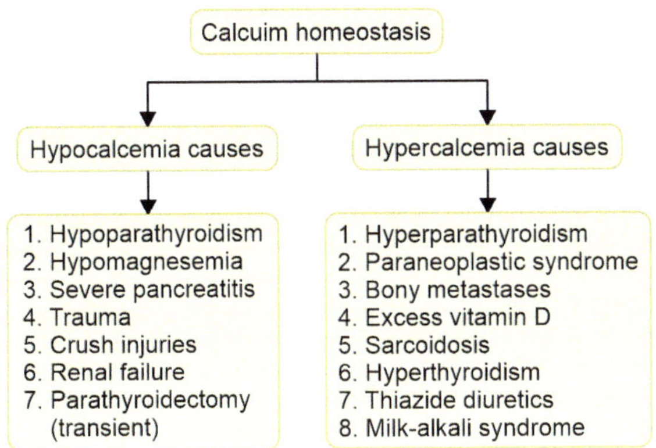

Figure 7: Causes of calcium abnormalities

Hypocalcemia

Clinical manifestations of hypocalcemia include lethargy, abdominal and muscle cramps, carpopedal spasm, and in severe cases convulsions. Important clinical signs to elicit are exaggerated tendon reflexes, Chvostek sign (spasm on tapping the facial nerve), and Trousseau's sign (spasm resulting from a blood pressure cuff applied to the upper limb). QT interval prolongation and T wave inversion are seen on the ECG. In severe cases conduction blocks and arrhythmias are seen.

Management initially involves investigating and correcting any pH abnormalities. In patients with an acute transient low calcium level, intravenous calcium gluconate or chloride can be given while monitoring the ECG. In patients with chronic low calcium, oral vitamin D and calcium supplements can be given. Malignancies associated with increased osteoclastic activity can result in hypocalcemia as a direct result of increased bone formation and in these cases the underlying cause of the hypocalcemia must be addressed.

Hypercalcemia

Clinical symptoms of hypercalcemia include fatigue, muscle weakness, depression, abdominal pains, constipation and nausea, and symptoms of renal calculi. Severe hypercalcemia (level >12 mg/dL) is a medical emergency as it can cause coma and death. ECG abnormalities include a shortened QT interval, prolonged PR and QRS, flattened T waves, and in severe cases conduction blocks and cardiac arrest. Malignancy and parathyroid abnormalities account for the majority of symptomatic hypercalcemia.

Treatment initially involves aggressive fluid replacement to enhance the excretion of calcium. If this is ineffective, then furosemide, IV pamidronate, and IV sodium sulphate are methods of reducing serum calcium. Management depends on the protocols within the local trust/hospitals. Corticosteroids can be used in patients where the cause is sarcoidosis, vitamin D intoxication, or Addison's disease. Plicamycin can be used in metastatic disease. Hemodialysis may be needed if there is refractory hypercalcemia or in renal failure patients with impaired excretion.

METABOLIC DISTURBANCES

Metabolic Acidosis

A metabolic acidosis is defined as a disturbance in the acid-base homeostasis resulting in acidosis. This can be due to overproduction of hydrogen ions, increased intake of acids, or an increased loss of bicarbonate ions. The physiological response is to counteract this and restore homeostasis. This is done by (1) hyperventilation in order to remove more CO_2 (Kussmaul respirations), (2) increased production or reabsorption of bicarbonate ions via the kidneys, and (3) increased secretion of hydrogen ions.

A lot can be determined by working out the anion gap in these patients. In normal individuals, there is an anion gap of <12 mmol/L, and it is usually due to albumin, thus the gap must be adjusted accordingly. Any value above this represents unmeasured ions, which is due to ingestion or generation within the body. The formula involves subtracting cations from anions:

$$\text{Anion gap} = (Na + K) - (Cl + HCO_3)$$

Causes of a High Anion Gap Acidosis include lactic acidosis, diabetic ketoacidosis, ingestion of acids (e.g., methanol, ethylene glycol), salicylate poisoning, and organic acid production in renal failure.

Causes of Normal Anion Gap Acidosis include medications such as acetazolamide, renal tubular acidosis, and loss of bicarbonate ions via the kidneys, gastrointestinal tract, or fistulae.

Of these causes, lactic acidosis and gastrointestinal tract losses post-surgery are the most common causes. Lactic acidosis develops as a result of reduced tissue perfusion, resulting in the production of lactic acid which can be corrected once perfusion is restored. Gastrointestinal tract losses are above the normal insensible losses that occur in the body, and bicarbonate ions are lost. The body maintains the anion gap by restoring chloride ions.

Metabolic Alkalosis

Metabolic alkalosis is a common problem amongst surgical patients as many of them are volume depleted postoperatively. In order to correct the metabolic alkalosis, it is pertinent to fluid resuscitate these patients with normal saline and adequately replace potassium via KCl solutions, as these patients are also chloride depleted. This will negate the need for the kidneys to reabsorb bicarbonate and will allow acid-base homeostasis. Figure 8 is an algorithm for diagnosing the source of the metabolic alkalosis.

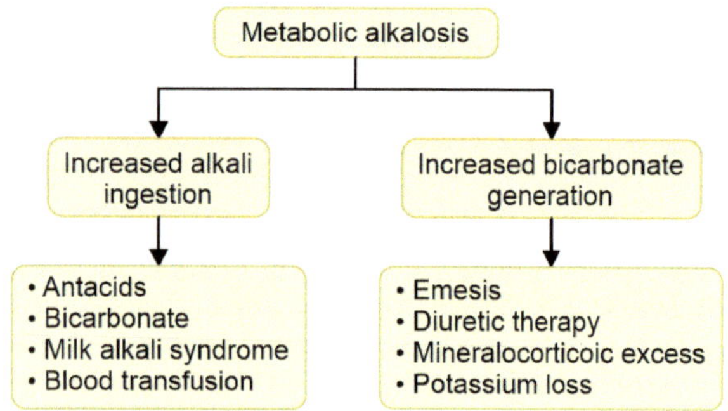

Figure 8: An algorithm for metabolic alkalosis

Respiratory Alkalosis

Hyperventilation and loss of CO_2 from the alveoli is the physiological phenomenon that results in respiratory alkalosis. It results in a high pO_2, low pCO_2 with or without metabolic compensation. This pattern of breathing can be seen in pain, anxiety, early stages of septicemia, neurological disorders (e.g., head trauma, meningitis), medications (e.g., salicylates), hypoxia, and thyrotoxicosis. Hyperventilation causes an electrolyte shift into cells, primarily potassium, and enhanced binding of calcium to albumin, resulting in symptomatic hypocalcemia and hypokalemia. Treatment generally involves correcting the underlying cause.[9]

Respiratory Acidosis

Any illness that causes the patient to hypoventilate will result in respiratory acidosis. This can be diagnosed by a high pCO_2, low pO_2, with or without metabolic compensation. The list below summarizes some of the causes of respiratory acidosis:

- Lung related: Effusion, atelectasis, pneumonia, mucus plug, COPD exacerbation.
- Postoperative pain: Intraabdominal or thoracic, preventing optimal lung expansion.
- CNS pathology.
- Abdominal distension or compartment syndrome.

Treatment involves correcting the underlying problem and optimizing lung expansion if possible. If medical therapy fails to recover the acidosis, then invasive ventilation should be considered in the context of the clinical case.

Types of Parenteral Solutions

Table 4: Types of parenteral solutions

Types of Infusion	Contents in mEq/L				
	Na	K	Cl	HCO_3	Osm
0.9% Saline	154	0	154	0	308
Ringer lactate	130	4	109	28	278
0.45% saline	77	0	77	0	407
3% saline	513	0	513	0	1026
5% dextrose	0	0	0	0	253
Normal body extracellular fluid	142	4	103	27	208

There are a number of different parenteral solutions used in practice. Ringer lactate and normal saline are isotonic solutions and are usually used to replace insensible losses. It is, however, important to bear a few points in mind when considering the type of fluid replacement including the volume deficit, the electrolyte abnormality present postoperatively, any potassium deficit, and replacement of any ongoing insensible loss.

Hypertonic solutions are reserved only in situations where there is severe hyponatremia. Care must be taken to correct sodium level slowly in order to prevent cerebral pontine myelinolysis.

Hypertonic saline solutions have been used in closed head injuries as has shown to increase the cerebral perfusion, reduce cerebral edema, and improve the overall outcome.[9-11] This is not the case for trauma patients as hypertonic saline solutions have not shown to be more beneficial than isotonic solutions.[12]

The other subset of parenteral therapy is colloids which includes albumin, gelatins, and dextrans. These are primarily used to expand intravascular volume in post-operative shock. Albumin is derived from blood, hence it can cause allergic reactions. Additionally, it has been shown in studies that it may cause renal and pulmonary failure when used during hemorrhagic shock.[13,14] Gelatins are derived from bovine collagen whereas dextrans are produced by bacteria grown on sucrose media. Both are volume expanders but dextrans are now only used to reduce plasma viscosity.

SPECIAL CONSIDERATIONS

Burns

Burns involve damage to the epidermis, dermis, or the subcutaneous tissue causing permanent disfigurement, pain, and electrolyte imbalance. The severity depends on the cause, degree of the burn, the body parts affected, and the presence or absence of inhalation injury.[15] The patient's age and co-morbidities can also influence the severity. There are four essential features in managing patients with thermal injury. These include prevention of burn shock by adequate fluid resuscitation, adequate ventilation, removal of necrotic tissue with wound closure, and metabolic support. In this section, we will concentrate on the fluid resuscitation needs.

Fluid resuscitation is a crucial step in managing a patient with thermal injury and an adequate fluid administration without causing overload can be difficult at times as these patients have burns associated edema which can be mistaken for overload to the inexperienced clinician. The physiological mechanism of adequate intravascular volume allowing optimal tissue perfusion can be disturbed in these patients.[16,17] Many texts describe urine output as the sole sensitive indicator in determining tissue perfusion. Lab studies have shown that kidneys are the first organs to experience hypoperfusion.[18] Therefore, renal function and urine output are useful indicators in assessing organ perfusion. The extent of burns is determined by the rule of nines, where body parts injured are expressed as a percentage (Figure 9), with 9% for each limb, 9% for the head and neck, and the remaining divided equally between the front and back of the body.

There are a number of resuscitation fluid formulae, but the commonly used regime is the modified Brooke formula.[19]

Figure 10 summarizes the management.

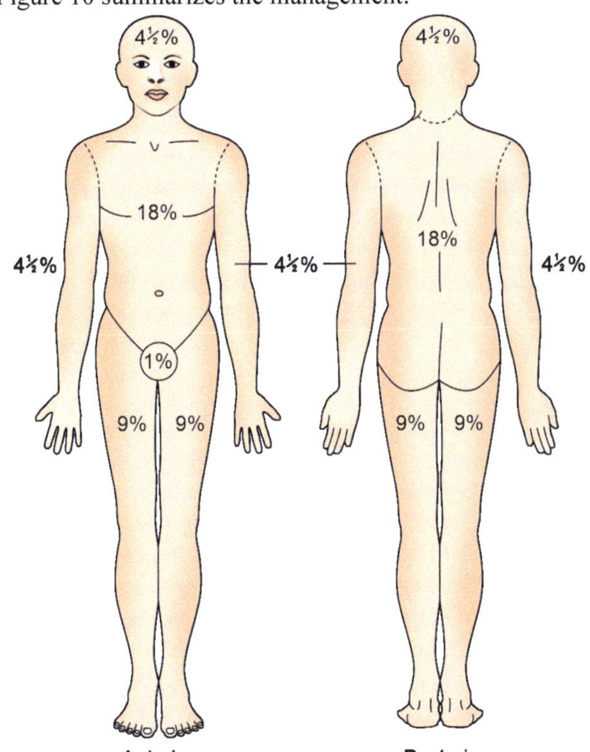

Figure 9: Rule of nines (Courtesy: Diagram taken from UW health website)

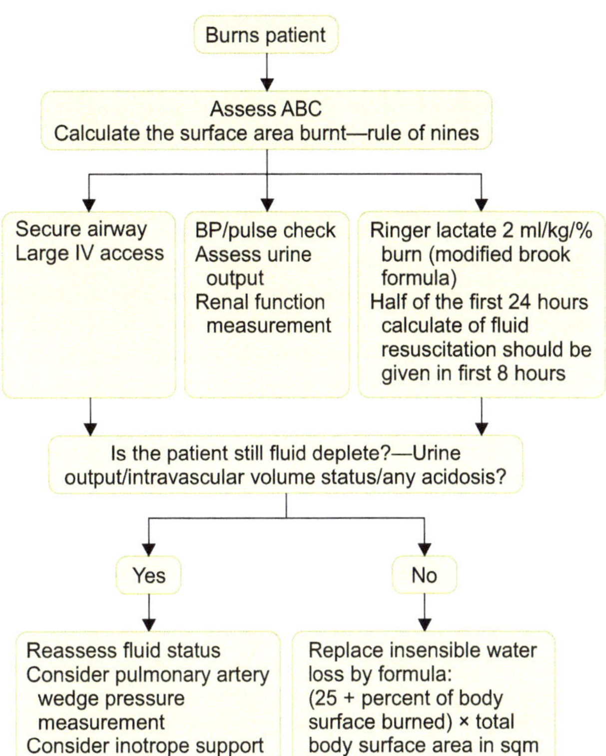

Figure 10: Management of burn patients

The electrolyte abnormalities in burn injury patients occur in phases which are categorized as below:[21-23]

1. Fluid accumulation phase: This occurs within 36 hours of the injury and causes fluid shift from the vascular compartment to the interstitial space causing high potassium, hyponatremia, hypovolemia, hypocalcemia, and metabolic acidosis.
2. Fluid remobilization phase: This usually occurs 2 days after the injury and causes fluid shift back to the vascular compartment causing low potassium, hypervolemia, hyponatremia, and metabolic acidosis.
3. Recovery phase: This may cause further electrolyte disturbance due to inadequate dietary intake or enteral feeding.

Burns patients are prone to infected wounds, pulmonary edema, airway compromise, and gastrointestinal complications such as Cushing's ulcer and paralytic ileus. Therefore, apart from correcting electrolyte abnormalities, one must undertake a thorough clinical assessment and manage any associated complications.

Gastric Outlet Obstruction

Gastric outlet obstruction is a pathological obstruction of the free flow of gastric contents into the duodenum. The causes include peptic ulcer disease, tumors, polyps, pyloric stenosis, or any extrinsic compression such as pseudocysts and gallstones.

Nausea and projectile vomiting are cardinal features of this surgical presentation. Additionally, there may be associated abdominal pain. The characteristic electrolyte abnormalities include increased urea and creatinine levels, low potassium which may be severe, and hyperchloremic metabolic alkalosis due to acid (HCl) loss from the stomach.

Definitive treatment involves correcting the underlying cause for gastric outlet obstruction; however, in the interim the electrolyte abnormalities must be corrected.

Biliary Fistula

Biliary fistulae are any abnormal communication with the bile duct system. They are usually internal as communication with the abdominal wall is rare. The fistulae are the result of chronic inflammation, adhesions, and erosions of the visceral surfaces. This communication is usually with the gastrointestinal tract and is usually caused by gallstones,[24] but can be due to bile duct malignancy, chronic cholecystitis, and inflammatory bowel disease.[25,26]

Patients with this fistula present with abdominal pain, nausea, dyspepsia, steatorrhea and rarely gallstone ileus. Frequently they can cause electrolyte abnormalities. These abnormalities include hyponatremia which can be profound in external biliary fistulae, hypokalemia, hypomagnesemia, and malabsorption of fat-soluble vitamins.

Colonic Diarrhea

Diarrhea is when there is a change in bowel habit where the stool becomes more loose and/or occurs more frequently. It is also defined as stool weight in excess of 200 g/day and having more than three bowel movements a day. It is a common problem, and its causes are vast. Diarrhea can be of acute or chronic in nature and is divided into the following types (with a few examples):

- Infective: Bacterial, viral, and protozoal
- Inflammatory: Autoimmune, radiation, and microscopic colitis
- Neoplastic: Colorectal, pancreatic, and VIPoma
- Metabolic: Thyrotoxicosis and carcinoid syndrome
- Drug related: Antibiotics, laxatives, and many other drugs have diarrhea as a side effect
- Malabsorption: Coeliac disease, Whipple's disease, and tropical sprue

Diarrhea results in a number of electrolyte disturbances along with dehydration if the total output exceeds the total fluid intake. This results in hypokalemia, hyponatremia[27], and metabolic acidosis due to bicarbonate loss.

These are the major electrolyte abnormalities. Replacement of the electrolytes should be prioritized by the severity of the disturbance and its effect on the body. Associated electrolytes such as magnesium levels can also be affected and therefore it is pertinent to check and correct these.

Liver Cirrhosis

Cirrhosis is a histological change of normal liver tissue into a fibrosed nodular liver as a result of chronic irreparable liver injury. There are a number of causes to chronic liver disease, however, alcohol and viral hepatitis are the leading causes worldwide.

Symptoms can develop and are usually a result of impaired hepatic synthetic function. This includes coagulopathy, hepatic encephalopathy, and variceal bleeding. Cirrhosis is a major problem worldwide and with scarcity of transplants, many of them have recurrent admissions with complications of their illness. One of the factors that warrant medical review is electrolyte disturbance. The electrolyte disturbances are divided into the cirrhosis phase and the post-liver transplant phase.

Cirrhosis phase: Cirrhosis impairs the normal synthetic function of the liver resulting in a scarcity of albumin. This in turn results in a reduced oncotic intravascular pressure. This causes a fluid shift into the extravascular space, resulting in ascites and peripheral edema. These patients have a number of electrolyte abnormalities resulting from the disease as well as the diuretic therapy:

1. Diuretic related hyponatremia, hyper/hypokalemia, renal impairment, hypomagnesemia, and hypocalcemia.
2. Hepatorenal syndrome causing renal impairment and refractory hyponatremia. Definitive treatment usually involved transplantation. Transjugular intrahepatic portosystemic shunting can be used (TIPS).
3. Raised ammonia levels resulting in hepatic encephalopathy. This is precipitated by infection, constipation, medications, variceal bleeding, renal failure, and a high protein diet.
4. Other abnormalities include uremia and hypoglycemia.

Liver transplantation phase: One must fulfill strict criteria in order to be eligible for a liver transplantation. Once eligible, the workup for transplantation involves minimizing any perioperative and postoperative complications. A number of electrolyte disturbances can occur, some of which are summarized below:

1. Calcium: Hypocalcemia is evident preoperatively; however, severe hypocalcemia is evident postoperatively as the new liver metabolizes citrate and there is massive blood transfusion during transplant which releases citrate. This is transient (36-48 hours) and should be

treated with intravenous fluid replacement.

2. Potassium: Hypokalemia is common preoperatively but immediately post-operative, the potassium level transiently rises due to reperfusion (10 minutes). Later on, hypokalemia may be a feature due to bile, ascitic, and nasogastric drainage loss.
3. Magnesium: Low magnesium is a feature throughout both the pre- and post-liver transplantation phases. Cyclosporin given postoperatively further increases renal magnesium loss.
4. Sodium: Hypernatremia is a feature intra- and post-operatively as blood products are frequently administered. Overzealous correction of this can cause neurological signs also known as central pontine myelinolysis.
5. Phosphate: Low phosphate levels are a feature post-operatively due to fluid administration, cyclosporine administration, and carbohydrate administration.

REFERENCES

1. Miller M. Syndromes of excessive antidiuretic hormone release. Crit Care Clin 2001;17:11.
2. Laureno R, Karp BI. Myelinolysis after correction of hyponatremia. Ann Med 1997;126:67.
3. Kapoor M, Chang G. Fluid and electrolyte abnormalities. Crit Care Clin 2001;17:571.
4. Adrogue HJ, Lederer ED, Suki WN, et al. Determinants of plasma potassium in diabetic ketoacidosis. Medicine 1986;65:163.
5. Kobrin SM, Goldfarb S. Magnesium deficiency. Sermin Nephrol 1990;10:525.
6. Aguilera IM, et al. Calcium and the anesthetist. Anesthesia 2000;55:779.
7. Wong ET, Rude RK, Singer FR, et al. A high prevalence of hypomagnesemia and hypomagnesemia in hospitalized patients. Am J Clin Pathol 1983;79:348.
8. Fisken FA, Heath DA, Somers S, et al. Hypercalcemia in hospital patients: clinical and diagnostic aspects. Lancet 1981;1:202.
9. Krapf R, et al. Chronic respiratory alkalosis. The effect of sustained hyperventilation on renal regulation of acid-base equilibrium. N Engl J Med 1991;324:1394.
10. Bushinsky DA, Monk RD. Calcium. Lancet 1998;352:306.
11. Gluck SL. Acid-base. Lancet 1998;353:474.
12. Moore FA, Mckinley BA, Moore EE. The next generation in shock resuscitation. Lancet 2004;363(9425):1988-96.
13. Shackford SR. Effects of small-volume resuscitation on intracranial pressure and related cerebral variables. J Trauma 1997;42:S48.
14. Moore EE. Hypertonic saline dextran for post-injury resuscitation: Experimental background and clinical experience. Aust NZ J Surg 1991;61:L732.
15. Wade CE, Kramer GC, Grady JJ, et al. Efficacy of 7.5% saline and 6% dextran-70 in treating trauma. A meta-analysis of controlled clinical studies. Surgery 1997;122:609.
16. Lucas CE. The water of life. A century of confusion. J Am Coll Surg 2001;192:86.
17. Lucas CE, Ledgerwood AM, Higgins RF, et al. Impaired pulmonary function after albumin resuscitation from shock. J Trauma 1980;20:446.
18. Shirani KZ, Pruitt BA Jr, Mason AD Jr. The influence of inhalation injury and pneumonia on burn mortality. Ann Surg 1987;205:82.
19. Horton JW, Baxter CR, White DJ. Differences in cardiac responses to resuscitation from burn shock, Surg Gynaecol Obstet 1989;168:201.
20. Cioffi WG, De Meules JE, Gamelli RL. The effects of burn injury and fluid resuscitation on cardiac function in vitro. J Trauma 1986;26:638.
21. Asch MJ, Mersol PM, Mason AD Jr, et al. Regional blood flow in the burned anaesthetized dog. Surg Form 1971;22:55.
22. Pruitt BA Jr. The burn patient: initial are. Curr Probl Surg 1979;16:23.
23. Harrison HN, Moncrief JA, Duckett JW, et al. the relationship between energy metabolism and water loss form vaporization in severely burned patients. Surgery 1964;56:263.
24. Noskin EA, Strauss AA, Strauss SF. Spontaneous internal biliary fistula: a review of literature and report of two cases. Ann Surg 1949;130:270.
25. Chandar VP, Hookman P. Choledocolonic fistula through a cystic duct remnant: a case report. Am J Gastroenterol 1980;74:179-81.
26. LeBlanc KA, Barr LH, Rush BM. Spontaneous biliary enteric fistulas. South Med J 1983;76:1249-52.
27. Pizzoti NJ, Madi JC, Iamanaca AI, et al. Hyponatremia: study of its epidemiology and mortality. Rev Hosp Clin Fac Med 1989;4:307-311.

❑❑❑

2

CHAPTER

Perioperative Cardiac Risk Stratification

Sanjay Gandhi, MD
Indreesh Ramachandra, MD
Magda Stawikowska, MD

2.1 INTRODUCTION

One of the guiding principles of surgery is "do no harm". Every surgeon wants to ensure that every patient has a successful outcome after the surgical procedure without any complications. In reality, there is always an inherent risk for potential complications with every procedure. The prudent surgeon tries to anticipate and, if possible, minimize the inherent risks to the greatest possible extent in the available time frame.

Nearly 100 million surgical procedures are performed worldwide annually. Approximately 1 million of these patients have cardiovascular complications.1 Cardiovascular complications impact mortality and morbidity in the short term, as well as up to 2 years in some studies. The incidence of major cardiovascular complications in patients undergoing elective major surgical procedures ranges from 1.9 to 4%, and accounts for 10–40% of all postoperative fatalities.

AIM OF PREOPERATIVE RISK STRATIFICATION

The purpose of preoperative evaluation is not to give medical clearance, but rather to (1) perform an evaluation of the patient's current medical status, (2) make recommendations concerning the evaluation, management, and risk of cardiac problems over the entire perioperative period, and (3) to provide a clinical risk profile that the patient, primary physician, non-physician caregivers, anesthesiologist, and surgeon can use in making treatment decisions. This is of importance as these decisions may influence short-term and long-term cardiac outcomes.

EVALUATION

Patient Characteristics – Identifying the High-Risk Patient

A great deal of clinical research has been focused on identifying this high-risk group and on strategies to minimize cardiovascular risk. Even in a group of high-risk patients, the majority of patients undergo surgical procedures successfully. The challenge is to identify the small group of patients at a high risk of cardiovascular complications in the perioperative period. This group has received great attention, and consequently consumes significant resources. Given that the background complication rate is low for the vast majority of patients, any strategy to identify a high-risk group has to be both highly sensitive and highly specific. In this regard, so far, the clinical history of the patient yields the greatest number of clues to help evaluate the magnitude of risk.

History

A good history is a crucial component of preoperative evaluation and provides the basis for assessment of peri-operative risk, further testing if required, and perioperative management. A focused history should be obtained to identify high risk cardiac conditions, specifically unstable coronary syndromes, decompensated heart failure, significant arrhythmia, or significant valvular heart disease (Table 1). The second important component of a history is assessment of the functional capacity of the patient which can be assessed with the Duke Activity Status Index (Table 2). The ability to perform a spectrum of daily tasks has been shown to correlate well with the assessment by more sophisticated treadmill testing and is an important prognostic marker for cardiovascular outcomes. A functional capacity of ≥4 metabolic equivalents (METs) is used in the preoperative algorithm. In more simple terms, if a patient is able to do light work around the house such as dusting or cleaning clothes or is able to walk up a hill or on level ground at 4 mph, they can exercise for ≥4 METs on a treadmill.

Table 1: Active conditions for which patients should undergo evaluation and treatment of cardiac conditions before non-cardiac surgery

Condition	Examples
Unstable Coronary Syndromes	Canadian Cardiovascular Society class III or IV angina, acute or recent myocardial infarction (>7 days but ≤ 30 days)
Decompensated Heart Failure	New York Heart Association class IV heart failure or new onset or worsening heart failure
Significant Arrhythmias	• High grade atrioventricular blocks-Mobitz II, 3rd-degree AV block • Symptomatic bradycardia • Supraventricular arrhythmias including atrial fibrillation with poorly controlled ventricular rate (HR >100 bpm at rest) • Symptomatic ventricular arrhythmias • New ventricular arrhythmia
Severe Valvular Heart Disease	• Severe aortic stenosis (aortic valve area <1.0 cm^2 or mean pressure gradient >40 mmHg or symptomatic) • Symptomatic mitral stenosis
Adapted from: ACC/AHA Guidelines on Perioperative Cardiovascular Evaluation and Care for Noncardiac Surgery[3]	

Table 2: Duke Activity Status Index (DASI)

Activity	Points
Is the patient able to	
Take care of themselves (i.e., eating, bathing, dressing, using the restroom)	2.75
Walk indoors	1.75
Walk on level ground for 1-2 blocks	2.75
Walk up a hill or up a flight of stairs	5.50
Run for a short distance	8.00
Accomplish light housework (i.e., dishes, laundry)	2.70
Accomplish moderate housework (i.e., sweeping, carrying groceries)	3.50
Accomplish heavy housework (i.e., scrub floors, moving furniture)	8.00
Accomplish yardwork	4.50
Have sexual relations	5.25
Participate in recreational activities (i.e., bowling, dancing)	6.00
Participate in strenuous activities (i.e., swimming, basketball)	7.50
Total is 0–58.2 points	
If points add up to ≥ 8 requires further investigation	

Following this, the history should include an assessment of modifiable risk factors and evidence for associated diseases including peripheral arterial disease or cerebral vascular disease. The cardiovascular evaluation must be undertaken within the framework of a patient's overall health including consideration for pulmonary disease, diabetes mellitus, renal insufficiency (serum creatinine level >2 mg/dL), and hematological disorders, as these co-morbid conditions have been shown to affect cardiovascular outcomes. In addition to perioperative management, this evaluation may provide an opportunity to affect the long-term management of patients with or at risk of cardiac disease.

Physical Examination

A focused cardiovascular examination including general appearance, vitals, peripheral pulse, and cardiac examination complements a good history. The examination provides clues to clinical evidence of heart failure (e.g., rales, elevated jugular venous pressure, peripheral edema, third heart sound), associated vascular disease (e.g., carotid bruit, decreased distal pulses) which heightens the suspicion for cardiac disease and murmurs suggestive of valvular heart disease.

Diagnostic Studies

The history and physical examination should guide the physician's decision to order further testing. These may include blood chemistries for metabolic or electrolyte disturbance, hematological tests for anemia, X-ray, and ECG.

1. Preoperative ECG: The current guidelines recommend a resting 12 lead ECG in patients with at least one clinical risk-factor who are undergoing vascular surgical procedures, or patients with known coronary heart disease, peripheral arterial disease, or cerebrovascular disease undergoing intermediate risk surgical procedures (Class I). However, a resting ECG is not recommended in asymptomatic persons undergoing low-risk surgical procedures.

2. Stress Test: Stress tests should only be considered in a limited subgroup of patients (Figure 1). These are patients with poor or uncertain functional capacity, with 3 or more clinical risk factors for CAD, and undergoing intermediate or high-risk surgery. The majority of patients undergoing noncardiac surgery do not need stress testing prior to surgery.

Figure 1: From the 2014 AHA/ACC guidelines, cardiac evaluation, and care algorithm for noncardiac surgery

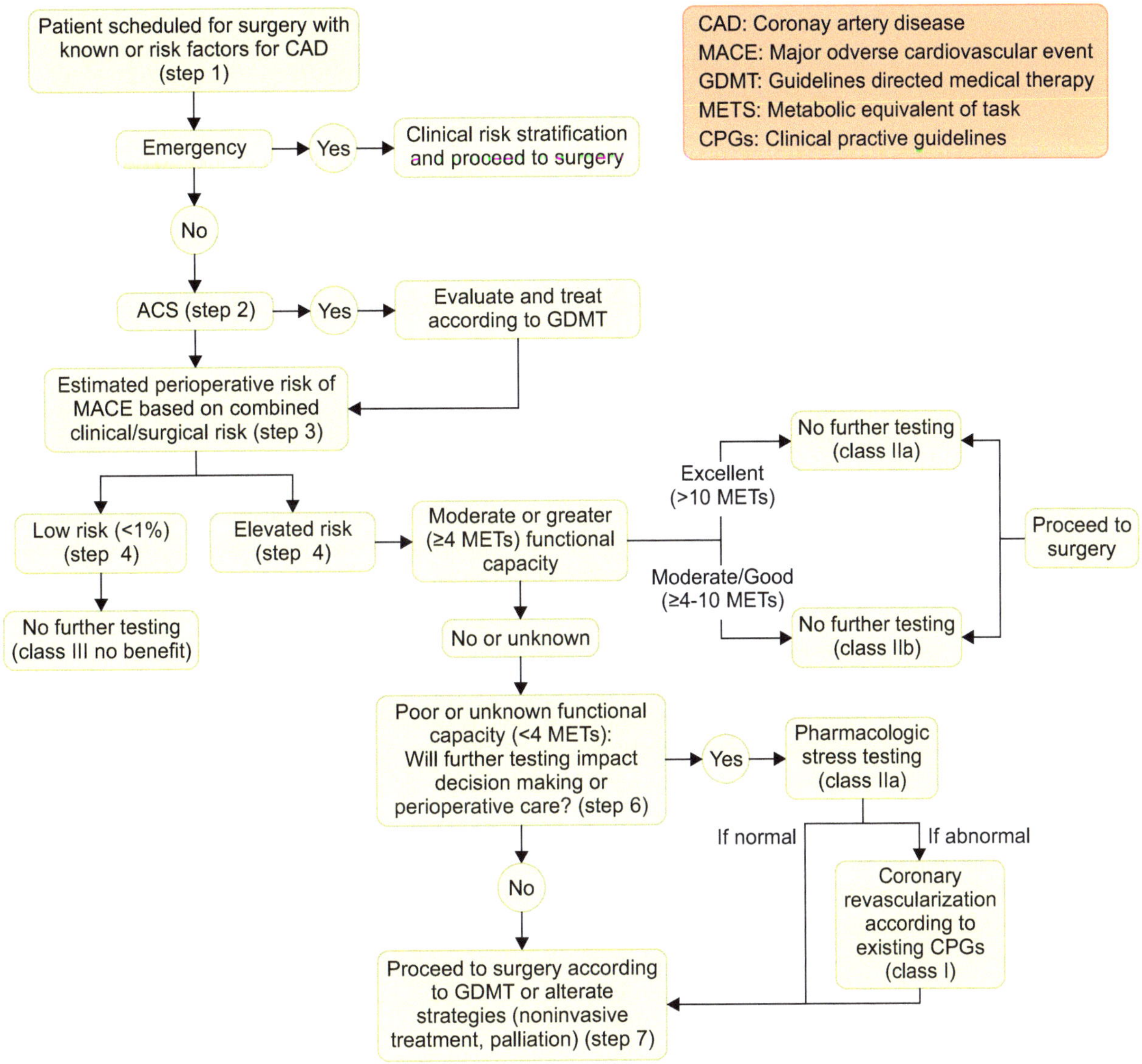

CAD: Coronay artery disease
MACE: Major odverse cardiovascular event
GDMT: Guidelines directed medical therapy
METS: Metabolic equivalent of task
CPGs: Clinical practive guidelines

Patient scheduled for surgery with known or risk factors for CAD (step 1)

Emergency → Yes → Clinical risk stratification and proceed to surgery

No

ACS (step 2) → Yes → Evaluate and treat according to GDMT

Estimated perioperative risk of MACE based on combined clinical/surgical risk (step 3)

Low risk (<1%) (step 4) → No further testing (class III no benefit)

Elevated risk (step 4) → Moderate or greater (≥4 METs) functional capacity

Excellent (>10 METs) → No further testing (class IIa)

Moderate/Good (≥4-10 METs) → No further testing (class IIb)

Proceed to surgery

No or unknown

Poor or unknown functional capacity (<4 METs): Will further testing impact decision making or perioperative care? (step 6)

Yes → Pharmacologic stress testing (class IIa)

If normal

If abnormal → Coronary revascularization according to existing CPGs (class I)

No

Proceed to surgery according to GDMT or alterate strategies (noninvasive treatment, palliation) (step 7)

(a) **Exercise Stress Test:** An exercise stress test can provide an objective measure of functional capacity, identify the presence of myocardial ischemia or arrhythmia, and estimate the risk for perioperative cardiovascular complications and long-term prognosis. The onset of myocardial ischemia at a low workload is associated with significantly increased risk for perioperative and long-term cardiac events (Table 3). In ambulatory patients this is the test of choice.

Table 3: Prognostic gradient of ischemic responses during an ECG monitored exercise test in patients with suspected or known coronary artery disease

Risk Level	Ischemic Response Gradient
High	Low-level exercise induced ischemia induced (<4 METs or HR <100 bpm; age-predicted HR <70%) with ≥1 of the following: • Horizontal or down-sloping ST depression >0.1 mV • ST-segment elevation >0.1 mV in non-infarct lead ≥5 abnormal leads • Persistent ischemic response, >3 min post-exertion • Typical angina • Exercise-induced decrease in systolic blood pressure by 10 mm Hg
Inter-mediate	Moderate-level exercise induced ischemia (4-6 METs or HR 100-130 bpm; age-related HR 70-85%) with ≥1 of the following: • Horizontal or down-sloping ST depression >0.1 mV • Persistent ischemic response, >1 to 3 min post-exertion 3-4 abnormal leads
Low	No ischemia or high-level exercise induced ischemia (>7 METs or HR >130 bpm; age-predicated HR >85%) with: • Horizontal or down-sloping ST depression >0.1 mV • 1-2 abnormal leads
Inad-equate Test	Was unable to reach an adequate target workload or HR response for age without an ischemic response. Results from patients who are undergoing noncardiac surgery unable to exercise to at least the intermediate risk level without ischemia should be considered an inadequate test.
bpm: beats per min; CAD: coronary artery disease; MET: metabolic equivalent of task; HR: heart rate	

(b) **Pharmacological:** Stress testing for patients who cannot exercise can be accomplished by a dobutamine stress echo (DSE) ordipyridamole/adenosine myocardial imaging with thallium-201 or technetium-99m. The DSE involves increased myocardial demand by pharmacological stimulation with dobutamine, while intravenous dipyridamole or adenosine induce a hyperemic response via vasodilatation. The overall sensitivity of DSE for prediction of perioperative death or MI is 85%, with a specificity of 70%. Beattie and colleagues2 examined the predictive value of stress testing with echocardiography versus nuclear perfusion imaging, including 25 studies with stress echo and 50 studies of stress nuclear imaging. The likelihood ratio for the primary endpoint of perioperative death or MI with a positive stress echo was twice that of a positive stress nuclear imaging. However, the finding of moderate to large ischemia by either pharmacological modality was highly predictive of perioperative death or MI, but such an abnormality was only present in 15% of all the patients tested.

c. Coronary angiography: Coronary angiography should only be considered if there is a clinical indication independent of the need for surgery. This would include patients with unstable angina or recent myocardial infarction, or patients in whom noninvasive evaluation reveals a large area of myocardial ischemia.

Surgery Characteristics

The risk of perioperative complications is due to an interaction between factors unique to the patient (e.g., age, CAD, valvular heart disease, renal disease, etc.), factors specific to the surgical procedure (e.g., endoscopic versus open, revascularization versus amputation, etc.), and the factors specific to the situation under which the surgery is being performed (e.g., emergently, academic center, rural hospital, etc.).

If adequate time is available to assess the patient prior to the surgery, the assessment may reveal factors that predict the short- and long-term outcomes for the patient. The ability to predict such outcomes may alter the decision for surgery.

For example, identifying the presence of significant left ventricular dysfunction may make the surgeon choose a laparoscopic approach over an open approach in a patient with chronic gallstone disease. The decision to operate on a patient with asymptomatic uterine fibroids discovered on an ultrasonogram may change to one of monitoring. The ability to predict long-term outcomes is important when the specific surgery is being per formed based on the expectation that the patient will live long enough to experience the benefit from the surgery, such as a hemicolectomy for multiple polyps in a patient with severe CAD.

Urgency of Surgery

Patients undergoing emergent surgery have a 2-to-4-fold higher mortality than patients undergoing elective surgery. This has been shown to be true for vascular surgery such as for abdominal aortic aneurysm (AAA) surgery. A patent with a ruptured aneurysm has >40% risk of mortality than elective AAA repair. Patients with an emergent medical condition need surgery immediately as a life-saving procedure. In this situation, there is usually little or no time for a formal cardiac evaluation. In some situations, surgery may be needed to be performed quickly, but not necessarily emergently such as in the case of a malignancy, limb gangrene, or acute cholecystitis due to a gallstone. In these situations, cardiac evaluation should be done rapidly, and optimization of medical therapy can be done. However, the delay due to additional cardiac testing should not delay thesurgical procedure to a point where it results in an overall worsening of prognosis.

Stepwise Approach for Perioperative Cardiac Assessment

Step 1: Urgency for non-cardiac surgery: if the surgery is deemed emergent, it may not allow for further cardiac assessment and in this case the role of the consultant would be to optimize perioperative medical management and post-operative follow-up. However, if the surgery is non-urgent, further evaluation can be done preoperatively.

Step 2: Evaluation for active cardiac conditions should be performed, including unstable coronary syndrome, arrhythmia, uncompensated heart failure, or severe valvular disease. If any of the above ispresent, it would require management by a cardiology consultant as per standard guidelines.

Step 3: Low risk surgery: if the cardiac risk from the proposed surgery is low, further testing usually does not add any incremental benefit and is not recommended.

Step 4: Patients functional capacity: if the patient has a functional capacity of≥4 METs without symptoms, management will rarely be changed by further testing. Therefore, it is appropriate to proceed with the planned surgery.

Step 5: If the patient has poor functional capacity, is symptomatic, or their functional capacity cannot be determined, further management is guided by the presence or absence of clinical risk factors. If a patient has no risk factors, it is appropriate to proceed with the planned surgery. If that patient has one or two risk factors, it might be appropriate in most patients to proceed with surgery. If the patient has 3 or more risk factors, further testing may be considered if a change in management follows.

In essence, the majority of patients undergoing non-cardiac surgery do not require stress testing. However, careful clinical evaluation of the patient in the context of the proposed surgery can guide further testing in moderate to high-risk patients where management is likely to change.

Anesthesia Consideration

All inhaled volatile anesthetic agents have adverse cardiovascular effects including myocardial depression and afterload reduction. However, in several clinical trials, the use of volatile anesthetics was associated with decreased troponin release, preserved LV systolic function, or decreased late cardiac events compared with the use of balanced anesthesia techniques with opiates. Isoflurane provides cardiac protection by preconditioning against ischemic injury. Regional or local anesthesia may be considered in high-risk patients. However, both epidural and spinal approaches cause sympathetic blockade with reduction in preload and afterload. For lower extremity or lower abdominal surgery, these may be considered. However, higher a dermatomal level of neuraxial anesthesia may result in hemodynamic consequences.

The MASTERS trial[6] (Multicenter Australian Study of Regional Epidural Anesthesia) randomized 915 patients undergoing abdominal surgery with epidural or general anesthesia. There was no difference in outcomes of death or MI in the two groups. However, there were fewer pulmonary complications in patients randomized to neuraxial anesthesia.

Medical Therapy to ReducePerioperative Cardiac Events

A variety of pathophysiologic mechanisms are triggered during the postoperative state including inflammatory cytokines, elevated circulating catecholamine, altered hemodynamic stress, hypercoagulability, and altered energy substrate metabolism. A single therapeutic intervention cannot alter the numerous, different potential triggers for myocardial ischemia and infarction. However, a combination of measures may reduce perioperative ischemia.

Perioperative Beta Blockade

It is widely believed that heightened sympathetic tone plays a significant role in perioperative cardiovascular complications, and that attenuation of this response will lead to improved outcomes. Based on several small and moderate sized studies, beta-blockers have gained wide acceptance for the reduction of perioperative cardiovascular complications in patients undergoing non-cardiac surgery despite limitations of these studies. The ACC/AHA/ESC guidelines regarding use of beta-blockers are provided in Table 4. The recent publication of the POISE trial,4 and a meta-analysis by Bangalore et al.5 have raised concerns about "automatic" or "universal" beta blockade use in the perioperative setting.

Table 4: AHA/ACC guidelines for beta-blocker use

CLASS I: Give Beta-Blockers
1. Patients who will undergo surgery and are currently taking beta-blockers to treat angina, hypertension, symptomatic arrhythmias, or other ACC/AHA class I guideline indications (Level of Evidence: C)
2. Patients who will undergo vascular surgery and they have a high cardiac risk, determined by findings of ischemia on preoperative testing (Level of Evidence: B)
CLASS IIa: Probably Recommend Beta-Blockers
1. Patients who will undergo vascular surgery and with a preoperative assessment that identifies CHD. (Level of Evidence: B)
2. Patients who will undergo vascular surgery and with a preoperative assessment that identifies high cardiac risk, >1 clinical risk factor is present (Level of Evidence: B)
3. Patients who will undergo vascular surgery or intermediate-risk surgery and with a preoperative assessment that identifies CHD or high cardiac risk, >1 clinical risk factor (Level of Evidence: B)
CLASS IIb: Uncertain Usefulness of Beta-Blockers
1. Patients who will undergo vascular surgery or intermediate-risk procedures and with a preoperative assessment that identifies one clinical risk factor (Level of Evidence: C)
2. Patients who will undergo vascular surgery and with no clinical risk factors, and are not already taking beta-blockers (Level of Evidence: B)
CLASS III: Avoid Beta-Blockers
1. Patients who will undergo surgery and have absolute beta blockade contraindications (Level of Evidence: C)
Adapted from: ACC/AHA Guidelines on Perioperative Cardiovascular Evaluation and Care for Noncardiac Surgery[3]

The POISE trial is the largest trial of perioperative beta blockade that used a fixed dose of long-acting metoprolol in patients 2 to 4 hours before undergoing noncardiac surgery. It demonstrated a significant reduction in nonfatal MI, but an overall increased risk of mortality and nonfatal strokes in the treatment group. A meta-analysis by Bangalore et al.5 of 33 trials, involving over 12000 patients, showed that perioperative beta-blockers were not associated with any significant reductions in all-cause mortality, cardiovascular mortality, or heart failure. Treatment of 1000 patients with beta-blockers results in 16 fewer nonfatal MI in survivors, but at the expense of 3 nonfatal disabling strokes and 104 hemodynamic events needing treatment.

Thus, trials have shown heterogeneity in the effects ofperioperative beta blockade on outcomes when beta blockade is administered to all patients. When effects of beta blockade were studied as stratified by surgical risk, those in the highest risk category had a 63-73% relative risk reduction compared to the intermediate risk category.

Hence, all patients cannot be treated as a homogeneous group. In addition, the beta-blockers studied included at enolol, bisoprolol, esmolol, and metoprolol. We recommend that beta-blockers should not be used for low-risk and intermediate-risk patients undergoing low-risk procedures if they do not have any other indication for beta-blockers. Further, beta-blockers, if indicated, should be commenced at least 1 week prior, and preferably even earlier in order to titrate the dose for the individual patient to achieve resting heart rates <70 beats per minute. This is based on the fact that the upregulation of beta receptors takes time and that lower heart rates are associated with greater protection. This period also allows for the detection of side-effects including bradycardia or hypotension. Ultra-short acting esmolol allows for rapid response to changes in the hemodynamic status of the patient in the intraoperative and immediate postoperative period. Once adequate stability has been established, and recovery is proceeding as expected, switch from IV to oral beta blockade should be made. Long-acting oral beta-blockers should be preferred at this time. In the long-term, beta-blockers should be continued if there is any indication for using a beta-blocker. If not, the beta-blocker should be gradually withdrawn over a period of weeks.

Perioperative Calcium Channel Blockers

The few studies of calcium channel antagonists demonstrated no significant reduction in mortality or cardiovascular eventsin patients undergoing noncardiac surgery. However, there were too few events in these studies to draw any meaningful conclusions. Withdrawal or discontinuation of calcium channel blockers may increase the risk for perioperative atrial arrhythmias.

Perioperative Alpha Agonists

A meta-analysis of 12 trials of central alpha2 adrenergic agonists showed a significant reduction in total mortality, and frequency of myocardial infarctions in patients undergoing vascular surgery. The results of this meta-analysis were primarily driven by the results of one trial of mivazerol. A trial of clonidine did not show any reduction in perioperative MI in patients undergoing noncardiac surgery but showed a trend towards reduction in mortality at 2 years. The trial however had very few events in the perioperative period.Thus, central alpha2 agonists may be added for hypertension control, or in a patient with hypertension and one clinical risk factor.

Perioperative Statins

Lipid lowering therapy using statins have shown to be beneficial in the secondary prevention of cardiovascular events. In addition, statins have been shown to stabilize atherosclerotic plaques, improve endothelial function, and alter inflammation. Observational and retrospective studies have suggested a statistically significant reduction inperioperative cardiac mortality in patients undergoing vascular surgery. One randomized study of statins in 200 patients undergoing noncardiac surgery showed a statistically significant reduction in cardiac events, and the composite endpoint of cardiac death, unstable angina, MI, and stroke. At this time available data suggests a beneficial effect of statins for reducing perioperative cardiac events in patients undergoing high and intermediate risk surgery.6

If the patient meets guidelines for statin therapy but isnot on a statin, the preoperative assessment should consider this as an opportunity to add statin therapy to reduce the lifetime risk of cardiovascular events. However, the dose and targets for statin therapy are unclear.

Table 5: AHA/ACC guidelines for statin use

ACC/AHA guidelines for statin therapy
Class I
For patients currently on statins (for CAD, diabetes mellitus, or hyperlipidemia), and scheduled for noncardiac surgery, the statin should be continued in the postoperative period.
Class IIa
For patients undergoing elective vascular surgery with and without clinical risk factors, it is reasonable to start a statin therapy.

Perioperative Nitroglycerin

Nitroglycerin causes systemic venodilation and reduces preload. It also reduces myocardial ischemia in patients with angina. In the perioperative setting, nitroglycerin can potentiate hypotension in conjunction with other anesthetic agents.

Nitroglycerin has not been shown to reduce cardiac events in patients undergoing noncardiac or cardiac surgery. It is reasonable to continue nitroglycerin in the postoperative period in patients who are on it preoperatively after taking into account potential hemodynamic effects of nitroglycerin. If nitroglycerin is needed perioperatively for controlling hypertension, it is reasonable to use a continuous infusion for a more predictable action than other routes.

Coronary Revascularization to Reduce Perioperative Cardiac Events

Routine coronary revascularization in patients with stable cardiac symptoms before noncardiac surgery does not significantly alter the short-term risk of death or MI, or the long-term outcome. In a large, randomized trial of coronary artery revascularization before elective major vascular surgery (CARP trial),[7] 510 patients with significant coronary artery disease (defined as one or major artery with at least 70% stenosis) among 5859 patients undergoing vascular surgery were randomly assigned to coronary revascularization or no coronary revascularization prior to surgery. Of the 225 patients in the revascularization group, 59% had PCI (PTCA and bare metal stent) and 41% had CABG. There was no difference in 30-day death (3.1% versus 3.4%), postoperative MI (12% versus 14%), or long-term mortality at 2.7 years (22% versus 23%) in the revascularization group compared with the non-revascularization group.

Preoperative CABG

The purpose of CABG prior to a surgery is not only to lower perioperative risk but also to provide long-term benefit. In a series of 1001 patients undergoing coronary angiography prior to elective vascular surgical procedures, 251 patients met the criteria for surgical revascularization.8 Of these216 patients underwent CABG, the mortality rate for CABG was 5.3% and the mortality rate after vascular procedures was 1.5%. The overall mortality rate for the entire cohort was 1.4% for patients with normal coronary arteries, 1.8% for patients with moderate CAD, 3.6% for patients with advanced CAD, and 14% for patients with severe, uncorrected, or inoperableCAD. However, patients undergoing low risk procedures such as skin, breast, or urological surgery have a very low mortality rate of less than 1% and may not benefit from preoperative revascularization. In a subset of patients undergoing higher risk surgical procedures, CABG reduces the rate of death (1.7% versus 3.3%) and nonfatal MI (0.8% vs.2.7%). This data suggests that patients undergoing low risk procedures are unlikely to derive benefit from CABG before low-risk surgery, but patients with multi-vessel disease or severe angina undergoing high risk surgery may benefit from revascularization prior to noncardiac surgery. Further, CABG may provide long-term benefit of survival in patients with three vessels CAD, especially those with low ejection fraction and diabetes as compared to medical therapy.

Preoperative Percutaneous Cardiac Intervention

The role of preoperative PCI to reduce perioperative events is very limited. Only patients with ST elevation MI, unstable angina, and non-ST elevation MI benefit from early invasive management. To date, the balance of evidence suggests that routine preoperative revascularization in patients with stable coronary artery disease is of no value in preventing perioperative death or MI.

Coronary revascularization is recommended in patientswith acute ST elevation, myocardial infarction, or in patients with high-risk unstable angina or non-ST elevation myocardial infarction. Coronary revascularization with coronary artery bypass graft surgery (CABG) or percutaneous intervention (PCI) before non-cardiac surgery is recommended for patients with stable angina who have significant left main disease, three vessel coronary artery diseases, or two vessel coronary artery disease with proximal left anterior descending artery involvement, especially if the ejection fraction is less than 50%.[3]

Management of Patients with CAD (Figure 2)

1. Patients with prior angioplasty (PTCA) without stent: It is recommended that in patients with recent PTCA without stent, the surgery be carried out at 2-8 weeks post-PTCA. Early surgery (2-4 weeks) should be avoided to allow for endothelialization at the site of angioplasty. Delayed surgery (>8 weeks) increases the risk of re-stenosis and is therefore not recommended.
2. Patients with PCI with bare metal stents: Bare metal stentthrombosis risk is highest in the first two weeks following stent implantation, is exceedingly rare after 4 to 6 weeks, and requires dual anti-platelet therapy (aspirin and thienopyridine) for at least 4 weeks. Therefore, it is reasonable to delay elective cardiac surgery for 4-6 weeks following implantation of a bare metal stent. Daily aspirin therapy should be continued perioperatively if possible.
3. Patient with drug eluting stents: Drug eluting stents are effective in reducing the risk of re-stenosis. However, due to effects of the drugs, the endothelialization is delayed. In addition to the risk of subacute stent thrombosis, there is a small but significant risk of late (up to 1 year) and very late (>1 year) stent thrombosis. The current guidelines recommend continuing dual anti-platelet therapy with aspirin and thienopyridine for at least 12 months. Therefore, any elective surgery should be delayed for at least one year. It is strongly recommended to continue with aspirin perioperatively. There is no evidence that use of heparin, anti-thrombin, intravenous anti-platelet agents, or coumadin will reduce the risk of stent thrombosis after discontinuation of oral anti-platelet agents.

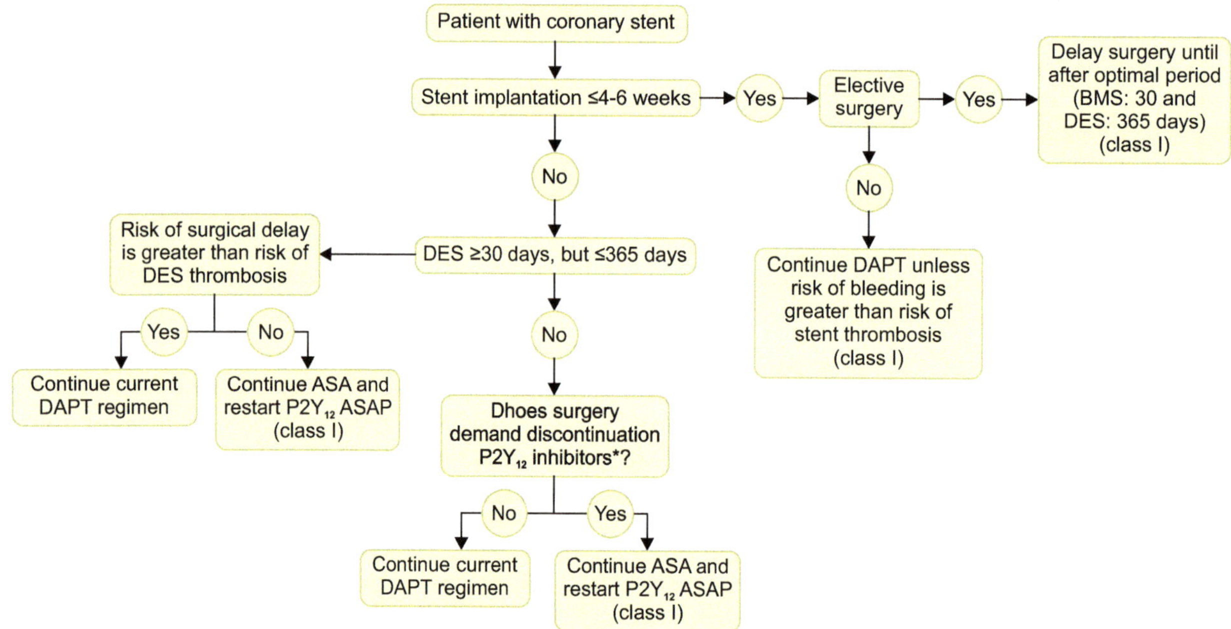

Figure 2. Anti-platelet management algorithm for patients with PCI and noncardiac surgery. ASA=aspirin, BMS=bare-metal stent, DES=drug-eluting stent, DAPT-dual antiplatelet therapy, PCI-percutaneous coronary intervention, and ASAP=as soon as possible.

MONITORING AND SURVEILLANCE

Detecting Perioperative MI

The diagnosis of perioperative MI is associated with 30 to 50% short-term mortality and reduced long-term survival. During the perioperative period, a myocardial infarction may go unrecognized. Most perioperative Misoccur during the first 72 to 96 hours after noncardiac surgery. During this period, patients may have an altered perception due to the post-surgical state, being in the unfamiliar ICU settings, or due to use of upload analgesics. Up to half of the patients with a perioperative myocardial infarction do not have typical symptoms.[1] A low index of suspicion is necessary to detect the infrequent perioperative MIs. There are no criteria established yet for the diagnosis of MIs following noncardiac surgery. However, Table 6 lists the criteria proposed by Devereaux et al.[1] Routine intra- and postoperative ST-segment monitoring can be useful in patients with known CAD, patients undergoing vascular surgery, or patients with single or multiple risk factors for CAD. A postoperative troponin measurement is recommended in patients with ECG changes and chest pain typical of acute coronary syndrome; however, its use is not well established in clinically stable patients. In patients with high or intermediate clinical risk factors with known or suspected CAD undergoing high or intermediate risk procedures, ECG should be done at baseline, immediately after surgery, and for the first 2 days after surgery. Cardiac specific troponin should be used to supplement the diagnosis in these symptomatic patients.

Table 6: Criteria for detecting perioperative myocardial infraction

At least one of the following:
Criterion 1:
Typical rise and fall of biomarkers (especially troponin) with the peak occurring after surgery in a patient without an alternative explanation. CK-MB should be used if a troponin assay is unavailable along with one of the following:
• New Q waves or ST wave changes of ischemia
• Symptoms compatible with ischemia
• Coronary artery intervention
• New wall motion abnormality on ECHO cardiographic imaging or new fixed defect on radionuclide imaging.
Criterion 2:
New pathologic Q waves if biomarkers were not obtained or were obtained at a time that an myocardial infraction could be missed.
Criterion 3:
Pathologic evidence of a new or healing myocardial infraction.

Role of Echocardiography

In patients with persistent hemodynamic instability, a bedside transthoracic echocardiogram can provide useful information about LV and RV function, wall motion, valvular function, and the status of the pericardium. If needed, despite transthoracic windows being suboptimal, a trans-esophageal echocardiogram can provide the necessary information which can guide therapy. There is minimal data regarding the utility or cost effectiveness of TTE or TEE in the perioperative setting for noncardiac surgery.

Role of Pulmonary Artery Catheter

The decision to place a pulmonary artery catheter must be weighed carefully in terms of the benefit versus the potential risks which include pulmonary embolism, infection, pneumothorax, and the potential for misinterpretation of the data leading to the wrong therapy. Studies have shown no role for the routine use of pulmonary artery catheters for hemodynamic monitoring in noncardiac surgery.

In specific patients with unstable hemodynamics, orthose with systolic LV dysfunction and coexisting renal dysfunction, pulmonary artery catheters may aid management if expertise in interpreting the hemodynamic data is available at the institution.

MANAGEMENT OF SPECIFIC SITUATIONS

Hypertension

Hypertension is common in patients undergoing noncardiac surgery. While long-term treatment of hypertension reduces morbidity and mortality, stage 1 or 2 hypertension (BP < 180/110) is not an independent predictor of perioperative cardiovascular complications. For patients on antihypertensive therapy, the medications should be continued perioperatively, especially beta-blockers and clonidine to avoid withdrawal hypertension. If the BP is<180/110, a delay in surgery is not recommended. However,for patients with BP ≥180/110, consideration should be given to improve blood pressure control prior to elective surgery. Beta-blockers appear to be an effective drug for blood pressure management in this setting. Oral antihypertensive medications should be restarted cautiously postoperatively, with care to avoid perioperative hypotension, especially in patients who have decreased vascular volumes. Patients taking angiotensin converting enzyme inhibitor (ACE-I) or angiotensin receptor blocker (ARB) for hypertension are at greater risk for intraoperatively sustained hypotension due to the ACE-I/ARB and anesthetic drug interaction resulting in the inability to compensate for hypovolemia. Except for patients with NYHA Class 3 or 4 CHF, it may be reasonable to hold ACE-Is or ARBs prior to surgery.

Valvular Heart Disease

Cardiac murmurs are commonly recognized in patients undergoing noncardiac surgery. A good history and physicalexamination to quantify the severity of the valvular disease is needed, and echocardiographic evaluation may be warranted for significant murmurs as per AHA/ACC guidelines.

1. Aortic stenosis:Severe aortic stenosis increases the risk of perioperative myocardial infarction. For patients with symptomatic severe aortic stenosis, aortic valve replacement should be considered prior to elective noncardiac surgery. For patients who are not candidates for aortic valve replacement, balloon angioplasty may be considered.
2. Mitral stenosis: Significant mitral stenosis increases the risk of heart failure perioperatively. Mitral balloon

valvuloplasty or open surgical repair should be considered in patients who would need these procedures independent of the need for noncardiac surgery, or in patients with severe mitral stenosis who are undergoing high risk surgery. Further, patients with mitral stenosis benefit from aggressive control of tachycardia to avoid pulmonary congestion.

3. Aortic regurgitation: In patients with severe aorticregurgitation, attention to afterload reduction and volume control is recommended to minimize the risk of pulmonary congestion.
4. Mitral regurgitation: Patients with severe mitral regurgitation also benefit from afterload reduction andjudicious use of diuretics.
5. Mechanical prosthetic valve: For patients who requireminimally invasive surgery (e.g., dental procedure, superficial biopsies), the recommendation is to briefly decrease the INR to a low therapeutic range and resume a normal dose of anticoagulation post-procedure. However, unfractionated heparin is recommended for patients with a high risk of thromboembolism, or for those undergoing surgery with a high risk of bleeding.
6. Antibiotic prophylaxis is no longer recommended formost procedures in patients with aortic and mitral stenosis or regurgitation unless the patient has a prior history of infective endocarditis or has a prosthetic cardiac valve.

VENOUS THROMBOEMBOLISM PROPHYLAXIS

The risk for venous thromboembolism (VTE) is increased in patients with the following risk factors: increased age, prolonged immobility, prior VTE, malignancy, major surgery (e.g., abdomen, pelvis, or lower extremity surgery), obesity, heart failure, myocardial infarction, fractures, and a hypercoagulable state. The choice of prophylactic therapy includes graded compression stockings, low dose subcutaneousheparin, low molecular weight heparin (LMWH), or intermittent pneumatic compression. These therapies should be considered depending on the risk of thromboembolism and the type of surgery (Table7).[9]

Table 7: Levels of thromboembolism risk in surgical patients and management

Level of Risk	Calf DVT %	Proximal DVT %	Clinical PE %	Prophylaxis	Example
Low	2	0.4	0.2	Early mobilization	- Minor surgery in <40-year-old
Moderate	10-20	2-4	1-2	LDUH every 12 hours, LMWH (<2400 units daily), GCS or IPC	- Minor surgery with risk factors - Surgery in 40-60-year-old with no risk factors
High	20-40	4-8	0.4-1	LDUH every 8 hours, LMWH (>3400 units daily) or IPC	- Surgery in >60-year-old with additional risk factors
Highest	40-80	10-20	0.2-0.5	LMWH (>3400 units daily), fondaparinux, oral vitamin K agonist or IPC/GCS plus LMWH/LUDH	- Surgery in patients with multiple risk factors - Hip or knee arthroplasty - Major trauma or spinal cord injury
Additional risk factors: Prior venous thromboembolism (VTE), cancer, and hypercoagulability.					
GCS: graduated compression stockings; IPC: intermittent pneumatic compression; LDUH: low dose unfractionated heparin; LMWH: low molecular weight heparin					

MANAGEMENT OF ANTICOAGULATION

Many patients are on long-term anticoagulation. The common reasons for long-term oral anticoagulation with vitamin K antagonists (warfarin and its derivatives) include prosthetic heart valves, atrial fibrillation, pulmonary embolism, and recurrent DVT.

Management of the anticoagulation regimen is important not only for reducing the risk of bleeding perioperatively, but also to minimize the risk of thromboembolism perioperatively. There is limited data available regarding specific management strategies. Most of the data is derived from the retrospective examination of patients who were on anticoagulation and underwent noncardiac procedures. The detailed recommendations derived from a consensus of expert opinion, and the limited data available have been published. Specifically, the risk of thrombosis on holding anticoagulation for 7 to 10 days has been extrapolated fromrandomized controlled trials of anticoagulation for atrial fibrillation, pulmonary embolism, and DVT. This has been balanced against the risk of bleeding during surgical procedures.

The specific recommendations include:

1. Indication for anticoagulation for each patient; theirrisk for thromboembolism should be carefully reviewed, and therapy should be tailored to the particular patient.
2. The oral anticoagulant (warfarin and its derivatives) should be withheld for a period of at least 3 to 5 days prior to the surgical procedure.
3. An INR should be measured on day 3 to day 5. If the INR<2.0, then the surgical procedure can be performed safely.
4. In patients who are at the highest risk of thromboembolic events, such as those with prosthetic mechanical valves, prior stroke, or having a homozygous genetic predisposition to thrombosis, oral anticoagulation should be substituted with either unfractionated heparin intravenously or LMWH subcutaneously. This is especially the case once their warfarin has been held and their INR is sub-therapeutic.
5. If unfractionated heparin is used, appropriate dosing guidelines should be followed with adjustment as per PTT values measured at 6-hour intervals. The intravenous unfractionated heparin should be discontinued 4 to 6 hours prior to the surgical procedure.
6. If LMWH is used, an appropriate weight-based dosing regimen should be used and corrected for estimated GFR (eGFR) values to minimize bleeding risk. The last dose of LMWH should be given 12 hours before the procedure. The last dose should be half the usual dose for the patient.
7. High-risk patients who are candidates for preoperative bridging with either unfractionated intravenous heparin or subcutaneous LMWH, are also likely to be appropriate candidates for postoperative bridging.
8. In the western world, the costs of hospitalization far outweigh the costs of subcutaneous LMWH, either self-administered or administered by a visiting nurse specialist. In the majority of cases in the developing world, postoperatively, most patients remain in the hospital until both the physician and patient feel reassured of the safety of being discharged home. In these circumstances, patients often stay long enough in the hospital such that a therapeutic level of anticoagulation can be achieved with oral vitamin K antagonists. Bridging can be achieved with intravenous unfractionated heparin using a weight-based regimen in most patients. The intravenous heparin should be commenced 12 to 24 hours after adequate hemostasis has been achieved. A loading dose is not recommended. Further adjustment of doses should be made using frequently monitored PTT levels.

Sub-cutaneously administered LMWH offers some advantages over continuous intravenous unfractionated heparin. It is easy for nurses to administer, it does not require frequent PTT monitoring, and the discomfort associated with frequent blood draws is avoided. Many hospitals may not be able to obtain PTT levels every 6 hours. If started in the hospital and if the patient is sub-therapeutic at the time of discharge, the patient is likely to find it easier to accept the need for subcutaneous twice daily injections, and therefore will continue it at home until therapeutic INR is achieved.

ARRHYTHMMIAS

Patients undergoing surgical procedures do not infrequently have arrhythmias. Both atrial and ventricular arrhythmias can occur. Along with pharmacotherapy, close attention should be paid to correction of electrolyte abnormalities (potassium and magnesium).

Acute supraventricular or atrial tachyarrhythmias that are hemodynamically unstable need to be immediately treated with electrical or pharmacological cardioversion. A consultation with a cardiologist may be needed for further arrhythmia specific management.

Premature atrial complexes (PACs), atrial bigeminy, or short runs of atrial tachycardia respond favorably to beta-blockers.

Patients with hemodynamically stable atrial flutter oratrial fibrillation need to have adequate control of the ventricular rate, usually achieved by beta-blockers. Other agents include calcium channel blockers and digitalis. Beta-blockers are the most effective, especially when given in regular 2-to-4-hour intervals. If beta-blockers are unable to control the ventricular rates, a cardiology consultation is needed to evaluate the patient for antiarrhythmic agents such as short-term amiodarone infusions.

Reentrant supraventricular tachyarrhythmia (SVT) can be treated either pharmacologically or with ablative therapy. The timing of therapy for the SVT should be based on the patient's symptoms and the reasons for the elective surgery. SVTs can be safely dealt with either before or after the elective surgical procedure.

Ventricular ectopics, bigeminy, complex ventricularectopy, and runs of non-sustained ventricular tachycardia, especially if asymptomatic, usually do not need additional therapy unless they are occurring in the setting of an underlying MI or decompensation of heart failure. Treatment directed to the underlying cause is usually all that is needed.

However, sustained ventricular tachycardia warrants consultation with acardiologist, and urgent electrical cardioversion is needed for hemodynamically unstable rhythms. The cause for sustained or symptomatic ventricular tachycardia must be searched for prior to the elective surgical procedure. These patients may need amiodarone in the perioperative period. Other useful agents for this include lidocaine or procainamide.

Bradyarrhythmia in the preoperative period maycontraindicate or limit the dose of beta-blockers that can be used in the perioperative setting. Asymptomatic sinus bradycardia, 1st degree AV block, right bundle branch block, bi-fascicular block, and left bundle branch block usually do not need any specific therapy in an asymptomatic patient.

In a patient with a more advanced conduction systemdisease such as 2nd degree or 3rd degree heart block, or in patients with syncope, the bradycardia would need to be addressed prior to the elective procedure. Patients may need a temporary pacemaker to help them get through thesurgery. Rarely do patients need a permanent pacemaker prior to their elective procedure. Once again, the timing is dependent upon the patient's symptoms and the reason for the surgical procedure.

PACEMAKERS AND DEFIBRILLATORS

Perioperative Management of Implantable Cardiac Devices

More patients are undergoing device implantation; pacemakers are inserted for symptomatic bradyarrhythmia, ICDs are used for primary or secondary prevention of sudden cardiac death, and biventricular devices are employed for heart failure. These same patients have significant co-morbidities putting them at risk for a variety of illnesses, some of which need noncardiac surgery (Table 8).

Table 8: Surgical checklist for implantable cardiac devices

Is patient pacemaker dependent	Yes	No
Has patient experienced shock for ventricular tachycardia/ventricular fibrillation	Yes	No
Has the device been evaluated in last 6 months	Yes	No
Any interval changes in cardiac status since last interrogation	Yes	No

Intraoperatively, the main issue confronting the surgeon is the potential interaction between diathermy and the device. Electromagnetic interference (EMI) of cardiac devices is an uncommon, but well-described phenomenon. Any external source capable of producing strong electromagnetic fields can potentially interfere with the implanted cardiac device. The interaction is unpredictable and can alter device programming temporarily or permanently. The result may be an inhibition of the device output or a triggering of the device output. Sometimes, it can result in overdrive pacing or even trigger the delivery of a shock.

For these reasons, the following recommendations have been made:

1. The output of the diathermy must be kept to the lowest effective signal. Diathermy should be used in short, intermittent bursts. These techniques minimize the number of far-field signals generated, lessening the likelihood of EMI.
2. The grounding patch of the diathermy device is usually placed far from the device. In abdominal surgeries, it is usually placed on the thigh. For head and neck surgeries, placing the patch on the scapular region opposite the side of the cardiac device directs the current vector away from the cardiac device. If that cannot be done, the grounding patch should be placed at a distance of atleast 10 cm or greater from the cardiac device. The strength of the electromagnetic field varies inversely with the square of the distance from the site of the flow of current. At distances >10 cm, and with the usual power settings of the diathermy device, the amount of EMI generated is likely to be small.
3. A magnet can be used to temporarily alter device programming. Placing a magnet over the device activates a reed switch that changes the pacing mode to asynchronous ventricular pacing in single chamber devices, or asynchronous dual chamber pacing in dual chamber devices. Asynchronous pacing refers to the device pacing the cardiac chambers, ignoring the underlying intrinsic rhythm. In the case of pacemakers, the effect of placing a magnet over the device during surgery may be all that is needed, however, the effects of an external magnet on pacemakers vary between manufacturers and even between models from the same manufacturer. It is best to contact the particular manufacturer to obtain accurate information.

   With regard to ICDs, almost all ICDs are reprogrammed to a monitor only mode when an external magnet is placed. Thus, the device would not shock or pace the patient, even in the case of a clinically significant ventricular tachycardia or ventricular fibrillation. The surgeon and anesthesiologist should be aware of this. These patients should be connected to an external defibrillator so that emergent defibrillation can be rapidly accomplished should the need arise.

   In biventricular devices, placing a magnet causes thedevice to pace asynchronously. If the device has defibrillation capacity as well, the magnet converts the device to a monitor mode only. These patients would need to be connected to an external defibrillator as well.
4. In addition, in some instances, reprogramming of the device should be considered prior to the surgery, especially if the anesthetist or surgeon is unfamiliar with perioperative device management.
5. Device function should be assessed, and all devices should be reset to their original programming mode postoperatively.

One important thing to recognize is that many monitoring devices count a pacer spike in calculating the heart rate. In this situation, if a patient is asystolic, the monitor will not detect asystole as it counts the pacing spikes as intrinsic cardiac electrical activity.

HEART FAILURE

Heart failure is increasing in prevalence throughout the developing and developed world. This is related to several factors including an aging population and the increasing prevalence of diabetes and hypertension in most parts of the world. Several studies have shown that these same patients are at the highest risk for perioperative complications during noncardiac surgery. Lee Goldman in his study in 1977 of factors that influence perioperative mortality, assigned the highest score to the physical finding of S3 on auscultation, which is a marker for decompensated heart failure. In the Revised Cardiac Index, a history of heart failure is a risk factor. The ACC guidelines consistently have suggested deferring elective noncardiac surgery in the presence of decompensated heart failure.

Recently, retrospective analysis of a large Medicaredatabase showed that patients who had a diagnosis of heart failure had a greater risk of complications in the perioperative period following noncardiac surgery, including mortality and readmission for heart failure. The magnitude of risk was higher than the magnitude of risk associated with known CAD in the same cohort. This fact, that even with current pharmacologic therapies, heart failure continues to be a significant risk factor is sobering. Unfortunately, there are no studies attempting to identify specific therapies or treatment strategies to manage heart failure in the perioperative setting.

In general, the conditions of these patients should be actively managed by a cardiologist with experience in the management of heart failure (Table 9). Fluid management with and without diuretics, doses of after load reducing agents, dose adjustments for any changes in renal function, as well as the hypotensive effects of narcotic agents are all challenges that require experience as well as a great deal of anticipation.

Table 9: Surgical checklist for heart failure

Any change in symptoms in the recent 2 weeks?	Yes	No
Any weight gain of >3 lbs over baseline in the last week?	Yes	No
Any change in medications in the last 2 weeks?	Yes	No
SBP <90/55 mmHg	Yes	No
BP >130/90 mmHg	Yes	No
Rales >1/4 of both lung bases	Yes	No
If the answer to any of these is yes, a consultation with a cardiologist should be obtained for managing any potential acute decompensation.		

If the answer to any of these is yes, a consultation with a cardiologist should be obtained for managing any potential acute decompensation.

Generally, perioperatively, it is better to cut down on the dose of diuretics and allow the patient to be mildly hypervolemic prior to the surgery in anticipation of fluid loss and shifts. Except for patients with a history of NYHA Class 3 of CHF, the dose of ACEI may be held on the morning of the surgery to minimize accentuation of the hypotensive response to anesthetic agents. Post-operatively, if patients are not able to take oral medications, then Intravenous enalapril every 6 to 8 hours can be used based on the blood pressure response. These patients benefit by the continuation of beta-blocker administration. It may be prudent to hold spironolactone to minimize hyperkalemia, which is frequently seen in this perioperative setting due to tissue injury. Discontinuing digoxin until the patient is able to take medications orally later on is prudent, and unlikely to cause any deterioration in the patient's cardiac condition.

A pulmonary artery catheter may be useful in managingpatients with severely compromised systolic function who are likely to experience significant fluid shifts. The risks and benefits have to be individualized for each patient. Even more useful is an accurate record of daily weight changes and frequent input/output monitoring. In general, trends in these changes are likely to give a clue to the shift in the patient's overall condition than any one-time value.

As soon as patients are capable of taking medications orally, their preoperative regimen should be reinstated. Usually, the medication doses are likely to be different from their immediate perioperative doses, but that is usually titrated over a period of weeks on an outpatient basis.

An important issue is the use of blood products in these patients. There is debate regarding the threshold for the transfusion of blood products. There is no absolute amount of hemoglobin for which transfusion is mandatory. Usually, many physicians will transfuse for a hemoglobin <8.0 g/dl, especially if the change is rapid or if the patient has symptoms that are likely to be ameliorated with transfusion. Small, randomized trials of transfusion in the perioperative setting have shown that patients who are transfused for symptoms are more likely to benefit compared to automatic transfusions triggered by a specific hemoglobin value.

Patients who have a history of heart failure with preserved systolic function are physiologically different from those with depressed systolic function. In these patients, the key to management is the adequate control of hypertension, heart rate, and appropriate fluid balance. Patients who have advanced pericardial disease or infiltrative diseases need active involvement of a cardiologist in the perioperative management for noncardiac surgery. These patients need adequate preload, and hence diuretics have to be used very cautiously.

SUMMARY

Perioperative risk assessment should be addressed both at the systems level, team level, and the patient level by the entire medical team.

1. All patients scheduled for elective procedures should have had a preoperative assessment of cardiac, pulmonary, and renal risk.
2. The patient's data should be appropriately color coded, so that providers are immediately alerted when certain high-risk features are present. If electronic charts are used, appropriate alerts should be triggered.
3. Specific alerts should trigger an automatic referral to aphysician with experience in perioperative cardiac management.
4. This risk assessment should be communicated during handoffs at every stage of care transition (i.e., from the clinic to the OR, OR to the ICU) and to the step-down units. In some institutions, standardized sign-out sheets have been used to reduce the risk of omission of data.
5. Internists or cardiologists should be involved early on in the postoperative period in the care of patients undergoing high-risk surgery, or in those with complex cardiovascular conditions.
6. Chain of Responsibility for care should be clearly established for the perioperative period.
7. Protocols for drug concentrations and dosages should be standardized for the hospital, and should ideally be identical between the OR, ICU, and step-down areas to minimize drug administration errors.
8. Protocols for use of perioperative medications such asbeta blockade, heparin, and analgesia should be established for nursing including cutoffs and indications for escalating therapy or alerting other team members.
9. Protocols for measuring biomarkers and performing ECGs should be well established.
10. Non-physician members should be allowed to escalate care if physicians are immediately unavailable.
11. Hospitals need to track the outcomes of surgery to detect patterns of care that may be improved through systems design.
12. Protocols for perioperative anticoagulation including indications for bridging, and postoperative resumption for anticoagulation should be established. The importance of following instructions regarding anticoagulants preoperatively, as well as postoperatively should be emphasized to the patient and their immediate family involved in the care of the patient. It is important to discuss the risks and benefits related to bleeding and anticoagulation. The need for any blood products should be discussed as well so that the patient and their family can make necessary arrangements for blood products.

At the team level, the greatest emphasis should be on complete communication during handoffs between providers and between stages of care.

Nurses and junior physicians should be familiar with the protocols at the institution so as to be able to give appropriate orders for the timely provision of care.

REFERENCES

1. Zhou X, Chen L, Su Z, Li Y, Tu M, Xiao J, Pan Z, Su D. Perioperative acute myocardial infarction in patients after non-cardiac surgery in China: Characteristics and risk factors. Medicine (Baltimore). 2019 Aug;98(34):e16929. doi:10.1097/MD.0000000000016929.PMID: 31441880; PMCID: PMC6716711.
2. Beattie WS, Abdelnaem E, Wijeysundera DN, Buckley DN. A meta-analytic comparison of preoperative stress echocardiography and nuclear scintigraphy imaging. Anesth Analg. 2006;102:8–16.
3. Fleisher LA, Fleis Chmann KE, Auesbach AD. 2014 ACC/AHA Guidline on Periperative Cardiovascular Evaluation and Management of patients undergoing noncardioc surgery. Circulation 2014 Dec; 130:24. https://doi.org/10.1161/CIR.0000000000000106
4. Devereaux PJ, Yang H, Guyatt GH, Leslie K, Villar JC, Monteri VM, Choi P, Giles JW, Yusuf S. Rationale, design, and organization of the PeriOperative ISchemic Evaluation (POISE) trial: a randomized controlled trial of metoprolol versus placebo in patients undergoing noncardiac surgery. Am Heart J. 2006 Aug;152(2):223-30. doi: 10.1016/j.ahj.2006.05.019. PMID: 16875901.
5. Bangalore S, Wetterslev J, Pranesh S, Sawhney S, Gluud C, Messerli FH. Perioperative β blockers in patients having non-cardiac surgery: a meta-analysis. Lancet. 2008;372:1962–76. doi: 10.1016/S0140-6736(08)61560-3.
6. Raju MG, Pachika A, Punnam SR, Gardiner JC, Shishehbor MH, Kapadia SR, Abela GS. Statin therapy in the reduction of cardiovascular events in patients undergoing intermediate-risk noncardiac, nonvascular surgery. Clin Cardiol. 2013 Aug;36(8):456-61. doi: 10.1002/clc.22135. Epub 2013 May 13. PMID: 23670940; PMCID: PMC6649547.
7. Santilli SM. The Coronary Artery Revascularization Prophylaxis (CARP) Trial: results and remaining controversies. Perspect Vasc Surg Endovasc Ther. 2006 Dec;18(4):282-5. doi: 10.1177/1531003506295144. PMID: 17351187.
8. Osswald BR, Blackstone EH, Tochtermann U, Thomas G, Vahl CF, Hagl S. The meaning of early mortality after CABG. Eur J Cardiothorac Surg. 1999 Apr;15(4):401-7. doi: 10.1016/s1010-7940(99)00029-9. PMID: 10371112.
9. Agnelli G. Prevention of Venous Thromboembolism in Surgical Patients. Circulation. 2004 Dec;110:24.doi: https://doi.org/10.1161/01.CIR.0000150639.98514.6c.
10. Hlatky MA, Boineau RE, Higginbotham MB, et al.. A brief self-administered questionnaire to determine functional capacity (the Duke Activity Status Index). Am J Cardiol. 1989; 64:651–4.

❑❑❑

3

CHAPTER

Surgical Genetics

Michael Jacobs, MD
Vijay K. Mittal, MD

INTRODUCTION

Genetics is a highly evolving field within the realm of healthcare. It is unique in that it allows the medical practitioner to treat not just the patient, but entire families afflicted with the disease. With the advent of the Human Genome Project, medicine has been able to unlock genetic information encoded within nucleated cells of the body and use the information to properly manage, prevent, and counsel families on their risks of malignant transformations.

Genetics in surgery has played an important role in collectively determining individuals at risk of the likelihood of a specific disease, the age of onset, and severity of disease. Genetic abnormalities have been identified in critical genes that undoubtedly play a role in the development of malignancy. Surgical oncologists have been able to offer prophylactic surgical therapies to prevent morbidity and decrease mortality among the population at large. This is particularly relevant to surgeons who may offer better long-term outcomes to patients afflicted with or who are at risk for developing cancer.

Basics of Genetics

Each human cell is composed of 46 chromosomes, each containing 23 pairs. The 23rd pair is designated as the sex chromosome, with XX for females and XY for males. Genes are those sections of the DNA that encode for proteins and different forms of genes are known as alleles. The genotype refers to the inherited DNA and is expressed in observable traits, known as the phenotype. Cells can have multiple chromosomal abnormalities including gain or loss of a chromosome, deletions, inversions, and translocations. Inheritance occurs through patterns of autosomal dominant, autosomal recessive, or sex-linked variations. An autosomal dominant pattern implies 50% inheritance, an autosomal recessive pattern results in a 25% inheritance pattern, and a sex-linked inheritance is determined by the presence of the X or Y chromosome. Penetrance refers to the likelihood that the gene will be expressed.

Normal and equal somatic chromosomal inheritance from each parent is referred to as diploid or disomy. Trisomy is the gain of a chromosome and loss of a copy is designated as monosomy. When a deletion occurs, a band, sub-band, or entire arm of a chromosome may be missing. Chromosomal rearrangements to either the same chromosome (inversion) or other chromosomes (translocation) are also seen. The karyotype refers to the appearance and number of chromosomes within the cell nucleus. In tumors, these abnormalities within the cells may result in multiple clonal cell populations with different abnormalities in their karyotypes.

DNA damage can occur as a result of normal metabolic byproducts or exposure to environmental factors. Free radicals are normal metabolic cellular byproducts that can lead to alkylation, oxidation, hydrolysis, and mismatch of DNA bases. Environmental factors, such as air pollution or cigarette smoke can also lead to inaccurate base matching, DNA strand cross-linking, or DNA strand breakage. This can further disrupt critical cell function or tumor suppressor activity. Thus, consistent DNA repair is critical to normal cellular function and is designed to reduce mutations that can lead to tumorigenesis or disrupted cell function. Thus, failure of DNA repair mechanisms can result in diseases or neoplastic conditions. Some examples of these disorders include Ataxia-telangiectasia; Bloom syndrome; Fanconi syndrome; TTP; and Xeroderma pigmentosum. Ataxia-telangiectasia is the result of a defective ATM gene on chromosome 11, thus preventing cell-cycle arrest or apoptosis. These patients are sensitive to double-stranded DNA breaks from ionizing radiation. Typical symptoms of this disease include decreased coordination of movements starting in childhood, enlarged capillaries, and recurrent respiratory infections. Bloom syndrome is a rare autosomal recessive disease with mutations in the BLM gene that encodes DNA helicases for repair and synthesis. Patients with Bloom syndrome have an increased risk of leukemia, lymphoma, and carcinoma. TTP is an autosomal recessive disorder that lacks normal nucleotide excision repair of UV damaged DNA, resulting in impaired growth, intellectual disability, and brittle hair. Xeroderma pigmentosum is a rare autosomal recessive disease that affects nucleotide excision repair (NER) and leads to an increased risk of cutaneous malignancies and premature aging secondary to extreme sensitivity to ultraviolet light.

Oncogenes and Tumor Suppressor

Proto-oncogenes are normal genes involved in the regulation of cell growth and differentiation. Oncogenes are altered forms of proto-oncogenes and play a critical role in neoplasia. Gene amplification, point mutation, and chromosomal translocation can cause oncogenes to become activated. Several oncogenes have been identified that can impact cell growth, differentiation, and signal transduction. They can be organized according to their cellular location and mechanism of action into a multitude of different categories including growth-factor receptors, G proteins, membrane-associated tyrosine kinases, growth factors, cytoplasmic threonine and serine kinases, nuclear factors, and cytoplasmic hormone receptors. For example, the Ras proto-oncogene normally encodes for G-proteins and GTP-binding proteins involved in signal transduction. The oncogenic mutant form is activated by a point mutation that leads to persistent signaling and can frequently be found in a significant number of lung, pancreatic, and colon cancers.

Tumor suppressor genes regulate the function and growth of cells. Mutations in tumor suppressor genes can result in loss of function and lead to neoplasia. These can be organized into genes that directly regulate the cellular growth and death cycle or maintenance of genomic stability. Examples of tumor suppressor genes that regulate cell growth and death include Adenomatous polyposis coli (APC), Familial adenomatous polyposis (FAP), and Retinoblastoma (Rb). Hereditary nonpolyposis colon cancer (HNPCC), Nucleotide excision repair (NER), and Xeroderma pigmentosum (XP) are examples of genes that are involved in maintaining genomic integrity.

Diagnostic and Pre-symptomatic Testing

Genetic testing can be used for pre-symptomatic patients vulnerable to inheritable diseases. It identifies changes in chromosomes, genes, or proteins that cause diseases associated with a characteristic genotype, phenotype, mutation, or karyotype. For example, BRCA testing is a common predictive and pre-symptomatic evaluation detailed later in the chapter.

Genetic Analysis

Genetic analysis refers to the evaluation and detection of abnormal DNA and genes that lead to diseases. In general, the process involves isolation of tumor mRNA, reverse transcription into complementary DNA (cDNA), and amplification of cDNA by the process of polymerase chain reaction (PCR). Through employing a specific primer, PCR can amplify specific genes. The PCR product undergoes gel electrophoresis, Southern Blotting, and sequencing; mutations p53 (tumor suppressor), and RAS (oncogene) can be easily detected. Further, this method can be used in tissues that are formalin fixed.

Role of Cytogenetic Analysis

Cytogenetic analysis has been an important screening method to detect some hematopoietic cancers. This tool has allowed for the detection of chromosome anomalies that occur as a consequence of incorrect chromosomal pair separation during mitosis. Thus, one chromosome may end up with an additional copy or short a copy. Both DNA damage and incorrect DNA repair are culprits leading to structural chromosomal derangements and cancers, however, these associations are not completely understood.

The Philadelphia Chromosome, discovered in 1960, was the first chromosomal abnormality found. This chromosomal aberrant occurs as a chromosomal translocation with chromosomes 22 and 9; it is often found in patients who have chronic myeloid leukemia. This translocation allows for fusion into the BCR-ABL gene. Scientists have since used cytogenetics to identify chromosomal abnormalities within other tumor suppressor genes, whereby the loss of such genes may explain some of the chromosomal irregularities found in carcinoma. This strategy has been successful in the identification of well-known genes such as the BRCA-1 and BRCA-2 genes that cause breast cancer.

Cytogenetics can also be used to identify the recurrence of specific diseases. Certain cytogenetic and molecular features can help diagnose tumor specifics. For cytogenetic analysis of intraoperative specimens, gross specimens should be fresh and transported in a quick, sterile manner. In the lab the specimens are cultured for analysis of chromosome content:[2] loss or gain of chromosomes, amplification, rearrangements, and deletions.

Another useful technique is Fluorescent in situ hybridization (FISH) as it can yield a great deal of information: chromosomal rearrangements, map loci, abnormalities, point mutations, and deletions. Further, the specimens can be paraffin-embedded, fresh, or frozen with quick analysis times. However, a suspicion for a particular genetic abnormality must be known before using FISH and histology must still be employed. Thus, the surgical team (pathologist, surgeon, cytogenetics specialist) needs to develop an appropriate approach for the suspected diagnosis for the patient to experience improved outcomes.

The genetic modifications that are characteristics of tumor cells become tumor markers. Expression of a tumor marker can occur from viral incorporation into cells, chromosomal translocations, DNA methylation pattern changes, and other genetic abnormalities (deletions and point mutations). When the distribution of methylation sites was evaluated in tumors, it was found that areas of hypomethylation increased gene expression and decreased chromosome stability. In contrast, hypermethylation can suppress gene transcription.

Common Cancers in Surgical Oncology

Breast Cancer

Hereditary breast cancer associated with the tumor suppressor genes BRCA 1 and BRCA 2 is rare, however, up to 950,000 individuals in the United States carry the mutated genes. The incidence of hereditary breast cancer is estimated to account for 5-10% to as much as 27% of all breast cancers. Women are predisposed to breast cancer if at least 5 of the genes are mutated; most genes exhibit autosomal dominant inheritance. Due to BRCA mutations, 100,000 cancer survivors are at risk for new malignancies. There is a 20-fold increase for early-onset breast cancer,[5] and a nine-fold increase for ovarian cancer.[6] Similarly, in males, the risk for breast cancer risk is also increased.[7] Amongst BRCA gene carriers, there is a 90% and 60% chance of developing breast cancer and ovarian cancer, respectively. Furthermore, when linked to BRCA-1 and BRCA-2, cancers afflict patients at a much younger age. For example, women that carry the mutation present with cancers in their 40's as opposed to their 60's with the sporadic forms of these diseases. There is a 50% chance that children of BRCA1/2 parents will inherit the mutated gene. Further, there is a high prevalence of BRCA1/2 genes amongst Ashkenazi Jews, where individuals are 10 times (2.65% of Ashkenazi Jews) more likely to have the gene (1995-96, studies). Amongst Ashkenazi women, 7% were found to have mutations in BRCA1/2. The following is a list of commonly associated genes linked to breast cancer:

BRCA-1 was identified in 1990 and was the first gene associated with breast cancer. It is located on the long arm of chromosome 17. It is a tumor suppressor gene, which may also increase the risk of cervical, uterine, pancreatic, and colon cancers. Additionally, it is associated with 10-15% of ovarian cancers in women.

BRCA-2 was identified in 1994 and was the second gene associated with breast cancer. It is located on the long arm of chromosome 13. It is more commonly associated with male breast cancer and is associated with an increased risk of testicular and prostate cancers. For all patients, it may also be associated with gastric, gallbladder, biliary cancers, and melanoma.

P53 is the most common mutation associated with cancer. It is a tumor suppressor gene. In breast cancer, it is associated with more aggressive disease and worse overall survival. In Li-Fraumeni Syndrome, TP53 mutations on 17p are associated with premenopausal breast cancer, childhood sarcoma, brain tumors, leukemia, and adrenocortical carcinoma.

CD1, cyclin CD1, is a key component of retinoblastoma and the MAPK pathway. It is overexpressed in 50% of human breast cancers. In animal studies, mice that are CD1 deficient are resistant to breast cancer development by activation of Ras oncogenes. This gene, also under current investigation, links to other cancers such as melanoma.

ATM, the ataxia-telangiectasia mutated gene is located on the long arm of chromosome 11. Breast cancer is associated amongst patients who only have one copy of the ATM gene, due to a deletion.

HER2 is a gene located on chromosome 17Q. It is also known as c-erb-2 (HER2/neu) or CD340. Typically, HER2 genes (two copies) are responsible for the production of HER2 protein, i.e., the human epidermal growth factor receptor. This receptor is involved in signal transmission pathways that affect cell growth and division. Increased levels of HER2 leads to constitutive activation of growth signals and subsequent uncontrolled growth and division. Amongst breast cancer patients, 25-30% have been found to have amplification of the HER2 gene. Such amplification has also been observed in tumors of the lung, intestines, prostate, and fallopian tubes. Detection of HER2 expression is done by immunostaining (IHC), ELISA, and FISH. Immunostaining is performed through employing antibodies labeled with dye. The tissue specimens are microscopically examined to assess intensity of the color reaction and the number of stained cells. Normal tissue cells are also used for immunostaining and serve as a control. ELISA (enzyme linked immuno-sorbent assay) analyzes serum samples and identifies the presence of HER2 receptor proteins on tumor cells. However, it does not detect the presence of amplification or overexpression.

FISH or fluorescence in situ hybridization incorporates antibodies that are labeled with fluorescent dye. Through this method, the number of copies of the HER2 gene can be ascertained. Upon application of the dye, fluorescence will radiate from copies of the HER2 gene, seen on fluorescent microscopy. Once these HER2 genes are detected, the drug trastuzumab (Herceptin), a monoclonal antibody that binds to HER2 receptors, can be used. Specific binding of the antibodies decreases the growth and cell division functions of the mutated HER2 gene.[9]

Colorectal Cancer

As one of the most common malignancies in the US and second deadliest after lung cancer, colon carcinoma genetic testing has proven beneficial in identifying common familial disease patterns. At least 2 major molecular events lead to colorectal cancer (CRC): 85% arise from chromosomal instability while 15% are due to events that result in microsatellite instability (MSI or MIN). Aneuploidy, alterations in chromosome number, or detectable losses at the molecular level of chromosome 5Q (APC), 18 Q (DCC), and chromosome 17p (TP53), and mutation of KRAS oncogene have been implicated. Although most causes of colon cancer are sporadic, there are two inherited types of CRC: Hereditary non-polyposis CRC (HNPCC) and Familial Adenomatous Polyposis (FAP).

HNPCC

HNPCC follows an autosomal dominant inheritance and is responsible for approximately 2-4% of all diagnosed cases of CRC per year. It is caused by a germline mutation in the genes responsible for DNA mismatch repair and is also associated with ovarian cancer, endometrial cancer, upper GI cancers, and transitional cell cancer of the ureter. Henry T. Lynch characterized the syndrome in 1966, whereby he observed a "cancer family syndrome," and is now known as Lynch syndrome. HNPCC can be divided into Lynch syndrome I (familial colon cancer) and Lynch syndrome II (HNPCC-associated with additional GI or reproductive system cancers). There are five genes involved in the pathogenesis of HNPCC: MSH2, MSH6, MLH1, PMS1, and PMS2. Ninety percent of the inherited mutations in HNPCC are in MSH2 or MLH1 (Table 1).

Table 1: Genes involved in the pathogenesis of HNPCC

GENE	CHROMOSOME LOCATION	% OCCURING IN HNPCC
MSH2	**Chromosime 2**	**60%**
MLH1	Chromosome 3	**30%**
PMS1	Chromosome 2	**5%**
PMS2	Chromosome 7	**5%**

The main feature of HNPCC is CRC which affects multiple family members, frequently at a younger age of average onset (45 years old). Each child of a parent with the HNPCC gene mutation has a 50% chance of inheriting the mutated gene. There is a predominance of right-sided or proximal tumors that tend to be poorly differentiated. There is also a reported higher average incidence of endometrial, ovarian, stomach, and intestinal cancers in families afflicted with HNPCC. These patients typically do not present with multiple polyps of the colon. They have been found to have an 80% risk of developing CRC. Genetic testing is recommended per the Amsterdam Criteria (Table 2). The original criteria helped determine the need for hereditary linkage analysis. The modified criteria was created to include pathology other than CRC (Table 3).

Table 2: Amsterdam Criteria for HNPCC Diagnosis

- CRC amongst at least 3 relatives, one of which is a first relative
- Exclusion of Familial adenomatous polyposis
- Observed in at least two successive generations, with at least one relative diagnosed with CRC before the age of 50 years

Table 3: Modified Amsterdam Criteria for HNPCC diagnosis

- At least three relatives should have HNPCC and its associated cancer
- One affected relative should be a first-degree relative of the other two
- Observed in at least two successive generations
- Before 50 years of age, at least one malignancy is diagnosed
- FAP excluded in CRC
- Tumors verified through pathologic examination

In 2007, the NCI published the Bethesda guidelines for identification of individuals who should receive genetic testing for Lynch syndrome related tumors (Table 4).

Table 4: Bethesda Criteria for MSI[6]

- Cancer amongst families that meet the Amsterdam criteria
- Patients with two HNPCC related cancers (this includes metachronous and synchronous CRC or associated cancers)
- Patients with CRC + a first-degree relative with CRC +/- HNPCC-related extracolonic cancer +/- colorectal adenomas; one of the cancers diagnosed at age <45 years, with adenoma diagnosed <45 years
- Patients with CRC or endometrial cancer diagnosed <45 years
- Patients with right sided CRC with an undifferentiated pattern on histopathology diagnosed <45 years
- Patients with signet ring cell type CRC diagnosed <45 years
- Patients with adenomas diagnosed <40 years

FAP

FAP is different from HNPCC in that it is exceedingly rare and that there are hundreds to thousands of precancerous polyps present at an early age. It is typical that 95% of patients have polyps by the age of 35, with most developing CRC by the age of 40. Most cases of FAP are due to mutations of the APC gene on chromosome 5Q21. APC is a tumor suppressor gene and genetic counseling is indicated in families where FAP has been diagnosed. Mutations in this gene follow an autosomal dominant inheritance pattern, where one copy of the mutated gene can result in disorder. Mutations can also occur in the MUTYH gene, which has an autosomal recessive inheritance pattern. Prenatal testing for this disease is possible if family members have been previously identified.

The "two hit hypothesis" suggests that, although initially these polyps are inherently benign, the often-mutated allele will accelerate generation of these polyps into cancerous growths. FAP patients who manifest extracolonic features such as soft tissue desmoids and epidermoid cysts, bone and dental abnormalities/osteomas, carcinoma of ampulla of Vater, papillary carcinoma of thyroid, and/or hepatoblastomas in childhood are further characterized as having Gardner syndrome. It is a subset of the APC gene mutations in FAP. Turcot Syndrome is another subset of APC gene mutations that includes CRCs and brain glioblastomas.

MEN Syndromes

Multiple endocrine neoplasia, or MEN syndromes, are inherited as autosomal dominant disorders and often used to characterize multiple endocrine tumors known to occur together. The presence of two or more tumor types does not automatically characterize individuals as having MEN, as there are sporadic forms of disease which may be responsible.

The MEN1 gene encodes a 610 amino acid named MENIN. MENIN is the gene mutation involved in 70-95% of patients with MEN1 syndrome, also known as Wermer's Syndrome. 50% of patients develop signs and symptoms by the age of 20 and greater than 95% have symptoms by the age of 40. Manifestations of the syndrome include tumors of the parathyroid glands, gastroenteropancreatic tract, and anterior pituitary. MEN1 is considered in endocrine tumor patients when 2/3 of the organs are affected, or where one organ is affected and there is a first degree relative diagnosed with MEN.[9]

MEN2 is further sub-classified into MEN2A (Sipple Syndrome) and MEN2B (papillary thyroid carcinoma pheochromocytoma and amyloid-producing medullary thyroid carcinoma). The common feature among both MEN 2A and 2B is the potential to develop into medullary thyroid carcinoma (MTC). Most cases of MEN2 derive from a variation in the RET proto-oncogene. The RET gene is involved in the TGF-beta signaling system that can affect numerous tissues throughout the body making this a gene that is often analyzed in genetic analysis. MEN2 generally results from a gain of function variant of the RET gene. MTC is the most frequent initial diagnosis of both MEN2A and MEN2B patients. In MEN2A, patients may also develop pheochromocytoma in 50% of cases and primary hyperparathyroidism in 5-20% of cases. However, MEN2B is characterized by MTC, mucocutaneous neuromas, and Marfanoid habitus.[9]

Cowden disease

PTEN, a 403-amino acid protein, is a tumor suppressor gene observed in glioma, breast, prostate, and renal cell carcinoma lines. The PI3K, involved in cell growth, is negatively controlled; this gene is implicated in Cowden's disease (Multiple Hamartoma Syndrome). There are other associated conditions: multinodular goiter, thyroid adenoma, hamartomatous GI polyps, and fibroadenoma of breast. A combination of major/minor criteria (International Cowden Consortium) can be used for diagnosis. However, it is important to note that Cowden's disease is associated with an increased risk of breast and thyroid cancers. In 81% of patients, PTEN mutations are identified.

Hereditary Malignant Melanoma

Genetic evaluations of primary melanomas have revealed inactivation of p16, a tumor suppressor gene that acts by aiding in cell cycle progression. With such mutations there is a 38-fold increased risk of developing melanoma. Twenty percent of familial melanoma cases are associated with the p16 mutation that occurs through either a point mutation, promoter methylation, or deletion of the gene.

Diffuse Gastric Cancer

Hereditary diffuse gastric carcinoma is a more recently identified autosomal dominant disorder that results from a germline mutation in the E-cadherin gene CDH-1. Patients with this mutation have a 70-80% increased risk of gastric carcinoma. E-cadherin is an adhesion molecule important in the function of epithelial cells and cell adhesion molecules. CDH-1 is also associated with lobular breast carcinomas, where the predominant mutation involves a premature stop codon of CDH-1 compared to gastric carcinomas where the mutation involves exon skipping and in-frame deletions.

REFERENCES

1. Fletcher C, Unni K, Mertens F. Soft tissue tumours: Epidemiology, clinical features, histopathological

typing and grading. In: *Tumours of Soft Tissue and Bone*. Lyon, France: IARC Press. 2002:12–17.

2. Sandberg A. Cytogenetics and molecular genetics of bone and soft-tissue tumors. *American Journal of Medical Genetics*. 2002;115:189–193.
3. Pfeifer J, Hill D, O'Sullivan J, Dehner L. Diagnostic gold standard for soft tissue tumours: morphology or molecular genetics? *Histopathology*. 2000;37:485–500.
4. Weitzel JN, McCahill LE. The Power of Genetics to Target Surgical Prevention. N Engl J Med, Vol. 344, No. 25 June 21, 2001.
5. Outcome of Preventive Surgery and Screening for Breast and Ovarian Cancer in BRCA Mutation Carriers American Society of Clinical Oncology. March 1, 2002 vol. 20 no. 5 1260-1268.
6. Lalloo F, Kerr BJ Risk Assessment and Management in Cancer Genetics.
7. Learoyd DL, Messina M, Zedenius J, Robinson BG. Molecular Genetics of Thyroid Tumors and Surgical Decision-making. World Journal of Surgery. August 2000, Volume 24, Issue 8, pp 923-933.
8. Dimitrios RH. Breast Cancer Outcomes: The Crucial Role of the Breast Surgeon in the Era of Personal Genetics and Systems Biology Annals of Surgery: June 2009 - Volume 249 - Issue 6 - pp 1067-1068.
9. Shapiro SE, Cote GC, Lee JE, Gagel RF, Evans DB. The Role of Genetics in the Surgical Management of Familial Endocrinopathy Syndromes Journal of the American College of Surgeons. Vol. 197, No. 5, November 2003.
10. Kouvaraki MA, Lee JE, Shapiro SE, et al. Genotype-phenotype analysis in multiple endocrine neoplasia type 1. Arch Surg 2002; 137:641–647.
11. Trump D, Farren B, Wooding C, et al. Clinical studies of multiple endocrine neoplasia type 1 (MEN1). Q J Med 1996;89:653–669.

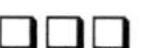

4

CHAPTER

Geriatic Surgical Care

Sulakshna Gandhi, MD
Dinesh Vyas, MD

INTRODUCTION

It is predicted that 21% of the world population will be greater than 60 years of age by 2050.[1] The older population, aged 65 years or older, comprised 12.9% of the United States population in 2009, and is expected to grow to be 19% of the entire population by 2030.[2] The population over 85 is projected to increase from 5.5 million in 2010 to 6.6 million in 2020. According to the National Hospital Discharge Statistics (NHDS) 2009, 38.6% of the total hospital discharges were for patients aged 65 years and over, with the average length of stay being 5.7 days. Amongst these, 41.3% of the discharges were with surgical procedures.[3] The most common domains of surgery utilized by the elderly were cardiothoracic surgery, neurosurgery, ophthalmology, urology, and orthopedic surgery.[4]

It is estimated that up to 50% of surgical emergencies and 75% of post-operative deaths are in elderly surgical patients.[5] These statistics indicate that there is an increasing demand being placed on the medical system, and more specifically on the surgery workforce. The general surgeon needs to have an in-depth understanding of the preoperative evaluation of geriatric patients, their potential comorbidities, and the impact of surgery on post-operative outcomes. The coexistence of multisystem disorders and declining physiologic reserves undoubtedly complexes the pre-operative assessment of the geriatric patient. Since there is a remarkable heterogeneity in the elderly population, the management plan needs to be formulated to meet specific demands in every individual.[6]

Finally, older patients are at increased risk of hospital-acquired complications, and these risks must be discussed with the patient and their family or caregiver. Complications which must be kept specifically in mind during pre-operative assessment in an elderly patient include postoperative risk of delirium, infections, pressure sores, malnutrition, and long-lasting functional impairment.

PREOPERATIVE ASSESSMENT

Careful and detailed assessment of elderly patients is paramount before undertaking surgery. Age, as an independent variable, is a minor contributor to perioperative morbidity and mortality, and postoperative outcomes are more likely to be influenced by the index illness, comorbidities, the effects of aging, and residual impairments from past diseases.[7] Presence of these variables increases with increasing age.

General Status:

The American Society of Anesthesiology (ASA) Physical status scale is an important tool to evaluate the preoperative general status of the patient.[8]

Table 1: Physical Status Classification by the American Society of Anesthesiologists

ASA Class	Disease State
1.	Healthy patient
2.	Mild, systemic disease
3.	Severe systemic disease, not incapacitating
4.	Severe systemic disease, threat to life
5.	Moribund, life expectancy <24 hours with or without an operation
6.	Organ donor
E (Modifier)	Emergency cases

Approximately 80% of patients aged 65 years or older fall into ASA class 3 or higher due to the presence of comorbidities.[10] This fact results in higher complication and mortality rates in the elderly population. The mortality rates after a major surgery in patients aged 65 years or more were 3.5% if they did not have any comorbid disease but rose to 10% if they had three or more comorbid conditions.[11]

Another prognostic system frequently used in critically ill patients is the Acute Physiology and Chronic Health Evaluation (APACHE) III score.[12] This system takes into account physiologic parameters, age, and chronic health status to predict perioperative mortality. Higher APACHE III scores have been associated with higher inpatient mortality rates.[12]

A major problem encountered in the geriatric population is the potential delay in surgical intervention, either due to misdiagnosis because of atypical presentation, or providers hesitation in performing elective procedures. Advancing age along with comorbid conditions and type of procedure are important predictors of postoperative morbidity and mortality.[5]

Functional Status

Frailty, although not a universal phenomenon, increases with age and encompasses a complex syndrome of loss of muscle mass, easy exhaustion, slow walking speed and reduced functional activity.[13] The assessment of frailty is important in determining the special post-operative strategies like delirium precaution, early ambulation, and minimization of medications. The Activities of Daily Living (ADL) scales predict surgical complications. Elderly patients who have lower activity levels have increased surgical risks when compared to elderly patients who are more active.[14]

Cognitive Status

Neuropsychological status evaluation is vital in the preoperative assessment of elderly patients and should be done through the mini mental status examination (MMSE). The presence of dementia preoperatively leads to increased chances of postoperative complications like delirium and poor functional outcomes six months after surgery.[6] The delirious state also places the patient at a high risk of falls and other life-threatening complications.

Nutritional Status

Malnutrition, indicated by more than 20% weight loss preoperatively and serum albumin levels less than 35 g/L, is an important predictor of postoperative morbidity and mortality.[15] Protein calorie malnutrition may occur in a short period in elderly, postoperative surgical patients. Immediate accurate nutritional support improves postoperative outcome and aids in wound healing.[16]

SPECIFIC ORGAN SYSTEM DISEASE FACTORS

Cardiovascular Disease

Cardiac complications such as myocardial infarction and congestive heart failure are the leading causes of mortality in all age groups. This is especially the case for the elderly who may have cardiac conditions as well as normal physiologic decline.[17] The risk of reinfarction is 30% if surgery is done within three months of an MI, 15% between three and six months, and 5% if the operation took place six months after an MI.[5]

The American College of Cardiology has categorized predictors of increased perioperative cardiovascular risk into major, intermediate, and minor risk factors.[18]

Table 2: Perioperative Cardiovascular Risk Factors

Major risk factors	Unstable coronary syndromes
	Decompensated heart failure
	Significant arrhythmias
	Severe valvular disease
Intermediate risk factors	Mild angina pectoris
	A past coronary event
	Compensated congestive heart failure
	Diabetes mellitus
Minor risk factors	Advanced age
	Abnormal electrocardiogram
	A rhythm other than sinus
	Low functional respiratory capacity
	Stroke
	Uncontrolled hypertension

Goldman Cardiac Risk Index (CRI) was the first prospective study to assign risk points for cardiac risk factors known in non-cardiac surgery.[19] This index was later simplified by Detsky et al. into six variables that identify preoperative cardiac risk.[20] According to this new model, an elderly patient with no risk factors has a cardiac morbidity rate of 0.5%. However, the risk increases with an increasing number of factors present. The mortality was 1.3% with one factor, 3.6 % with two factors, and 9.1 % with three factors.

Table 3: Original and Revised Goldman Classification[21,22]

Original Goldman Classification	Points	Revised Goldman Classification	Points
Age >70 years	5	History of heart failure	1
Myocardial infarction in previous six months	10	History of ischemic heart disease	1
Presence of S_3 gallop or jugular venous distension	11	History of cerebrovascular disease	1
Valvular aortic stenosis	3	Preoperative insulin therapy	1
ECG rhythm other than normal sinus	7	Preoperative serum creatinine > 2 mg/dL	1
Presence of >5 PVC_s/min	7	High-risk surgery	1
Poor general health status	3		
Intra-abdominal, intrathoracic, or aortic procedure	3		
Emergency Surgery	4		
Total possible points	53	Total possible points	6

Preoperative risk assessment

The history, physical examination and ECG are indispensable for a rational assessment of the risk of myocardial infarction, and can be used to quickly sort patients into groups according to the level of risk.[23] Non-invasive cardiac testing like dipyridamole-thallium scintigraphy or dobutamine stress echocardiography might be useful in intermediate- or high-risk patients but have limited use in low-risk patients undergoing non-cardiac surgery.[24] A combination of clinical evaluation and dipyridamole-thallium imaging appears to be the most appropriate approach for the prediction of adverse postoperative cardiac events.[25] Perioperative beta-blocker agents have been shown to reduce the risk of in-hospital death among high-risk, but not low-risk patients.[26] If a patient is susceptible to bacterial endocarditis, preventative measures should be taken using standard protocols.[27]

Pulmonary Disease

Pulmonary disease leading to postoperative complications accounts for 40% of total complications and 20% of preventable deaths.[14] The American College of Physicians has identified the following risk factors associated with a high probability of post-operative complications: cigarette smoking, COPD, site of operation, heart failure, ASA class 2 or higher, age, general anesthesia, duration of anesthesia, and preoperative respiratory infection.[28] Age alone is not an independent risk when adjusted for variables like physical status and pulmonary function.[29] The site of the surgery is the greatest risk factor, the higher risk surgical interventions being those of the upper abdomen, aorta, and peripheral vascular interventions.[29]

Baseline chest radiograph must be obtained for elderly patients undergoing major surgery.[5] For patients undergoing lung resection, preoperative spirometry and arterial blood gasses (ABG) are clearly indicated. Findings suggestive of postoperative pulmonary complications include VC <50% of predicted value, FEV_1 <50% of predicted value, or substantial hypoxemia or hypercapnia.[30] Preoperative pulmonary testing is not recommended routinely except for patients who are smokers or have lung disease.[30] When preoperative pulmonary testing reveals abnormal results, respiratory therapy should be offered in the form of intermittent positive pressure breathing, bronchodilators, and incentive spirometry.[31]

Renal Disease

Elderly patients experience a decline in renal function, evidenced by a decrease in GFR (1 mL/min every year after 40 years of age) and a decrease in urinary concentrating ability. This increases their susceptibility to renal ischemia perioperatively and to nephrotoxic agents.[32] Perioperative renal failure has a mortality of 50% and is higher in the elderly.[32] Poor prognostic indicators include oliguria, urine sediment abnormalities, and a rise of serum creatinine of 3 mg/dL or greater.[33]

The most predictable preoperative risk factors for postoperative renal failure include elevated serum creatinine or BUN, advanced age, and cardiac failure.[34] Therefore, all elderly patients must undergo basic urinalysis, and have electrolyte panels before any surgical intervention. Any underlying abnormalities found should be promptly corrected.[32] Perioperative renal management in elderly patients should include intravascular volume repletion and avoidance of nephrotoxic drugs.

As there is a high association of known and silent comorbid conditions in the geriatric population, routine screening or baseline workup is recommended. The following flow diagram shows an overview of the pre-operative workup in geriatrics patients (Figure 1). It is a guide and not a rule, and the workup should be tailored to the individual patient.

Figure 1: Flowchart for preoperative surgical evaluation of geriatric patients

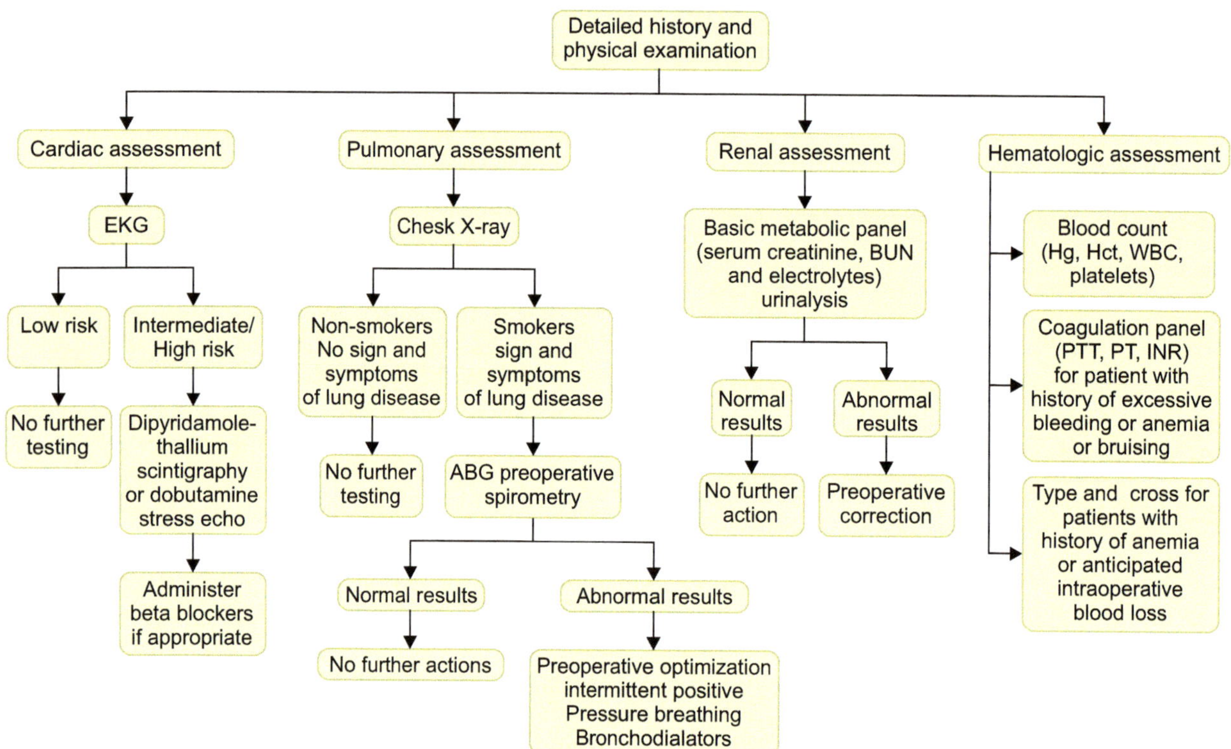

TYPE OF SURGERY

Two major factors to be considered while determining postoperative risks are the emergent nature of surgery and the site of surgery.

Emergency Versus Elective Procedure

The surgical risk increases tremendously in an emergency procedure, especially in an elderly patient.[6] The rate of postoperative complications is considerably higher in emergency surgeries (59%) as compared to elective surgeries (39%).[35]

Body Cavity versus Non-body cavity Surgery

Geriatric patients can undergo elective surgery that avoids the body cavity with relatively lower risk. However, mortality is greatly increased if the geriatric patient undergoes a thoracic or abdominal procedure.[6]

Specific Considerations

Minimal Access Laparoscopic Surgery

The number of laparoscopic surgeries performed has increased tremendously over the past years due to its advantages over the conventional open procedure. Laparoscopic surgeries result in decreased postoperative complications including atelectasis, ileus, and wound infection. Amongst the elderly, such complications can lead to pneumonia, electrolyte imbalances, and even sepsis.[36] In the elderly population, the decreased physiological reserve and multiple co-morbidities make the surgical procedure even more challenging.

However, the benefits of laparoscopic surgery must be balanced against the adverse effects of increased intra-abdominal pressure caused by CO_2 insufflation, and pneumoperitoneum and cardiopulmonary effects such as increased peripheral vascular resistance and decreased venous return. Hypercarbia and acidosis are direct myocardial depressants. It is imperative to maintain adequate preoperative and intraoperative volume control and careful mechanical ventilation to control hypercarbia and acidosis to allow safe application of minimally invasive procedures in the elderly.[36]

Breast Surgery

Postmenopausal women, aged 55 years and older, account for approximately 66% of incident cases of breast cancers and experience 77% of breast cancer mortality.[37] Ironically, the screening for breast cancer is less widespread in women older than 65 than in women younger than 65.[38] Physicians should strongly consider recommending annual screenings until the age of 75, after this age, screening should be performed yearly or even at 3-year intervals. However, prior to taking hormone replacement therapy, patients of any age should undergo mammogram screening. Additionally, in terms of screening, an important factor to consider is life expectancy; however, it is important to note that comorbid, progressive conditions (i.e., NYHA III and IV, severe diabetes, CHF, steroid or oxygen-dependent COPD, malignancy, and terminal condition) affect the screening outcomes.

It is recommended that clinical breast examinations be performed annually. Further, to increase awareness, it is recommended that one performs self-examinations monthly; however, it is important to note that this can be difficult for those who have conditions such neuropathy or arthritis within the hands. In such patients, annual clinical breast examination is of great importance.[39]

In terms of determining surgical candidacy for the elderly, it is recommended that Preoperative Assessment of Cancer in the Elderly (PACE) be employed. It predicts the individualized risk of cancer surgery and the post-operative complications.[40] Interestingly, both younger patients and patients over 70 years of age should be offered the same surgery. However, there are a few procedures that are often performed including breast conserving surgery, whole breast radiotherapy, and mastectomy (with or without postoperative radiotherapy). A mastectomy should be performed for large or multifocal tumors that cannot be treated with conservative excision. Axillary Lymph Node Dissection (ALND) should be performed if there are nodes that are present or highly suspected on a physical exam. In clinically node negative disease, axillary staging by Sentinel Lymph Node Biopsy (SLNB) with completion ALND for tumor positive SLNB should be completed. Tamoxifen treatment is only indicated for ER-positive tumors in the elderly with a short life expectancy of less than two to three years and who are not surgical candidates after optimization of medical conditions, or if the patient refuses surgery.

Chemotherapy tends to have greater effects on patients who are hormone negative but have positive nodes. Specifically, in such patients, anthracycline is commonly administered. In addition, trastuzumab can be given to HER2-positive patients with no underlying cardiac disease. However, if older women have metastatic ER-positive cancer, then hormone treatment should be offered.[41]

Thyroid and Parathyroid Surgery

The incidence of thyroid cancer increases with age. Elderly patients will most often present with cardiac symptoms related to hyperthyroidism (i.e., atrial fibrillation). Surgical intervention for a thyroid nodule depends on the characteristic of the nodule such as the nodule being benign, malignant, euthyroid, or thyrotoxic. If the nodule increases in size and leads to symptoms of compression, surgery is needed. For elderly thyroid cancer patients, surgery has an increased risk of mortality.[42] The incidence of papillary carcinoma decreases with age, however elderly patients have an increased risk of local recurrence and distant metastases.[43] The risk of mortality from follicular carcinoma increases with age due to a higher prevalence of vascular invasion and extracapsular extension.[42] Anaplastic carcinoma occurs primarily in the elderly patients and rapid local invasion may lead to airway blockage, dysphagia, or cervical tenderness. Surgical resection of the tumor is usually not attempted for cure due to poor prognosis of the tumor, however, surgical palliation or tracheostomy may be done to alleviate respiratory distress.[44]

In the geriatric population, there is convincing evidence of improved quality of life after surgery for primary hyperparathyroidism.[45] The symptoms of hyperparathyroidism usually encountered in elderly patients are a dementia-like state and osteoporosis.[46] Limited parathyroidectomy without bilateral neck dissection is a viable option in patients with multiple comorbidities. A drop in the intraoperative levels of PTH can be used to confirm the removal of a suspected hypersecreting parathyroid gland.[45]

Cardiovascular Surgery

Coronary Artery Bypass Grafting (CABG)

The number of elderly patients undergoing cardiovascular surgery has been increasing over the years. An improvement in preoperative assessment and patient selection has led to decreased morbidity and mortality rates in the elderly after cardiac surgery.[47] Amongst the elderly, CABG is associated with increased mortality rates due to depressed left ventricular function, postoperative stroke, the need for a preoperative or postoperative intra-aortic balloon, previous CABG, postoperative adult respiratory distress syndrome, and mediastinitis.[48] The elderly group has a significantly higher incidence of comorbid conditions such as COPD, cerebrovascular disease, and renal dysfunction. Elderly patients have a higher chance of having triple-vessel disease due to poor ejection fraction, left ventricular hypertrophy, significant valvular disease, and a previous history of myocardial infarction compared to their younger counterparts.[47] In addition, there is a higher probability for the geriatric population to be classified as NYHA class III or higher, and for their condition to be more emergent. Despite these risk factors, octogenarians can undergo CABG with a favorable outcome when done electively in patients with normal to moderately depressed left ventricular function.[49] The overall mortality rate is approximately 3% in elective cases, 13.5% in urgent cases, and 33% in emergent cases.[49]

Valve Replacement Surgery

It has been found that many elderly patients often present with valvular disease with the most common one being senile calcific aortic stenosis, followed by ischemic regurgitation of the mitral valve.[47] The operative mortality rates are 5.3% for aortic valve replacement and 20.4% for mitral valve replacement.[50] Additional coronary artery bypass grafting increases the mortality rate in patients >70 years of age to 8% for aortic valve replacement.[51] The most common complication after any valve surgery is a neurological problem. This could be due to an embolus from the diseased valve, a thrombus in the atrium, or an ascending aortic disease.[47] Long-term complications to be anticipated after valve surgery include thromboembolism, anticoagulant related hemorrhage, hemolysis, infections, and valve dysfunction. Bioprosthetic valves are preferred over mechanical valves whenever possible to avoid life-long anticoagulation.

Geriatric Trauma

The aging population has led to an increase in geriatric trauma, accounting for approximately 23% of hospital trauma admissions.[52] Elderly patients do not tolerate trauma as well as younger patients because of severe pre-existing comorbid conditions. The decreased physiological reserve in the geriatric trauma patient could result in a downward spiral of complications, organ dysfunction, and death.[53] In elderly patients, standard injury scoring systems including the Injury Severity Score (ISS) is generally a worse predictor than in younger patients.[54] Geriatric patients are at an increased risk of delayed death from trauma (> 24 hours), with the most common cause of death being multiple organ failure and sepsis.[53] Falls and syncope are the two most common causes of injury in the elderly.[55] Patients more than 80 years of age tend to have an increased morbidity and mortality from blunt thoracic trauma which can lead to rib fractures and pneumonia.[56] An aggressive and multidisciplinary approach to the treatment of an elderly trauma patient is warranted.[53] Although the majority of elderly injury survivors achieve independent living, long-term follow-up indicates significant residual disability in quality of life.[57]

Special Concerns in the Terminally Ill Patients

Gastrointestinal Disturbances

Nausea and vomiting cause much physical and psychological discomfort for terminally ill patients and their families. The main syndromes identified for nausea and vomiting include gastric stasis, medications, chemotherapy, raised intracranial pressure, mechanical bowel obstruction, ileus, or anxiety induced emesis.[58] It is important to have a thorough history and physical examination to measure the severity of the symptoms and find an underlying etiology.[59] Drugs are the mainstay of treatment and the oral route is the best option for prophylaxis prior to chemotherapy. However, if a patient cannot tolerate oral treatment, they may require suppositories or injections.[58] Special attention should be made to prevent dehydration or malnutrition that may be due to poor oral intake.

Diarrhea and constipation are common gastrointestinal disturbances in terminal patients. Constipation can be caused by narcotics, intestinal obstruction, metabolic abnormalities, and dehydration. Patients should be well hydrated and can be treated with stool softeners and laxatives to alleviate constipation.[60] Diarrhea, although less frequent than constipation, has a multifactorial etiology ranging from drugs, radiotherapy, chemotherapy, or the disease process itself. Treatment should be directed at maintaining hydration and therapies for symptomatic improvement such as bulk-forming agents, opioids, and octreotide.[60]

Malignant Bowel Obstruction

Malignant bowel obstruction can result from advanced gastrointestinal malignancy or from the extrinsic compression of bowel loops from progressive tumor burden. Patients typically present with cramping abdominal pain, nausea, and vomiting.[61] Conservative therapy includes NPO, IV fluids, and nasogastric decompression. Medical palliation includes antiemetics, antispasmodics, and octreotide.[60] Surgical palliation may offer permanent relief from obstruction but is associated with higher perioperative morbidity and mortality. Patients with ascites, multiple sites of obstruction, poor functional status, and poor nutrition with serum albumin levels <3g/dL are unlikely to benefit from palliative surgery.[61]

Depression and Asthenia

Asthenia encompasses symptoms of fatigue not relieved by rest, decreased mental capacity, and decreased overall functioning.[62] Depression and asthenia are common causes of an impaired quality of life in terminally ill patients. In cancer patients, overactivity of the hypothalamic-pituitary-adrenal axis along with increased levels of IL-6 have been implicated as the causes of depression.[63] Treatment of depression should be individualized. Patients with intense stress reactions should be offered psychotherapy. Pharmacotherapy is the choice of treatment for patients with major depressive disorder.[63] Psychostimulants are effective in the management of asthenia.

Anorexia and Cachexia

Anorexia and Cachexia (i.e., wasting syndromes) may be caused by systemic illnesses such as chronic organ failure, AIDS, infections, and cancer.[62] Elevated levels of cytokines like IL-6 and TNF may play an important role in the metabolic alterations leading to wasting syndromes.[61] However, with cancer/hypermetabolism, wasting syndrome is often not reversible with commonly employed nutrition strategies. In the absence of an underlying correctable cause, dexamethasone and prednisone may be beneficial because they can increase the patient's appetite and improve their quality of life.[61]

Pain Management

Pain is present in 89% of patients referred to palliative care.[64] An initial pain assessment should include the severity of pain, aggravating/relieving factors, and other qualitative features often used to describe pain. Therapy should then be individualized for every patient. Drugs commonly used for the treatment of pain include nonopioid analgesics such as acetaminophen and nonsteroidals. These can be combined with opioids to improve efficacy. Opioids include weaker compounds like codeine or stronger agents such as morphine, oxycodone, methadone, hydromorphone, and fentanyl.[61]

Patients with intermittent pain receive immediate-release medications on an as-needed basis. Patients with constant pain receive around-the-clock or sustained release medications. Dose can be escalated reasonably according to the patient's report of pain. Transdermal fentanyl patches are helpful for chronic pain management in terminally ill patients. Morphine is the drug of choice and is the reference point for all the other opioids that are used. Short-acting drugs like Demerol should be avoided for chronic use as they can lead to CNS toxicity. NSAIDs are helpful in managing mild to moderate somatic pain but have a "ceiling effect".[61] NSAIDs are particularly useful in managing pain from bony metastases.

The most common side effect of opioids is constipation, so patients need to be prescribed laxatives along with opioids. Lactulose is the best choice for a laxative, as it is both a stool softener and an evacuant. Another concern while prescribing high doses of opioids is respiratory depression, but tolerance to respiratory depression develops within 36 hours and thus large doses of morphine can be safely prescribed in terminally ill patients. Providers should not be deterred from prescribing pain medication due to addiction because terminally ill patients require analgesics to improve their quality of life. Further, such patients rarely demonstrate symptoms of addiction.[61]

Palliative Surgery

Palliative surgery for advanced cancer patients involves complex decision making for caregivers and patients. It focuses on providing the maximum benefit to the patient with the least invasive intervention so as to improve the quality of life in terminal disease states.[65] Surgical palliation may range from extensive debulking surgeries to less invasive procedures to alleviate symptoms like intractable vomiting.

Palliative care shifts the focus from curing a disease to quality. It often employs a multidisciplinary approach involving chemotherapy, hospice, radiotherapy, and surgical intervention. However, risks and benefits must be carefully considered upon practicing surgical interventions.[66]

Studies have shown that age should not be considered as a criterion in decision making for palliative surgery. Data supports equivalent outcomes from palliative surgery for older patients with good functional status when compared to younger patients.[67]

Medication Use in Elderly Patients

The American Geriatric Society (AGS) has updated the Beers Criteria in 2012. This criteria separates major medications or classes of mediations into three categories: (1) potentially inappropriate medications and classes of medication to avoid in the elderly, (2) potentially inappropriate medications and classes of medication to avoid in the elderly who have specific diseases and syndromes due to the risk of causing an exacerbation, and (3) medications to use with caution in the elderly.[68] The criteria urge to avoid the use of anticholinergics, antispasmodics, antiparkinsonian agents, and antithrombotic agents in elderly patients. There is evidence to avoid the use of NSAIDs COX-2 inhibitors, diltiazem, verapamil, and thiazolidinediones (i.e., pioglitazone and rosiglitazone) in patients with heart failure. Alpha blockers and tricyclic antidepressants should be avoided in patients with a history of syncope. Anticholinergics, benzodiazepines, and antipsychotics should be avoided in patients with dementia and cognitive impairment. Aspirin, antipsychotics, carbamazepine, tricyclic antidepressants, and vasodilators should be used with caution in older adults.

Ethical Considerations

End-of-life care dilemmas have gained attention amongst terminally ill patients. Straightforward and open communication with the patient and family is the key to effective and compassionate end-of-life care.[69] Physicians are not required to provide futile life-sustaining treatments. The decisions of the patient or surrogate decision maker take precedence over a physician's judgment of what is the most appropriate care.[65] To avoid conflict between the family and patients, communication must be emphasized; diagnosis, treatment plans, and transition to palliative care must be discussed at length.[67]

REFERENCES

1. United Nations. Dept. of Economic and Social Affairs. Population Division., World population ageing, 1950-20502002, New York: United Nations. xlix, 483 p.

2. Aging Statistics. 09/01/2011; Available from: http://www.aoa.gov/aoaroot/aging_statistics/index.aspx.
3. Number, percent distribution, rate, days of care with average length of stay, and standard error of discharges from short-stay hospitals, by sex and age: United States, 2009. 2009; Available from: http://www.cdc.gov/nchs/data/nhds/2average/2009ave2_ratesexage.pdf.
4. Etzioni DA, et al. The aging population and its impact on the surgery workforce. Ann Surg, 2003. 238(2): p. 170-7.
5. Ergina PL, Gold SL, Meakins JL. Perioperative care of the elderly patient. World J Surg, 1993. 17(2): p. 192-8.
6. Thomas DR, Ritchie CS. Preoperative assessment of older adults. J Am Geriatr Soc, 1995. 43(7): p. 811-21.
7. Preston SD, et al. Geriatric surgery is about disease, not age. J R Soc Med, 2008. 101(8): p. 409-15.
8. Dripps RD, Lamont A, Eckenhoff JE. The role of anesthesia in surgical mortality. JAMA, 1961. 178: p. 261-6.
9. Muravchick S. Preoperative assessment of the elderly patient. Anesthesiol Clin North America, 2000. 18(1): p. 71-89, vi.
10. Hosking MP, et al. Outcomes of surgery in patients 90 years of age and older. JAMA, 1989. 261(13): p. 1909-15.
11. Seymour DG, Vaz FG. A prospective study of elderly general surgical patients: II. Post-operative complications. Age Ageing, 1989. 18(5): p. 316-26.
12. Knaus WA, et al. The APACHE III prognostic system. Risk prediction of hospital mortality for critically ill hospitalized adults. Chest, 1991. 100(6): p. 1619-36.
13. Audisio RA, et al. Preoperative assessment of surgical risk in oncogeriatric patients. Oncologist, 2005. 10(4): p. 262-8.
14. Seymour DG, Pringle R. Post-operative complications in the elderly surgical patient. Gerontology, 1983. 29(4): p. 262-70.
15. Seltzer MH, et al. Instant nutritional assessment. JPEN J Parenter Enteral Nutr, 1979. 3(3): p. 157-9.
16. Mullen JL, et al. Reduction of operative morbidity and mortality by combined preoperative and postoperative nutritional support. Ann Surg, 1980. 192(5): p. 604-13.
17. Miller DL. Perioperative care of the elderly patient: special considerations. Cleve Clin J Med, 1995. 62(6): p. 383-90.
18. Eagle KA, et al. ACC/AHA Guideline Update for Perioperative Cardiovascular Evaluation for Noncardiac Surgery--Executive Summary. A report of the American College of Cardiology/American Heart Association Task Force on Practice Guidelines (Committee to Update the 1996 Guidelines on Perioperative Cardiovascular Evaluation for Noncardiac Surgery). Anesth Analg, 2002. 94(5): p. 1052-64.
19. Wertheim WA. Perioperative risk. Review of two guidelines for assessing older adults. American College of Cardiology and American Heart Association. Geriatrics, 2000. 55(7): p. 61-6; quiz 69.
20. Detsky AS, et al. Predicting cardiac complications in patients undergoing non-cardiac surgery. J Gen Intern Med, 1986. 1(4): p. 211-9.
21. Goldman L, et al. Multifactorial index of cardiac risk in noncardiac surgical procedures. N Engl J Med, 1977. 297(16): p. 845-50.
22. Lee TH, et al. Derivation and prospective validation of a simple index for prediction of cardiac risk of major noncardiac surgery. Circulation, 1999. 100(10): p. 1043-9.
23. Goldman L. Assessment of perioperative cardiac risk. N Engl J Med, 1994. 330(10): p. 707-9.
24. Mangano DT, et al. Dipyridamole thallium-201 scintigraphy as a preoperative screening test. A reexamination of its predictive potential. Study of Perioperative Ischemia Research Group. Circulation, 1991. 84(2): p. 493-502.
25. Eagle KA, et al. Combining clinical and thallium data optimizes preoperative assessment of cardiac risk before major vascular surgery. Ann Intern Med, 1989. 110(11): p. 859-66.
26. Lindenauer PK, et al. Perioperative beta-blocker therapy and mortality after major noncardiac surgery. N Engl J Med, 2005. 353(4): p. 349-61.
27. Dajani AS, et al. Prevention of bacterial endocarditis. Recommendations by the American Heart Association. JAMA, 1997. 277(22): p. 1794-801.
28. Mohr DN, Jett JR. Preoperative evaluation of pulmonary risk factors. J Gen Intern Med, 1988. 3(3): p. 277-87.
29. Smetana GW. Preoperative pulmonary assessment of the older adult. Clin Geriatr Med, 2003. 19(1): p. 35-55.
30. Crapo RO. Pulmonary-function testing. N Engl J Med, 1994. 331(1): p. 25-30.
31. Zibrak JD, O'Donnell CR, Marton K. Indications for pulmonary function testing. Ann Intern Med, 1990. 112(10): p. 763-71.
32. Beck LH. Perioperative renal, fluid, and electrolyte management. Clin Geriatr Med, 1990. 6(3): p. 557-69.
33. Hou SH, et al. Hospital-acquired renal insufficiency: a prospective study. Am J Med, 1983. 74(2): p. 243-8.
34. Novis BK, et al. Association of preoperative risk factors with postoperative acute renal failure. Anesth Analg, 1994. 78(1): p. 143-9.

35. Keller SM, et al. Emergency and elective surgery in patients over age 70. Am Surg, 1987. 53(11): p. 636-40.
36. Stewart BT, Stitz RW, Lumley JW. Laparoscopically assisted colorectal surgery in the elderly. Br J Surg, 1999. 86(7): p. 938-41.
37. Yancik R, et al. Effect of age and comorbidity in postmenopausal breast cancer patients aged 55 years and older. JAMA, 2001. 285(7): p. 885-92.
38. Costanza ME. The extent of breast cancer screening in older women. Cancer, 1994. 74(7 Suppl): p. 2046-50.
39. Breast cancer screening in older women. American Geriatrics Society Clinical Practice Committee. J Am Geriatr Soc, 2000. 48(7): p. 842-4.
40. Pasetto LM, Lise M, Monfardini S. Preoperative assessment of elderly cancer patients. Crit Rev Oncol Hematol, 2007. 64(1): p. 10-8.
41. Biganzoli L, et al. Management of elderly patients with breast cancer: updated recommendations of the International Society of Geriatric Oncology (SIOG) and European Society of Breast Cancer Specialists (EUSOMA). Lancet Oncol, 2012. 13(4): p. e148-60.
42. Mueller-Gaertner HW, Brzac HT, Rehpenning W. Prognostic indices for tumor relapse and tumor mortality in follicular thyroid carcinoma. Cancer, 1991. 67(7): p. 1903-11.
43. McConahey WM, et al. Papillary thyroid cancer treated at the Mayo Clinic, 1946 through 1970: initial manifestations, pathologic findings, therapy, and outcome. Mayo Clin Proc, 1986. 61(12): p. 978-96.
44. Har-El G, et al. Thyroid cancer in patients 70 years of age or older. Retrospective study of 50 patients. Ann Otol Rhinol Laryngol, 1987. 96(4): p. 403-10.
45. Irvin GL. 3rd and D.M. Carneiro, "Limited" parathyroidectomy in geriatric patients. Ann Surg, 2001. 233(5): p. 612-6.
46. Sheldon DG, et al. Surgical treatment of hyperparathyroidism improves health-related quality of life. Arch Surg, 2002. 137(9): p. 1022-6; discussion 1026-8.
47. Aziz S, and Grover FL. Cardiovascular surgery in the elderly. Cardiol Clin, 1999. 17(1): p. 213-31.
48. Khan SS, et al. Interaction of age and preoperative risk factors in predicting operative mortality for coronary bypass surgery. Circulation, 1992. 86(5 Suppl): p. II186-90.
49. Ko W, et al. Isolated coronary artery bypass grafting in one hundred consecutive octogenarian patients. A multivariate analysis. J Thorac Cardiovasc Surg, 1991. 102(4): p. 532-8.
50. Davis EA, et al. Valvular disease in the elderly: influence on surgical results. Ann Thorac Surg, 1993. 55(2): p. 333-7; discussion 337-8.
51. Zaidi AM, et al. Good outcomes from cardiac surgery in the over 70s. Heart, 1999. 82(2): p. 134-7.
52. Richmond TS, et al. Characteristics and outcomes of serious traumatic injury in older adults. J Am Geriatr Soc, 2002. 50(2): p. 215-22.
53. Perdue PW, et al. Differences in mortality between elderly and younger adult trauma patients: geriatric status increases risk of delayed death. J Trauma, 1998. 45(4): p. 805-10.
54. Oreskovich MR, et al. Geriatric trauma: injury patterns and outcome. J Trauma, 1984. 24(7): p. 565-72.
55. Rubenstein LZ, Josephson KR. The epidemiology of falls and syncope. Clin Geriatr Med, 2002. 18(2): p. 141-58.
56. Bergeron E, et al. Elderly trauma patients with rib fractures are at greater risk of death and pneumonia. J Trauma, 2003. 54(3): p. 478-85.
57. Inaba K, et al. Long-term outcomes after injury in the elderly. J Trauma, 2003. 54(3): p. 486-91.
58. Glare PA, et al. Treatment of nausea and vomiting in terminally ill cancer patients. Drugs, 2008. 68(18): p. 2575-90.
59. Markowitz AJ, Rabow MW. Management of intractable nausea and vomiting in patients at the end of life: "I was feeling nauseous all of the time . . . nothing was working". JAMA, 2008. 299(15): p. 1826.
60. Cherny NI. Taking care of the terminally ill cancer patient: management of gastrointestinal symptoms in patients with advanced cancer. Ann Oncol, 2004. 15 Suppl 4: p. iv205-13.
61. Dunn GP, et al. Palliative care by the surgeon: how to do it. J Am Coll Surg, 2002. 194(4): p. 509-37.
62. Ross DD, Alexander CS. Management of common symptoms in terminally ill patients: Part I. Fatigue, anorexia, cachexia, nausea and vomiting. Am Fam Physician, 2001. 64(5): p. 807-14.
63. Hinshaw DB, Carnahan JM, Johnson DL. Depression, anxiety, and asthenia in advanced illness. J Am Coll Surg, 2002. 195(2): p. 271-7; discussion 277-8.
64. Glare P, Walsh D, Sheehan D. The adverse effects of morphine: a prospective survey of common symptoms during repeated dosing for chronic cancer pain. Am J Hosp Palliat Care, 2006. 23(3): p. 229-35.
65. Sullivan DJ, Hansen-Flaschen J. Termination of life support after major trauma. Surg Clin North Am, 2000. 80(3): p. 1055-66.

66. Galante JM, et al. Experience and attitudes of surgeons toward palliation in cancer. Arch Surg, 2005. 140(9): p. 873-8; discussion 878-80.
67. McCahill LE, et al. Decision making in palliative surgery. J Am Coll Surg, 2002. 195(3): p. 411-22; discussion 422-3.
68. American Geriatrics Society updated Beers Criteria for potentially inappropriate medication use in older adults. J Am Geriatr Soc, 2012. 60(4): p. 616-31.
69. Burns JP, et al. End-of-life care in the pediatric intensive care unit: attitudes and practices of pediatric critical care physicians and nurses. Crit Care Med, 2001. 29(3): p. 658-64.

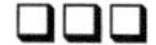

5
CHAPTER

Clinical Research

Ashir Kumar, MD

INTRODUCTION

Clinical research has contributed to significant changes in the practice of medicine. Following the Second World War, when the experiments on humans that were carried out in the concentration camps by physicians in Germany were brought to light, and later when it was discovered that unethical research practices were also common in western countries, the need for universal guidelines addressing the ethical principles for human research became clear. The Nuremberg Code was drafted in August 1947, and since then has served as the foundation for human subject research. This was followed by the Declaration of Helsinki in 1964.[1] In the United States; the Belmont Report was formulated in 1979 by the National Commission for the Protection of Human Subjects of Biomedical and Behavioral Research.[2]

Today in the 21st century, surgeons engage in a wide variety of research activities which have clinical implications. These include experiments on laboratory animals, basic science research, utilizing blood or tissues from human subjects, retrospective chart reviews, utilizing surgical techniques in an experimental manner, use of medical and surgical devices, utilizing tissues or organs obtained from other species for human beings, and patient surveys, etc. It is beyond the scope of this chapter to elaborate on steps necessary for planning and developing each of these research areas. However, it is essential that all research should have sound planning and undergo critical review by a team that includes a statistician, as well as experienced and qualified clinicians and scientists. A poorly designed research proposal which lacks the potential to answer a valid scientific question is not worth carrying out as it produces risks to human subjects without the potential of any benefit to society or individuals.

It is essential to consider the boundaries between biomedical research and the practice of medicine since research and practice often overlap. The 'practice of medicine' is defined as a commonly accepted procedure or intervention that is designed to positively contribute to the well-being of a person. Research is defined as a systematic investigation to test a hypothesis or to contribute to generalizable knowledge. For regulatory purposes, investigators should consider any activity involving human beings as research if there is any component of research present; this is the case even if there is an overlap with the 'practice of medicine.' The Nuremberg Code, which focuses on the basic rights of study subjects, and the Declaration of Helsinki, which defined the responsibility of researchers to the study subjects, provided the basis for current regulations.[3] In the United States, Federal regulations are based upon the Belmont Report which summarizes the general ethical principles that should underlie the conduct of research involving human subjects.[1-5]

These principles are (1) respect for persons, (2) beneficence, and (3) justice

1. **Respect for Persons**: This principle is divided into two moral requirements, the requirement to acknowledge autonomy and the requirement to protect those with diminished autonomy. Thus, it demands that subjects are enrolled only after they voluntarily consent. A person who is not able to fully comprehend the nature of the research should not be a research subject in most instances. In the case of incapacitated individuals, it may require protecting them while they are incapacitated.[2]
2. **Beneficence**: This can be summarized as first do no harm, and then maximize possible benefits and minimize possible harms. For physicians this is not new. The Hippocratic Oath, do no harm, has been a basic principle of medical ethics across the globe. Investigators, in conjunction with Ethics Board, should determine the best way to reduce risks and maximize benefits when a specific research activity may not provide benefit to the research subject, but may offer the potential of benefit to other patients or society at large.[2]

3. **Justice**: This requires fairness in the selection of patients in medical research and should be applicable at both the individual and societal level. The ethical selection of research patients requires that only poor patients, minorities, or patients living in institutions not be systematically selected. Similarly, conducting specific research studies in countries which are unlikely to benefit, either because of lack of medical resources or because of the medical practices in the population, would be unethical. Ethics boards reviewing the research application often collaborate either with community ethics boards or with representatives from the tribe to assure that this principle is not overlooked.[2]

To assure that the principles outlined in the Nuremberg Code, the Declaration of Helsenki and the Belmont Report are followed, various international organizations and government and research institutions (i.e., hospitals, universities, and clinics) have developed regulations for investigators to abide with. Institutional Review Boards (IRB), medical ethics boards, or other designated bodies conduct the review of the research to assure that the investigators are meeting local and governmental regulations before any subjects are enrolled.[5-9] Most scientific journals require authors to attest that the research paper being considered consists of research data collected only after the research protocol was duly approved by an IRB. Several government agencies require that clinical trials be listed on websites open to the scientific community and public at large before research is carried out. Similarly, funding agencies require that IRB approval be sought before funds can be utilized for research.

The Consent Process

The Consent Process is the cornerstone of ethical research.[2,5] Table 1 lists important elements of the consent document. It is essential to have a\n adequate consent document developed specifically for the subject population and the nature of research. This requires that the document be easily comprehended by the study subjects. It should clearly describe the nature of research study, study procedures, potential risks, and anticipated benefits, if any. In medical research, it is essential that subjects be informed if alternative treatment options are available to them if they refuse to participate in the research. Research physicians should be aware that as researchers and physicians, they often have an inherent advantage when a patient is being treated in any setting where the patient expects that the treating physician will only offer the best. Depending upon the societal norms and hierarchy, the patient may feel that they are in a position where they cannot challenge or ask questions to the treating physician or their staff. It is essential that all researchers understand that signatures on a consent form should not be considered valid if the research subject did not comprehend the research study or did not agree to place their signature under duress. Obtaining consent is not merely having signatures on a piece of paper but following a well-developed process where the patient has no reason to feel coerced and thus has the freedom to decline to participate without any implication on their future relationship with the physician researcher or the medical institution. Further, the subject should be provided information regarding who should be contacted to obtain additional information about the research study, to understand the rights as a human subject of research, to report any adverse events, and to register any complaints or irregularities about the research itself.

Table 1: Important Components of Consent Document[2,5,10]

• Statement that study involves research
• Appropriate alternative procedures/treatment so that a subject does not believe that participation in the research activity is the only option
• Purpose of research study
• Expected duration of subject's participation
• Procedures (in lay person's language, avoiding medical jargon) to be followed
• Risks to study participant
• Potential benefits to the study subject or others (do not over promise, if there were well accepted benefits why would you be testing it further)
• Confidentiality of research records and subject's privacy
• Any compensation to the subject
• Contact information of individual(s) who will answer any questions related to the research
• Persons or agencies to contact for research related injury or other adverse outcomes
• Persons or agencies who are responsible for providing care in the event of a bad outcome/injury, and person or agencies who will be responsible for payment/fees
• Persons or agencies to contact to understand the rights of the research subject or to lodge a complaint or concern about the research investigator's conduct
• An explicit statement that participation in research activity is voluntary
• An explicit statement that refusal to participate will involve no penalty, or loss of benefits for the subject
• An explicit statement that the research subject may discontinue participation at any time during the course of the study, without penalty or loss of benefits. If there are consequences for the subject's decision to withdraw, list those.
• A place for the subject's name, signatures, and date

Human Subject Research Related Regulations

It is beyond the scope of this chapter to discuss fine points of all research regulations. Researchers should be aware that there are International Standards and country specific regulations. In the United States, research is regulated under 45 Code of Federal Regulations (CFR), and 46 by the Office of Human Research Protection (OHRP) under the United States Department of Health and Human Services. Besides these federal regulations, there are state and local regulations dealing with specific issues (e.g., stem cell research).[8-10] In India, the Medical Council of India (MCI) and the Indian Council of Medical Research (ICMR) have guidelines for physicians and other medical researchers to follow.[8,9]

Researchers should also be aware that there may be tribal customs or religious edicts that may interfere with certain research. In the United States there are the Food and Drug Administration's (FDA) regulations that researchers and institutions need to comply with. Approved drugs and medical devices fall within these regulations. The FDA also requires that all clinical trials be listed on a specific website. Similarly in India, The Clinical Trials Registry, India (CTRI) hosted at the ICMR's National Institute of Medical Statistics is an online public record system for registering clinical trials being conducted in India.[11] The ICMR has also published guidance for investigators for collaborative medical research in India. Researchers based in the United States should be cognizant that approval from government and other regulatory bodies abroad may take additional time for review and approval, and therefore should work closely with their collaborators abroad to assure that all necessary regulations are met. Over the past two decades, newspaper headlines and journal articles have vividly described research where the researchers from abroad, including the United States based researchers, did not follow the guidelines, or a particular research study offered no benefit to the local population. Due diligence in dealing with local regulatory and human ethical issues is essential if one does not want to be a subject of such exposure on the internet or other media. It is the responsibility of the principal investigator, being the team leader, to assure that all members of the research team are knowledgeable about research regulations and are sensitive to the needs of research subjects.[12-15]

Research Categories and the Review Process[10]

Depending upon the risk to the human subjects, OHRP classifies research into three categories: exempt from review, expedited review category, and full review category.

Exempt from Review: A research project is classified as exempt if it involves no more than the minimal risk to the human subject and the research falls within six defined categories. Minimal risk means that the probability and magnitude of anticipated harm or discomfort in research are not greater than those ordinarily encountered in daily life, or during the performance of routine physical or psychological examination or tests. Just because the research falls within the "exempt" from review category does not mean that it requires no review by an IRB or another independent body. Researchers should familiarize themselves with institutional regulations to avoid being misled by the title 'exempt from review,' and then find themselves in non-compliance with the regulations.

Expedited Review Category: Research belonging in this category also involves no more than minimal risks to subjects but does not fall into any of the six exempt categories. Nine categories are identified for expedited review when certain specific guidelines are met for each subcategory.

Full Review Category: Any research where the potential of risk is more than minimal, falls under the full review category. All full review category research requires that it be approved at a convened board meeting with ample opportunity for prior review, and that there is adequate time for discussion by members at the meeting.

The IRB and research institutions set their own procedures, though fulfilling the OHRP guidance, to review and approve research projects falling in the Exempt and Expedited category.

Research Involving Vulnerable Populations

Institutional Review Boards and regulatory agencies often require that investigators identify if the study population will purposely include subjects that may be considered high risk, vulnerable, or susceptible to undue influence by researcher (e.g., minors, institutionalized persons, low income individuals, prisoners, patients with mental impairments, cognitively impaired individuals, wards of state or other agencies, students, pregnant women, women of child bearing age, patients with HIV infection, or subjects with certain other conditions that may make them more vulnerable). The rationale for obtaining this information is to assure that the review process takes into account steps necessary to protect human subjects, and that the required regulations are followed. If research protocol includes subjects who need additional protection, investigators should pay particular attention to the nature of vulnerability and describe measures taken during the consent process and the conduct of the research to minimize potential risks.[10,12-16] Table 2 lists the characteristics of research protocols that require additional scrutiny by the investigators and the IRBs.

Table 2: Study Protocols That Require Additional Scrutiny by Investigators and Regulatory Boards

• Conducting research in a developing country
• Conducting research in a population with a different language or dialect
• Conducting research in subjects with high illiteracy rates
• Conducting research in a population where research procedures/treatments have no potential to provide any benefit
• Obtaining tissue/blood and storing it for future research
• Potential for tissue/blood to be distributed to other institutions or colleagues who were not a part of the original research team
• Materials obtained from subjects that have potential to be patented and/or provide financial gains to investigators, institutions, or funding agencies
• Research using codes but not de-identified data
• Research on materials/data previously collected for research

How to Prepare For and Navigate the Review Process Successfully

Experienced researchers as well as young investigators often dread preparing an application for review by the IRB and then the review process that follows. Although the prime responsibility of the IRB or ethics committees is to protect human subjects, the committee members and the administrative staff also want to facilitate the conduct of ethical research. It is the responsibility of the principal investigator to set the tone for the research team, to assure that all team members are familiar with the existing regulations, and to work diligently to assure subjects safety. Table 3 summarizes the measures that investigators can take to facilitate review of their research protocol and successful completion of the work. Investigators should also be aware that regulations change frequently. Furthermore, it is essential to know how some regulations are interpreted and that IRBs differ across institutions. Therefore, when relocating to a new institution, one should not presume that regulations existing at the previous institution will still be adequate. Even if one is an experienced researcher, it would be prudent to discuss the nature of the research protocols with the IRB staff or chair. Clarifying issues and getting familiar with local requirements will save investigators valuable time and unnecessary correspondence.

Table 3: Measures that Investigators Should Take to Facilitate Compliance with Regulations.

• Assemble a dedicated research team sensitive to the issues related to human subject research
• Contact IRB to clarify issues that you consider may require additional review by the IRB
• Contact IRB to clarify issues that you consider may require additional review by the IRB
• While preparing an application, consult the IRB guidelines and consent requirements
• Submit a complete application with necessary attachments
• The PI and co-investigator should work closely with the research team in responding to queries during the review process
• Promptly submit any documents from the sponsors to the IRB for review. Add your comments to clarify the issues
• Good record keeping
• Submitting all revision and renewal materials at least 4 weeks before the lapse of approval to provide the IRB adequate time for review
• Inform the IRB of any correspondence regarding audits from the sponsor or other regulatory agencies
• Regularly meet with research staff to assure good communication

Acknowledgement: Jude Dye and Lydia Robinson provided valuable assistance in the preparation of this manuscript.

Note: Since this chapter discusses research regulations and historical documents related to the development of research regulations, several statements from the regulations and historical documents are included verbatim here.

REFERENCES

1. WMA Declaration of Helsinki – Ethical Principles for Medical Research Involving Human Subjects. Accessed at (7/2/2012): http://www.wma.net/en/30publication/10policies/b3/index.html.
2. The Belmont Report: Ethical Principles & Guidelines for the Protection of Human Subjects of Research. Accessed at (7/2/2012): http://www.hhs.gov/ohrp/humansubjects/guidence/belmont.html.
3. Shuster, Evelyne. Fifty Years Later: The Significance of the Nuremberg Code. N. Engl. J Med 1997; 337: 1436-1440.

4. International Ethical Guidelines for Biomedical Research Involving Human Subjects, Geneva: Council for International Organizations of Medical Sciences, 1993.
5. National Institute of Health, Office for Protection From Research Risks, Protection of Human Subjects, 45CFR.46, 1991.
6. International Compilation of Human Standards. Accessed at (7/2/2012): http://www.hhs.gov/ohrp/international/intlcompilation/intlcompilation.html.
7. Steinbrook, Robert. Improving Protection for Research Subjects. N. Engl. J Med 2002; 346: 1425-1430.
8. Vashishtha, Vipin M. MCI's New Code of Ethics for Medical Professionals: An Exercise in Vain or a Welcome More Indian Pediatrics. 2010; 47: 329-330.
9. Thatte UM, Bavdekar SB. Clinical Research in India: Great Expectations? J Postgrad Med. 2008; 54: 318-323.
10. Biomedical and Health Institutional Review board (BIRB), Michigan State University; Human Research Protection Program. Accessed at (10/4/2012) http://humanresearch.msu.edu/birb.html.
11. Clinical Trials Registry – India National Institute of Medical Statistics. (Indian Council of Medical Research). Accessed at (6/3/2012): http://ctri.nic.in/clinicaltrials/loginphp.
12. Ballantyne, Angela J. How to Do Research Fairly in an Unjust World. Amer J. Bioethics 2010; 10: 26-35.
13. Fitchett JR. Ethical Consideration of Clinical Trials in the Developing World. Trans R Soc Trop Med Hyg 2009; 103: 756-760.
14. Emerson CI, Singer PA, Upshur RE. Access & Use of Human Tissues from the Developing World: Ethical Challenges and a Way Forward Using a Tissue Trust. BMC Med Ethics 2011; 25:2.
15. Blom E, DeVries R. Towards Local Participation in the Creation of Ethical Research Guidelines. Indian J Med Ethics 2011; 8: 145-147.
16. Halila R. Assessing the Ethics of Medical Research in Emergency Settings: How Do International Regulations Work in Practice. Sci Eng Ethics 2007; 13: 305-313.

6

CHAPTER

Rural Surgery

Lauren Smithson, MD
Vijay Mittal, MD

1.1 INTRODUCTION

The art of being a true general surgeon is slowly fading with increasing sub-specialization and the explosion of surgical technology. Where this art remains is in the pockets of rural areas worldwide where individual surgeons are the sole providers of surgical care. There, trauma, gynecology, otolaryngology, obstetrics, orthopedics, all fall within the scope of practice. The rural surgeon is the general surgeon. The trends towards sub-specialization threaten the existence of the generalist surgeon, however. In 2012, 88% of US residents entered fellowships (ABS data). Not only are there fewer surgeons going into general practice, but there are also even less moving to rural communities to work.

The decline of rural surgery began to draw attention almost 30 years ago in America, and since then, many people have commented on the increasing need and critical shortage of general surgeons in rural practice. It has become a dilemma that has yet to find a solution. No suggestions to date have provided a lasting solution that provides general surgeons for an ever-present rural population. Surgical education also enters the discussion on the direction of rural surgery. Debates from as far back as 1994 have discussed the concept of rural surgery tracts or fellowships for general surgery residents interested in exploring the opportunities in community surgery, but opinions on the effectiveness and implementations still differ. Whatever the conclusions may be, the end point is that the disappearance of the general surgeon directly affects the number of rural practitioners, rural residents, and the communities that form the foundations of our collective societies. Although this chapter focuses primarily on rural surgery in the United States, the problem is experienced worldwide.

The loss of broad-based training, the desire for specialization, and the lack of exposure to rural options has had a significant impact on surgery in the rural communities, causing America to reach a critical point in the delivery of healthcare to nearly 60 million Americans. General surgery is indeed a primary care service, as crucial to the life of the community as it is to the lives of the patients. It is part of the general shift in our society away from the pastoral and towards the urban, but that does not negate its value. This chapter aims to outline the scope of rural practice, the changes in education, and the need for political advocacy that will help to rejuvenate a fundamental necessity at risk of extinction in the delivery of healthcare in the 21st century.

Rural Communities and Physician Distribution

As early as the 1960s, concern began to grow about the possibility of a physician shortage in rural communities.[1] At the beginning of the 20th century, 40% of America's population lived and worked on farms. As of 2005, this number dropped to 2%.[2] Despite the significant reduction in agriculture as a way of life, nearly 62 million Americans still live in areas that are deemed 'rural'. Many formats are available for the subdivision of the land into urban or rural, but most literature quotes the division of land into areas based on census information and commuting data. These 'areas' devised from the Rural-Urban Commuting Area (RUCA) codes include urban, large rural, and small rural or isolated rural areas.[1] Table 1 defines the population sizes in each area. RUCA was developed by the Washington, Wyoming, Alaska, Montana, Idaho Rural Health Research center (WWAMI), and is the accepted federal definition of rural communities.[3] According to these codes, 2,052 counties in the United States are considered rural. These commuting areas, however, do not always predict medical or surgical catchment geography accurately. Another population division based on a surgical education model describes small rural communities as <10,000, large rural communities as 10,000-50,000, and urban communities as >50,000.[4] Similar models for the division of territories or populations into rural sizes exist for Canada, Australia, and Northern Scotland.[5] These countries, among others, have also expressed concern over the loss of physician coverage in more rural areas, with coverage reaching a critical low in the last 10-20 years. In Canada, for example, the centralization of surgical services has resulted in a nearly 50% decrease of small volume surgical sites.[6]

Table 1: Division of Rural-Urban Commuting Areas (RUCA)[7]

RUCA	Population
Urban	>50,000
Large Rural	10,000-50,000
Small Rural or Isolated Rural	2,500-10,000

General surgeons are the second most common physician in rural areas after family practitioners. Family practitioners are evenly distributed between the RUCA populations, but general surgeons are most often found in large rural or urban areas. Isolated rural communities have a significant reduction in availability of surgeons per 100,000 people. Overall, since 1981, there has been a reduction by about 25% in the general surgery workforce in America; the population has been growing while the number of general surgeons has been declining. Where there were 1,047 general surgeons in 1981, 2008 had 1,032, which is approximately 5 per 100,000.[2] Between 1996 and 2006, the number of active general surgeons decreased by 2.3%.[8] The total number of practicing general surgeons is failing to keep up with the needs of the national population. This shortage is acutely felt in isolated areas. From 1981-2005, small rural areas showed a decline in practicing physicians of 16 to 35%.[7] In 2005, isolated rural areas were struggling to manage with 4.67 general surgeons per 100,000 whereas large rural areas had 7.71 per 100,000.[7] In North Carolina, 47 counties experienced a decline in the number of general surgeons from 1995-2005; four counties lost all their surgeons, and 18 had none.[2] Although variable between states, this trend of vacated counties is nationwide.

The increasing efficacy of emergency medical services and transport could lead to the conclusion that a loss of the general surgery workforce in the rural communities is acceptable, but this is false. Rural communities, both in America and abroad, appreciate having general surgery services closer to home.[9] People prefer individualized care in a familiar environment as it addresses their emotional, psychological, and cultural needs as well as their surgical needs.[6] Besides the contentment of the population, the role of the rural surgeon in triage for trauma in isolated areas is also indisputable.[10,11] At the American College of Surgeons meeting in October 2012, data was presented that indicated 69% of rural people have general surgery services less than 30 minutes away, and 95% of patients live within one hour of a general surgery service (ACS unpublished data). Regardless, there is not enough access. There are currently 1,250 to 1,400 critical access hospitals, but the number is dropping.[12] Not all of these critical access hospitals have surgical facilities. For example, 365 rural counties in America have operating room facilities available, but no operating surgeon.[12] As of 2009, 353 critical access hospitals in the United States have no surgeon in the county.[13] The Scottish Department of Health realized in the 1990s that some of the characteristics of remote communities in Scotland favored the continued provision of emergency surgical services.[14] Emergency care is at the heart of acute services in rural areas. The loss of surgical services has a spiraling effect, more than just emergency care. Maternal and fetal medicine in rural areas are both heavily reliant on general surgery. Without access to cesarean section, only 40% of women can deliver locally, whereas 85% delivered locally when a surgical service was available.[15] The presence of a surgical program stabilizes the delivery of emergency medicine, maternity care, and acute care, along with the recruitment and retention of health care staff.[16] These critical access hospitals, which are central to smaller communities, need surgeons to not only provide a necessary primary care service, but also for the financial stability of the community.

In the late 1980s and early 1990s, a closure of many community hospitals resulted in the loss of general surgeons in those rural environments, for, unlike general practitioners, surgeons require a hospital in order to manage their trade. The situation becomes somewhat of a 'chicken or egg' question. A general surgeon is an economic benefit to a medical center. Surgeons bring between 1 and 2.5 million dollars per year in revenue to the hospital where they practice.[12] In other words, surgeons bring in 40% of total revenue in ancillary services and 50% of inpatient services.[17] This often makes the difference between a critical access hospital remaining open or closing due to lack of financial viability. So, is it the closure of the hospitals that results in a decrease in rural surgery, or is it the loss of surgeons that results in the closure of hospitals? In a recent survey on the impact of surgeons on rural community hospitals, 87% of administrators thought surgery was critical to hospital viability, with 40% believing that the hospital would have to close if the general surgery service was lost.[11] Surgical patients are a valuable component to rural hospital occupancy rates, and the loss of this resource financially jeopardizes community hospitals further.[18] This interdependent relationship is at the heart of the issue. The financial aid brought to a community by a general surgeon is undeniable, but the likelihood of a surgeon being able to maintain a practice in a community is dependent on multiple intrinsic and extrinsic factors.

Just as the decreasing distribution of general surgeons in rural areas is of concern, so too are the physician demographics (Table 2). Close to one third of practicing surgeons in rural communities are over the age of 55 (ACRS unpublished data). Most are male or foreign graduates.[7] There are a variety of factors contributing to this bottleneck age effect. Current rural surgeons have typically had an established practice in their community for decades. Even when new surgeons choose to move to rural communities, they often do so at a later age. The decline in rural surgeons under the age of 40 occurred more in rural areas than urban ones, and there was an increase in those over 50.[7] The basic rate of attrition in surgery is contributing to the decline in numbers of rural practitioners.[4] The other demographic that is found in rural practice is foreign medical graduates. In Canada, 60% of rural surgical providers were foreign trained, serving a required return of service agreement.[19] Similar statistics are noted in Australia and New South Wales. The United States physician workforce is approximately 25% foreign medical graduates.[20] At present, foreign graduates are still accepted into surgical residencies, but this may be altered in the near future as policies change. Restricting foreign graduate entry into surgical residency would result in a further reduction of potential rural surgeons.

Table 2: Current demographics of rural surgeons

Male sex
Age >50
Foreign graduate
Raised in rural environment
History of previous urban practice
Spouse from a rural environment
No physicians in the family

Another demographic issue that has been raised amongst rural practitioners is the sex bias. Women now make up 60% of the medical student classes. From 1981 to 2005, the number of women in general surgery has gone from 1.4 to 13.4%. The number of women in general surgery is now approximately 25%. It has been noted that only 6.1% of rural practitioners in large rural areas are women, compared to 11.7% of surgeons in urban areas.[7] This may reflect the fact that most rural surgeons are older, and the number of women in surgery has only begun to increase in the last 20 years. Regardless of the reason, the discrepancy will be felt unless more women are encouraged to go rural. This is especially important as women are more likely to go into general practice than fellowship. This makes female surgeons a valuable commodity in an era where specialization is normal.[9] If there are more women entering general practice after residency, then exploring their interest in rural medicine should be undertaken. Few women are currently choosing to practice rural surgery.[1] Changing this statistic could open up an entirely new pool of available general surgeons, especially if there is a reduction in the number of foreign trained or rurally raised surgical trainees.

Those surgeons who do choose to go into rural practice are influenced by a number of personal factors. People from rural backgrounds more frequently chose to enter rural practice. As fewer people are dwelling in rural areas, the potential source of physicians is dwindling. Other physicians who choose to go to rural areas have had exposure to rural medicine during their training. Relatively few programs in America offer rural rotations or tracts for medical students or residents. Those who have spouses from rural areas are more likely to return to rural practice.[3,21] The influence of a spouse was among the three most important factors in the practitioners' decision-making paradigm.[22] Many surgeons are deterred from entering rural practice if no employment exists for their spouse. A further effect is family. Surgeons who do not have a physician in the family are more likely to choose rural practice. Those with a parent or sibling who was a physician are typically not inclined to pursue rural options.[21]

Issues in the Practice of General Surgery in Rural Communities

The life of a rural surgeon is a strange juxtaposition of satisfaction and frustration. Although approximately 85% of rural surgeons are pleased with their jobs, 25% planned to leave rural surgery within 5 years.[23] Considering the impact of these practitioners in rural communities, both from a medical and economic standpoint, it would seem that maintaining their presence is paramount. Many studies have been conducted to determine the factors that affect the decisions of rural surgeons to either commence or continue in rural surgery. Forty to fifty percent of rural surgeons are concerned over government intervention and the closure of rural hospitals affecting their practices.[18] The loss of control over practice and the financial concerns drives surgeons to more central areas. Thirty-one percent of surgeons that go to rural areas move within 5 years to either another location or back to fellowship.[13] The pleasure of an independent rural practice is often undermined by financial concern and fatigue.

One of these concerns is financial stability. Recent graduates from surgical residency carry between $150,000 and $400,000 in medical school debt. It is difficult to risk further financial strain in rural practice if there is little assurance of continuity, risk of hospital closure, or not enough work. Practicing rural surgeons who are not financially stable move to an urban practice. In Canada, many surgical practitioners feel that rural hospitals provide low volumes and low complexity due to limited support services. Employment at larger centers was necessary for financial survival, with rotations in rural hospitals.[24] Internationally, the lack of investment and commitment to surgeons and surgical infrastructure in rural areas has led surgeons to migrate to large cities and university centers, where the financial support is adequate.[20] In the United

States, however, there seems to be less difference in salaries between rural and urban surgeons, with rural surgeons making slightly less.[4] Rural reimbursement, however, is often lower than in urban environments.[25] There is concern over practice limitations from a financial perspective. The shift in medicine from a humanitarian approach to a business approach has resulted in fixed budgets and health care restrictions, which often undermines the delivery of health care. This unfortunate imbalance is furthered by the exponential increase in the cost of medical technology and pharmaceuticals that can be limited to rural hospitals. One example is the recent introduction of intravenous acetaminophen, which costs about 8 to 10 dollars for a 1-gram dose. The argument that it reduces opioid use and cost has been debated, and the cost of oral acetaminophen is a fraction of the expense.[26] Recent studies have shown that hospitalization costs of a laparoscopic appendectomy to be higher than that of an open surgery in uncomplicated cases.[27] Health care cost is quickly outstripping the ability to pay for it. One suggestion to counteract this financial concern is a hospitalist approach to surgical care, where the surgeon is employed by the institution, which has shown to have modest increases in net incomes for the general surgeon.[8] This is a format of employment in some US hospitals but is not mainstream practice. Other methods to reduce costs should be explored, such as protecting medical finances to divert towards maintaining critical access hospitals and employing surgeons for vacant rural operating rooms.

Health care restrictions also affect the availability of qualified staff. At an open forum of the American College of Surgeons, one young surgeon in solo rural practice remarked that, although he loved his life, it was somewhat impractical to "perform a partial colectomy for perforated diverticulitis in the middle of the night when your only assistant is a septuagenarian scrub nurse with crippling carpal tunnel syndrome". Ancillary staff is the backbone of safe and successful surgical care. Although the rural surgeon is typically the critical care intensivist, enterostomal therapist, and wound specialist, they cannot also be the respiratory therapist, scrub nurse, certified anesthetist, and postoperative care nursing staff. A lack of these elemental services means a non-functioning operative practice. Even the more peripheral non-surgical services are essential; for example, the radiology technologist and ultrasound technician are needed to maintain both the operative equipment and radiology equipment. Although a majority of these services are available in rural hospitals, the lack of them or the threat of their loss is a detrimental factor in providing adequate surgical care. The loss of general-practitioner (GP)-anesthetists in rural hospitals in Canada often results in the permanent loss of surgical and maternal services.[28] Consider intensive care, if a patient requires a procedure that would put them in the ICU postoperatively, but that ICU has no appropriately trained nursing staff or respiratory therapist, what is the alternative course for the surgeon? Either the surgeon stays and becomes both the intensivist and respiratory therapist or that patient gets referred to a tertiary center. It becomes the limitations of the system and not the limitations of the surgeon which affect the cases performed. The presence of an experienced and competent surgical team can be the determining factor towards favorable outcomes in emergent cases.[29] In surgical training, a 'systems-based practice' is emphasized. If that system is not available, then there is ultimately no role for the surgeon either. It is a dilemma of many rural surgeons, and one that many graduates interested in rural surgery would prefer to avoid.

Another element of rural practice is the breadth of its scope. Rural practitioners are often the only practitioners in the area and are responsible for the care and/or triage of patients and cases that they might not have faced in their training. One example is the proportion of gynecological procedures to general surgery procedures (Table 3). Many of the job postings currently seeking general surgeons require experience in cesarean sections and hysterectomies, along with the colectomies, cholecystectomies, and endoscopy requirements. Even in 1997, it was noted that endoscopy and gynecology made up a majority of the procedures performed in rural America.[9] In Australia, one study of a rural hospital with two general surgeons showed that they performed nearly 8,400 procedures in 5 years, with 46% of those outside the scope of what is typically considered 'general surgery cases'.[5] Orthopedics made up a majority of those cases including closed fractures, amputations, dislocations, and internal fixations.[5] In Canada, routine appendectomies, D&C, endoscopy, cesarean sections, obstetric repair, herniorrhaphies, and wound care are performed by general practitioner (GP)-surgeons, as permanent general surgeons are often not available.[30] Emergent surgery and triage fall to the rural surgeon, even if the hospital has rotators in subspecialties. This requires the ability to perform procedures that are well outside the field of general surgery.[5] These include vascular emergencies, multisystem trauma, cesareans, craniotomies, and peritonsillar abscesses. If elective procedures in these areas are shifted to regional centers, the skill set allowing a rural practitioner to perform emergent procedures safely is threatened.[19]

Table 3: Common procedures seen in rural surgery practices[5,9]

General Surgery (44% of total cases)*	Hernias Breast Colorectal Biliary Endocrine – thyroid, pancreas, adrenal
Endoscopy (29% of total cases)**	Colonoscopy Upper endoscopy PEG insertion Bronchoscopy
Orthopedics (12% of total cases)	Closed fracture reduction Internal fixation Amputations
Gynecology	Cesarean section Hysterectomy
Neurosurgery	Carpal Tunnel Emergent craniotomy and/or Burr hole
Thoracic	Thoracotomy Decortications Tracheostomy
Otolaryngology	Tonsillectomy Adenoidectomy
Urology	Vasectomy Circumcision Orchiectomy/Orchiopexy Nephrectomy
*Percent of total cases taken from cases seen in rural practice in Australia[5] **Endoscopy listed in Landercasper as most frequently performed cases in rural practice[9]	

Considering the role of the surgeon in emergency care, the concern over work hours comes to the forefront. Call overload and physician burnout are issues common to all practitioners in rural areas including anesthetists, intensivists, and family practitioners. It is a situation that adds considerable mental stress to an already rigorous position. Call schedules vary depending on the number of surgeons in the area, but are typically onerous.[31] In Australia, a 1:2 call schedule violates the safe-working guidelines of the Royal Australasian College of Surgeons and the Australian Medical Association, but there is no easy solution to this relatively frequent state of affairs.[5] Difficulty finding coverage is another concern that rural doctors face. Solo practice leaves a practitioner alone by definition. Burnout affects 40 to 50% of surgeons, and the effect is worse in solo practice.[32] Multispecialty groups and partnerships may provide more physicians to share workload, but often the call schedules extend 3 to 5 days.[25] The lack of peer support and strenuous call can also be daunting for young surgeons just starting out, and could be a deterrent to rural practice.[1] The inability to find coverage and manage call schedules offsets the joy of independence and being an integral part of the community.[33] Aging practitioners also struggle to find partners who are willing to work in rural areas because of the strained work-life balance.[34]

Financial concerns and the support of qualified staff are just two of the professional issues that exist in rural practice. The availability of other specialists to supplement surgical services is a limiting factor in the type and amount of surgery that can be performed. The commitment required for strenuous call schedules, sometimes 24 hours 7 days a week for those surgeons in solo practice, is a deterrent to many residency graduates who might consider rural practice. Investment into developing more sustainable work schedules and support systems for young practitioners is necessary.

Surgical Education and Rural Surgery

A greater majority of graduating residents in surgery enter fellowship. This number has been increasing steadily over the past decade, and the reasons for this increasing subspecialization are multifold. Three main concerns are implicated in the extension of training for these graduates: (1) gaining expertise allows surgeons to specialize and not experience the workload or work hours of the general surgeon, (2) to survive in the work environment, a more specialized talent is required to interest prospective employers, (3) uncertainty and a lack of confidence at the end of a 5-year training program to enter into practice. Combined, these factors have contributed to the reduction in graduates willing to practice rural medicine. It is not only the graduates who are affecting this change, but also the attitudes and structures of the residency programs.

There is a belief in the academic surgical community that it is 'unreasonable to expect urban students in tertiary centers to complete training and pursue a rural practice'.[18] It seems contradictory that programs training general surgeons will graduate residents who are not prepared for general practice. As rural surgery is the last bastion of general surgery, a graduate of a general surgery residency should theoretically be a prime candidate for rural practice. Unfortunately, even as recently as 2007, there were general surgery programs that strongly disagreed with the notion that they were training general surgeons to practice in a rural environment, even though they indicated awareness of the surgeon shortages in rural areas.[35] It was more likely that smaller community programs were intent on a more broad-base general surgery training.[35] With the focus so ardently placed on academic medicine, or 'incubation', there is a resultant decline in those interested in rural practice. Despite this 'tertiary care' thought process, some training programs both in America and abroad have realized the importance of tailoring surgical training for those interested in pursuing rural medicine. Attempts have been made to incorporate neurosurgery, orthopedics, and gynecology into American residency models, but as this is a suggestion and not a requirement, the implementation is varied.[36]

Many studies have been conducted to determine the factors influencing a physician's decision for practice location. As previously mentioned, rural surgeons are often from rural origins, but another noted factor in influencing practice location was exposure to rural practice during their training. Thirty years ago, studies showed that more rural surgeons had completed a rural rotation. Those who entered urban practice often had not been exposed to rural medicine during residency.[21] In a study by Steinwald and Steinwald, urban-reared participants in rural training programs chose rural practice almost two times as often as those who did not participate in rural training programs.[37] After the inception of the rural surgery rotation in Tennessee, the percentage of residents entering rural surgery increased from 37 to 58%. Rural rotations also offer the benefit of exposure to cases not frequently seen in academic or urban centers. Trainees frequently choose to practice where they feel competent and comfortable.

Exposure to rural medicine should begin even before medical school (Figure 1). Medical students who completed their secondary school education in rural areas are more likely to pursue rural lifestyles. Students who participate in rural health placements prior to medical school are also more likely to go into rural practice.[38] Undergraduate college or university students who experience rural medical environments prior to entering general surgery residency are more likely to practice in a similar setting.[39] It is imperative at this fundamental level to identify those applicants who profess an interest in rural medicine and provide them with the necessary educational support to prepare them for practice, starting with a position in medical school.[3]

Medical student rotations add to the development of burgeoning physicians, but their interests are generally still malleable. Many students who enter medical school with a planned specialty find their interests changing as they experience various rotations. The broad range of skills required for rural practice appeals to a greater majority of students.[10] Most students get more hands-on, clinical and practical experience when they do a rural rotation, which in more likely to engage them and draw their interest. The importance of mentorship at this level is crucial, and to showcase rural surgery by exposing these future doctors to the holistic nature of rural health systems would be of great benefit. Forty percent of rural surgeons had rural exposure in medical school, whereas 11% had the same exposure in residency.[1]

Figure 1. Levels of influence in identifying and encouraging interest in rural surgery

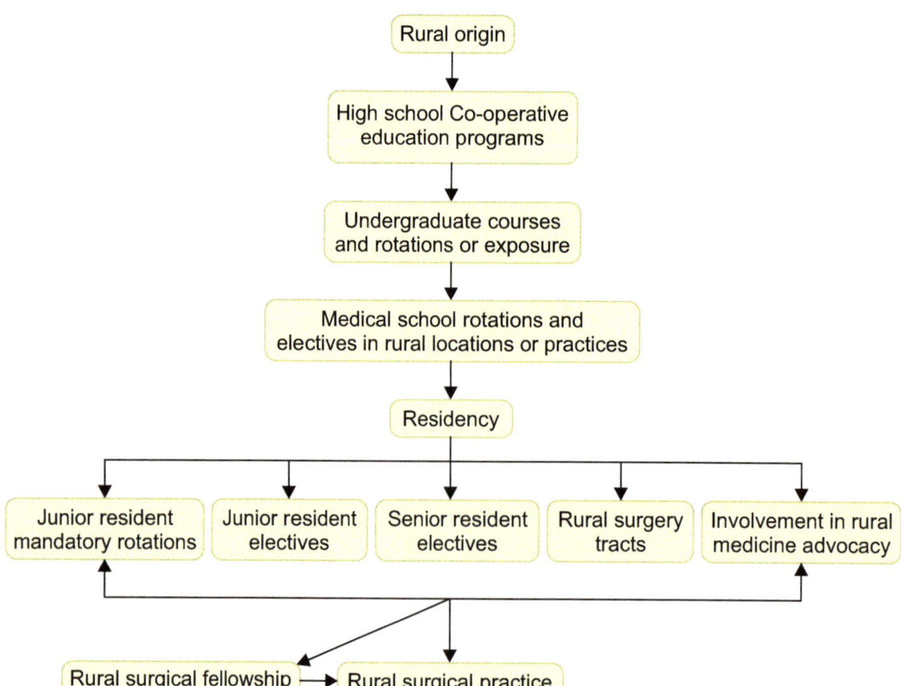

Residency training is the final common pathway to guide trainees into practice. It is also the point in training which is less flexible for elective rotations and more demanding in terms of educational, research, and administrative duties. In addition to rigorous schedules, very few programs in the country offer rural tracts or rotations for residents. General surgeons practicing in rural areas often include gynecology and orthopedics in their practice, but only half the surgery residency programs in the United States offer these subspecialty rotations. Wong reported in 2003 that a greater exposure to subspecialties occurs in rural rotations.[40] Many administrators argue that with limited hours and increasing educational and administrative demands, the inclusion of a rural surgery rotation is implausible. In direct opposition to the sentiment is that of the resident. Most residents given the opportunity to practice rural medicine during training have positive experiences. In Kentucky, residents assigned involuntarily to a rural rotation were eager for the opportunity because of the quantity and variety of surgical experience available.[21] Working in rural hospitals has proven to be beneficial to residents from both a surgical and endoscopic perspective because there are no fellows, more autonomy, and fewer residents to compete for cases. There is greater operative and endoscopic experience in rural rotations.[5] In Tennessee, a 3-month rural surgery rotation resulted in more total cases for residents than its urban counterpart. This included more endocrine, pancreas, spleen, and trauma cases.[4] There is a clear benefit to residents in terms of training and there is a concurrent benefit to the communities by establishing relationships with future surgeons and encouraging them to consider rural practice.

Current administrative thought is to make a rural rotation mandatory during surgical residency training. Within that dictum, the level of training when the resident would obtain optimal benefit remains undecided. Where should the emphasis be placed? Does exposure to rural medicine as a medical student affect the field that a potential surgeon might choose? Does a junior resident receive the full benefit of the varied case exposure? Is it too late to put a senior resident, with other administrative and service obligations, into a rural stream to influence their imminent decisions? Both models have been attempted, with evidence that while junior residents have the opportunity to greatly develop technical skills and patient management, senior residents also benefit from exposure to practice models and business or financial concerns.[21] A longer term in a rural hospital for mid-level or senior residents improves knowledge of the business of medicine as well as how to communicate effectively with referring providers.[34] A mandatory rotation for junior residents will expose them to more procedures and independence, while creating an elective for senior residents who can tailor their education towards their own goals may optimize the benefits of the rotation.[41]

The length of rural training rotations is also under debate. In Australia, a 6-month rotation established after initial resident reports suggested that at least 3 months was needed.[39] North Dakota places residents in remote hospitals for a month in both their first and second years of residency.[42] In Oregon, the rural surgery model allows residents to work in a smaller community hospital for one year. The residents completing this training often return with 250 to 300 major surgical procedures as well as experience in gynecology, urology, and orthopedics.[34] Many residents who participate in rural tracts are interested in a life of international medicine, which is comparable to the work of a rural surgeon. Other options include a rural rotation for fourth year residents of a variable length, depending on their career interests.[33] An international elective in a medically underserved area is another option that provides exposure to and performance of a number of general surgery cases which may influence a graduate's decision to pursue rural medicine.[33]

More residents are entering fellowship after residency. It is becoming the 'rule' rather than the 'exception.'[8] One factor causing this shift is the fear that graduates will not be able to compete in the job market without specialization. In terms of rural surgery, that is a contradiction in terms. Those who do complete fellowships in subspecialties often require large referral bases or extensive intensive care facilities that are not applicable to rural settings, thus effectively eliminating them from seeking rural employment. Rural surgery requires a broader scope of practice for physicians to be successful after residency. Consequently, educational programs must be better positioned to meet the needs of the communities these surgeons intend to serve. At present, current training regimens for general surgeons may not properly prepare general surgery residents to practice in rural communities.[4]

In order to embark on the 'return to general surgery' in general surgery training, the breadth of training should be expanded. Collaboration in interventional radiology, ultrasound performance and interpretation, bronchoscopy and endoscopy, and specific treatments of geriatric and pediatric populations has been suggested.[8] In one study, only 52% of general surgery training programs had rotation in obstetrics-gynecology.[9] What is needed is for governing bodies of resident education to allow more flexibility in training.[42] Residency programs must consider placing greater emphasis on significant experience in areas of orthopedics, hand/plastics, otolaryngology, urology, gynecology, obstetrics, and endoscopy.[3] Without this exposure, surgical residents graduating in the current environment will not have the exposure necessary to replace the retiring rural surgeons. A change in the case exposure of residents during their accredited program should be sufficient without having to create a fellowship for rural surgery. This is however, another consideration for encouraging graduates towards rural practice.

The format of this fellowship is still a subject of debate. Should the focus be on volume, exposing the fellow to high yield general surgery cases, or should the focus be on those types of cases and emergencies that are seen by the rural surgeon but missed in residency? Another concern is adding to the length of surgical training. For sure an additional year of training, with more autonomy and independent decision making would be of benefit, but at the cost of prolonging one of the longest residency programs and increasing trainee indebtedness.[43] It may end up as more of a deterrent than an attraction for continuing in general surgery.[8]

Another concern that pushes residents into fellowship is the feeling of being unprepared for general surgery.[8] This has been a growing problem due to two factors: (1) increasing administrative and logistical demands from educational governing bodies and (2) limited work hours. The adoption of duty hour restrictions has narrowed the scope of clinical experience for residents.[25,44,45] This feeling is not limited to trainees in the United States. The European Union limited their trainee doctors even more strictly. The limited hours, though attempting to combat resident/trainee fatigue and improve quality of care, means that cases of educational benefit are often missed. Overnight call, which has the benefit of exposing trainees to the urgent decision-making and independent thought, has been reduced, if not removed entirely from the junior resident curriculum. It is a process that limits the education of trainees, especially those interested in continuing as general surgeons instead of entering fellowships. In an attempt to combat this concern in Australia, the Royal Australasian College of Surgeons implemented a rural surgical training program that gives not only specialty posts in rural surgery, but also links trainees with surgical mentors who can teach them the management of more foreign cases.[5]

The training of surgeons is the most important resource available for increasing the numbers of rural surgeons. Fundamental skills and exposure to subspecialty cases will help prepare the general surgeon for emergency and triage work. Rural rotations will benefit not only the resident in their training and confidence, but also the community who may be able to bring a new surgeon to their hospital if a good rapport is established. Whether the creation of a rural surgical fellowship is successful or not, the flexibility in residency programs will be the foundation to creating awareness of rural practice as an alternative to specialization after graduation.

Quality of Care and Public Perception

The perceived 'loss of quality' that accompanies a loss of specialization is another issue that plagues the general surgeon. This suspected reduction in the quality of care has been proven repeatedly to be a false assumption. Several studies have demonstrated that high-quality surgical care can be achieved in the rural environment with excellent outcomes.[46,47] In one rural community, reported hospital stays were found to be marginally higher, but in-hospital mortality was lower than the national average.[10] With regards to colectomies, rural hospitals have been found to have lower volumes but better mortality outcomes. This directly negates the popular opinion that high volume always relates to high quality.[48] There is a perception amongst urbanites that subspecialist medical care means 'better' medical care. Local populations, however, are usually satisfied with their care.[10] Other surgical professionals suggest withdrawing local surgical services based on the impression of insufficient workload to maintain skills, professional isolation, lack of replacements, and inability to properly care for more serious surgical problems. The advent of the 'Center of Excellence' has had an impact on the practice of rural surgery. Certain centers are qualified to perform certain procedures after obtaining a set number of cases and are given this new moniker. In some cases, centers of excellence are being initiated in rural areas.[42] It is more common that low volume centers in rural areas are prevented from doing certain procedures because of the restriction to centers of excellence.[48] Quality outcome measures that determine the concept of a center of excellence focus on procedural volume. The prime example of this is the American College of Surgeons National Surgical Quality Improvement Program (ACS-NSQIP) data. NSQIP allows hospitals and surgeons to track their surgical outcomes, but it is expensive and time-consuming to implement, as well as based on procedural volume.[1] This is not feasible in rural hospitals. Typically, rural centers have high quality outcomes without the volume. There are programs available that use process-based outcome measurements against measured surgical benchmarks. Another method of quality improvement in smaller hospitals would be to have rural surgeons keep logs to document experiences and share them with larger centers.[42] The best defense for surgeons with low or moderate procedural volume is knowledge of their own outcomes data.[33] The traditional morbidity and mortality meetings of surgical teams are less applicable in small centers where there might be only one surgeon, but they are still important in maintaining quality of care.[48] These meetings need to be adapted for rural practices, perhaps incorporating other practitioners or surgical team members including nurses and surgical staff, or developing telecommunications with a tertiary center to present and discuss cases. These models of quality outcomes may properly represent the care being received in rural centers, and thus permit them to continue with restricted procedures.

Due to the isolation of practicing rural surgery, there is a concern that continuing medical education and physician quality suffers. Varying opinions have been noted on the exposure to, and quality of continuing medical education (CME) for rural surgeons. In Canada and Australia, it has been noted that CME is limited either by availability of courses or availability of coverage whilst away on conference.[31] In the United States, rural doctors are satisfied (86%) with the CME available to them.[18] Secondary to the isolation of the rural surgeon, concerns have been raised with regards to the technological advancement and standard of care being limited. This consideration is based on reduced financial capital in local hospitals and lack of available training.[48] This is an unfounded concern. When laparoscopic cholecystectomies were introduced, the dissemination of knowledge to, and acceptance of practice in community hospitals matched that of urban centers.[49] This is now the accepted standard of care in urban and rural centers. With regards to more recent advances in surgical technique, specifically robotic surgery, single port site laparoscopy, and natural orifice surgery, there are limited general surgery uses even in urban practice. Patients who received care in rural hospitals are generally satisfied with their treatment, noting no disparity in the skill and knowledge of their practitioners.

The foundation of surgical care is the patients. Rural patients are different from urban patients. Reports from rural patients experiencing surgical care both in a local hospital and in a center of excellence found their own community surgical services superior.[6] Similar experiences have been noted in maternity data. Surgical patients are under considerable stress and undergo emotional, financial, social, and cultural costs if forced to seek general surgical services outside their communities.[6] Local services mean a heightened sense of community at a time of personal crisis. Strong relationships with health care providers and individualized care that gives the patients a better sense of control over their own health are of paramount importance in rural populations.[50] There is an impersonal nature to regional surgical care as well as unfamiliar communication styles. Familiarity and trust become more important than many other elements of medical care to rural inhabitants.[6] The effect of locally delivered health care on patients and their families is undeniable. Rural residents are not demographically different from their urban counterparts, but they desire a culturally different style of surgical care which is irreplaceable. In considering 'quality surgical care,' a holistic view must be employed. For rural patients, local services and support provide this overall wellness model better than do subspecialty services at regional centers. Not only is wellness directly related to local care, but local residents believe that non-emergent medical conditions should be treated by their local practitioners and should not require travel to distant specialists.[11] Some patients will even forgo treatment if it requires travel.

Quality outcomes are currently a major area of interest in surgical practice. They are being used not only for determining the skill and competency of surgeons, but also the financial reimbursements of hospitals and individual practitioners. Quality measures that look at procedural volumes define certain sites as centers of excellence, a title that low volume rural centers may not be able to achieve, thus deepening the bias against the community hospital. Low volume centers do not necessarily mean low quality, and the number of rural residents who profess satisfaction in their local surgical care is testament to that fact. Surgeons must work to maintain skills and remain updated with current operative technologies, but as telecommunication improves, this has been facilitated. CME and technological advancements are not impediments to good practice in rural areas. Keeping logs and personal accountability to standards of care is the best method for rural surgeons to examine their own practice.

Resources, Support, and Advocacy

The isolation of the rural practitioners can in part be alleviated by good communication. Where once communication about patients or concerns was nearly impossible, current video and telecommunication developments have altered this circumstance. Rural communities are linked to tertiary centers for consultation on malignancy multidisciplinary meetings and tumor boards.[10] Opening up rural practice to the consultant opinions of tertiary care via video conference is a resource that should be exploited further. This could provide rural practitioners with a form of mentorship and professional development that would be beneficial in reducing the sense of isolation.[31] Video teleconferencing has been used to carry out weekly ward rounds between remote and tertiary sites with the benefit of discussing and directing day-to-day care.[51] This has the potential to not only benefit the patients, but also the practitioner, who can develop patient management skills and also professional relationships with tertiary centers where they could participate in surgeries that have to be referred due to complexity.[51]

Another support mechanism for isolated practices is the support of contemporaries who face the same issues. With new social media advancements, the international and rural worlds are getting smaller. Other support groups meet in person. In Europe, the Viking Surgeons group is an example of how rural surgeons come together to support one another.[10] Surgeons from Scotland, Norway, and Finland, amongst other northern European nations, come together for social and scientific retreats. They discuss advances in surgery, share experiences, and talk about individual practices in various countries. There is a sense of camaraderie that helps alleviate some of the isolation that can be a component of rural practice. In the United States, there is a new committee from the American College of Surgeons that not only brings together rural surgeons at the annual American College of Surgeons meeting, but also meets throughout the year to address issues in rural surgery and brings them to the attention of the College. The collegialities these organizations bring are important to both drawing awareness to the issues in rural surgery and to develop relationships and communication between professionals.

In order to provide effective surgical services, a surgeon is only as capable as the resources available to them. The infrastructure of the hospital is critically important. Necessary resources include radiology, pathology, technologist services, and nursing care. Surgical care is limited by a lack of support staff rather than by the ability of the surgeon. This includes not only the surgical team of anesthetists and nurses, but also those providers who supply pre- and post-operative care. Other professionals in the rural community are of synergistic value when surgical practice becomes isolated. Family practitioners are the largest component of rural practitioners, with general surgeons a close second. Family practitioners often staff the hospital and the emergency room in rural communities. The interdependence of family practitioners and surgeons can be seen in pre- and post-operative care, as well as in hospital care and emergency triage. They also assist in the operating room and are known to provide some basic surgical and gynecological services such as vasectomy, dilatation and curettage, endometrial biopsies, infant circumcision, and flexible sigmoidoscopies. In urban areas, there has been a decline in the number of family practitioners assisting in the operating room over the past decade, but this fall may be less in rural communities.[11] Cooperation becomes paramount for a functional medical practice. A closer relationship between medical and surgical practitioners means more awareness of the need for surgical evaluation and management which can be very helpful in avoiding unnecessary midnight calls for a surgeon that may already be on a very taxing call schedule.

This synergy has more than just an effect on the solo surgeon. It will affect rural medicine as a whole. There seems to be a growing awareness of the issues in rural healthcare at the federal level worldwide. Regardless, the focus of their concern is not on surgery alone, but rather on all critical services, and implementation is not occurring at a quick pace. Administrative circles in medicine are developing an understanding of the power of a collective approach to improving rural health care. A unified voice for rural practice has more political advantage. Advocacy at the federal level for more funding and support will be considered if there is a unified front including anesthesia, radiology, surgery, medicine, and nursing factions. In a symposium sponsored by the Center for Rural Health Research of British Columbia in 2010, a combined group of rural practitioners determined that an alignment of anesthetists, general surgeons, and operating room nurses would provide a collective voice for the problems facing rural medicine.[31] A mutually beneficial political merger with family medicine would help to ensure hospital availability for family practice while also providing a working environment for a general surgeon.[8] This would remove the handicap imposed on family practitioners in need of hospital resources, and give rural surgeons a more stable work environment.

Changes in First-World International Rural Surgical Practices

The United States is not the only first world nation to be affected by the changes in surgical practice. Since the 1950s and 1960s, other countries have noticed a similar loss in the utility and presence of general surgeons. Many have developed new models of health care administration, with government policy affecting change, and medical boards actively recruiting for rural practice (Table 4).

Table 4: Changes in international models of rural practice

	Education	Rural Practice	Administration
Canada	• Rural and Island tracts in established medical schools • Development of new medical school focused on rural medicine • Cooperative educations programs for high school students	• GP-surgeons and GP-anesthetists • Nurse practitioners have increased scope of practice • Telecommunication and aeromedical retrieval	• Community directed financial incentives • Focus on rural surgery through journals and CME • Online support • Society for Rural Surgeons • Center for Rural health research developed
Australia	• Flexibility in resident training schemes for rural exposure • Rotations in rural facilities • Mandatory and elective rotations	• General practitioners as surgeons with supplementation from visiting surgeons and subspecialists • Shared practice • Rotating academic surgeons from nearby university programs • Emergency and locum reliefs established between urban and rural centers	• Government funded programs for rural medical training • Aeromedical retrieval at national level
United Kingdom (Scotland)	• Rural training for postgraduates in medicine	• Remote sites are linked to tertiary center • Video links and telecommunication for consultation • Collegiality (groups such as Viking Surgeons) • Subspecialists visit rural centers	• National Health Service (NHS) involvement in determining quality of care in isolated areas • Improved communication and connection to tertiary centers • Requisite number of practitioners to maintain facilities • Rural surgery recognized as a formal specialty • Government based splinter groups addressing issues in rural medicine

Australia

The problem of rural recruitment and retention is also an issue in Australia, with many practices being a solo or two-man team, or without a resident surgeon at all. Many of the current rural practitioners are nearing retirement.[39] In smaller communities, excellent elective and emergent surgical care has been provided by general practitioners as opposed to surgeons. Visiting surgeons and subspecialists have supplemented these efforts, but due to the paucity of subspecialties, general surgeons who do practice in rural communities have developed a broad skill base. An aeromedical retrieval service under the Royal Flying Doctor Service has provided a safety net for the rural communities, but the need for immediate care has not been replaced.[51] Australia has approached this problem from a national level. There is an awareness of the workforce issues in medicine, and government funded programs have been instituted to encourage rural surgical training schemes.[39] Many medical schools now incorporate both mandatory and voluntary rural training rotations.[52] The Royal Australasian College of Surgeons has encouraged flexibility for trainees pursuing training in subspecialties to better benefit the community where they intend to practice.[51] Some communities have developed a rotation of surgeons from a larger center who practice in the rural locale for one week; this has proved functional for over fifteen years.[51] These models of 'shared practice' also allow for weekend coverage in other nearby rural practices and locums to give some respite. Overall trends are attempting to relieve some of the main concerns of surgeons in remote areas such as grueling call schedules and professional isolation, and also allows for trainees to be introduced into the rural practice, providing more exposure to the needs and benefits of working in remote locations.

Canada

Due to a small population compared to its land mass, as well as fewer residency training programs and available physicians, Canada has had to make adjustments. Twenty-two percent of Canada's population lives in communities under 10,000. These communities are often without a resident surgeon. Because 99% of Canada's land mass is considered rural, it is a near impossibility to provide enough rural surgical care from board certified general surgeons. Canada has had a long history of family practitioners (GP) and nurse practitioners (NP) with specialized training acting as the resident surgeon in most small communities. GP-surgeons and GP-anesthetists have been given additional training after finishing a 2-year residency program in family practice. These practitioners are qualified to operate or deliver anesthesia and are often the only practitioners in rural environments.[30] They are, however, dwindling in numbers as well, with continued training being limited by costs.[24,28] The introduction of the Northern Ontario School of Medicine (NOSM) in 2005 was intended to specifically train doctors interested in rural medicine. It was the newest medical school created in Canada in 30 years. British Columbia also has a rural medicine program, as well as an island medicine program as components of their medical school. These have been established for much longer than NOSM, with the intention to care for the remote communities of northern British Columbia and Victoria. At least two well-known Canadian journals focus on discussing issues in rural practice that are available online and in print. Options for online CME are available through both sources. The Society of Rural Physicians of Canada (SRPC) has been established to connect rural practitioners (http://www.srpc.ca/). Founded in 1992, the SRPC works on behalf of its 3,000 members and the Canadian public to perform, to develop, and to advocate for health delivery, support rural doctors and communities in crisis, offer CME, research rural health issues, and foster communication among rural physicians.

Scotland

Ninety percent of Scotland's population is classified as rural. More than half of the rural population has driving times over an hour to reach a population center of 30,000 or more.[10] One of the major concerns in Scotland is the loss of health services in the Isles, which are relatively inaccessible in bad weather, and where over 100,000 people reside.[10] Scotland, however, under the National Health Service (NHS), has a strong desire to supply health care to rural communities. Resident surgical services were maintained in regions with two surgeons, early identification of trainees to potentially serve, strong links with main hospitals, proper transfer arrangements for specialist treatments, good radiology and laboratory services, two anesthesiologists, and video links with major emergency department with orthopedic services had to be available.[10] In 2000, the Scottish Executive realized that rural medicine had to continue due to the remote nature and inaccessibility of many communities. A working group set up by the executive concluded that rural surgery should be a formalized specialty, that all remote surgical units should be linked to a tertiary hospital. A minimum of three locally based surgeons were necessary to sustain these units. Acute care specialists had to be available if the surgeon was not. Adequate patient transport, electronic communications, and site-specific training for locum surgeons working in remote areas were required.[10] The Scottish Government still helps determine the needs of remote communities with regards to medical care, including surgery, and has developed a number of splinter groups to address issues for the survival of rural surgery. The Rural General Health (RGH) model was established to define what care was needed, and it included requisite anesthesia services, core surgical services, and specialties services that could be provided by visiting surgeons. Also addressed by a separate tripartite group was the need for rural medical training pathways in general practice, general medicine, general surgery, and anesthesia.[10] The importance of a multilevel approach to improving and providing health care and health care professionals in remote and rural communities is evident in Scotland. Currently local surgical care is provided in an RGH or community hospital, and if referral is necessary after consultation, the patient can travel to a larger city hospital. Specialty services are usually provided by subspecialist surgeons who travel from larger centers. What is important to glean from the Scottish awareness of rural medicine is that the involvement of the Scottish government and health service has been crucial. Similar involvement of governing bodies in North America may be of benefit.

Increasing Surgeon Interest in Rural Medicine

In order to change the direction in which rural surgery seems to be headed in most first world countries, modifications must be made from the most fundamental unit, the individual burgeoning doctor, to the most complex, the government. To increase surgeon interest in rural medicine, improvements have to make the workplace a challenging but rewarding environment that has more benefits than frustrations. Good, qualified professional and financial support with adequate development opportunities and reliable assistance from tertiary facilities is mandatory. These elements of the workplace have to be addressed at the administrative level, not only from the surgical governing bodies, but also from the non-medical administration. This will serve to increase the appeal of working in rural communities. It does not, however, address the individual workforce issue.

Increasing surgeon interest in rural medicine starts before the medical school level, and interactive programs for high school students include co-operative education programs.[52] Foundations in rural surgery at the level of undergraduate education are almost more effective at attracting potential rural practitioners than at the graduate school level.[39] Early identification of students who wish to enter rural practice can help to guide their training. In Australia, quotas have been created in medical schools for those high school students coming from rural areas who wish to return home to practice.[39] Reserving medical school positions for people who wish to practice rurally would identify and encourage applicants. Rural rotations during medical school will further expose students to community practice. Those medical students interested in rural surgery could be identified and supported, perhaps even financially compensated. Increasing the quota of residents intending to remain in general surgery would help offset the numbers entering fellowship.[8] Mandatory rural surgery rotations in American residencies may prove beneficial for the residents and the communities, as they have in Australia. Rural tracts, as are seen in Canada and Oregon, for those residents who intend to go into remote practice, should be increased and encouraged. Fewer tertiary level rotations, such as transplant and burn rotations, and more subspecialty exposure such as in otolaryngology, obstetrics, gynecology, urology, and orthopedics, would broaden general surgery training. In Scotland and Australia, partnerships between academic and rural centers have provided not only a solid training opportunity but have also created professional relationships that could expand into practice opportunities between rural surgeons and trainees. Those rural surgeons also benefit from visiting professionals assisting in operations and alleviating some of the strain of call schedules and lack of leave. Links between rural and tertiary centers are the key to assuring the interest and development of the general surgeon in rural medicine. To have professional and personal support lessens the feeling of isolation and improves the quality of care by looking at outcomes, having consultations services, and developing a trust for referrals. Commitments from larger institutions are needed in order to keep rural practices going.[51] Tertiary centers have to acknowledge the value of the rural general surgeon in order to develop a strong working relationship.

Other models have been suggested to increase the desire of practitioners to go to rural areas. Incentives such as tax exemption and debt relief have been suggested.[18] In Canada, communities have taken it upon themselves to offer financial incentives for surgeons to come to their area. Subsidies for rural living have also been suggested, not only for surgeons but for other necessary professions such as nursing, anesthesia, and radiology.[8] Governmental aid has been noted in northern communities in the form of a northern living allowance to increase physician interest. A viable lifestyle, one that does not involve 24/7 call, is becoming necessary to attract young physicians. It was reported that, due to the shifting mentality of work-life balance, every retiring surgeon in remote communities likely must be replaced by two new doctors.[51] A strong relationship with a tertiary hospital can provide occasional professional relief, but another option is practice sharing.[7] This model has been used with success in family practice models in Canada; however, financial concerns would have to be addressed, as the amount of work would have to be able to sustain two practitioners.

Governing bodies related directly to surgery such as the Royal Australasian College of Surgeons, the Royal College of Surgeons of Edinburgh, and the American College of Surgeons (ACS) have started to make changes to better serve remote areas. In 2012, the ACS addressed the issues in rural surgery by introducing the Advisory Council on Rural Surgeons (ACRS), the first new advisory council in 50 years. This committee includes policy makers, rural surgeons, program directors, medical students, and residents who meet to discuss and address issues in rural surgery in an effort to affect change (Table 5). The development of communication and education are amongst their highest priorities. One of the most important issues that has come to light in their discussions is advocacy at the federal level, and the determination that this can be best achieved through solidarity between all rural practitioners: nurses, nurse anesthetists, anesthesiologist, physician's assistants, family practitioners, rural hospitalists, radiologists, and surgical and radiology technicians. Only through commitment to rural medicine can rural surgery be improved. This then becomes a federal issue, and health advocacy is the last level of improving surgeon's interest in rural practice. If the financial and ancillary support is there to create a thriving practice and a good life, then the trainees will be more inclined to venture toward it. Without that, more centralization and the loss of rural medicine are certainties.

Table 5: Examples of American Board of Surgery (ABS) efforts for improved awareness in rural surgery

Task force on General Surgery (TAGS)	January 2012	• Consider issues in general surgery training and practice • Appointed advisory committee
General Surgery Advisory Council (GENSAC)	June 2012	• Discussion of long-standing problems in general surgery practice and training • Standardized curriculum for medical students for surgical skills • Surgical curriculum modifications for residency • Developing models of post-residency training
ACS Advisory Council on Rural Surgery (ACRS)	June 2012	Communication with and between rural surgeons • Discussion of issues pertaining to rural surgery and training • Bringing issues in rural surgery to the attention of the ACS • Addressing medical schools and residencies to affect more rural exposure • Supporting the creation of a documentary film on rural surgery

Another method of assuring that there is an influx of work into rural communities is a return of service agreement. One suggestion would be to assure a position in an academic or urban institution after a requisite number of years in rural practice.[51] Other models have made it mandatory that foreign graduates practice in remote or rural areas for a given length of time before being allowed the freedom to choose their area of practice. This has even been implemented with some success by communities who pay for the training of an individual with the understanding that the practitioner will return to that community.[24] Financial incentives would attract young surgeons with considerable debt.

As rural medicine is intimately knit to the quality of the support, improvements in ancillary services need to be addressed. Rural nurses are as necessary as physicians, and interest could be influenced by offering incentives for nurses willing to practice in rural areas. Scholarships for people from small towns going into nursing, surgical technology, radiology technicians, or physician assistant programs could be given with the stipulation that these people return to practice in their communities. Local medical secretarial and administration courses could be offered for rural residents seeking to improve professional skills or further their careers. Work visas could be offered to foreign trained nurses, or exchange programs created for nursing and support staff to increase the interest in rural medicine. More effort into the development of sustainable ancillary services in rural communities needs to be made in order to attract physicians to remote communities. In doing so, the community will grow financially while developing local surgical services. This broad scale approach to improving rural medicine does, however, require considerable input from a federal level.

Summary

General surgeons are an integral and sustaining component of a rural community. They bring quality and effective medical care to local residents while concurrently increasing financial benefit. Currently, however, rural surgery is waning in most first world nations. More than 80% of surgical residents are entering specialist training and remaining in urban centers. This is due to a combination of changes in surgical residency programs, and the increasing notion that volume-based outcomes equate to superior care. It has been noted that exposure to rural medicine, and the cultivation of people from rural areas are the major factors in recruiting physicians to rural areas; however, many surgical programs in the United States, approximately 65%, do not have rural electives or tracts for their residents, or do not believe that rural training is a priority. In order to affect change, there needs to be input from every level. Communities have to get actively involved in recruitment, tertiary or urban centers have to develop relationships with their rural counterparts, resident programs have to increase exposure to the benefits of rural surgery, governing bodies have to put forth an effort to save rural medicine, and federal governments have to be willing to invest financially in their remote populations. There have been many recent steps made to affect change, but it is a slow process, and more commitment has to be put into developing sustainable solutions to deliver effective and quality surgical care to the 60 million rural Americans who still look to their local practitioners, and more specifically local surgeons, first.

REFERENCES

1. Doty B, Zuckerman R. Rural Surgery: Framing the issues. Surg Clin N Am 2009;89:1279-84.
2. Zuckerman R, Doty B, Gold M, et al. General surgery programs in small rural New York State hospitals: a pilot survey of hospital administrators. J Rural Health. 2006;22:339-42.
3. Doty B, Heneghan S, Gold M, et al. Is a broadly based surgical residency program more likely to place graduates in rural practice? World J Surg 2006;30:2089-93.
4. Milligan JL, Nelson HS, Mancini ML, et al. Rural surgery rotation during surgical residency. The American Surgeon 2009;75:743-6.
5. Campbell NA, Kitchen G, Campbell IA. Operative experience of general surgeons in a rural hospital. ANZ J Surg 2011;81:601-3.
6. Humber N, Dickinson P. Rural patients' experiences accessing surgery in British Columbia. Can J Surg 2010;53:373-8.
7. Lynge DC, Larson EH. Workforce issues in rural surgery. Surg Clin N Am 2009;89:1285-91.
8. Polk HC, Bland KI, Ellison EC, et al. A proposal for enhancing the general surgical workforce and access to surgical care. Annals of Surgery 2012;255:611-7.
9. Landercasper J, Blintz M, Cogbill TH, et al. Spectrum of General Surgery in Rural America. Arch Surg 1997;132:494-7.
10. Sim AJW, Grant F, Ingram AK. Surgery in Remote and Rural Scotland. Surg Clin N Am 2009;89:1335-47.
11. Pathman DE, Ricketts III TC. Interdependence of General surgeons and primary care physicians in rural communities. Surg Clin N Am 2009;89:1293-1302.
12. Drucker PF. Post-capitalist society. New York: Harper Business/HarperCollins; 1993.
13. Sheldon GF, Milligan JL, Nelson HS, Mancini ML, et al. Rural surgery rotation during surgical residency. The American Surgeon 2009;75:743-6.
14. Acute Services Review. Scottish Office Department of Health. Edinburgh: Scottish Office Publications; 1998.
15. Centre for Rural Health Research. Sustaining intrapartum services in communities with no local cesarean section. In: Policy Briefs: Issues in Rural Maternity Care Series. 1.4. Vancouver (BC): The Centre; 2008.
16. Klein M, Christilaw J, Johnston S. Loss of maternity care: the cascade of unforeseen dangers. CJRM 2002;7:120-1.
17. Kane RL, Olsen D, Neuman J, et al. Giving and getting surgery in Utah: An urban-rural comparison. Surgery 1978;83:375-81.
18. Stevick JA, Nullis EN, Connally SR, et al. Perspectives of Rural Surgical Practice in Georgia. The American Surgeon 1994;60:703-6.
19. Humber N, Frecker T. Rural surgery in British Columbia: Is there anybody out there? Can J Surg 2008;51:179-84.
20. Pollock JD, Love TP, Steffes BC, et al. Is it possible to train surgeons for rural Africa? A report of a successful international program. World J Surg 2011;35:493-9.
21. Asher EF, Martin LF, Richardson JD. Rural rotations for senior surgical residents. Arch Surg 1984;119:1120-4.
22. Parker RC, Tuxill TG. The attitudes of physicians towards community practice. J Med Educ 1967;48:885-95.
23. Movassaghi H, Kindig D. Medical practice and satisfaction of physicians in sparsely populated rural counties of the United States: results of a 1988 survey. J Rural Health 1989;5:125-36.
24. Barry AW. Meeting the Challenge: Providing anesthesia services in rural hospitals. Can Med Assoc J 1995;153:1455-6.
25. Hamar SK. Impact of restriction of work hours-A rural perspective. Surgery 2003;134:27-8.
26. Hiller A, Helenius I, Nurmi E, et al. Acetaminophen improves analgesia but does not reduce opioid requirement after major spine surgery in children and adolescents. Spine 2012;15:37.
27. Cárdenas-Salomon CM, Cervantes-Castro J, Jean-Silver ER, et al. Hospitalization costs of open vs. laparoscopic appendectomy: 5-year experience. Cir Cir. 2011;79:534-9.
28. Chiasson PM, Roy PD. Role of the general practitioner in the delivery of surgical and anesthesia services in rural western Canada. Can Med Assoc J 1995;153:1447-52.

29. Bhattacharyya R. Operative experience of general surgeons in a rural hospital (Re: ANZ J. Surg. 2011;81:601-3). ANZ J Surg 2012.
30. Humber N, Frecker T. Delivery models of rural surgical service in British Columbia (1996-2005): Are general practitioner-surgeons still part of the picture? Can J Surg 2008;51:173-8.
31. Gryzbowski S, Prinsloo L, Kilpatrick N. Professional isolation in small rural surgical programs: the need for a virtual department of operative care. Can J Rural Med 2011;16:103-5.
32. Bittner JG IV, Khan Z, Babu M, et al. Stress, burnout and maladaptive coping: Strategies for surgeon well-being. Bulletin of the American College of Surgeons. 2011;96:17-22. Accessed online at www.womensurgeons.org/aws_library/surgeonburnout.pdf. January 14, 2013.
33. Cogbill TH, Cofer JB, Jarman BT. Contemporary issues in rural surgery. Curr Probl Surg. 2012 May;49(5):263-318. doi: 10.1067/j.cpsurg.2012.01.002. PMID: 22500672.
34. Deveney K, Hunter J. Education for rural surgical practice: the Oregon Health & Science University model. Surg Clin N Am 2009;89:1303-8.
35. Burkholder HC, Cofer JB. Rural Surgery Training: A survey of program directors. J Am Coll Surg 2007;204:416-21.
36. Sheldon GF. Surgical Practice in Rural Areas: Introduction. Surg Clin N Am 2009;89:xvii-xix.
37. Steinwald B, Steinwald C. The effect of preceptorship and rural training programs on physicians' practice location decisions. Med Care 1975;13:219-229.
38. Jones AR, Oster RA, Pederson LL, et al. Influence of a rural primary care clerkship on medical students' intentions to practice in a rural community. J Rural Health 2000;16:155-61.
39. Bruening MH, Anthony AA, Maddern GJ. Surgical rotations in provincial South Australia: the trainees' perspective. ANZ J Surg 2003;73:65-68.
40. Wong K, Birks D. Operative experience in the Victorian general surgical training programme. ANZ J Surg 2003;73:1036-40.
41. Borgstrom DC, Heneghan SJ. Bassett Healthcare rural surgery experience. Surg Clin N Am 2009;89:1321-3.
42. Antonenko DR. Rural Surgery: The North Dakota experience. Surg Clin N Am 2009;89:1367-1372.
43. Naylor RA, Reisch JS, Valentine RJ. Factors related to attrition in surgery residency based on application data. Arch Surg. 2008;143:647-51.
44. Rotondo MF, Milligan JL, Nelson HS, Mancini ML, et al. Rural surgery rotation during surgical residency. The American Surgeon 2009;75:743-6.
45. Warshaw AL, Sarr MG. The now and future world of restricted work hours for surgeons. Surgery 2003;134:1-2.
46. Reeve TS, Curtin A, Fingleton L, et al. Can total thyroidectomy be performed as safely by general surgeons in provincial centers as by surgeons in specialized endocrine surgical units? Making the case for surgical training. Arch Surg. 1994;129:834-6.
47. Birks DM, Gunn IF, Birks RG, et al. Colorectal surgery in rural Australia: scars; a surgeon-based audit of workload and standards. ANZ J Surg. 2001;71:154-8.
48. Finlayson SRG. Assessing and Improving the Quality of Surgical care in rural America. Surg Clin N Am 2009;89:1373-1381.
49. Kemp JA, Zuckerman RS, Finlayson SR. Trends in adoption of laparoscopic cholecystectomy in rural versus urban hospitals. J Am Coll Surg. 2008;2006:28-32. Epub 2007 Sep 17.
50. Hogue CJ, Hoffman S, Hatch MC. Stress and preterm delivery: a conceptual framework. Paediatr Perinat Epidemiol. 2001;15 Suppl 2:30-40.
51. Bruening MH, Maddern GJ. Rural Surgery: the Australian experience. Surg Clin N Am 2009;89:1325-33.
52. Hickner JM. Training for rural practice in Australia 1990. Med J Aust. 1991;154:111-8.

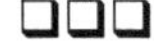

7

CHAPTER

Respiratory Failure and Ventilator Management

Nitin Puri, MD, FCCP
Vinod K. Puri, MD, FCCM

INTRODUCTION

Mechanical Ventilation

Positive pressure mechanical ventilation (MV) has fundamentally altered the practice of medicine and surgery. It has allowed patients to be treated who prior to just a few decades ago would not have been offered many modern treatments. The purpose of this chapter is to familiarize the reader with mechanical ventilation and the basic concepts behind its use. A more thorough understanding of the history of ventilation, its nomenclature, its physiologic effects, and its associated co- morbidities will enable the reader to provide better care for their patients. The decision to initiate and discontinue mechanical ventilation is complex and cannot be taken lightly. This chapter is meant to supplement the knowledge learned at a patient's bedside and enhance the care of surgical patients.[1]

Brief History of Mechanical Ventilation

The concept of assisted ventilation is ancient, with a reference to the Prophet Elisha in the Old Testament performing mouth to mouth resuscitation on a child in 800 BC (Book of Kings Verse 4:34). In Western Europe, the first attempts at assisted ventilation were the use of Fire Bellows connected to patient's mouths in the 16th century. This crude form of ventilation was improved upon over the next three centuries, but never widely adopted. Negative pressure ventilation (NPV) decreases intrathoracic pressure to create gradient between the atmosphere and the thorax was a significant advancement in the 19th century. The primary mode of NPV was the Iron Lung and later the cuirass, an iron vest around the patient's chest. The Iron Lung was used to ventilate patients, but it had significant disadvantages. These limitations included its size, lack of utility in patients with unstable airways and the venous pooling of blood in patients due patient immobility. These problems created an opportunity for innovation during the polio epidemic of 1952 in Copenhagen, Denmark. Bjorn Ibsen, an anesthesiologist, recommended positive pressure ventilation with a tracheostomy and demonstrated a substantial decrease in mortality. His method required continuous manual ventilation during which medical students were enlisted to manually ventilate the patients at bedside and thus created the impetus for modern mechanical ventilation.

The first volume ventilator to be widely used was the Engstrom, which provided a constant volume powered by pistons. It delivered a preset volume without regard to the pressure applied to the lungs. Pressure based ventilation was advanced by both Bird and Bennett. These ventilators delivered a preset pressure to the patient's lungs without regard to volume delivered. These advances enhanced scientists' understanding of pulmonary physiology. New syndromes were elucidated such as Acute Respiratory Distress Syndrome (ARDS) as physicians tried to grasp their inability to oxygenate patients. This led to the development of Positive End Expiratory Pressure (PEEP) valves and pressure waveforms which helped clinicians treat advanced lung disease. Further advances in mechanical ventilation were the addition of more ventilatory modes and refining the concept of weaning patients off the respirator. Downs, an anesthesiologist, invented two different modes of mechanical ventilation, the first was Intermittent Mandatory Ventilation, which he developed to help wean patients off respiratory support. Later on, he also introduced Airway Pressure Release Ventilation. Intermittent Mandatory Ventilation mode was revolutionary as it allowed patients to take breaths between mandatory ventilation. Norlander furthered this concept in the 1980s with the development of Pressure Support Ventilation. The latter mode allows patients to control their own respiratory rate and it augments the patient's inspiratory effort. The next major advancement in ventilators was the development of microprocessors enabling real time graphics and internal safety alarms. Graphics enhanced physicians' understanding of dyssynchrony leading to new modes of ventilation which responded to patient's respiratory demands and changes in lung physiology. Older models were altered and used for new applications to ventilate patients with refractory hypoxemia. Positive pressure ventilation is in the midst of a new era where ventilators may need less instruction, but a greater understanding by clinicians to make sure they are ventilating patients appropriately.[1]

Indications for Mechanical Ventilation

One of the most important aspects of mechanical ventilation is knowing when to institute it, as no specific value of oxygen (O_2) or carbon dioxide (CO_2) necessitates mechanical ventilation. Instead, the overall clinical picture guides when it should be initiated. Respiration is a complex physiologic process which requires interaction of the nervous system, the upper airway, the lower airway, thorax, pleura, cardiovascular system, and the lungs. Specific indications to intubate patients have been proposed such as patients who cannot protect their airway or patients with increased work of breathing. These decisions need to be made by a practitioner at the bedside. The primary reason to intubate a patient is acute respiratory failure which has been characterized as Type 1 Lung Failure, an oxygenation failure or Type 2 Pump failure, a ventilation failure (Figure 1, Table 1).[2]

Figure 1: A classification of respiratory failure based on function.

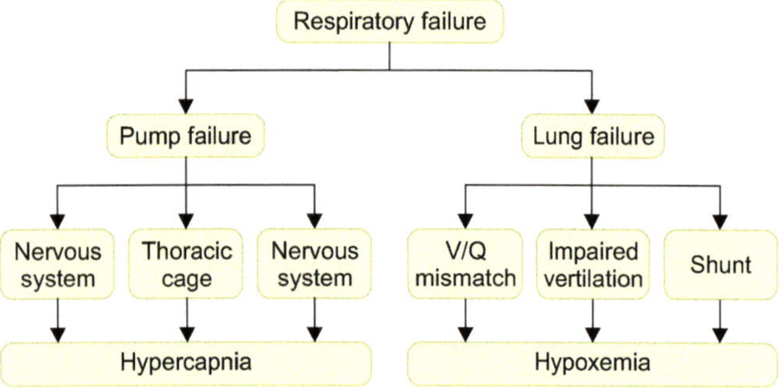

Table 1: Common Indications for Mechanical Ventilation (MV)

Ventilation	Normal	MV Indication
$PaCO_2$ mm Hg	33-45	>55
V_d/V_t	0.25-0.4	>0.6
Oxygenation		
FiO_2	0.21	1.0
PaO_2 mmHg	75-100	<70 mask
A-aDO_2 mm Hg	25-65	>450
Lung mechanics		
Respiratory Rate – breaths/min	12-30	>35
Vital Capacity-ml/kg	65-70	<15
Forced Expiratory Volume-1 sec (FEV1) ml/kg	50-60	<10
Inspiratory Force (IF)-Cm/H_2O	75-100	<25
*This table lists indications for mechanical ventilation based on arterial blood gasses and lung mechanics. However, clinicians are justified in interpreting data in the context of a patient's disease and the stage at which they are asked to intervene. It is appropriate to remind when a patient meets these parameters, they may be ready to be weaned off the ventilator.		

Glossary of Terms and Definitions:

- **Acute Respiratory Distress Syndrome (ARDS):** Advanced lung disease associated with severe hypoxia
- **Auto Positive End Expiratory Pressure**: Inappropriate development of positive end expiratory pressure due to insufficient expiratory time in a ventilated patient
- **Compliance**: The elasticity of the lung, defined as pressure divided by volume
- **Cycling:** The process of the ventilator switching from inspiration to passive expiration
- **Dead Space**: Area of lung which is ventilated, but not perfused
- **Inspiratory Pause**: Pause at end inspiration to measure used to measure plateau pressure
- **Minute Ventilation**: Total Volume of gas exchanged in one minute, defined as respiratory rate multiplied by tidal volume
- **Positive End Expiratory Pressure (PEEP):** Pressure left in the lower airway after passive exhalation in a mechanically ventilated patient
- **Plateau Pressure**: Pressure applied to small airways and alveoli
- **Peak Pressure**: Pressure of the whole respiratory system
- **Tidal Volume**: Amount gas inhaled and exhaled during one respiratory cycle
- **Spontaneous Breathing Trial (SBT)**: A weaning trial for patients while they are on the ventilator
- **Trigger**: Mechanism to alert ventilator to deliver a breath

- **Ventilator Associated Pneumonia**: A pneumonia which occurs in a patient after they have been on the ventilator for 48-72 hours

Table 2: Common Breath Types of Ventilators

Breath Type	Trigger	Target	Cycle
Volume Control	Elapsed time (rate/min)	Flow (1 L/sec)	Volume 500 mL
Volume Assist	Patient effort	Flow	Volume
Pressure Control	Elapsed time	Pressure (20 cm H_2O)	I Time 0.8 sec
Pressure Assist	Patient effort	Pressure	I Time
Pressure Support Ventilation	Patient effort	Pressure (10 cm H_2O)	Reduction of flow in circuit

Type 1 Respiratory Failure

Common Causes of Hypoxemic Respiratory Failure

1. Alveolar Hypoventilation
2. Diffusion Abnormalities
3. Shunt
4. Ventilation/Perfusion Mismatch

This type of respiratory failure is characterized by hypoxemia which occurs primarily by the four basic mechanisms listed above. Alveolar hypoventilation is characterized by insufficient respiratory effort to support a patient's oxygen requirements and, as a consequence, a patient's CO_2 will increase. An example of this is a postoperative surgical patient who had received excessive narcotics which suppresses his or her central respiratory drive. Increases in $PaCO_2$ would result in hypoxemia as predicted by the alveolar gas equation (Table 3). A decrease in PAO_2 secondary to a decrease in O_2 in inspired air is an obvious cause of hypoxemia.

Table 3: Equation for Alveolar Oxygen concentration, gradient and pulmonary shunt.

1. Alveolar Oxygen tension (PAO_2) = FiO_2 (Pb-PH_2O)-0.8 ($PaCO_2$) pb = Atmospheric pressure in mmHg (Normal 760 mm Hg at sea level) pH_2O = Water vapor pressure in mmHg (Normal 47 m Hg at sea level) FiO_2 = Fraction of inspired O_2 (Normal 0.21)
2. Alveolar-arterial O_2 gradient (A-aDO_2) = PAO_2-PaO_2 Normal varies with FiO_2 = <10 mm Hg on room air, < 50 mm Hg on FiO_2 1.0 or 100% A-aDO_2 > 300 mm Hg on FiO_2 indicates significant pulmonary shunt
3. Arterial O_2 content = Hemoglobin x 1.34 SaO_2/100 + (PaO_2 x 0.0031) Mixed venous O_2 content = Hemoglobin x 1.34 SvO_2 + (PvO_2 x 0.0031) Pulmonary end capillary O_2 content = Hemoglobin x 1.34 + (PAO_2 x 0.0031)
4. Pulmonary shunt (Qs/Qt) = Pulmonary end capillary O_2 content-Arterial O_2 content Pulmonary end capillary O_2 content-Mixed venous O_2 content X100 Normal <5%

Diffusion impairment is characterized by the impeded flow of oxygen from alveoli to the capillaries which surround them. An example of this would be a patient with fibrotic lung disease. In these patients, hypoxemia will be the defining characteristic as patients have an increased ventilatory drive often causing the CO_2 to be normal or low.

One of the primary goals of positive pressure ventilation is to reduce shunt. Shunt refers to ventilated, but non- perfused areas of the lung. Shunt is part of the cardiac output that returns to the left heart without exposure to ventilated alveoli. All patients have a small percentage of pulmonary shunt, so called physiologic shunt which is the reason that PAO_2 (Alveolar Oxygen) is higher than PaO_2 (Arterial oxygen) in normal individuals. Pulmonary shunt termed anatomical shunt can have cardiac origin, for example in a patient with an arterial septal defect or ventricular septal defect. An example of clinically significant pulmonary shunt is a patient with Acute Respiratory Syndrome (ARDS) or multilobar pneumonia with dense consolidation of the lung. Mechanical ventilation is useful in reducing shunt by recruiting partially or fully collapsed alveoli. However, a side effect of mechanical ventilation may also cause over distention of compliant parts of the lung causing redistribution of pulmonary blood flow to poorly ventilated sections of the lung.

For actual measurement of pulmonary shunt, simultaneous sampling of mixed venous blood from the tip of the properly placed pulmonary artery catheter and arterial blood is required. Calculation of arterial and mixed venous O_2 content and pulmonary end capillary O_2 content as given in equations 3 will allow the use of equation 4. If shunt exists there will be a significant difference between the alveolar and arterial partial pressures of oxygenation. This difference between the two is called the Alveolar Arterial gradient (Table 1, equation 2). To determine the patient's cause of hypoxia, clinicians can increase the fractional inspiration of oxygen (FiO_2) to 1.0 and patients with shunt will have non-linear improvement in their oxygenation.

As opposed to those with shunt, patients with ventilation/perfusion (V/Q) mismatch oxygenation will improve except in extreme cases by an increased FiO_2. The most common mechanism of hypoxemia encountered in clinical practice is V/Q mismatch. In postoperative surgical patients, atelectasis is the common cause of relative hypoxemia relieved by O_2 supplement.

With the ideal ratio of alveolar ventilation to perfusion (VA)/(Q) being 1. The alveolar ventilation to perfusion ratio varies in different parts of the lung. In normal upright human beings, ventilation is highest at the apex of the lung and perfusion is highest at the base. V/Q mismatch can occur for a variety of reasons, such as postoperative atelectasis, or bronchospasm secondary to asthma. In these patients, ventilation (VA) is compromised but perfusion (Q) is normal. The body's mechanism of dealing with this type of V/Q mismatch is hypoxic vasoconstriction. The alveolar arterioles will constrict in an area of relative hypoxia and thereby divert blood flow to well ventilated areas.

Type 2 Respiratory Failure

Type 2 respiratory failure is characterized by inadequate ventilation and a subsequent rise in PCO_2. Hypercapnia is due to three possible mechanisms:

1. Increased CO_2 production
2. Increased dead space
3. Decreased tidal volume

Increased CO_2 production is a direct result of hypermetabolism which could be caused by burns, sepsis, or trauma in a surgical patient. Hypermetabolic production of CO_2 is an unusual cause of hypercapnia as most patients are able to increase their effective alveolar ventilation in response to the decreased pH due to the elevated PCO_2. Surgical patients may suffer this type of respiratory compromise when they have coexisting morbidities such as neuromuscular disease.

Excessive dead space ventilation can increase PCO_2. Dead space refers to the area of the lung, which is ventilated, but not perfused. All ventilated patients have anatomic dead space comprised of the conducting airways of the respiratory system. Alveolar dead space refers to areas of the lung which are ventilated, but under perfused. Patients with increased dead space will have higher PCO_2 and need to increase their alveolar ventilation to blow off the excessive CO_2.

A common example is in surgical patients undergoing abdominal surgery who have increased dead space ventilation, with rapid shallow breathing and low tidal volumes. This is referred to as wasted ventilation since patients with abnormally high VA/Q ratios are ineffective in eliminating PCO_2.[1] Patients with pulmonary embolisms or those with high positive end expiratory pressure also may have increased dead space ventilation.

Decreased tidal volume ventilation can increase a patient's PCO_2 due to their inability to take adequate breaths. This may occur in a patient who is splinting post operatively after thoracic surgery. The key to treating these types of patients is to adequately treat their pain without suppressing their respiratory drive. If excessive narcotics are given hypoventilation may ensue due to depression of the central nervous system depression.

Mechanics and Nomenclature of Mechanical Ventilation

The key to understanding mechanical ventilation and its nomenclature is developing a working knowledge of how ventilators work.

Physiologic Effects of Mechanical Ventilation and nomenclature

This section will deal with the effects of positive pressure ventilation and define the nomenclature which will be used throughout the chapter. At the beginning of a breath ambient and alveolar pressure are equal at zero. Positive pressure ventilation generates positive pressure inside the thoracic cavity. A spontaneously breathing person generates negative pressure compared to ambient pressure inside the thoracic cavity upon inhalation which allows atmospheric air to flow into the lungs. A negative pressure gradient is generated through diaphragmatic and intercostal muscles working in conjunction to expand the rib cage. This pressure gradient reverses with diaphragmatic and intercostal muscle relaxation and exhalation occurs. At end-inspiration and end-expiration the atmospheric pressure is equivalent to the alveolar pressure. Tidal Volume is the amount of gas inhaled and exhaled during one respiratory cycle. Tidal Volume in a patient who is mechanically ventilated is the amount of gas inspired during one respiratory cycle. Minute ventilation is the amount of tidal volume exchanged over one minute. In a patient who is mechanically ventilated, tidal volume and respiratory can be manipulated as necessary for the patient's benefit.

The ease of ventilating a patient often depends on the compliance of the lung. The compliance of a mechanical ventilated patient's lungs is reflected by the plateau pressure (Figure 2). Plateau pressure is the pressure applied to the small airways and alveoli and peak inspiratory pressure is the pressure of the whole respiratory system. Plateau pressures can be measured at end inspiration with an inspiratory pause during mechanical ventilation. Inspiratory pause of 10 seconds causes a temporary stoppage of gas flow between the ventilator and the patient. In a healthy patient there should be minimal difference between PIP and plateau pressures. The difference between the PIP and plateau pressure is the pressure required to overcome the resistance in the conducting airways. An obstruction in the endotracheal tube will increase the gradient between the plateau and peak inspiratory pressure.

The PIP and plateau pressure will be elevated in a patient with multilobar pneumonia, but the gradient between the two pressures will be normal. Mean airway pressure is the average of pressure applied in the respiratory cycle during ventilation. These concepts and definitions are important when trying to ventilate a patient (Table 4).

Figure 2: Airway pressure that is more important is plateau Pressure (Ps) measures with applying an inspiratory pause. During MV it is recommended to be kept below 35 Cm H_2O.

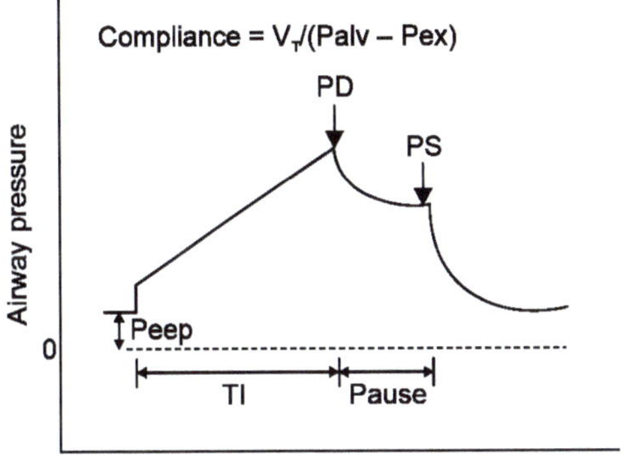

Table 4: Normal values of lung volumes and pressure

- Tidal Volume 5-8mL/kg
- Minute Ventilation 6-7 Liters/minute at rest
- Compliance Normal 0.1L/cm H_2O
- Peak Inspiratory Pressure (PIP) -modified equation = Flow x Resistance + Volume/Compliance
- Gradient Between Peak Inspiratory Pressure (PIP) and Plateau Pressure =5 mmHg

Types of Breaths

A mechanically ventilated patient can take four types of breath. Spontaneous breaths are those that are initiated and terminated by the patient and not supported by the ventilator. Mandatory breaths are defined by a ventilator initiated or terminated act of inspiration. Although some disagreement exists about the classification of assisted and supported breaths, assisted breaths for the purpose of this text are defined as a mandatory breath that is initiated by the patient and delivered by machine. Supported breaths are breaths initiated by the patient but supported by the ventilator.

Trigger

The mechanism to alert the ventilator to deliver a breath is triggering. This is either time-cycled or initiated by the patient. The two common mechanisms of triggering are pressure and flow. Pressure triggering requires patients to generate a preset negative inspiratory pressure. This threshold to deliver a breath is known as sensitivity. Usually, a negative pressure of 2 cm H_2O is sufficient to generate a ventilator breath. Flow-sensing triggering is when the patient generates a preset inspiratory flow signaling to the ventilator to trigger a breath. This mode of triggering was developed to reduce the dyssynchrony between the patient and ventilator. Flow triggering was a more sensitive signal than pressure triggering, reducing the interval between the patient's signal for a breath and the ventilator's delivery of a breath. The sensitivity difference between both triggering mechanisms is now minimal. Two common problems associated with triggering are auto-triggering and ineffective triggering. Auto-trigger which occurs when the sensitivity for triggering is set too low (Figure 3). Breaths are delivered to the patient without the patient actually causing the changes required for breath delivery. Two examples of noise that cause auto-triggering are leaks or water in the ventilator circuit. The opposite of auto-triggering is ineffective triggering where the sensitivity is set too high, and patients are unable to signal to the ventilator that a breath is needed (Figure 4). Patients with obstructive pulmonary disease who are ventilated often suffer from this problem due to auto-positive end expiratory pressure (Auto-PEEP), a phenomenon explained below.

Figure 3: Double Triggering, a form of auto-triggering

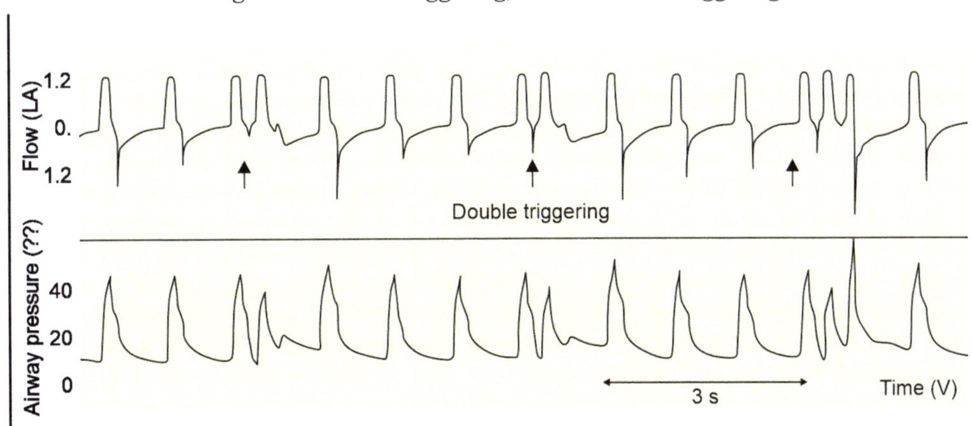

Fig. 3. Flow and airway pressure recording showing double-triggering, defined as two consecutive ventilator cycles separated by an expiratory time less than one-half the mean inspiratory time. Double-triggering occurs when the ventilator inspiratory time is shorter than the patient's inspiratory time. The patient's effort is not completed at the end of the first ventilator cycle and trigger's a second ventialtor cycle

Figure 4: Ineffective Triggering

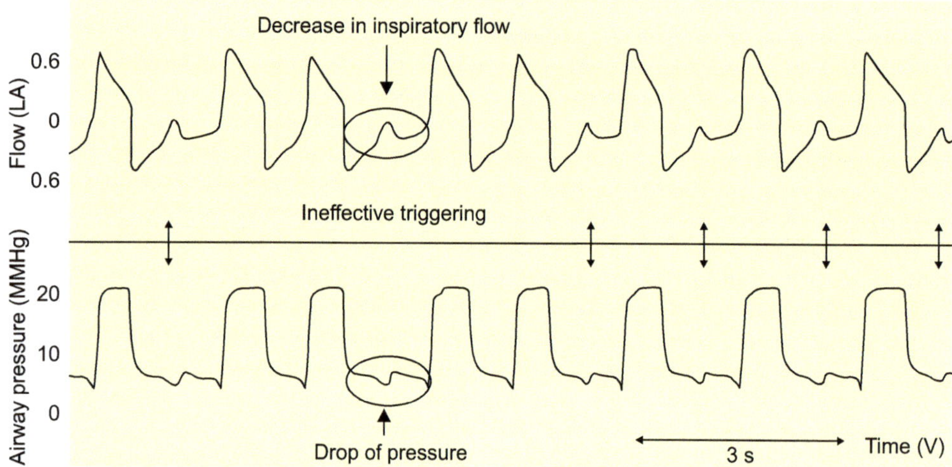

Fig. 1. Flow end airway pressure tracings showing inffective triggering, i.e., a wasted effort, defined as an airway pressure drop simultaneous to a flow decrease during the expiratory period and not followed by a ventialtor cycle, indicating that the patient's effort was not detected by the ventilator (arros)

Inspiratory Limit

Ventilators are programmed to deliver pressurized air to a specific limit. The three variables are volume, pressure, and flow. Volume directed ventilation delivers a particular tidal volume independent of lung mechanics leading to possible alveolar overinflation and iatrogenic lung injury. Pressure directed ventilation delivers a tidal volume to a preset pressure or a preset inspiratory time independent of lung mechanics and may lead to insufficient minute ventilation. In flow-specific ventilation tidal volume delivered will not exceed preset flow.

Cycling

Cycling means the switch from inspiration to passive expiration. The three variables that define cycling are time, volume, and flow. Volume-cycled breaths deliver a preset tidal volume in closed circuit ventilation. Once the total volume is delivered, the patient switches to passive exhalation. An important caveat of volume-cycled ventilation is the pressure relief valve which opens as a safety mechanism if the pressure in the ventilator circuit is excessive. This allows an appropriate early termination of the inspiratory cycle. In time-cycled breaths inspiration occurs during a preset time then passive exhalation occurs. Pressure control ventilation is defined by this type of cycling with a constant pressure delivered during the preset interval. The patient's tidal volume is determined by the pressure applied and the patient's intrinsic lung characteristics. This is an important difference between time-cycled ventilation and volume-cycled ventilation as tidal volume is not guaranteed. If the clinician is concerned with elevated airway pressures, this mode may be advantageous. Flow-cycled breaths change from inspiration to passive expiration when the patient's inspiratory flow decreases to a preset value. Patients have to initiate their own breaths in flow cycled ventilation. The patient determines their tidal volume by their inspiratory effort and lung mechanics. Pressure support ventilation is defined by this type of cycling pattern. A time-based safety mechanism exists to terminate the inspiratory cycle in flow-cycled breaths in case there is a leak in the airway circuit (Figure 5).

Figure 5: Breath cycling, difference between patient-initiated breath and ventilator-initiated breath

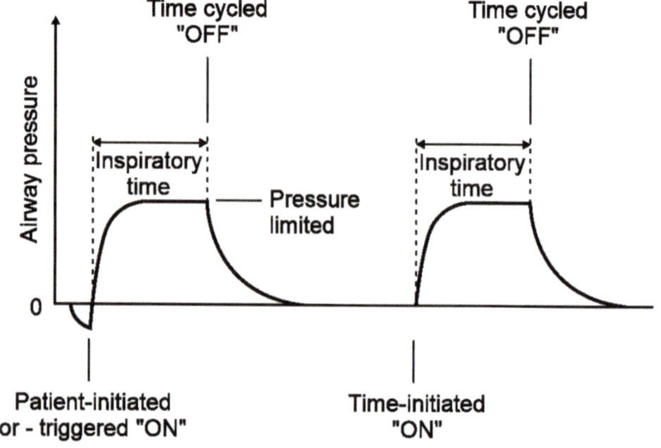

Parameters Set in Common Ventilation Modes

Positive End Expiratory Pressure (PEEP) and Continuous Positive Airway Pressure (CPAP)

Positive End Expiratory Pressure refers to the pressure left in the lower airway after passive exhalation in a mechanically ventilated patient. Continuous positive airway pressure (CPAP) is almost identical to PEEP, except that CPAP is the term applied when a patient is spontaneously breathing without ventilatory assistance. This pressure is maintained by a constant gas stream which provides a level of pressure inside the patient's lungs which is above atmospheric pressure. Applied PEEP is set by clinicians in multiple modes of mechanical ventilation and a basic understanding of its utility and possible harms are required for anyone who manipulates ventilators. The first well-known application of PEEP with mechanical ventilation was the Engstrom Ventilator in the 1950s. Its utility was demonstrated by Frumin et al., using it to improve oxygenation. It was the recognition of the syndrome of ARDS, a disease of severe lung parenchymal injury which further piqued clinicians' interest in PEEP. Positive End Expiratory Pressure is useful in patients with decreased lung compliance to help patients overcome alveolar collapse. The applied positive pressure can open collapsed diseased alveoli and in turn increase functional residual capacity. Functional residual capacity is the volume of air in the lung parenchyma at end-expiration. Determining the optimal level of PEEP is difficult as the amount of PEEP required to recruit and keep alveoli open in one area of the lung may not be the same in another area of the lung. This is one of the challenges of ventilating a patient with heterogeneous lung disease as over distention of alveoli can lead to iatrogenic injury amongst other harms. To determine optimal PEEP for inspiratory pressure volume curves can be constructed to determine the lower inflection point which is the average alveolar pressure to open alveoli which close during expiration. The upper inflection point represents the overdistention of alveoli without increase in volume and a flattening of the pressure volume curve (Figure 6). Studies have shown a significant limitation to the use of inflection points, but titrating PEEP blindly in patients with severe lung disease is inadvisable. Early studies of PEEP in surgical patients indicated that in almost one fourth of the patients expected decrease in intrapulmonary shunt did not occur. [8] Moreover, A-aDO_2 was not always a good predictor of shunt. 8If used properly some of the benefits of PEEP are decreased left ventricular afterload, increased lung compliance, reduced shunt by multiple mechanisms including recruitment of collapsed alveoli and increase of functional residual capacity. Positive end expiratory pressure also increases intrathoracic pressures and can cause iatrogenic injury including barotrauma, hypoxia by increasing shunt and decreased cardiac output (Table 5).

Figure 6: Demonstration of inspiration Lower Inflection Point and Upper Inflection Point and the effect of Distending Pressure (PEEP)

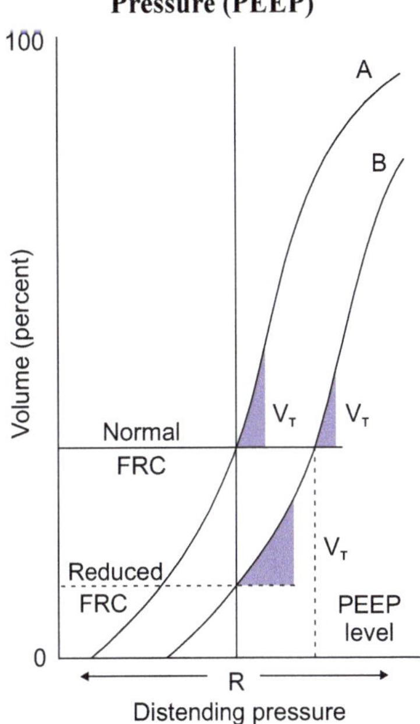

Table 5: Common Possible Advantages and Disadvantages to Positive End Expiratory Pressure

Advantages	Disadvantages
Improves Oxygenation	Decreased Venous Return
Improves Functional Residual Capacity	Decreased Cardiac Output
Improves Lung Compliance	Barotrauma
Decreases Shunt	Increases Shunt

Fractional Inspiration of Oxygen (FiO_2)

The fractional inspiration of Oxygen (FiO_2) is the admixture of oxygen delivered to patients and can be set anywhere from 21% to 100%. Ambient air has 21% oxygen and pressure of oxygen is 760 mmHg at sea level, with decreasing pressures of oxygen as a person travels above sea level (Table 1).

Common Modes of Mechanical Ventilation

Mode of ventilation refers to how the ventilator has been set to interact with patients.

Assist Control Pressure Control

The clinician sets the inspiratory time and the pressure limit (peak pressure) in this mode of ventilation. Breaths are initiated either by the patient or the ventilator. The ventilator breaths are time-cycled and pressure limited. As discussed above, a constant pressure is applied during the time-cycle and tidal volume will vary with lung mechanics. Graphically, the flow waveform for this type of ventilation is decelerating (Figure 7). Flow is highest at the beginning of inspiration and gradually decreases throughout the inspiratory phase till ventilator cycles to passive expiration. This is due to slowing flow as the pressure limit is reached in the inspiratory phase. Gas flows along a pressure gradient until the preset pressure is reached inside the thorax and then pressure is maintained till the ventilator cycles to the expiratory phase. One possible advantage of this mode of ventilation is the limitation of alveolar distention due to preset pressure limits.

Figure 7: Example of Pressure Control Waveform

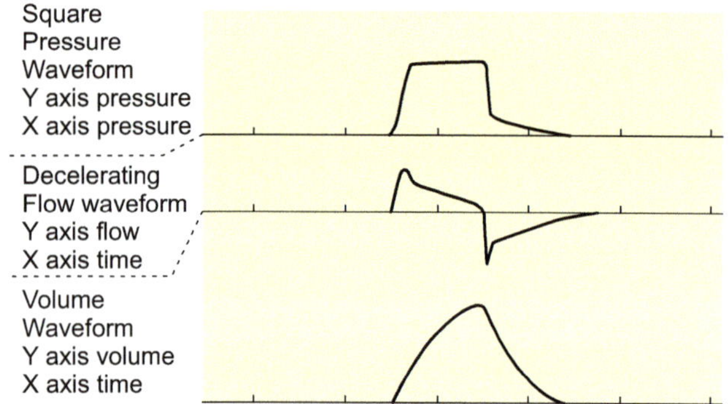

Assist Control Volume Control

The clinician sets the tidal volume and flow in this mode of ventilation. Breaths are initiated either by the patient or the ventilator. The ventilator breaths are volume cycled and either flow or volume limited. Graphically, the flow waveform for volume-cycled ventilation depends on how the clinicians set up the ventilator. The decelerating waveform of pressure-control ventilation can be used, but also a sinusoidal or square waveform (Figure 8). One advantage of assisted volume control ventilation is that patients can be ventilated with different flow patterns, which may enhance their comfort. Another is that due to guaranteed tidal volume ventilation is assured. Important limitations of this mode are possible alveolar over distention with excessive tidal volumes and unnecessary hyperventilation.

Figure 8: Example of Volume Control Waveform

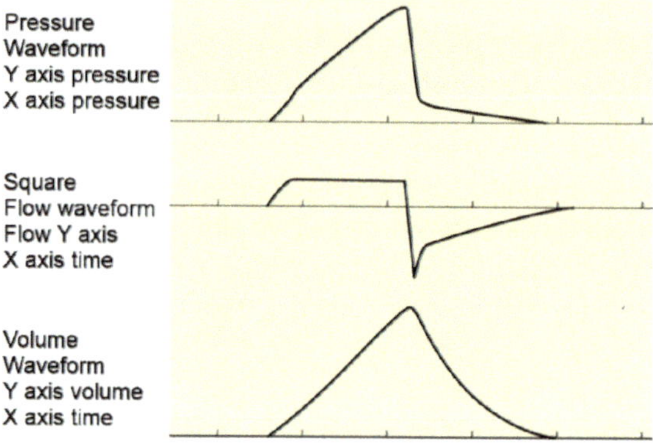

Pressure Support Ventilation (PSV)

The clinician sets the level of support to augment inspiration in this mode of ventilation. Patients must have an intact respiratory drive because the patient initiates all breaths. Breaths are flow cycled and have no specific limit. The flow waveform is decelerating (Figure 9). Pressure support can be used as an independent mode of ventilation, or it can be used in conjunction with other modes. During inspiration, the ventilator will adjust flow to augment the patient's inspiratory effort to the preset pressure mandated by the clinician. This does not guarantee a specific tidal volume and patients with changing lung mechanics can also have changing minute ventilation. The level of pressure support can be increased to augment tidal volume. The clinician needs to be cognizant that PSV should not be used in patients with depressed respiratory drive and used with caution in those with changing lung compliance due to possible decreased tidal volumes. The mode is currently being used in almost 50% of patients for weaning them from ventilator support.

Figure 9: Example of Pressure Support Waveform with PEEP

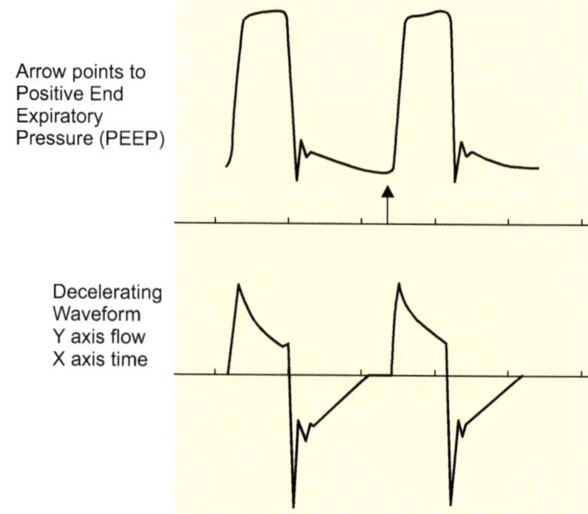

Synchronized Intermittent Mandatory Ventilation (SIMV)

This form of ventilation was first described in 1973 in a case series. It was designed to help facilitate the weaning of patients off ventilators. Clinicians set respiratory rate, PEEP level, volume, cycling mechanism and flow pattern for mandatory breaths. Patients are able to take spontaneous breaths of a variable nature in addition to mandatory breaths due to a demand valve in the ventilator circuit without mechanical assistance (Figure 10). A much feared but eventually theoretical consideration of "breath-stacking" was overcome with microprocessor technology which allowed patients respiratory effort to be synchronized with the ventilator. However, studies documented persistent respiratory alkalosis in patients ventilated with SIMV.[9] The second significant limitation was the increased work of breathing due to the resistance caused by breathing through the endotracheal tube. In a study where SIMV and PEEP were used as primary mode of weaning in ARDS patients, we found a failure rate of 28% due to increased respiratory distress.[10] SIMV as a mode of ventilation is still favored by many clinicians including surgeons and anesthesiologists. At ventilator rates greater than 8/minute, SIMV is very similar to A/C mode. At lower rates i.e., 2-4/minute, higher levels of PEEP for improving oxygenation may be possible.

Figure 10: SIMV Volume Control

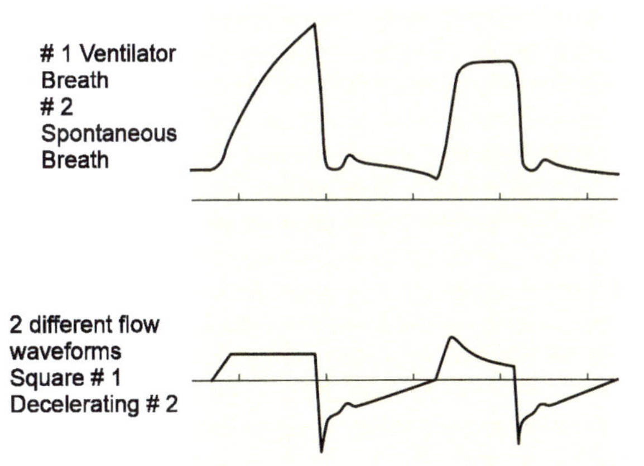

Pressure Regulated Volume Control (PRVC)

In this form of ventilation, the machine adjusts pressure attempting not to compromise tidal volume. This is an example of closed loop ventilation as opposed to open-loop ventilation in which the machine does not alter its breath delivery based on feedback. In this mode, the clinician sets a pressure limit, respiratory rate, and desired tidal volume. The breaths are time-cycled and patient or machine triggered. An initial breath is delivered after settings are determined by the clinician and the compliance of the respiratory system is calculated. The next three breaths are delivered at 75% of the pressure limit set by the clinician in an attempt to deliver the desired tidal volume. In fact, if the settings remain static, clinicians will be able to observe decreased inspiratory pressures as the patient's disease process improves.

Continuous Mandatory Ventilation

This mode of ventilation will not be detailed extensively, because of its limited use. The patient is unable to initiate breaths on their own and their breaths are given by pressure control or volume control. This mode can lead to significant patient discomfort unless they are heavily sedated or paralyzed due to dyssynchrony with the ventilator. This mode of ventilation was the initial mode of ventilation used prior to the development of assist control ventilation.

Alternative Modes of Mechanical Ventilation

These modes of ventilation are less commonly used in adults, but maybe used more in centers that have more expertise. Our purpose is to describe the modes for the reader to develop familiarity with them.

Inverse Ratio Ventilation

Is a mode of ventilation where the inspiratory time exceeds the expiratory time. A normal inspiratory to expiratory ratio is between 1:2 to 1:4, this mode will change the inspiratory time to double the expiratory time. This strategy of ventilation purposely creates auto-PEEP and has been associated with improved oxygenation in ARDS patients but has not consistently shown any other benefit. This mode further requires paralysis or heavy sedation as it is uncomfortable for patients.

Airway Pressure Release Ventilation (APRV)

In patients who are difficult to oxygenate, alternative modes of ventilation have been explored. Patients with ARDS are sometimes ventilated with Airway Pressure Release Ventilation (APRV) as a salvage mode of ventilation. In APRV clinicians can increase the patients mean airway pressure. Clinicians set a high pressure (P_{High}), a low pressure (P_{Low}), a time level at P_{High} (T_{High}) and a time at low pressure (T_{Low}). Patients' breath above the ventilator spontaneously, while the ventilator cycles between P_{High} and P_{Low}. Carbon dioxide is eliminated with the patient's spontaneous breathing and with the changes between P_{High} and P_{Low}. To increase carbon dioxide elimination, clinicians can increase the frequency of intervals of P_{High} with shorter T_{Low} times. To increase oxygenation, clinicians can increase P_{High} pressure and Thigh time, at the expense of carbon dioxide elimination. As with any significant changes made on mechanically ventilated patients, obtaining a blood gas within the first hour is advisable. Unlike patients in ACVC where the plateau pressure can be measured with an inspiratory hold, patients cannot have their plateau pressure measured accurately in APRV. Since patients are breathing over the ventilator, transpulmonary pressure would be a more accurate description of the pressures felt by a patient's alveoli. Transpulmonary pressure is the difference between the alveolar pressure and the intrapleural pressure in the lungs. It can more accurately be assessed by placement of an esophageal balloon to estimate pleural pressure. Besides not being able to accurately estimate alveolar distending pressure, two frequently cited disadvantages of the APRV are its predilection for hypercapnia and concern for barotrauma due to the elevated peak airway pressures.

Adaptive Supportive Ventilation (ASV)

It is based on the mathematical principle that alveolar ventilation can be done more efficiently than with other forms of ventilation. It uses closed loop ventilation to achieve minute ventilation goals by manipulating pressure limits, the inspiratory and expiratory ratio and respiratory rate. The clinician provides the patient's ideal body weight, PEEP, FiO_2, pressure limit and trigger level for assisted cycles. Also, the clinician provides a minute volume target usually of 0.1L/kg/min for adults. The ventilator determines the patient's respiratory mechanics from a test breath and then gives the patient a target tidal volume and respiratory rate based on the clinician settings. This mode of ventilation gives time-cycled, pressure controlled, or pressure supported breaths and can be the mode of ventilation for a patient who goes from apnea to being weaned off the ventilator.[11]

Proportional Assist Ventilation (PAV)

This is also another form of closed loop ventilation in which the ventilator measures elastance and resistance in individual breaths to determine support needed by the patient to overcome the work of breathing. Proportional Assist Ventilation is patient triggered, pressure limited, pressure controlled, and flow cycled. The primary difference between this mode and PSV, is that it adjusts support given to the patient based on the patient's lung mechanics. Clinicians set the PEEP, FiO_2 and the percentage of work they would like the ventilator to do to overcome the elastance and resistance required for effective ventilation.

High Frequency Ventilation (HFV)

This category of ventilation includes two different modalities, oscillators, and jet ventilators. The difference between the two types is beyond the scope of this text. They both operate differently than conventional mechanical ventilation. Conventional ventilation delivers tidal volume with bulk flow as opposed to high frequency ventilation which delivers breaths through non-convective gas transport. To be termed a high frequency ventilator for an adult, the respiratory rate needs to be greater than 300 breaths per minute. Most of the data supporting this type of ventilation exists in the pediatric and neonate literature, however, this modality found increased use in the H1N1 crisis. Potential advantage of HFV is the high mean airway pressures with less dramatic swings in pressures leading to less lung injury. Potential disadvantages are iatrogenic harm inadvertently caused by clinicians' unfamiliarity with this mode of ventilation, inspissated secretions and hypercapnia. It is not supported for use in adult ARDS but may have use in specific clinical situations.[27]

Neurally Adjusted Ventilatory Assist (NAVA)

This unique form of ventilation uses neural stimulus to trigger respiratory effort through sensing electrical activity of the diaphragm (EAdi) with electrodes on a nasogastric tube. The signal from the diaphragm to the ventilator also helps the ventilator determine the level of respiratory support required by the patient. Theoretically, this is a significant advancement as triggering mechanisms are not needed and this has the potential to reduce patient-ventilator dyssynchrony.[1]

Weaning Patients from Mechanical Ventilation

Equally as important as initiating mechanical ventilation, is the decision to relieve a patient from mechanical ventilation. The weaning process usually takes 40–50% of the overall ventilation time. Weaning success is defined as spontaneous breathing for 24 hours or more without the need for mechanical assistance. Before the decision is made to wean a patient from a ventilator two fundamental questions need to be asked. Has the condition which required the patient to be mechanically ventilated been resolved? Does the patient have other medical comorbidities which may interfere with their ability to spontaneously breathe? Extensive objective criteria exist to help clinicians liberate patients from mechanical ventilation, but some measurements are easier to obtain than others (Table 6). These measurements and observations can provide useful information about patients, but individually none have proven to be accurate enough to predict weaning success.[13] A better method of predicting weaning success is a spontaneous breathing trial (SBT). A SBT is a formal examination of a spontaneously breathing mechanically ventilated patient with minimal ventilatory support for anywhere between 30 to 120 minutes. Importantly, there is no data to support SBT greater than 120 minutes. Minimal ventilatory support has different definitions, but a CPAP level of 5 mmHg to prevent airway collapse with or without 5-8 mmHg PS to overcome upper airway resistance provided by the endotracheal tube (ETT) is commonly used. Higher levels of CPAP and PS can be used and is up to the clinician's discretion. Another SBT method is to do a T-piece weaning trial which involves the patient being disconnected from the ventilator and only receiving a flow of oxygen through the ETT. Due to the lack of ventilatory support to overcome the increased airway resistance from the ETT, this SBT method is more challenging than doing a trial with PS and CPAP. No single parameter should be used to determine a patient's success or failure of an SBT, but rather an integrated assessment of the patient's clinical status. The integral components of this assessment are the patient's hemodynamics status, their gas exchange, their oximetry, clinical signs of increased work of breathing and their mental state. A patient's vitals should be stable during an SBT without labile blood pressure or significant tachyarrhythmias or bradycardic events. Similarly, the patient should not become significantly tachypneic or apneic during an SBT. Desaturation events and or physical examination signs of increased work of breathing like accessory muscle use would be a possible harbinger of failure. Patients who are unprepared to be liberated can become both anxious and agitated or if their cardiopulmonary system is inadequate to the task, they may become diaphoretic. Clinicians have to carefully observe patients during SBT as a multitude of clinical signs both objective and subjective if seen can help predict a patient's ability to be successfully weaned from mechanical ventilation.

Table 6:[1] Adapted from MacIntyre NR Discontinuing Mechanical Ventilation

Causes of Weaning Failure	Explanation
Respiratory Drive Failure	Inability of patient to generate reliable respiratory drive due to CNS injury or medications
Oxygenation Failure	Inability to oxygenate due to loss of PPV or FiO_2
Cardiovascular Failure	Cardiac failure due to loss of PPV
Muscle Failure	Due to weakened muscles secondary weakened, fatigued, or metabolically disturbed muscles
Psychological Factors	Patient due to delirium or primary CNS condition is unable to handle spontaneous ventilation

Once a patient passes an SBT, clinicians must assess whether a patient can protect their airway without the ETT. Patients with significant secretions may not be able to expectorate them after being liberated from mechanical ventilation. Different criteria have been proposed, but a generally agreed upon practice pattern is the need for suctioning less than every 2 hours. The ability to clear secretions and protect one's airway lies in the patient's ability to cough, which should be determined adequate prior to liberation. Another contentious point is a patient's mental status prior to extubating. The literature is inadequate as to whether patients with altered mental status who pass an SBT with an adequate cough and secretion load should be able to be extubated. A large randomized controlled trial with a uniform definition of altered mental status is needed before definitive recommendations on this subject can be offered. However, clinicians should hesitate to extubate patients who were intubated primarily due to an inability to protect their airway if their altered mental status has not shown significant improvement. Patients with difficult airways should always be treated with caution when the decision to extubate them is made. If anesthesia and the tools needed for a problem are available, they should be present at the bedside. If clinical uncertainty exists about whether to extubate a patient with a difficult airway, it is better to wait until the clinician is more confident, they will be liberated successfully.

Not all patients pass SBT and determining the cause of their failure can be difficult, but it is important. The failure to wean can be classified into five broad categories (Table 7). It is important that clinicians address these limitations, otherwise patients will continue to fail in the weaning process. Clinicians are not alone in trying to wean patients as protocols, which allow respiratory therapists, and nurses to actively participate in SBT have been shown to decrease patient's length of ventilation. An organized approach to the weaning process is important as subjective decisions made by physicians alone can lead to unnecessarily prolonged ventilation.[1]

Table 7: Clinical Findings and Ventilator Signs of Tension Pneumothorax

Clinical Findings of Tension Pneumothorax
Deviated trachea away from tension pneumothorax side
Decreased breath sounds
Distended neck veins
Increased dullness to percussion
Ventilator Signs of Tension Pneumothorax
Elevated Peak and Plateau Pressures
Vitals signs
Decreased blood pressure
Increased heart rate
Decreased oxygenation saturation

Failing Extubation

The precise percentage of patients who need to be reintubated after extubation is unclear, with a wide range cited of between 2-25.[15] Even further disagreement exists upon an acceptable number of re-intubations to occur in an ICU. The optimal reintubation rate would be zero, however an ICU with a low reintubation rate is likely being overly cautious and one with a high reintubation rate is likely being overly aggressive. Unnecessarily prolonged intubation can lead to increased costs, increased length of stay, exposure to more sedatives, increased infectious risks and the harmful physiologic effects of positive pressure ventilation. While the premature discontinuation can lead to significantly increased mortality, higher risk of nosocomial pneumonia and possible airway loss.

The most common causes for reintubation in the ICU are respiratory failure, congestive heart failure, aspiration or excess pulmonary secretions, and upper airway obstruction. Upper airway obstruction deserves closer examination as 1-4% of the general ICU population requires reintubation due to it. It is caused by laryngeal edema secondary to mechanical trauma to the larynx due to the ETT. Laryngeal edema has a wide variety of presentations with the worst cases requiring reintubation with a technically difficult laryngoscopy or cricothyroidotomy. A majority of patients will develop symptoms anywhere within 5 to 30 minutes of extubation. Most will specifically develop post-extubation inspiratory stridor, which is a whistle like sound produced due to airflow through an edematous narrowed airway. Patients with laryngeal edema as the cause of their reintubation have a lower mortality rate than other clinical causes, but clinicians still need to be vigilant to determine which patients are at risk for the phenomenon. Epidemiological studies have cited female gender, large ETT to trachea and prolonged ventilation as risk factors, but disagreement about the relevance of these findings exists. The presence of a cuff leak of greater than 110cc accurately predicts patients will not have post-extubation stridor. Cuff leaks are performed by suctioning the secretions around the ETT cuff, lowering the cuff, and measuring the expiratory tidal volumes. Expiratory tidal volumes should be less than 110 cc than inspiratory tidal volumes. The lack of a presence of a cuff leak, however, does not accurately predict patients who will develop post-extubation stridor. Prior to extubation if a clinician suspects laryngeal edema steroids can be given prophylactically. If a patient is extubated and they develop stridor steroids, racemic epinephrine, non-invasive ventilation, and heliox all have been used. None has been proven to alter patient outcomes, but the potential benefit in individual cases often warrants a trial of these modalities. The use of non-invasive ventilation may delay reintubation which can be associated with increased mortality, therefore this adjunct needs to be used with extra caution. All therapies for patients with post-extubation stridor need to be used with caution as if laryngeal edema progresses patients may not be able to be reintubated requiring an emergent tracheostomy or cricothyroidectomy.[16]

Tracheostomy in Intensive Care Unit

Tracheostomies are one of the most important and commonly performed procedures in the ICU. The benefits of placing a tracheostomy for patients who will require prolonged mechanical ventilation are multifold including reduced exposure to sedatives, improved comfort, enhanced communication, decreased ventilator associated infections, and theoretically decreased work of breathing. In a European survey, 10% of ICU patients received tracheostomies and the median day of placement was day twelve. The risk factors for tracheostomy in this study was the duration of mechanical ventilation, reintubation, coma, and neuromuscular disease.[1] Surprisingly little consensus exists about the optimal timing and indication for this commonly performed procedure. The medical literature does not clearly support early or late placement of tracheostomy in patients who will require prolonged mechanical ventilation (>21 days). Patients with tracheostomies create a significant health burden and the procedure has its own associated morbidities as it should be noted that half of patients who are critically ill who receive tracheotomies are dead within one year.[28] The most common adverse postoperative events associated with placing tracheostomies are stoma inflammation, stoma infection and bleeding.[14]

Common Encountered Problems in Mechanical Ventilation:

Mechanically ventilated patients are subject to multiple medical comorbidities due to being on PPV. These morbidities are due to a loss of host defenses secondary to the penetration of the oropharynx barrier, an exposure to pharmacological agents used to keep patients sedated and the general physiologic effects of PPV.

Ventilator Associated Pneumonia (VAP)

Ventilator Associated Pneumonia refers to a pneumonia that arises more than 48-72hrs after intubation. It occurs in 9-27% of all intubated patients. A wide variation about the attributable mortality due to VAP exists with ranges quoted between 0-70%.1 It is important to know in surgical patients' specific factors that may predispose them to VAP. A review of a colectomy database with 48,247 adults showed that postoperative pneumonia was significantly more common in patients undergoing emergent versus elective surgery 11.1% vs 2.9%.[18] A variety of pathogens cause VAP, with the most common gram negative multidrug resistant organism is Pseudomonas Aeruginosa. Other common gram-negative organisms include Klebsiella and Acinetobacter. Multiple gram-positive organisms cause VAP, but Multidrug Resistant Staphylococcus Aureus (MRSA) is a primary concern as few antibiotics can treat it. Anaerobes and viruses cause few VAP, but viruses and opportunistic pathogens can cause VAP in immunocompromised hosts. Preventing VAP would be ideal, but few interventions appear to have made a difference. Preventing intubation or reintubation are the primary mechanisms to avoid a VAP. A continuous subglottic suction system as part of an ETT and raising the head of the bed 45 degrees appear to be the most effective interventions. In specific patient populations other interventions have proven useful, such as the use of chlorhexidine oral antiseptic in coronary artery bypass surgery patients. Selective decontamination of the digestive tract with antibiotics did not make a difference and is not recommended. The prevention of VAPs remains an elusive goal and strategies are continuing to evolve.[19]

Equally as difficult is the diagnosis of VAP. Both the Infectious Disease Society of America and American Thoracic Society recommend cultures prior to initiation of antibiotic therapy. Cultures should be quantitative endotracheal aspirate, protected brush specimen or a bronchoalveolar lavage. A clinical strategy emphasizes the need for a new or evolving infiltrate on a chest radiography, plus two other criteria. The variables are a fever greater than 38 degrees Celsius, purulent sputum and leukocytosis or leukopenia. Requiring each of these criteria to be present increases specificity but decreases sensitivity. If reliable cultures are negative, the antibiotics can be discontinued. Antibiotics should not be delayed if cultures cannot be obtained in a reasonable period or if patients are hemodynamically unstable.[18] It should be noted that the Centers for Disease control is currently changing the definition of VAP to a broader category of Ventilator Associated Events (VAE). This change is to address the subjectivity in defining VAP. VAEs are triggered by increases in FiO_2 by more than 10% or PEEP by greater than 2 mmHg for greater than two calendar days. These events can occur for a variety of reasons including, but not limited to pulmonary edema, mucous plugging, and infection. If it is due to a respiratory infection that meets the criteria for VAP.

Auto-PEEP

Auto-PEEP is the inappropriate development of PEEP due to insufficient expiratory time on a ventilated patient. Auto-PEEP is seen in patients with obstructive airway diseases (Asthma, COPD) who require prolonged expiratory times, patients with elevated respiratory rate, those dyssynchronous with the ventilator and patients inappropriately short inspiratory times. Three important consequences of Auto-PEEP are hemodynamic compromise due to high intrathoracic pressures secondary to decreased cardiac return, patient difficulty triggering the ventilator for breath initiation and barotrauma. The treatment for Auto-PEEP is the prolongation of expiratory times and this can be done by a multitude of mechanisms. It can be corrected by decreasing respiratory rate, decreasing tidal volume, and increasing the inspiratory flow. In patients with obstructive airway disease, it is important to use bronchodilators to relieve obstruction as this will help Auto-PEEP.

Ventilator Induced Lung Injury (VILI)

Ventilator Induced Lung Injury (VILI) can involve microscopic to gross trauma, leading to a multitude of morbidities.[20] We now know VILI can be in four different ways including biotrauma, atelectrauma, volutrauma, and barotrauma. Biotrauma is inflammation due to ventilator driven lung injury and can contribute to VILI. Atelectotrauma is cyclic opening and closing of collapsed alveoli leading to inflammation. Volutrauma is airway injury due to excessive distending volumes and barotrauma is airway injury due to excessive airway pressures. The incidence of barotrauma according to a large multinational survey was 2.9% in all patients and 0.5% in post-operative patients according to an earlier study. Barotrauma was an independent predictor of increased mortality, increased ICU length of stay and increased number of days on the ventilator.[20] The results of both volutrauma and barotrauma can be both microscopic with inflammation, but also gross with alveolar rupture. Alveolar rupture leads to extra-alveolar air which can migrate to the peritoneum, the vascular circulation, and the subcutaneous skin. The most common and clinically relevant complications are pneumothorax, pneumomediastinum and subcutaneous emphysema.

Pneumothorax are defined as a presence of air in the pleural cavity with collapse of the lung. Pneumothoraces are divided into primary and secondary events. Those which occur on the ventilator are secondary pneumothoraces because they are due to mechanical ventilation and or underlying disease. A tension pneumothorax is an extreme form pneumothorax in air builds up in the pleural space due to a ball and valve like effect where air enters the pleural cavity but is not allowed to escape. Eventually, the excess pressure causes the lung to collapse and causes a hemodynamically significant stoppage in venous return. Patients can develop cardiac arrest if clinical signs are not heeded, and treatment is not offered (Table 8, Figure 10).

Table 8: Modifiable Risk Factors for Delirium

Modifiable Risk Factors for Delirium
Mimic circadian rhythm
Brain ischemia
Hypoxemia
Modify the administration of psychoactive medications,
Aggressively treat infection and the manifestations of severe sepsis
Reducing unnecessary sedatives
Reducing unnecessary pain med
Treating pain
Treating anxiety
Ensuring adequate sleep hygiene – limiting interruptions
Ensuring adequate sleep hygiene – limiting interruptions, reducing noise, fluctuating light to mimic circadian rhythm

Miscellaneous conditions associated with Mechanical Ventialtion

Venous Thromboembolism (VTE)

Venous thromboembolism remains a significant concern in critically ill patients not only due to their increased incidence of VTE events, but also due to the patient's limited cardiopulmonary reserve. The incidence of VTE has been cited up to 60% in trauma patients.[1] Mechanical ventilation is one of the primary risk factors for developing VTE due to patient immobility. In one study 23.6% of ICU patients developed DVT despite adequate prophylaxis and half of those patients have pulmonary embolism. It is important that patients have adequate DVT prophylaxis when they are mechanically ventilated unless a specific contraindication exists.[21]

Stress Ulcers

Stress Ulcers are a significant cause of morbidity in critically ill patients and mechanical ventilation greater than 48 hours is a primary risk factor. If a patient is likely to be ventilated for more than 48 hours, gastrointestinal prophylaxis should be instituted. In one study of 847 patients the other significant risk factors were coagulopathy defined by platelets < 50,000 or INR > 1.5. Patients who were mechanically ventilated greater than 48 hours or had coagulopathy had a 3.7% of clinically significant risk of gastrointestinal bleeding.[22]

Delirium in Mechanically Ventilated Patients

Delirium is a sudden onset of a significant disturbance in the cognitive abilities of a patient resulting in confused thinking. In a landmark study on delirium in mechanically ventilated patients 81.7% of studied patients developed delirium and this had dire consequences.[23] Of the patients who developed delirium they had higher mortality at 6 months 34% versus 15%, delirious patients spent a median 10 days longer in the hospital and those who survived to hospital discharge were 9 times more likely to have cognitive impairment than non-delirious patients.

The first step to treating delirium is recognizing it, both in its hyperactive and hypoactive forms. The CAM-ICU screen is one method as half of intubated patients have intense anxiety and 40% percent suffer from the fear of dying (Figure 11).[23] It is important to treat these symptoms without oversedation of patients with opiates and benzodiazepines. The treatment of delirium with antipsychotics has not been proven to be beneficial in randomized control trials and should be done as a last resort.[29]

Figure 11: Tension pneumothorax

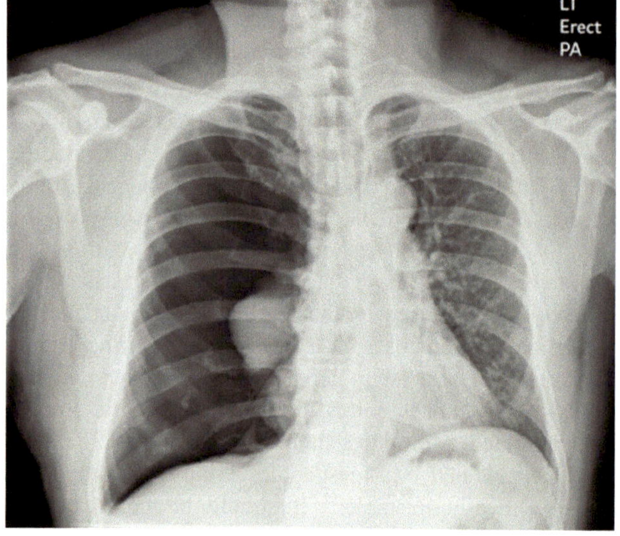

Acute Respiratory Distress Syndrome (ARDS)

Acute Respiratory Distress Syndrome was first described in 1967 in a case series by Ashbaugh and Petty. The twelve patients were hypoxic, had stiff lungs and had opacification on their chest radiographs. The pathophysiology of the syndrome can be characterized by three phases. Early ARDS is defined by the exudative phase characterized by acute inflammation leading to protein rich fluid flooding the alveoli due to increased capillary and alveolar permeability. This is followed by a proliferative phase of uncontrolled fibroblasts with fibroblastic deposition. In some, a fibrotic third stage can occur leading to less compliant lungs and prolonged ventilation perfusion mismatches. The mortality for ARDS has decreased since its initial description but has remained steady at approximately 40% over the last two decades.[25] Specifically, in surgery patients preoperative risk factors for ARDS development includes an American Society of Anesthesiologist status 3-5, emergent surgery, renal failure, chronic obstructive pulmonary disease, number of anesthetics during the admission and male sex. Significant intraoperative risk factors included fraction inspired oxygen, crystalloid administration in liters and packed red blood cell transfusion can lead to postoperative ARDS.[26]

A common definition for ARDS was agreed upon in 1994 and refined again in 2012 (Table 9).[26] Defining ARDS has been one of the difficulties encountered in clinicians' ability to decrease the mortality associated with it. Significant advancements have occurred in the treatment of ARDS, including the use of low tidal volume ventilation, prone positioning, and the use of steroids in early disease. Prone positioning has a multitude of benefits including the recruitment of the lungs and the redistribution of blood flow to improve ventilation-perfusion mismatch, thus improving oxygenation. Early steroids improve mortality and should be started in patients when ARDS is recognized. Therapeutic paralysis in the first forty-eight hours of ARDS was initially thought to improve mortality, but a second clinical cast doubt on this hypothesis. Paralytics are still used in ARDS, but associated side effects should limit their use. The driving pressure is the plateau pressure minus the PEEP. A retrospective analysis of ARDS net patients showed that patients with a driving pressure <15 had improved clinical outcomes, but this has not been prospectively validated. Esophageal balloons to measure intrathoracic pressure have limited prospective clinical data behind their use but have not been widely adopted. Inhaled vasodilators have been widely used for the treatment of ARDS and are associated with improved oxygenation through improvements in ventilation-perfusion mismatching but have not been shown to affect mortality. Similarly, no clinical trial shows that the use of Extracorporeal Membranous Oxygenation (ECMO) improves outcomes for patients with ARDS, but transfer to a regional ARDS center can improve outcomes.[30]

Table 9: International Definitions of ARDS

American-European Critical Care (AECC) 1994 Definition
1. Acute Presentation
2. Arterial Partial Pressure Oxygen to Fractional Inspiration Oxygen < 200 (PaO_2/FiO_2 < 200)
3. Bilateral Infiltrates on Chest Radiograph
4. Pulmonary Capillary Wedge Pressure < 18 mmHg
Berlin Definition
1. Acute, Presentation within 1 week of a known clinical insult or worsening respiratory symptoms
2. Bilateral opacities on chest radiograph not fully explained by effusions, lung collapse or nodules
3. Origin of edema respiratory failure not fully explained by cardiac failure or fluid overload
4. Oxygenation as defined
Mild: PaO_2/Fio_2 between 200-300 mmHg with PEEP or CPAP greater than or equal to 5 cm H_2O
Moderate: PaO_2/FiO_2 between 100-200 mmHg with PEEP or CPAP greater than or equal to 5 cm H_2O
Severe: PaO_2/FiO_2 less or equal 100 mmHg with PEEP or CPAP greater than or equal to 5 cm H_2O

Covid

Over five million people have died from Covid, but the mortality is far lower than the Spanish flu of 1919 due to modern medical infrastructure, advancement in therapeutics, and quick clinical trials. The quoted mortality for mechanically ventilated Covid patients ranges from 40% to 80% which is higher than ARDS, but through the use of mechanical ventilation, lives have been saved. COVID-19 enters the alveoli through angiotensin receptor two cells, often leading to a cytokine storm and pulmonary fibrosis. The use of steroids and interleukin-6 inhibitors has decreased mortality, but no specific mode of mechanical ventilation has improved patient outcomes. Management of COVID-19 patients with respiratory failure mirrors best practices for patients with ARDS.[31]

SUMMARY

Positive pressure ventilation has been a tremendous boon to the practice of medicine, but its use is fraught with complications. A thorough understanding of the indications for its use, its physiologic effects and the nomenclature used to describe it is necessary to optimize its utility. Understanding the parameters for breath delivery and different modes of ventilation allows clinicians to choose the optimal mode for their patient. Weaning patients from mechanical ventilation is an evolving art but doing it in a timely manner can help avoid complications associated with prolonged mechanical ventilation. Our increased knowledge of mechanical ventilation has allowed us to better define disease processes not recognized prior to the positive pressure ventilation era. As positive pressure ventilation becomes more sophisticated, it remains important that clinicians understand the fundamentals to provide care for their patients.

REFERENCES

1. Goligher E, Ferguson N, Kenny L. Core competency in mechanical ventilation: Development of educational objectives using the Delphi technique Crit Care Med 40:2012;2828-2832.

2. Puri N, Puri V, Dellinger R.P. History of Technology in the Intensive Care Unit. Critical Care Clinics, 25 (1);185-200.
3. Roussos C. Respiratory muscle fatigue and ventilatory failure. Chest. 1990;97:89S-96S.
4. Ventilation-Perfusion Relationships In West J Respiratory Physiology eds, 8th edition. Baltimore, MD: Lippincott Williams & Wilkins 2008.
5. Chatburn RL, Branson RD. Classification of Mechanical Ventilators. In: MacIntyre NR, Branson RD, eds. *Mechanical Ventilation.* 2nd edition. St. Louis, MO: Elsevier.
6. Thille AW, Rodriguez P, Cabello B, et al. Patient-Ventilator Asynchrony During Assisted Mechanical Ventilation. Intensive Care Med 2006;32:1515-1522.
7. Mergoni M, Volpi A, Bricchi C, Ross A. Lower inflection point and recruitment with PEEP in ventilated patients with acute respiratory failure. JAP 91:2001;441-450.
8. Powers SR, Mannal R, Nelclerio M, et al. Physiologic consequences of positive end-expiratory pressure (PEEP) ventilation. Ann Surg 1973;178:265-72.
9. Culpeper JA, Rinaldo JE, Roger RM. Effect of mechanical ventilator mode on tendency towards respiratory alkalosis. Am Rev Respir Dis 1985;132:1075-1077.
10. Jeyakumar P, Puri VK. Weaning from mechanical ventilation in adult respiratory distress syndrome. Indian J anaesth. 2003;47:33-36.
11. Conti G, Costa R. Technological development in Mechanical Ventilation. Current Opinion in Critical Care 2010;16:16:26-33.
12. Stewart NI, Jagelman AJ. Webster NR Emerging modes of ventilation in the intensive care unit BJA 107(1):2011;74-82.
13. MacIntyre NR. Discontinuing Mechanical Ventilation. MacIntyre NR, Branson RD, eds. Mechanical Ventilation. 2nd edition. St. Louis. Mo–elsevier:2009:320.
14. Epstein SK. Decision to extubated. Intensive Care Med 2002:28:535-546.
15. Kollef MH, Shapiro SD, Silver P, et al. A randomized, controlled trial of protocol-directed versus physician-directed weaning from mechanical ventilation. Crit Care Med 1997;25:567–574.
16. Frutos-Vivar F, Estavan A, Apezteguia C, et al Outcome of mechanically ventilated patients who require a tracheostomy. Crit Care Med 33;2005:290-298.
17. Terragni PP, Antonelli M, Fumagalli R, et al. Early vs. Late Tracheotomy for Prevention of Pneumonia in Mechanically Ventilated Adult Patients. JAMA 2010;303:1483-1489.
18. Bekaert M, Timisit JF, Vansteelandt S, et al. Attributable mortality of ventilator-associated pneumonia: A reappraisal using causal analysis Am J Respir Crit Care Med 2011;184:1133-1139.
19. Guidelines for the management of adults with hospital-acquired, ventilator-associated and healthcare-associated pneumonia. Crit Care Med 2005;171:388-416.
20. Attia J, Ray JG, Cook DJ, Douketis J, Ginsberg JS, Geerts WH. Deep vein thrombosis and it prevention in critically ill adults. Arch Intern Med 2001;161:1268–1279.
21. Cook DJ, Fuller HDm, Guatt GH, et al. Risk factors for gastrointestinal bleeding in critically ill patients. Canadian Critical Care Trial Groups N Engl J Med 1994;330:377-381.
22. Attia J, Ray JG, Cook DJ, et al. Deep vein thrombosis and its prevention in critically ill adults. Arch Intern Med 2001;161:1268-1279.
23. Pochard F, Lanore JJ, Ferrand J, et al. Subjective psychological status of severely ill patients discharged from mechanical ventilation. Clin Intensive Care 1995;6:57-61.
24. Walkey AJ, Summer R, Alkana P. Acute Respiratory Distress Syndrome: Epidemiology and management approaches. Clin epidemiology 2012;6:159-169.
25. Blum MJ, Stentz MJ, Dechert R, et al. Preoperative and intraoperative predictors of postoperative Acute Respiratory Distress Syndrome in general surgical population. Anesthesiology. 2013;118:19-29.
26. The ARDS Definition Task Force JAMA 2012;307:2526-2533.
27. Ferguson ND, Cook DJ, Guyatt GH, et al. High-frequency oscillation in early acute respiratory distress syndrome. N Engl J Med. 2013;368(9):795-805.
28. Bice T, Nelson JE, Carson SS. To Trach or Not to Trach: Uncertainty in the Care of the Chronically Critically Ill. Semin Respir Crit Care Med. 2015;36(6):851-858. doi:10.1055/s-0035-1564872.
29. Devlin JW, Skrobik Y, Gélinas C, et al. Clinical Practice Guidelines for the Prevention and Management of Pain, Agitation/Sedation, Delirium, Immobility, and Sleep Disruption in Adult Patients in the ICU. Crit Care Med. 2018 Sep;46(9):e825-e873. doi: 10.1097/CCM.0000000000003299. PMID: 30113379.
30. Fernando SM, Ferreyro BL, Urner M, Munshi L, Fan E. Diagnosis and management of acute respiratory distress syndrome. CMAJ. 2021 May 25;193(21):E761-8.
31. Su WL, Lu KC, Chan CY, Chao YC. COVID-19 and the lungs: A review. Journal of infection and public health. 2021 Nov 1;14(11):1708-14.

❑❑❑

8

CHAPTER

End of Life Care

Vinod Puri, MD, FACS
Nitin Puri, MD, FCCP

INTRODUCTION

It is estimated that 20% of the deaths in the United States occur in the hospital. Many of these patients die in the intensive care units (ICU). In North America 40-70% of ICU deaths follow decisions to forgo CPR. End-of-life care has become an essential part of the practice of critical care medicine. A thorough understanding of the ethical principles, legal concepts and social norms is expected of the physicians directing care at the end of life. In addition to an as accurate as possible prediction of prognosis of various diseases and their complications, the physician is required to guide patients, families, and medical colleagues during discussions related to limitations of life support. It is understandable that laws may differ in various countries. Moreover, religious beliefs and cultural practices of the patients deserve respect.

The remarkable technological advances in medicine in the twentieth century has brought with it the realization that prolonging life at the end has the potential to cause unnecessary suffering. It has been documented that 50% of the patients dying in the ICU receive mechanical ventilation and 25% undergo an attempted cardiopulmonary resuscitation (CPR). By the early 1980s, several investigators observed that survival statistics for hospitalized patients who underwent CPR had not improved in the previous twenty years.[1-3] This was despite the widespread promotion and adoption of CPR techniques. Of the better outcomes 12-14% survival had been reported, whereas survival as low 2-3% had also been reported. In the face of improved initial "successful" with resuscitation being from 30 to 40%, it is discouraging to note the lack of improved hospital survival. It is also estimated that fewer than 10% of patients who have CPR, leave the hospital in a functional state. Thus, the role of providing limited care to critically ill patients had become acceptable.

Analyzing the causes of poor survival, one is struck with a heterogeneous patient population and underlying causes of cardiac arrest. The conclusion was inescapable, that universal CPR in patients dying in the hospital as a policy, needed to be moderated. The Do Not Resuscitation Orders (DNR) which had become commonplace by that time were either made late or not at all. We found that patients designated 'No CPR' or DNR had survival as good as or somewhat better than patients receiving full CPR.[3] More recently, Heyland et al. analyzed whether patients with and without cancer have different perspectives on CPR decision making.[4] They included patients over 55 years old, suffering from terminal COPD, NHA class IV heart failure, or cirrhosis Child's C and were compared to patients with cancer with metastasis or stage IV lymphoma. With a 6-month mortality of 57.4% at least 45.6% of the patients had an end-of-life designation (e.g., DNR) order. Only 3% of the patients had accurate knowledge of the outcome of CPR and 37% of the patients were not open to end-of-life decisions. There was no difference in patients with and without cancer about their understanding of CPR. The dilemmas posed by allegiance to duty, to preservation of life needs to be counterbalanced by principles of informed consent and freedom of choice. We have reviewed the evolution of DNR orders in the United States.[5] In the early 1960s hospitals en mass adopted CPR practices for all patients dying in the confines of the hospital. It is noteworthy that there was no edict from health care bodies or the government. An attorney has commented on the confusion amongst the physicians as CPR was fostered and embraced by them. Presumptive CPR became the standard of care and physicians abetted by hospital attorneys were unwilling to change practices. One observer has even compared universal CPR to a perceived birthright!

A basic belief that CPR can work has persisted. DNR orders were a reaction to these policies to avoid CPR in a patient who was going to die anyway. A number of shortcomings of DNR policies are recognized as they have been implemented. By now, several organizations such as the American College of Surgeons, American Society of Anesthesiologists, and Association of Operating Room Nurses have all condemned automatic cancellation of DNR orders in the preoperative period. It is estimated that 15% of patients with DNR orders undergo surgical procedures. Two thirds of anesthesiologists assumed reversal of DNR orders without discussing the matter with the patient or surrogates. Therefore, new recommendations require discussion with the patient or family members.

In additional inputs such as Living Wills or Advanced directives (ADRs), Durable Power of Attorney have been devised. It is estimated that only 10-20% of patients have ADRs, and 60-70% of ICU patients are unable to speak for themselves. Ethicist Paul Ramsey has put patients' directives in perspective by pointing out that it is wrong to simply talk about a patient's right to refuse treatment.[6] That sole guide to action cannot find medical or logical reason to distinguish physician's actions between the dying and those with terminal illness. A belief that autonomous choice makes the moral difference between life and death decisions, which then are imposed on the physician or technician is neither reasonable nor sensible. He pointed out that we do not confer dignity on the dying by simply withdrawing tubes and stopping the respirator! "If the dying die with a degree of nobility it will be mostly their own doing in doing their own dying." Ramsey had tried to de-romanticize the 'Death with Dignity' movement.

In general, the studies reveal dissatisfaction with end-of-life care.[6] Palliative care is distinct from end-of-life care as provided in the ICU. The critical care specialists take responsibility for relief of pain and suffering as they struggle with decisions about limitations of care. If a patient is a candidate to transfer out of the ICU to a step-down unit or discharged home, the palliative care team is consulted, and care is assumed by the team of physicians and nurses.

The goal in medicine is to make good moral choices versus right or perfect choices. Ramsey emphasizes that problems in medical ethics are not simply technical problems on which an expert or physician has an opinion but are rather the problems of human beings in situations where medical care is needed. They are moments in every human life.[6a] Applied ethics deals with imperfect persons, options, and circumstances. The ancient edict "to cure sometimes, to relieve often, to comfort always" is the guiding principle. What follows is a brief history of ethics as medicine has evolved, a discussion of legal principles, and a reference to a few famous cases.

Relief of Pain and Suffering

Historically, little attention had been paid in medicine to the relief of pain in the dying. Lynn et al. referred to the only significant study published by William Osler in 1908.[8] Osler reported that he was convinced that only 90 of 486 deaths he studied at Johns Hopkins felt pain at the time of death. Unfortunately, Osler himself did experience pain. He described six weeks of enduring sharp pleuritic pain with bouts of coughing. Additionally, he had two operations to drain empyema under general anesthesia and died two weeks later. In Osler's case, pneumonia had not been the "friend of the aged." Nuland observed," By and large dying is a messy business.[9]" Relief of suffering has always been one of the most important obligations in medicine. Reflecting on the nature of suffering, Cassel points out that its relation to organized medicine has been rarely addressed.[10] Suffering is experienced by persons, not merely by bodies, and at its source has challenges that threaten the intactness of the person. He points out that a physician's failure to understand suffering can result in medical intervention that, though technically adequate, only fails to relieve suffering and becomes suffering itself. Suffering also has a temporal element as it influences a person's perception of future events. There are other dimensions of personhood, and it would not exist if the future events were not a major concern. Suffering can occur when physicians do not validate a patient's pain. As the patient has had experience of illness and medical care, it influences present illness and medical care. Cassel lists fear, confidence, physical symptoms, and anguish as important factors that intermingle with the current illness. A complex set of roles is to be expected of a person. Even a dying patient wishes to retain some vestiges of those personas. In Cassels's elegant words, "No person exists without others; there is no consciousness without a consciousness of others, for the speaker without a hearer, and no act that somehow does not encompass others."

Disease can alter a patient's perception that his own body is perceived as not friend but enemy. This phenomenon can happen suddenly without warning. And yet we all perceive a future. Hope dwells in the perception that there is a future. Religion and mystic beliefs of the patient may find some incoherent expression. Others have indicated suffering as an unfinished narrative of a life i.e., story. At the end of life, a patient may be anxious to complete that story. Thus, compassion, which literally means to 'suffer along', may be as important as the powerful analgesics and sedatives that we administer to the dying patient.

Oaths, Covenants, and Contracts: A History

Robert Veatch has reviewed the topic of the professional codes of conduct.[11] The Hippocratic Oath is recognized by both physicians and lay persons as the basis of medical ethics. Though of uncertain origin, it can be traced to ancient Greece. In the 5th century B.C., a group of physicians headed by Hippocrates produced scientific and ethical writings. Hippocratic Corpus was the collection of various writings. The Oath is the most important historical writing which has been the foundation of ethics for Western physicians.

The Oath consists of two parts, the first initiates the students into a Greek cult. It includes a covenant about sharing knowledge and honoring the teacher. The second part, often referred to as the code of ethics, is separate from the first part. The pledge by physicians to apply measures, the most important being, "for the benefit of the sick according to my ability and judgment." The 4th century B.C. Oath is not relevant to modern times.

John Gregory (1724-1773) lectures on the 'Duties and Qualifications of a Physician' was influenced by Scottish philosophers David Hume and Frances Hutcheson. Thomas Perceval prepared Medical Ethics in 1789. It deals with institutional relationships with physicians. The American Medical Association (AMA) founded in 1847 also drew up a Code of Medical Ethics. Its emphasis was on duties of physicians to their patients and their colleagues. Revisions of this document occurred every few years. Then, in 1957, Principle of Medical Ethics appeared as ten brief statements. In 1980, revision of this document resulted in the statement of seven principles. Emphasis had shifted to respect for the patient's dignity and a duty not to deceive the patient when imparting information.

The Judicial Council of the AMA has provided periodic updates of their opinions. The World Medical Association has also adopted two codes of ethics. Veatch listed 41 associations of physicians and other medical professionals with their codes of ethics. Professional codes of ethics are viewed as a set of rules appropriate to medical decision makers. The AMA acknowledges that codes are not laws but are intended as guides to responsible professional behavior. The Nuremberg Code originating from the World War II trials has the status of international law.

The 1983 President's Commission on the Study of Ethical and Behavioral Research may not have the force of law, but it represents the collective wisdom of the American population. As such, the recommendations of the Commission have been immensely influential in dictating institutional policies. For the first time, the Commission found no particular treatment including such 'ordinary' hospital treatments as parenteral nutrition or hydration, antibiotics, and transfusions to be universally warranted and thus obligatory for patients to accept.

Covenant

The covenant has its roots in historical events. The Hippocratic Oath taken by a young physician is an example of a covenant. The obligations he undertakes regarding dealing with patients is a Code. Patients play no role in specifying the moral duties of the novice physician or his teachers.

Contract

The contract involves agreement in which two parties calculate their own interests and agree upon some joint project. William May's views on contracts seem to follow contemporary legal business models. However, 'the social contract' does not have the same connotations. Veatch points out the fallacy of a physician providing treatments he considers beneficial to a patient who does not want them. Thus, a unilateral code developed by medical professionals may become burdensome to the patient. Traditional views expressed in the Hippocratic group that only persons with specialized knowledge or training such as physicians can know the ethical truths have been rejected by modern society. Acceptance of the framework that layperson and physician together can make medical ethics work for the benefit of the patient is the basis for the Ethics Committees legitimacy.

Relevance to Surgery

The following considerations listed in Table 1 bear scrutiny.

Table1: Surgical Patients

1. Concept of postoperative mortality?
2. What is special about 30-day mortality?
3. Are trauma patients different than other surgical patients?
4. Are cardiac surgery and neurosurgery patients different?
5. Do referring physicians know their patients better than the surgeons?

The surgical patients are as likely to require end-of-life care as non-surgical patients. Yet, the surgical texts have devoted little space to the consideration.[12] The barriers to the surgeons' involvement in end-of-life care have to do with the emphasis on surgical skill mastery and often an overly optimistic estimate of surgical procedure success. Confusion also exists as to the difference between obtaining informed consent for surgery and for subsequent provision of interventions such as mechanical ventilation, feeding tubes etc. Eason et al. reviewed four textbooks of surgery.[13] They concluded that texts provide little information about breaking bad news to the patient or surrogates or information about advance care planning, mode of death, effect on surrogates, and symptom management. The authors concluded that discussions of surgical deaths must include death from both acute and chronic disease. The end-of-life topic is essentially absent in surgical literature. As an example, a well-known textbook discussing ethics in ICU and in the context of futility concludes, "We do not offer ongoing medical care to a patient who meets criteria for brain death.[12]" Nelson, a physician with a law degree, identified three factors as barriers to high quality palliative care in the ICU.[14]

1. Cultural context-denial of death
2. Prognostic uncertainty
3. 'Silos' of disciplines

Family members often do not know what life saving measures mean. Their unrealistic expectations may be made worse by physicians with insufficient training in communication. Failure to identify the appropriate goals on the part of the physicians may pose a greater barrier.

An important recent study emphasizes the need to focus on all patients receiving surgical procedures.[15] The investigators reviewed 1,802,029 patients over the age of 65 who died in 2008. They calculated the proportion of patients who had surgery within the year before death and adjusted for age, sex, race, and income. They found that 31.9% of patients underwent an inpatient surgical procedure the year before death, 18.1% during the last month before death. Eight percent or 144,162 underwent a procedure in the last week of life. Regions of the country with a high number of hospital beds had a high calculated End of Life Intensity Score as did regions with high total Medicare spending.

One fifth of the elderly in United States die in ICUs, half receive mechanical ventilation, and one fourth receive CPR. There was a reduction in the number of admissions, hospital days, and ICU days in patients without surgery. The resource utilization points to a need for better planning of end-of-life care in surgical patients.

The fact is that even elective surgery is currently performed in many chronically ill patients with multiple risk factors. Advances in anesthesia and postoperative care have resulted in the classic contraindication to surgery (i.e., poor general conditions become almost obsolete). Moreover, the complex high risk cardiac, neurologic, or cancer surgery is often undertaken in elderly or feeble patients. Most preoperative consultations or 'clearances' are narrowly focused on the specialty of the consultant. Though global risk assessment has been introduced, none entail the considerations of often prolonged painful periods spent in the ICUs or nursing homes. Since 30-day mortality is part and parcel of surgeons' mental make-up, their insistence on invasive and unlimited care is the cause of conflict with colleagues who wish to focus on patient comfort. Agencies such as Medicare no longer insist on indexing 30-day mortality but instead wants to record any hospital mortality.

It stands to reason that a family physician or internist who has known the patient for many years may know the patients' wishes and personality better than the surgeon. Thus, the informed consent obtained for the purpose of surgery may have a limited role when end-of-life care issues emerge. It is fair to say that patients with multiple traumas who may have required an operation are no different than other patients in regards to eliciting their wishes for end-of-life care.

Bioethical Principles

There has been a long tradition in Judeo-Christian religious thought where the second half of the twentieth century was inspired by liberal political philosophy. Veatch emphasizes the secular thinkers such as Lock and Jefferson. The American Bill of Rights has also influenced our reasoning.[11] Thus, medical ethics has moved away from strict boundaries of the Hippocratic Oath. Self-determination as a legal principle has dominated legal case-law in the United States. The following four principles are accepted as the foundation of ethical discussions:

1. Autonomy: an obligation to respect the wishes of the competent patient.
2. Non-maleficence: an obligation not to harm persons under our care.
3. Beneficence: an obligation to benefit others.
4. Justice: an obligation to distribute benefits and harms fairly.

Veatch in 1981 and Beauchamp and Childress in 1983 recognized the primary principles and detailed their views on several derivative principles or rules.[11] The derivative rules such as veracity, respect for privacy, patient-doctor relationship confidentiality, and avoidance of conflict of interest are part and parcel of medical ethics. Figures 1 and 2 identify how the above principles have attained equal importance.

Figure 1: Traditionally, physicians were dominant in making medical decisions and patients deferred to them.[11]

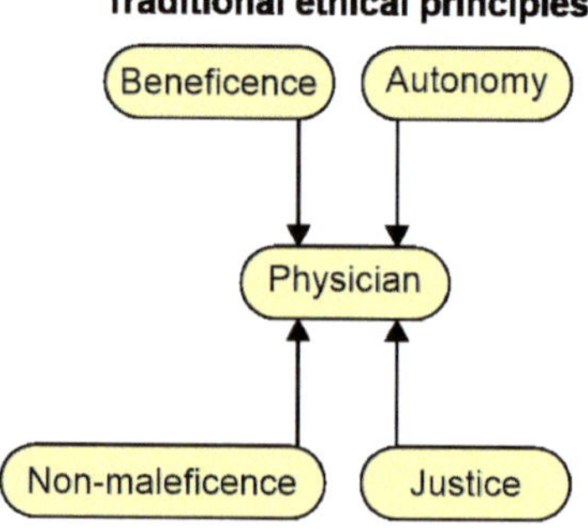

Figure 2: By the early Eighty's, physicians adjusted to giving equal importance to patient's right of self-determination or autonomy.[11]

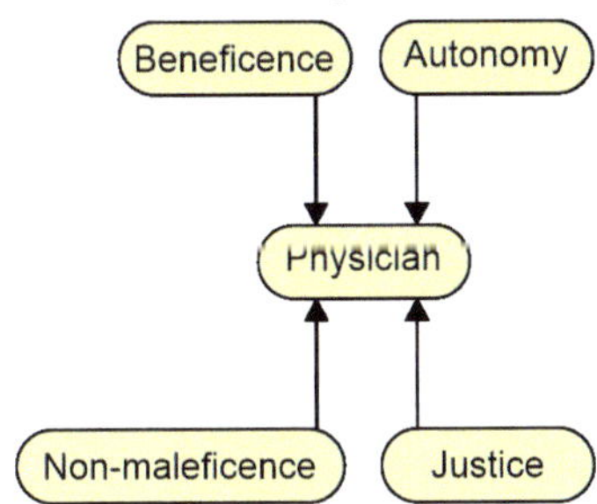

Autonomy

This brief description of autonomy is from James and Childress.[11] Derived from Greek autos (self) and nomos (law or rule) as applied to human beings that a person chooses and acts freely and rationally out of his own life plan. This does not mean that the life plan is not informed by family or friends. Autonomy is rooted both in society and history. Inspiration for the life plan may be a religious tradition such as prohibiting blood transfusion for Jehovah Witnesses. The individual while exercising autonomy is still interested in the effect of his decisions on others. Since a person should be competent to exercise autonomous decisions, the patient in question is presumed competent. A broad view of capacity to make decisions is presumed. It is also recognized that decision-making capacity may be intermittent. For obvious reasons, children are not considered autonomous. A principle of assent is often used for adolescents.

Caveats

In practice, autonomy or principle of self-determination has dominated discussion of actual cases. However, it would be a mistake to ignore subtleties and nuances in the interpretation of autonomy. Though accepted as a supreme principle as a negative right, autonomy does not bestow a right to a specific treatment. The surrogates similarly do not have the absolute right to demand treatments on behalf of the patient. In this context, it is better not to consider one principle (i.e., autonomy) as trumping all other moral principles. Using legal terms, none of the principles are considered absolute but only prima facie binding. In actual cases, we need to strike a balance. For moral reasoning, Veatch emphasizes prudence or discernment of the situation.

Non-Maleficence

The Hippocratic Oath enjoins physicians to do what benefits the patient. "Do No Harm" expressed in Latin as '*primum nocere'* is considered the primary principle of medical ethics. Though often cited by physicians, Jonsen feels that neither philosophers nor physicians have pressed it very far as a principle of ethical analysis.[11] Medicine is considered a moral enterprise in many cultures. Jonsen provides examples from Greek inscriptions, Hindu religious texts, and Chinese code to document injunction against doing harm and helping those in need.[11a]

The legal principle of 'due care' is derived from the ethical precept to provide benefit to the patient. In this context, lack of education, information, or skill may harm the patient.

Risk benefit ratio due care requires analysis of collected data and reasonable estimates of benefits and harm to the patient. Since every intervention in critical care has the chance to harm instead of benefiting the patient, these considerations are important in introducing new therapies or even continuing current treatment.

Beneficence

The obligation to benefit others arises out of the duty outlined in non-maleficence. The prominence of Commands, "Thou shall not kill" and "Thou shall not bear false witness" are in early Judaic code, as Decalogue formed the bedrock of medical ethics. Ross considers duty of non-maleficence as distinct and as prima-facie more binding.[11] A conundrum often faced by physicians in ICUs is how to balance the duties of beneficence and non-maleficence while providing analgesics and sedatives in large doses to the dying patients. These drugs may hasten the demise of the patient. Besides a societal duty to provide comfort and relieve pain, physicians and nurses may invoke the double effect concept. A derived rule, the 'Double Effect' was proposed as a religious concept in medieval times, it is applicable in end-of-life care. The fact that some well-intentioned acts such as relief of pain and suffering may hasten death have to be defended based on good intentions. The object of the direct intention must be good or at least morally indifferent. The concept of positive and negative duties may determine the justification for a harmful effect. Thus, the benefit determinant equation considers not only harm but some determinant of benefit.

Obligation to Prolong Life

The Hippocratic Oath in fact does not imply an obligation on the part of the physician to prolong life. There are more recent Christian sources which seem to imply such a duty. Ethicists may argue that life should be considered useful, productive, happy, and healthy for such an obligation. In ancient times, the question of whose life would arise as would the idea of duty. In Greek and Roman cultures, euthanasia was accepted and the help of surgeons to 'open up the veins' is described.

In current practice, if the patient objects to prolongation of life, the meaning of duty to prolong life is questionable. Similarly, the idea of professional ethics was imprecise. It may still be questionable in different cultures, systems of medicine, and jurisdictions as to what that duty entails. One rule mentioned in the Hippocratic Corpus is to refuse treatment to those overwhelmed by their disease. This was an instance when medicine was powerless. Physicians treating such patients were open to criticism in society. Platonists, cynics, and stoics considered suicide an honorable alternative to hopeless illness.

Justice

The final principle in bioethics is problematic as its application to an individual patient is rarely immediate. This, despite the advice by Buchanan that continued the development of both bioethics and of theorizing about justice in general, necessitates the exploration of the problems of justice in healthcare. Theories of justice arise from the concept of utilitarianism which is a comprehensive moral theory. Briefly, *act utilitarianism* defines rightness with respect to acts, an act is right if it maximizes utility._

Rule Utilitarianism

With respect to rules of action, rightness of action is judged. The rule should maximize utility and falls under a particular rule. It allows us to judge institutions. However, resource utilization and futility arguments have been considered incendiary and should not be made by individual physicians or hospital standards committees. This is in the public domain to devise adequate policies.

Rights founded on consideration of utility may be called derivative. John Rawls' theory of Justice considers it as fairness. It enjoins:

1. The principle of greatest equal liberty
2. The principle of equality of fair opportunity
3. The difference principle. Social and economic institutions must be arranged to maximally benefit those who are worst off.

The basic structure of society is justice since it exerts a pervasive and profound influence on an individual's life prospects. A reference to *Social Contract* is in order. It is an object of rational collective choice, basic commitment and principles agreed upon that may be rightly enforced. Voluntary agreement requires willing cooperation of all members of society, including those who are worse off. Kant's identification of autonomy with rationality also justifies Rawls's principles of justice which are distinct from utility. Rawls's principles of justice generate rights. His Principle of Equality of Fair Opportunity has crucial influence on healthcare or lack of it upon individual development. Nozick's Libertarian Theory on the other hand proposes that coercion may only be used to prevent or punish physical harm, theft, and fraud to enforce contracts. The right to private property is fundamental in his view and individuals have a property right in their person.

The theories are germane to the practice of critical care as ICU resources are finite. This is even truer of societies in emerging economies. The classic question as to who gets the last ICU bed cannot be resolved by instantly increasing ICU beds. Thus, end-of-life care becomes important as framed in the principle of distributive justice.

As ethical rules are applied to end-of-life care, certain moral distinctions emerge and will be discussed briefly.

Moral Distinctions

1. Active versus passive acts: In care of the dying, though societal acceptance of passive acts is more acceptable, the ethicists find no difference between the two. In omission of a treatment, harms and benefits may be as significant as commission of the treatment.
2. Withdrawing and withholding: Justification for not commencing a treatment is also sufficient for ceasing it. A reluctance to initiate mechanical ventilation is often cited because we may not be able to stop it once started. Sometimes the physicians may resolve this conundrum by using the concept of time trials. By initiating a treatment with the understanding that it will be stopped if sufficient improvement in a patient's condition does not occur over a finite period of a few days, an agreement may be reached with family members and colleagues.
3. Pain relief versus killing: It is the socially accepted duty of the physicians and nurses to relieve pain. The intentions of the caregivers are of vital importance, as alluded to in the concept of double effect.
4. Ordinary versus extraordinary: Sotto, a Christian priest in 1582 used the terms 'obligatory' versus 'non-obligatory' to define the responsibilities of the patient during an illness. Bonez, another priest in 1595 used the terms 'ordinary' and 'extraordinary' for the same purpose. By 1978, ethicist Paul Ramsey pointed out that these terms were no longer useful. Some of the early formulations emphasized the use of ordinary means of life support such as intravenous fluids versus extraordinary means such as a respirator. The reasons for underlying the therapy are more important. The current terminology of burdens benefits refers to the patient and not to the caregivers.
5. Killing versus allowing to die: Though the latter implies

approval, the ethicists find no difference between the two. It is important to recognize that what kills the patient is the underlying disease.

6. Food and water: Hydration and feeding when provided artificially are in the category as other treatments. There is no additional obligation other than helpful hand feeding to a dying patient. Gastric tube feedings in patients with dementia have not shown any survival benefit. Aspiration and pneumonias are not reduced with tube feedings. In many cultures, it is considered quite honorable for a person to starve themself to death. Studies have shown that simple measures such as moistening the lips are more helpful than providing intravenous hydration, which may increase dyspnea in a dying patient.

Catastrophic Neurological Conditions

Familiarity with three neurologic conditions is useful to all clinicians including surgeons.

1. Brain death: All 50 states in the United States have adopted brain death laws. Permanent absence of all brain functions, including brain stem, apnea, loss of brain stem reflexes, and cranial nerve functions are needed for making the diagnosis of brain death. Precautions to avoid hypothermia and sedative/muscle relaxants before making the diagnosis of brain death are in order. Various institutions have somewhat differing policies, many insisting on two examinations from 6 hours to 24 hours apart. One of the clinicians usually is a neurologist or a neurosurgeon. Additional tests such an EEG and blood flow studies of the brain have been used but many institutions do not insist on these. Since brain death is the same as traditional cardiopulmonary death, its declaration is followed by removal of life support systems.
2. Persistent Vegetative State (PVS): A multi-society task force defined PVS as a clinical condition of complete unawareness of self and the environment, accompanied by sleep wake cycles with either complete or partial preservation of hypothalamic and brain stem functions. These patients show no evidence of sustained, reproducible, purposeful, or voluntary behavioral responses to visual, auditory, tactile, or noxious stimuli, no evidence of language comprehension or expression. They are also bladder and bowel incontinent and have variously preserved cranial nerve and spinal reflexes. The diagnosis of PVS requires at least a month in this condition after acute traumatic or non-traumatic brain injury. Recovery of consciousness from PVS is unlikely after one year.

   The significance of PVS is related to ethical considerations as to what treatments are appropriate besides respectful hygiene care as guided by the family. Hospital admissions or even surgical procedures when performed at the insistence of the surrogates raise many ethical questions.

   Caveat: A common mistake especially in less advanced societies is to label a patient in PVS as 'brain-dead'. This results from poor understanding of the public and persons writing or talking about the patient in question. The distinction between brain death and PVS must always be maintained by physicians and the public alike.
3. Locked-in Syndrome: A state with consciousness and cognition retained but movement and communication are impossible because of paralysis of voluntary motor systems. Compared to the first two, this is a rare occurrence.

Euthanasia

The term in Greek means a 'good death' or 'easy death'. Accepted in ancient Greek and Roman cultures, it has strong prohibition in Catholic theology. Subsequent variations have resulted in terms such as 'voluntary' and 'involuntary' euthanasia. Intentional killing of innocent human beings is prohibited in all religions. In the context of end-of-life care, terms such as 'active' and 'passive' euthanasia are often discussed. Only Netherlands and lately Belgium have legalized active euthanasia. There is an ongoing debate as to the morality and abuses of the practice. Thirty seven of the 50 states have laws against euthanasia.

In 1991, Timothy Quill, wrote about one of his patients, the case of 'Diane'.[16] Quill had prescribed barbiturates to a patient suffering from myelogenous leukemia for which the patient had refused treatment. The case eventually reached the United States Supreme Court, which held that here was no constitutional right to assisted suicide. Jack Kevorkian, a retired Michigan pathologist gained enormous notoriety by assisting more than 30 patients to commit suicide. The state passed a special law to prohibit his actions. He was prosecuted and spent several years in jail before his death.

In United States, the state of Oregon was the first to legislate what became known as 'assisted suicide'. A patient with terminal illness is free to request medicines in doses which would cause his death. But the doctors are prohibited from administering any drugs to cause death. The follow-up after many years has shown that many patients never take the drugs but are in general at peace that they have control of their death.[16] Subsequently, Washington State has enacted a similar law and Montana had a court ruling to permit the practice. Several other states have considered similar laws. In Oregon, 311 patients have died in eleven years after the enactment of the assisted suicide law which accounts for 1 in 1,000 recorded deaths. It is also reported that 1 in 50 dying patients have discussed assisted suicide with their physicians and 1 in 6 with their families.

Any discussion of euthanasia in the environment of an ICU is beside the point. Working in a team with accountable practices and documentation, an abuse of authority by the physicians or nurses will arouse suspicion and enquiry.

Law and the End-of-Life Care

We will consider applicable laws and a few note-worthy cases decided by the courts in the United States. A summary of the usual misconceptions about law and removal of life support summarized by a lawyer are listed in Table 2.[18]

Table 2: Common myths about terminating life support.

1. Anything that is not specifically permitted by law is prohibited.
2. It is murder or suicide to terminate life support.
3. For life support to be stopped, patients must be terminally ill.
4. Withholding treatment is permissible, but it must be continued once started.
5. Legally, tube feeding is different from other treatments.
6. Life support termination requires going to court.
7. Living wills are not legal.

In general, it needs to be pointed out that courts do not wish to 'practice' medicine and physicians are free to practice their profession according to prevalent state laws and hospital policies.

Karen Ann Quinlan: Karen was a 22-year-old woman who fell into a coma after an overdose of sleeping pills and alcohol. She remained in a PVS. After 10 months, no improvement was observed, and the family requested to discontinue the respirator. Physicians worried about the legality of discontinuing the ventilator approached the court. In 1976, the New Jersey Supreme court decided that artificial life support can be discontinued as she had previously expressed a specific wish not to have her life maintained with a machine. She was removed from the ventilator, but tube feedings were continued. She lived for another 10 years in a nursing home.

Key points: this was the first case to reach the courts and was widely discussed in medical journals, ethics publications, and lay press. It also made the public aware of the neurologic condition of PVS.

Nancy Beth Cruzan: Nancy was a 33-year-old woman who suffered severe brain damage after an automobile accident. She was in PVS and maintained tube feeding. Four years later, the family requested removal of the feeding tube. The Missouri Supreme Court refused the request, and the case eventually reached the United States Supreme Court. The Court found 'a constitutional right to refuse medical care, including feeding tubes.'

Judge Anton Scalia wrote, "I would have preferred that we announce, clearly and promptly that Federal Courts have no business in this field, the point at which life becomes 'worthless' and the point at which means necessary to preserve it become 'extraordinary or 'inappropriate' are neither set forth in the constitution nor known to nine judges of this court."

However, the state of Missouri required 'clear and convincing evidence' of a patient's wishes. It took seven years till 1990 for the family to gather enough evidence from friends before the court ruled in favor of the family. The feeding tube was removed, and she died two weeks later.

Key points: The state courts initially refused to accept the testimony of friends that Nancy Cruzan had made statements to the effect she would not like to be maintained by artificial means. The young people may make casual remarks in conversation with family or friends. It was felt that more people would start to make living wills or execute advance directives (i.e., clear, and convincing evidence). Whether such a purpose has been served especially amongst the young remains unknown.

Helga Wanglie: Helga was an 85-year-old woman who fell and broke her hip in December 1989. She was treated at a county hospital in Minneapolis, MN. After a bout of pneumonia, she became ventilator dependent. For 5 months, attempts were made to wean her off the ventilator but failed. In May 1990, she was transferred to a subacute hospital for ventilator dependent patients. She suffered a cardiac arrest, was revived, and sent back to the county hospital. She was in a PVS, supported with a ventilator and tube feedings.

Her husband, a retired lawyer who had earlier admitted the patient had never discussed life in coma or her wishes for end-of-life care, now insisted on continuing all treatments. He did accept a DNR decision. Her doctors concluded that it was not in her best interests to keep her alive. After her second admission, the lead of the hospital ethics committee filed a case in the court to appoint an independent conservator. The court ruled narrowly in favor of the husband to appoint him the conservator. The patient died 3 days after the court's verdict at the age of 87.

Key points: This was the first case filed with courts by the hospital and doctors to limit end-of-life care of the patient. The hospital held that the family cannot demand that physicians continue to give treatment that is not in the best medical interests of the patient. This case was extensively discussed in the medical and ethics journals as a new kind of 'right to die', the patient's request for treatment, the physician's obligations, and even the public policy implications.[18,19] The hospital had not requested the court to stop any kind of treatment but to appoint a conservator independent from the family. The total cost of $800,000 for the care of this patient was paid in full by the insurers. The following statement appeared in the Minneapolis Star Tribune in May 1991 "The hospital's plea is born of realism, not hubris -- It advances the claim that physicians should not be slaves to technology, any more than patients should be its prisoners. They should be free to deliver, and act on an honest and time-honored message: 'Sorry, there is nothing more we can do.'"

Terri Shciavo: Terri was a 26-year-old woman who collapsed at home in 1990. She suffered from bulimia and a potassium disorder was suspected as the cause of cardiac arrest. She lapsed into PVS, though this diagnosis was later contested by her parents. In 1991, her husband flew her to California for experimental treatment with no improvement. In 1993, the husband of the patient won 1.3 million dollars in malpractice settlement. Terri's husband and her parents were initially on good terms, but their relations became increasingly fractious. Her father tried to remove the husband as the legal guardian and leveled various accusations. Terri's parents tried again in 1998 and failed.

In 2000, ten years after Terri's collapse, the husband approached the court to remove Terri's feeding tube. The feeding tube was removed and reinserted according to court orders as her parents joined in litigation. In 2003, Florida Governor Jeb Bush stepped in, and a special Terri's law was passed by the state legislature. By now the case had caught the imagination of the nation and various pro-life groups had started to be agitated. On television, endless images of Terri following a balloon were shown, casting doubt on the diagnosis of PVS. Later, it became clear that these were carefully edited video images. Terri's Law was struck down by the Florida State Supreme Court. The case was heard in the Federal Court in Atlanta, but the United States Supreme Court refused to hear the case. Even the United States Congress and President George Bush got involved in the case. In 2005, Terri died after removal of the feeding tube. An autopsy showed that Terri had suffered severe damage to her brain causing cortical blindness and confirmed the diagnosis of PVS.

Key points: When the families cannot agree on the proper course to pursue in the care of a patient, the physician's job becomes difficult. The help of pastoral care professionals is justifiably sought. However, the extraneous issues of control and even finances are a recipe for a messy outcome. A similar case in Michigan involved a paralyzed patient whose wife and mother fought in courts for years for removal of the feeding tube. A disability payment appeared to be at the root of the dispute. It is still appropriate that the majority of the family disagreements get resolved by focusing on the patient's expressed wishes and comfort.

Lawsuits

Reviewing the experience of actual lawsuits filed in the United States courts since 1975, and related to stopping life-support, Meisel identified 60 reported appellate court cases.[20] One case of criminal liability from California was dismissed. A case of civil damages in New Jersey resulted in the hospital paying the brain-dead patient's family. This case involved keeping the patient on the ventilator to obtain organs for transplantation. The State of New Jersey also amended its brain death law. Another case in California resulted in the hospital not being paid for the ventilator care that the patient had refused. On the other hand, a wrongful 'life' case in Ohio in a patient who received CPR despite DNR designation was dismissed without damages.

Decision Making

Physicians play the dominant role in making treatment decisions even in the model of shared decision-making. Cook et al. reported that in 851 mechanically ventilated patients from 15 ICUs and 5 countries, 63.3% were successfully weaned, 17.2% died in the ICU, and 19.5% had the mechanical ventilator withdrawn.[21] They analyzed the reasons for withdrawal and in each of the reasons listed below, the physicians' perception and opinion mattered.

1. Cognitive function impaired
2. Likelihood of survival less than 10%
3. Patient did not want life support
4. Need for vasopressors and inotropes

Akerman has posed some familiar questions that physicians face and are listed in Table 3. The answer to all of them is in the negative.[22]

Table 3: Withholding and withdrawing life sustaining treatment

1. Are physicians legally required to provide all possible life-sustaining treatments?
2. Is withholding or withdrawing treatment the same as euthanasia?
3. Is removing the ventilator considered killing?
4. Are you killing the patient if you treat pain?
5. Does treatment of symptoms constitute euthanasia?
6. Is it illegal to prescribe large doses of opioids to relieve pain, breathlessness, or other symptoms?

For a competent patient able to speak for themself, there is little debate that they should be asked about initiating life sustaining treatments. Focusing on the individual is the norm in Western societies. During treatment, ethicists hold that the physician is obligated to the patient and no one else. Surrogates such as family members become decision makers when a patient is incompetent or rendered so by disease or drugs. The notion of competence is not a strict psychiatric evaluation but expressed as the patient's decision-making capacity. Institutions give wide latitude to the patient to express their wishes, even with a gesture. In African American and Hispanic patients, traditionally family members assume a greater role. We also need to be aware of non-traditional family configurations. Divorce, distance, or non-availability of any family or friends may make the task of the medical professional difficult. It is not uncommon to deal with court appointed legal guardians in patients suffering from dementia or severe disability. Our experience is that often these legal guardians also know very little about their clients' wishes and routinely insist on full resuscitation orders. Though one needs to engage the legal guardian in discussion for appropriate treatment, it would be a misrepresentation to say that the treatments are mandated by the court. It has been pointed out that autonomy is not transferable to the family members. When withdrawing treatments at the end of life, conflicts with family or surrogate decision makers is not unusual. It is a misconception that the family speaks for the incompetent patient with the same authority that a competent patient would.[7a] Two special categories of decision-making have been proposed.

1. Best interests: The surrogate makes a choice for the patient to protect the patient's interests. These include relief of suffering, preservation, as well as restoration of function, quality, and extent of life sustained.
2. Substituted Judgment: The well-being and self-determination of the patient is protected. The surrogate attempts to reach the same decision as the incapacitated patient if he could choose. The limitation is that the patient must be competent. Substituted judgment emerged during the discussion on Karen Ann Quinlan's case and becomes relevant when discussing patients in PVS.

Futility Argument

It was argued in the mid-eighties that certain treatments such as CPR may be futile in some patients and should not be offered. Many hospitals defined categories of futile treatments and adopted policies against unlimited care. In 1987, the Hastings Center published guidelines for stopping futile treatments. Unfortunately, the same guidelines talk about physiologically futile treatments that may offer some psychological benefit. This is a weak argument. For this and other reasons, these policies have had a limited impact on patient care. The value-laden term is considered pejorative by many family members and has been opposed by many physicians and ethicists.

In Texas, an elaborate mechanism has been set up by the cooperating hospitals and was subsequently approved by the legislature to provide the orderly discontinuation of treatments.[23] A follow-up review indicated some success and an optimistic outlook on conflict resolution. Without involving the courts, we have argued for an enhanced role of ethics committees.[7a] It is worthwhile to point out that no case in the United States has gone to jury trial for withholding or withdrawing treatment. In more paternalistic systems, physicians dominate decision-making. However, a balance between compassionate delivery of healthcare and the interpretation of ethical principles is required.

How to Proceed?

There has been a concerted effort to improve Education for Physicians on End-of-life Care (EPEC) with curriculum development, training sessions, and conferences funded by the Robert Wood Johnson Foundation.[24] It has been emphasized that educational efforts should occur in the out-patient setting of primary care physician offices. Unfortunately, the medical crisis dictates the discussion of the issues in the crowded hallways and waiting rooms of the ICUs. It is suggested to approach one family member, accepted by others as a spokesperson. Serial discussions are invariably required with the ability to change plans as the patient's condition changes. Life-sustaining treatments should be discussed in simple terms, avoiding medical jargon. Involvement of nurses and pastoral care representatives is quite helpful during the family meeting. If the family members desire the presence of a referring physician or specific consultant, that should be arranged. Table 4 lists the suggested eight-step protocol to engage in discussion regarding the end-of-life issues with the patient and surrogates.

Low Resource Societies and End-of-Life Issues

Table 4: Protocol to Discuss Withholding and Withdrawal of Treatment

1. Familiarity with institutional policies and state laws
2. Find a private and appropriate setting for discussion
3. Ask the patient and family what they understand
4. Discuss patient's values and general goals of care
5. Establish discussion's context
6. Discuss preferences in specific treatments
7. Respond to emotions
8. Establish and implement the plan

End-of-life issues is a fairly new phenomenon in many emerging countries as intensive care is becoming more available and established. For the time being, it is difficult to assess the problem's magnitude. However, it is certain that these issues will affect many patients and families. Currently, approaches in Western countries aimed to prepare patients and the public in topics (e.g., living wills and durable power of attorneys) have not been very effective. Therefore, reliance on these tools may not always be useful. The changing religious and social attitudes are likely to have a profound effect on end-of-life issues. Currently, the lack of education in bioethics and the paucity of case law are obstacles in promoting policies that depend on the principles of autonomy or self-determination and resultant informed consent. For example, we observed the contradictory judgments issued in a case by the Indian Supreme Court.[5b] For a woman in PVS, the court decided that the right to live cannot be interpreted to include the right to die an unnatural death curtailing the natural life span. It is a stretch of imagination for the court to consider a PVS patient supported by a ventilator as having a 'natural life span'. For example, the 1994 Brain-Death law is limited to potential organ donors. This is an error in the Indian law that needs to be corrected. Many medical professionals believe and proclaim that it is 'illegal' to discontinue mechanical ventilation in dying patients. Yet, it is not unusual to observe abrupt discontinuation of life-support systems when a patient's family cannot pay for the medical care.[5c]

The practice of taking a dying patient home seems too common in many societies. A peculiar designation 'Left Against Medical Advice' (LAMA) is pointed out by Mani to be the unilateral withdrawal of care by the family based on lack of financial resources.[25] In many cases, physicians are complicit in this decision banking on a strong sense of fatalism. Barnett and Aurora report in a physician survey that the majority of pulmonary and critical care physicians did not use DNR orders.[26] They felt that their institutions did not allow it, yet 35% had performed withdrawal of life support. The contrast with Western European physicians' attitude was stark.[27] Only 6% of physicians in Europe did not use DNR orders compared to 59% in India. Amongst the European physicians, 77% would withdraw therapy versus 30% of Indian physicians. Similarly, 40% of European physicians were willing to use large doses of opioids versus 3% of Indian physicians. This points out a remarkable shortfall in the end-of-life care in India. The authors also expressed surprise that LAMA has never been considered withdrawal of care. A plea to consider this special category was made. The perceived legal restraint and absence of institutional policies were the barriers. Moreover, a lack of social networks, hospice facilities, and reliance on families to provide home care are reasons for the approach that many Western societies would find hard to accept. These conditions are likely to change in the future and the need for integrated systems of support for dying patients will emerge.

The effect of availability and the embracement of life-support technology in the developing world may result in the uncontrolled escalation of treatment when it is no longer beneficial. Of major importance from a practical point of view is the fact that in many societies equitable medical systems do not exist to provide intensive care to all their citizens. The lack of medical insurance, underfunded public hospitals, and the absence of basic facilities such as electricity and refrigeration are huge obstacles to the provision of intensive care.

Medical professionals have a responsibility to use new technology wisely, compassionately, and honestly, and must recognize their limitations. The ethical and legal constraints may be weak or non-existent. Paternalism is very much in evidence, where the physicians may make most of the decisions to continue or stop life support. If the only criteria for the delivery of end-of-life care is whether a patient can pay for it, the abuse by institutions and practitioners can be imagined. Case law is meager and physicians may be fearful of the criminal charges often brought against them by unsatisfied relatives or vengeful persons. Thus, the tendency to continue painful, expensive, and ineffective treatments exist. In these circumstances, a physician is not likely to advocate withdrawal or withholding treatment even when indicated. However, it remains paramount to guide patients and their families through the initiation and withdrawal of treatments with the goal of relieving pain and suffering. Table 5 lists some suggestions for physicians and institutions in emerging economies from experience gained by clinicians in developed countries.

Table 5: Suggestions for alternative policies in low resource societies

1. Universal CPR in all patients dying in the hospital is not necessary
2. Allow unilateral DNR decisions, insist on disclosure and written justification
3. Apply brain death laws based on clinical written criteria for all patients
4. Establish ethics committees in academic and large teaching hospitals
5. Be mindful of DNR and futile care policies
6. Curriculum for medical students and residents should include end-of-life care
7. Create professional societies to educate the judiciary and legislature

SUMMARY

In a critique of DNR policies, we raised the question whether our policies have resulted in more humane care.[5] The answer at best would be a qualified yes. Advance directives are still executed by a small minority of the population. The self-determination law passed in the late 1990s is adhered to by the hospitals in a perfunctory manner. The large 1977 Study to Understand Prognoses and Preferences for Outcomes and Risks of Treatment (SUPPORT) pointed out some salient facts.[6] The investigators interviewed surrogates of the elderly or seriously ill patients who had died within one year of hospitalization. They found out that 60% of the patients would have preferred comfort care. In 10% of the patients, care was contrary to the preferred approach. The 11% rate of attempted resuscitation was almost four times higher than the 3% rate reported a few years later in a Canadian study by Heyland et al.[4] They advocated strategies to improve patient's understanding of CPR, foster a willingness to discuss CPR, and involve patients, family members, and physicians in decision making. It has been argued that treating every age-related change as a disease or a form of deviance is foolish. It is not always a problem to solve and does not require recruiting a salvage expert (specialist!) for each struggling system. DNR discussions provide an opportunity to discuss other common therapies, often introduced at the end of life (e.g., dialysis, artificial feeding by stomach tubes, and mechanical ventilation). A promise to provide adequate pain relief and avoid suffering should be explicitly made to the conscious patient and to the family members.

Out of control treatments leave many patients and families fearful. Callahan has pointed out the illusion that we could control our medical choices, "Yet there is hardly below the surface a remarkable and rising anxiety about dying-not necessarily death as such, but a combination of an extended critical illness gradually transformed into extended dying".[28]

New challenges arose with the COVID-19 pandemic. Patients with COVID-19 induced acute respiratory distress syndrome (ARDS) did not survive CPR in the ICU.[29] Provision and continuation of highly invasive and expensive therapies such as Extra Corporeal Membrane Oxygenation (ECMO) in COVID-19 ARDS has raised ethical issues of enormous consequences.

REFERENCES

1. Bedell SE, Delbanco TL, Cook EF, et al. Survival after cardiopulmonary resuscitation in the hospital. N Engl J Med. 1983; 309:569.
2. Hershey CO, Fisher L. Why outcome of cardiopulmonary resuscitation in general wards is poor. Lancet 1982; i:31.
3. Kyff J, Puri VK, Raheja R, et al. Cardiopulmonary resuscitation in hospitalized patients: Continuing problems of decision-making. Critical Care Med 1987; 15:41.
4. Heyland DK, Frank C, Groll D, et al. Understanding cardiopulmonary resuscitation decision making. Perspectives of seriously ill hospitalized patients and family members. Chest 2006; 130:419-28.
5. Puri VK. DNR policies in North America: A procedural morass-resuscitation policies revisited. Indian J Crit Care Med 2006; 10:35-9.
   a. Puri VK, Weber LJ. Limiting the role of the family in discontinuation of life sustaining treatment. J of Medical Humanities. 1990; 11:91-98.
   b. Puri VK. End-of-life issues for a modern India-Lesson learnt from the West. Indian J Crit Care Med 2005; 9:81-85.
   c. Puri VK. Death in the ICU: Feelings of those left behind. (Editorial) Chest 2003; 124:11-2.
6. Ramsey P. The indignity of 'Death with Dignity'. On Moral Medicine. Eds Lammers SE, Verhey A. Pub William B Erdman's Publishing Company, Grand Rapids, Mi 1983-185.
   a. Ramsey P. *Preface to The Patient as Person.* On Moral Medicine. Eds Lammers SE, Verhey A. Pub William B Erdman's Publishing Company, Grand Rapids, Mi 1983-41.
7. The SUPPORT Principal Investigators: A controlled trial to improve care for seriously ill hospitalized patients. The study to Understand Prognosis and Preferences for Outcomes and Risks of Treatment (SUPPORT). JAMA 1995; 274:1591-8.
8. Lynn J, Teno JM, Phillips RS, et al. Perspectives by family members of the dying experience of older and seriously ill patients. Ann Intern Med 1997; 126:97-106.
9. Nuland SB. How we die: Reflections on life's final chapter. New York, NY: Vintage Press 1993;141-142.
10. Cassel EJ. The nature of suffering and the goals of medicine. N Engl J Med. 1982; 306:640-645.
11. Veatch RM. The History of Medical Ethical Systems-p7. Medical Ethics 1989, Ed Veatch RM, Jones, and Bartlett Publishers.
    a. Veatch RM. Cross Cultural Perspectives in Medical Ethics: Readings 1983 Ed Veatch RM, Jones, and Bartlett Publishers.
12. Nathans AB, Mair RV. Greenfield's Surgery-Eds Mullholand MV, Mair RV –p 212 Critical Care. 2006 5th Edition. Pub Williams and Wilkins.
13. Easson AM, Crosby JA, Librach SL. Discussion of death and dying in surgical textbooks. Am J Surg. 2001; 182:34-9.

14. Nelson J. Identifying and overcoming the barriers to high quality palliative care in the intensive care unit. Crit Care Med 2006;34: Supplement 324-31.
15. Kwok AC, Semel ME, Lipsitz SR, et al. The intensity and variation of surgical care at the end of life: a retrospective cohort study. Lancet 2011; 378:1408-13.
16. Quill TE." Death and Dignity". N Engl J Med 1991; 324:691-94.
17. Julian JZ, Prokopetz BA, Lehman MD. Redefining physicians' role in assisted dying. N Engl J Med 2012; 367:97-99.
18. Cranford R. Helga Wanglie's ventilator, Rie M-Limits of a wish, Ackerman F-The significance of a wish, Callahan D-Medical futility, medical necessity: the problem without a name. Hasting Center Report 1991 July-Aug 23-25.
19. Angell M. The case of Helga Wanglie-A new kind of "Right to Die": Informed demand for non-beneficial treatment. N Engl J Med 1991; 325:511-15.
20. Meisel D. Common myths about terminating life support. Archives Int. Med 1991; 151:1487.
21. Cook D, Rocker G, Marshall J, et al. Withdrawal of mechanical ventilation in anticipation of death in the intensive care unit. N Engl J Med 2003; 349:1123.
22. Halevy A, Body BA. Multi-institution collaborative policy on medical futility. JAMA 1996; 276:571-4.
23. Ackerman RJ. Withholding and withdrawing life-sustaining treatment. Am Family Physician 2000; 62:1555-1560.
24. Emanuel LL, von Gunten CJ, et al. Education for physicians on end-of-Life Care Trainer's Guide, Module 11, withholding, withdrawing therapy. EPEC Project, The Robert Wood Johnson Foundation, 1999.
25. Mani RK, Amin P, Chawla R, et al. Limiting life-prolonging interventions and providing palliative care towards the end-of-life in Indian intensive care units. Indian J Crit Care Med 2005; 9:96-107.
26. Barnett VT, Arora VK. Physician beliefs and practice regarding end-of-life care in India. Indian J Crit Care Med 200812:109-115.
27. Vincent JL. Forgoing life support in western European intensive care units: The results of an ethical questionnaire. Crit Care Med 1999; 27:1626-33.
28. Callahan D. The troubled dream of life: living with mortality. New York, NY: Simon & Schuster.1993.
29. Shah P, Smith H, Olarewaju A, et al. Is cardiopulmonary resuscitation futile in Coronavirus Disease 2019 patients experiencing in-hospital cardiac arrest? Crit. Care Med 2021; 19:201-208.

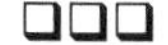

9

CHAPTER

Interventional Radiology

Proot Singh Kang, MD

INTRODUCTION

Interventional radiology is a specialty devoted to advancing patient care through the integration of clinical and imaging-based diagnosis with minimally invasive therapy. Since the advent of interventional radiology in the late 1960s, this field has evolved into a specialized branch with an ever-expanding role in current day medicine and surgery.

Interventional radiology uses X-rays, fluoroscopy, ultrasound, CT, or MRI for diagnoses and treatment of diseases with minimally invasive techniques. Presently, many conditions that once required surgery can be treated using interventional radiology-based treatments, offering less risk, less pain, and shorter recovery time. In many disease conditions, interventional radiology can be complimentary to surgical management to improve patient care and outcomes. This is applicable to patients with multiple comorbidities or high-risk situations where interventional radiology procedures can help stabilize or prepare the patient for definitive surgical management at a later time. Advances in procedural techniques and the addition of newer devices have greatly expanded the role of interventional radiology.

PRINCIPLES

Broadly, there are two types of interventional radiology techniques. The first technique the underlying disease process through a direct percutaneous puncture using a needle and/or a catheter introduced via the Seldinger technique under fluoroscopic, ultrasound, CT, or MR guidance to reach the target, which can be within any visceral cavity or solid organ. The Seldinger technique is a multistep procedure whereby a thin needle is introduced in a tubular structure (i.e., artery or hollow viscera) or cavity through which a guidewire can be placed. The needle is removed while holding in the guidewire. This is followed by the placement of a long diagnostic or drainage catheter, or a variety of ostomy tubes depending on the indication. Using a direct needle technique, aspiration or biopsy of a solid lesion could be performed with image guidance, seen in Figures 1A and 1B. Alternatively, a needle or a catheter could be placed for fluid collection and drainage, or removal of pus as seen in Figures 2A to 2C. Additionally, a special needle (i.e., thermal ablation needle) can be placed percutaneously into a neoplasm of the liver, kidney, or lung for radiofrequency ablation or cryoablation as shown in Figure 3. All of these procedures can be performed with imaging guidance, allowing the avoidance of vital structures with minimal risk to the patient.

The second technique is using percutaneous access into tubular channels (i.e., arterial system, venous system, urinary system, gastrointestinal system or the biliary system) in order to treat specific disease processes. The catheter is introduced via the Seldinger technique and guidewires are used to navigate under fluoroscopic guidance into specific locations, providing therapy. Once the catheter reaches a specific site, therapeutic devices can be introduced over a guidewire to open a blockage using angioplasty balloons, deliver stents, or stent grafts shown in Figures 4A and 4B. In case of bleeding or leakage of urine or bile, catheter-based procedures can be used to seal or exclude the disease process. The catheter can deliver therapeutic medications such as thrombolytic or chemotherapy to specific sites, thereby avoiding the risk of exposure to remote organs. Embolo-therapy via a percutaneous catheter is another major advancement in technique, especially with the addition of microcatheters to treat bleeding from remote sites, seen in Figure 5.

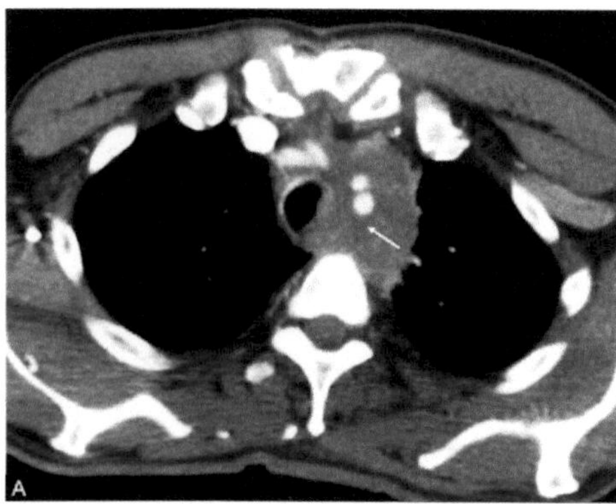

Figure 1A: Axial CT scan with iodine contrast showing a left upper lobe and mediastinal mass encasing the aortic arch vessels (arrow).

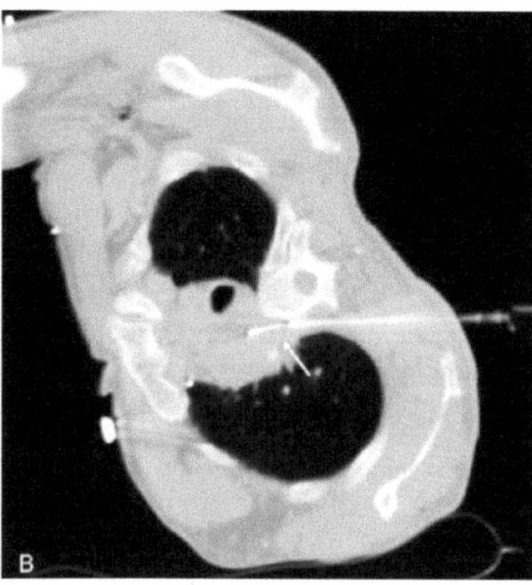

Figure 1B: Axial CT image of the same patient in prone oblique position with a trucut biopsy needle (arrow) introduced in the mass via the left paravertebral posterior approach, using iodine contrast enhanced CT guidance.

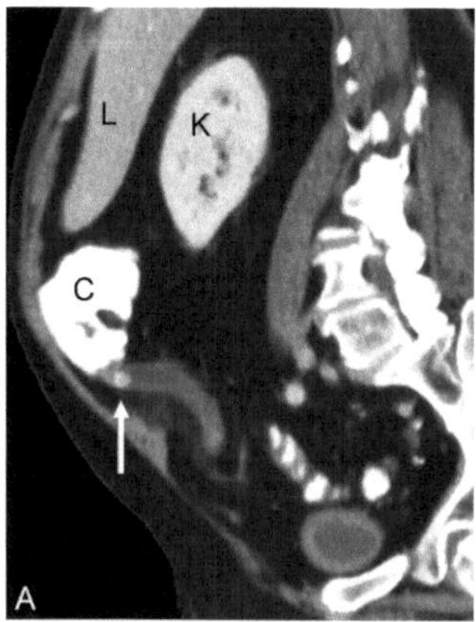

Figure 2A: CT scan reconstructed sagittal oblique image, obtained with oral and intravenous contrast, showing an enlarged inflamed appendix with an appendicolith at its junction with the cecum (C). The patient underwent laparoscopic appendectomy. Liver (L), Right Kidney (K).

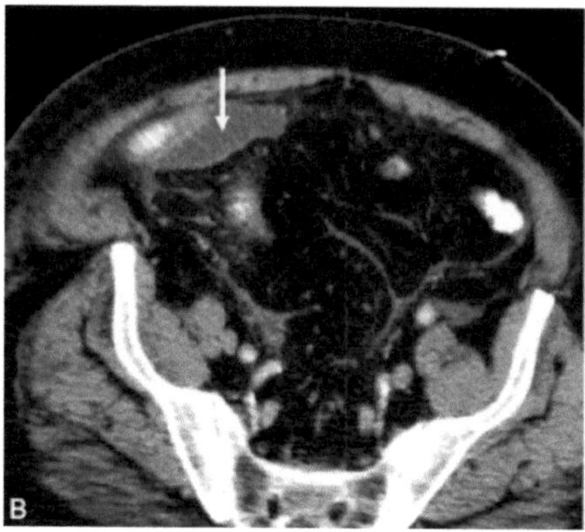

Figure 2B: Two weeks post-appendectomy CT scan shows fluid collection with peripheral enhancement. (arrow) This patient had lower abdominal pain and increased white blood cell count.

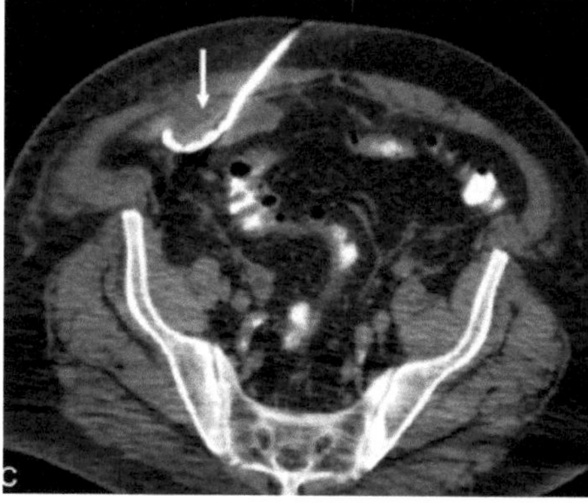

Figure 2C: CT scan demonstrating the drainage of postoperative abscess with 8 Fr pigtail catheter (arrow) placed under CT guidance.

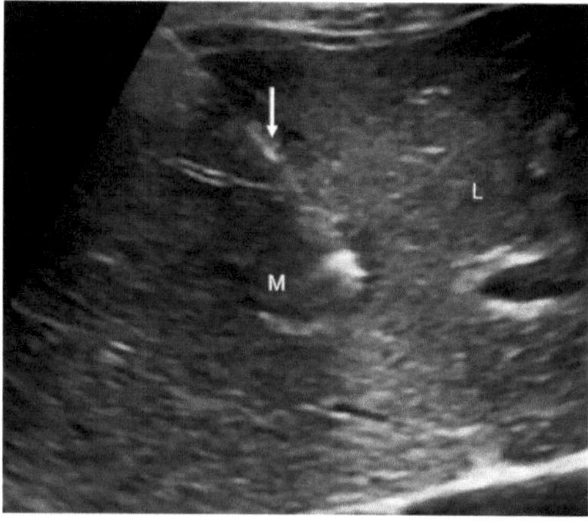

Figure 3: Axial ultrasound image of the liver (L), showing a radiofrequency ablation needle (arrow) guided into a hepatocellular carcinoma mass lesion (M) for treatment. The mass (M) had previously been biopsied using a percutaneous needle

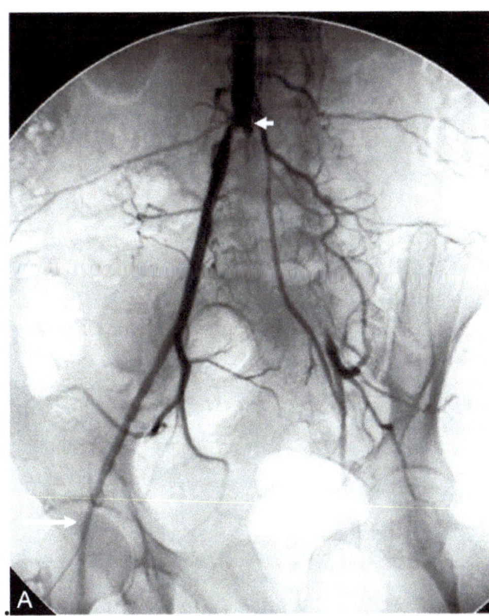

Figure 4A: Pelvic angiogram showing an occluded left iliac artery at the aortic bifurcation (arrowhead) and significant stenosis of the proximal right common iliac artery. Percutaneous catheter placed via right common femoral artery (arrow).

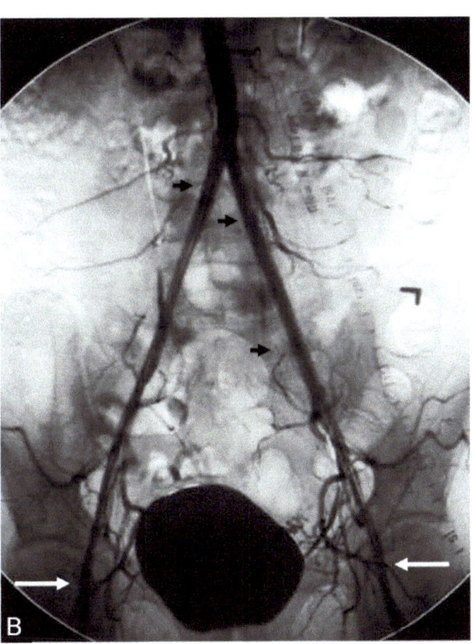

Figure 4B: Postintervention pelvic angiogram following revascularization of the left iliac artery with balloon expandable stent and placement of "kissing" aortic bifurcation stents (arrowheads) using bilateral femoral artery access (arrows).

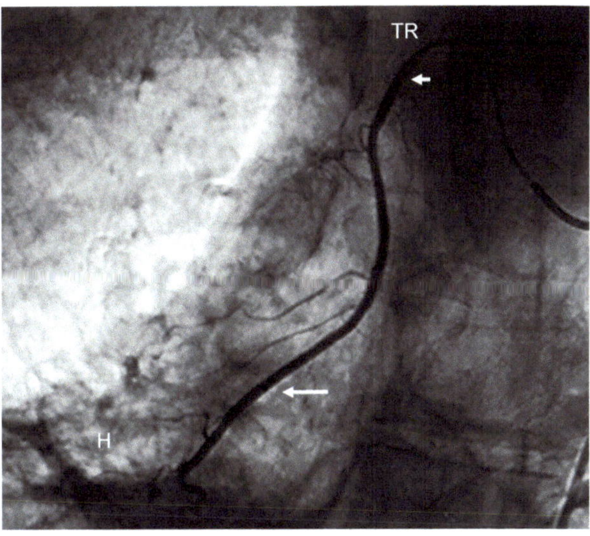

Figure 5: Right bronchial artery (arrowhead) angiogram, with microcatheter tip (arrow) is a distal location prior to embolization of hemoptysis (H) with polyvinyl alcohol particles. Trachea (TR).

PATIENT EVALUATION AND PREPROCEDURE REQUISITES

The evaluation of the patient requires understanding of their clinical condition, checking appropriate lab tests such as complete blood cell count with platelets, coagulation profile, and basic electrolytes including renal function. Assessment of patient allergies and current medications is necessary. Since most of the interventional radiology procedures involve the use of iodine-based contrast media, a history and risk of contrast reactions should be addressed. In a patient with prior history of contrast reaction, premedication with steroids and antihistamines is performed. Most of the procedures are done under conscious sedation using short-acting intravenous benzodiazepines and opioid medications in combination with a local anesthetic. General anesthesia is rarely necessary. In any case, an optimal patient outcome depends on close communication and consultation between the surgeon and the interventional radiologist. This is paramount in postoperative cases where a specific interventional procedure may avoid a second immediate surgery. An example of this situation is basket retrieval of retained common bile duct stones post-cholecystectomy via the T-tube tract.

SCOPE OF INTERVENTION RADIOLOGY IN SURGERY

Interventional radiology procedures are used in the management of diseases affecting a majority of the body organs and systems such as gastrointestinal, hepatobiliary, cardiovascular, thoracic, obstetrics and gynecology, urinary and surgical infectious diseases, trauma, oncologic, and transplant medicine. To illustrate the various interventional radiology procedures, case examples are presented as they are discussed in the following sections. These will be discussed in two broad groups, nonvascular interventions and vascular interventions.

A. Nonvascular Interventions

Percutaneous sampling and/or drainage of fluid collections, abscess within solid organs, and pleural or peritoneal cavity is commonly performed for initial diagnosis or for postoperative patients. Percutaneous sampling could be performed using needle aspiration most commonly under ultrasound or CT scan guidance shown in Figure 6. Based on the gross and laboratory assessment of the fluid removed, further treatment can be planned. If the diagnosis of an abscess is suspected or already established, percutaneous catheter placement ranging from 6 to 18 French size could be performed within intra-abdominal abscess cavities, acute cholecystitis (Figures 7A and 7B), liver abscess (Figures 8A to 8C), lung abscess, pyothorax, pneumothorax, hydronephrosis, tubo-ovarian abscess, etc. Noninfected fluid collection such as pleural effusion, pericardial effusion or ascites can also be drained by simple aspiration. These can be easily repeated without significant risk in cases of recurrent ascites in cirrhotic patients.

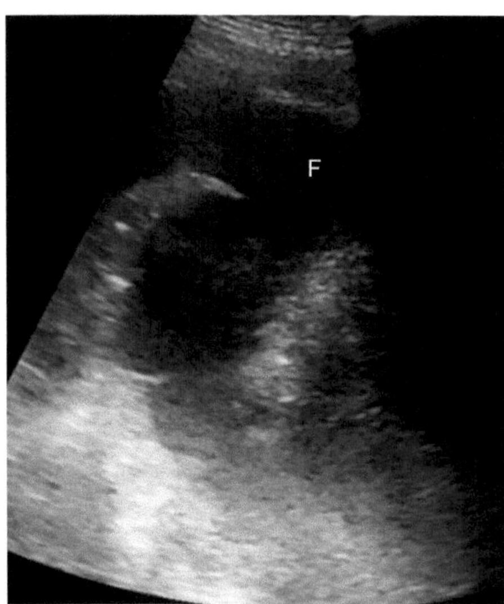

Figure 6: Ultrasound image of pleural effusion (F), showing the edge of the atelectatic lung (arrow) to be avoided, during guided thoracentesis of the fluid.

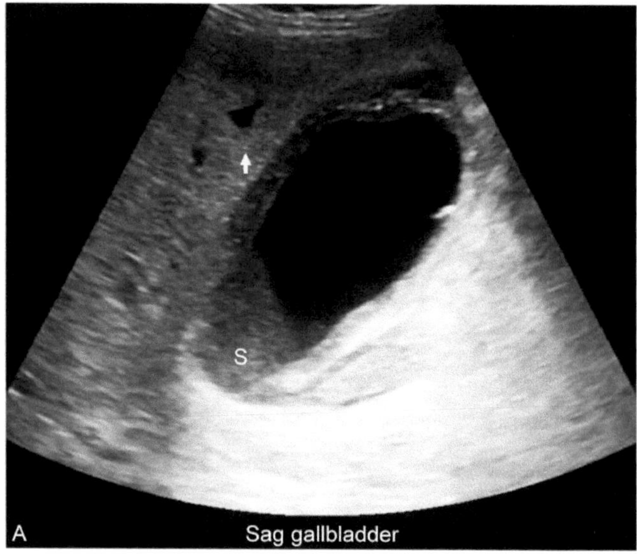

Figure 7A: Longitudinal ultrasound image of a distended gallbladder with wall thickening (arrowhead) and dependent sludge/pus (S), consistent with acute acalculous cholecystitis.

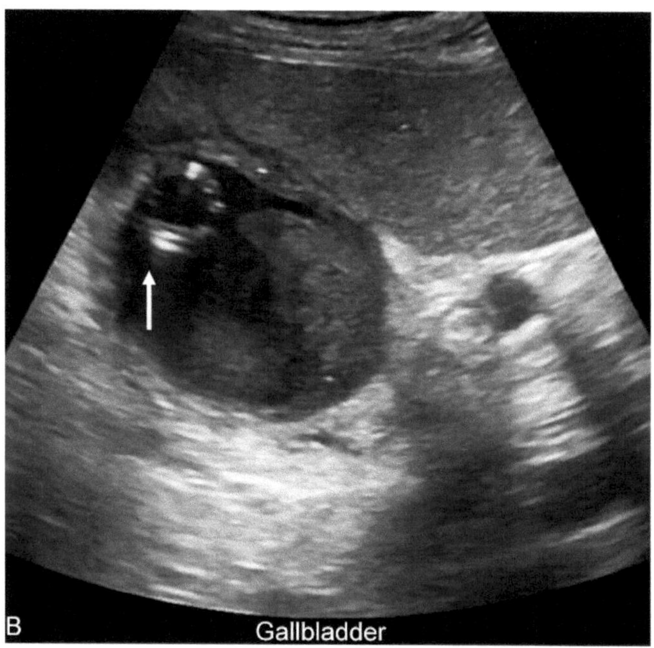

Figure 7B: Ultrasound guided percutaneous transhepatic pigtail 8 Fr drainage catheter (arrow) placed within the gallbladder with removal of infected bile.

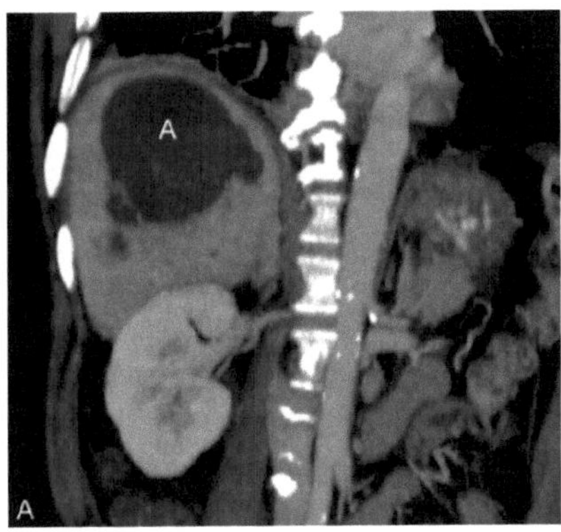

Figure 8A: Coronal CT scan image showing a large irregular abscess (A) in the right lobe of the liver in a patient with fever, abnormal liver function tests, and increased white cell count.

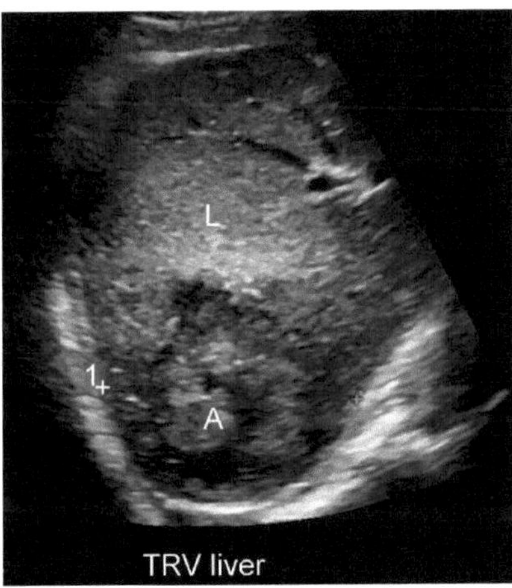

Figure 8B: Ultrasound image of the liver (L), obtained during guided placement of a percutaneous 10 Fr pigtail drainage catheter to remove thick pyogenic material from the abscess (A).

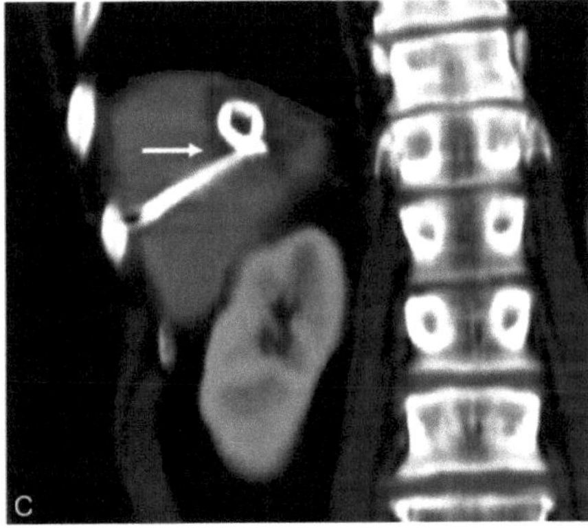

Figure 8C: Coronal CT scan image at two weeks follow-up, showing near complete resolution of the abscess with the pigtail catheter (arrow) in position. The catheter was removed due to negligible output at this point.

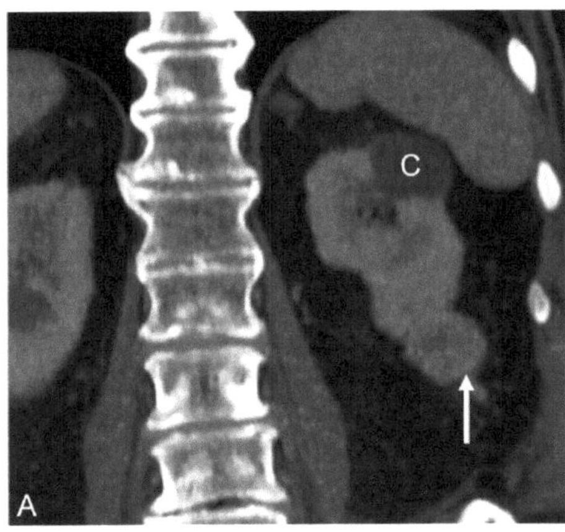

Figure 9A: Coronal CT scan image of the left kidney demonstrating a solid 3 cm enhancing mass lesion (arrow) at the lower pole. Incidental note made of a cortical renal cyst (C) at the upper pole.

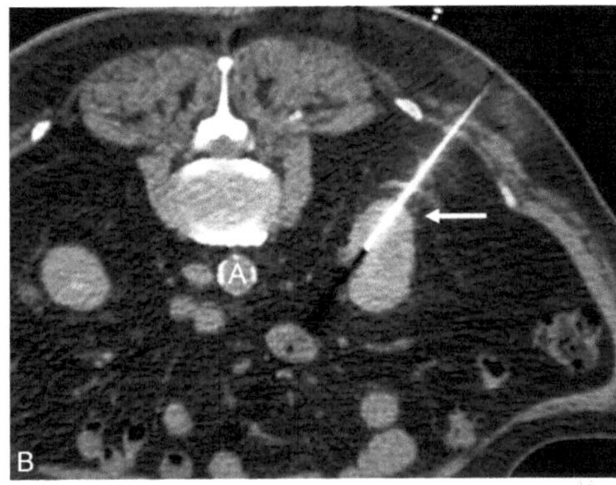

Figure 9B: Axial prone CT scan during image guided percutaneous biopsy and radiofrequency ablation of the lower pole mass (arrow) in this patient with high surgical risk. Biopsy revealed clear cell renal carcinoma. Aorta (A).

Malignant recurring pleural effusion can be managed by the placement of implanted tunneled pleural cuffed catheters to facilitate fluid removal as necessary. This can significantly improve patient quality of life. Additionally, sclerosing agents can be introduced via the pleural catheter to cause pleurodesis and prevent recurrent fluid accumulation.

Percutaneous biopsy is commonly performed for pulmonary nodule, pulmonary masses, mediastinal lymph nodes, abdominal or retroperitoneal masses, lymph nodes, and viscera of the abdomen and pelvis. These are typically performed using ultrasound or CT scan for guidance. Alternatively, fluoroscopy guidance or rarely MRI can be used for large pulmonary lesions. Various biopsy techniques include aspiration for cytology or histology as well as core biopsy to obtain larger samples. In patients with a high risk of bleeding due to low platelets or elevated prothrombin time, a trans-jugular biopsy of the liver or kidney can be obtained. This can help with essential diagnosis as well as staging of the neoplasm for preoperative planning.

Recent innovations in thermal ablation techniques have advanced the application of interventional radiology procedures for the management of renal cell carcinoma, nonsurgical hepatocellular carcinoma (HCC), and nonsurgical lung neoplasm. One of the methods available is heat ablation using radiofrequency or microwave technology seen in Figures 9A to 9C. The other method of tumor treatment is cryoablation which essentially causes tissue death by freezing. These techniques consist of specialized needles which are introduced percutaneously under imaging guidance and placed accurately within the tumors for thermal ablation. Chemical ablation of HCC with absolute alcohol injection is a viable option in select cases. These nonsurgical ablative techniques are usually performed in patients who are not surgical candidates or need to be downgraded in terms of tumor burden to become eligible for surgical treatment.

In the gastrointestinal tract, esophageal dilatation of benign strictures can be performed under fluoroscopic guidance. In case of malignant obstruction, esophageal, gastric, or colonic stenting can be performed for palliative management of symptoms. Percutaneous gastrostomy tube placement is also feasible. In case the patient has a risk of aspiration, the gastrostomy tube can be combined with an additional coaxial jejunostomy tube to safely feed the patient.

Percutaneous transhepatic biliary access is useful in the management of postoperative bile leak or obstruction. Dual percutaneous biliary access and catheter drainage is performed for the Klatskin type of neoplasm shown in Figure 10A and 10B. In case of malignant biliary obstruction, percutaneous biliary catheter drainage and/or biliary stenting can be performed for palliative therapy of neoplasms such as unresectable pancreatic carcinoma or cholangiocarcinoma, shown in Figures 11A and 11B. The frequency of biliary interventions has decreased with advances in endoscopic biliary interventions. However, if the ERCP is unsuccessful or difficult to perform due to prior surgery, percutaneous transhepatic biliary access is a viable option. This allows for bile sampling as well as a brush or forceps biopsy of an obstructing mass.

Benign biliary strictures can be treated with balloon angioplasty and long-term external biliary catheters. Percutaneous biliary access can sometimes be combined with endoscopic intervention using a rendezvous guidewire snare technique for optimal patient care by collaboration.

Percutaneous cholecystostomy catheter drainage for acute cholecystitis is useful in otherwise sick or unstable patients who are unable to undergo cholecystectomy. Patients with retained common bile duct stones, following cholecystectomy and T-tube, can undergo stone extraction using a basket catheter placed via an established T-tube tract, thereby avoiding a second exploration.

Celiac plexus block using absolute alcohol in widespread pancreatic or upper abdominal malignancy causing intractable pain, deserves special mention as it can be accurately performed under CT guidance, using minimal contrast media for confirming location seen in Figure 12. A total of 30 to 50 mL of absolute alcohol can be injected with a local anesthetic for a good response.

In the urinary system, a simple procedure such as percutaneous nephrostomy, can be the initial access to a variety of interventions shown in Figures 13A to 13C. Some of the indications are relief of infection, stone disease, urinary diversion for distal obstruction, fistula, or injury. Percutaneous nephrostomy also provides access for percutaneous nephrolithotomy, double J ureteral or nephron-ureteral stent, and ureteral stricture dilatation. In case of an inoperable malignant urinary obstruction, long-term bilateral nephrostomy drainage provides palliative relief. Some of the inoperable urinary fistulas may be managed by bilateral ureteral occlusions using coils and gel foam, combined with bilateral nephrostomy drainage catheters as seen in Figures 14A and 14B.

B. Vascular Interventions

Within the arterial system most diagnostic information can be obtained by high resolution CT or MR angiography. Most of the invasive arterial procedures are now combined with interventions. Peripheral arterial diseases such as arterial stenosis, occlusions, or aneurysms can be treated using angioplasty, stent, and/or stent graft placement. This is applicable in a wide variety of anatomical sites such as aorto- iliac, femoral-popliteal, aortic arch vessels, carotid, renal, and more. Thrombolysis using percutaneous methods can significantly decrease the morbidity and mortality in peripheral arterial disease as shown in Figures 15A to 15D. In the pulmonary arterial system, thrombolysis can be performed for massive pulmonary embolism using either mechanical thrombectomy tools or pharmacological thrombolytics. In several cases where open surgery has high morbidity and mortality, an endograft can achieve comparable results as in the repair of abdominal aortic aneurysm or thoracic aortic

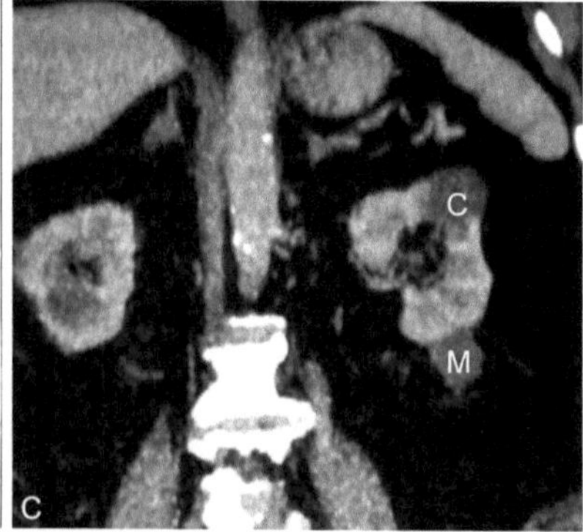

Figure 9C: Coronal CT image at 6 months follow-up post-radiofrequency ablation. Shows shrinking left renal lower pole mass (M) without significant enhancement, consistent with successful treatment. Cortical renal cyst (C).

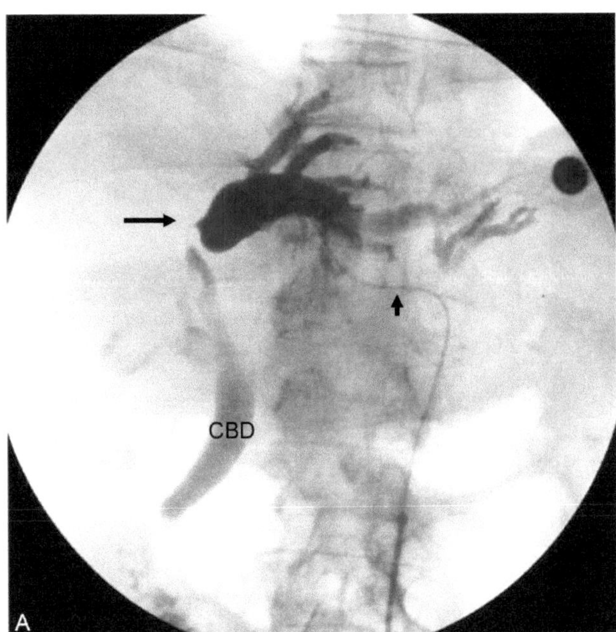

Figure 10A: Percutaneous transhepatic cholangiogram from a left ductal approach (arrowhead) showing a Klatskin lesion causing severe stenosis at the confluence of intrahepatic ducts (arrow) with slow flow into the common bile duct (CBD). No communication with right ductal system seen.

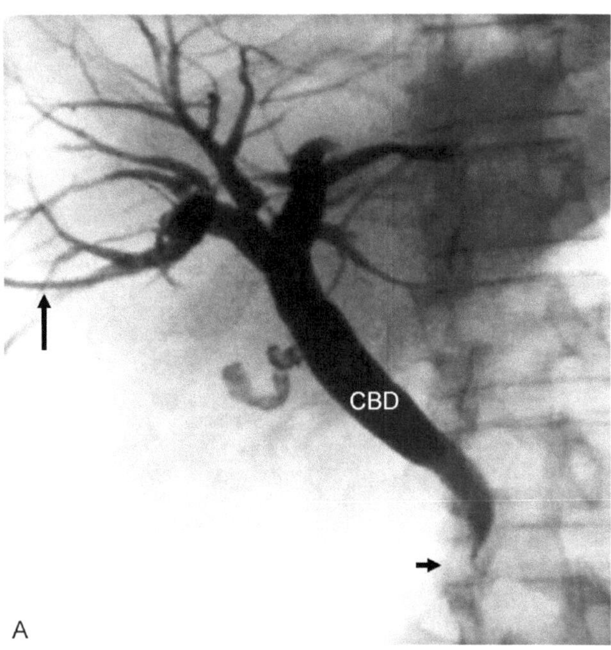

Figure 11A: Percutaneous transhepatic cholangiogram from right sided access (arrow), shows severe stricture (arrowhead) of the common bile duct (CBD), caused by a nonresectable pancreatic carcinoma.

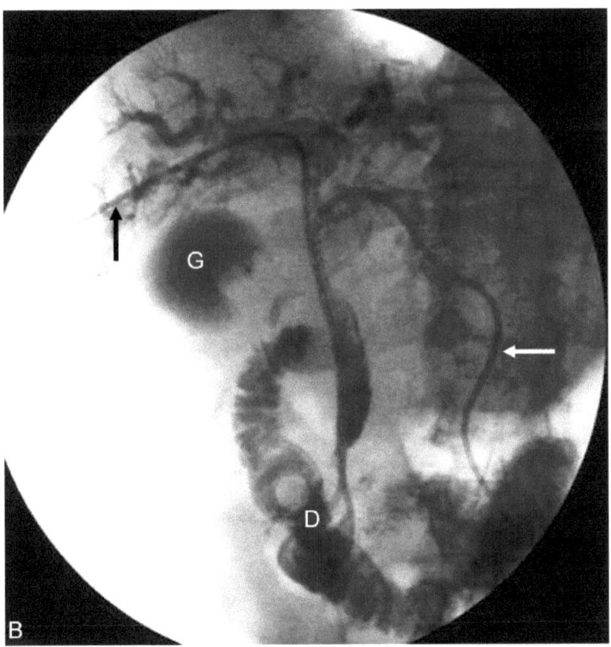

Figure 10B: Cholangiogram image showing bilateral transhepatic biliary access (arrows) with placement of internal/external drainage catheters ending in the duodenum (D). There is a small amount of retained contrast in the gallbladder (G).

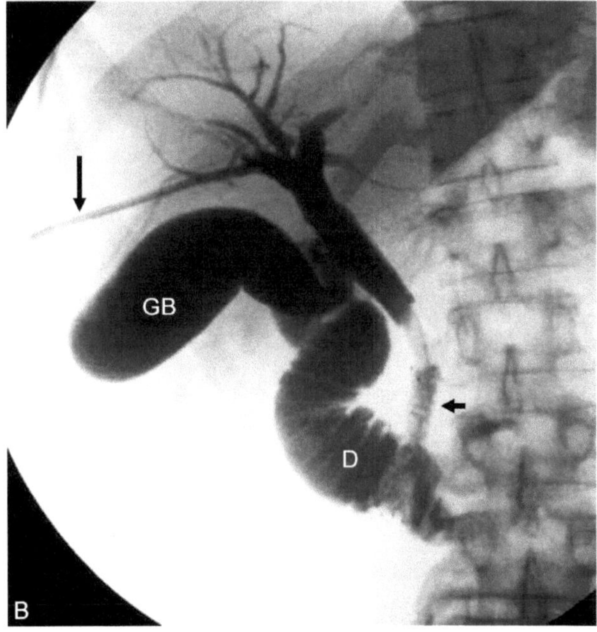

Figure 11B: Cholangiogram image via right sided access (arrow), showing internal metal stent (arrowhead) across the mass lesion with contrast flow into the duodenum (D). Gallbladder (GB).

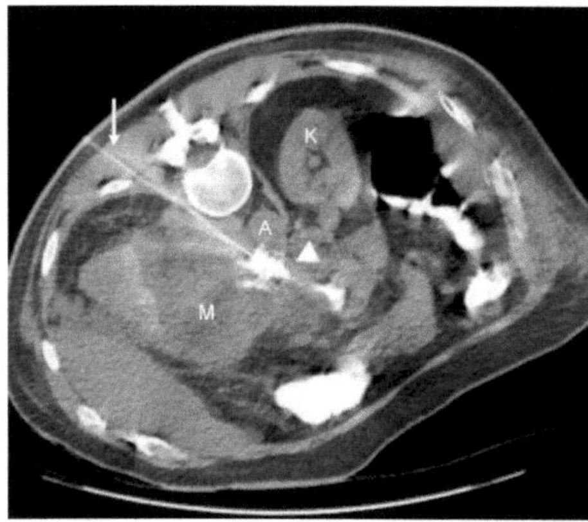

Figure 12: Celiac plexus block using CT guidance. Percutaneous needle (arrow) placed via paravertebral trajectory into the mass (M) encasing the celiac plexus region as confirmed with a small amount of contrast (arrowhead) prior to injection of absolute alcohol. Left Kidney (K), Aorta (A).

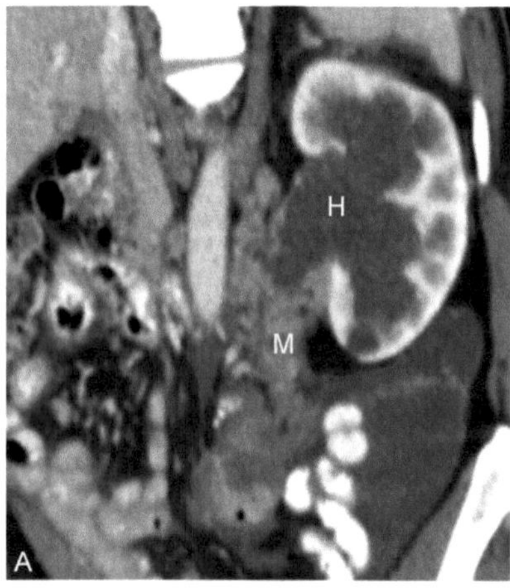

Figure 13A: Coronal CT image showing severe left hydronephrosis (H), caused by malignant retroperitoneal mass (M).

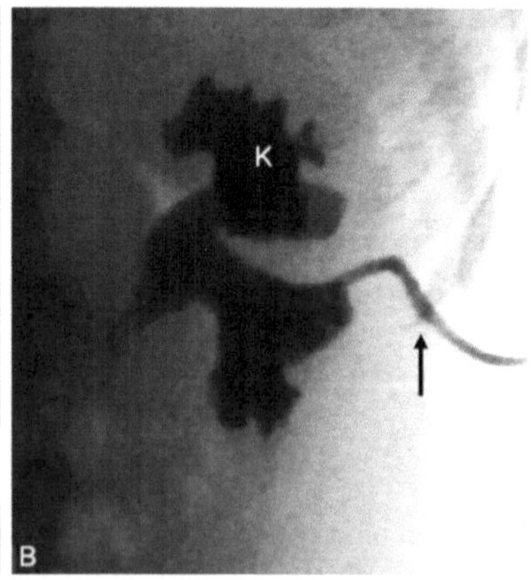

Figure 13B: Nephrostogram obtained during placement of percutaneous 8 Fr pigtail catheter (arrow) into the collecting system of the left kidney (K), via lower pole calyx, using ultrasound for access guidance.

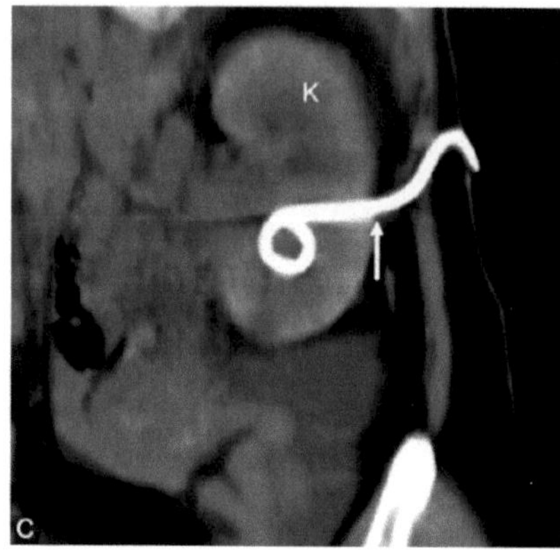

Figure 13C: Coronal CT scan obtained in follow-up during treatment shows relief of left kidney (K) hydronephrosis with a nephrostomy catheter in position (arrow).

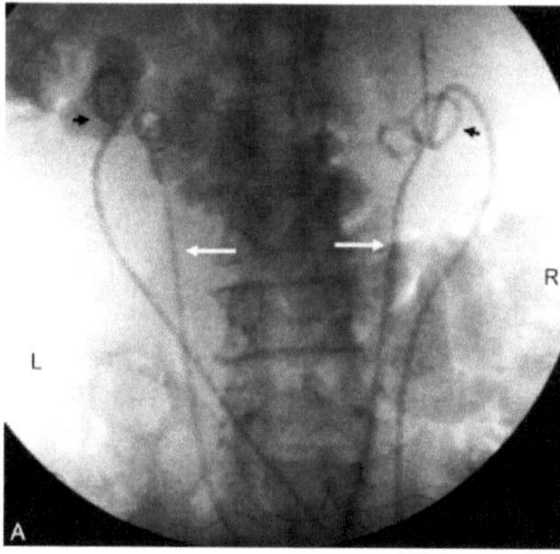

Figure 14A: Fluoroscopic spot image of a patient with malignant recto-vesicular fistula, initially managed with placement of bilateral diverting percutaneous nephrostomy catheters (arrowheads) and double J stents (arrows).

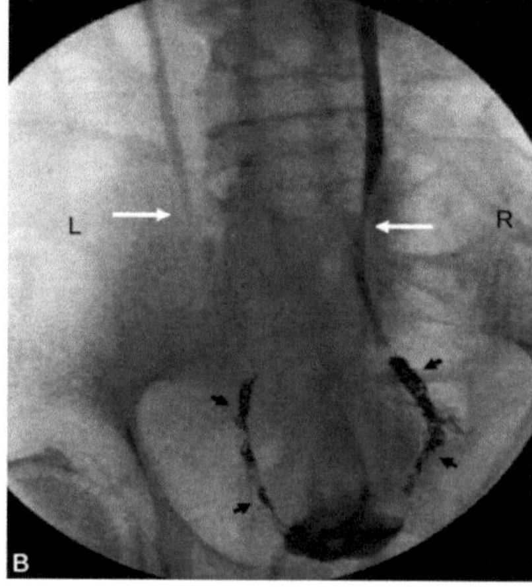

Figure 14B: Following unsuccessful resection of rectal cancer and persistence of the urinary fistula, both double J stents were removed from the ureters (arrows) via nephrostomy access using the snare technique. Both distal ureters were occluded using embolization coils with permanent diverting bilateral nephrostomy catheters.

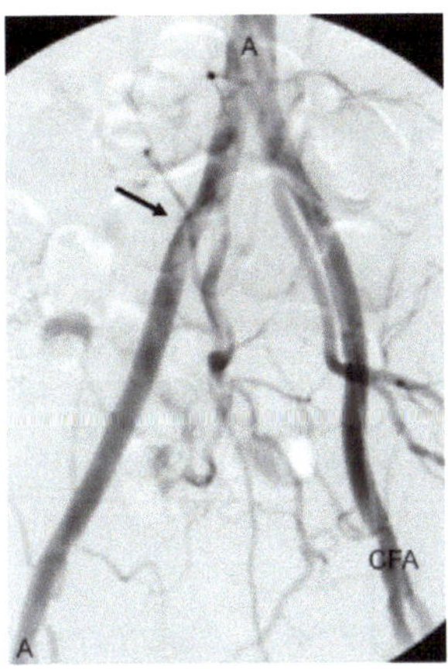

Figure 15A: Pelvic arteriogram showing significant stenotic lesion in the right iliac artery (arrow) causing distal thrombo-embolism as seen on the next image (Figure 15B). Percutaneous access obtained via the left common femoral artery (CFA). Aorta (A).

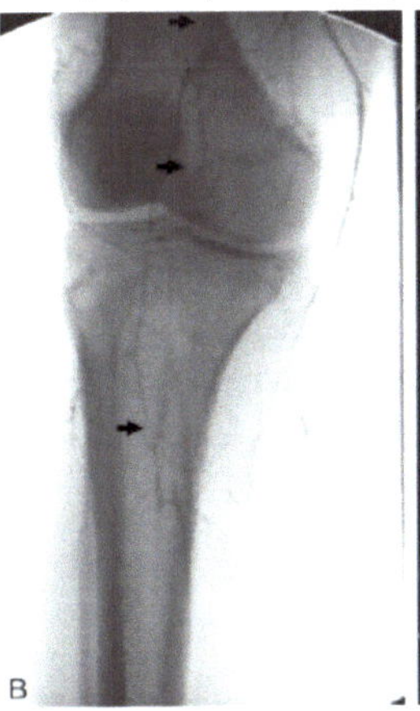

Figure 15B: Arteriogram of the right leg below the knee, demonstrating absence of flow in the right popliteal artery and tibial branches (arrowheads) consistent with thrombo-embolism in this patient with a cold ischemic right foot.

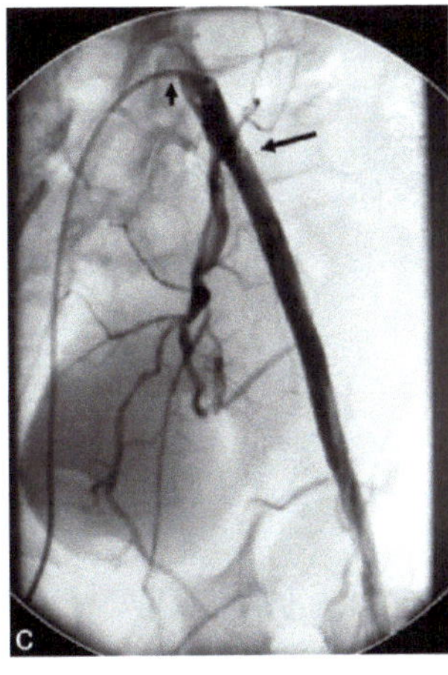

Figure 15C: Postintervention arteriogram shows patent right iliac artery after stenting (arrow), performed via a sheath over the aortic bifurcation (arrowhead).

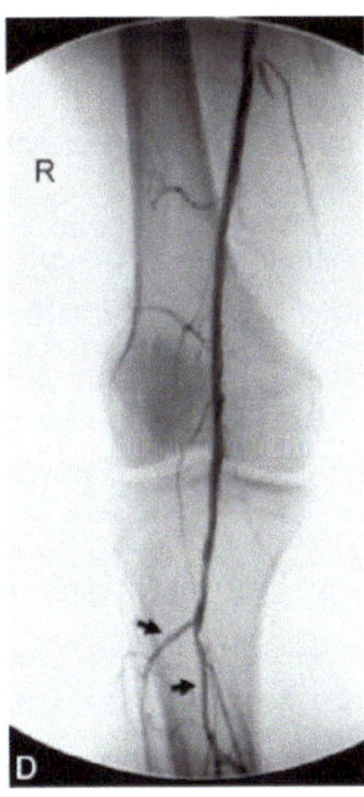

Figure 15D: Right leg arteriogram following 24 hours thrombolysis via infusion catheter showing patent right popliteal artery (arrow) and tibial arteries (arrowhead). Foot amputation was averted in this patient.

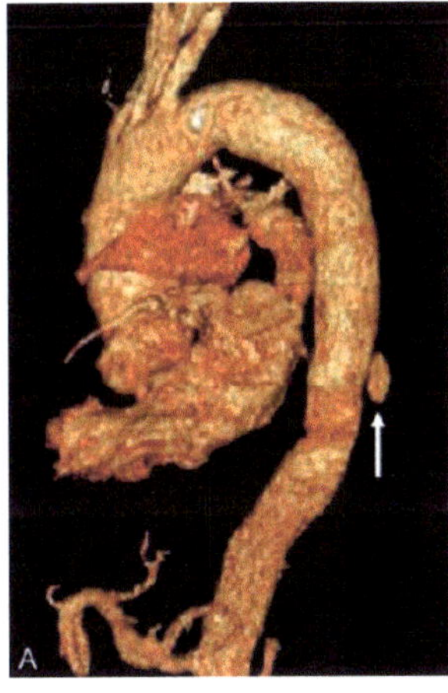

Figure 16A: CT scan 3D image of the thoracic aorta showing a leaking thoracic aneurysm (arrow) presenting with chest pain and left hemothorax.

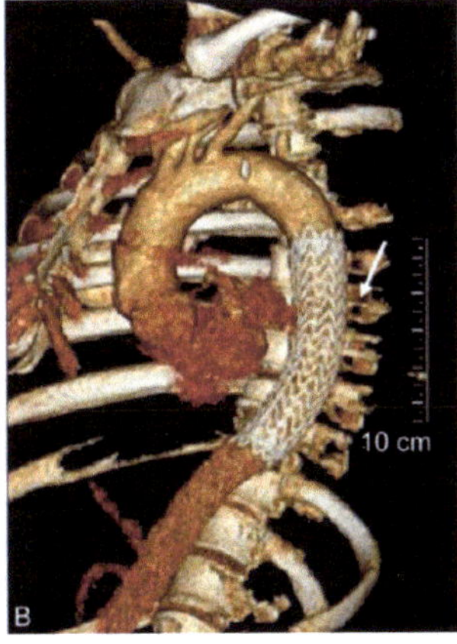

Figure 16B: CT scan 3D image following thoracic aortic endograft (arrow) showing successful exclusion of the aneurysm.

aneurysm, seen in Figures 20A and 20B, with minimally invasive techniques. Intracranial aneurysms can now be successfully treated via percutaneous embolization methods by neuro-interventionalists.

Treatment of various types of bleeding with the use of percutaneous transcatheter embolo-therapy is a highly developed field especially with the advancement of microcatheter techniques and the development of embolic material such as polyvinyl alcohol particles, micro-coils and glue.

Hemoptysis from chronic conditions such as bronchiectasis, tuberculosis, or less commonly lung malignancies can be managed using bronchial artery embolization. Embolization can be performed in cases of pulmonary artery malformations, aneurysm, or injury selective branch.

Symptomatic fibroids are now commonly treated with uterine artery embolization, thereby avoiding a hysterectomy for treating a benign disease, seen in Figures 17A and 17B. A similar embolization procedure can be used in the treatment of postpartum hemorrhage.

Treatment of gastrointestinal bleeding requires the detection of the source and possible intervention for its management. Examples include embolization of the gastroduodenal artery for bleeding duodenal ulcers, detection, and embolization of bleeding from diverticular disease, vascular malformation, or complication following colonoscopy procedures. Some of these are managed entirely using interventional radiology procedures and, in other cases, a critical patient can be stabilized for definitive surgical management later, seen in Figures 18A and 18B. Vascular complication of pancreatitis can lead to pseudoaneurysm formation, which is best treated using percutaneous embolization if accessible as seen in Figures 19A to 19C.

Portal hypertension from liver disease can cause complications of gastrointestinal bleeding commonly from varices or result in severe ascites and abdominal distension. The creation of a trans-jugular intrahepatic portosystemic shunt by interventional radiology techniques can significantly relieve the portal hypertension and control the recurrence of bleeding and ascites, shown in Figure 20.

Life-threatening hematuria from renal cell carcinoma can be effectively managed with percutaneous embolization shown in Figures 21A to 21C. Some surgeons routinely prefer to have the renal tumor embolized preoperatively for facilitating surgical excision and decreasing blood loss during surgery. Postoperative complications resulting in hemorrhage and pseudoaneurysm can at times be successfully treated with percutaneous catheter embolization as shown in Figures 22A to 22C, a case of partial nephrectomy.

There has been significant development in the management of liver neoplasms, especially HCC. Nonsurgical patients with HCC can undergo trans-arterial chemoembolization (TACE) with improvements in both survival and outcome. Selective patient can be downgraded following TACE and/or selective portal vein embolization to eventually undergo definitive surgical therapy such as liver transplant or resection as seen in Figures 23A to 23D. Recurrence of hepatocellular carcinoma in post-resection cases can be treated with TACE. Hepatic metastases from carcinoid or intestinal adenocarcinoma in selected cases are sometimes a candidate for TACE or other trans-arterial embolization procedures. Close cooperation between liver physicians and surgeons can have a significant impact on patient survival.

Venous procedures and interventions performed by interventional radiology have come to play a dominant role in patient care. These consist of central venous access such as placement of non- tunneled or tunneled catheters and implanted ports. Hemodialysis access maintenance involving angioplasty, de-clot, and management of arteriovenous fistulas or grafts are routinely performed. Superior vena cava (SVC) syndrome can result from mediastinal involvement from inflammation or neoplasm resulting in SVC and/or brachiocephalic vein obstruction with and without thrombosis. Stenting and/or thrombolysis of central venous occlusions due to a benign or malignant etiology can be performed, shown in Figures 24A to 24C. Placement of vena cava filters as well as the retrieval of filters no longer indicated has a significant role in the management of venous thromboembolic disease, seen in Figures 25.

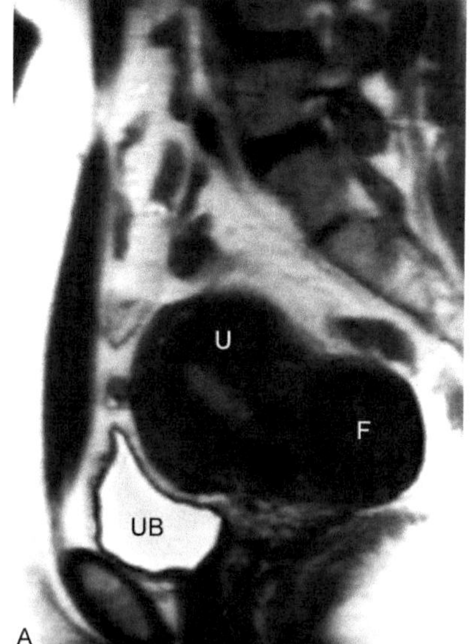

Figure 17A: Sagittal MRI image of the pelvis demonstrating an enlarged uterus (U), with an additional large posterior fibroid (F) in this patient with lower abdominal pain, excessive vaginal bleeding, urinary frequency, and anemia. Urinary Bladder (UB).

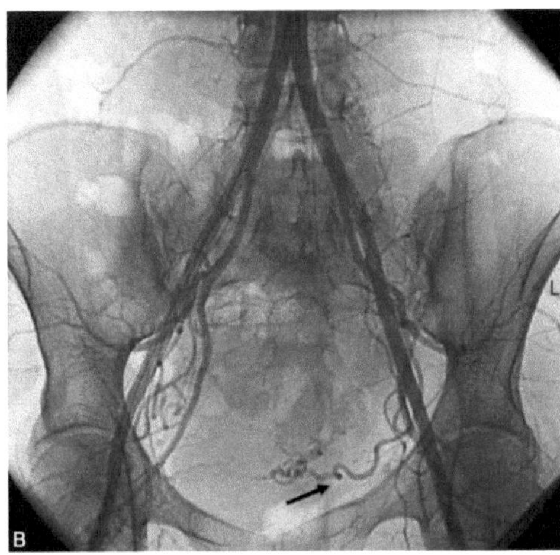

Figure 17B: Pelvic arteriogram image obtained during uterine artery (arrow) embolization using polyvinyl alcohol particles. Successful relief of symptoms in 2 to 3 months.

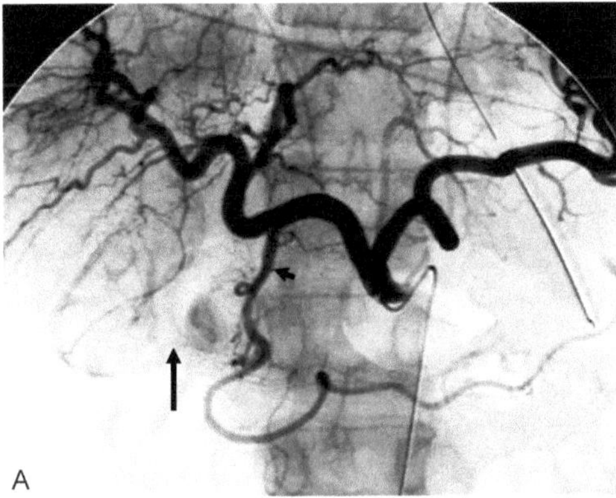

Figure 18A: Celiac axis arteriogram (C) in a patient with recurrent hematemesis following unsuccessful endoscopic treatment of a bleeding duodenal ulcer. Contrast extravasation (arrow) seen arising from a gastroduodenal artery (arrowhead) branch.

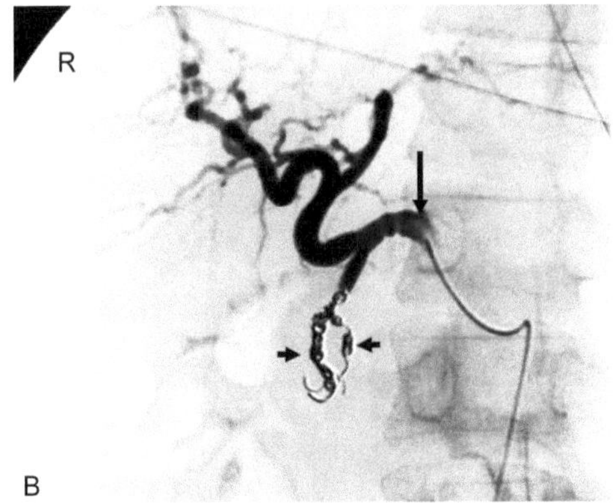

Figure 18B: Hepatic arteriogram (arrow) after successful coil occlusion of gastroduodenal artery bleeders (arrowheads). This allowed for the critical patient to recover for a subsequent definitive surgical management.

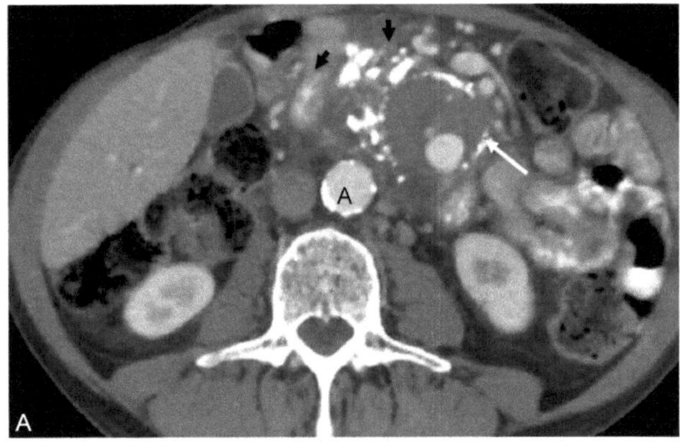

Figure 19A: Axial CT scan of the abdomen demonstrating a pseudocyst of the pancreas with a pseudoaneurysm (arrow), in a patient presenting with hematemesis. Multiple pancreatic calcifications (arrowheads) are seen. Endoscopy revealed bleeding from the ampulla. Aorta (A).

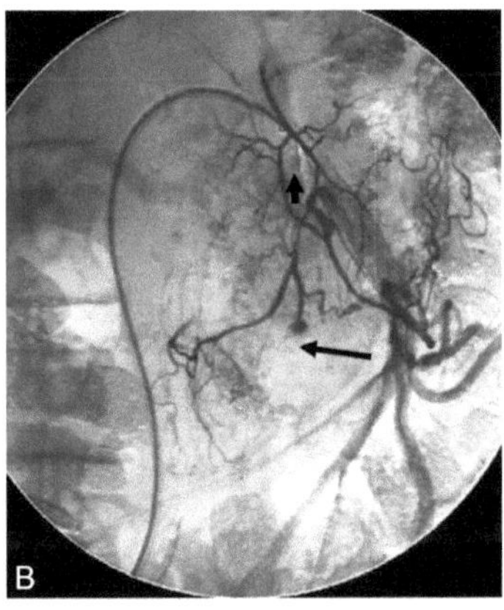

Figure 19B: Arteriogram of the superior mesenteric artery (SMA) showing a branch (arrowhead) feeding the pseudoaneurysm (arrow).

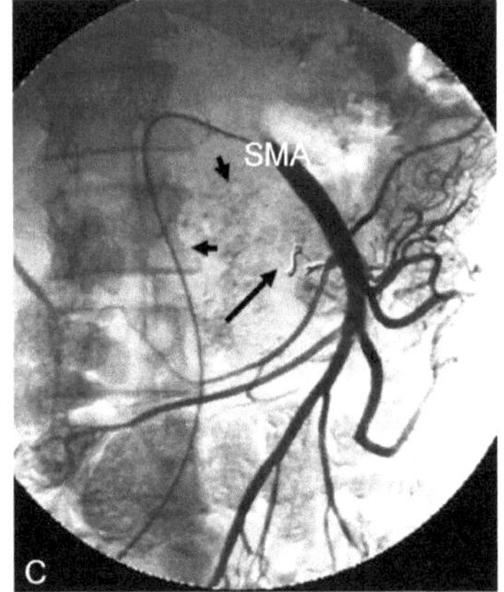

Figure 19C: Superior mesenteric arteriogram (SMA) following successful coil embolization of the pseudoaneurysm (arrow), thereby avoiding a high-risk open surgery. Scattered pancreatic calcifications are seen (arrowheads).

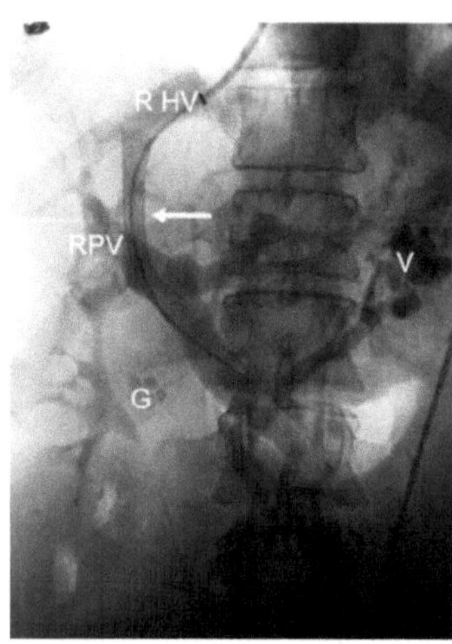

Figure 20: Angiogram obtained during creation of a transjugular intrahepatic portosystemic shunt (TIPS), from the right hepatic vein (R HV) to the right portal vein (R PV) using a metal stent (arrow). Also noted are gastroesophageal varices (V) and gallstones (G).

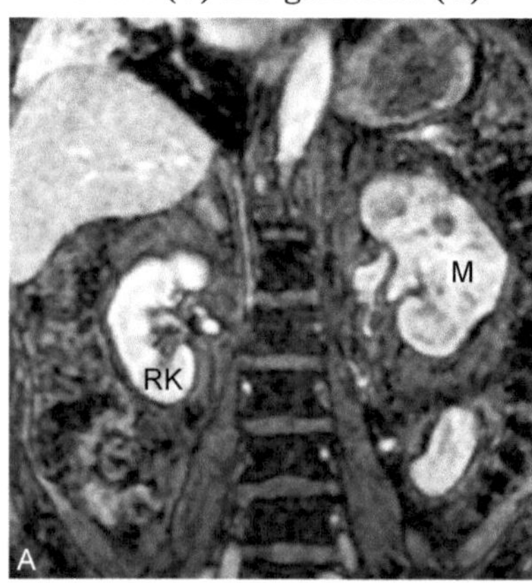

Figure 21A: Coronal MRI scan with gadolinium contrast showing a large enhancing mass (M) in the left kidney of patient with hematuria. Normal right kidney (RK) is seen.

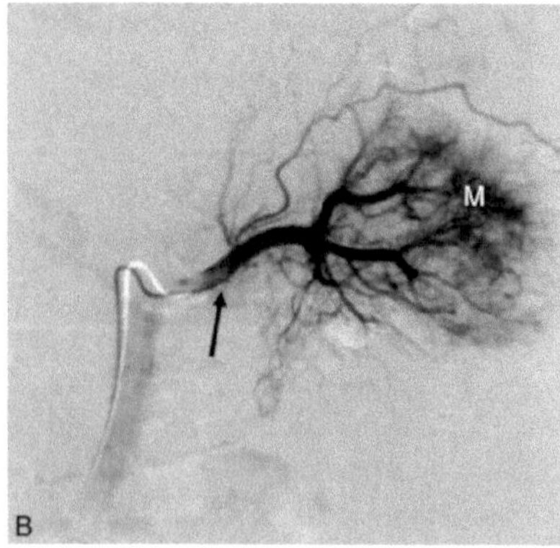

Figure 21B: Arteriogram of the left kidney (arrow) obtained when the hematuria exacerbated to become life-threatening. The large enhancing mass (M) seen is consistent with renal cell carcinoma.

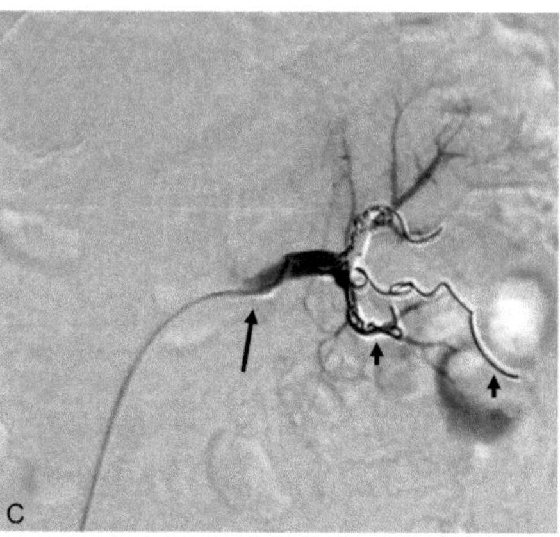

Figure 21C: Postembolization arteriogram of the left kidney (arrow) following occlusion of the left renal artery with polyvinyl alcohol particles and coils (arrowhead). The hematuria was emergently controlled, and the patient subsequened a nephrectomy.

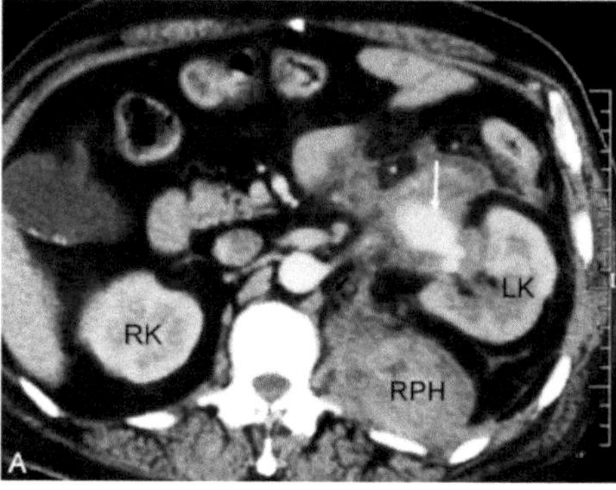

Figure 22A: Axial CT scan image with intravenous contrast showing left sided retroperitoneal hemorrhage (RPH) in a patient with recent partial nephrectomy of the left kidney (LK) for an upper pole neoplasm. Also seen is a large pseudoaneurysm (arrow) on a branch of the left renal artery (arrowhead).

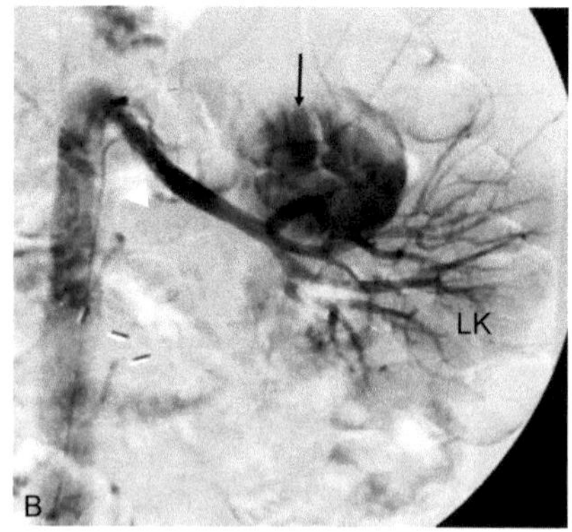

Figure 22B: Arteriogram image with a catheter in the left renal artery (arrowhead) showing a large pseudoaneurysm in the partial nephrectomy site and the preserved lower half of the left kidney (LK).

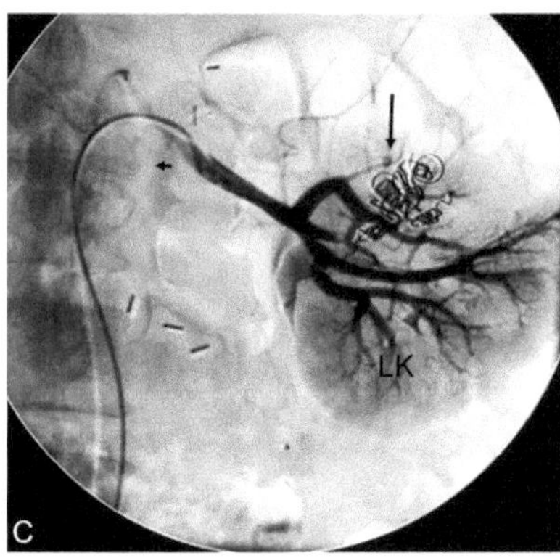

Figure 22C: Arteriogram of the left renal artery (arrowhead) following successful coil embolization of the pseudoaneurysm (arrow) and its feeding branches. The lower half of the left kidney (LK) was preserved.

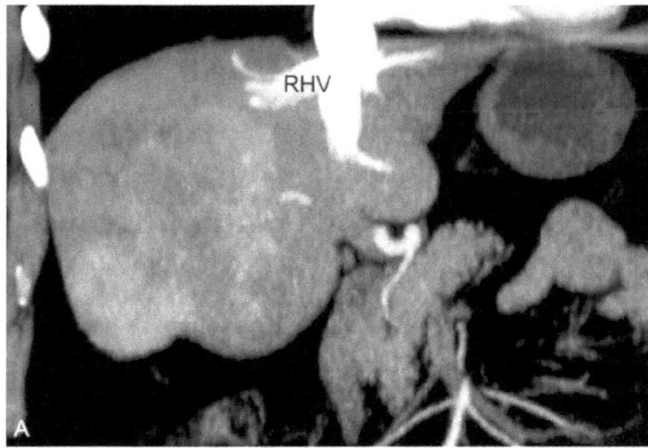

Figure 23A: Coronal CT image of the liver showing a large enhancing mass (arrow) occupying most of the right lobe. Percutaneous biopsy proved a diagnosis of hepatocellular carcinoma. Right Hepatic Vein (RHV).

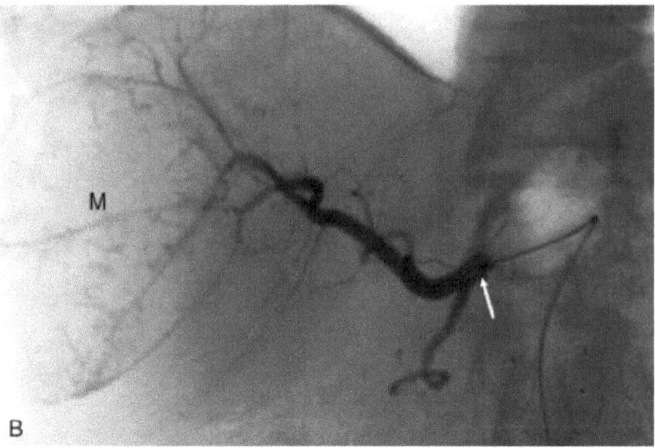

Figure 23B: Hepatic arteriogram (arrow) image performed during trans-arterial chemoembolization (TACE) shows the large mass (M) in the right lobe with tumor blush and displaced hepatic arterial branches. Cisplatin, mitomycin, and doxorubicin admixed with ethiodol was injected followed by polyvinyl alcohol particles.

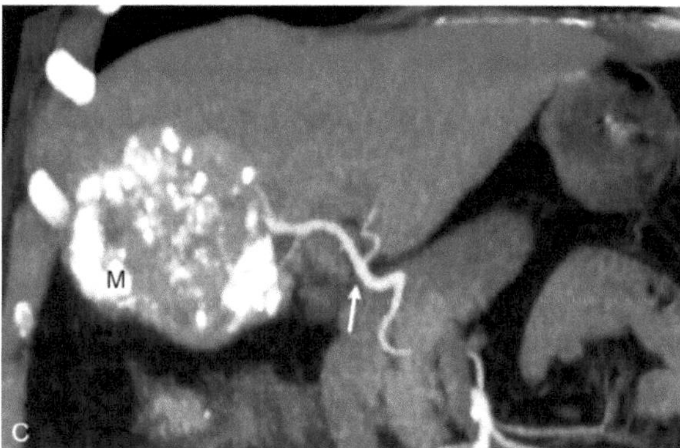

Figure 23C: Coronal CT image, one month following TACE shows significant reduction in the ethiodol stained mass (M) with compensatory hypertrophy of the unaffected left lobe. Note preserved main hepatic arterial supply (arrow).

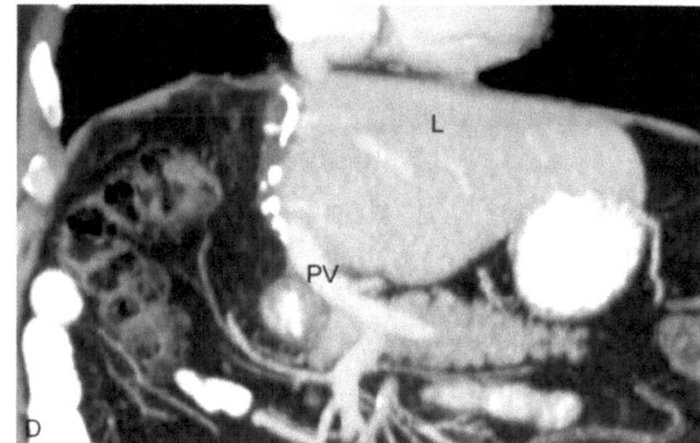

Figure 23D: Coronal CT image post right hepatectomy showing a normal appearing hypertrophied left lobe liver (L), and patent main and left portal venous system (PV).

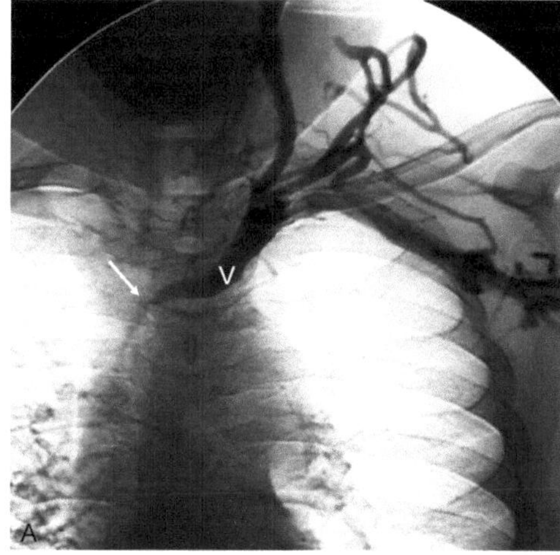

Figure 24A: Central venogram of the chest from left brachial vein percutaneous access in a patient with left arm and facial swelling due to superior vena cava (SVC) syndrome. Occlusion at the upper SVC (arrow) and medial left brachiocephalic vein (V) seen with multiple venous collaterals in the left upper chest and neck.

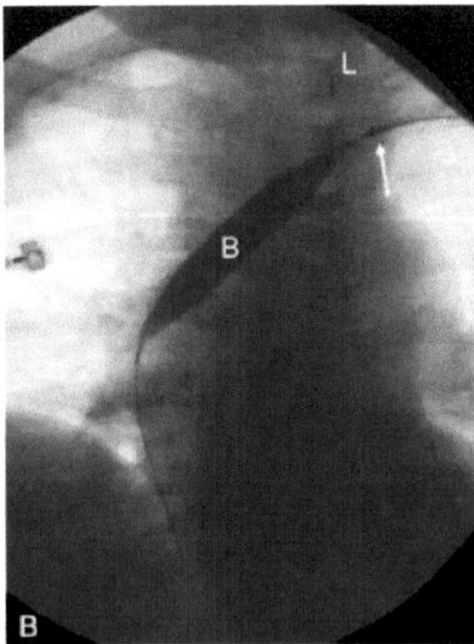

Figure 24B: Fluoroscopic image during large diameter (12 to 16 mm) percutaneous transluminal balloon (B) angioplasty of the occlusion following guidewire crossing via a vascular sheath (arrow).

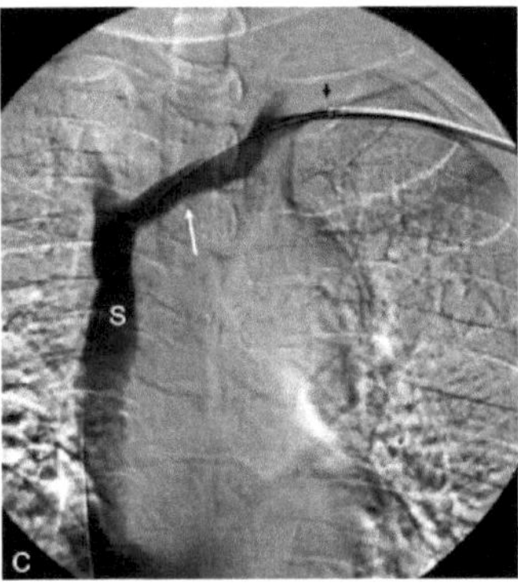

Figure 24C: Postintervention venogram via sheath (arrowhead) injection shows patent left brachiocephalic vein with stent (arrow) and patent superior vena cava (S).

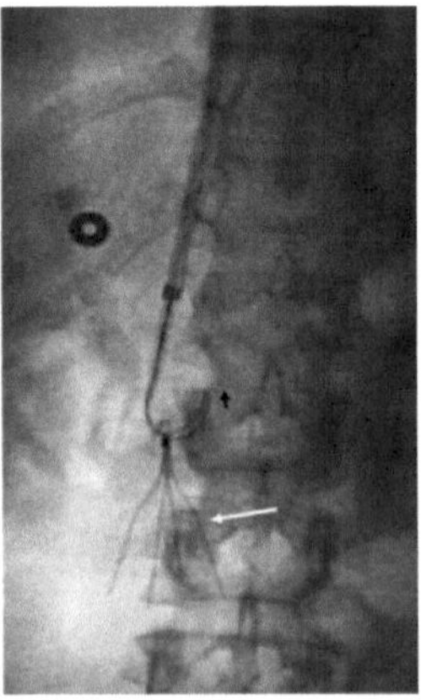

Figure 25: Fluoroscopic image of an inferior vena cava filter (arrow) in a patient with lower extremity deep venous thrombosis and a short-term indication to stop anticoagulation to undergo major surgery for gynecological malignancy. The filter was retrieved via percutaneous snare (arrowhead) following successful recovery from surgery and resuming anticoagulation.

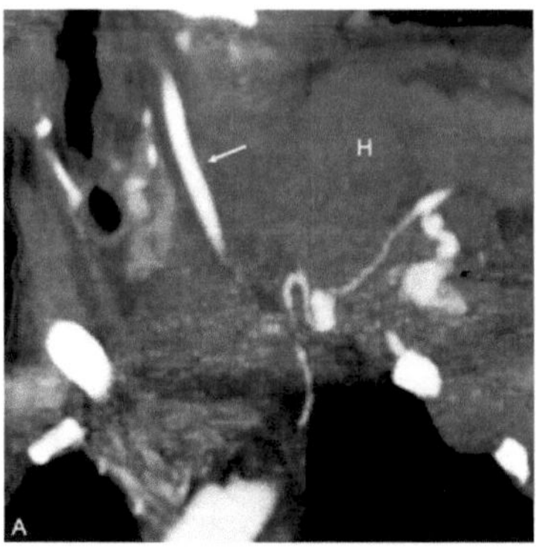

Figure 26A: Coronal CT angiogram reconstructed image of the left upper chest and neck in a stab injury showing large displacing hematoma (H) arising from laceration of the left subclavian artery branches (arrowhead). Patent left common carotid artery (arrow).

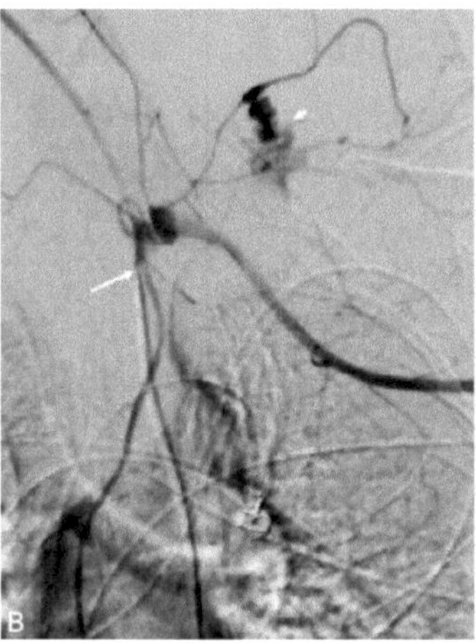

Figure 26B: Emergent arteriogram of the left subclavian artery (arrow) showing patent left vertebral and left internal mammary artery. Active bleeding (arrowhead) with extravasating contrast seen from costo-cervical branch.

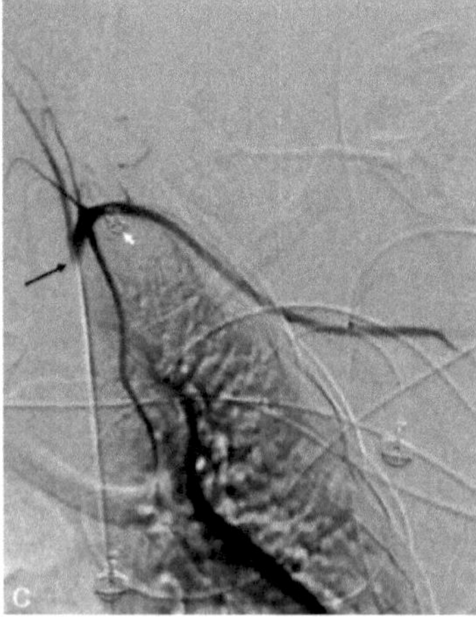

Figure 26C: Post-coil embolization (arrowhead) arteriogram of the left subclavian artery (arrow) following successful treatment of the bleeder.

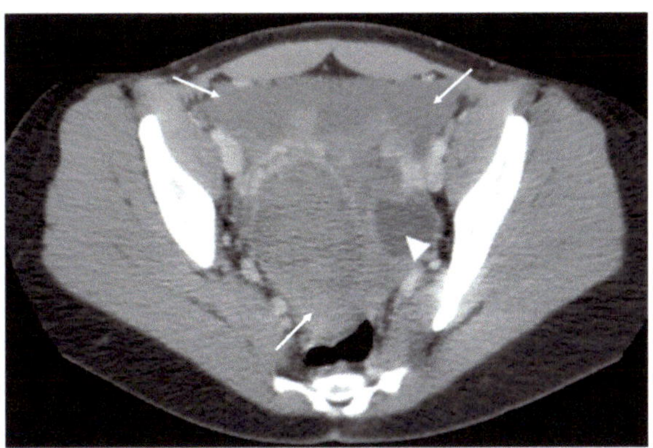

Figure 27: CT pelvis axial image in a 25-year-old female with history of blunt trauma showing high density free fluid (arrows} consistent with hemorrhage. Low density ovarian cyst (arrowhead) noted on the left side.

Retrievable vena cava filters placed for high thromboembolic risk surgical patients can be later removed once the patient can be anticoagulated or they no longer need caval filtration. Common conditions, such as symptomatic varicose veins in the lower extremity, can be sclerosed with a percutaneous endogenous laser or a radiofrequency technique. Varicocele causing infertility or scrotal pain can be embolized via percutaneous transvenous access with sclerosing agents or coils.

The role of interventional radiology in trauma deserves special mention as clinical and radiological assessment of injured patients can help triage them into appropriate management pathways. Significant injury to solid viscera such as the liver, spleen, or kidney can now be treated with interventional radiology embolic techniques and avoid the need of a laparotomy. There is an emerging role of endograft for thoracic aortic injuries. Other specific sites such as bleeding from a pelvic fracture, intercostal or epigastric arterial bleeding, etc. can be selectively or sub-selectively embolized using percutaneous trans-arterial catheters with embolic material such as gel foam, coils, or polyvinyl alcohol particles. Bleeding from high-risk areas such as epistaxis or neck injuries can be effectively treated with percutaneous transcatheter embolization as seen in Figures 26A to 26C.

SUMMARY

Interventional radiology offers a wide variety of procedures based on innovations and the continual development of minimally invasive techniques over the past 35 years. Currently many disease conditions have the option of benefiting from interventional radiology interventions for both the presurgical and postsurgical management of patients. The best patient outcome requires close cooperation between the interventional radiologist and the surgeon in order to select the most appropriate form of treatment. Current data, availability, and best evidence should factor in the decision making of optimizing patient care.

REFERENCES

1. Kandarpa K, Aruny JE. Handbook of Interventional Radiologic Procedures, 2002.
2. Kaufman JA, Lee MJ. Vascular and Interventional Radiology: The Requisites, 2004.

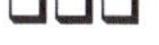

10

CHAPTER

Surgical Infections

Puja Van Epps, MD
Gopala K. Yadavalli, MD

1.1 INTRODUCTION

Joseph Lister revolutionized the surgical landscape and gave birth to the modern surgical era with his use of carbolic acid to reduce germs and subsequently refining the use of aseptic principles in surgery. Over 140 years later, despite the widespread use of antisepsis and modern antimicrobials, surgeons cannot escape the need to not only be aware of surgical infections, but also to know how to treat them and continue their efforts to reduce these infections.

Surgical infections can be categorized into two main groups: infections that occur postoperatively in a surgical site and infections that require surgical treatment. Of these, surgical site infections (SSI) are a major cause of morbidity and mortality around the world.[1] In 1999, the Center for Disease Control and Prevention (CDC) reported that between 14% to 16% of all nosocomial infections were related to surgical sites, making SSIs the third most common type of nosocomial infection.[2] Similarly, most studies report a comparable impact on the Indian healthcare system. Reported rates of SSIs in Indian hospitals have varied from 3% to 40%.[3,4]

Staphylococcus aureus remains the most common isolated surgical wound in India and around the world. A growing proportion of these isolates are methicillin-resistant *S. aureus* (MRSA), which is of concern due to its impact on morbidity and mortality.[5] Surgical patients are not immune to the emergence of virulent and resistant strains of bacteria, viruses, and fungi. With the ubiquitous use of antibiotics and the increasing complexity of patients including immunosuppressed patients, surgeons must become familiar with both basic knowledge as well as new challenges that are arising in the practice of infectious diseases in surgical patients. This chapter will include a discussion on the setting of infection, its immune basis, host factors, common infections and pathogens encountered in surgical patients, their management, and the role of infection control.

INFLAMMATION AND THE IMMUNE BASIS OF INFECTION

Surgical intervention is associated with disruption of barrier defenses and with acquired lesions in innate and adaptive immunity.[6] Incisions, placement of indwelling catheters, and implantation of hardware can facilitate entry of microorganisms and allow establishment of infection in the early postoperative period. An extensive study of patients undergoing accidental trauma, thermal burns, and significant surgical intervention has demonstrated that immunosuppression is a common feature in these individuals.[7,9] Deactivation of monocytes and depletion of circulating dendritic cells has been observed in cardiac and non-cardiac surgery settings.[10] Impairment of cytokine secretion is an immunological hallmark of surgical injury and can involve both innate (e.g., NK cell) and adaptive (e.g., T cell) pathways. The use of extracorporeal circulation (e.g., cardiopulmonary bypass) and corticosteroids intra- and perioperatively can further exacerbate these immune defects.[11]

HOST FACTORS

Microorganisms contaminate virtually all surgical wounds, but only a minority of them cause disease. The development of infection depends on the interplay between the immune system of the host, procedure related risk factors, as well as the microbe and its ability to adhere to and invade the host tissue. A number of host factors can increase the patient's risk of developing an infection, including diabetes, malnutrition, malignancy, hypoxemia, immunosuppression due to transplantation, and hypothermia. In surgical patients with the above risk factors or other states of immunodeficiency, care must be taken to correct or control the underlying condition to prevent wound infection.

Diabetes is a known risk factor for impaired wound healing and increased infections. It is thought to be a result of both long-term effect of diabetes on macro and microvasculature as well as impaired functioning of complement and antibodies due to hyperglycemia in the acute setting. Hyperglycemia in post-surgical patients has been shown to be associated with an increased rate of SSIs. Recent evidence suggests that tight glucose control in the preoperative period, even in non-diabetics, is associated with a reduced frequency of infections.[12] Optimizing nutritional status in the perioperative period may also reduce the risk of infection. Low serum albumin levels have been associated with increased rates of infections. In a 2006 meta-analysis looking at 17 trials studying the use of specialized nutritional support with immune-modulating nutrients in the pre-, peri-, and postperative settings, it was found that improving the nutritional status was associated with a 39% to 61% reduction in infectious complications.[13]

Although it is presumed that increased oxygen availability is a positive host factor in terms of reducing infection, studies on the use of supplemental oxygen in surgical patients have been conflicting. While initial studies on patients undergoing colon surgery indicated a 50% reduction in SSIs in patients receiving 80% supplemental oxygen compared to 30%,[14] recent data by Pryor and colleagues suggests there are much higher rates of infection in patients receiving high FiO 2 in the perioperative setting.[15] Currently, the use of supplemental oxygen is recommended with the goal of maintaining adequate oxygenation and not to provide hyperoxia.

MICROBIOLOGY

Surgical site infections

SSIs by definition is an infection that occurs at any site related to and after a surgical procedure. As discussed above, the impact of SSIs on healthcare in both the resource-limited and well-resourced nations is far reaching. An Indian study looking at 1,125 surgeries, showed that not only was there an almost two-fold increase in expenditures associated with SSIs, but the rate of mortality was also higher at 12.8% in patients who developed SSIs compared to 3.8% in those who did not.[16] SSIs are categorized based on the anatomic level of infection as seen in Table 1.

The risk of wound infection is in part determined by the degree of contamination present in a wound. Surgical wounds are classically divided into (1) clean, (2) clean, contaminated, (3) contaminated, and (4) dirty. Risk of infections, as predicted by the National Nosocomial Infection Surveillance (NNIS) score is directly related to, but not limited to, the degree of contamination.[2] The ranges of infection rates are around 3% to 5% for clean wounds, and upward of 27% for dirty wounds.[4] The risk factors for developing an SSI are listed in Table 2.

Table 1: Surgical site infections: categorized based on the anatomic level of infection

Incisional
Superficial: infection of the skin or the subcutaneous tissue
Deep: deeper infection involving the tissue beneath the superficial layer, fascia, and muscles
Organ/space
Infection involving any part of the body manipulated during a surgical procedure other than the body wall

Table 2: Risk factors for surgical site infections

Patient Factors	Procedure related
Diabetes/hyperglycemia	Recent or prolonged hospitalization
Age	Wound class
Malnutrition	Preoperative shaving
Malignancy	Contamination of operating room/personnel
Steroid or other immunosuppressive use	Prolonged hypotension
Prior contamination, colonization, or infection	Improper antimicrobial prophylaxis
Cigarettes smoking	Poor postoperative wound care

Surgical wound infections typically present within the first or second week of surgery. Patients may complain of pain at the surgical site or may simply present with postoperative fever. The key is to thoroughly inspect the wound for signs of inflammation including edema, erythema, and abscess formation. Presence of fluctuance, tenderness, or purulence may indicate subcutaneous tissue infection. Deep space infections in the absence of superficial signs can be more challenging to diagnose. In such cases, imaging such as CT scan, if available, may be necessary. The definitive treatment of an established SSI is drainage and wound debridement. Culture of the site should be performed to identify the etiology and aid in the proper antibiotic selection.

The microbiology of surgical infections is typically polymicrobial and isolates are increasingly resistant to commonly used antibiotics. In a study of 117 surgical infections, between 67% to 80% of non-abscess related infections were polymicrobial.[17] According to much of the published data, *S. aureus* is the most commonly isolated microorganism in the Indian setting. Rates of MRSA range from 20% to 40% in various studies done in India looking at SSIs.[3,5] Other gram-positive bacteria of clinical importance are coagulase-negative *Staphylococci*, *Enterococcus sp.* and *Streptococcus sp.* The most common gram-negative isolates are *Pseudomonas aeruginosa*, *E. coli*, and *Klebsiella sp. Bacteroides fragilis*, *Peptostreptococcus*, and *Clostridium sp.* are important anaerobes that cause disease in surgical patients. The antibiotic management of these infections will be discussed later in this chapter.

Community Acquired Infections

Infections requiring surgical treatment are also an important category of infections that surgeons need to be aware of when assessing a patient. These include skin and soft tissue infections (SSTIs), cutaneous abscesses, and intra abdominal infections. There will also be a brief discussion on tetanus in this section.

SSTIs range from cellulitis to diffuse necrotizing infections, including fasciitis and myositis. Most superficial skin infections are easily treated with wound care and antibiotics. However, infections involving deeper layers of tissue, including muscle and fascia can cause systemic illness and prove to be rapidly fatal. These infections generally require aggressive surgical debridement along with antimicrobials. Cellulitis is easily diagnosed based on clinical findings, which include localized erythema, tenderness, and edema. Risk factors for developing cellulitis include diabetic neuropathy, peripheral vascular disease, and alcoholism among others. *Staphylococcus sp.* and *Streptococcus sp.* are the most commonly implicated infections, and gram-negative bacilli play an important role in immunocompromised or hospitalized patients. In a large study at the All-India Medical Institute of Medicine Sciences, researchers looked at over 5,000 samples from SSTIs. *S. aureus* was found to be the most common isolate.[18] MRSA was found to be over 38% of isolates. Additionally, over 66% of gram-negative isolates were extended-spectrum beta-lactamase producers. On the other hand, necrotizing infections can be difficult to diagnose, and they spread rapidly. Clinical findings can include the presence of cellulitis, open wounds, necrotic tissue, intense pain, crepitus, and signs of systemic illness including fever, tachycardia, or hypotension. Plain film may reveal the presence of gas in an extremity. *Clostridium perfringens* causes necrotizing cellulitis as well as myositis or myonecrosis, often termed as gas gangrene. The organism usually enters open wounds from contaminated soil. As soon as this diagnosis is suspected, radical tissue-saving debridement should be performed. Non-clostridial infections include necrotizing fasciitis and can be either due to mixed, synergistic flora from the peritoneum or perineum, or caused by Group A *Streptococci*. Although both gangrene and fasciitis require surgical treatment, an important distinction is that fasciitis often only requires removal of dead skin and fascia, and it generally does not require amputation. In terms of antimicrobial therapy, broad-spectrum antibiotics are usually clinically indicated. Coverage should include activity against gram-negative, gram-positive, and anaerobic bacteria.

The mainstay treatment for a subcutaneous abscess is drainage of the infected area. Abscess formation is characterized by an infectious process resulting in necrotic tissue composed of dead or dying cell components and bacteria. Clinically this presents as localized tenderness and signs of inflammation. Treatment requires drainage of the pus. Furuncles usually begin in infected hair follicles or skin glands. These are the most common type of surgical infection and typically only require incision and drainage. Carbuncles occur when an infection of furuncles spreads through the subcutaneous tissue resulting in multiple connecting tunnels. This gives the appearance of multiple small openings in the skin, usually draining pus. These not only require adequate drainage and often excision of sinus tracts, but also require antibiotics with coverage against *Staphylococcus sp.* and *Streptococcus sp.* Hidradenitis suppurativa is abscess formation within apocrine sweat glands. Treatment varies depending on the extent of infection. It can range from draining individual abscess, to excising and grafting large, affected areas. Perirectal abscesses result from infection of the crypts of the anorectal canal. These can extend into the pelvis as well as the genitourinary tract and can cause significant morbidity in immunocompromised patients. These require adequate drainage and antibiotic coverage against gram-negative and gram-positive organisms. Lastly, diabetic foot ulcers or abscesses typically result from repetitive injury to compromised tissue. These are also typically mixed flora infections and require both debridement and excision of dead tissue including bones. Osteomyelitis is a common complication of foot infections and should be evaluated in any patient presenting with a diabetic foot ulcer.

Tetanus

Despite being a largely vaccine-preventable illness, tetanus continues to cause havoc in the developing world. There are 1,000,000 cases of tetanus per year worldwide and about 300,000 deaths as a result.[17] Clostridium tetani gains entry through contaminated wounds and infects the nervous system.

Tetanus is a clinical diagnosis, as confirmatory tests are not usually available. Although the mean incubation period is seven days, tetanus can occur in one day to several months postexposure. Once the diagnosis is suspected, the mainstay therapy is neutralization of the toxin with tetanus immunoglobulin, proper wound management, and IV antibiotics. Immunization recommendations for tetanus are listed in Table 4.

Intra-abdominal and/or retroperitoneal abscesses can carry with them a significant amount of morbidity and mortality. Aside from some specific exceptions, most of these infections usually require percutaneous drainage. Patients with these infections typically present with systemic signs of illness including fever, abdominal pain, and sepsis or frank shock. Diagnosis often requires imaging such as a CT scan or abdominal ultrasound. Infections that do not typically require surgical intervention are spontaneous bacterial peritonitis, salpingitis, diverticulitis for the first two to three episodes, and amebic liver abscesses. Most of the remaining intra-abdominal infections not only require empiric antibiotic coverage against gram-negatives and anaerobic bacteria, but also need surgical debridement or drainage. The key to treating these infections is source control that can only be effectively achieved in the operative setting. The etiology of these infections can often be polymicrobial. The fluid or tissue obtained in the operating room must be sent for culture to determine the exact organism for targeted therapy.

Postoperative fever

Hospital acquired infections in surgical patients are an important component of this discussion. Although fever is a common occurrence in the postoperative setting, not all fevers are infectious in nature and not all infections will result in a fever. It is helpful to think of the 5 "W's" when trying to determine the cause of a postoperative fever as seen in Table 3.

The most frequent non-surgical infections in this setting are urinary tract infections, pneumonia, and invasive catheter related infections. The diagnosis is usually through the physical exam, culture, and laboratory data or plain film of the chest. Empiric antibiotic coverage should be based upon the suspected site of infection, common pathogens, and drug resistance data at each individual institution. If the initial investigation is negative, further imaging with a CT or MRI of the operative site may be indicated. Abdominal ultrasound is a less costly alternative to CT when an abscess is suspected. The likelihood of an SSI increases the longer the postoperative fever remains undiagnosed. The key is to promptly determine the need for surgical intervention, including debridement, drainage, and/or removal of hardware. In the era of frequent antibiotic use, *C. difficile* colitis is an important emerging infection in both surgical and medical patients. A surgical patient presenting with diarrhea, abdominal pain, fever, or leukocytosis should be started on empiric coverage against *C. difficile* with metronidazole and, where available, a stool sample should be sent for toxin or antigen testing.

Table 3: 5 "W's": determine the cause of a postoperative fever

Wind	Water	Wound	Walk	Wonder drugs
Pneumonia Pulmonary embolus Atelectasis	Urinary tract infection	Surgical site infection Infected hardware/ catheter	Deep venous throm-bosis	Drug fever Trans-fusion related fever

Table 4: Tetanus immunization: quick review

Indication	Immunization/prophylaxis
Routine adult immunization	Td 0.5 mL every 10 years
Clean Minor Wounds	
Unknown or incomplete immunization	Td 0.5 mL, no TIG needed
Complete immunization	No Td or TIG needed
Tetanus Prone Wounds	
Unknown or incomplete immunization	Td 0.5 mL and 250 units TIG given IM
Complete immunization	Td 0.5 mL (unless last dose <5 years ago)

Td = adult tetanus-diphtheria vaccine; TIG = tetanus immune globulin

MANAGEMENT OF SURGICAL INFECTIONS

The decision to initiate antimicrobial therapy in a patient depends on several factors, including the clinical condition of the patient, the presumed identity of the pathogen, and the site of suspected infection. The goal of therapy is to achieve control of the infection so that host defenses can clear it. Achieving this goal not only depends on the choice of antimicrobial but also on the ability to exceed the minimum inhibitory concentration of the antibiotic at the site of infection against suspected or proven pathogens. Table 5 lists some common infections encountered in surgical patients and suspected pathogens. Once empiric antibiotics have been initiated, the key is to observe for a therapeutic response in the patient and follow the appropriate cultures for identification and sensitivity patterns. Failure to respond to therapy could be due to a variety of reasons including inappropriate initial choice, inadequate levels of antibiotics, presence of a secondary infection, failure to adequately drain a pocket of infection, or development of drug resistance. Antimicrobial drug resistance is a major concern for medical and surgical patients alike. Antimicrobial drug resistance in the Indian healthcare settings is rising steadily, including the spread of extended spectrum beta-lactamase and carbapenems producing organisms.[18]

In a study looking at surgical infections in northern India, between 22% to 53% of gram-negative isolates were multidrug-resistant.[17] Overuse of antimicrobial therapy has repeatedly been implicated in the spread of these drug resistant bacteria. The judicious use of antibiotics not only involves the appropriate choice of agent but also the duration of treatment. Infection control strategies such as strict hand washing between patient interactions and contact precautions also play a critical role in minimizing the development of multidrug-resistant organisms.

Fungal infections are an increasing cause of morbidity in surgical patients. *Candida sp.*, especially *C. albicans*, are the most commonly identified fungal pathogens. While the recovery of *Candida sp.* from open wounds or sputum usually reflects colonization rather than true infection, fungemia or intra-abdominal fungal abscesses almost always represent an invasive infection and warrant therapy. Amphotericin B is the most commonly used antifungal; however, due to its toxicity careful dosing is required. Lipid-complex or liposomal preparations of amphotericin B are generally better tolerated than conventional, deoxycholate preparations, but are considerably more costly, limiting their utility for many patients. Fluconazole is the appropriate antibiotic choice for *C. albicans* infections, however non- *C. albicans* species such as *C. glabrata, C. krusei,* and fungi are exhibiting increased levels of resistance to fluconazole and require therapy with an alternate antifungal such as voriconazole or caspofungin. The selection of the appropriate antimicrobial therapy for resistant pathogens, both bacterial and fungal, is best done in close consultation with a clinical microbiologist and, if available, a clinical infectious disease specialist.

Infection Control

While most risk factors for the development of infection cannot be eliminated, there is abundant data to suggest that perioperative antisepsis practices as well as antimicrobial prophylaxis reduces the risk of surgical infections. Although various sources of potential bacterial contamination of a surgical wound exist, including operating room staff and poor air quality, the patient's endogenous flora is believed to be the major source of infection. For instance, nasal colonization of patients with *S. aureus* is believed to be a risk factor for the development of postoperative infection. The data on the routine use of topical mupirocin to reduce this risk, however, has been conflicting. There have been several studies showing a reduction in *S aureus* with the use of mupirocin; however, a randomized controlled trial involving around four thousand patients failed to show a significant decrease in *Staphylococcal* SSIs.[19] Additionally, there has been concern regarding the development of mupirocin resistance in *S. aureus* when used routinely.

Table 5: Common pathogens for various sites

Site of Infection	Suspected Pathogen
Skin/soft tissue	Staphylococcus, streptococcus
Gas gangrene	Clostridium
Biliary tract infections	E. coli, Klebsiella, Enterococcus
Peritonitis/intra-abdominal abscess	E. coli, Pseudomonas, anaerobes
Hospital acquired colitis	Clostridium difficile
Urinary tract infection	E. coli, Klebsiella
Hospital acquired pneumonia	Staphylococcus (suspect MRSA), Pseudomonas, Klebsiella, Acinetobacter
Catheter related infection, Infection control	Staphylococcus, Enterobacteriaceae

However, preparation of the operative site using antiseptic agents is not a matter of debate. The site should be prepped with a thorough wash to remove any visible contaminants followed by the application of an antiseptic agent for disinfection. These agents have evolved since Lister's carbolic acid, with alcohol or iodine containing products being among the most inexpensive and readily available. Chlorhexidine gluconate has greater antimicrobial activity when compared to these products, but it may not be readily available in resource limited settings. There have been numerous studies showing an increased risk of SSIs with preoperative shaving. And despite CDC recommendations against shaving with a razor, this practice remains ubiquitous. It is believed that the nicks and cuts caused by a razor mobilize the patient's endogenous flora and can result in infection. If hair needs to be removed, it is recommended to use electric hair clippers immediately before the operation. In a large 10-year study, the risk of infections was the highest when hair was removed using a razor (2.5%), as compared to electric clipper (1.4%) or no hair removal (0.9%).[20]

Preoperative antisepsis of surgical team members is also a key component in reducing surgical infections. Using surgical hand scrubs is a well-established practice across the world. Alcohol based products are the most commonly used germicidal agents in Europe and the developing world. An effective hand scrub should be about 2 to 3 minutes long and does not have to involve scrubbing with a brush.[21] Nails should be kept short to avoid colonization and achieve proper bacterial load reduction during scrubbing. Aside from these, universal precautions to maintain sterility should be maintained throughout the operation. The operating room should be a controlled environment with proper ventilation, sterilized instruments, as well as proper surgical attire that reduces bacterial shedding during a procedure.

Antimicrobial Prophylaxis

Antimicrobial prophylaxis refers to a short course of antibiotics given in the pre-operative (one hour before incision) and peri-operative (24 hours after surgery) setting, to reduce the risk of SSIs. The principle behind the use of prophylaxis is to eliminate, or at least reduce, the bacterial load that may be inoculated into the surgical wound at the time of the surgery. Despite the presence of evidence and proper guidelines for the use of antimicrobial prophylaxis, numerous studies have shown improper timing and choice of antibiotic usage in India.[22] A 2006 study looking at challenges in adherence to guidelines of antimicrobial prophylaxis identified a lack of familiarity as the number one barrier to proper antimicrobial use in this setting.[23] As the study discusses, there are several areas of improvement when it comes to this issue in the Indian setting.

Cephalosporins are the mainstay of prophylaxis when it comes to surgical procedures. Which also means that there is an increasing prevalence of resistant organisms, the most concerning of which is *S. aureus*. As mentioned previously, this is the most commonly isolated organism in surgical infections, and the incidence of MRSA, including cephalosporin-resistant staphylococci, has increased between 30% to 40% in the Indian setting.[5] Additionally, the incidence of multidrug-resistant gram-negative bacilli, and resistant fungal pathogens is also on the rise. There is an urgency to realize the prevalence of fungal infections in the Indian setting. The timing of antibiotic administration is also important. Generally, the initial dose of antibiotics should be at the onset of the procedure. For long surgical procedures, antibiotics may have to be redosed to achieve adequate levels during the procedure. The duration of prophylaxis remains up for debate. There have been studies leaning both ways when it comes to short versus long courses of antibiotics. Currently, a first-generation cephalosporin such as cefazolin is recommended for most procedures. In abdominal surgeries, where there is a risk of a ruptured viscous, addition of an aminoglycoside such as gentamicin or clindamycin is often warranted. Metronidazole in combination with cephalosporin is also occasionally used. In surgeries where there is a high risk of MRSA infection, vancomycin may be considered. It should be noted that because of the aforementioned issues, these recommendations will not remain static.

REFERENCES

1. Kirkland KB, Briggs JP, Trivette SL, Wilkinson WE, Sexton DJ. The impact of surgical-site infections in the 1990s: attributable mortality, excess length of hospitalization, and extra costs. Infect Control Hosp Epidemiol 1999;20:725-30.
2. National Nosocomial Infections Surveillance (NNIS) System report, data summary from January 1990-May 1999, issued June 1999. Am J Infect Control 1999;27:520-32.
3. Kamat U, Ferreira A, Savio R, Motghare D. Antimicrobial resistance among nosocomial isolates in a teaching hospital in goa. Indian J Community Med 2008;33:89-92.
4. Lilani SP, Jangale N, Chowdhary A, Daver GB. Surgical site infection in clean and clean-contaminated cases. Indian J Med Microbiol 2005;23:249-52.
5. Kownhar H, Shankar EM, Vignesh R, Sekar R, Velu V, Rao UA. High isolation rate of Staphylococcus aureus from surgical site infections in an Indian hospital. J Antimicrob Chemother 2008;61:758-60.
6. Yadavalli GK, Auletta JJ, Gould MP, Salata RA, Lee JH, Heinzel FP. Deactivation of the innate cellular immune response following endotoxic and surgical injury. Exp Mol Pathol 2001;71:209-21.
7. Hershman MJ, Cheadle WG, Appel SH, et al. Comparison of antibody response with delayed hypersensitivity in severely injured patients. Arch Surg 1989;124:339-41.
8. Livingston DH, Appel SH, Wellhausen SR, Sonnenfeld G, Polk HC, Jr. Depressed interferon gamma production and monocyte HLA-DR expression after severe injury. Arch Surg 1988;123:1309-12.
9. Polk HC Jr., George CD, Wellhausen SR, et al. A systematic study of host defense processes in badly injured patients. Ann Surg 1986;204:282-99.
10. Yadavalli GK, Chien JW, Wener KM, et al. Interleukin 12 and interferon-gamma synthetic deficiency is associated with dendritic cell cytopenia after cardiac surgery. Shock 2005;24:26-33.
11. Butler J, Rocker GM, Westaby S. Inflammatory response to cardiopulmonary bypass. Ann Thorac Surg 1993;55:552-9.
12. Van den Berghe G. Insulin therapy for the critically ill patient. Clin Cornerstone 2003;5:56-63.
13. Waitzberg DL, Saito H, Plank LD, et al. Postsurgical infections are reduced with specialized nutrition support. World J Surg 2006;30:1592-604.
14. Greif R, Akca O, Horn EP, Kurz A, Sessler DI. Supplemental perioperative oxygen to reduce the incidence of surgical-wound infection. Outcomes Research Group. N Engl J Med 2000;342:161-7.
15. Pryor KO, Fahey TJ the 3rd, Lien CA, Goldstein PA. Surgical site infection and the routine use of perioperative hyperoxia in a general surgical population: a randomized controlled trial. Jama 2004;291:79-87.
16. Suchitra JB, Lakshmidevi N. Surgical site infections: Assessing risk factors, outcomes and antimicrobial sensitivity patterns. African J Microb Res 2009;3:175-179.
17. Saini S, Gupta N, Aparna, Lokveer, Griwan MS. Surgical infections: a microbiological study. Braz J Infect Dis 2004;8:118-25.
18. Mohanty S, Kapil A, Dhawan B, Das BK. Bacteriological and antimicrobial susceptibility profile of soft tissue infections from Northern India. Indian J Med Sci 2004;58:10-5.

19. Kalmeijer MD, Coertjens H, van Nieuwland-Bollen PM, et al. Surgical site infections in orthopedic surgery: the effect of mupirocin nasal ointment in a double-blind, randomized, placebo-controlled study. Clin Infect Dis 2002;35:353-8.
20. Tanner J, Woodings D, Moncaster K. Preoperative hair removal to reduce surgical site infection. Cochrane Database Syst Rev 2006;3:CD004122.
21. Loeb MB, Wilcox L, Smaill F, Walter S, Duff Z. A randomized trial of surgical scrubbing with a brush compared to antiseptic soap alone. Am J Infect Control 1997;25:11-5.
22. Srishyla MV, Rani MA, Damodar S, Venkataraman BV, Jairam N. A preliminary audit of practice—antibacterial prophylaxis in general surgery in an Indian hospital setting. Indian J Physiol Pharmacol 1994;38:207-10.
23. Khan SA, Rodrigues G, Kumar P, Rao PG. Current challenges in adherence to clinical guidelines for antibiotic prophylaxis in surgery. J Coll Physicians Surg Pak 2006;16:435-7.

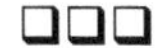

11

CHAPTER

Treatment of Surgical Infections

Asha Shah, MD
Vijay K. Mittal, MD, FACS

SURGICAL INFECTION

The human body has several barriers that protect against infection including the skin, immunoglobulin A in the respiratory tract, the acidic pH of the stomach, and the normal gut flora. When these barriers are violated, infection can set in. And although many situations can be managed conservatively, there are instances in which surgical intervention is required. An understanding of specific infections that require surgical intervention, infections due to surgery, and antimicrobial therapy is resourceful for all surgeons.

DISEASE SPECIFIC INFECTIONS

INTRA-ABDOMINAL INFECTION

Peritonitis is inflammation of the mesenchymal cell lining of the abdominal cavity. Primary peritonitis occurs in the absence of a definitive intra-abdominal source. Rather, the process occurs due to hematogenous or lymphatic spread of microorganisms including *S. pneumonia*, *E. coli*, and *K. pneumonia* among many other organisms. Primary peritonitis is monomicrobial in nature and it is rare to require surgical intervention. Primary peritonitis most commonly occurs in cirrhotic patients with ascites. Low serum sodium levels, Child-Pugh stage C, and elevated polymorphonuclear neutrophilic leukocyte (PMN) counts in ascitic fluid are considered independent risk factors.[1] The clinical presentation is variable amongst patients, some present with asymptomatic ascites and others having abdominal pain, fever, and leukocytosis. The diagnosis is established by performing paracentesis with both microbial and cytological evaluation of the ascitic fluid. Again, primary peritonitis will most often exhibit single morphotype on gram stain and culture and have PMN counts greater than 250 cells/mL. In addition to paracentesis, patients suspected of having bacterial peritonitis should have blood and urine cultures. Treatment of primary peritonitis should be initiated immediately upon presentation to optimize patient outcome. Ideally, antimicrobial therapy should begin after ascitic fluid has been obtained for analysis. Most studies suggest broad-spectrum coverage with third generation cephalosporin until cultures finalize. Suggested regimens include Cefotaxime administered 2g IV every 8 hours, Ceftriaxone 1g IV every 12 hours, or 2g every 24 hours for a total of 5 days.[2,3]

Secondary peritonitis is more common than primary peritonitis and is due to perforation of the bowel due to a neoplasm, infection, or other intra-abdominal infectious pathology including appendicitis, diverticulitis, and several other entities. Although different microbes will be implicated with a perforated gastric ulcer versus a perforated colon pathology, broad-spectrum antibiotics covering both aerobes and anaerobes should be initiated until the etiology of peritonitis is established. Aside from broad-spectrum antimicrobial coverage, source control will be key in the management of secondary peritonitis.[4] Therefore, unlike in primary peritonitis, surgical management is usually indicated in secondary peritonitis.

There are different definitions for tertiary peritonitis throughout the literature.[71] Perhaps the most precise definition is that tertiary peritonitis is an intra-abdominal infection that persists or recurs 48 hours following adequate surgical source control of secondary peritonitis.[72] The most commonly implicated organisms include *Enterococcus, Candida, Staphylococcus epidermidis,* and *Enterobacter.*[73] Risk factors include old age, malnutrition, and immunosuppression. The diagnosis of tertiary peritonitis is often difficult and non-specific. Patients may display persistent leukocytosis, fever, or have an inadequate response to antimicrobial therapy.

Although, this may also be present in cases of inadequate source control in secondary peritonitis (i.e., missed bowel injury).[71] Management includes optimizing resuscitation and appropriate anti-microbial therapy. Intervention is not always in the form of surgery. For example, in the presence of intra-abdominal abscess, image guided drainage can be performed.

SKIN AND SOFT TISSUE INFECTIONS

Skin and soft tissue infections can range from mild to severe with selected cases requiring surgical intervention. Erysipelas and cellulitis are most commonly due to *Staph* and group A Strep species. These infections occur due to a break in the skin from a minor trauma, which allows bacteria to enter. Once diagnosed, antibiotic therapy is the mainstay of therapy and should be initiated promptly to prevent progression of infection to systemic manifestations. Cutaneous abscesses, carbuncles, and furuncles may require surgical incision and drainage if spontaneous drainage does not occur. The purulent fluid expelled should be sent for gram stain and culture. Mild cases can be managed with incision and drainage alone, whereas moderate and severe cases with presence of systemic inflammatory response syndrome (SIRS) will likely also require administration of antibiotics.[5]

Necrotizing soft tissue infections involving either the skin, subcutaneous tissue, fascia, or muscle, are perhaps the most clinically important for a surgeon to recognize, as the mortality rates are high if left untreated.[6] Risk factors include diabetes mellitus, immunosuppression due to chronic illness or steroid use, peripheral vascular disease, and renal failure. The most commonly affected areas include the extremities, perineum, and trunk. Patients may present with skin changes and pain out of proportion to exam findings. The diagnosis is usually based on clinical exam findings including skin discoloration, crepitus, and drainage of thin grayish, "dishwater" type fluid. Patients may also have systemic manifestations including fever, leukocytosis, hypotension, and tachycardia. Although not necessary, radiographic imaging can be undertaken in cases where the diagnosis in uncertain. Subcutaneous gas can be seen on plain films and air tracking through the soft tissues can be seen on computed tomography (CT) scan. These infections can be either polymicrobial or monomicrobial (e.g., group A strep, *P. aeruginosa*, or *C. perfringens*). Treatment should begin promptly with fluid resuscitation, blood glucose control, and the initiation of broad-spectrum antibiotics. For mixed infections, Piperacillin-Tazobactam (3.37g IV every 6-8 hours) plus Vancomycin (30mg/kg/d in two divided doses) is suggested. For monomicrobial group A Strep infection, penicillin (2-4 million units IV every 4-6 hours) plus Clindamycin (600-900 IV every 8 hours) is recommended.[5] Once the patient is adequately resuscitated, early surgical debridement is necessary. All devitalized tissue should be debrided, and the patient should be counseled that more than one debridement may be necessary. Once debridement is complete and the infection has cleared, negative pressure wound therapy can assist to facilitate wound closure, as large defects may be present.

POST-OPERATIVE INFECTIONS

In the early 90's the National Veterans Affair Surgical Risk Study (NVASRS) was undertaken to assess pre-operative risk factors with post-operative outcomes due to increased mortality seen in VA hospitals in the 1980's. Due to the success of this study, in 1994 the National Surgical Quality Improvement Program (NSQIP) was created to reduce the number of surgical complications. Currently, studies have shown that each year, the average participating hospital prevents 250 to 500 complications, saves 12 to 36 lives, and reduces costs by millions of dollars.[74]

SURGICAL SITE INFECTIONS

Surgical Site Infections (SSI) occur in 2% to 5% of patients undergoing an inpatient surgical procedure and impose a significant financial burden on the healthcare system.[7] The Centers for Disease Control (CDC) lists three basic categories based on depth of involvement which are (1) superficial incisional, in the skin and subcutaneous tissues, (2) deep incisional, penetrating to the muscle and fascia, and (3) organ and/or space. Surgical wounds are classified into four main classes based on the estimated bacterial load for that specific procedure.

Table 1: Surgical wound class

Wound Class	Example of surgical procedure
Class I (clean)	Breast biopsy, ventral hernia repair
Class II (clean-contam-inated)	Cholecystectomy, elective colectomy
Class III (contaminated)	Penetrating chest or abdominal trauma
Class IV (dirty)	Perforated viscus, necrotizing fasciitis (Figure X)

Pathogens involved can be both endogenous meaning the pathogen is patient related (i.e., skin flora or gut flora) and exogenous (i.e., surgical personnel, operating room equipment). The most commonly implicated pathogen is *Staphylococcus aureus*, others include coagulase negative staphylococci, enterococcus, and *E. coli.* The focus of SSI should be on prevention rather than treatment. Several measures have been studied to reduce the incidence of SSIs. Preoperative measures include clipping hair, skin prep in the operating room, and antimicrobial prophylaxis. Shaving or clipping hair the night before has been associated with higher incidences of SSIs than clipping hair the day of surgery. The use of depilatory agents may provide even greater benefit than clipping, however it is associated with adverse skin reactions in some patients. Several different antiseptic solutions are available for skin preparation in the operating room including povidone-iodine, alcohol-containing products, and chlorhexidine gluconate. Although each has its advantages and disadvantages, all agents should bc applied in circular motion starting at the proposed incision site. The Surgical Care Improvement Project (SCIP) was added in 2006 and is a national partnership of organizations that works to reduce surgical complications. The guidelines for antimicrobial prophylaxis include (1) administration of prophylactic antibiotic within one hour prior to incision and two hours for Vancomycin or Fluoroquinolones, (2) the appropriate selection of antibiotics based on the type of procedure, and (3) discontinuing all antibiotics within 24 hours of surgery end time and 48 hours for cardiac surgery patients because prolonged administration does not improve outcomes and can be responsible for *Clostridium difficile* infections.[8]

Table 2: Approved antibiotics for specific surgical procedures

Surgical Procedure	Approved Antibiotics (dose based off of patient's weight in kg)
Coronary Artery Bypass Graft or Other Cardiac Surgery or Vascular Surgery	Cefazolin, Vancomycin, or Cefuroxime If β-lactam allergy: Clindamycin or Vancomycin
Hip or Knee Arthroplasty	Cefazolin, Vancomycin, or Cefuroxime If β-lactam allergy: Clindamycin or Vancomycin
Colon Surgery	Cefotetan, Cefoxitin or Ampicillin/Sulbactam or Ertapenem Metronidazole + – Cefazolin or – Cefuroxime or – Ceftriaxone If β-lactam allergy: Clindamycin + – Aminoglycoside or – Quinolone or – Aztreonam or Metronidazole + – Aminoglycoside or – Quinolone
Abdominal Hysterectomy or Vaginal Hysterectomy	Cefazolin, Cefotetan, Cefoxitin or Cefuroxime or Ampicillin/Sulbactam If β-lactam allergy: Clindamycin + – Aminoglycoside or – Quinolone or – Aztreonam or Metronidazole + – Aminoglycoside or – Quinolone or Vancomycin + – Aminoglycoside or – Aztreonam or – Quinolone
Abdominal Hysterectomy with another Procedure Code of Colon Surgery or Vaginal Hysterectomy with an Other Procedure Code of Colon Surgery	Cefazolin, Cefotetan, or Cefoxitin or Cefuroxime or Ertapenem or Ampicillin/Sulbactam If β-lactam allergy: Clindamycin + – Aminoglycoside or – Quinolone or – Aztreonam or Metronidazole + – Aminoglycoside or – Quinolone or Vancomycin + – Aminoglycoside or – Aztreonam or – Quinolone

Regarding antimicrobial prophylaxis, it is important to re-dose the antibiotic at three-hour intervals for procedures lasting longer than three hours. Other measures to reduced SSIs includes maintaining normothermia immediately post-operative, control of blood glucose levels especially important for cardiac surgery patients, limiting operating room traffic, and maintaining sterile dressings post-operative for 24 to 48 hours.

PNEUMONIA

Post-operative pulmonary complications include pneumonia, unplanned intubation, and failure to wean from the ventilator as defined by the National Surgical Quality Improvement Program (NSQIP). The incidence of these pulmonary complications ranges from 2.7% to 4.4% for all patients undergoing noncardiac surgery,[9,10] specifically the incidence of post-operative pneumonia at academic NSQIP hospitals, which are hospitals with greater than 500 beds, ranges from 1.4 % to 1.7%. Post-operative pneumonia can be divided into three main categories: non-ventilator associated pneumonia, ventilator associated pneumonia (VAP), and aspiration-associated pneumonia.

Non-ventilator-associated pneumonia

Atelectasis is defined as the collapse of alveoli leading to impaired clearance of mucous and ultimately entrapping bacteria and facilitating their growth. Risk factors associated with increased incidence of developing pneumonia include tobacco use, chronic obstructive pulmonary disease (COPD), malnutrition, and immunosuppression. The most common sign of atelectasis post-operatively is fever within the first 24 hours. This occurs due to the activation of alveolar macrophages that release IL-1. Once atelectasis is suspected, the focus should be on preventing progression to pneumonia by taking measures to re-expand the alveoli. The I COUGH program was implemented at Boston Medical Center to prevent non-ventilator-associated pneumonia. The components included: incentive spirometer use, coughing and deep breathing, oral care, patient education, getting out of bed, head elevation, and post-operative pain control. In this study, the incidence of post-operative pneumonia declined from 2.6% to 1.6%.[11] Diagnosis of pneumonia as per NSQIP includes: chest radiograph with infiltrate, one sign of pneumonia (i.e., fever, leukocytosis, or altered mental status), and one microbiologic laboratory finding (i.e., positive cultures from blood, bronchoalveolar lavage, or pleural fluid specimens) or two symptoms (i.e., purulent sputum, worsening cough, dyspnea, rales or rhonchi, or worsening gas exchange).[12]

Ventilator associated pneumonia

Ventilators are an important adjunct in post-operative management of selected patients (i.e., after prolonged operation requiring a large amount of fluids). However, intubation and mechanical ventilation puts patients at an increased risk for developing pneumonia and therefore efforts should be made to use noninvasive ventilation such as face masks.[13] Patients on mechanical ventilation have several risk factors putting them at risk including stenting the glottis open allowing bacteria direct access, loss of cough reflex and ability to clear secretions, and bacteria that can harbor within the ventilator circuit.

Table 3: Methods to reduce risk for VAP[13]

Methods
Use of orogastric tubes to prevent sinusitis
Frequent aspiration of subglottic secretions
Endotracheal cuff pressure >20 cm H_20 to prevent bacterial leaking around the cuff
Use of sedation protocols to facilitate and accelerate weaning
Adequate staffing in ICU to reduce duration of ventilator use
Careful elimination of condensation from ventilator circuit
Avoiding reintubation

Aspiration pneumonia

Aspiration occurs in patients with altered mental status. Aspiration pneumonitis (Mendelson's syndrome) occurs when sterile gastric contents are aspirated into the lower respiratory tract whereas aspiration pneumonia refers to the aspiration of colonized oropharyngeal secretions.[14] The most common organisms implicated in aspiration pneumonia include *S. pneumoniae, S. aureus, H. influenzae,* Enterobacter, and *Pseudomonas aeruginosa*. Treatment follows that of ventilator associated pneumonia. Preventative strategies include good oral hygiene, avoiding excessive use of narcotics and/or sedatives, and elevating the head of the bed.

Table 4: Treatment guidelines for non-ventilator and ventilator associated pneumonia[13]

Patients	Treatment
Patients who do not have known risk factors for multidrug resistant (MDR) pathogens, early onset, and any disease severity	Ceftriaxone or Ciprofloxacin or Ampicillin/sulbactam or Levofloxacin, moxifloxacin, or Ertapenem
Patients who do have known risk factors for multidrug resistant (MDR) pathogens, late onset, and any disease severity	For *Pseudomonas aeruginosa*, *Klebsiella pneumonia*, and Acinetobacter species Cefepime, ceftazidime or Piperacillin-tazobactam plus ciprofloxacin or Imipenem or meropenem or Levofloxacin or Tobramycin plus linezolid or Amikacin, gentamicin or Vancomycin For MRSA Linezolid or Vancomycin

URINARY TRACT INFECTIONS

There are several host defense mechanisms that normally prevent the development of urinary tract infections (UTI). These include long urethra in males, urine flow, transitional epithelium, urethral IgA, and urethral mucus. When an indwelling catheter is used, these mechanisms are compromised. Catheter-associated urinary tract infection's (CAUTI) are the most common hospital associated infection.[15] It is estimated that over 25% of patients with an indwelling catheter for up to 2 to 10 days will develop bacteremia and of these patients, about a quarter will go on to develop CAUTI.[16] The most commonly implicated organism is *E. coli*.[17] Others include *Enterobacter*, *Enterococci*, coagulase negative *Staphylococcus*, *Pseudomonas aeruginosa*, and *Candida*.[18] Diagnosis can be aided by the clinical picture including presence of a fever and pyuria. However, microbiologic analysis of urine samples definitively makes the diagnosis of CAUTI. The sample should be obtained directly from the tubing either from the collection port or by puncturing the tubing with a needle.[17] A number of preventative strategies have been examined and include use of sterile technique, using the smallest gauge catheter, a closed drainage system, avoiding irrigation, and avoiding excessive replacement.[19] However, the single most important preventative strategy is limiting catheter use and duration.

SUPPURATIVE PAROTITIS

Suppurative parotitis is especially common in elderly postoperative patients. Risk factors include poor oral hygiene, dehydration, malnutrition, and agents that thicken oral secretions such as anticholinergics.[20] The most common microbes implicated are *Staphylococcus aureus* and anaerobic bacteria. The predominant anaerobes include gram-negative bacilli including Prevotella and Porphyromonas, Fusobacterium, and Peptostreptococcus.[21] The classic symptoms include pain and hyperemia in the parotid region. Physical exam findings include edema, induration, and tenderness to palpation due to inflammation of the parotid parenchyma. Imaging studies such as ultrasound or CT scan can aide in diagnosis. Treatment includes broad-spectrum antibiotics, incision, and drainage if an abscess is present. If left untreated, acute suppurative parotitis can lead to osteomyelitis and mediastinitis.[12]

SPECIAL CONSIDERATIONS

CAT, DOG, AND HUMAN BITES

The exact incidence of animal bites is unknown because it is underreported. However, there is an estimated incidence 3 to 6 million animal bites per year with 80% to 90% being from dogs, 5% to 15% from cats, and the remainder from other animals.[23] Dog bites tend to inflict a crushing type of wound due to the pressure their jaws exert and cat bites tend to be puncture type wounds allowing for bacterial entry into deep tissue spaces.[24,25] Both aerobic and anaerobic bacteria are usually isolated from dog and cat bite wounds, with the most common organism being *Pasteurella multocida* and *septica*.[26] Several different antibiotics can be used to treat infections related to dog and cat bites, with varied coverage. Amoxicillin-clavulanate, doxycycline, and TMP-SMX are some of the more commonly used oral agents.[5] Human bites can range from lacerations to puncture wound but are primarily limited to the subcutaneous tissues and most commonly involve the hands. The three most commonly isolated organisms are Streptococcus species especially *Streptococcus anginous*, *S. aureus*, and *Eikenella corrodens*.[27] Amoxicillin-clavulanate and doxycycline are the main oral agents used in the treatment of infected wounds.[5] Prophylactic use of antibiotics for noninfected wounds is recommended for patients who are immunocompromised, asplenic, have advanced liver disease, have moderate to severe disease, or have invasion into the joint space or periosteum.[5] Whether it is a dog, cat, or human bite, these wounds should not be closed primarily. Rather copious irrigation and debridement of necrotic tissue should be undertaken with delayed primary or secondary closure.[28] An exception to this is facial wounds, which after irrigation and debridement can be closed primarily with good healing rates.[29]

PERITONEAL DIALYSIS CATHETER INFECTION

The leading cause of peritoneal dialysis (PD) catheter infections is peritonitis. Peritonitis is the most common reason that patients ultimately discontinue PD and switch to hemodialysis (HD). Exit-site (tunnel) infections clinically manifest as erythema over the tunnel, purulence, and tenderness. Erythema alone is not indicative of infection, as newly placed catheters can cause this type of skin reaction. The most common organisms involved are *S. aureus* and *Pseudomonas aeruginosa*.[30] Staph infections should be treated with oral antibiotics for two weeks and longer for Pseudomonas. If there is no resolution with antibiotic therapy, it should be considered to remove and replace the catheter, which can be done in the same setting.[31] Exit-site or tunnel infections can progress to peritonitis which will present with cloudy, effluent, and abdominal pain.[32] To make the diagnosis, one liter of dialysate should be allowed to dwell for one to two hours and then collected for analysis. A PMN count >50% is indicative of peritonitis.[30] Once suspected, empiric intraperitoneal (IP) antibiotic therapy should be initiated which consists of first-generation cephalosporin or vancomycin for gram-positive coverage, and third generation cephalosporin or aminoglycoside for gram-negative coverage. A minimum dwell time of six hours is recommended. Although more commonly employed in cases of hemoperitoneum, fibrin can form within the catheter. Thus, it may be beneficial to add heparin to the dialysate.[30] Refractory peritonitis is defined as effluent that does not clear within five days of antibiotic therapy.[33] These cases should be managed with catheter removal to preserve peritoneum integrity for future PD use.[34] Catheter removal should also be considered for cases of fungal and mycobacterium peritonitis.

LINE INFECTIONS

There are two terms to describe line infections: central-line associated bloodstream infections (CLABSI) and catheter-related bloodstream infections (CRBSI). Use of vascular catheters is important in both the inpatient and outpatient setting. In the inpatient setting, central venous access can provide reliable access to administer fluids and blood products, and it can serve as a method for hemodynamic monitoring. In the outpatient setting, dialysis catheters can be used in the renal failure population. In the United States, it is estimated that 300 million catheters are used yearly, with 3 million of these being central venous catheters (CVC).[35] In the United States, 250,000 CLABSIs occur annually in both ICU and non-ICU settings.[36] The different type of CVC used depends on the patient's needs and includes non-tunneled catheters, tunneled catheters, implantable ports, and peripherally inserted central catheters (PICCs).[37] Potentially, modifiable risk factors of CLABSI include multiple CVCs, increased duration of use, multi-lumen CVCs, parenteral nutrition administration, and femoral or internal jugular access.[38] CVCs can be infiltrated with microorganism by two routes: extraluminally from the patient's skin organisms and intra-luminally from direct contamination of the catheter.[39] Gram-positive organisms are the most common causative microbes, with coagulase negative *Staphylococcus* being the most common. Other organisms implicated include *S. aureus* with MRSA accounting for up to 50% of cases, Enterococcus, and Candida.[40,41] The Michigan Keystone Intensive Care Unit Project was the first statewide effort to improve ICU quality and patient safety.[42] The Michigan Health and Hospital Association partnered with a team from John Hopkins to reduce the rate of CLABSIs.[43] Five evidence-based interventions were grouped and consisted of[44] hand hygiene, use of full barrier precautions, chlorhexidine skin preparation, avoiding line placement in the femoral vein, and prompt removal of the CVC. This led to decreased rates of CLABSI, from a mean of 7.7 to 1.3 over the course of 16 to 18 months.

ANTIBIOTICS: MECHANISM OF ACTION AND RESISTANCE

Affects cell-wall or plasma membrane

β-lactams are the oldest and perhaps the most widely used antibiotics. These are bactericidal drugs that work by inhibiting cell-wall synthesis. The antibiotics in this group include penicillin-related, cephalosporins, monobactams, and carbapenems. The cell wall consists of peptidoglycan, which is synthesized by enzymes located within the plasma membrane.[45] These enzymes that bind penicillin are termed penicillin-binding proteins (PBP) with each bacterial group possessing its own variety.[46] The antibiotics bind to these enzymes ultimately preventing cell wall synthesis. There are three primary mechanisms of β-lactam resistance which are reduced access to the PBPs, reduced PBP binding affinity, and enzymes that bind and hydrolyze β-lactams.[47] To overcome the latter, several agents that block the enzyme B-lactamase have been manufactured including clavulanic acid, sulbactam, and tazobactam. A non-enzyme mediated form of resistance is seen in methicillin-resistant *Staphylococcus aureus* (MRSA) infections. Resistance here is mediated by the mecA gene, which is a PBP.

Vancomycin, although not considered a β-lactam, also interferes with cell wall synthesis by binding to the terminal d-alanine residues of the peptidoglycan chain.[45] Vancomycin resistant enterococci (VRE) resistance occurs by modifying or removing the binding target for the drug.[48]

With the presence of vancomycin and methicillin resistant gram-positive organisms, there has been a demand to develop new antimicrobial agents. Daptomycin does not inhibit cell wall synthesis but rather directly binds to the plasma membrane and causes rapid depolarization resulting in bacterial cell death.[49]

There are antifungal agents that also affect the cell wall via different mechanisms. Imidazole derivatives including ketoconazole, fluconazole, itraconazole, and voriconazole affect ergosterol synthesis and causes cell lysis.[50] Amphotericin B binds to sterols within the plasma membrane which compromises the integrity of membrane permeability.[51] Echinocandins including caspofungin, micafungin, and anidulafungin inhibit the enzyme 1,3 B-glucan-synthase which blocks cell wall synthesis.[52]

Affects protein synthesis

The antibiotics in this class bind to a ribosomal subunit and prevent protein synthesis. Ribosomes contain both a 30S and 50S subunit, and the drugs are divided accordingly. 30S subunit inhibitors, including tetracycline and aminoglycosides, prevent protein synthesis by blocking mRNA binding to the tRNA subunit.[53] Aminoglycosides, however, irreversibly bind to the ribosome making it bactericidal. The main resistance mechanisms against aminoglycosides are either a decreased uptake of the drug or the bacterial expression of enzymes that modify the antibiotic and make it inactive.[54] Two types of resistance mechanisms predominate for tetracycline efflux and ribosomal protection, both of which can be found on plasmids.[55]

50S subunit inhibitors, including chloramphenicol, macrolides (i.e., erythromycin), and clindamycin, prevent protein synthesis by interfering with tRNA function. Resistance to both erythromycin and clindamycin can occur through transformation of the binding sites of the ribosomal subunit.[56]

Affect Nucleic Acids

These classes of antibiotics have different effects on nucleic acids and include Rifampin, Fluroquinolones, and Metronidazole. Rifampin belongs to a group termed rifamycin antibiotics. They were discovered in 1957 as a product of *Streptomyces mediterranei* fermentation.[57] Rifampin specifically works by inhibiting RNA polymerase which is the enzyme responsible for DNA transcription.[58] The fluroquinolones are the only antibiotics that directly inhibit DNA synthesis.[59] They have two target enzymes DNA gyrase and topoisomerase IV, each of which have different physiologic consequences.[60] Although it was initially indicated for the treatment of protozoal infections, Metronidazole is also successfully used in the treatment of anaerobic bacterial infections such as Bacteroides, fusobacteria, and clostridia. Although the exact mechanism of action is not fully understood, Metronidazole works by inhibiting DNA synthesis and causing DNA damage by oxidation.[61] The mechanism of resistance to Metronidazole differs among different organisms (i.e., anaerobes vs. protozoa), but the common theory is that there is reduced activation of the drug leading to decreased uptake.[61] Lastly, acyclovir is an antiviral drug that inhibits DNA polymerase. It is used against herpes simplex virus and varicella-zoster virus.[62]

Affects metabolic pathways

Sulfonamides are generally considered to be bacteriostatic drugs that interfere with the utilization of the PABA substrate, ultimately preventing the synthesis of dihydrofolic acid.[63] Trimethoprim works by blocking the reduction of dihydrofolate to tetrahydrofolate.[64]

COMPLICATIONS

Clostrium Difficile Associated Diarrhea (CDAD)

Clostridium difficile is responsible for up to 25% of antibiotic associated diarrhea (AAD) cases. Other, rare causes include *S. aureus*, *Clostridium perfringens*, *Salmonella* species, and *Klebsiella oxytoca.*[65] *C. difficile* is a gram-positive, spore forming anaerobe, capable of producing mild diarrhea to fulminant colitis.[66] Risk factors include old age, hospitalization, immunosuppression, and antibiotic use. Surgical patients are at increased risk for developing CDAD because of the use of prophylactic and therapeutic antibiotics in this group.[66] Antibiotics, both long- and short-term, that are more commonly implicated include clindamycin, cephalosporins, B-lactams, and fluroquinolones.[67] Antibiotics ultimately alter the colonic bacterial environment allowing *C. difficile* to proliferate. *C. difficile* strains that produce toxin A and B are the ones that are pathogenic.[66] Toxin A and B are encoded by the tcdA and tcdB genes and are considered proinflammatory and cytotoxic. Both are responsible for disrupting the actin cytoskeleton and tight junctions leading to damage of intestinal cells.[68] The diagnosis should be suspected in patients with a known history of antibiotic use and have fever, cramps, abdominal pain, and diarrhea. There are many different types of stool tests with varying sensitivities and specificities, but in the United States most hospitals use EIA because it is inexpensive, rapid, and technically easy to perform.[65]

Table 5: Stool tests available for diagnosing *C. difficile*[65]

Test
Cell cytotoxicity assay
Stool culture
Enzyme immunoassay (EIA) for toxin A and B
Glutamate dehydrogenase (GDH) test
ELISAs for toxins A or toxins A and B
Immunochromatography for toxin A
Polymerase chain reaction (PCR) for toxins

Computed tomography (CT) can be obtained which may reveal colonic wall thickening but is especially helpful in diagnosing pseudo-membrane colitis or fulminant colitis. Endoscopy can also be undertaken, and visualization of pseudo-membranes is considered diagnostic. Once suspected, even if stool testing is negative, empiric treatment with antibiotics should be initiated because, if left untreated, the morbidity and mortality are high. Treatment with antibiotics is dependent on disease severity. Addition of probiotics has not been proven and therefore is not recommended as per the Society of Healthcare Epidemiology of America (SHEA) and Infectious Disease Society of America 2010 guidelines.[69]

Table 6: Antimicrobial therapy recommendations based on disease severity[69]

Disease severity	Recommended regimen
Initial episode: mild-to-moderation	Metronidazole 500mg, PO, TID for 10-14 days
Initial episode: severe	Vancomycin 125mg, PO, QID for 10-14 days
Severe, complicated	Vancomycin 500mg, PO, QID and Vancomycin 500mg/100ml per rectum Q6h (as retention enema) and Metronidazole 500mg IV Q8h
First recurrence	Treat with same regimen as initial episode, based off disease severity
Second recurrence	Treat with different regimen

Fidaxomicin is another antimicrobial agent that can be used against *C. difficile*. It is a macrocyclic antibiotic that is considered bactericidal. It has been reported to eradicate

C. difficile as effectively as vancomycin, with lower rates of recurrence.[70] Surgical intervention should be considered in patients that are severely ill with rising white blood cell counts, and with persistence or progression of disease despite adequate antimicrobial therapy.

Clostridium difficile infection can progress to fulminant disease in 3% to 5% of cases.[76] Determining which patients should undergo surgical management in cases where acute abdomen infection is not present, is still a matter of debate. Cases of persistent or worsening leukocytosis, lactic acidosis, and failure to respond to antimicrobial therapy should be considered for surgical intervention. In cases of perforation or toxic megacolon, subtotal colectomy with ileostomy is the standard of care. Segmental colectomy or ileostomy/colostomy alone have been shown to have higher mortality rates.[75] Alternatives to surgery have been described with varied success, including diverting loop ileostomy with colonic lavage using eight liters of warm polyethylene glycol intraoperatively, followed by 10 days of vancomycin antegrade enemas.[77]

REFERENCES

1. Schwabl P, Bucsics T, Soucek K, et al. Risk factors for development of spontaneous bacterial peritonitis and subsequent mortality in cirrhotic patients with ascites. Liver Int. 2015 Feb 2.
2. Runyon BA, McHutchison JG, Antillon MR, Akriviadis EA, Montano AA. Short-course versus long-course antibiotic treatment of spontaneous bacterial peritonitis. A randomized controlled study of 100 patients. Gastroenterology. 1991 Jun; 100(6):1737-42.
3. Alaniz C, Regal RE. Spontaneous Bacterial Peritonitis: A Review of Treatment Options. Pharmacy and Therapeutics. 2009;34(4):204-210.
4. Wittmann DH, Schein M, Condon RE. Management of secondary peritonitis. Annals of Surgery. 1996;224(1):10-18.
5. Stevens, D et al. Practice guidelines for diagnosis and management of skin and soft tissue infections: 2014 updated by the Infectious Diseases Society of America. Clin Infect Dis. June 18, 2014.
6. Anaya DA, Dellinger EP. Necrotizing soft-tissue infection: diagnosis and management. Clin Infect Dis. 2007 Mar 1;44(5):705-10. doi: 10.1086/511638. Epub 2007 Jan 22. PMID: 17278065.
7 Fry DE. Surgical Site Infections and the Surgical Care Improvement Project (SCIP): Evolution of National Quality Measures. Surg Infect 2008;9(6):579-84.
8. Dimick JB, Chen SL, Taheri PA, Henderson WG, Khuri SF, Campbell DA Jr. Hospital costs associated with surgical complications: a report from the private-sector National Surgical Quality Improvement Program. J Am Coll Surg. 2004;199(4):531-537.
9. Smetana GW. Postoperative pulmonary complications: an update on risk assessment and reduction. Cleve Clin J Med. 2009;76:4: S60-S65.
10. Cassidy MR, Rosenkranz P, McCabe K, Rosen JE, McAneny D. I COUGH: Reducing Postoperative Pulmonary Complications With a Multidisciplinary Patient Care Program. JAMA Surg. 2013;148(8):740-745.
11. McNelis J, Castaldi M. "The National Surgery Quality Improvement Project" (NSQIP): a new tool to increase patient safety and cost efficiency in a surgical intensive care unit. Patient Safety in Surgery. 2014;8:19.
12. Guidelines for the Management of Adults with Hospital-acquired, Ventilator-associated, and Healthcare-associated Pneumonia. Am J Respir Crit Care Med Vol 171. pp 388–416, 2005.
13. Marik PE. Aspiration pneumonitis and aspiration pneumonia. N Engl J Med, Vol. 344, No. 9 · March 1, 2001.
14. Saint S, Chenoweth CE. Biofilms and catheter-associated urinary tract infections. Infectious Disease Clinics of North America, 2003 June; 17(2):411-432.
15. Rebmann T, Greene, LR. Preventing catheter-associated urinary tract infections: An executive summary of the Association for Professionals in Infection Control and Epidemiology, Inc. Elimination Guide. American Journal of Infection Control, 2010 October; 38(8):644-646.
16. Hooton TM, Bradley SF, Cardenas DD, Colgan R, Geerlings SE, Rice JC, Saint S, Schaeffer AJ, Tambyah PA, Tenke P, Nicolle LE: Diagnosis, prevention and treatment of catheter-associated urinary tract infection in adults; 2009 international clinical practice guidelines from the Infectious Diseases Society of America.
17. Nicolle LE. Urinary catheter associated infections. Infect Dis Clin North Am 2012, 26:13.28.
18. Lo E, Nicolle LE, Coffin SE, Gould C, Maragakis LL, Meddings J, Pegues DA, Pettis AM, Saint S, Yokoe DS. Strategies to prevent catheter-associated urinary tract infections in acute care hospitals: 2014 update. Infect Control Hosp Epidemiol. 2014 May;35(5):464-79. doi: 10.1086/675718. PMID: 24709715.
19. Krippaehne W, Hunt M, Englebert J. Acute Suppurative Parotitis: A study of 161 cases. Annals of surgery 1962. 156 (2): 251-257.
20. Brook I. Acute bacterial suppurative parotitis: microbiology and management.J Craniofac Surg. 2003 Jan;14(1):37-40.
21. Fattahi TT, Lyu PE, Van Sickels JE. Management of acute suppurative parotitis. J Oral Maxillofac Surg.

2002 Apr;60(4):446-8. doi: 10.1053/joms.2002.31234. PMID: 11928106.

22. Gilchrist J, Sacks JJ, White D, Kresnow MJ. Dog bites: still a problem?. Inj Prev. Oct 2008;14(5):296-301.
23. Chambers GH, Payne JF. Treatment of dog bite wounds. Minn Med. 1969;52:427-430.
24. Dire DJ. Cat bite wounds: risk factors for infection. Ann Emerg Med. Sep 1991;20(9):973-9.
25. Talan DA, Citron DM, Abrahamian FM, Moran GJ, Goldstein EJ. Bacteriologic analysis of infected dog and cat bites. Emergency Medicine Animal Bite Infection Study Group. N Engl J Med. 1999 Jan 14;340(2):85-92.
26. Talan DA, Abrahamian FM, Moran GJ, et al. Clinical Presentation and Bacteriologic Analysis of Infected Human Bites in Patients Presenting to Emergency Departments. Clin Infect Dis. (2003) 37 (11): 1481-1489.
27. Patil PD, Panchabhai TS, Galwankar SC. Managing human bites. Journal of Emergencies, Trauma and Shock. 2009;2(3):186-190.
28. Donkor P, Bankas DO. Study of primary closure of human bite injuries to the face. J Oral Maxillofacial Surg. 1997;55:479–81.
29. Li PK, et al. Peritoneal Dialysis catheter-related infections recommendations: 2010 update. Peritoneal Dialysis Internation. Vol 30 pp 393-423.
30. Posthuma N, Borgstein PJ, Eijsbouts Q, ter Wee PM. Simultaneous peritoneal dialysis catheter insertion and removal in catheter-related infections without interruption of peritoneal dialysis. Nephrol Dial Transplant 1998; 13: 700–3.
31. Rocklin MA, Teitelbaum I. Noninfectious causes of cloudy peritoneal dialysate. Semin Dial 2001; 14:37–40.
32. Choi P, Nemati E, Banerjee A, Preston E, Levy J, Brown E. Peritoneal dialysis catheter removal for acute peritonitis: a retrospective analysis of factors associated with catheter removal and prolonged postoperative hospitalization. Am J Kidney Dis 2004; 43:103–11.
33. Szeto CC, Chow KM, Wong TY, Leung CB, Wang AY, Lui SF, et al. Feasibility of resuming peritoneal dialysis after se- vere peritonitis and Tenckhoff catheter removal. J Am Soc Nephrol 2002; 13:1040–5.
34. The Joint Commission. Preventing Central Line–Associated Bloodstream Infections: A Global Challenge, a Global Perspective. Oak Brook, IL: Joint Commission Resources, May 2012.
35. Maki DG, Kluger DM, Crnich CJ. The risk of bloodstream infec- tion in adults with different intravascular devices: A systematic review of 200 published prospective studies. Mayo Clin Proc. 2006 Sep;81(9):1159–1171.
36. Kelly LJ. The family of vascular access devices. J Infect Prev. 2009 Sep;10 Suppl 1:s7–12.
37. Safdar N, Kluger DM, Maki DG. A review of risk factors for catheter-related bloodstream infection caused by percutaneously inserted, noncuffed central venous catheters: Implications for pre- ventive strategies. Medicine (Baltimore). 2002 Nov;81(6):466–479.
38. Crnich CJ, Maki DG. The promise of novel technology for the prevention of intravascular device-related bloodstream infection. I. Pathogenesis and short-term devices. Clin Infect Dis. 2002 May 1;34(9):1232–1242.
39. O'Grady NP, Alexander M, Burns LA, Dellinger EP, et al. Healthcare Infection Control Practices Advisory Committee (HICPAC). Guidelines for the prevention of intravascular catheter–related infections. Clin Infect Dis. 2011 May;52(9):e162–193.
40. Wisplinghoff H, Bischoff T, Tallent SM, Seifert H, Wenzel RP, Edmond MB. Nosocomial bloodstream infections in US hospitals: Analysis of 24,179 cases from a prospective nationwide surveil- lance study. Clin Infect Dis. 2004 Aug 1;39(3):309–317.
41. Pronovost PJ, Berenholtz SM, Goeschel C, et al. Improving patient safety in intensive care units in Michigan. J Crit Care. 2008 Jun;23(2):207–221.
42. Pronovost P. Interventions to decrease catheter-related blood- stream infections in the ICU: The Keystone Intensive Care Unit Project. Am J Infect Control. 2008 Dec;36(10):S171.e1–5.
43. Pronovost PJ, Berenholtz SM, Goeschel CA, et al. Creating high reliability in health care organiza- tions. Health Serv Res. 2006 Aug;41(4 Pt 2):1599–1617.
44. McManus MC. Mechanisms of bacterial resistance to antimicrobial agents. Am J Health Syst Pharm, 54 (1997), pp. 1420–1433.
45. Ghuysen JM. Serien B-lactamases and penicillin binding proteins. Annual Reviews in Microbiology. 1991. 45: 37-67.
46. Rice LB. Mechanisms of Resistance and Clinical Relevance of Resistance to β-Lactams, Glycopeptides, and Fluoroquinolones. Mayo Clinic Proceedings. 2012;87(2):198-208.
47. Courvalin P. Vancomycin Resistance in Gram-Positive Cocci. Clin Infect Dis. (2006) 42 (Supplement 1): S25-S34.
48. Straus S. Mode of action of the new antibiotic for Gram-positive pathogens daptomycin: Comparison with cationic antimicrobial peptides and lipopeptides. Biochimica et Biophysica Acta (BBA)-Biomembranes. Vol 1758, Issue 9, September 2006 1215-1223.
49. Borgers M. Mechanism of action of antifungal drugs, with special reference to the imidazole derivatives. Rev Infect Dis. 1980 Jul-Aug;2(4):520-34.

50. Baginski M, Czub J. Amphotericin B and its new derivatives - mode of action. Curr Drug Metab. 2009 Jun;10(5):459-69.
51. Sucher AJ, Chahine EB, Balcer HE. Echinocandins: the newest class of antifungals. Ann Pharmacother. 2009 Oct;43(10):1647-57.
52. Weisblum B. Antibiotic Inhibitors of the Bacterial Ribosome.Volume 32, Issue 4. Bacteriologic Reviews. 1968. 493-528.
53. Mingeot-Leclercq MP, Glupczynski Y, Tulkens PM. Aminoglycosides: Activity and Resistance. Antimicrobial Agents and Chemotherapy. 1999;43(4):727-737.
54. Speer BS, Shoemaker NB, Salyers AA. Bacterial resistance to tetracycline: mechanisms, transfer, and clinical significance. Clinical Microbiology Reviews. 1992;5(4):387-399.
55. Steward CD, Raney PM, Morrell AK, et al. Testing for induction of clindamycin resistance in erythromycin-resistant isolates of Staphylococcus aureus. J Clin Microbiol. 2005 Apr;43(4):1716-21. doi: 10.1128/JCM.43.4.1716-1721.2005. PMID: 15814990; PMCID: PMC1081368.
56. Wehril W. Actions of Rifamycins. Bacteriological Reviews. 1971. Vol 35, Issue 3. P 209-309.
57. Wehril W. Rifampin: mechanisms of Actions and resistance. Clin Infect Dis. (1983) 5 (Supplement 3): S407-S411.
58. Hooper DC. Mechanisms of Action of Antimicrobials: Focus on Fluoroquinolones. Clin Infect Dis. (2001) 32 (Supplement 1): S9-S15.
59. Drlica K. Mechanic of fluroquinolone action. Curr Opin Microbiol. 1999 Oct;2(5):504-8.
60. Löfmark S, Edlund C, Nord CE. Metronidazole Is Still the Drug of Choice for Treatment of Anaerobic Infections. Clin Infect Dis. (2010) 50 (Supplement 1): S16-S23.
61. Gnann JW Jr, Barton NH, Whitley RJ. Acyclovir: mechanism of action, pharmacokinetics, safety and clinical applications. Pharmacotherapy. 1983 Sep-Oct;3(5):275-83.
62. Henry RJ. "The mode of action of sulfonamides." Bacteriological reviews 7.4 (1943): 175.
63. Gleckman R, Blagg N, Joubert DW. Trimethoprim: mechanisms of action, antimicrobial activity, bacterial resistance, pharmacokinetics, adverse reactions, and therapeutic indications. Pharmacotherapy. 1981 Jul-Aug;1(1):14-20.
64. Bartlett JG, Gerding DN. Clinical Recognition and Diagnosis of *Clostridium difficile* Infection. Clin Infect Dis. (2008) 46 (Supplement 1): S12-S18.
65. Efron P, Mazuski JE. Clostridium difficile Colitis. Surgical Clinics of North America. Volume 89, Issue 2, April 2009, Pages 483–500.
66. Bartlett JG. Clinical practice: antibiotic-associated diarrhea. N Engl J Med 2002;346:334-9.
67. Carter GP, Rood JI, Lyras D. The role of toxin A and toxin B in *Clostridium difficile*-associated disease: Past and present perspectives. *Gut Microbes*. 2010;1(1):58-64. doi:10.4161/gmic.1.1.10768.
68. Cohen SH, et al Clinical Practice Guidelines for Clostridium difficile Infection in Adults: 2010 update by the Society of Healthcare Epidemiology of America (SHEA) and Infectious Disease Society of America (IDSA). Infection Control and Hospital Epidemiology. Vol 31: 5. 431-455.
69. Louie TJ, Miller MA, Mullane KM, et al. Fidaxomicin versus Vancomycin for *Clostridium difficile* Infection. N Engl J Med 2011; 364:422-431.
70. Mishra SP, Tiwary SK, Mishra M, Gupta SK. An introduction of Tertiary Peritonitis. *Journal of Emergencies, Trauma, and Shock*. 2014;7(2):121-123. doi:10.4103/0974-2700.130883.
71. Calandra T, Cohen J. The international sepsis forum consensus conference on definitions of infection in the intensive care unit. Crit Care Med. 2005;33:1538–48.
72. Nathens AB, et al. Tertiary peritonitis: clinical features of a complex nosocomial infection. World J Surg. 1998 Feb;22(2):158-63.
73. Malagoni MA. Evaluation and management of tertiary peritonitis. 74Am Surg. 2000 Feb;66(2):157-61.
74. Seltman AK. Surgical Management of *Clostridium difficile* Colitis. *Clinics in Colon and Rectal Surgery*. 2012;25(4):204-209.
75. Neal MD, Alverdy JC, Hall DE, Simmons RL, Zuckerbraun BS. Diverting loop ileostomy and colonic lavage: an alternative to total abdominal colectomy for the treatment of severe, complicated *Clostridium difficile* associated disease Ann Surg 20112543423–427.427, discussion 427–429.

❑❑❑

12

CHAPTER

Acute Kidney Injury

Abhishek Swami, MD

1.1 INTRODUCTION

Perioperative kidney injury is a significant problem that is associated with considerable mortality, morbidity, and increased length of hospital stay. Recovery from acute kidney injury is often incomplete even if baseline renal function is normal; with only roughly 15% of patients with perioperative acute renal failure (ARF) fully recovering. Mortality is high in patients who develop ARF, and may be as high as 50% in patients who develop perioperative ARF. Presently, our ability to detect early kidney injury is limited and, with the present means, we are only able to detect renal dysfunction once the damage has already been done. Therefore, a detailed evaluation in the perioperative period should include a thorough assessment of the risk for renal injury and measures should be instituted to prevent renal damage where possible.

Definition and Incidence

Broadly, acute kidney injury (AKI) is defined as an abrupt decline in kidney function, typically occurring over hours to days. The risk of kidney injury varies with different studies because of variations in the study populations and the definition of renal failure. Traditionally, the term ARF is broad and incorporates a heterogeneous collection of definitions, ranging from an increase in serum creatinine of 25% to the need for renal replacement therapy. It is known that even small changes in renal function that do not necessarily cause organ failure can have an impact on patient outcomes, and this knowledge has prompted a change in terminology from ARF to AKI. Recognizing the need for a uniform definition of ARF, a few standard definitions and classifications of AKI have been developed. The most recent definition was proposed by Kidney Disease: Improving Global Outcome (KDIGO) and is the preferred definition.

The KDIGO guideline definition of AKI is as follows: "Increase in serum creatinine by $\geq$0.3 mg/dL ($\geq$26.5 micromol/L) within 48 hours, or increase in serum creatinine to $\geq$1.5 times baseline, which is known or presumed to have occurred within the prior seven days, or urine volume <0.5 mL/kg/hour for six hours).

Other standard definitions comprise the RIFLE criteria (Risk of renal dysfunction; Injury to kidney; Failure of kidney function; Loss of kidney function; and End-stage kidney disease) and a subsequent modification proposed by the Acute Kidney Injury Network (AKIN). These classification systems have been validated in numerous settings.[1]

The reported incidence of postoperative AKI has ranged between 5% to 25%. Studies using the RIFLE criteria have reported the postoperative AKI incidence to be about 20% to 25%. A few studies have also looked at the risk of mortality in patients with postoperative AKI. In a recent retrospective study from a single center that looked at around 40,000 patients undergoing non-cardiac surgery, the incidence of postoperative AKI was noted to be around 6 % utilizing the KDIGO criteria. It was also noted that the risk of death increased 2 folds in patients with AKI. It has been observed that the risk of mortality in patients with postoperative AKI is high and proportionate to the degree of renal injury. In patients undergoing cardiac surgery, the risk of 90-day mortality has been reported to be 32% in the more severe category of RIFLE-F (failure) compared with the less severe categories of RIFLE-R (risk) at 8% and RIFLE-I (injury) at 21%. The RIFLE classification was found to be an independent risk factor for mortality in these studies.

Etiology

The etiology of AKI in the perioperative period is multifactorial. The traditional classification of AKI into prerenal, intrinsic, and postrenal causes should be applied for the evaluation of perioperative AKI as well. Prerenal AKI occurs due to renal hypoperfusion from any cause, this can be reversed if the hypoperfusion is corrected promptly. If lack of perfusion is severe or prolonged, then injury may progress to ischemic acute tubular necrosis (ATN), which is the most common cause of perioperative AKI. The intrinsic causes of AKI can be more broadly categorized as vascular, glomerular, tubular, or interstitial. The postrenal causes of AKI are due to bladder or ureter obstruction.

Risk Factors

There are no specific guidelines for identifying risk factors for AKI and preoperative renal risk stratification; furthermore, the data about risk factors in the literature is not uniform. The reason for this is a lack of a standardized definition and a paucity of accurate biomarkers to detect AKI. Several predictive models have been developed to risk stratify patients undergoing cardiac surgery, but only limited studies have looked at the noncardiac surgery population. The risk factors can be broadly divided into those that can be identified preoperatively and those that occur intraoperatively, detailed in Table 1.

Preoperative Risk Factors

Several preoperative factors are predictive of postoperative AKI. The most important modifiable risk factors are hypovolemia and hemodynamic instability. Elevated creatinine and chronic kidney disease are also substantial risk factors. Some studies have demonstrated that elevated creatinine is associated with exponential increases in postoperative ARF. Other diseases like chronic obstructive pulmonary disorder (COPD) requiring bronchodilators, chronic liver disease, uncontrolled hypertension, coronary artery disease (CAD), peripheral vascular disease (PVD), and congestive heart failure (CHF) have been reported to confer kidney injury in those undergoing surgery. There is an association between obesity and ARF after cardiac and noncardiac surgery, which is independent of comorbidities including hypertension and diabetes. Women have an increased risk of developing ARF compared to men at every baseline serum creatinine level. Some evidence suggests that there is a genetic basis for increased renal risk, where patients with the epsilon-4 allele of apolipoprotein develop AKI less than patients with other alleles.[1]

Table 1: Risk factors for acute kidney injury

Preoperative risk factors	Intraoperative risk factors
• Advanced age • Female • Obesity • Elevated preoperative BUN and SCr • History of renal dysfunction • Left ventricular dysfunction • Hemodynamic instability • PVD/CAD • Septicemia • Comorbidities: diabetes, COPD, uncontrolled HTN, liver disease • Severity of illness • Medications: diuretics, vasopressors, NSAIDs, antibiotics, IV contrast • Genetic	• Emergency surgery • Cardiac surgery: CABG, CPB • Vascular surgery • Liver transplantation • Hemodilution/anemia • Medications: diuretics, vasopressors, NSAIDs, antibiotics, aprotinin • General anesthesia

The use of diuretics and vasopressors can decrease renal perfusion and potentiate AKI. There is no evidence with the limited available data that angiotensin-converting enzyme inhibitors (ACE-I) increase the risk of AKI; however, several clinicians choose to withhold ACE-I before surgery as these can impair renal autoregulation and can compromise GFR in the face of other insults. There are several other medications administered commonly in the perioperative period such as nonsteroidal anti-inflammatory drugs, antibiotics, and contrast dyes that can be nephrotoxic. There is the widespread use of herbal medications and alternative forms of medicines in the developing world which are potentially nephrotoxic, and one should always inquire about their use since such information is not always forthcoming.

Intraoperative Risk Factors

Surgery itself leads to a reduction in GFR. Surgery causes a release of various stress response hormones including angiotensin, catecholamines, rennin, and arginine vasopressin, all of which can lead to a redistribution of renal blood flow and a decrease in GFR.[1] Additionally, general anesthesia results in hemodynamic compromise and depresses cardiac function, which further causes ischemic renal injury.

Emergency surgeries confer greater risk as these patients are usually more ill and hemodynamically compromised.

Furthermore, there is no opportunity to stabilize their volume status and optimize medical treatment preoperatively.

Certain types of surgery such as vascular surgery, cardiac surgery, or liver transplantation are more likely to affect renal blood flow. AKI risk post liver transplant has been reported to be greater than 50%. Low serum albumin and intravascular volume depletion are predisposing factors. There appears to be a greater risk of AKI with prolonged duration of cardiopulmonary bypass (CPB) and aortic cross clamping time,[10] in addition to procedures that are more complex (i.e., combined CABG and valve surgery). Hemodilution or anemia on CPB also increases the risk of AKI significantly; however, the mechanism is not clear. Vasoconstrictor hormone release (i.e., angiotensin and epinephrine) and inflammatory cytokines may be responsible. Cardiac and vascular surgeries can also induce AKI from athero-embolism.

Diuretics and vasopressors are commonly used during surgeries and cause a reduction in GFR. Aprotinin is a protease inhibitor that has been used to reduce perioperative bleeding in CABG, orthopedic surgeries, and liver transplant surgeries. An association between aprotinin administration and postoperative AKI has been described. It is suspected that intrarenal hemodynamics are affected via activation of kinin pathways due to aprotinin. Aprotinin was banned in November 2007.

Preoperative Risk Prediction Scores

Noncardiac Surgery

There is a lack of validated risk predictor scores for patients who undergo noncardiac surgery whereas there are a variety of predictive models described for these patients. Kheterpal et al. recently studied about 15,000 patients with normal preoperative renal function undergoing noncardiac surgery in a prospective observational study in an attempt to identify risk profiles for ARF (defined as GFR of ≤50 ml/min within the first seven days postoperative) in the general surgical population. They identified seven independent preoperative predictors and developed propensity scores related to specific preoperative risk factors as seen in Table 2 and 3.[7] This score might help predict the risk of developing ARF after surgery. The model needs further validation, but it may prove useful in allowing timely interventions to prevent kidney injury and can act as a guide for preoperative discussions with patients.

Table 2: Preoperative predictors of postoperative ARF

- Age, year (59 years or greater)
- Emergent surgery
- Liver disease
- BMI in kg/m2 (32 kg/m2 or greater)
- High risk surgery (intrathoracic, intraperitoneal, supra-inguinal, vascular, surgeries, with large loss of blood or fluid shifts)
- PVD, occlusive
- COPD necessitating bronchodilator therapy

Table 3: Frequency and hazard ratio of ARF in relation to the number of preoperative risk factors

Preoperative risk class	Acute renal failure %	Hazard ratio
Class I (0 risk factors)	0.3	
Class II (1 risk factor)	0.5	2
Class III (2 risk factors)	1.3	4.7
Class IV (3 or more risk factors)	4.3	16

Cardiac Surgery

One useful risk-prediction scoring model was developed by Thakar et al. It is based on their study of about 33,000 patients undergoing open-heart surgery, regardless of preoperative renal function. The scoring model was developed on 15,838 randomly selected test subjects and was validated on the remaining patients. In this system, points are awarded based on risk factors, seen in Table 4, and patients can be assigned to one of four risk categories of increasing severity. The risk of ARF requiring dialysis in these risk categories ranged between 0.5% to 22%.[11]

Table 4: ARF score

Risk factor	Points
Female	1
CHF	1
Left ventricular ejection fraction of less than 35%	1
IABP preoperative use	2
COPD	1
Diabetes requiring insulin	1
History of a previous cardiac surgery	1
Emergency surgery	2
Only having valve surgery (reference to CAGB)	1
Valve surgery + CABG (reference to CAGB)	2
Other cardiac surgeries	2
Preoperative creatinine 1.2 to <2.1 mg/dL	2
Preoperative creatinine 2.1	5
*0 = minimum score; 17 = maximum score	

Risk categories based on score	Frequency of ARF requiring dialysis
0-2	0.4%
3-5	1.8%
6-8	7.8%
9-13	21.5%

Measures to Prevent Kidney Injury

1. Assess the risk: Using the tools described above, the degree of overall risk should be assessed based on the patient's individual risk and the characteristics of the procedure. This will help identify the high-risk patients. These tools can easily be used in limited-resource settings, as the parameters are mostly clinical and incorporate simple diagnostic tests.
2. Calculate estimated GFR: This calculation should use the modification of diet in renal disease (MDRD) equation. This will help establish preoperative renal dysfunction (GFR <60 ml/min). Patients with GFR ≤60 ml/min should be considered high risk regardless of other risk factors.
3. Adjust medications: Based on the renal function (eGFR using the MDRD equation) ascertain which medications need a dose adjustment. Avoid medications such as ACE-I, angiotensin receptor blockers, NSAIDs, aminoglycosides, aprotinin, or excessive diuretic use, especially if the patient has preexisting renal dysfunction.
4. Assess and optimize volume status: A thorough clinical assessment should always be done to look for signs of dehydration or decreased volume status such as orthostatic hypotension, tachycardia, decreased skin turgor, collapsed peripheral veins, or low urine output. A physical exam may be useful, but it is not very sensitive in detecting volume status. High blood urea nitrogen (BUN) or uric acid, metabolic alkalosis, or sodium disorders may provide further clues. Central venous pressure (CVP) measurements can be reliably used to assess and monitor volume status. If there is evidence of hypovolemia, it should be corrected before surgery. Uncorrected hypovolemia may lead to renal medullary hypoxia and ischemic ATN. The ideal fluid for correcting hypovolemia and hypotension is controversial. There is no evidence that colloids are better than crystalloids. Colloids are expensive and hence their use is not justified. The amount of crystalloids administered should be directed according to hemodynamic parameters, urine output (UO), and invasive monitors including CVP. Mean arterial pressure (MAP) should be maintained >65 to 70 mmHg, UO >0.5 cc/kg/hr, and CVP 10 to 15 mmHg.[12] It may be harmful to provide excessive fluid resuscitation, and monitor patients closely for volume overload.
5. Preserve renal perfusion: Hypotension should be prevented. Any antihypertensive medication can result in renal injury because of lowered blood pressure. In patients with long-standing hypertension, acute lowering of blood pressure to values even in the normal range should be avoided. ACE-I and angiotensin receptor blockers can decrease renal perfusion due to vasodilation of the efferent arteriol. These medications can affect renal autoregulation and should not be given to patients until they have a restored fluid volume. Additionally, patients who are at risk of AKI should not be given hypotensive anesthesia. Abdominal insufflation for laparoscopic procedures may compromise renal perfusion; thus, patients at risk of AKI should consider having lower pressures (<15 mmHg) or gasless laparoscopy.
6. Limit the use of contrast agents: Contrast-induced nephropathy (CIN) can occur in patients with chronic renal insufficiency, dehydration, diabetes mellitus, congestive heart failure, high contrast volume, and high osmolar contrast. If a patient needs contrast, a low osmolar nonionic agent is preferred. Intravenous fluids such as normal saline are important for increasing urine flow, and thus should be used before and after procedures. To decrease the chances of developing CIN for at-risk patients, adequate intravenous volume expansion with isotonic crystalloid is needed. This consists of an expansion rate of 1.0 to 1.5 ml/kg per hr for 3 to 12 hours prior to the procedure and continued for 6 to 24 hours post-procedure. However, there is insufficient data comparing oral fluids to intravenous volume expansion in CIN prevention measures. Patients may also be given sodium bicarbonate infusion to reduce CIN risk. The role of acetylcysteine is controversial and there have been both positive and negative studies. The benefit may be undefined, but it is certainly harmless and should be used in high-risk patients. Prophylactic hemodialysis and hemofiltration have not been validated as effective strategies. Follow-up serum creatinine should be measured in all high-risk patients, at no less than 24 hours or no more than 72 hours after contrast exposure.[13,14]
7. Optimize hematocrit levels: Some evidence suggests that low hematocrit levels are associated with increased mortality in dialysis patients. Furthermore, cardio-pulmonary bypass hemodilution is associated with a higher AKI likelihood. Hematocrit should be maintained at >24%.

8. Identify AKI: The KDIGO criteria is a reasonable tool to assess kidney injury. Timely identification of AKI is very important as early intervention may reverse the injury. Urine output and creatinine should be monitored closely in the perioperative period. There have been enormous efforts directed towards finding prevention or pharmacotherapeutic AKI treatments. Promising treatments in experimental models or initial studies oftentimes have failed to have clinical success. Renal dose dopamine has not shown any benefit. Fenoldopam (dopamine-1 receptor antagonist), loop diuretics, anaritide (recombinant atrial natriuretic peptide), and calcium channel blockers have been tried and have not shown consistent benefit. Further studies are needed and some of these agents may show promise in the future.

SUMMARY

AKI is an abrupt decrease in kidney function. This new definition is more sensitive in detecting AKI. Mortality secondary to perioperative AKI is often greater than 50%, with even small SCr changes resulting in significant increases in mortality. Major risk factors include prior renal dysfunction, an elevation in SCr, hemodynamic insult, dehydration, decrease in cardiac function, and cardiac and vascular surgery. Most importantly, perioperative interventions aim to maintain euvolemia, preserve renal perfusion, and avoid nephrotoxins.

CHRONIC KIDNEY DISEASE: PERIOPERATIVE EVALUATION OF PATIENTS WITH KIDNEY DISEASE

Chronic kidney disease (CKD) occurs when there is damage to the kidney resulting in a GFR of <60 ml/min 1/1.73 m2 for ≥3 months. The damage may present as abnormalities in the histology, urine, or radiological imaging. Once CKD is identified, it should be assigned a stage based on the level of kidney function, irrespective of diagnosis and according to the KDOQI CKD classification (Table 5).

Table 5: KDOQI CKD Classification

Stage	Description	GFR (mL/min/1.73m2)
1.	Kidney damage including normal or increased GFR	Greater than 90
2.	Mild decrease in GFR	60 to 89
3.	Moderate decreae in GFR	30 to 59
4.	Severe decrease in GFR	15 to 29
5.	Kidney failure	Less than 15; or patient is on dialysis

Preoperative Assessment

CKD increases the risk for postoperative cardiovascular complications. In regards to increased perioperative cardiovascular risk, patients at intermediate risk have a creatinine level ≥2 according to the updated American College of Cardiology/American Heart Association (ACC/AHA) guidelines on perioperative cardiovascular evaluation of noncardiac surgery. Futhermore, patients who have advanced kidney disease have electrolyte and acid-base abnormalities which can be further aggravated by the effects of surgery and anesthesia. Anesthesia should be avoided in patients with CKD with a serum potassium level above 5.5 mEq per L.

Patients with advanced CKD are predisposed to anemia and are at an increased risk of worsening anemia with blood loss. They are also at an increased risk for excessive bleeding during surgery from defects in platelet aggregation due to uremia. Optimization of hemoglobin before surgery is helpful. To decrease the bleeding risk, desmopressin (DDAVP) can be administered before surgery in select patients who have advanced renal failure with high BUN levels. Patients who are adequately dialyzed do not warrant any therapy.

Preoperative diagnostic testing in patients with CKD should include serum electrolytes, BUN, SCr, calcium, complete blood count, and chest radiograph. Patients who are on dialysis are advised to undergo dialysis a day before surgery to avoid any electrolyte disturbances.

Patients with CKD oftentimes will have pre- and intra-operative hypertension. Most patients with hypertension and kidney disease should continue their antihypertensive therapy during the surgical period, with a few exceptions.

Postoperative assessment

CKD is an independent risk factor for postoperative death and cardiovascular events after elective, noncardiac surgery. CKD increases the risk for multiple postoperative complications, including acute renal failure, hyperkalemia, acid-base disturbances, volume overload, infections, drug toxicity, and more. All of these impact surgical morbidity and affect postoperative outcomes.

Fluid, Electrolytes and Acid-base Disturbances

Patients with advanced CKD (CKD Stage 4 and 5) are unable to concentrate and dilute urine; including a decreased ability to excrete sodium. With less sodium excreted, patients are predisposed to volume overload and hyperchloremic metabolic acidosis, when they are given large volumes of saline solution. Hyponatremia may occur from hypotonic fluids due to an inability to excrete free water with low GFR, these patients are also predisposed to excessive and inappropriate secretion of antidiuretic hormone.

Patients with advanced CKD Stage 5 and patients with diabetic nephropathy (Type 4 RTA) cannot excrete a potassium load. These patients can have a metabolic acidosis due to a reduction in ammonia synthesis and a decreased ability to excrete hydrogen ions. It is important to avoid a potassium load unless significant hypokalemia exists. Hyperkalemia can occur during transfusions, tissue breakdown, acidosis, ACE-I, heparin, beta-blockers, rhabdomyolysis, and the use of Ringer lactate solution as a replacement fluid. Another common situation leading to hyperkalemia in the perioperative period is the fasting state that causes low insulin secretion and a shift of potassium from inside cells and out into the plasma.

Acute Renal Failure

CKD increases patients' risk of developing ARF. ARF is an independent risk factor for increased postoperative morbidity and mortality. Attention to fluid balance is paramount. Avoiding medications that can potentiate ARF are best avoided. NSAIDs are contraindicated. ACE-I are best avoided in the immediate postoperative setting unless there is a compelling reason. Radiocontrast agents and antibiotics such as aminoglycosides should not be used unless necessary.

Pharmacology

CKD affects both the pharmacokinetics and the pharmacodynamics of many drugs. This effect predisposes these patients to adverse side effects. Attention should be given to medication dose adjustments when managing surgical patients with kidney disease. The effect of altered clearance must be addressed, and dose adjustments should be done based on the estimated GFR to avoid unwarranted toxicity. Patients with ARF estimated GFR is a poor predictor of true renal clearance and adjustments should be made based on the severity of the renal failure.

Dialysis Access

Dialysis access care is important in patients with end-stage renal disease. Vascular access can be termporary or permanent. Temporary vascular access consists of tunneled and non-tunneled catheters. Permanent access includes native arteriovenous fistulas and grafts, and peritoneal dialysis catheters. Avoiding intravenous lines in the arm with fistulas and grafts is important. When new catheters are placed, the subclavian vein should be avoided, due to a high risk of stenosis after catheterization. If a femoral vein is cannulated, it is best to utilize it for the short-term. Also, the catheter should be changed to the internal jugular vein because the risk of infection is much higher with a femoral Quinton.

AKI Management in the Perioperative Period

All efforts should be made to prevent AKI in the perioperative period by identifying at-risk patients. Potential nephrotoxic insults should be eliminated, and volume status and electrolyte imbalances should be corrected to minimize the risk of AKI.

Once AKI has occurred, it should be promptly identified. Attention to urine output in the postoperative period is paramount as creatinine levels may not be reliable. Elevation in creatinine may occur late, which can delay the diagnosis of AKI. In the early period, AKI may be reversible with the correction of hemodynamic status, correction of volume status, and removal of nephrotoxic insults. Management of established AKI is largely supportive as mentioned above. Renal replacement therapy (RRT) is indicated for refractory metabolic and volume derangements. The indications for dialysis or RRT in AKI are outlined in Table 6:

Table 6: Indications for Dialysis or RRT in AKI

Indications
Classic Indications: – Uremic complications: encephalopathy, pericarditis – Refractory hyperkalemia and acidosis – Refractory hypervolemia. – Progressive azotemia
Potential Indications: – Electrolyte imbalances – Volume disturbances – Sepsis – Increased intracranial pressure – Toxicities/poisonings

RENAL REPLACEMENT THERAPY

Principles of renal replacement therapy (RRT)

1. Diffusion: This refers to the movement of solutes through a semipermeable membrane across a concentration gradient from blood to the dialysate. Uremic solutes, potassium, etc move from higher concentrations in the blood to lower concentrations in the dialysate fluid. This type of solute transport occurs in HD and continuous venovenous hemodialysis.
2. Hemofiltration or convection: This consists of the movement of solutes with the plasma water through the membrane pores in response to transmembrane pressure applied from the blood compartment of the hemofilter. This results in the movement of all solutes along with plasma water out of the blood into the effluent compartment. Fluid along with physiologically useful electrolytes are infused back as replacement fluid

into the blood either pre-filter or post-filter. The amount of replacement fluid can be titrated depending upon the amount of ultrafiltration needed. This type of transport is utilized in Continuous Veno Venous Hemofiltration (CVVH).

Continuous Veno Venous Hemodiafiltration (CVVHD) combines both types.

Modalities of Renal Replacement Therapy

1. Intermittent hemodialysis (IHD): Also referred to as the conventional modality, involves intermittent therapy with higher blood and dialysate flows. IHD offers rapid clearance of solutes and ultrafiltration during brief treatments of 3 to 5 hours.
2. Continuous renal replacement therapies (CRRT): These include Continuous Veno Venous Hemofiltration (CVVH) or Continuous Veno Venous Hemodiafiltration (CVVHD). CRRT provides a more gradual removal of fluid and solute and is indicated for prolonged treatment times, generally 24 hrs/day. However, due to system clotting or other diagnostic/therapeutic procedures, the therapy is often interrupted.
3. Prolonged intermittent renal replacement therapy (PIRRT): These treatments generally last from 8 to 16 hours. They have slower rates of clearance of solute and ultrafiltration compared to IHD, but are more rapid than CRRT
4. Peritoneal dialysis (PD): Dialysate fluid is instilled and left to dwell into the peritoneal cavity via a catheter that is inserted into the peritoneum. The peritoneal membrane has a rich blood supply and acts as a semipermeable membrane, facilitating the diffusion of solutes from blood to the dialysate. While PD is a well-established modality for renal replacement in end-stage renal disease patients, it is rarely used as an acute modality. In patients with AKI, it is reserved for resource-poor situations such as unavailability of equipment and skilled nursing to perform CRRT or HD. PD is a simpler modality that is less labor-intensive, cost-effective, and does not require complex machines. PD may also be used in patients who are unable to get vascular access or are at high risk for such access. In these patients, the peritoneal catheter can be placed at the bedside and PD promptly initiated.

The Optimal Modality for RRT

Multiple studies have not shown any benefit of CRRT over iHD in patients with AKI requiring renal replacement therapy in the ICU. Intermittent hemodialysis and continuous renal replacement therapy are equally effective. Continuous modalities such as CVVH or CVVHD are preferred in patients with hypotension or tenuous hemodynamic status. Whereas iHD is preferred in cases of severe hyperkalemia, and toxicities where rapid clearance is required.

REFERENCES

1. Schreiber MJ. Minimizing perioperative complications in patients with renal insufficiency. Cleve Clin J Med. 2006;73 Suppl 1:S116-20.
2. Bellomo R, Ronco C, Kellum JA, Mehta RL, Palevsky P. Acute renal failure - definition, outcome measures, animal models, fluid therapy and information technology needs: the Second International Consensus Conference of the Acute Dialysis Quality Initiative (ADQI) Group. Crit Care. 2004;8(4):R204-212.
3. Hoste EAJ, Kellum JA. Acute kidney injury: epidemiology and diagnostic criteria. Curr Opin Crit Care. 2006;12(6):531-37.
4. Kuitunen A, Vento A, Suojaranta-Ylinen R, Pettilä V. Acute renal failure after cardiac surgery: evaluation of the RIFLE classification. Ann. Thorac. Surg. 2006;81(2):542-6.
5. Lombardi R, Ferreiro A. Risk factors profile for acute kidney injury after cardiac surgery is different according to the level of baseline renal function. Ren Fail. 2008;30(2):155-60.
6. Mehta RL, Kellum JA, Shah SV, et al. Acute Kidney Injury Network: report of an initiative to improve outcomes in acute kidney injury. Crit Care. 2007;11(2):R31.
7. Kheterpal S, Tremper KK, Englesbe MJ, et al. Predictors of postoperative acute renal failure after noncardiac surgery in patients with previously normal renal function. Anesthesiology 2007;107(6):892-902.
8. Chew ST, Newman MF, White WD, et al. Preliminary report on the association of apolipoprotein E polymorphisms, with postoperative peak serum creatinine concentrations in cardiac surgical patients. Anesthesiology 2000;93(2):325-31.
9. Wagener G, Brentjens TE. Renal disease: the anesthesiologist's perspective. Anesthesiol Clin 2006;24(3):523-47.
10. Rosner MH, Okusa MD. Acute kidney injury associated with cardiac surgery. Clin J Am Soc Nephrol 2006;1(1):19-32.
11. Thakar CV, Arrigain S, Worley S, Yared J, Paganini EP. A clinical score to predict acute renal failure after cardiac surgery. J Am Soc Nephrol 2005;16(1):162-8.

12. Vincent J, Gerlach H. Fluid resuscitation in severe sepsis and septic shock: an evidence-based review. Crit. Care Med 2004;32(11 Suppl): S451-54.
13. Solomon R, Deray G. How to prevent contrast-induced nephropathy and manage risk patients: practical recommendations. Kidney Int. Suppl. 2006;(100):S51-53.
14. McCullough PA, Stacul F, Becker CR, et al. Contrast-induced Nephropathy (CIN) Consensus Working Panel: executive summary. Rev Cardiovasc Med 2006;7(4):177-97.
15. Mathew, et al. Chronic kidney disease and postoperative mortality: A systematic review and meta-analysis International 2008;73:1069–81.
16. Palevsky et al., "KDOQI US Commentary on the 2012 KDIGO Clinical Practice Guideline for Acute Kidney Injury."

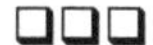

13

CHAPTER

Laparoscopic, Endoscopic, and Robotic Techniques

Vijay K. Mittal, MD
Ananya Das, MD
Nirupa Gopinath, MD
Arpit Aggarwal, MD
Jasneet Bhullar, MD

INTRODUCTION

Since the start of the 21st century, great advancements began taking place at a rate never seen before opening both opportunities and challenges to the surgical community. This rapid pace of technological progress, when combined with the aging of the American population and increasing shortage of general surgeons, has consequently generated a unique responsibility for surgeons globally.

The coalescences of major science and technology advances since the turn of the century has transformed human civilization. Recently, achievements including the invention of microchips and miniaturization have yielded a boom of information technology. In the medical field, the National Science Foundation funded research in medical robotics and femto-second lasers has resulted in the development of less invasive, more intricate, and cost-effective surgical devices.

Innovation within Minimally Invasive Surgery (MIS) has yielded in significant improvements in clinical outcome and perioperative recovery for surgical patients. Global incorporation of endoscopy, laparoscopy, and robotic MIS is truly evolving surgical field at a great pace never seen before.

ENDOSCOPIC SURGERY GASTROINTESTINAL ENDOSCOPY

Endoscopy means "looking inside" and typically refers to looking inside the human body for medical reasons using an instrument called an endoscope (Figure 1). Endoscopy is a minimally invasive diagnostic and interventional technique in which a tube-like device is inserted into a body orifice allowing physicians to assess the inner lining the GI tract. The endoscope can be rigid or flexible. Diagnostic uses can be conducted with rigid or flexible endoscope, and it allows for inspection of mucosal surfaces, narrow-band imaging, and photography. On the other hand, interventional capabilities can only be done with a flexible endoscope, and procedures include biopsies, foreign body retrieval, stent placement and dilation. Most diagnostic endoscopic procedures are done with or without minimal sedation. In some facilities, endoscopists have the option of administering sedation with fentanyl/midazolam and proceeding with the procedure. More commonly, propofol based deep sedation is increasingly administered in hospitals by certified nurse anesthesiologists. Unlike general anesthesia required for laparoscopic and robotic operations, sedation in endoscopy is limited to mild to moderate anesthesia with rudimentary monitoring of patients during the procedure. EGD and colonoscopy are visibly integral components of gastrointestinal minimally invasive surgery.

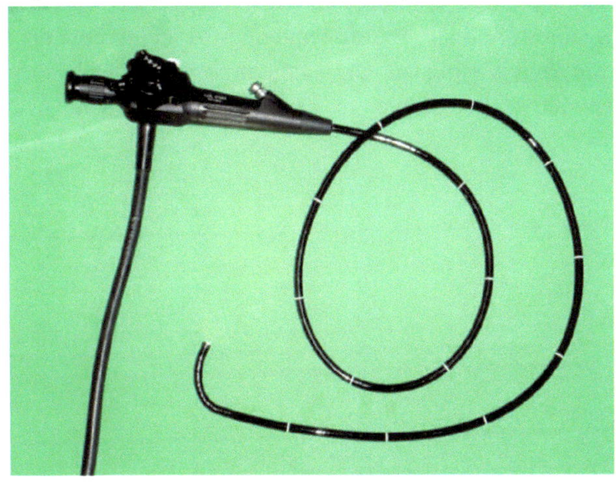

Figure 1: Endoscope

There are two kinds of endoscopy that are commonly performed on the gastrointestinal tract:

1. Esophagogastroduodenoscopy to visualize the esophagus, stomach and duodenum shown in Figure 2.
2. Colonoscopy to visualize the colon (large bowel) and rectum shown in Figure 7.

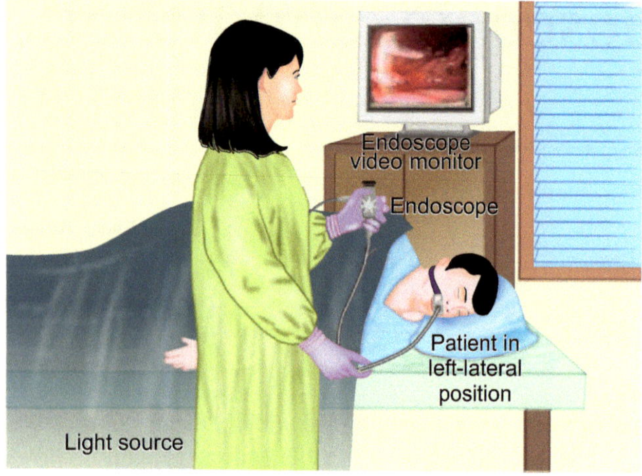

Figure 2: Endoscopy procedure

ESOPHAGOGASTRODUODENOSCOPY (EGD)

The patient lies on their left side with their head resting on a pillow. The endoscope is then passed over the tongue and into the oropharynx. Quick and gentle manipulation under vision guides the endoscope into the esophagus. The endoscope is slowly moved through the esophagus as the physician notes any pathology. It then passes through the stomach quickly, past the pylorus, and into the first and second parts of the duodenum for examination. After reaching the second part of the duodenum, the endoscope returns to the stomach for a more thorough examination. At this stage, any necessary procedures are done. Before removing the endoscope, air in the stomach is aspirated. During the procedure, the physician often takes photographs to later show the patient while explaining any findings.

The endoscope can simply be used to inspect the digestive tract lining and is oftentimes all that is needed. However, the endoscope is particularly valuable because it can obtain a biopsy. To obtain small biopsies, a pincer (biopsy forceps) is inserted into and passes through the scope. The pincers can take 1 to 3 mm samples of tissue under direct vision. The intestinal mucosa heals quickly from such biopsies.

Then the pathologist can histologically examine the biopsy tissue with light microscopy and/or immunohistochemistry. Biopsied material can also be tested on urease to identify Helicobacter pylori.

Esophagus

The esophagus is routinely examined during diagnostic esophagogastroduodenoscopy (EGD) (Figure 3). Gastroesophageal reflux disease (GERD), particularly with a suboptimal response to proton pump inhibitor-based therapy, is a very common indication for diagnostic EGD. Dysphagia, particularly experienced with solid food and with a progressive course, is an alarming symptom and should be promptly evaluated by EGD. Commonly performed therapeutic procedures are esophageal dilations using both boogie and balloon dilators. Caustic strictures are quite common in certain parts of the country because of ingestion of lye and other caustic chemicals.

Initial endoscopic evaluation in such patients, usually in the first 24 hours, is indicated to grade severity and extent of injury. The treatment of caustic esophageal strictures is often complicated by frequent recurrence and may benefit by endoscopic injection of a steroid at the site of the stricture. Esophageal varies, often acutely bleeding, are frequently encountered in patients with chronic liver disease. Although current data is overwhelmingly in favor of variceal banding in terms of safety and efficacy, esophageal sclerotherapy is more prevalent in developing countries primarily for economic reasons.

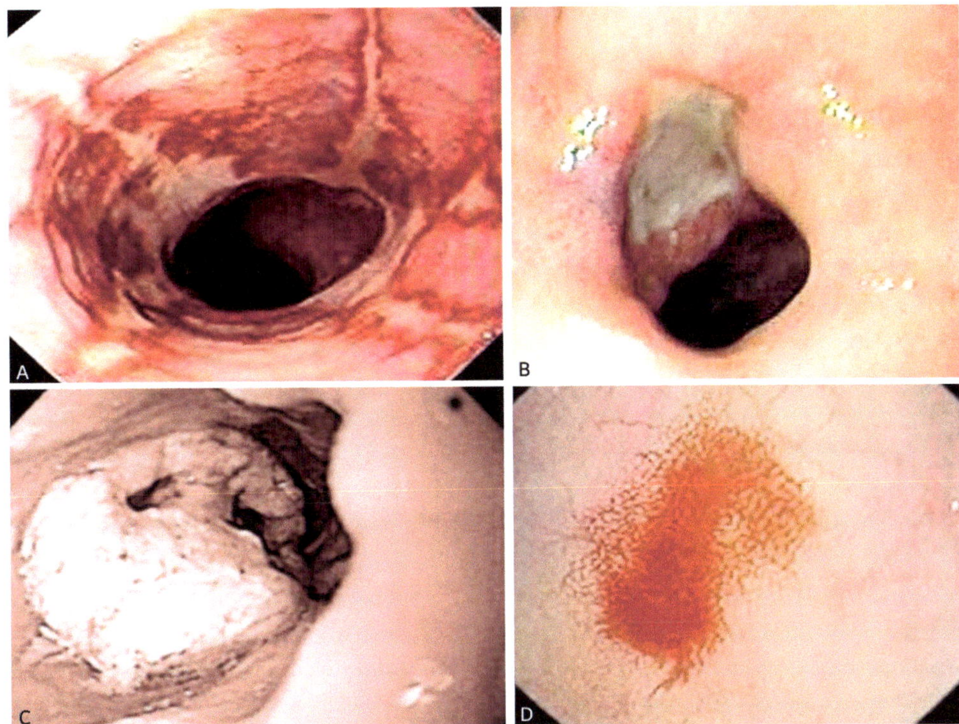

Figure 3: Endoscopic images of commonly seen upper gastrointestinal pathology. (A) Erosive esophagitis due to reflux. (B) A duodenal ulcer of peptic etiology. (C) A squamous cell esophageal cancer with partial luminal obstruction by the ulcerated mass. (D) An angio-ectasia (arteriovenous malformation) commonly seen in the small intestine as a bleeding lesion

Stomach

Peptic ulcer is very common globally, and EGD is most performed for evaluation of dyspepsia. Functional dyspepsia, often with gastroparetic symptoms of bloating and early satiety, is widely prevalent in the population and it is difficult to distinguish from organic dyspepsia. The judicious use of diagnostic endoscopy is critical in the appropriate work-up of these patients. H. pylori is a bacterium that infects the mucus lining of the stomach and duodenum. It is often the cause of peptic ulcers, gastritis, and duodenitis. Today, many stomach ulcers are treated with antibiotics effective against H. pylori. Gastric varices are common and seen in cirrhosis and noncirrhotic portal hypertensive diseases such as extrahepatic portal vein obstruction. Gastric outlet obstruction is an additional complication of peptic ulcer disease and endoscopic interventions include balloon dilation and stent placement.

Small Intestine

With the advent of newer endoscopic techniques such as balloon-assisted enteroscopy, endoscopic evaluation of the small intestine is quickly shifting from radiological studies to direct endoscopic evaluation. With the use of balloons incorporated on the endoscopes and over-tubes (in case of double-balloon endoscopes), the mechanical hurdle of looping and consequent non-progression has been greatly reduced allowing for further assessment of the small intestine, via either transoral or transrectal route. Non-specific intestinal ulcerations of indeterminate etiology are the cause of bleeding in many patients presenting with overt obscure gastrointestinal bleeding. Besides intestinal bleeding, infectious disorders such as intestinal tuberculosis are common clinical indications for enteroscopy. The availability of wireless capsule endoscopy is still very limited outside teaching hospitals.

Large Intestine

Interestingly, neoplastic diseases of the colon are distinctly less common in regions such as sub-Sahara Africa and unlike western countries, screening colonoscopy is not routinely indicated. Europe and the US share similar rates of chronic inflammatory bowel disease and their diagnostic, and therapeutic rates of intervention. There are growing reports of increasing prevalence of Crohn's disease in South East Asia. Furthermore, anorectal disorders are globally common and treatments of hemorrhoids such as rubber band ligation and transanal hemorrhoidal deartelization Doppler procedure utilize rigid proctoscopes.

Hepatopancreatobiliary System

Endoscopic cannulation of the pancreaticobiliary system in conjunction with fluoroscopic guidance allows for diagnosis and therapy of gallstone disease and gallbladder cancer (Figure 4). Although many physicians practice diagnostic ERCP, in most communities, only a few select endoscopists perform therapeutic ERCP. They often perform endoscopic sphincterotomy and place bile duct stents.

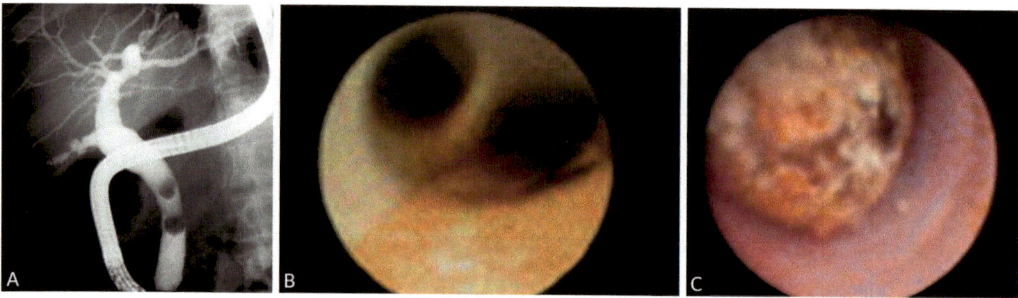

Figure 4: (A) Retrograde cholangiogram showing two bile duct stones shown as filling defects. (B) Cholangioscopy is a useful technique to visualize the endoluminal aspect of the biliary tree for direct visualization of pathologic lesions such as a stone or (C) tumor.

Biliary ascariasis is a unique disorder often seen in South East Asian countries, requiring ERCP and endoscopic removal of degenerated round worms. With the dissemination of laparoscopic cholecystectomy to smaller cities and towns, bile duct injury is commonly encountered and prompt endoscopic therapy with placement of biliary prosthesis is crucial. Pancreatic endotherapy such as pancreatic sphincterotomy, or pseudocyst drainage is less commonly performed. Invasive surgical procedures are still the mainstay treatment of many biliopancreatic disorders, which are typically treated in the west by endoscopic or at least by minimally invasive surgery.

Endoscopic ultrasonography (Figures 5 and 6) is expensive, and there is a lack of trained physicians, especially within rural settings. There is a perception that practices have advanced, but expensive technologies such as EUS may not be economically viable in some regions.

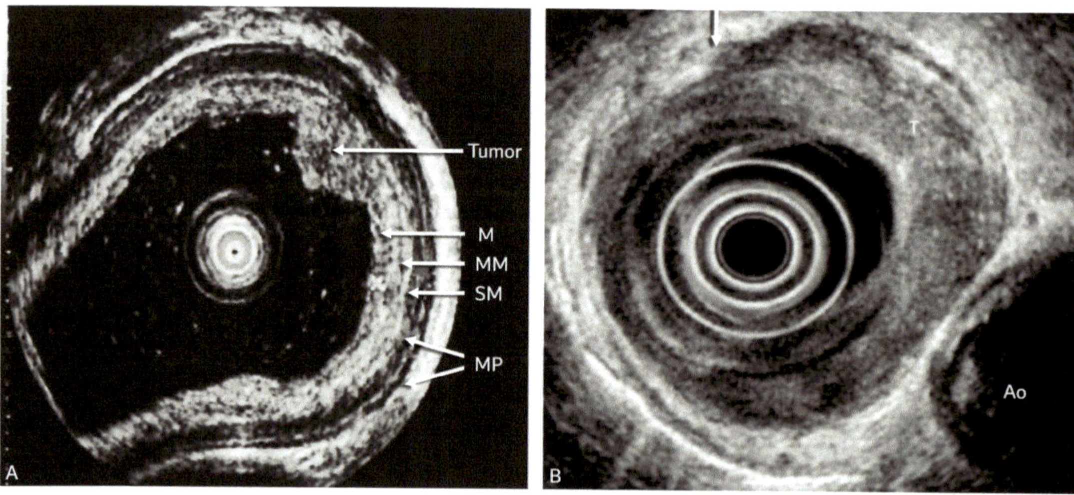

Figure 5: (A) Endoscopic ultrasonographic image obtained by a high frequency catheter probe of an early esophageal cancer limited to mucosa and amenable to endoscopic resection. m represents mucosa; mm, muscularis mucosa; sm submucosa; mp muscularis propria. (B) EUS image of a locally advanced esophageal cancer that has progressed through the muscularis propria into periesophageal tissue (T3 category tumor). The tissue plain between the tumor and the descending aorta (Ao) remains intact

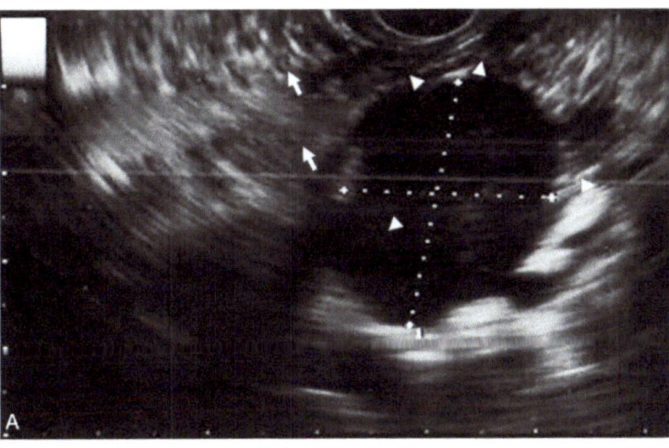
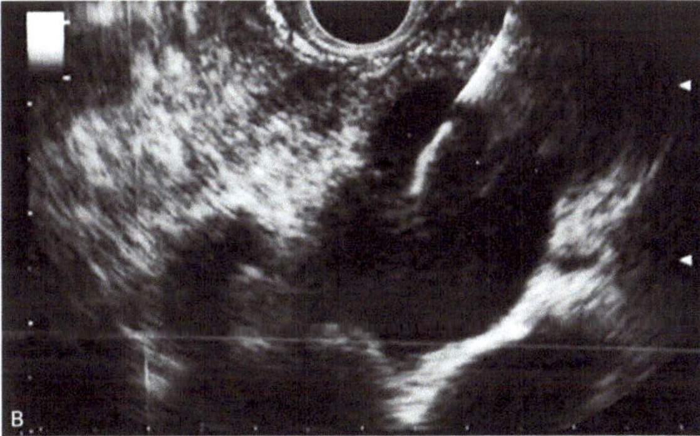

Figure 6: (A) EUS image of a malignant appearing celiac lymph node in a patient with esophageal cancer. (B) EUS guided fine-needle aspiration is being performed for confirmation of nodal metastasis.

Gastrointestinal cancer has distinctly different incidence patterns in the Eastern hemisphere compared to the Western hemisphere. In fact, the so-called esophageal cancer belt spans across the Asian continent and account for 75% of esophageal cancer diagnosis. In the absence of established endoscopic screening programs, most esophageal cancers are diagnosed late in their clinical course, and with very limited opportunity for curative treatment. Utilization of palliative measures such as endoscopic stent therapy and endoscopic gastrostomies are low. With the initial reports of radiofrequency based endoscopic ablative therapy of early squamous cell cancer and precancerous high-grade dysplasia, there may be an opportunity for institutions to incorporate endoscopic screening programs in hopes of reducing incidence of this morbid cancer.

Late diagnosis is typical for other common concerns as well such as gastric and gallbladder cancer. Access to endoscopic palliation is very limited and is often not pursued for financial reasons. Colorectal cancer is uncommon, although in some reports an increasing incidence has been reported in more affluent segments of society.

COLONOSCOPY

Colorectal cancer is the second leading cause of cancer deaths in the United States. Studies have shown that removing polyps, which may develop into cancer, decreases the risk of colorectal cancer. Thus, screening studies looking for cancer before a person has symptoms is extremely important. Screening is helpful in finding cancers at early stages, enabling more simple treatment compared to finding the cancer after symptoms appear and potential spread. The most effective method for colon and rectal cancer screening is the colonoscopy, recommended to be done every 10 years starting at the age of 45 for average risk patients. Patient with a personal or family history of colorectal polyps, inflammatory bowel disease or colorectal cancer are considered high risk and should have earlier and more frequent surveillance colonoscopies.

Colonoscopy is the minimally invasive endoscopic examination of the colon, where an endoscope is passed through the anus. It may provide a visual diagnosis and grant the opportunity for biopsy or removal of suspected lesions. Colonoscopy allows the doctor to visually see whether polyps or cancer are present (Figure 7). When obtaining a biopsy, biopsy forceps are inserted through a channel in the colonoscope, then the forceps remove a small tissue sample that is sent off for microscopic examination. The introduction of air into the colon may be necessary for better visibility.

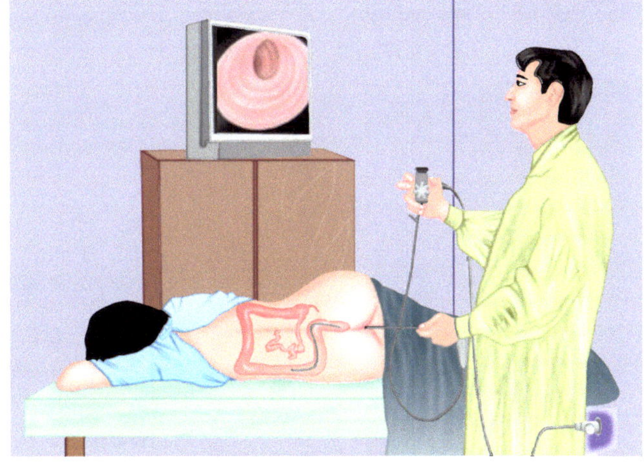

Figure 7: Colonoscopy procedure

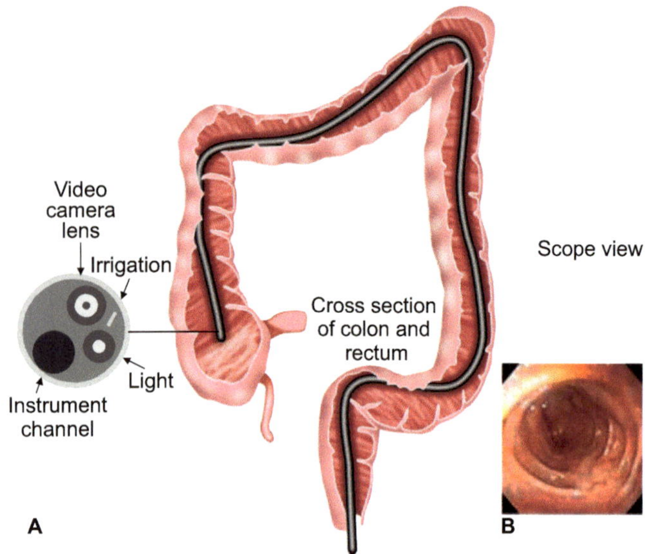

Figure 8: How an endoscope travels through the colon and generates an image viewed by the physician.

A polyp is an abnormal growth of tissue (tumor) projecting from the inner lining of the bowel into the lumen. Colon polyps are uncommonly associated with symptoms. Colon polyps are a concern because they can potentially have microscopic portions of colon cancer difficult to detect and they pose a risk of transforming with time into colon cancer. Since most polyps are asymptomatic, they are usually discovered at the time of colon cancer screening with colonoscopy.

Most polyps can be completely removed safely during colonoscopy. Polyps are removed with biopsy forceps shown in Figure 9 or snare resection shown in Figure 10, with or without cautery.

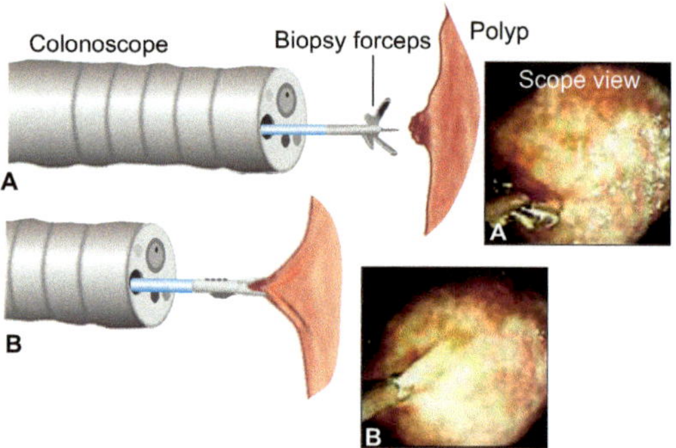

Figure 9: Biopsy forceps used to remove a polyp.

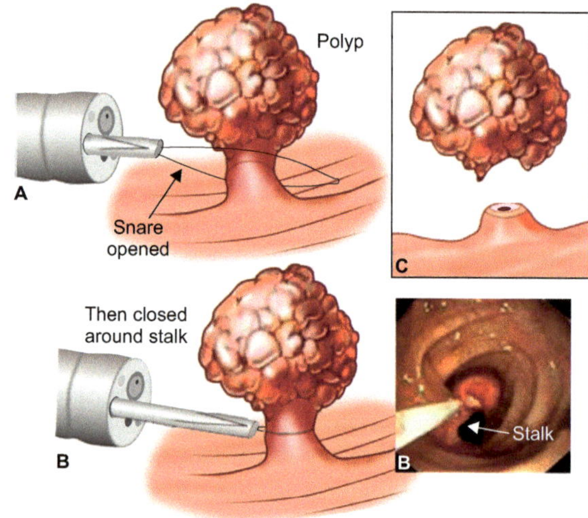

Figure 10: Snare resection of a polyp.

Some polyps which do not have a stalk require special techniques. Saline is injected into the surrounding area to elevate the polyp and facilitate removal by snare.

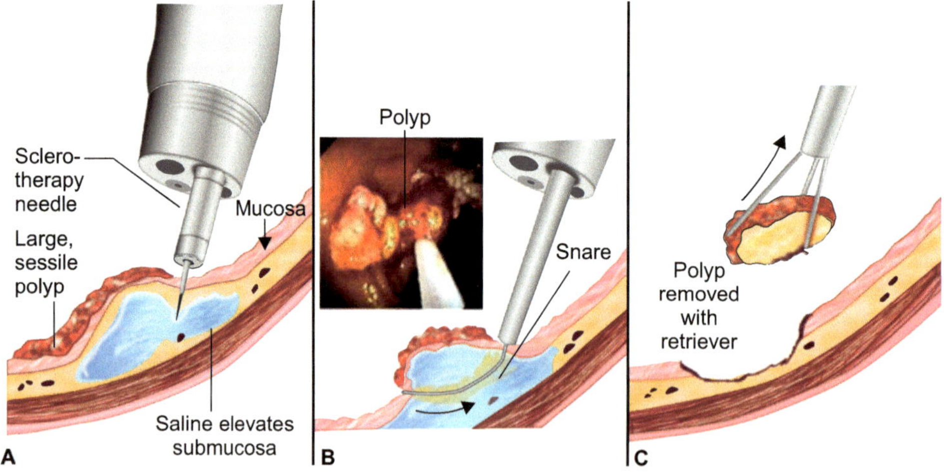

Figure 11: A polyp without a stalk, requiring saline injection to lift the polyp so it can be removed by snare resection.

Snare and cautery current can resect large polyps by piecemeal. If the polyp cannot be successfully resected, the patient must undergo surgery. Large polyps may require marking of the polypectomy site with India ink. Such site tattooing is helpful in localizing the area of interested in subsequent colonoscopies and future surgeries.

Endoscopic Training and Competency

Advancements in endoscopic diagnostic and therapeutic evaluation has yielded the need standardize didactic knowledge and technical understanding for procedures. In response in 2004, the Society of American Gastrointestinal and Endoscopic Surgeons (SAGES) introduced the Fundamentals of Endoscopic Surgery (FES) course. The FES program consists of two components: a web-based didactic curriculum and a validated virtual-reality assessment to evaluate fundamental technique. To complete the course, participants need to pass a written test of knowledge and hands-on skills test. It's effective, reproducible, and standardized content led the American Board of Surgery (ABS) to mandate FES as a pre-requisite for board certification.

FES Didactic Curriculum [64]

Module 1	Technology	• Characteristics of Endoscopes • Equipment Setup/Care • Troubleshooting
Module 2	Patient Preparation	• Informed Consent • Anesthesia Risk Assessment • Bowel Preparation • Prophylactic Antibiotic Therapy • Management of Anticoagulation
Module 3	Sedation & Analgesia	• Monitoring • Sedation Recovery • Alternative Sedation • Small Caliber Endoscopy
Module 4	Upper Gastrointestinal Endoscopy	• Indications • Preparation • Diagnostic EGD • Complications
Module 5	Lower Gastrointestinal Endoscopy	• Indications • Preparation
Module 6	Performing Lower GI Procedures	• Colonoscopy, Rigid Endoscope • Important Considerations
Module 7	Lower GI Anatomy, Pathology, Complications	• Pathology Recognition • Complications
Module 8	Didactic ERCP	• Indications • Performance of ERCP • Complications
Module 9	Hemostasis	• Non-thermal Techniques • Thermal Techniques
Module 10	Tissue Removal	• Resective Techniques • Sampling Techniques • Ablative Techniques
Module 11	Enteral Access	• Indications • PEG • Procedures with PEJ • Replacement • Complications
Module 12	Endoscopic Therapies	• Dilation • Foreign Body Removal • Transgastric Laparoendoscopy • Choledochoscopy • Tumor Localization

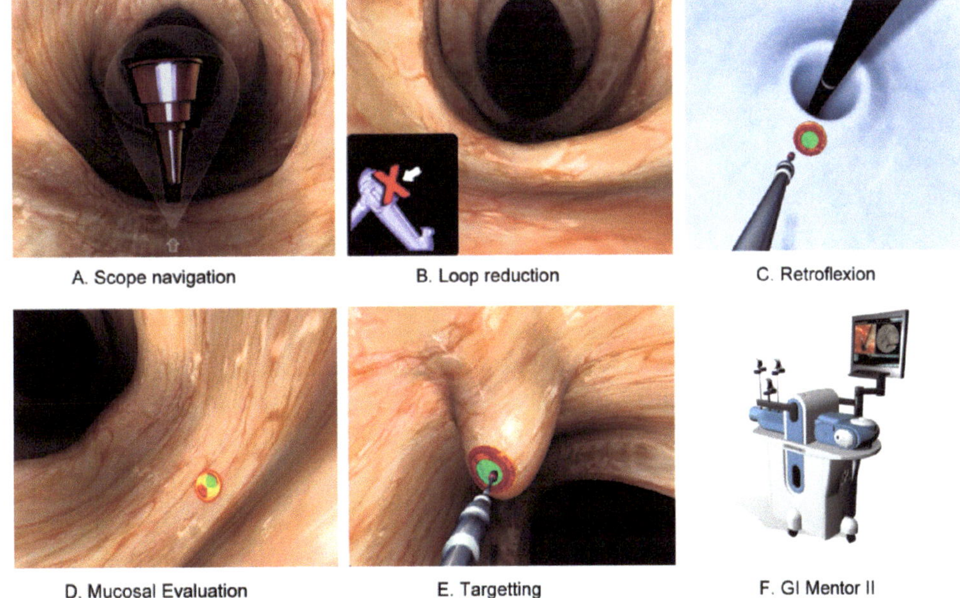

Figure 12: FES Skills Examination[65]

Minimally invasive endoscopy and surgery is clearly a cornerstone to diagnosis and treatment of many gastrointestinal and hepatopancreatobiliary disorders. However, it is important to recognize that access to health care technology varies globally because health care costs in many developing countries are based on out-of-pocket expenses. Economic constrains may therefore influence medical decisions. In southeast Asia for example, more than 80% of the endoscopic facilities are provided by the private health care sector, and in the government health sector the endoscopic diagnostic facilities are often underdeveloped or nonexistent. Global accessibility of medical devices such as endoscope will require the ongoing and persistent medical advocacy by medical providers and global leaders. With recognition of the importance of this discipline by health care institutions and governments, minimally invasive surgery may have the potential to improve clinical outcomes in a cost-effective manner.

LAPAROSCOPIC SURGERY

Traditionally, surgical operations are performed with large incisions over the skin to access the relevant body areas and cavities. Minimally invasive surgery not only offers a more cosmetic appeal, but it also improves clinical outcome measures and hospital cost-effectiveness. Laparoscopic/thoracoscopic surgeries are now widely adopted by thoracic, abdominal, and pelvic surgeons.

Benefits of minimally invasive or laparoscopic procedures are:

- Less postoperative discomfort since the incisions are much smaller.
- Quicker recovery times.
- Shorter hospital stays.
- Earlier return to full activities.
- Much smaller scars.
- Less internal scarring.
- Smaller chance of developing hernias through the abdominal incision.

Minimally invasive surgeons make a few small incisions about half an inch long in the abdomen and introduces a small video camera through one of these incisions to visualize the organs of the abdominal cavity. The video camera is connected to a television monitor which helps guide the surgeon's actions. The surgeon performs the surgery using thin, long instruments also introduced through the small incisions. The main difference in laparoscopic surgery to conventional surgery is that the surgeon, instead of looking at the organ directly, is looking at the video monitor. The video camera becomes the surgeon's eyes in laparoscopy surgery, since the surgeon uses the image from the video camera positioned inside the patient's body to perform the procedure. The currently available high-definition cameras and monitors provide greatly magnified and accurate images of the relevant body parts. But the challenge for the surgeon is to develop the hand-eye coordination skills needed to perform these surgeries.

Almost every abdominal, pelvic, and thoracic operation has been done through laparoscopic minimally invasive technique. Still, regardless of open or MIS approach, technical precision and understanding comes with comprehensive, repetitive, and focused training. Laparoscopic surgery poses unique challenges because it relies on a two-dimensional view, limited rotational dexterity, and is labor intensive for operators. A moment of inattention could lead to unforgiving complications. Surgeon must be trained to perform traditional operations through contemporary and state-of-the-art medical

Laparoscopic colon surgery is becoming increasingly popular due to advantages (relative to open surgery) including:

- A quicker normalization of colon function.
- Shorter hospital length of stay and faster recovery time.
- Decreased postoperative pain.
- The ability to return to normal activities more quickly.
- A smaller scar.

General anesthesia and safe positioning are paramount to both laparoscopic and robotic MIS. Insufflation of the peritoneal cavity, called pneumoperitoneum, requires the neuromuscular paralysis and deep sedation achieved through the induction of general anesthesia. Laparoscopic and robotic instruments are introduced within the space created after carbon dioxide gas insufflation a surgical space. However, insufflation of the abdominal/pelvic cavity may result in changes in cardiorespiratory status and musculoskeletal. Other less common but notable mechanical failure include: *device failure leading to iatrogenic trauma, burn, disassembly, and misfiring of instruments and staplers. Other complications included neurologic injuries like visual loss, and corneal ulceration. Neuromuscular injuries like compartm*ent syndrome in the legs, rhabdomyolysis, nerve injuries, and pressure ulcers.[6,8,9,10] Pulmonary complications like acidosis, pulmonary edema, barotraumas, atelectasis, pneumothorax, capnothorax. carbon dioxide embolization, pneumomediastinum, and subcutaneous emphysema. Cardiovascular complications include arrhythmia, hemorrhage, hypotension, and bradycardia due to increased vagal tone.[11-15]

Training and Competency

As technology continues to be adopted, rapid training of future surgeons will become an essential part of surgical residencies. In 2004, the Society of American Gastrointestinal and Endoscopic Surgeons (SAGES) launched the validated Fundamentals of Laparoscopic Surgery (FLS) curriculum and with the American College of Surgeons (ACS), promoted FLS to be a minimum standard before a surgeon should be allowed to independently perform laparoscopic procedures. Like FES, FLS consists of a free didactic curriculum and testing of knowledge and manual skills. Passing the cognitive component of the skills portion consisting of back and forth peg transfer, cutting a marked circle penalty for deviation outside, placing a secure knot with a pre-tied ligating loop or endoloop at a marked area, and needle driving and intracorporeal and extracorporeal suturing. [67] (Figure 13) Dexterity and relaxed laparoscopic skills are developed through practice and repetition. Advanced laparoscopic skills that essential for complex gastrointestinal operations are gradually perfected by training surgeons through simulation practice and operative application (Figure 14)

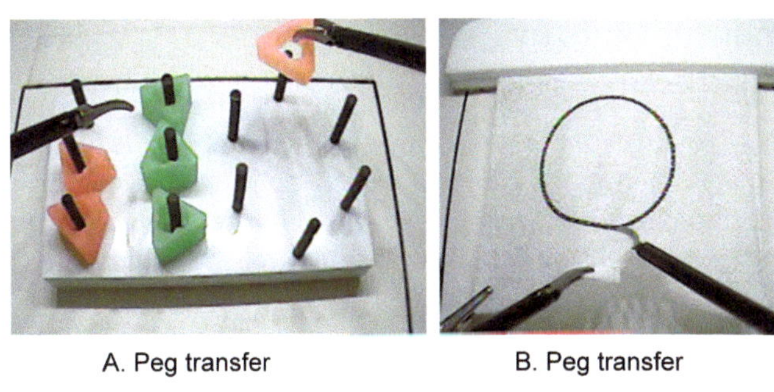

A. Peg transfer B. Peg transfer

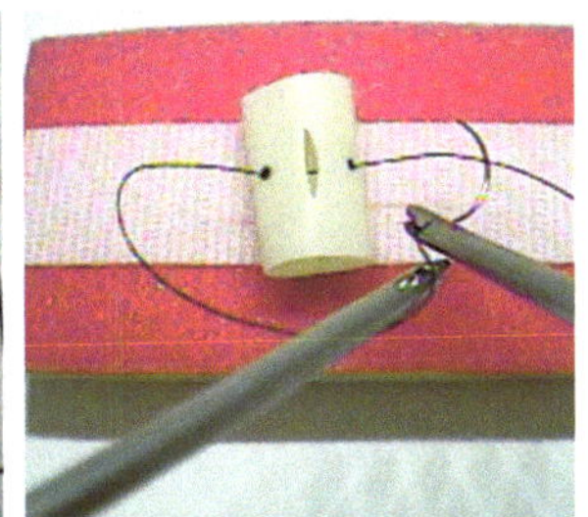

C. Ligating loop D. Suture knot

Task	Task name	Proficiency level*	Second	Allowable errors	Repetitions**
1.	Peg transfer	mean	48	no drops outside field of view	
2.	Precision cutting	mean +2 s.d.	98	all cuts between 2 circles of the training gauze	2 consecutive
3.	Ligating lopp	mean +2 s.d.	53	up to 1 mm accuracy error al-lowed	2. consecuive
4.	Suture wit extracorporeal knot	mean +2 s.d.	136	up to 1 mm accuracy error al-lowed	2 consecutive
5.	Suture with intracorporeal knot	mean +2 s.d.	112	up to 1 mm accuracy error al-lowed	2 consecutive +10 nonconsecutive
* Based on expert-derived peformance ** Maximum number of repetitions is 80					

Figure 13: FLS skills task and assessment

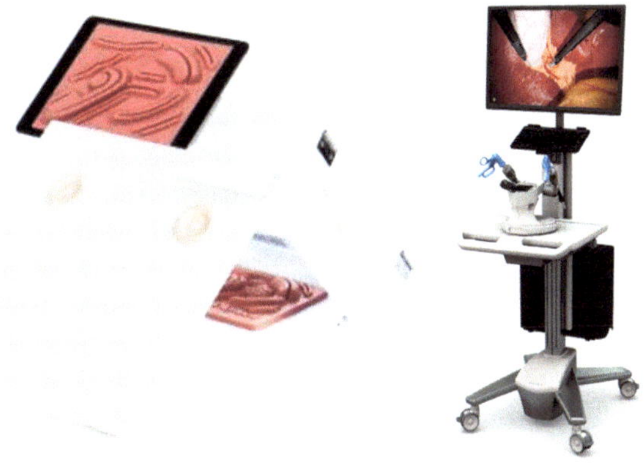

Figure 14 [68-69] : Laparoscopic simulators

ROBOTIC SURGERY

Initially FDA approved in 2000, the use of robotic minimally invasive surgery has rapidly expanded and evolved the field of surgery. The robotic platform gained exceptional popularity with urologists because of its utility within the deep confines of the pelvis. In 2012, 2,500 da Vinci robotic systems had been sold across the world, 2,000 alone in the United States, with 450,000 robotic procedures performed. The industry has grown from one FDA approved manufacturer to eight in the USA-five were registered in 2021. Today, robots expanded role is exemplified through its applications within abdominal wall, hepatobiliary, colorectal, and even transplant surgery. Concurrently, it is imperative that surgeons utilizing the technology understand its limitations.

Definitions and Evolution of Robotic Systems

Robot: a machine capable of carrying out a complex series of actions automatically.

Robotic Surgery: a technique where a surgeon performs surgery using a computer that remotely controls small instruments attached to a robot.

Definition by SAGES: "a surgical procedure or technology that adds a computer technology enhanced device to the interaction between a surgeon and a patient during a surgical operation and assumes some degree of control heretofore completely reserved for the surgeon.[1]"

History of the Robot

Robotic surgery is deemed the modern revolution in the field of medicine, and its use continues to be developed and published. The term 'robot' is derived from the Czechoslovakian word robota meaning forced labor. In 1495, the first robot was developed by Leonardo da Vinci. This robot imitated human movements and was named the Metal plated Warrior. In 1920, early robots were designed to perform simple tasks such as moving materials, parts, tools etc.[2] In medicine, robotics started as the voice-recognition system called HERMES, after which several computer-assisted robots have been developed. In 1985, the first robotic-assisted surgery was performed by Kwoh et al. for Neurosurgery by a robot named Puma 560. In 1991, Davies et al, performed a transurethral resection of the prostate by a robot named Probot. For a period, further development of robotics continued, but nothing was approved by the Food and Drug Administration (FDA). Finally, in 1993, Automated Endoscopic System for Optimal Positioning (AESOP) became the first surgical robotic device to gain FDA approval, and thus began the era of robotics in surgery. In 2003, two systems, Zeus, and da Vinci, merged to become the da Vinci Surgical System. Since then, the da Vinci has been the only commercially available telerobotic system to be used in the world.[2-6]

Advantages and Disadvantages of Robotic Minimally Invasive Surgery

Compared to traditional operating room devices, surgical robots are much more complex, both electrically and mechanically. Additionally, they involve both direct external and internal contact with the patient. These are important features that differentiate surgical robots from other equipment including traditional operating room instruments, intraoperative imaging devices, and operating microscopes.

There are many advantages of robotic surgery, especially for the patients. The surgeon has better defined anatomy with magnification and 3-D stereoscopic visualization. For example, robotic visualization and dissection within the deep narrowed pelvic male during a prostatectomy has improved clinical outcomes. The patient experiences less pain, minimal blood loss, faster recovery, less risk of infection, shorter stay in the hospital, less scarring, a less invasive procedure, and a quicker return to normal activities.

As with any technology, there are also disadvantages. The disadvantages of robotic surgery include their expense to obtain and maintain, a loss of tactile feedback, and the need for special surgical team training on the operation of the robot. For the patient robotic surgery carries the same risk of any surgery such as heart attacks, stroke, and death. Furthermore, each surgery will have its own complications. Side effects of impotence and incontinence may result from nerve damage from dissection or nature of disease. [7]

Prolonged Robotic Surgery and Second Time-Out

In 2008, the World Health Organization (WHO) published a surgical checklist to promote patient safety. The checklist addressed three phases of an operation; first before the induction of anesthesia (sign-in), second before the incision of the skin (time-out), and finally before the patient leaves the operating room (sign-out). The checklist was designed to minimize the most common and avoidable risks to surgical patients. The WHO checklist also addressed open and minimally invasive surgery. Then, with advancements in technology, robotic surgery was adopted and has since grown at a rapid pace. This new technology and inexperienced surgeons and surgical teams exposed patients to prolong surgery and complications. Thus, to minimize the reversible adverse events, Joseph B. Song et al developed a second time-out checklist for these lengthy robotic surgeries. This checklist is to be conducted three to four hours after the start of surgery in attempts to enhance perioperative patient safety and quality of care. The checklist focuses on the increased risk from position related complications and other adverse events. Other injuries including increased intraocular pressure, neuropathy and blindness, pneumoperitoneum, ventilation-perfusion perfusion mismatch, and Laryngeal edema have been reported.[16]

Legal and Ethical Issues of Robotic Surgery

Over the past two decades, physicians have been trained to perform robotic surgery on the job at certified training centers. However, privileges for robotic surgery vary widely because there is no universal guideline that exist for training and credentialing robotic surgery. Developing and maintaining robotic surgical skills requires frequent practice. Two studies conducted by experienced advanced laparoscopic surgeons evaluating the adaptation the robotic platform was done. After an initial phase of training, both studies demonstrated that a minimum of 50 robotic cases were necessary to start becoming consistent, and greater than 75 cases were necessary to become proficient.[22] There are several studies assessing learning curves for robotic MIS including pelvic surgery specialties like urology and gynecology.[23-34] A lack of case volume in robots often resulted in longer operating room times, increased complications, and increased costs to the medical system. Robotic surgeons should therefore undergo rigorous training and proctored assessment prior to independent use of the robotic platform.

Moreover, medical legal implications are not clearly defined for robotic surgery and currently no standardized credentialing system exists to evaluate surgeon competency and patient safety with robotic surgery performance. Zorn KC et al. anticipates that in the future, there will be discussion to initiate regulatory oversight of surgeon certification and proctorship.[17] Such an oversite is needed because critics allege that the number of complications from robotic surgeries are underreported and, currently, no national registry for robotic surgery related complications exists. In the future, we can anticipate an increase in lawsuits on defective robotic system, inexperienced surgeons, inadequate training, etc. Patients who suffer from complications after robotic surgery will not only have the potential to sue surgeons, and hospitals but also the robotic manufacturer and telecommunications company.[21] We must also consider important ethical issues from robotic surgeries such as equipment safety and reliability, provision of adequate information, and maintenance of confidentiality. Additionally, we must consider the issue of the expense of a robotic system, underfinanced hospital systems, affordability issues to patients leading to specialist shortage in underdeveloped regions.[18] And there is also liability exposure for surgical robotic instructors.[19,20]

Training and Competency

During the initial rise of robotic MIS, training standards and credentials for robotic surgery is largely left to individual hospitals and residency programs. State and national accreditation and regulatory bodies have developed tools that define, assess, and assure maintenance of physician competence.[57] SAGES and Minimally Invasive Robotic Association introduced a structured course around 2012, and they recommended institutions develop a formalized curriculum which includes hand-on training, observation of live cases, and proctored formal assessment of competency. Similar to FES and FLS, minimally invasive surgeons are required to obtain Fundamental of Robotic Surgery (FRS) certification for robotic surgery privileges. Its success was evidenced when a study published in 2021 demonstrated clear skill development through such a formalized curriculum and increased console time. [63] It is not surprising that its implementation has expanded to over 75% of surgical training problems around the US. Robotic certification, achieved during or after residency training, includes a didactic curriculum, team training/communication module, and skill development simulation tasks. Providers must be trained in the unique technical portions of robotic platform such as device preparation including port placement, targeting, and arm maneuverability. Providers must show proficiency in fundamental exercises like clutching, needle driving, energy devices, and control of multiple arms. More advanced and also expensive devices can simulate surgeries like hysterectomy, inguinal hernia repair, and colectomy.

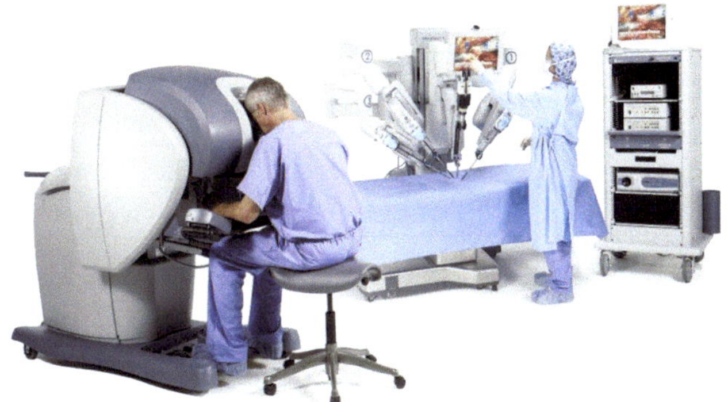

Figure 14: Surgeon console with inbuilt simulation module, patient cart, and vision cart[59]

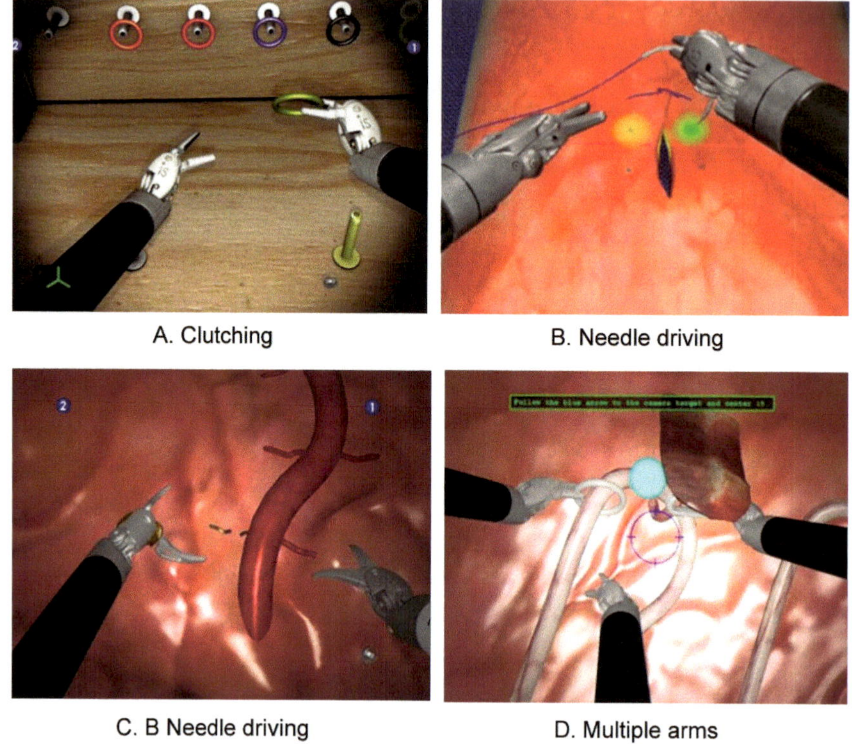

A. Clutching B. Needle driving

C. B Needle driving D. Multiple arms

Figure 15 da Vinci Xi Robot Skills[6]

Many residency and fellowship training programs across the US use a similar robotic curriculum to certify their trainees. Providers who have limited robotic training have ample opportunity to attend day or weekend long skill training courses hosted by manufacturers. Although variable credentialing pathways for individual hospital systems exist, all new robotic surgeons must have their first five cases reviewed. For the resident/fellow surgeon-in-training, proficiency must be validated by program director verifying at least 20 robotic console cases, 10 bedside cases, and a 6-month case volume log. New users must complete Intuitive Clinical Pathway course and complete two proctored cases which are reviewed by Robotic Director.

Table: Requirements and Pathways for Robotic certification of graduating residents

Pathways:	Requirements
Graduates of a Residency or Fellowship:	10 bedside cases, 20 console cases AND letter of robotic proficiency from Program Director
Surgeon WITHOUT Robotic Experience:	Complete robotic surgery course with 8 hours of hands-on training AND 5 proctored cases with letter attesting competency by proctoring surgeon
Surgeon WITH Robotic Experience:	Letter of prior credentialing AND 6-month case volume

The incorporation of advanced minimally invasive endoscopy and surgery in clinical practice requires addition fellowship and continued medical education. For instance, skills for advanced endoscopic procedures such as ERCP for hepatobiliary pathology, submucosal resection for large polyps, and gastroplasty for weight loss are attained through complex flexible endoscopy fellowship programs. Similarly, advanced gastrointestinal laparoscopic and robotic fellowship training to conduct operations involving bariatrics, hepatopancreaticobiliary, foregut, colorectal, and abdominal wall. The integration of technology with the intricacies of complex pathology clearly necessitates sufficient experience and training. While completion of accredited residency programs may be appropriate for basic minimally invasive endoscopy and surgery, complex pathology and advanced procedures require further technical and cognitive development. It is essential for minimally invasive surgeons and health care institutions to safely integrate advanced technology with a pursuit for continued medical excellence to achieve the highest level of care for patients.

REFERENCES

1. Herron DM, et al. A consensus document on robotic surgery: prepared by the SAGES-MIRA robotic surgery consensus group, 2007by SAGES.
2. M. Albani JM. The role of robotics in surgery: A Review, Science & Technology Review, 166 Missouri Medicine March/April 2007 Vol 104 No 2.
3. Patel VR, Chammas MF Jr, Shah S. Robotic Assisted Laparoscopic Radical Prostatectomy: A Review of the Current State of Affairs, Int J Clin Pract. 2007; 61(2):309-314.
4. Weinberg L, Roa S, Escobar PF. Robotic Surgery in Gynecology: An Updated Systematic Review, Obstetrics and Gynecology International, vol 2011 article ID 852061.
5. Wedmid A, Lukhani E, Lee DI. Future perspectives in robotic surgery, BJU International vol 108, 1028-1036.
6. Lanfranco AR, Castellanos AE, Desai JP, Meyers WC. Robotic Surgery, A Current Perspective, Annals of Surgry,2004; 239: 14-21.
7. Barry MJ, Gallagher PM, Skinner JS, Fowler FJ. Adverse effects of robotic-assisted laparoscopic versus open retropubic radical prostatectomy among a nationwide random sample of medicare-age men; JCO February 2012 vol 30 no5 513-518.
8. Ou YC, Yang CR, Wang J, Yang CK, Cheng CL, Patel VR, Tewari AK. The learning curve for reducing complications of robotic-assisted laparoscopic radical prostatectomy by a single surgeon, BJU Int 2011Aug; 108(3):420-5.
9. Sarma J. Robot-assisted Pelvic Surgery: Pathphysiological Considerations for Patient selection (in press).
10. Mills JT, Burris MB, Warburton DJ, Conaway MR, Schenkman NS, Krupski TL. Positionong injuries associated with robotic assisted urological surgery, J Urol. 2013 Aug; 190(2):580-4.
11. Kaushik D, High R, Clark CJ, LaGrange CA. Malfunction of the Da Vinci robotic system during robot-assisted laparoscopic prostatectomy: an international survey; J Endourol 2010 Apr;24(4):571-5.
12. Campos JA, Ueda K. Update on anesthetic complications of robotic thoracic surgery, Minerva Anestesiol, 2013 Jul 23(Epub ahead of print).
13. Gupta K, Mehta Y, Sarin Jolly A, Khanna S. Anaesthesia for robotic gynaecological surgery, Anaesth Intensive Care 2012 Jul; 40(4):614-21.
14. Gainsburg DM. Anesthetic concerns for robotic-assisted laparoscopic radical prostatectomy, Minerva Anesthesiol 2012 May; 78(5):596-604.
15. Fuller A, Pautler SE. Complications following robot-assisted radical prostatectomy in a prospective Canadian cohort of 305 consecutive cases, Can Urol Assoc J. 2012 Mar 2:1-6.
16. Song JB, Vemana G, Mobley JM, Bhayani SB. The second" time-out": a surgical safety checklist for lengthy robotic surgery, Patient safety in surgery 2013, 7:19.
17. Zorn KC, et al. Training, credentialing, proctoring and medico legal risks of robotic urological surgery: recommendations of the society of urologic robotic surgeons. J Urol. 2009 Sep; 182(3) 1126-32.
18. Mavroforou A, Michalodimitrakis E, Hatzitheo-Filou C, Giannoukas A. Legal and ethical issues in robotic surgery; Int Angiol 2010 Feb:29(1) 75-9.
19. Lee YL, Kilic G, Phelps JY. Liability exposurefor surgical robotics instructors; J Minim Invasive Gynecol. 2012 May-Jun; 19(3): 376-9.
20. Lee YL, Kilic G, Phelps JY. Medicolegal review of liability risks for gynecological stemming from lack of training in robot-assisted surgery: J Minim Invasive Gyyneco 2011 Jul-Aug: 18(4):512-5.
21. T McLean. The complexity of litigation associated with robotic surgery and cybersurgery: Int J Med Robotics Compu Assist Surg 2007; 3:23-29.
22. Lenihan JP. Navigating, credentialing, privileging, and learning curves in robotics with an evidence and experienced-based approach, Journal of clinical obstetrics and gynecology; 2011 Vol 54, number 3, 382-390.
23. Hernandez JM, Dimou F, WeberJ, et al. Defining the learning curve for robotic-assisted esophagogastrectomy; J Gastrointest Surg 2013 Aug 17(8): 1346-51.
24. White HN, Frederick J, Zimmerman T, Carroll WR, Magnuson JS. Learning curve for transoral robotic surgery: a 4-year analysis. JAMA Otolaryngol Head Neck Surg 2013 Jun;139(6):564-7.
25. Fung AK, Aly EH. Robotic colonic surgery: is it advisable to commence a new learning curve? Dis colon Rectum 2013 Jun;56(6):786-96.
26. Hong YM, Sutherland DE, Linder B, Engel JD. "Learning curve" may not be enough: assessing in the oncological experience curve for robotic radical prostatectomy: J Endourol. 2010 Mar;24(3):473-7.
27. Jimenez-Rodriguez RM, Diaz-Pavon JM, de la Portilla de Juan F, Prendes-Sillero E, Dussrt HC, Padillo J. Learning curve for robotic-assisted laparoscopic rectal cancer surgery. Int J Colorectal Dis. 2013 Jun;28(6):815-21.

28. Chandra V, Nehra D, Parent R, Woo R, Reyes R, Hernandez-Boussard T, Dutta S. Surgery. 2010 Jun;147(6):830-9.
29. Sng KK, Hara M, Shin JW, Yoo BE, Yang KS, Kim SH. The multiphasic learning curve for robot-assisted rectal surgery, Surg Endosc. 2013 Mar 19 (in print).
30. Tasian GE, Wiebe DJ, Casale P. Learning curve of robotic assisted pyeloplasty for pediatric urology fellos: JUrol. 2013 Feb 11(in print).
31. Cela V, Freschi L, Simi G, Ruggiero M, Tana R, Pluchino N. Robotic single-site hysterectomy: feasibility, learning curve and surgical outcome. Surg Endosc. 2013 Jul: 27(7): 2638-43.
32. Madhuri TK, Hamzawala I, Tailor A, Butler-Manuel S. Robotic assisted surgery in gynaecologic oncology-starting a program and initial learning curve from a UK tertiary referral center: the Guilford perspective: Int J Med Robot. 2012 Dec;8(4):496-503.
33. Gross ND. Commentary: is robotic surgery thyroid surgery worth the learning curve? Otolaryngol Head Neck Surg. 2012 Dec;147(6):1047-8.
34. Philippou P, Waine E, Rowe E. Robot-assisted laparoscopic prostatectomy versus open: comparison of the learning curve of a single surgeon; J Endourol. 2012 Aug;26(8): 1002-8.
35. Chitwood WR Jr, Nifong LW, Chapman WHH, et al. Robotic surgical training in an academic institution; Annals of Surgery: Vol 234, No 4, 475-486.
36. Moles JJ, Connelly PE, Sarti EE, Baredes S. Establishing a training program for residents in robotic surgery; Laryngoscope, 2009, 119:1927-1931.
37. Lucas SM, Gilley DA, Joshi SS, Gardner TA, Sundaram CP. Robotics training program: Evaluation of the satisfaction and the factors that influence success of the skills training in a resident robotics curriculum; Journal of Endourology Vol 25, NO 10, Oct 2011; 1669-1674.
38. Jenison EL, Gil KM, Lendvay TS, Guy MS. Robotic Surgical Skills: Acquistion, Maintenance, and Degradation: JSLS 2012 Apr-Jun; 16(2) 218-228.
39. Dulan G, Rege RV, Hogg DC, Gilberg-Fisher KM, Arian NA, Tesfay ST, Scott DJ. Developing a comprehensive, proficiency-based training program for robotic surgery; Surgery 2012 Sep 152(3):477-88.
40. Menhadji A, Abdelshehid C, Osann K, et al. Tracking and assessment of technical skills acquisition among urology residents for open, laparoscopic, and robotic skills over 4 years: is there a trend? J Endourol. 2013 Jun; 27(6): 783-9.
41. Curry M, Malpani A, Li R, et al. Objective assessment in residency-based training for transoral robotic surgery. Laryngoscope. 2012 Oct; 122(10): 2184-92.
42. Geller EJ, Schuler KM, Boggess JF. Robotic surgical training program in gynecology: how to train residents and fellows. J Minim Invasive Gynecol. 2011 Mar-Apr; 18(2):224-9.
43. Buchs NC, Pugin F, Volonte F, Morel P. Learning tools and simulation in robotic surgery: State of the Art. World of Surg. 2013 May 3 (in print).
44. Smith AL, Scott EM, Krivak TC, et al. Dual-console robotic surgery: a new teaching paradigm. J Robot Surg. 2013 June; 7(2): 113-118.
45. Abboudi H, Khan MS, Aboumarzouk O, Guru KA, Challacombe B, Dasgupta P, Ahmed K: Current status of validation for robotic surgery simulators – a systematic review; BJU International 2012; 111, 194-205.
46. Liss MA, Abdelshehid C, Quach S, et al. Validation, correlation, and comparison of the da Vinci Trainer and the da Vinci surgical skills simulator using the mimic software for urologic robotic surgical education; Journal of Endourology 2012 Dec: 26(12): 1629-1634.
47. Alzahrani T, Haddad R, Alkhayal A, et al. Can: Validation of the da Vinci surgical simulator across three surgical disciplines: A pilot study: Urol Assoc J 2013;7(7-8): e 520-9.
48. Perrenot C, Perez M, Tran N, Jehl JP, Felblinger J, Bresler L, Hubert J. The virtual reality simulator Dv-Trainer is a valid assessment tool for roboyic surgical skills: Surg Endosc. 2012 Sep;26(9):2587-93.
49. Lyons C, Goldfarb D, Jones SL, Badhiwala N, Miles B, Link R, Dunkin BJ. Which skills really matter? Proving face, content, and construct validity for a commericial robotic simulator: Surg Endosc. 2013 Jun;27(6):2020-30.
50. Lee JY, Mucksavage P, Kerbl DC, Huynh VB, Etafy M, McDougall EM. Validation study of a virtual reality robotic simulator – role as an assessment tool? J Urol. 2012 Mar;187(3): 998-1102.
51. Gavazzi A, Bahsoun AN, Haute WV, et al. Face, content and construct validity of a virtual reality simulator for robotic surgery (SEP Robot); Ann R Coll Surg Eng J 2011; 93: 152-156.
52. Hung AJ, Patil MB, Zehnder P, Cai J, Ng CK, Aron M, Gill IS, Desai MM. Concurrent and predictive validation of a novel robotic surgery simulator: a prospective, randomized study. J Urol. 2012 Feb; 187(2):630-7.

53. Kesavadas T, Stegemann A, Sathyaseelan G, et al. Validation of robotic surgery simulator (RoSS); Stud Health Tecnol Inform. 2011; 163:274-6.
54. Seixas-Mikel SA, Stegemann A Kesavadas T, Srimathveeravalli G, Sathyaseelan G, Chandrasekhar R, Wilding G, Peabody JO, Guru K. Content validation of a robotic surgical simulator; BJU Int. 2011 Apr;107(7):1130-5.
55. Kenney PA, Wszolek MF, Gould JJ, Libertino, Moinzadeh A. Face, content, and construct validity of Dv-trainer, a novel virtual reality simulator for robotic surgery: Urology. 2009 Jun;73(6):1288-92.
56. Sethi AS, Peine WJ, Mohammadi Y, Sundaram CP. Validation of a novel virtual reality robotic simulator: J Endourol. 2009 Mar;23(3):503-8.
57. Levine AI, Schwartz AD, Bryson EO, DeMaria S Jr. Role of simulation in US Physician Licensure and Certification; Mount Sinai Journal of Medicine 79:140-153, 2012.
58. Lendvay TS, Hannaford B, Satava RM. Future of robotic surgery; The cancer Journal 2013 Mar/Apr: 19(2):109-119.
59. Densford, F. (2017, September 15). *11 surgical robotics companies you need to know* . The Robot Report. Retrieved November 8, 2022, from https://www.therobotreport.com/11-surgical-robotics-companies-you-need-to-know/2/
60. Lee JY, Mucksavage P, Sundaram CP, McDougall EM. Best practices for robotic surgery training and credentialing. J Urol. 2011 Apr; 185(4) 1191-7.
61. Wang, G., Zeng, Y., Sheng, X. (2021). Instructions for Use of Da Vinci Surgical Robots. In: Wang, G., Zeng, Y., Sheng, X. (eds) Robotic Surgery and Nursing. Springer, Singapore. https://doi.org/10.1007/978-981-16-0510-9_2
62. DeHaven, Mary E MD; Bowman, Daman DO; Monroe, Natalie DO; Seton, Tristan MD; Protyniak, Bogdan MD, FACS. Fundamentals of Robotic Surgery: An Objective and Easily Trackable Curriculum for General Surgery Residency Robotics Training. Journal of the American College of Surgeons: November 2022 - Volume 235 - Issue 5 - p S220-S221 doi: 10.1097/01.XCS.0000894728.27045.d1
63. Doster, D.L., Collings, A.T., Stefanidis, D. et al. The American Board of Surgery flexible endoscopy curriculum prepares individuals to pass the fundamentals of endoscopic surgery manual skills test. Surg Endosc *(2022).* https://doi.org/10.1007/s00464-022-09559-2 64. https://www.fesprogram.org/fes-didactic/
65. *Vassiliou, M.C., Dunkin, B.J., Fried, G.M.* et al. *Fundamentals of endoscopic surgery: creation and validation of the hands-on test.* Surg Endosc ***28****, 704–711 (2014). https://doi.org/10.1007/s00464-013-3298-4*
66. Julian D, Tanaka A, Mattingly P, Truong M, Perez M, Smith R. A comparative analysis and guide to virtual reality robotic surgical simulators. Int J Med Robot. 2018 Feb;14(1). doi: 10.1002/rcs.1874. Epub 2017 Nov 10. PMID: 29125206.
67. *Revised Manual Skills Guidelines*. https://www.flsprogram.org/wp-content/uploads/2014/03/Revised-Manual-Skills-Guidelines-February-2014.pdf.
68. Jetpack. *Lap Tab Trainer*™, 3-DMed, 6 Apr. 2021, https://www.3-dmed.com/product/lap-tab-trainer/?gclid=Cj0KCQiA4OybBhCzARIsAIcfn9nlifk-uF9evbiDL6wc0hNGWhw_Nu9vqa3Xk1dCBTWuQOHfiZY51QwaAlUrEALw_wcB#&gid=1&pid=1.
69. "Lap Platforms." *Simbionix*, 21 June 2022, https://simbionix.com/simulators/lap-mentor/platforms/.

❑❑❑

14

CHAPTER

Animal and Human Bites

Neha Varshney MD FCAP
Jasnet Singh Bhullar MD

INTRODUCTION

Animal bites are a major public health problem in children and adults all around the world. 17.4 million animal bites are reported annually.[1] Factors such as the health and species of the animal, the age and health of the person bitten, and the ease of access of high-quality health care, all play a role in the health impact of the animal bite. While many animal species can theoretically bite humans, the most common and important species include dogs, cats, and snakes. Animal bites can cause lacerations, avulsions, punctures, or scratches, and can introduce microorganisms into the wound. These infections can be caused by microorganisms from the environment, the victim's skin, or from the "normal" flora of the biter. They are often mistakenly considered innocuous by both patients and physicians. Although 80% of patients never seek medical care, there has been a trend of increasing awareness of the severity of infectious complications.

Dog Bites

It is estimated that 95% of total animal bites are from dogs. Most fatalities occur in younger children of below 10 years of age, the greatest risk of death is for victims younger than 4 years. Also, in the elderly of greater than 50 years of age, it could be quite fatal. Dog bites can cause anything from minor wounds like scratches and abrasions to major wounds like deep open lacerations and puncture wounds, tissue avulsions, and crush injuries. The jaws of large dogs can exert a strong force that may inflict serious injury. Lethal injuries, although rare, usually involve the head and neck, or direct penetration of vital organs in young children. The extremities, particularly the dominant hand, are the most frequent site of dog bites for older children or adults.

Infection occurs most commonly from bites of the extremity, when there is a delay in treatment, or when the patient is at extremes of age. They are usually associated with Pasteurella, Eikenkella, and Capnocytophaga canimorsus.[2]

Rabies

In developing countries, dogs account for 90% or more of rabies cases transmitted to humans. The remaining incidences occur by other wild animals like raccoons, rats, skunks, foxes, etc. Unprovoked dog bites increase the likelihood of rabies. Once the disease is contracted, it is 100% fatal. The incubation period for rabies can be up to one year; therefore, follow-up is extremely crucial. A prodrome of 2 to 10 days is seen and includes fevers and paresthesia at the bite site. Neurologic changes can also be noted and include aphasia, paralysis, hypersalivation, and myoclonus.[4]

Cat Bites

Injury from cat bites is somewhat different from dog bites in their potential for infection and injury to deeper tissues and organs. A puncture wound is typical of a cat bite because cats have long, slender, sharp teeth. However, abrasions and lacerations involving the hand and upper extremities may also occur.

The most frequently encountered pathogens are Pasteurella multocida and Pasteurella septica (found in almost 75% of cases), but Streptococci, Staphylococci, Bacteroides, and Moraxella can also be seen.[2] Cat bites can also transmit Bartonella henselae, the organism responsible for the cat-scratch disease. Even minor cat scratches can cause wound infections and abscesses by P. multocida. The wound infections commonly present earlier than that of typical skin organisms and cause rapidly progressive cellulitis, which will be noticeable within six hours and readily identifiable within 24 hours. Presenting symptoms include discoloration, tenderness, swelling, often purulent drainage, and adenopathy. Additionally, it can lead to the formation of joint infections, tenosynovitis, and osteomyelitis at the wound location and can cause arthritic joint and prosthetic valves, leading to infection at distant sites. Rarely, pericarditis and meningitis caused by P. multocida have also been reported in the literature.

Table 1: Commonly encountered bacterial isolates from dog and cat[2]

Pasteurella multocida	Micrococcus luteus
Pasteurella canis	Neisseria canis
Pasteurella dagmatis	Actinobacillus
Capnocytophaga canimorsus Eikenella corrodens	Corynebacterium spp. Bacteroides tectum
α and β Hemolytic Streptococci	Peptostreptococcus
Enterococci	Fusobacterium nucleatum
Staphylococcus aureus	Moraxella spp.
Staphylococcus epidermidis	Prevotella zoogleoformans

Snake Bites

Venomous snakes, usually Vipers, lead to considerable morbidity and mortality worldwide. Only 10% to 15% of snakes are venomous. Snakebites disproportionately affect the poor population in rural areas; commonly two patterns are seen viz. bites to the arm, ankle, foot, or lower leg. Often this can occur when farmers working in the fields accidentally disturb the snake, or when the patient is sleeping on the ground and is exposed to a nocturnal species. Snake venom contains several potentially dangerous substances, such as hemolysis toxin, neurotoxin, cardiotoxin, and proteolytic enzymes. Some of these can sometimes result in a neuromuscular blockade.

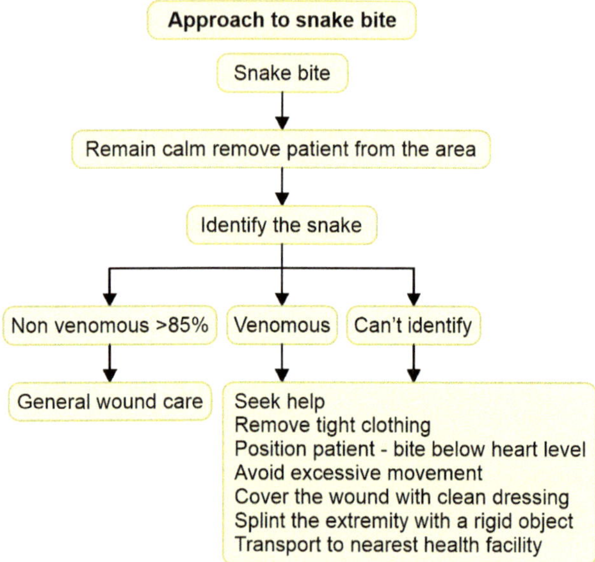

Figure 1: Management of snake bite

The two most important factors that affect the pathophysiology of the bite are the venom's toxicity and the victim's response. The most reliable signs of envenomation are extreme local pain, swelling, and discoloration developing within half an hour of the bite. Some venom can directly cause acute kidney injury, which is commonly accompanied by hypotension and rhabdomyolysis secondarily. The rest of the signs and symptoms depend on the type of toxin involved.[5]

Table 2: Differences between Non-Venomous and Venomous Snakes

	Non-Venomous Snakes	Venomous Snakes
Head	Rounded	Triangle except for cobra
Fangs	Not present	Present
Pupils	Rounded	Elliptical pupil
Anal Plate	Double row of plates	Single row of plates
Bite Mark	Row of small teeth	Fang marks

Human Bites

The human bite may present as a semi-circular or circular area of erythema with or without bruising and usually involves the hand or upper extremity in almost 70% of cases. Overall, the infection rate for human bite wounds and their complications is much higher than for animal bites. The fight bites or closed fist injuries are associated with a much-increased incidence of infectious complications. Wounds of the lips and paronychia, and infections of the structures more frequently seen in children account for self-inflicted fight wounds. Self-inflicted bites may be associated with psychiatric illness or metabolic disease. If a bite mark has an inter-canine distance >3 cm, it probably came from an adult and may indicate child abuse. The high infection rate in human bites is due to the microbiology of the human mouth, the relatively poor vascular supply to structures in the hand, the position of the hand when the injury occurred, the intensity of the injury, and delay in care-seeking.

The closed fist fight injuries (patient hitting another human in the mouth using a closed fist), usually manifest as a minor laceration on the back of the hand which may involve injuries to the metacarpophalangeal joint, extensor tendon sheath, tendon, and sometimes even bone. "Chondral" fractures can result from a tooth hitting the articular surface of the joint and chipping off fragments of the articular cartilage. Involvement of the joint space may even lead to the destruction of the joint tissues.[6]

Bacteriologically, the dirtiest bites are the human bites. The oral flora of humans contains a high concentration of pathogenic organisms. Infected wounds are usually polymicrobial. Group A Streptococci followed by Staphylococcus and Eikenella are frequently seen.[2]

Human bites may result in the transmission of Hepatitis B, Hepatitis C, Tetanus, Syphilis, Tuberculosis, and Herpes. Although HIV can be secreted in the human saliva (low viral titers), it is not considered to be transmitted, unless there is exposure to blood.

Spider Bites

Most spiders do not pose a threat to humans. Mammalian tissues see almost no effect from the venom of most spiders. Only a few spider species' bites are powerful enough to pierce human skin. The spiders most likely to inflict any medically important bites in humans are black widow spiders and recluse spiders.

Usually, a spider bite manifests acutely as a single papule, pustule, or wheal with a halo of erythema. Some envenomation can cause systemic symptoms, particularly those of widow spiders, funnel-web spiders, and recluse spiders. Allergic reactions are usually not caused by bites, however, and are typically caused by contact with spiders.[7]

Bee Stings

The majority of people develop only a minor local reaction, but patients allergic to venom are at a much higher risk for systemic allergic reactions (i.e., anaphylaxis), which can be particularly severe, and are the leading cause of anaphylaxis fatalities. There are also several uncommon and delayed types of reactions that may develop after stings, such as serum sickness. Local reactions consist of symptoms that are confined to the tissues which are contiguous with the sting and are usually mild and transient, although some patients develop large local reactions or secondary bacterial infections.

INVESTIGATIONS

Laboratory Studies: Aerobic and anaerobic blood cultures with antibiotic sensitivity are needed before antibiotic therapy, especially in patients with an infected bite wound and signs of systemic infection. A complete white blood cell count, erythrocyte sedimentation rate, and C-reactive protein may be elevated in patients with cellulitis, joint infection, osteomyelitis, or sepsis.

Wound Culture: Wound cultures of uninfected bite wounds may not be useful. In infected wounds, Gram stain and aerobic and anaerobic cultures must be obtained before the initiation of antibiotics. The laboratory requisition should mention that an animal or human bite wound is the source of the culture.

Plain Radiographs and Ultrasound: Deep bite wounds near joints warrant radiographs to evaluate for disruption of joints or bone, and evidence of foreign bodies such as embedded teeth. Plain radiographs are also indicated in markedly infected wounds to detect bony and soft tissue injury, subcutaneous gas, and changes associated with osteomyelitis. Ultrasound can be useful in identifying abscess formation and locating radiolucent foreign bodies in infected wounds.

Head Computed Tomography: Dog bites to the head, seldom, penetrate the skull, which may result in a depressed fracture, local infection, and brain abscess. A head computed tomographic (CT) scan is pertinent in patients with a deep dog bite to the scalp, including puncture wounds, especially in infants less than two years of age.

GENERAL MANAGEMENT

Stabilization

Direct pressure must be applied to actively bleeding wounds and a neurovascular assessment should be performed in areas distal to the wound. Deep wounds to vital structures should be considered and treated as major penetrating trauma.

History and Examination

Once the patient is stable, a detailed history should be performed to make a preliminary assessment. There are some medical conditions, such as diabetes mellitus and anything which causes immunosuppression, which can put the patient at a higher risk of infection from a dog bite. Any information which will help determine the patient's risk of infection, including time of injury, whether or not the animal was provoked, and the overall health and immunization status (e.g., tetanus) of the patient, needs to be mentioned. Important information such as ongoing medications and allergies should be mentioned in the patient record. The physical examination should include measuring and classifying the wound (i.e., laceration, puncture, crush, or avulsion), and examining the range of motion of the relevant proximal areas. Other pertinent negative findings like nerve, vascular, and motor function should also be recorded.

Wound Preparation

Meticulous wound care is one of the most important steps in treating a laceration due to an animal or human bite, more so in case of puncture wounds. Appropriate local anesthesia may facilitate adequate wound cleansing. Cleaning with 1% povidone-iodine or 1 % benzalkonium chloride, and pressure irrigation with abundant amounts of saline would help in decreasing the count of bacteria. Debridement of devitalized tissue is crucial to remove any nidus for infection. The wound should be thoroughly examined to identify any injury to deep structures and the possibility of a foreign substance. Wounds near joints should be looked at carefully to assess for damage to the underlying tendon sheath, fascia, joint capsule, and bone. Appropriate imaging should be ordered if a potentially deep bite occurs close to bone or if a foreign body might be present.

Wound Closure

Primary closure

The approach to wound closure varies depending on the site of the injury and the type of wound. A clinician may perform primary wound closure of simple lacerations due to dog bites. In contrast, most cat or human bites are left unclosed to heal by secondary intention.[4] Infection of wounds on the face is uncommon, mostly due to the robust vascular supply to the scalp and face. Moreover, cosmesis is crucial in such cases, so the experienced clinician may choose to close promptly.

Indications for primary wound closure of open lacerations are:

- Clinically uninfected laceration
- Less than 12 hours old for the body, 24 hours for the face
- Locations except for hands and feet.

Proper wound care is necessary for better healing and reducing infection risk in patients after wound closure. Upon suturing of bite wounds, abundant irrigation, debridement, avoidance of deep sutures (if possible), administration of prophylactic antibiotic therapy, and close follow-up must be done.

Wounds at high risk for developing infection should not be closed initially include:

- Crush injuries
- Puncture wounds
- Wounds older than12 hours on the body, 24 hours on the face
- Bites involving the hands and feet
- Human or cat bites, with the exception of those to the face
- For bite wounds in compromised hosts like diabetes mellitus, immunocompromised, absent spleen or splenic dysfunction, venous stasis, the wounds should be irrigated generously, dressed, left open to drain, and examined every day.[10]

Surgical Management

Surgical management may be necessary for the following:

- Complicated facial lacerations
- Deep wounds that impact tendon, bone, joints, or other major structures
- Wounds with complex infections (e.g., abscess formation, osteomyelitis, or joint infections)
- Wounds associated with compromised neurovascular structures

Antibiotic Prophylaxis

Prophylactic antibiotics decrease the infection rate of select animal bites, especially cat bites. Antibiotic prophylaxis is discouraged, but it is indicated in certain high-risk wounds as follows:

- Deep puncture wounds, especially cat bites
- Wounds near areas of underlying venous and/or lymphatic compromise
- Crush injury
- Wounds on the face, hand(s), genitalia, or close to a bone or joint
- Bite wounds in compromised hosts

Tetanus Prophylaxis

Tetanus prophylaxis is warranted in all cases of animal bites.

Table 3: Tetanus prophylaxis[8]

	Previous doses of Tetanus Toxoid	
	< 3 or unknown	> or equal to 3 doses
Clean and minor wound		
Tetanus toxoid containing vaccine	Yes	Yes, if last dose > 10 years
Human Tetanus Ig	No	No
All other wounds		
Tetanus toxoid containing vaccine	Yes	Yes, if the last dose > 5 years
Human Tetanus Ig	Yes	No

SPECIFIC MANAGEMENTS

Dog Bite

Just 15% to 20% of total dog bite wounds become infected, but prophylactic antibiotic administration for three to seven days is recommended regardless. If there is evidence of frank cellulitis, a 10-to-14-day treatment is usually recommended. Amoxicillin-clavulanate potassium (Augmentin) is the preferred antibiotic for dog bites. Unless the patient is a pregnant woman or is under 8 years old, doxycycline is the recommended alternative for patients who are allergic to penicillin.

To address the risk of a rabies infection, the dog owner is asked to provide current documentation to prove the animal's immunization against the rabies virus. If the dog's vaccination is up-to-date, the dog should remain in the owner's home. If the dog cannot be quarantined for 10 days, the patient must be given rabies immunization starting within 48 hours of the time of the bite. The immunization can be stopped if the animal is discovered to be rabies free.

Table 4: Rabies post-exposure prophylaxis (PEP) schedule[9]

Vaccination status	Intervention	Regimen*
Not previously vaccinated	Wound cleaning	All PEP should start with immediate complete cleaning of all wounds with soap and water. If obtainable, a virucidal agent, such as a povidone-iodine solution, should be used to irrigate the wounds.
	Human rabies immune globulin (HRIG)	Give 20 IU/kg of body weight. If physically possible, the entire amount should be applied around and in the wound(s), and any leftover volume should be dispensed at a location (intramuscular [IM]) far away from vaccine administration. Additionally, HRIG should not be given via the same syringe as the vaccine. Since HRIG may somewhat decrease active synthesis of rabies virus antibody, administration should not exceed the recommended dose.
	Vaccine	Human diploid cell vaccine (HDCV) or purified chick embryo cell vaccine (PCECV) 1.0 mL, intramuscular in the deltoid area†, 1 each on days 0,§ 3, 7 and 14.¶
Previously vaccinated**	Wound cleaning	All PEP should start with immediate complete cleaning of all wounds with soap and water. If obtainable, a virucidal agent such as povidone-iodine solution should be administered to irrigate the wounds.
	HRIG	HRIG should not be given.
	Vaccine	HDCV or PCECV 1.0 mL, intramuscular in the deltoid area†, 1 each on days 0§ and 3.

* These regimens are viable for individuals of all age groups, including children.

† The deltoid is the sole allowable vaccination site for adults and older children. For younger children, the lateral side of the thigh can be used. The gluteal area is never used.

§ Day 0 is the day the first dose of vaccine is given.

¶ For immunosuppressed patients, rabies PEP should be dispensed using all 5 doses of vaccine on days 0, 3, 7, 14, and 28.

** Any individual with a history of pre-exposure vaccination with HDCV, PCECV, or rabies vaccine adsorbed (RVA); prior PEP with HDCV, PCECV or RVA; or any prior vaccination with another rabies vaccine and a documented history of antibody response to the vaccination.

Cat Bite

Wound care is the most important thing in cat bites. Just like a dog bite, Amoxicillin-clavulanate potassium (Augmentin) is also the preferred antibiotic for a cat bite.

Human Bite

Human bites are the dirtiest bites, they require extensive irrigation and debridement in the operation room. Prophylaxis for HIV and Hep B should be given. Any anti-HBs antibody negative patient bitten by an anti-HBsAg positive individual should be given both hepatitis B immune globulin (HBIG) and the hepatitis B vaccine.

Bee Stings

The limb should be elevated if the sting is on an extremity. Cold compresses are soothing acutely. Oral prednisone reduces significant swelling and NSAIDs reduce pain. Pruritus can be treated with oral antihistamine and applied at high potency until the itching subsides. Epinephrine is the drug of choice to avoid fatal anaphylactic reactions.

Spider Bites

For the Brown widow spider, the antidote is IV calcium gluconate. Muscle relaxants can be used as well. Dapsone is helpful in Brown recluse spider bites. Surgical debridement is only required if extensive damage is present.

Snake Bite

Blood for type and crossmatch, coagulation studies, liver, and renal functions should be ordered in snake bites. A compression bandage can be applied. Treatment is antivenom, dosage of which depends on the amount of the envenomation and not the size of the patient. Hypotension can be managed with fluids.

REFERENCES

1. Planning Commission of the Government of India. Report of the Working Group on Disease Burden for the 12th five-year plan. http://planningcommission gov.in/aboutus/ committee/ wrkgrp12/health WG_3_1communicable.pdf.
2. Goldstein EJ, Citron DM, Wield B, et al. Bacteriology of human and animal bite wounds. J Clin Microbiol 1978; 8:667.
3. Stevens DL, Bisno AL, Chambers HF, et al. Practice guidelines for the diagnosis and management of skin and soft tissue infections: 2014 update by the infectious diseases society of America. Clin Infect Dis 2014; 59:147.
4. Hemachudha T, Laothamatas J, Rupprecht CE. Human rabies: a disease of complex neuropathogenetic mechanisms and diagnostic challenges. Lancet Neurol 2002; 1:101.
5. Warrell DA. Snake bite. Lancet 2010; 375:77.
6. Brook I. Human and animal bite infections. J Fam Pract 1989; 28:713.
7. Isbister GK, Fan HW. Spider bite. Lancet 2011; 378:2039.
8. Centers for Disease Control and Prevention (CDC). Updated recommendations for use of tetanus toxoid, reduced diphtheria toxoid and acellular pertussis (Tdap) vaccine from the Advisory Committee on Immunization Practices, 2010. MMWR Morb Mortal Wkly Rep 2011; 60:13.
9. Manning SE, et al. "Advisory Committee on Immunization Practices Centers for Disease Control and Prevention (CDC). Human rabies prevention—United States, 2008: Recommendations of the Advisory Committee on Immunization Practices." MMWR Recomm Rep 57.RR-3 (2008): 1-28.
10. Dire DJ. Emergency management of dog and cat bite wounds. Emerg Med Clin North Am 1992; 10:719.

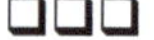

15

CHAPTER

Coagulation and Anticoagulation

Madan Mohan Reddy Paluru, MD
Kayla K. Umemoto, BA
Vijay Mittal, MD

INTRODUCTION

Hemostasis is a complex, physiological process with the purpose of limiting bleeding through the formation of a blood clot at the site of vessel injury. Hemostasis is divided into primary and secondary hemostasis. Primary hemostasis involves platelet aggregation and formation of the platelet plug. Secondary hemostasis consists of the coagulation cascade resulting in the deposition of insoluble fibrin, which results in the formation of a mesh in and around the platelet plug, strengthening and stabilizing the clot. Primary and secondary hemostasis occur simultaneously and work in tandem. Another important component of hemostasis is the fibrinolysis pathway. This process can be dysregulated and result in pathological thrombus formation (thrombosis) manifesting as pathological bleeding.[1] This chapter discusses steps involved in hemostasis, bleeding disorders, and commonly used anticoagulants in practice.

PRIMARY HEMOSTASIS

During primary hemostasis, a weak platelet plug is formed. It consists of four phases: first there is vasoconstriction of the damaged vessel, then there is platelet adhesion, platelet activation, and platelet aggregation. With vasoconstriction, the damaged endothelium synthesizes and releases endothelin-1, a potent vasoconstrictor. Other factors involved in vasoconstriction that are released during platelet aggregation include thromboxane A2 (TXA2) from platelet membranes and serotonin (also known as 5-hydroxytryptamine or 5-HT). The damaged endothelium then exposes subendothelial collagen and von Willebrand factor (vWF), it also releases inflammatory mediators and ATP. During platelet adhesion, platelets first roll along the vessel wall, then they adhere to the exposed subendothelial collagen, and their glycoprotein (Gp) Ib-IX receptor bind to vWF, thus resulting in platelet activation.

Thrombin stimulates platelet granule release, thus activating platelet activation. The platelet granule consists of platelet activating factor, serotonin, and adenosine diphosphate (ADP). Once released, the ADP can bind to P2Y1 and P2Y12 receptors on the platelet membrane. When P2Y1 is bound, it induces the platelet to form a pseudopod shape, aiding in platelet aggregation. When P2Y12 is bound, it helps induce the clotting cascade. These activated platelets result in platelet aggregation. Another receptor expressed after activation is the Gp IIb/IIIa receptor which binds to vWF and fibrinogen. Fibrinogen is a molecule found in circulation and binds to Gp IIb/IIIa once it is exposed. It is then responsible for the interconnection between platelets, ultimately forming a weak platelet plug.[2] Platelet aggregation is reversible. Heparin is not involved with the formation of a platelet plug and therefore hemostasis can occur in patients who are heparinized.

SECONDARY HEMOSTASIS

The platelet plug alone is not enough to achieve hemostasis and it is therefore necessary to form a clot at the site of injury. The process of clot formation is known as the clotting cascade. It is dependent on several clotting factors, designated by roman numerals I through XIII, which activate each other. The clotting cascade results in the formation of fibrin (an insoluble plasma protein) from fibrinogen (a soluble plasma protein). These fibrin proteins form the clot by sticking together. To add complexity, the clotting cascade consists of two pathways, the intrinsic and the extrinsic pathway which converge through a common pathway in the end to form the clot (Figure 1).

INTRINSIC PATHWAY

When there is trauma inside the vascular system, the intrinsic pathway is activated. This consists of being activated by platelets, collagen, exposed endothelium, or chemicals. The components of the intrinsic pathway are Hageman Factor (Factor XII), Factor XI, Factor IX, and Factor VIII. First, Factor XII contacts the exposed subendothelial collagen and is activated, becoming Factor XIIa. Then, Factor XIIa activates Factor XI to Factor XIa and Factor XIa activates Factor IX to Factor IXa. Factor IXa then works with Factor VIIIa, activating Factor X. Once Factor X is activated, the cascade is now part of the common pathway.

EXTRINSIC PATHWAY

When there is external trauma resulting in blood escaping the vascular system, the extrinsic pathway is activated. The protein called tissue factor (TF) present on the cell membranes of all human cells except endothelium and red blood cells, binds to Factor VII and thus activates it to Factor VIIa and forms the TF-Factor VIIa complex. This complex then activates Factor X to Factor Xa and is now part of the common pathway. This complex also has the ability to work in the intrinsic pathway via activation of Factor IX, this is known as the alternate pathway.

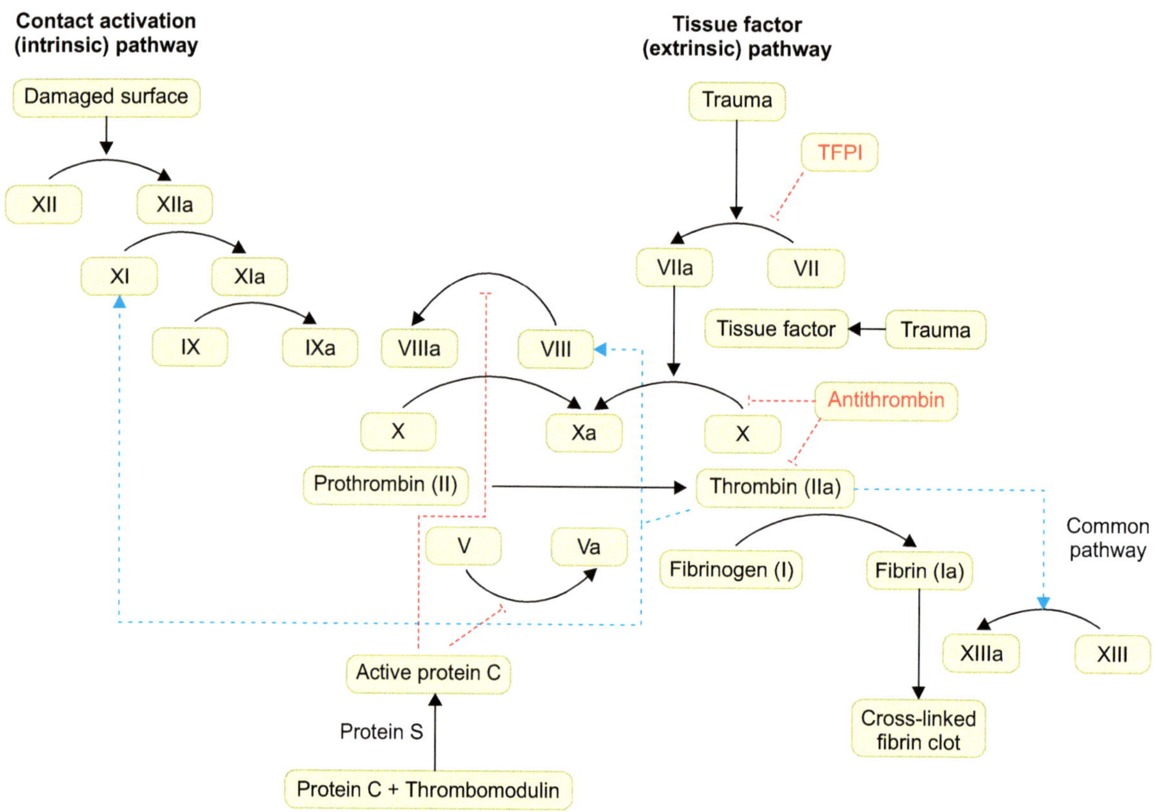

Figure 1: The clotting cascade in overview

COMMON PATHWAY

When Factor Xa is formed, the common pathway is initiated. Factor Xa binds to Factor Va and calcium present on the surface of phospholipids, thus forming a prothrombinase complex which can then activate prothrombin (Factor II) into thrombin (Factor IIa). Prothrombin is cleaved into thrombin by serine protease. Now activated, thrombin can activate Factor XIIIa which is responsible for crosslinking with fibrin and forming a clot that is stabilized.

REGULATION OF HEMOSTASIS

Uncontrolled hemostasis can result in increased clot burden and propagation of clots beyond the site of injury. Thrombomodulin secreted by the endothelium forms a complex with thrombin, making thrombin unavailable to cleave fibrinogen. This process can also activate protein C (APC) which inhibits Factors V and VIII, thus further reducing the generation of thrombin. Additionally, the endothelium releases tissue plasminogen activator (tPA) after injury. Tissue plasminogen activator can cleave plasminogen, initiating fibrinolysis. Fibrinolysis begins at the same time as clot formation, allowing blood flow restoration and the healing phase after trauma.

COAGULATION DISORDERS

HEMOPHILIA

Hemophilia results from a Factor VIII clotting factor deficiency (hemophilia A), a Factor IX deficiency (hemophilia B), or a Factor XI deficiency (hemophilia C) resulting in a bleeding tendency. Hemophilia A is the most common form. These are congenital disorders which are inherited in an X-linked recessive pattern; thus, males are much more commonly affected. Severity is classified by plasma factor levels of mild (levels of 5%-30%), moderately severe (1%-5%), and severe (less than 1%). Platelet function is normal in patients with hemophilia; therefore, they have normal primary hemostasis and normal platelet plug formation. Thus, these patients do not necessarily bleed immediately after an injury. Severe hemophilia can result in spontaneous bleeding into joints which often leads to severe arthropathies. Other features include retroperitoneal hematomas, intramuscular hematomas, intracranial bleeding, and gastrointestinal and genitourinary bleeding episodes. Patients who have moderately severe hemophilia will spontaneously bleed less but are likely to severely bleed following surgical procedures or trauma.

Coagulation work-up will show prolonged PTT due to an intrinsic factor deficiency in all types of hemophilia (Factors VIII, IX, XI) during basic bleeding workup. Both bleeding time and PT will be normal. For initial testing, a mixing study is the best test. In a mixing study, the patient's plasma is mixed with normal plasma. If the PTT is normal after mixing, the patient may have hemophilia because the clotting factor deficiency will be corrected. For a more accurate test, specific clotting factor assays can be performed.

Patients with hemophilia are best managed with giving them specific recombinant factors. Thirty to forty percent of clotting factor levels should be restored in patients with mild hemorrhage, 50% for patients with severe bleeding, and 80% to 100% for patients with life-threatening bleeding.[3] If recombinant factors are not immediately available, cryoprecipitate can be used temporarily for severe bleeding and desmopressin can be used for minor bleeding. Desmopressin is useful because it releases Factor VIII from endothelial cells.

VON WILLEBRAND DISEASE

Von Willebrand factor (vWF) is a molecule that endothelial cells and megakaryocytes synthesize. vWF is responsible for carrying Factor VIII and is responsible for platelet adhesion during primary hemostasis. A vWF and Factor VIII deficiency results in von Willebrand Disease (vWD), the most common inherited bleeding disorder. There are three types of vWD; type 1 vWD is a partial quantitative vWF deficiency and is the most common type. Type 2 vWD is a qualitative vWF defect. Type 3 vWD is a total vWF deficiency. Type 1 and 2 are autosomal dominant diseases, while type 3 is autosomal recessive.

Patients usually present in childhood, manifesting as recurrent, prolonged mucosal bleeding such as epistaxis and menorrhagia. Additionally, children tend to bleed after surgical or dental procedures. Diagnosis is by a Ristocetin cofactor assay which measures the vWF's capacity to agglutinate platelets, thus detecting vWF dysfunction. Decreased agglutination seen on the Ristocetin cofactor assay is diagnostic of vWD. For patients who have type 1 and type 2 vWD, desmopressin (DDAVP) can be used for bleeding episodes. DDAVP is a useful treatment because it induces increased plasma levels of vWF. Since patients with type 3 vWF have a total vWF deficiency, they are usually unresponsive to DDAVP and thus need vWF concentrates for treatment.

PLATELET DISORDERS

Platelet disorders cause easy bruising, epistaxis, petechiae, and purpura. Major platelet disorders are due to surface protein abnormalities and include Bernard-Soulier syndrome and Glanzmann thrombasthenia. Bernard-Soulier syndrome is due to a Gp Ib receptor defect, the receptor responsible for binding vWF and is needed for platelet adhesion to the subendothelium. Glanzmann thrombasthenia is due to a dysfunctional platelet Gp IIb/IIIa complex, leading to defective platelet aggregation.

Treatment for platelet disorders is platelet transfusion. Uremia with BUN >60 to 80 mg/dl, usually seen in ESRD patients, can result in inhibition of platelet function by inhibiting vWF release. First-line treatment is hemodialysis, DDAVP is the treatment for an acute reversal, and cryoprecipitate is the treatment for moderate to severe bleeding.

DISSEMINATED INTRAVASCULAR COAGULOPATHY (DIC)

DIC is microvascular thrombosis in a nonspecific location arising due to activation of intravascular coagulation.[4] The etiology of DIC is varied and includes sepsis, severe trauma (i.e., surgery), and as a pregnancy complication. Due to the diseased state of the patient, excess thrombin, a procoagulant, is stimulated resulting in thrombosis and since the diseased state is not localized, the thrombosis can occur throughout the vasculature. Additionally, with the excessive use of thrombin, there is consumption of platelets and coagulation factors resulting in bleeding.

Laboratory findings consistent with DIC are a prolonged aPTT and PT/INR due to the consumption of coagulation factors, a decrease in platelets and fibrinogen, and elevated fibrin degradation products (i.e., D-dimer).[4]

Treatment consists of treating the underlying etiology and replacing deficient components to a level that can support the control of spontaneous bleeding. Prophylactic transfusions of blood components should be given based on has finding to percent serious complications like DIC.[4]

HYPERCOAGULABILITY DISORDERS

FACTOR V LEIDEN MUTATION

In order to maintain balance in hemostasis, thrombin is inhibited by activated protein C (APC). It forms a complex with its cofactor, protein S, and cleaves Factors Va and VIIIa, thereby preventing them from participating in the coagulation cascade. In patients with a Factor V mutation, the factor is resistant to APC cleavage resulting in hypercoagulation. This is the most common congenital hypercoagulability disorder. Patients are usually young Caucasians in their mid-forties, and they will most likely have a personal and family history of thrombosis such as multiple VTEs starting at a young age and are unusually located. Venous thrombosis treatment includes anticoagulation with heparin, then warfarin therapy. Lifelong anticoagulation is typically not required.

ANTIPHOSPHOLIPID ANTIBODY SYNDROME

Antiphospholipid antibodies are antibodies that target antigens on platelet and endothelial cell phospholipids. The targeted phospholipids include cardiolipin in the mitochondria and lupus anticoagulant in the cell membrane. Antiphospholipid antibody syndrome is often associated with SLE and rheumatoid arthritis. Patients are predisposed to arterial and venous thrombi formation and spontaneous abortion. Diagnostic workup can reveal prolonged PTT which cannot be corrected with FFP. Additionally, patients often have a positive Russell viper venom time and false-positive syphilis RPR test. Treatment includes heparin and warfarin for anticoagulation. Patients may require lifelong anticoagulation.

ANTICOAGULATION AGENTS

UNFRACTIONATED HEPARIN

Heparin is an indirect anticoagulant that activates plasma antithrombin III. The heparin-antithrombin III complex can then bind and inhibit clotting factor proteases, including thrombin (Factor IIa), IXa, and Xa.[5] Heparin has a half-life of 60 to 90 minutes. It is cleared initially by the reticuloendothelial system and later by the kidneys. Since heparin does not cross the barrier of the placenta, it can be used during pregnancy. Dosage for therapeutic anticoagulation (a bolus is 80 µ/kg) is followed by infusion at 18 µ/kg/hr; the therapy is adjusted to target a PTT of 60 to 80 seconds. A bolus should be avoided during the immediate postoperative period. Protamine is the reversal agent. A protamine reaction is rare, but can cause hypotension, bradycardia, and decreased heart function.

A rare, but well-known complication of Heparin is Heparin-induced thrombocytopenia (HIT). In HIT, there is the formation of anti-heparin antibodies (IgG heparin-PF4 antibody) which leads to platelet destruction and thrombocytopenia. Additionally, there is platelet aggregation that leads to thrombosis. HIT should be considered when platelet levels drop to <100k, when platelets drop by a factor of >50% from admission levels, or thrombosis develops while a patient is on heparin. HIT is diagnosed by ELISA for heparin antibodies and a serotonin release assay. Treatment includes stopping heparin immediately when HIT is considered and starting the patient on argatroban, a direct thrombin inhibitor, for anticoagulation.

LOW MOLECULAR WEIGHT HEPARIN (LMWH)

LMWH acts by selectively inhibiting Factor Xa and has little effect on Factor IIa. Additionally, LMWH has a better subcutaneous bioavailability (70 to 90%) when compared to unfractionated heparin (20 to 30%). The half-life of LMWH is 4 to 6 hours and is primarily metabolized by the kidney and is thus contraindicated in patients with renal failure. Compared to unfractionated heparin, LMWH has a smaller effect on aPTT and whole blood clotting time, relative to activity of Factor Xa. Thus, laboratory monitoring of aPTT is not required. Enoxaparin is the commonly used agent. Fondaparinux is another Factor Xa inhibitor with similar properties. Protamine is usually not effective and there is no known reversal agent.

WARFARIN

Warfarin inhibits the enzyme vitamin K epoxide reductase and is responsible for the prevention of the vitamin K-dependent decarboxylation of glutamic residues on the Factors II, VII, IX, X, and proteins C and S. The anticoagulant effect develops gradually over 5 to 7 days and needs bridging with heparin initially. Warfarin has a recommended INR of 2 to 3 for prophylaxis and treatment of thrombotic diseases. Warfarin-induced skin necrosis occurs when patients are given warfarin without first being heparinized. Since protein C and S have a short half-life, their levels decrease before the pro-coagulation factors; thus, resulting in a relative hyper-thrombotic state. If a patient has a relative protein C deficiency, they are particularly susceptible to these side-effects. If a patient does have skin necrosis, they should be treated with heparin. Also, this side effect can be prevented by giving the patient heparin prior to starting warfarin. Warfarin does cross the placental barrier and should not be used during pregnancy. If a patient must undergo warfarin reversal, they should first stop the warfarin, then immediate reversal can be achieved with IV vitamin K and Fresh Frozen Plasma (FFP) or a Prothrombin Complex Concentrate (PCC) transfusion.

ORAL DIRECT FACTOR XA INHIBITORS

Oral Xa inhibitors include apixaban, rivaroxaban, and edoxaban. These drugs have a rapid onset of action and a shorter half-life. They can be given to patients at fixed doses and do not require monitoring. Andexanet alfa was recently approved by the FDA as reversal agent, and hemodialysis was tried with limited success. Direct factor Xa inhibitors act as a competitive Factor Xa "decoy" molecule.

DIRECT THROMBIN INHIBITORS

Direct thrombin inhibitors directly bind to the active site of thrombin and inhibit the coagulation cascade downstream compared to indirect thrombin inhibitors such as heparin and LMWH. Parenteral forms include Hirudin, Lepirudin, Bivalirudin, and Argatroban. The only oral direct thrombin inhibitor available for use is Dabigatran. Idarucizumab, recently approved by the FDA, is an anticoagulant reversal agent that binds to dabigatran and is made of a humanized monoclonal antibody Fab fragment.

Table 1: Antiplatelets and Reversal Agents

Antiplatelet Agent	Mechanism	Antidote	Duration to be off the medication prior to surgery[6,7]
Aspirin	COX-1 platelet inhibitor preventing thromboxane A2 synthesis which is needed for platelet activation	Platelets Desmopressin	7 -10 days
Clopidogrel/Prasugrel	$P2Y_{12}$ inhibitor an ADP receptor. This receptor is needed for platelet activation	Platelets Desmopressin	5-7 days
Abciximab/Eptifibatide	GpIIb/IIIa inhibitor which is the final step of platelet activation	Platelets FFP or PCC	>12 hours
Heparin	Binds and activates antithrombin III, thus binds and inhibits thrombin faster	Protamine sulfate	4-6 hours (if receiving continuous IV infusion); one dose (if intermittent, subcutaneous dosing)
Dabigatran	Direct thrombin inhibitor	Idarucizumab	2-5 days (depending on renal function)
Apixaban/Betrixaban	Direct inhibitor of factor Xa	Andexanet alpha PCC	2-3 days (depending on renal function)

FFP: fresh frozen plasma; PCC: prothrombin complex concentrate; PFA: platelet function analyzer

REFERENCES

1. Gale AJ. Continuing education course #2: current understanding of hemostasis. Toxicol Pathol. 2011 Jan;39(1):273-80. doi: 10.1177/0192623310389474. Epub 2010 Nov 30. PMID: 21119054; PMCID: PMC3126677.
2. Garmo C, Bajwa T, Burns B. Physiology, Clotting Mechanism. [Updated 2021 Sep 8]. In: StatPearls [Internet]. Treasure Island (FL): StatPearls Publishing; 2022 Jan-. Available from: https://www.ncbi.nlm.nih.gov/books/NBK507795/?report=classic.
3. Kulkarani R. Comprehensive care of the patient with hemophilia and inhibitors undergoing surgery: practical aspects. Hemophilia. 2013;19(1):2-10.
4. Boral BM, Williams DJ, Boral LI. Disseminated Intravascular Coagulation, American Journal of Clinical Pathology, Volume 146, Issue 6, December 2016, Pages 670–680, https://doi.org/10.1093/ajcp/aqw195.
5. Harter K, Levine M, Henderson SO. Anticoagulation drug therapy: a review. West J Emerg Med. 2015 Jan;16(1):11-7. doi: 10.5811/westjem.2014.12.22933. Epub 2015 Jan 12. PMID: 25671002; PMCID: PMC4307693.
6. O'Riordan JM, Margey RJ, Blake G, O'Connell PR. Antiplatelet Agents in the Perioperative Period. Arch Surg. 2009;144(1):69–76. doi:10.1001/archsurg.144.1.69.
7. Baumann-Kreuziger L, Slawski B, Foy P, Pfeifer K, Jung B, Hardman J. Guideline: Management of Anticoagulant Medication in the Periprocedural and Surgical Settings. March 2019.

❑❑❑

16

CHAPTER

Quality Improvement and Patient Safety

Jasneet Singh Bhullar MD
Marine Bolliet MD
Laurence Cheung MD
Vijay K. Mittal MD

INTRODUCTION

Across the world, different types of healthcare programs are in place. It has been reported that despite the healthcare programs being in place and being periodically upgraded, the target populations continue to have limited access to the recommended healthcare. There are numerous differences between the ideal pattern of care and the reality of care.[1-5] While over 130 million major operations are performed annually in the United States, and with advances in perioperative care, there are still significant variations in surgical outcomes. Hospital care including preventative medicine, regardless of patient acuity, can be significantly improved.[1-3] Patient safety has always been at the core of healthcare,[6,7] resulting in increased research and advocacy work in the area. This has led to initiatives focused on protecting patients and improving patient care and safety. The attention to this topic has further led hospitals to reflect on their performance and to find ways to assess the quality of the care received at their institution. To adequately assess the care they provide, and to ultimately improve it, hospitals must have data that is pertinent, meaningful, and valuable so that changes can be implemented.

The Centers for Medicare & Medicaid Services (CMS) and the Joint Commission on Accreditation of Healthcare Organizations (JCAHO) developed indicators of quality based on practice guidelines and current evidence with the aim of improving healthcare quality. The indicators are objective measures of hospital performance and are a uniform way to highlight areas for improvement.[8-11] Although, practice guidelines are meant to improve patient outcomes, variations, and disparities in the quality of care.[5,8,12-15]

The Joint Commission on Accreditation of HealthCare Organizations in the United States has defined an indicator as "a quantitative measure that can be used to monitor and evaluate the quality of important governance, management, clinical, and support functions that affect patient outcomes." Such indicators should be timely, reliable, comparable, valid, and responsive to change.[16,17] However, the indicators themselves do not evaluate quality, but are meant to bolster quality improvement initiatives. While tools like the indicators can lead to significant benefit to a system, they are also at risk of being manipulated and used inappropriately.

In recent years, indicators that demonstrate negative findings are being emphasized to compare and diminish hospitals and the care they provide. However, the publishing of mortality rates within hospitals by organizations such as Medicare,[18] may not aid in quality improvement, and instead may result in adverse effects.[19,20]

MARYLAND HOSPITAL ASSOCIATION (MHA) QUALITY INDICATOR PROJECT (QI)

Dating back to the 1980s, hospitals in Maryland, USA started to question how well they were doing. In fact, the Maryland Hospital Association (MHA), an organization that focuses on initiatives at Maryland hospitals and works closely with trustees, created an initiative dedicated to establishing quality indicators.[21,22]

Initially, indicators were locally developed and implemented in state hospitals. This meant that the indicators were, and still are, developed and adapted to the needs of the participating hospitals. The indicators were clearly defined to ensure that the information collected was comparable and useful.

While there was no external party to oversee the development of the MHA QI project, the organizers emphasized that it was up to the hospitals to use the indicators to implement their own quality improvement initiatives. The indicators were to be used for continued improvements and were not meant to be used punitively. Thus, the overall aim of the MHA QI Project was centered on providing clear and valuable information to further develop strategies for quality improvement for hospitals. The project organizers further suggested a framework (Figure 1) hospitals could use to help analyze the data and guide the improvement initiatives.

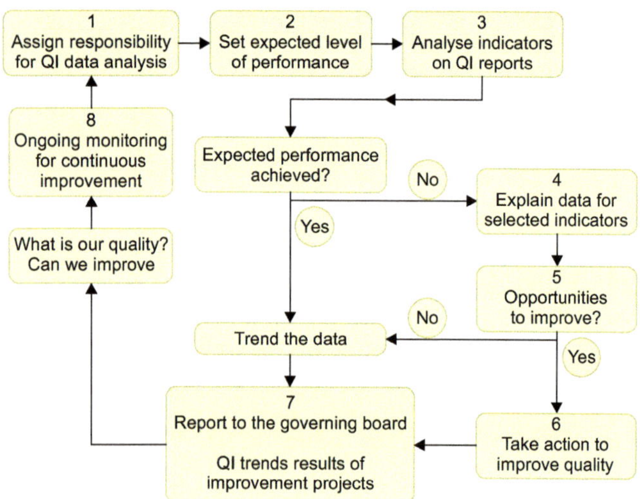

Figure 1: The flowchart shows the approach to analysis of and response to indicator data suggested in the MHA QI Project.

In 1986, the project advanced to a new phase of development after being awarded a research grant from the Robert Wood Johnson Foundation. Due to the grant, the project spread from Maryland to the rest of the United States. In the year following the advancement and spread of the project, 40 hospitals became involved, and data was being collected from 10 indicators. In 1996, further expansion led to participation from 1,100 hospitals not just in the United States, but also the United Kingdom, Japan, and Canada.

Due to the increase in participation, five additional indicators were created for outpatient and day cases (Table 1). In 1996, the MHA developed the project and associated indicators to include four areas: long term, psychiatric care, pediatric care, and process of care.

Participating hospitals attempted to acquire data for the 15 available indicators, although not all indicators were required to participate. The data was then collected and collated followed by being entered into a specially designed software that allowed the data to be graphically demonstrated.

Table 1: Shows the inpatient and outpatient indicators.

Inpatient Indicators (Implemented in 1986)
Infections:
1. Hospital acquired
2. Surgical wound
Mortality:
3. Inpatient
4. Neonatal
5. Peri-operative
6. Caesarean sections
Unplanned:
7. Readmissions
8. Admissions after ambulatory procedures
9. Returns to an ICU
10. Returns to the OR
Outpatient or Day Case Indicators
1. Unplanned return to accident and emergency <72 hours
2. Patients in accident and emergency >6 hours
3. Change in patient management due to a discrepancy between the initial and final X-ray reports
4. Prior to completing treatment, patients leaves accident and emergency
5. Day-of cancellation of a day case procedure

A coordinator responsible for systems, collected coded data from local hospitals and submitted them to the QI project. The QI project central office further collated and analyzed the data, producing detailed reports for participating hospitals. This allowed the hospitals to compare their individual results against the remainder of the project. In addition, the graphics software created through the project was provided to the hospitals and the system coordinators so that local analyses and comparisons could take place.

The strengths of the MHA QI Project can be summarized as follows:

1. Indicator validity is determined by their ability to promote change and create a sustainable quality improvement cycle; this has been useful in many collated studies due to the continued recruitment and participation of hospitals in the project.
2. The validity is enhanced by hospitals acting as both the recipients and users of data.
3. The reliability is ensured by regular surveys through the project that allows for frequent feedback to help further guide the quality improvements by the hospitals.
4. Anonymous data that protects patient confidentiality mitigates issues involving tabling of the league and external judgements.
5. Through internal use of indicators, risk adjustment becomes minimized.

The Surgical Infection Prevention (SIP) Project

Despite advances in perioperative care, significant variation in surgical outcomes still exists.[23-30] Postoperative complications range from 6% to 130% for noncardiac surgery patients[23,24] and high-risk surgery patients, respectively.[25,26] The following are common postoperative surgical complications: postoperative sepsis, surgical site infections (SSIs), respiratory complications, cardiovascular complications (including myocardial infarction), and thromboembolic complications.[23-30]

These complications have effects that extend beyond the complication itself, such as increased hospitalization length, increased costs, and increased mortality.[27] On average, for patients with a postoperative complication, their hospitalization is extended by 3 to 11 days compared to complication free patients.[24-25,27-29] Numerous initiatives focused on inpatient care improvement have been implemented by the Centers for Medicare and Medicaid Services (CMS).[30]

In 2002, the Centers for Disease Control and Prevention (CDC) and the CMS, launched the National SIP Project to emphasize prophylactic antimicrobials including the type and timing to ultimately decrease SSIs and their associated morbidity and mortality.[31,32] The project direction was informed by prior work (Medicare Quality Improvement Organization and National Nosocomial Infection Surveillance System) conducted by the CDC.[33-38]

In this project three performance measures were employed to determine quality improvement and national surveillance:

1. Percentage of patients receiving parenteral antimicrobial prophylaxis (one hour after incision time) or fluoroquinolones and vancomycin (within two hours).
2. Percentage of patients receiving antimicrobial prophylactic regimen per pre-established guidelines.
3. Percentage of patients with antimicrobial prophylaxis is discontinued (appropriately) 24 hours after the surgery.

Due to the association with decreased SSIs, antimicrobial timing and selection were chosen as specific quality improvement measures. Duration of antimicrobial prophylaxis was chosen due to the increase in bacterial resistance associated with unnecessary antimicrobial use. The three SIP Project performance measures (ORYX core set) have been employed by the Joint Commission on Accreditation of Healthcare Organizations (JCAHO[39]); the measures, via the Hospital Quality Alliance, have been included in hospital performance reporting (Hospital Compare Website).[40]

The Surgical Care Improvement Project (SCIP)

In April 2003, the CMS and many organizations including the VA, American Society of Anesthesiologists, and the CDC convened to assess the issue of surgical complications and mortality. Through this meeting SCIP, a joint initiative among organizations committed to improving surgical safety via postoperative complications was created.[41] In addition to the 10 organizations initially involved in its development, 130 more organizations joined.[41]

The SCIP collaboration assesses quality in four general areas where there is a high incidence of complications and associated cost, making these areas ideal targets for improvement and prevention measures. SCIP outcome measures and processes of care are summarized in Table 2 and 3.

1. **SSIs** are a common surgical complication, accounting for 14% to 16% of hospital-acquired infections, 2% to 5% of patients post-clean extra-abdominal operations, and up to 20% of intra-abdominal surgical patients.[42] Additionally, there are measures focused on postoperative blood glucose amongst patients undergoing cardiac surgery,[43,44] preoperative hair removal,[45] and normothermia maintenance in patients undergoing colorectal surgery.
2. **VTE**, without prophylaxis, can result in deep vein thrombosis in 25% of operations, pulmonary embolism in 7% of operations. In major orthopedic surgeries, the rates are higher at 50% and 30% respectively. However, audits have found that despite the existence of evidence-based guidelines, VTE prophylaxis is underused.[48] Appropriate VTE prophylaxis based upon operation type is a target for SCIP process measures.[49]
3. **Adverse cardiac events,** such as sudden cardiac death, acute myocardial infarction, and pulmonary edema, can occur in up to 30% of vascular surgery patients, and 2% to 5% of noncardiac surgery patients. Perioperative cardiac events have a mortality rate of 60%, weight higher financial costs, and increased length of hospital stay.[50-52] With regards to SCIP, new process measures are focused on continuing critical home medications such as beta-blockers for patients with conditions including arrhythmias, angina, and hypertension.[53]
4. **Respiratory complications**. Amongst intubated patients, 9% to 27% experience ventilator associated pneumonia. Up to 90% of associated pneumonias are found while patients are mechanically ventilated in intensive care units.[54] Patients who are mechanically ventilated are not only at increased risk for pneumonia, but also at increased risk for stress ulcers and gastrointestinal bleeding. Some proposed quality improvement measures include elevating the bed, prophylaxis for stress ulcers, and ventilator weaning protocols such as decreasing the duration of mechanical ventilation.

Table 2: Proposed process of care performance measures for the National Surgical Care Improvement Project.

Category	Performance Measures
Infection prevention	Prophylactic antimicrobials: Received within an hour prior to surgical incision[a] Consistent with current published guidelines Discontinued within 24 hours of post-surgery[b] Additionally, controlled blood glucose levels for cardiac surgery patients, proper removal of hair with clippers or no hair removal, maintaining normothermia in colorectal surgery patients.
VTE prevention	Consistent with the current guidelines and is administered within 24 hours before or after surgery
Cardiac event prevention	Perioperative beta-blockers provided to patients on beta-blockers prior to arrival
Respiratory complications prevention	For patients requiring mechanical ventilation: Elevate the bed's head at least 30 degrees Stress ulcer disease prophylaxis Document the standard weaning protocol

VTE: venous thromboembolism.

a. For patients requiring fluoroquinolones or vancomycin during surgical prophylaxis, the antimicrobial should be received within 2 hours before incision.

b. For cardiac surgery patients, antimicrobials should be discontinued within 48 hours.

Table 3: Outcome measures for the National Surgical Care Improvement Project.

Category	Outcome Measure(s) during Index Hospitalization
Infection[a]	Rates of postoperative surgical site infection
Venous thromboembolism[a]	Intra- or postoperative pulmonary embolism (or diagnosed within 30 days post-surgery) Intra- or postoperative deep vein thrombosis (or diagnosed within 30 days post-surgery)
Cardiac events[a]	Intra- or postoperative acute myocardial infarction. (or diagnosed within 30 days post-surgery)
Prevention of respiratory complications[a]	Rates of postoperative ventilator-associated pneumonia
Global measures	Within 30 days post-surgery: 1. Risk-adjusted Medicare patient mortality 2. Risk-adjusted readmission of patient

a. There have been several proposed outcome measures. It should be noted that these measures are useful for a hospital's internal quality improvement efforts, not for public accountability

SUMMARY

There is an unwavering international commitment to evaluate the outcomes and processes involved in surgical care. Different types of policies and projects have been implemented in different countries with the focus on improving patient care and outcomes. Though there are broad national and international partnerships, hospitals worldwide should participate in activities and projects aimed at reducing surgical complications, which then translates to improved patient care.

REFERENCES

1. Jencks SF, Huff ED, Cuerdon T. Change in the quality of care delivered to Medicare beneficiaries, 1998–1999 to 2000–2001. JAMA 289: 305–312.
2. McGlynn EA, Asch SM, Adams J, Keesey J, Hicks J, et al. (2003) The quality of health care delivered to adults in the United States. N Engl J Med 348: 2635– 2645.
3. Kerr EA, McGlynn EA, Adams J, Keesey J, Asch SM (2004) Profiling the quality of care in twelve communities: results from the CQI study. Health Aff (Millwood) 23: 247–256.
4. Schuster MA, McGlynn EA, Brook RH (2005) How good is the quality of healthcare in the United States? 1998. Milbank Q 83: 843–895.
5. Asch SM, Kerr EA, Keesey J, Adams JL, Setodji CM, et al. (2006) Who is at greatest risk for receiving poor-quality health care? N Engl J Med 354: 1147– 1156.
6. Kohn LT, Corrigan JM, Donaldson M, eds. To err is human: building a safer health system. Committee on Quality of HealthCare in America, Institute of Medicine. Washington DC: National Academies Press, 2000.
7. Committee on Quality of Healthcare in America, Institute of Medicine. Crossing the quality chasm: a new health system for the 21st century. Washington DC: National Academies Press, 2001.

8. Peterson ED, Roe MT, Mulgund J, DeLong ER, Lytle BL, et al. Association between hospital process performance and outcomes among patients with acute coronary syndromes. JAMA 295: 1912–1920.
9. Peterson ED, Shah BR, Parsons L, Pollack CV Jr, French WJ, et al. Trends in quality of care for patients with acute myocardial infarction in the National Registry of Myocardial Infarction from 1990 to 2006. Am Heart J 156: 1045–1055.
10. Maeda JL. Evidence-based heart failure performance measures and clinical outcomes: a systematic review. J Card Fail 16: 411–418.
11. Tu JV, Khalid L, Donovan LR, Ko DT. Indicators of quality of care for patients with acute myocardial infarction. CMAJ 179: 909–915.
12. Hasnain-Wynia R, Baker DW, Nerenz D, Feinglass J, Beal AC, et al. Disparities in health care are driven by where minority patients seek care: examination of the hospital quality alliance measures. Arch Intern Med 167: 1233–1239.
13. Bernheim SM, Spertus JA, Reid KJ, Bradley EH, Desai RA, et al. Socioeconomic disparities in outcomes after acute myocardial infarction. Am Heart J 153: 313–319.
14. Kosiak B, Sangl J, Correa-de-Araujo R. Quality of health care for older women: what do we know? Women's Health Issues 16: 89–99.
15. Correa-de-Araujo R, Stevens B, Moy E, Nilasena D, Chesley F, et al. Gender differences across racial and ethnic groups in the quality of care for acute myocardial infarction and heart failure associated with comorbidities. Women's Health Issues 16: 44– 55.
16. Joint Commission on Accreditation of HealthCare Organizations. Primer on indicator development and application. Chicago: JCAHO, 1990.
17. Anonymous. Characteristics of clinical indicators. Quality Review Bulletin 1989;15:330-9.
18. Blumenthal D. Quality of health care. part 1: quality of care - what is it? N Engl J Med 1996;335:891-3.
19. Smith P. Outcome related performance indicators and organizational control in the public sector. British Journal of Management 1993;4: 135-51.
19. McKee M, Hunter D. Mortality league tables: do they inform or mislead? Quality in Health Care 1995;4:5-12.
20. Kazandjian VA, Wood P, Lawthers J. Balancing science and practice in indicator development: the Maryland Hospital Association Quality Indicator (Q1) Project. Int 7 Qual Health Care 1995;7:39-46.
21. Kazandjian VA, Thomson RG, Law WR, Waldron K. Do performance indicators make a difference? The Joint Commission Journal on Quality Improvement 1996;22:482-91.
22. Dimick JB, Chen SL, Taheri PA, Henderson WG, Khuri SF, Campbell DA Jr. Hospital costs associated with surgical complications: a report from the private-sector National Surgical Quality Improvement Program. J Am Coll Surg 2004; 199:531–7.
23. Khan NA, Quan H, Bugar JM, Lemaire JB, Brant R, Ghali WA. Association of postoperative complications with hospital costs and length of stay in a tertiary care center. J Gen Intern Med 2006; 21:177–80.
24. Dimick JB, Pronovost PJ, Cowan JA, Lipsett PA. Complications and costs after high-risk surgery: where should we focus quality improvement initiatives? J Am Coll Surg 2003; 196:671–8.
25. Dimick JB, Pronovost PJ, Cowan JA Jr, Lipsett PA, Stanley JC, Upchurch GR Jr. Variation in postoperative complication rates after high risk surgery in the United States. Surgery 2003; 134:534–40.
26. Zhan C, Miller MR. Excess length of stay, charges, and mortality attributable to medical injuries during hospitalization. JAMA 2003; 290: 1868–74.
27. Collins TC, Daley J, Henderson WH, Khuri SF. Risk factors for prolonged length of stay after major elective surgery. Ann Surg 1999; 230: 251–9.
28. Fleischmann KE, Goldman L, Young B, Lee TH. Association between cardiac and non cardiac complications in patients undergoing non cardiac surgery: outcomes and effects on length of stay. Am J Med 2003; 115:515–20.
29. Khuri SF, Henderson WG, DePalma RG, Mosca C, Healey NA, Kumbhani DJ. Determinants of long-term survival after major surgery and the adverse effect of postoperative complications. Ann Surg 2005; 242: 326–41.
30. Surgical Infection Prevention homepage. Available at: http://www .medqic.org/sip. Accessed 11 January 2006.
31. Bratzler DW, Houck PM. Antimicrobial prophylaxis for surgery: an advisory statement from the National Surgical Infection Prevention Project. Clin Infect Dis 2004; 38:1706–15.
32. Gaynes R, Richards C, Edwards J, et al. Feeding back surveillance date to prevent hospital-acquired infections. Emerg Infect Dis 2001; 7:295–8.
33. Gaynes RP, Culver DH, Horan TC, et al. Surgical site infection (SSI) rates in the United States, 1992–1998: The National Nosocomial Infections Surveillance System basic SSI risk index. Clin Infect Dis 2001; 33(2 Suppl):S69–77.

34. National Nosocomial Infections Surveillance System. National Nosocomial Infections Surveillance (NNIS) System report, data summary from January 1992 to June 2002, issued August 2002. Am J Infect Control 2002; 30:458–75.
35. Jencks SF,Wilensky GR. The healthcare quality improvement initiative: a new approach to quality assurance in Medicare. JAMA 1992; 268: 900–4.
36. Jencks SF, Cuerdon T, Burwen DR, et al. Quality of medical care delivered to Medicare beneficiaries: A profile at state and national levels. JAMA 2000; 284:1670–6.
37. Jencks SF, Huff ED, Cuerdon T. Change in the quality of care delivered to Medicare beneficiaries 1998–1999 to 2000–2001. JAMA 2003; 289: 305–12.
38. Joint Commission on Accreditation of Healthcare Organizations. Surgical infection prevention core performance measures for national implementation. Available at: http://www.jcaho.org/pms/core+measures/10asipmeaslistpop.pdf.
39. US Department of Health and Human Services. Hospital compare. Available at: http://www.hospitalcompare.hhs.gov.
40. Surgical Care Improvement Project homepage. Available at: http:// www.medqic.org/scip.
41. Bratzler DW, Houck PM, Richards C, et al. Use of antimicrobial prophylaxis for major surgery: baseline results from the National Surgical Infection Prevention Project. Arch Surg 2005; 140:174–82.
42. Alexander JW, Fischer JE, Boyajian M, Palmquist J, Morris MJ. The influence of hair-removal methods on wound infections. Arch Surg 1983; 118:347–52.
43. Kjonniksen I, Andersen BM, Sondenaa VG, Segadal L. Preoperative hair removal: a systematic literature review. AORN J 2002; 75:928–38.
44. Kurz A, Sessler DI, Lenhardt R. Perioperative normothermia to reduce the incidence of surgical-wound infection and shorten hospitalization. Study of Wound Infection and Temperature Group. N Engl J Med 1996; 334:1209–15.
45. Geerts WH, Heit JA, Clagett GP, et al. Prevention of venous thromboembolism. Chest 2001; 119(1 Suppl):132S–175S.
46. Kleinbart J, Williams MV, Rask K. Prevention of venous thromboembolism. In: Making health care safer: a critical analysis of patient safety practices. Evidence Report/Technology Assessment 43. AHRQ publication no. 01-E058, July 2001. Rockville, MD: Agency for Healthcare Research and Quality, 2001. Available at http://www.ahrq.gov/ clinic/ptsafety/chap31a.htm.
47. Geerts WH, Pineo GF, Heit JA, et al. Prevention of venous thromboembolism. Chest 2004; 126:338S–400S.
48. Bratzler DW, Raskob GE, Murray CK, Bumpus LJ, Piatt DS. Underuse of venous thromboembolism prophylaxis for general surgery patients: physician practices in the community hospital setting. Arch Intern Med 1998; 158:1909–12.
49. Auerbach AD. Beta-blockers and reduction of perioperative cardiac events. In: Making health care safer: a critical analysis of patient safety practices. Evidence Report/Technology Assessment 43. AHRQ publication no. 01-E058, July 2001. Rockville, MD: Agency for Healthcare Research and Quality, 2001. Available at http://www.ahrq.gov/clinic/ ptsafety/chap25.htm.
50. Selzman CH, Miller SA, Zimmerman MA, Harken AH. The case for b-adrenergic blockade as prophylaxis against perioperative cardiovascular morbidity and mortality. Arch Surg 2001; 136:286–90.
51. Lindenauer PK, Pekow P, Wang K, Mamidi DK, Gutierrez B, Benjamin EM. Perioperative beta-blocker therapy and mortality after major noncardiac surgery. N Engl J Med 2005; 353:349–61.
52. Fleisher LA, Beckman JA, Brown KA, et al. ACC/AHA 2006 guideline update on perioperative cardiovascular evaluation for noncardiac surgery: focused update on perioperative beta-blocker therapy. Available at: http://www.acc.org/clinical/guidelines/perio/periobetablocker.pdf.
53. Niederman MS, Craven DE, Bonten MJ, et al. Guidelines for the management of adults with hospital-acquired, ventilator-associated, and healthcare-associated pneumonia. Am J Respir Crit Care Med 2005; 171:388–416.

❑❑❑

17
CHAPTER

Simulation in Surgery

Vijay K. Mittal, MD
Binit Katuwal, MD
Jasneet Singh Bhullar, MD
Gokulakkrishna Subhas, MD

INTRODUCTION

Since there has been a reduction in training hours and of opportunities due to patient safety concerns, simulation training has rapidly evolved.[1] Simulation is a training modality that enables achieving technical competency, without the jeopardization of patient care. Simulation is an exercise or device that enables one to recreate, under test conditions, situations likely to be faced in clinical practice.[2] A long list of state-of-the-art devices is being made to teach and attain objective evaluations of the trainee's technical abilities which might enable detection and evaluation of near miss events or errors before risking the patient. As with the flight simulation in aviation industry, the ability to detect near misses can anticipate a potential error before it occurs, thus preventing unwanted complications.[3] Patient safety should be the utmost priority and it should not be compromised to train or test a student's skills, therefore simulators are very valuable because they can achieve this goal with complete safety.[3]

Simulation exercises in medicine attempt to recreate events which are common in clinical practice and are important for students to know and understand. Simulators consist of the technologies used to imitate various specific tasks. High-fidelity simulators can reproduce the clinical environment with a lot of detail and precision and include virtual reality or laparoscopic simulators.[4] Low fidelity simulators are rudimentary or incomplete clinical environments and include pelvic or chest manikins, most often used for surgical and obstetric training.[4]

Surgical advancements have created unique challenges for education, questioning the efficacy of the old surgical skill training model "see one, do one, teach one".[5] Different barriers to progression have been identified, which includes less available time for faculty to teach, limited institutional resources, limited instructions, and potentially the most important barrier is the lack of a uniform objective technical skills assessment.[6] Restriction on duty hours as mandated by the ACGME for trainees, which was implemented to decrease fatigue and errors, might also be responsible in decreasing the amount of time students have for hands-on learning. This is an example of a dissociation of the traditional model of "apprentice and master" introduced in the late 1800s by Osler and Halsted. This reduction had led to concern over the insufficient development of new student's technical skills that are acquired in the operating room and requires learning and practice outside of patient care, thus highlighting the importance of simulation exercises.[6]

HISTORY OF SIMULATION

Simulation is not a new concept. Medical simulation has been practiced for centuries, albeit in primitive forms. The first simulators in the medical field consisted of human patient models, varying from different cultures and geography. In this regard, the efforts in the late 20th century were a major step towards modern simulation. There were also huge lessons learnt from other fields outside of medicine. Simulation training is well established in the non-medical community like military, aviation, nuclear power, gaming industry, racing etc. Civil aviation requires certification, annual recertification, and intensive simulation training to pilot different aircraft. The Military uses simulation for training soldiers and military medical personnel to teach and maintain skills. However, in the medical world, there was a long delay in accepting simulation due to skepticism, lack of communication, and the burden of proof.[7] In medicine, simulator development started with Anesthesiology, with further advancements in the last ten years after the Institute of Medicine (IOM) report. Today the medical world has acknowledged that simulation is the future of medical education and multiple articles have been written in the last decade envisioning how simulation can revolutionize medical education, patient care, and patient safety.

ADVANTAGES OF SIMULATION

As mentioned before, restrictions in resident hours have made efficiency during residency training necessary. There is a steep learning curve for many surgical procedures. There is a probability that the resident could complete training without actually having enough experience to safely perform these procedures.[8] There are many other reasons for the need of simulation in medicine. These include patient safety, ethical issues, training, warm-up, and preoperative planning. It has been proven in several studies that virtual reality-based (VR) simulation in medicine has many benefits including exchangeable scenarios, automated assessment, fully controllable environments, unlimited repetitions, and more.[9] Additionally, there are programs that can help strengthen teamwork and communication skills and identify issues in the system that impair optimal patient care. Simulation programs are therefore helpful in improving both individual and team performance.[4]

One barrier in effective learning could be limited resources in instruction. First, there is limited availability of cadaveric material, which used to be the gold standard for practicing surgical techniques outside of patient care. Second, there is limited availability of faculty expertise. With pressures of increasing productivity in increased clinical duties, many faculty have less time to teach, especially for critical assessment during a resident's formative development which needs considerable time. The pressure to increase clinical productivity to maintain income has resulted in reduced numbers of teaching faculty. Therefore, simulation can mitigate this impact of having limited instructional resources.[6]

When done systematically, simulation enables a standardized objective evaluation of performance. They can act as refresher courses and introduce new technology for experienced physicians. With proper validation, they can eventually be a tool to show a surgeon's proficiency, helping with credentialing and certification.[4]

REDUCE MEDICAL ERRORS

Confucius once said, *"Tell me, and I will forget. Show me, and I may remember. Involve me, and I will understand."* In November 1999, the Institute of Medicine (IOM) released a report: To err is human: building a safer health system. The report read, "Health care in the United States is not as safe as it should be - and can be. At least 44,000 people, and perhaps as many as 98,000 people, die in hospitals each year as a result of medical errors that could have been prevented." According to the report, medical errors can be defined as the failure of a planned action to be completed as intended, or the use of a wrong plan to achieve an aim.

Students are taught of potential errors they will face and how to avoid them, in a uniform and comprehensive manner. The key to simulation is the ability to detect near misses and prevent related errors and complications. Thus, the reporting of near misses is stressed during aviation simulation training and is one of the industry's strengths.[3]

Simulation is clearly a great way to address both risk management and patient safety. Physician can learn how to avoid error in a safe and engaging environment, where patients cannot be harmed.[10] Additionally, they expose residents to rare events that might not be encountered during training. Thus, an opportunity to practice and learn from mistakes without harming patients.[4]

MEDICAL AND SURGICAL DISCIPLINES

Simulation based education has been used by medical educators in various medical disciplines to improve quality of care. Simulation enables trainees to gain valuable clinical skills in a safe, forgiving environment, and provides an opportunity to gain critical feedback on their performance from trained faculty supervisors. Oftentimes, residents must insert central venous catheters for resuscitation of critically ill patients, even if they do not have adequate preparation and training. This is dangerous because this procedure is associated with serious complications such as arterial puncture, pneumothorax, and catheter-associated bloodstream infections. This is one of the many examples why the American Board of Internal Medicine recommends internal medicine residents to receive simulation training prior to performing such invasive procedures on patients.[11]

Surgery has a broad catalog of invasive medical treatments that involves the cutting of a body for a specific reason, such as the removal of diseased tissue or to repair a tear or breakage. Thus, most parts of the training are focused on procedures. Surgery was traditionally learnt by repeated practice on patients. During the early stages of learning technical skills, the residents should not be in the operating room; they must practice until they have achieved automaticity in the basic skills. The mastery of basic skills outside of the operating room allows trainees to focus on more complex issues, both technical and nontechnical, in the operating room. Deliberate practice is a crucial part of the process to develop mastery or expertise.[12]

Traditionally, a surgical resident's training and evaluation has been a subjective process; an assessment of their technique, skill, dexterity, and insight. It is important to have an objective measure of a resident's progress since competence and safety are crucially important.[3] The training of a surgeon includes the acquisition of several characteristics. These include a solid knowledgebase, decision making abilities, and other attributes that can be measured with objective testing. However, the most critical to the surgeon are probably the core technical skills.[3] Simulation plays a big role in achieving this purpose. Across the country, there have been various preparatory training programs for new trainees beginning residency, with the aim of improving the clinical orientation process for new postgraduate year (PGY)-1 residents, Baystate Medical Center, Massachusetts was the first to develop such a program. They have created an intensive curriculum that incorporates cognitive and procedural skills, and essential training activities for early PGY-1 clinical duties. This PGY-1 Boot Camp is a preparatory simulation-based training that starts at the beginning of a resident's internship to introduce the necessary skills for basic surgical patient problem assessment and management; including simulated patient care encounters and technical skills training.[13]

Simulators are increasingly becoming an indispensable tool in gastroenterology for both the novice and advanced endoscopist.[14] Simulation-based educations are also available to address the competencies for professionalism, collaboration, communication, management, and leadership.[15]

VIRTUAL REALITY SIMULATORS

Virtual reality simulators that use interactive computer graphics have greatly impacted military and commercial pilots' skill levels, and similar training can be promising for the medical field.[3] Virtual-reality simulation has been important in early resident training for laparoscopic, plastic, gastrointestinal, dermatologic, ophthalmologic, and some laryngology procedures.[3]

Virtual-reality simulators are used in many laparoscopic surgical training programs for psychomotor skill training required for this type of surgery. It has been proven that training basic laparoscopic skills in a skills-lab setting improves performance in the operating room.[16] Advancements in this area have enabled residents to practice surgical cases in an environment immersed in great quality in auditory, visual, and haptic feedback. In the fields of laparoscopic surgery, anesthesia, radiology, ophthalmology, interventional cardiology, and obstetrics and gynecology, there is growing evidence that virtual-reality simulation is an effective methodology to gain technical skills in many important procedures.[2]

The availability of patient-specific virtual-reality rehearsal can improve carotid artery stenting procedures for interventional endovascular performance. Using a generic module is also potentially valuable in the endovascular field, similarly to that proven in the laparoscopic field. With virtual-reality simulation, medicine would be following the path other high-stakes industries have used, enabling the minimization of complications during standard and more complex procedures, thus improving overall patient safety.[17]

COST

Fortunately, state-of-the-art simulation is not necessary and low technology solutions can be both effective and cost effective. Thus, expense is not always a barrier.[10] However, not all simulation programs are created equal and poorly constructed and executed simulations can actually be detrimental by reinforcing bad habits. Many institutions unfortunately spend a lot of money on simulations before even developing their programs.[4]

COST OF SURGICAL TRAINING

Trainee surgeons tend to be slower, reducing operating theater throughput. Additionally, may have more complications, increasing hospital stay and costs. Bridges and Diamond calculated that the cost of training a surgical resident in the operating room for 4 years was nearly $50,000. In 1997, the annual cost of training a surgical resident in the operating room was totaled to be around $53 million. This high cost indicates a need for digital skills, selection criteria, the development of training curriculum and resource facilities, the pre-operating room need for basic surgical techniques, and the acquisition of virtual surgery training modules.[18]

A study conducted by the Penn Medicine Clinical Simulation Center showed a cost of $4.2 million to implement; the cost included initial construction to renovate existing space and the purchase of equipment. The annual operational cost was $476,000. The study was focused on the 38 first year residents for a 4-week simulation rotation. The annual cost per resident was $12,516 which does not include the cost of teaching. The conclusion of this study was that there is a significant cost involved in implementing the ACS/APDS Curriculum.[19]

TRANSLATION INTO PATIENT CARE

It is important to demonstrate the value of new training methods before adopting them. Multiple studies demonstrate improved skills in the operating room amongst trainees who used a simulated environment to practice laparoscopic skills. Other studies show that simulation training improves operating room performance including improvements in parameters such as decreases in operative time and intraoperative errors. Important clinical improvements in patient outcome include less patient discomfort during colonoscopy, decreased mortality rates for cardiopulmonary resuscitation, and fewer costs and complications in central venous catheters placement and thoracocentesis.[8]

Meta-analysis has shown that simulators provide better training in skills for laparoscopic surgery compared to the traditional apprenticeship approach. Adoption of simulators in surgical residency programs is highly encouraged for teaching laparoscopic surgery skills to residents.[20]

In a prospective randomized controlled trial, 25 surgical residents were allocated to receive either conventional residency training or a comprehensive training curriculum for laparoscopic colorectal surgery. Participation in a comprehensive ex-vivo training curriculum for laparoscopic colorectal surgery results in improved technical knowledge and improved performance in the operating room compared with conventional residency training.[21]

Using laparoscopic simulation training, trainees were able to significantly improve their advanced laparoscopic skills to a level comparable to expert surgeons. More importantly, these learned skills were transferred to a more complex live animal model.[22]

SIMULATION TRAINING CURRICULUM

A comprehensive simulation training curriculum must be made. This curriculum must provide objective metrics to assess residents' technical skills, including complementary simulation tools and several perceptual and spatial ability test instruments.[3] Surgical performance is monitored by identifying, qualifying, and using technical errors; the metrics then undergo outcome analysis. Metrics that have been validated include errors, time-to-completion, psychomotor tracking, and economy of motion.[3] The use of innovative simulation devices that train surgical tasks and basic skills through repetitive proctored challenges may lead to better detection and analysis of potential surgical errors. Surgical trainees exposed to such a curriculum can potentially achieve a great amount of pre-patient expertise, thus providing healthcare of higher quality throughout their career.[3] The simulator records task-specific scores and overall scores on the residents' performance. Components of the score include the time required to finish a task and accuracy relative to optimal performance. The score receives a penalty if the residents require excessive time to finish a task, or for hitting "hazards," anatomical areas that surgeons should take care to avoid.[3]

Complications are prevented primarily by the attending surgeon intervening. The attending surgeon assesses the resident's performance through briefing, debriefing, and over-the-shoulder evaluation. Additionally, the resident's performance is assessed via the use of predetermined metrics, objective simulator responses, and via the resident's observations.

Strong programs to improve patient safety consist of didactics, simulations, and debriefing sessions. Participants gain a baseline knowledge of the subject matter through the didactic portion. It should be hand in hand with the simulation exercises and have benefits whether done before or after a simulation session. When didactics are completed before the simulation, participants' fears of looking unprepared during the simulation should be allayed. When didactics are completed after the simulation, participants should have the opportunity to gain practical experience to apply the didactic knowledge.

The simulation gives residents practical, hands-on experience. This is particularly valuable because learners generally retain more from doing rather than from during lecture.[4] Debriefing is potentially the most important portion because it gives a framework for open communication between team members without the pressure and stress of explaining any poor outcomes. Digitally recorded simulations enable an unbiased look at what occurred. Participants are often surprised due to a disconnect between their perception of events compared to the recorded documentation. Therefore, debriefing gives attendees an opportunity to evaluate their performance and discuss system issues that may have interfered with a more optimal outcome.[4]

The number of programs that have invested in simulators continue to expand. In a study by Ehdaie et al., they noticed that despite having laparoscopic simulator access, residents often do not use them. If the program includes a laparoscopic curriculum, however, the residents report using surgical simulators more often compared to programs without curriculum. Hence creation of a curriculum is important, and incorporating stimulators enhances education.[5] With such rapid changes in the healthcare environment and surgical technology, surgical education must also evolve to develop a robust surgical skills curriculum incorporating surgical simulators.[5]

Currently, there are no uniform and objective standardized metrics to assess technical skills. Without these metrics, programs cannot measure technical proficiency and provide uniform formative feedback during training.[6] It is also suggested by more recent literature that it is more important to reach a predefined level (criterion-based training), over completing an arbitrary number of procedures, repetitions of tasks, or hours practicing with the simulator (time-based training). Criterion-based training also supposedly boosts the motivation of residents.[16]

When educators provide more information to trainees which forces them to multitask, the educator must pay extreme attention to the trainees' skill level. An effective strategy is to pause the technical skill performance, explain the relevant point, and then continue the technical performance. This teaching strategy should give the trainee a better comprehension of the relevant point, resulting in better retention and recall of the information.[23]

5 W'S FOR SETTING UP TRAINING CURRICULUM

The "Five W's" can help guide the initiation of a simulation program. First, there is the "who," who the program is directed to, whether it is the experienced physicians, house staff, or the entire team involved in patient care. Second, is the "what," including the topic and the type of simulation. There are many simulation programs to choose from. Third, is the "where." When choosing a location, it is important to consider space and equipment constraints. Remember that on-site and off-site drills can achieve different aims. The advantage of off-site drills is having the undivided attention of the participants since they cannot be preoccupied with clinical responsibilities. The advantages of on-site drills are having valuable learning opportunities and the ability to test the hospital systems and response times. Fourth, is the "when," with simulations ideally occurring both during scheduled and unscheduled sessions. Scheduled sessions must occur to ensure all staff attend and are exposed to the entire program without interruptions. Impromptu on-site sessions enable testing of the system, allowing participants to reinforce good practices in a realistic setting. Fifth, is the "why," it is important to establish clear expectations with the staff so that they understand the value and purpose of the simulation, though it may not be realized immediately. Generally, new initiatives face resistance. Establishing mutual goals early allows the participants to better understand any potential benefits of the simulation.[4]

SIMULATION ASSESSMENT

Simulators are used for training and assessment. This process includes assessment of models/simulators and assessment of learners.

ASSESSMENT OF THE MODELS/SIMULATORS

The assessment of the models/simulators includes verification and validation of models. Validation is the process of determining whether we have built the right model, whereas verification is designed to see if we have built the model right. Some assessment models come with built-in assessment tools that can be used to certify the competency of learners, creating an environment where learners train-to-proficiency rather than to an arbitrary number of repetitions.[25]

ASSESSMENT OF LEARNERS

Evaluating performance in the operating room is difficult and efforts have focused on techniques that standardize the assessment process outside the operating room.

1. OSATS (Objective Structured Assessment of Technical Skills): Global assessment score and task specific checklist.[12]
2. HMA (Hand Motion Analysis): This uses kinesiology, the study of human movement. With the use of electromagnetic markers, HMA can assess and follow clinical parts in relation to joint movement (e.g., depth perception, hand direction, finger visual tracking of moving objects, finger-pressure coordination, finger strength, spatial visualization, speed of movements, finger dexterity, and fine-control precision). This helps assess the resident's surgical skills using simulation.
3. OSCE (Objectively Structured Clinical Examination): This is a type of examination designed to test clinical skill performance and competence.
4. Simulated operating rooms assess surgical competence in an environment that is realistic. Skills assessed include decision-making, communication, crisis management, and leadership.

NEW CONCEPTS

A newer popular concept is the idea that video games may improve operating ability, particularly endoscopic procedures. Video game users have been shown to acquire endoscopic techniques faster, and video game training seems to improve performance.[1] Playing video games involves the 3-dimensional (3D) manipulation of objects through a 2D screen, requiring wrist and hand dexterity. These skills appear similar to the newer surgical techniques (i.e., laparoscopy).[1] Additionally, residents with extensive video game experience have stronger visuospatial ability. Under similar thought, the younger surgeons appear to achieve laparoscopic skills more easily than their older colleagues, one potential explanation being the increased video game usage amongst this population.[1]

It is likely that the virtual-reality simulator generation will create a virtual surgical environment using data from individual patient anatomy (e.g., CT images) by downloading and superimposing radiology images into the simulator. This technology can be a visual and mental rehearsal used to help the surgeon prior to the real surgery. Thus, the surgeon can anticipate hazards and risks, and note them on radiology images to be used during the real surgery. Over the next few years, the surgical simulators will reach a performance level making them suitable to test and certify surgeons.[3]

SURGICAL SKILLS CURRICULUM

The ACS/APDS National Surgical Skills Curriculum: The American College of Surgeons through the Association of Program Directors in Surgery, jointly developed a standardized skills curriculum for residents in three phases. Phase I (Table 1) includes 20 modules that address basic surgical skills designed with first- and second-year residents. There are videos and assessment tools available. The assessment tool is based on the Objective Structured Assessment of Technical Skills (OSATS). Phase II consists of 15 modules that include advanced skills and procedures. Phase III includes 10 modules that address team-based skills. For Phase II (Table 2) and Phase III (Table 3), ACS is currently working on developing the assessment tools, using technology to develop simulators.

Table 1: Sample plan to use simulators and equipment needed for training on each module of Phase 1 Basic / Core Skills and Tasks from ACS/APDS Curriculum

	Module	Simulators	Instruments
1	Basic Laparoscopic Skills	Box Trainer, Instructional video with FLS tasks	Stopwatch, Endo graspers, Endo shears, Endo dissectors Endo needle holders, Silk suture, Endo loop Knot pusher
2	Advanced Laparoscopic Skills	Simbionix LapMentor II Mentice MIST	
3	Airway management	Pig, Cadaver or Mannequin (Laerdal SimMan 3G) Immersion Endoscopy Accut-ouch System	Endotracheal tube Tracheostomy set Tracheostomy tubes
4	Asepsis and Instrument Identification	Abdominal mannequin	Instrument tray
5	Bone Fixation and Casting	Leg Skeleton model (Sawbones) Standardized patient	Splints undercast padding plaster bandages Splint, Large basin, Water source, Hare / Sager traction splint, Sling
7	Central line insertion and Arterial Lines	Task trainers from (blue phantom, simulab, enasco, limbs and things) Laerdal Arterial Line Simulator Ultrasound machine NEJM Clinical videos	Central line kits Arterial line kits
8	Chest Tube and Thoracentesis	Blue Phantom Thoracentesis Trainer Beef/pork rib model with 1L saline bags and Chux TraumaMan® System (Simulab) Anesthetized animal Cadaver	Chest tubes, Chest tube insertion tray, Kelly and tonsillar clamps, Suture, Dressings, Underwater seal drainage system
9	Colonoscopy	SIU Colonoscopy model Colonoscope Immersion Endoscopy Accut-ouch System	Light source Monitor Suction and irrigation setups

	Module	Simulators	Instruments
10	Handsewn Gastrointestinal Anastomosis	Pig or Veal Intestine Single & double-layer bowel model (Limbs & Things, syn-cadaver, simulab) Foam bowel and stomach	Instruments Suture
11	Inguinal Anatomy	Cadaver Inguinal hernia trainer (Limbs & Things) Peanut dissectors Websurg video	Polypropylene mesh, blade scalpel, Tissue forceps Weitlaner retractor, Metzenbaum scissors, Suture material Needle holder, Penrose drain, Kelly clamps
12	Knot Tying	Tying board, Tying rope Covidien knot tying video	Silk ties, Needle driver, Suture scissors, Forceps
13	Laparotomy Opening and Closure	Limbs & Things Laparotomy Trainer SIU Laparotomy model	Laparotomy tray, Adson forceps, DeBakey forceps blade scalpel, Metzenbaum scissors Sutures: Vicryl Polypropylene, Skin stapler
14	Stapled Gastrointestinal Anastomosis	Pig intestine Foam bowel & stomach Single- & double-layer bowel model Limbs & Things	Autosuture GIA, TA, CEEA, EEA
15	Surgical Biopsy	Medium size orange Chicken thigh with implanted olive Chicken thigh with wire Pig's foot, Blue Phantom ultrasound models Skin pads, ACS breast biopsy videos Ultrasound machine	Syringe with needle, Needle driver, blade scalpel Adson forceps, suture, Punch biopsy instrument Glass slides, Fixative spray, Specimen container +/- FNA biopsy gun & tubing
16	Suturing	Synthetic skin pads or Pig's foot	Scalpel blade, Needle driver, Adson forceps Suture scissors, Suture
17	Tissue Handling, Dissection, and Wound Closure	Cadaver forearms (including elbow joint) Synthetic skin pads	Blade scalpel, Needle driver, Adson forceps, Suture scissors, Suture, Hemostats, Kelly clamps, Wound retractors, Vessel loops, Subcutaneous and subcuticular suture
18	Upper Endoscopy	SIU Upper endoscopy model Simbionix GI Mentor II Open PEG box model	
19	Urethral and Suprapubic Catheterization	Catheterization Models (Limbs & Things)	Suprapubic catheter set Foley catheter set
20	Vascular Anastomosis	PTFE graft Packing foam Dasie (Dog Abdominal Surrogate for Instructional Exercises) Gore-Tex® vascular graft Penn AAA simulator Limbs and Things	Replacement AAA and Core vascular skills set DeBakey forceps, #11 blade scalpel, Castro needle drivers Potts scissors, Metzenbaum scissors 5-0 and 6-0 Prolene double-armed suture

Table 2: Sample plan to use simulators and equipment needed for training on each module of Phase 2 Advanced procedures from ACS/APDS Curriculum

	Module	Simulator
1	Gastric Resection and Peptic Ulcer Disease	Symbionix LapMentor Box trainer Websurge video
2	Laparoscopic Appendectomy	Cadaver Porcine model Simbionix LapMentor II (laparoscopic only) Websurg video
3	Laparoscopic Inguinal Hernia Repair	Cadaver Porcine model Symbionix LapMentor II Websurg video
4	Laparoscopic Right Colon Resection	Live animal Limbs & Things double-layer bowel model Foam bowel
5	Laparoscopic Sigmoid Resection	Simulab CBDE model
6	Laparoscopic Nissen Fundoplication	Symbionix LapMentor Porcine model Box model with mesh Websurg video
7	Laparoscopic Ventral Hernia Repair	Inanimate model made of Gore-Tex® Surgical Science LapSim Websurg video
8	Laparoscopic Ventral/Incisional Hernia Repair	Anesthetized pig Websurg video Box model with Limbs & Things double-layer bowel model and endo-stitch
9	Laparoscopic/Open Bile Duct Exploration	ACS SLN biopsy video
10	Laparoscopic/Open Cholecystectomy	Cadaver Limbs & Things Open Inguinal hernia trainer Websurg video (femoral and inguinal hernias)
11	Laparoscopic/Open Splenectomy	Cadaver Pig
12	Open Inguinal/Femoral Hernia Repair	Cadaver torso Video
13	Open Right Colon Resection	Cadaver torso, Symbionix LapMentor II (lap), Surgical Science LapSim, Box model with Simulab gallbladder model, Websurg video
14	Parathyroidectomy/Thyroidectomy	Cadaver torso, Foam stomach, Autosuture GIA, TA, CEEA, EEA, Websurg video
15	Sentinel Node Biopsy and Axillary Lymph Node Dissection	Cadaver, Limbs & Things, Hemostasis Pad adapted over an upper airway model and Knot tying board with deep hook

Table 3: Sample plan to use simulators and equipment needed for training on each module of Phase 3 Team-Based Skills from ACS/APDS Curriculum

	Module	Simulator
1	Laparoscopic crisis	Simulated abdomen, Cadaver, Pig
2	Laparoscopic Troubleshooting	Simulated abdomen, Cadaver, Pig
3	Latex Allergy Anaphylaxis	SimMan 3G
4	Patient Handoff	SimMan 3G
5	Postoperative Hypotension,	SimMan 3G
6	Postoperative MI (Cardiogenic Shock)	SimMan 3G
7	Postoperative Pulmonary Embolism	SimMan 3G
8	Preoperative Briefing	SimMan 3G
9	Retained Sponge on Postoperative Chest X-Ray	SimMan 3G, Abdominal mannequin
10	Trauma Team Training	SimMan 3G

TYPES OF SURGICAL SIMULATORS

HUMAN SIMULATION

Standardized Patient and OSCE: A lay person (actor) functioning as a simulated patient. The students take a history, conduct a physical examination, communicate with the patient, order, and interpret investigations, and write management plans.

Cadaver: A fresh frozen cadaver is used for teaching anatomy and practice procedures. Preserved human cadavers do not have the same tissue elasticity as fresh cadavers do.

The visible human dataset: The National Library of Medicine provides a high-fidelity 3D virtual model of a human cadaver that was derived from patient specific data, utilizing artificial intellgence.

ANIMAL SIMULATION

Dogs, pigs, goats, and sheep are commonly used in medical training. They can be used either alive, under anesthesia, as parts, or as fresh cadavers. Pig labs are commonly used for open and closed surgical procedures and are performed on live pigs under anesthesia (Figure 1). They provide a high-fidelity non-patient environment and allow students to develop the psychomotor and cognitive skills in an operating room setting. This requires an animal care facility and veterinary staff. Animal parts can be used for practicing certain procedures. For example, pig feet are used for suturing and knot tying (Figure 2), chicken or turkey breast is used for ultrasound guided breast biopsy, and pig intestine is used for bowel anastomosis.

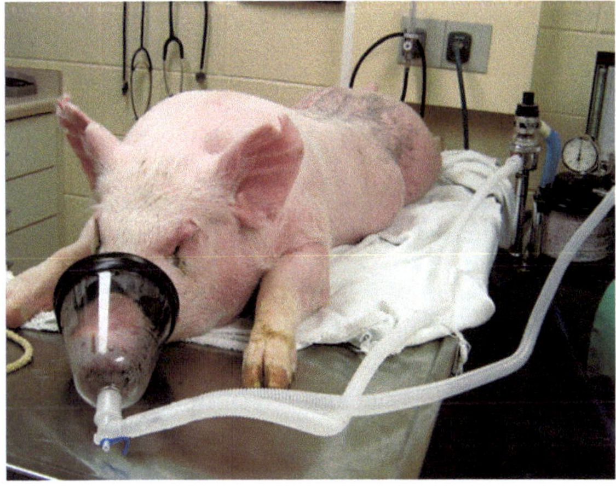

Figure 1: Pig under anesthesia

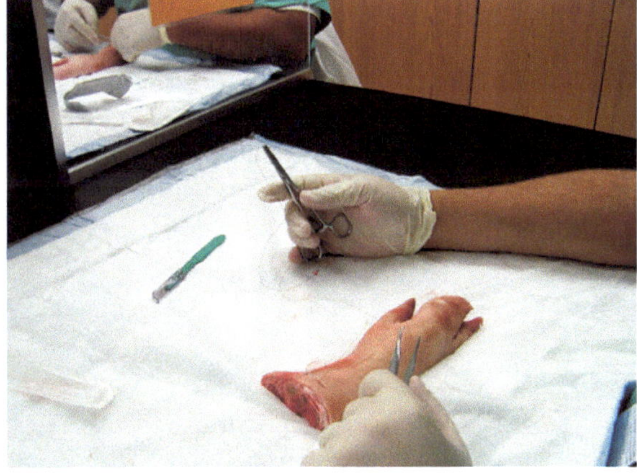

Figure 2: Pig feet used for suturing and knot tying practice

MECHANICAL SIMULATION

Mechanical simulators are widely used and are well-known forms of surgical simulators. These models are valuable for medical students and residents to practice and hone important skills. A few commonly used simulators are shown in Figures 3 through 9. Figures 3 through 6 show basic procedural training skills models and Figures 7 through 9 show advanced procedural skills models.

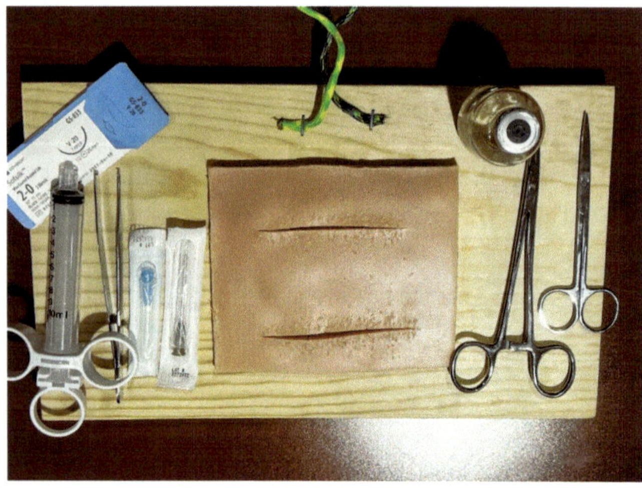

Figure 3: Suturing and knot tying models

To practice suturing and knot tying techniques, one can use an orange skin, a pig foot available in supermarkets, or commercially available boards from various manufacturers. There is also expired suture material available at esuture.com.

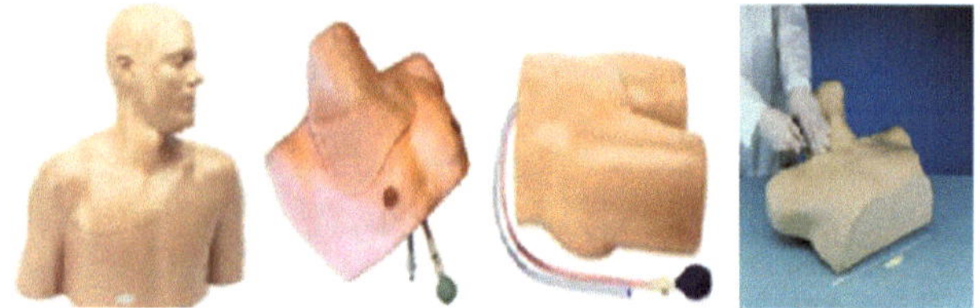

Figure 3: Task trainers for central line catheterization. Some models are ultrasound compatible with landmarks

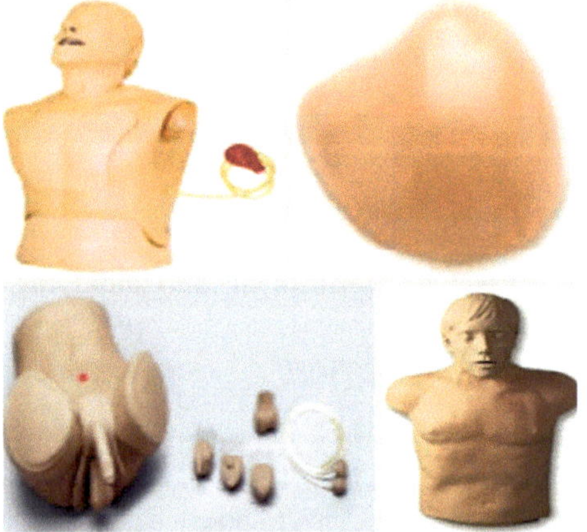

Figure 4: Task trainers for different procedures. Below are nasogastric tube placement, breast biopsy, bladder catheterization, and BLS training models

Laparoscopic simulator

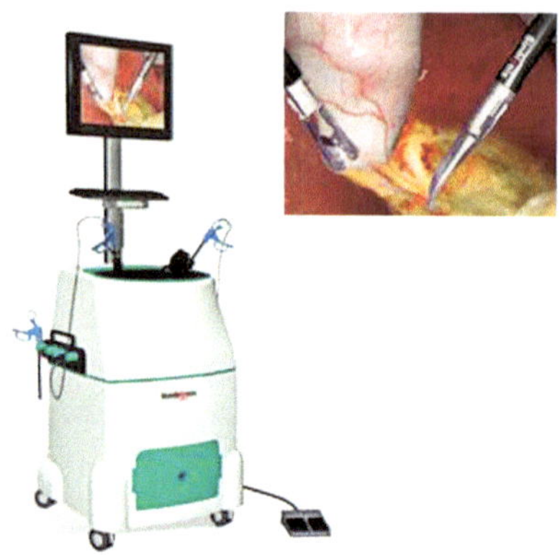

Figure 5: The virtual reality simulators are high fidelity visual, audio, touch cues and actual tools integrated with computers focused on simple and complex task training on some procedure modules. The virtual reality simulators offer both basic and advanced training skills

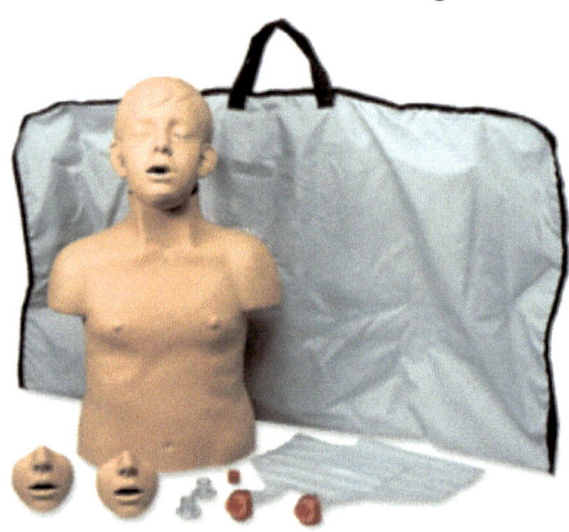

Simulaid Mannequin and Equipment

Figure 6: Simulaid mannequin and SimMan 3G mannequin for trauma training, interprofessional team training, and disaster training. The full body human simulators come with advanced features and a wide range of scenarios and patient cases

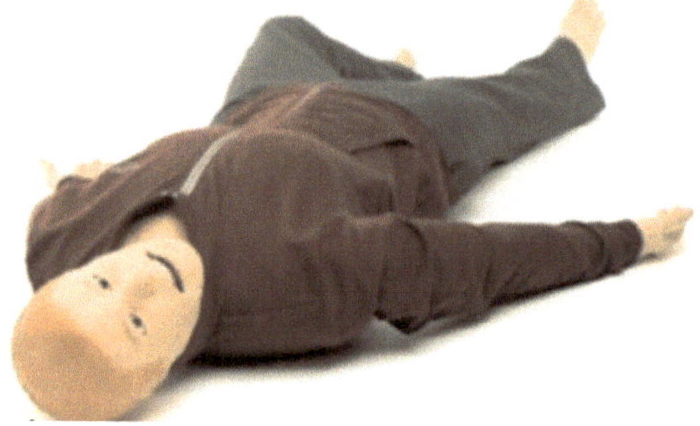

SimMan 3G Mannequin and Equipment

Figure 7: Virtual reality robotic surgical simulators. There are currently four robotic simulators: the dV-Trainer and da Vinci Skills simulators

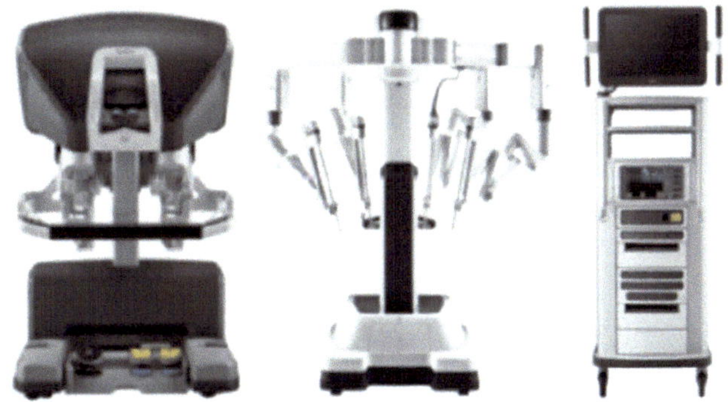

da Vinci Robot. Surgeon console (left), patient cart (middle), vision cart (right)

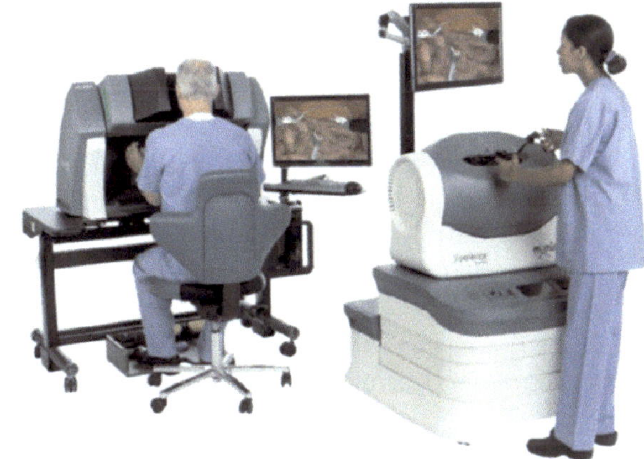

dV-Trainer Robot

THE FUTURE OF SIMULATION IN SURGICAL TRAINING

It is no longer acceptable to practice on a patient, the old saying "See One, Do One, Teach One," has changed to "See One, Practice Many, Do One, Teach One." The American College of Surgeons has a major role in developing and implementing the surgical skills curriculum through the Division of Education into residency programs. In 2003, ACGME mandated the implementation of six competencies to be taught, measured, and certified in residency training: Patient Care, Medical Knowledge, Practice-Based Learning, and Improvement, Interpersonal and Communication Skills, Professionalism, and System-Based Practice. In 2008, ACGME mandated that all surgical residency programs must have access to simulation and skills laboratories and must focus on patient safety. Technical and non-technical skills competency must be achieved in the skills center through simulation. In 2009, ABS mandated that all graduating surgical residents must pass the FLS examination before qualifying for the American Board of Surgery Certifying Examination. ACS launched a patient education program consisting of simulation for patients and their families. It includes training patients and their families to take care of ostomies, drains, tubes, and more using simulation. In 2012, SAGES and ACS recommended that all surgeons who practice laparoscopic surgery be certified through the Fundamentals of Laparoscopic Surgery Program (FLS). Since greater than one million minimally invasive surgeries are performed annually, SAGES and ACS also recommend that institutions that credential surgeons for laparoscopic surgery should potentially be required to have FLS certification are part of their credentialing process. In 2014, FES Fundamentals of Endoscopic Surgery was mandated for surgical residents.

Questions for the Future of Simulation[14]

Can simulators:

- Be used to assess procedural competency in credentialing or recredentialing?
- Provide a quicker skills assessment than analyzing multiple clinical cases?
- Be used to develop new complex skills (i.e., endoscopic submucosal dissection)?
- Act as a procedural experience repository?

SUMMARY

Simulation has the potential to promote ongoing training with a consistently reproducible process, enabling periodic surgical skill assessments while at the same time improving patient safety and reducing surgical errors by screening would-be physicians. It also improves overall efficiency by cultivating proficiency through rehearsing complex, patient specific procedures.[26] Similar to the success of simulation in the aviation industry, simulation technology and methodology in medicine can be used to improve the quality of surgical training for procedures.[3]

REFERENCE

1. Lynch J, Aughwane P, Hammond TM. Video games and surgical ability: a literature review. *J Surg Educ* 2010;67(3):184-9.
2. Francis HW, Malik MU, Diaz Voss Varela DA, Barffour MA, Chien WW, Carey JP, et al. Technical skills improve after practice on virtual-reality temporal bone simulator. *Laryngoscope* 2012;122(6):1385-91.
3. Fried MP, Satava R, Weghorst S, Gallagher A, Sasaki C, Ross D, et al. The Use of Surgical Simulators to Reduce Errors. In: Henriksen K, Battles JB, Marks ES, Lewin DI, editors. *Advances in Patient Safety: From Research to Implementation (Volume 4: Programs, Tools, and Products)*. Rockville (MD), 2005.

4. Argani CH, Eichelberger M, Deering S, Satin AJ. The case for simulation as part of a comprehensive patient safety program. *Am J Obstet Gynecol* 2012;206(6):451-5.
5. Ehdaie B, Tracy C, Reynolds C, Cung B, Thomas K, Floyd T, et al. Evaluation of laparoscopic curricula in American urology residency training. *J Endourol* 2011;25(11):1805-10.
6. Wiet GJ, Stredney D, Wan D. Training and simulation in otolaryngology. *Otolaryngol Clin North Am* 2011;44(6):1333-50, viii-ix.
7. Buck GH. Development of simulators in medical education. *Gesnerus* 1991;48 Pt 1:7-28.
8. Zendejas B, Cook DA, Bingener J, Huebner M, Dunn WF, Sarr MG, et al. Simulation-based mastery learning improves patient outcomes in laparoscopic inguinal hernia repair: a randomized controlled trial. *Ann Surg* 2011;254(3):502-9; discussion 09-11.
9. Ullrich S, Kuhlen T. Haptic palpation for medical simulation in virtual environments. *IEEE Trans Vis Comput Graph* 2012;18(4):617-25.
10. Walsh K. Simulation is the way to bring risk management and patient safety together. *Acad Med* 2011;86(10):1193; author reply 93-4.
11. Barsuk JH, Cohen ER, Feinglass J, McGaghie WC, Wayne DB. Unexpected collateral effects of simulation-based medical education. *Acad Med* 2011;86(12):1513-7.
12. Reznick RK, MacRae H. Teaching surgical skills--changes in the wind. *N Engl J Med* 2006;355(25):2664-9.
13. Fernandez GL, Page DW, Coe NP, Lee PC, Patterson LA, Skylizard L, et al. Boot cAMP: educational outcomes after 4 successive years of preparatory simulation-based training at onset of internship. *J Surg Educ* 2012;69(2):242-8.
14. Aslanian HR. Ain't nothing like the real thing? Simulators in endoscopy training. *Gastrointest Endosc* 2012;75(2):261-2.
15. Bearman M, O'Brien R, Anthony A, Civil I, Flanagan B, Jolly B, et al. Learning surgical communication, leadership and teamwork through simulation. *J Surg Educ* 2012;69(2):201-7.
16. Brinkman WM, Buzink SN, Alevizos L, de Hingh IH, Jakimowicz JJ. Criterion-based laparoscopic training reduces total training time. *Surg Endosc* 2012;26(4):1095-101.
17. Willaert WI, Aggarwal R, Daruwalla F, Van Herzeele I, Darzi AW, Vermassen FE, et al. Simulated procedure rehearsal is more effective than a preoperative generic warm-up for endovascular procedures. *Ann Surg* 2012;255(6):1184-9.
18. Bridges M, Diamond DL. The financial impact of teaching surgical residents in the operating room. *Am J Surg* 1999;177(1):28-32.
19. Danzer E, Dumon K, Kolb G, Pray L, Selvan B, Resnick AS, et al. What is the cost associated with the implementation and maintenance of an ACS/APDS-based surgical skills curriculum? *J Surg Educ* 2011;68(6):519-25.
20. Al-Kadi AS, Donnon T, Oddone Paolucci E, Mitchell P, Debru E, Church N. The effect of simulation in improving students' performance in laparoscopic surgery: a meta-analysis. *Surg Endosc* 2012.
21. Palter VN, Grantcharov TP. Development and validation of a comprehensive curriculum to teach an advanced minimally invasive procedure: a randomized controlled trial. *Ann Surg* 2012;256(1):25-32.
22. Varas J, Mejia R, Riquelme A, Maluenda F, Buckel E, Salinas J, et al. Significant transfer of surgical skills obtained with an advanced laparoscopic training program to a laparoscopic jejunojejunostomy in a live porcine model: feasibility of learning advanced laparoscopy in a general surgery residency. *Surg Endosc* 2012.
23. Dubrowski A, Brydges R, Satterthwaite L, Xeroulis G, Classen R. Do not teach me while I am working! *Am J Surg* 2012;203(2):253-7.
24. Evans LV, Gusberg RJ. Creating a surgery clerkship in a changing environment: reality, simulation, and the rules of engagement. *Yale J Biol Med* 2012;85(1):143-52.
25. Gallagher AG, Ritter EM, Champion H, Higgins G, Fried MP, Moses G, et al. Virtual reality simulation for the operating room: proficiency-based training as a paradigm shift in surgical skills training. *Ann Surg* 2005;241(2):364-72.
26. Healy GB. The college should be instrumental in adapting simulators to education. *Bull Am Coll Surg* 2002;87(11):10-1.

❑❑❑

18

CHAPTER

Surgical Education

Gokulakkrishna Subhas, MD
Amanpreet K. Bhullar, MD
Simarnjit Singh, MD
Jasneet Singh Bhullar, MD
Vijay K. Mittal, MD

INTRODUCTION

Learning is a complex process. The level of surgical training and competence is indicative of the level of care a patient receives.[1] Surgical residency programs are designed to develop competent surgeons in a safe and educationally efficient environment.[2] The training of surgeons has evolved dramatically throughout the millennia since the birth of the art of surgery.[3] For more than a century, our fundamental model of surgical education has remained constant. However, this model is being challenged by significant training environment changes. Increased intolerance for error, reduction in trainee independence, increasingly difficult technology advancements, and an adequate emphasis on patient safety have significantly altered the nature of surgical training.[2]

Attempts to improve surgical education began nearly a millennium ago; these were the first minuscule steps in a long process of advancing training in the art of surgery.[3] The modern surgeon, in addition to a lifelong commitment to learning and honing their craft, is also required to fulfill their role as a teacher and a manager.

William Halsted established the surgical residency program at Johns Hopkins University in the early twentieth century. At the time, surgeons did not have formal sub-specialization or differentiation, and they conducted operations on a variety of anatomical structures and organ systems. With the advancement of surgical knowledge and the diversification of feasible operations, the tree of surgery began to sprout branches. Nonetheless, they all remained connected to the tree's trunk for a long time.[6]

Surgical Training

While technical proficiency is critical for a successful outcome, additional characteristics of a skilled surgeon include intellectual talents, personality traits, communication abilities, and a commitment to practice.[2] Optimizing educational experiences is critical in a variety of sectors, not the least because of the limits imposed by few resources such as time and staff. Medical school and residency education, in specific, are stressed by a lack of resources compared to the massive amount of material that students and residents must understand. Additionally, this must occur in an environment with considerable time constraints.[8]

There is a changing picture of general surgical training due to a proliferation of fellowships in surgical subspecialties, as well as the increasing desire of these sub-specialties to be recognized as independent specialties. The proliferation of advanced fellowships in surgical oncology, endocrine surgery, breast surgery, gastrointestinal surgery, and other general surgery subspecialties has worn down the experience of a general surgery residency, creating a system where residents now recognize the importance of pursuing advanced training to gain further experience. This results in the proliferation of fellowships, eroding the value of core training. Laparoscopic fellows are increasingly performing procedures that were formerly performed by general surgeons on a routine basis, such as fundoplication and partial.[6]

Training in the United States of America

In the United States, around 312 hospitals offer general surgery residency training; approximately half of these are "university hospitals", meaning they are part of a medical university, the remaining programs are at "community" or regional hospitals affiliated to a university. The Accreditation Council for Graduate Medical Education (ACGME), a non-governmental, not-for-profit organization, determines the maximum surgical residents that can be trained at a single hospital. The ACGME is responsible for residency program quality and accrediting the surgery programs through the Residency Review Committee for Surgery (RRC). The RRC conducts on-site visits to residency programs every five years, and more frequently if deficiencies are identified. Around 1,400 medical graduates choose to pursue graduate studies in general surgery each year. All of these residents eventually finish a five-year residency in general surgery and subsequently enter the practice of surgery. In addition to these are additional training opporations for one to two years to presure carrersin various subspecialties.[6]

Surgical residency training programs encounter numerous obstacles in their efforts to develop competent surgeons. The Accreditation Council for Graduate Medical Education (ACGME) mandates that residents undergo training in six competencies (Table 1), and programs must meticulously document residents' achievement of those competencies. These are meant to ensure both competent trainees and high-quality patient care.[9] Teaching patterns in most of the residency programs across the US include weekly grand rounds, didactics covering core curriculum, and morbidity and mortality discussions held weekly (Table 2). In 2006, the Surgical Council on Resident Education (SCORE) partnership formed between the major surgical education organizations in the United States. SCORE's purpose is to improve general surgery resident education in the United States by developing a national standard curriculum for general surgery residency training.

Morbidity and mortality (M&M) meetings aim to improve the standards of surgical care and are required in all hospitals responsible for training junior surgical staff. M&M meetings must be carefully planned and well organized. They are essentially peer reviews of errors made during patient care. The goals of a well-run M&M conference are to learn from complications and errors, to alter behavior and judgment in light of prior experiences, and to avoid repetition of errors that result in complications. Meetings should be non-punitive in nature and should be centered on the objective of improving patient care. Additionally, they highlight recent cases and provide recommendations for professionals involved in the case. Meetings are also critical for detecting system concerns (e.g., out-of-date policies, changes in patient identification methods, and arithmetic errors) that affect patient care.

Table 1: ACGME competencies

Surgical Education Resident Requirements
1. Patient Care Treat health problems and promote health by providing compassionate, appropriate, and effective patient care.
2. Medical Knowledge Demonstrate and apply knowledge of established and evolving epidemiological, biomedical, clinical, and social-behavioral sciences.
3. Practice-Based Learning and Improvement Demonstrate competence during investigation and analysis of patient care, to appraise and assimilate scientific evidence, and to continuously improve patient care through self-evaluation and lifelong learning.
4. Interpersonal and Communication Skills Demonstrate interpersonal and communication skills for successful exchange of information and collaboration with patients, their families, and the health care team.
5. Professionalism Demonstrate consistent professional responsibility and an ethical code of conduct.
6. Systems-Based Practice Demonstrate an understanding of and responsiveness to the greater context and system of health care, as well as the ability to effectively utilize other system resources to offer optimal health care.

Table 2: Typical teaching schedule in surgical residency

Weekly		
Tuesday	7am to 8am	Morbidity and mortality meeting
Wednesday	7am to 8am	Grand rounds with an expert
Speaker Wednesday	8am to 11am	Core topics in surgery discussion
Thursday	7am to 8am	(Alternate) video conference teaching in core topics in surgery on consortium basis
Thursday	9am to 10am	Teaching rounds
Friday	7am to 8am	Multidisciplinary tumor board meeting
Friday	11am to 12am	Meeting of program director with senior
Residents Saturday	8am to 10am	(Not fixed) grand rounds with an expert
Speaker Tuesday/ Thursday	2pm to 4pm	Skills lab/gross anatomy dissection

Monthly		
1st Monday	4pm to 5pm	
1st Monday	5pm to 6pm	
4th Wednesday	6pm to 8pm	
4th Friday	8am to 10am	

Physicians must have the required abilities to keep up with a large amount of available information as the volume of medical literature continues to grow. The journal club provides a platform for residents to stay current on current literature while also teaching them how to critically analyze it. The organizers will conduct periodic evaluations of this conference to determine whether the resident and faculty goals align. Additionally, formal evaluation is important in providing an objective assessment of the knowledge obtained by house staff through participation in journal club. Journal clubs have evolved into a platform for members to learn critical appraisal techniques, thereby expanding their knowledge of the medical literature. Additionally, they have evolved as a tool for promoting evidence-based medicine practice. It is important to design a format that is both educational and stimulating for its members. During journal club, participation is important for further educating its participants via the constant exchange of ideas and interactions amongst members.

Table 3: Journal Club

Holistic Surgery

Structure:

- Conveniently fit journal club into the residency schedule
- Select one or two residents in advance to facilitate the discussion.
- Select an article >3 weeks prior to the scheduled presentation
- Assigned resident(s) and faculty advisors should meet prior to the presentation to plan the areas of focus and the discussion
- Distribute the articles to participants >2 weeks prior to meeting
- Encourage participants to be prepared for discussion by reading the article before journal club

Article:

- Select articles that emphasize different aspects of experimental design
- Create a controversy-utilizing debate format
- Select classic articles
- Meticulously analyze single article
- Use problem-based learning methods

Evaluation:

- Conduct periodic written surveys to measure participants' goals and overall satisfaction.
- If resident attendance is not optimal, survey them to potentially make a meeting schedule change and/or meeting duration change
- Evaluate additional knowledge gained by the participants through self evaluation surveys or objective measures such as a pretest/posttest format.

Tumor boards are an essential component of cancer patient care. Tumor Board is an approach to treatment planning that includes discussions of current medical and surgical oncology cases. Imaging, pathology, and treatment options are all addressed. As cases become available, residents are expected to post and present them. The tumor board incorporates factors such as' assessing learning needs, interacting among provider-learners with opportunities to practice the skills learned, and sequenced and multifaceted educational activities.

The teaching of basic surgical science principles is an important part of surgical residency training. A formal, didactic core curriculum is used to accomplish this. Most programs administer the core surgical curriculum through a weekly teaching conference attended by all resident levels. Residents present here, and in addition to fundamental surgical principles, an enhanced focus is now being placed on leadership, professionalism, and communication, as well as systems-based practice.

Ethics

Ethics in surgery dates back 400-500 years. Indian surgery is renowned for its empathy, overall efficiency, and recognition. Ancient India made significant contributions to ethics and surgical training. They have enormous relevance nearly 3,000 years later, despite widespread concerns about the disintegration of long-held value systems and cherished norms of medical practice.[11]

Many surgeons face profound ethical issues as part of their daily work. An ethics curriculum would certainly meet most components of professionalism. Residents are expected to exhibit compassion, respect, and integrity; an overriding commitment to the needs of patients and society over self-interest; accountability to patients, profession, and the society; and a commitment to ongoing professional development and excellence. They should show a commitment to ethical norms relating to the provision or withholding of clinical care, patient information confidentiality, business practice, and informed consent. Additionally, they should display responsiveness and sensitivity to patients' gender, age, and disabilities,[12] which are part of six competencies laid down by ACGME.

Working Hours

Historically, extensive work hours have always been believed to be an essential component of resident education and have become the public face of a profession that needs dedication and hard work. Long working hours for surgical residents is a time-honored tradition of presumed merit but is the one that has recently come under scrutiny and criticism.[13]

The widespread push to shorten surgical trainees' working hours is motivated by concerns about patient safety and surgical residents' quality of life. This is being implemented in the west. The European working hour directive caps the average work week at 48 hours, including overtime, and requires a minimum of 24 hours of uninterrupted rest per week and 11 hours per day.[2,14] The difficulty will be to accomplish the same educational objectives of a surgical residency in less hours. Newer training formats such as the "mentorship model, "case-based model," and "night float model" provide novel concepts for increasing the efficacy of surgical residency training while accommodating the 80-hour workweek in the USA. While following these approaches, caution should be exercised to avoid optimizing resident training at the expense of patient care.[15] However, there is a growing concern that this will result in lengthened training programs, decreased complexity, and volume of operative experience, and narrowing of surgical skill. Finally, there is a growing consensus that graduating residents are less proficient than their teachers (Table 5).[2]

In contrast to western countries, surgical residents in India are not restricted in their work hours. He may work for an endless number of hours each day and still feel that his patient care is incomplete. As he moves through his first to third years of residency, his patient care responsibilities and operative experience expand.[1] Additionally, many programs retain a fairly rigorous hierarchical structure to training, which frequently relegates junior residents to performing several mundane chores, resulting in a significant amount of educational time being wasted among this group of trainees.[2]

STRUCTURED CURRICULUM

The purpose of a structural curriculum especially in surgery enables skill development with defined objectives.

Operative elective dedicated supervised training lists, day surgery and emergency lists will all continue, as will the maintenance of a surgical logbook detailing experience, outpatient clinics and on-call duties.[4] We need to refocus on the service to education ratios for all of our trainees, trying to optimize educational opportunities where possible. We require a structured training program that facilitates the rapid ascension to technical competence. The program must demonstrate that residents perform a broad range of challenging procedures in order to graduate as qualified surgeons. Residents must concurrently enter their operative experience in the ACGME case log system for each year of residency. A total of at least 750-850 major cases should be logged in by the resident at the time of graduation. This should include 200 Major cases logged in as a chief resident (Table 6).

Feedback must be timely and consistent. Expert feedback, when presented in a pedagogically sound manner, has been shown to shorten learning curves.

By clearly defining important modules for general surgery with clear expectations, clear educational objectives, and competency assessment, the training process has the potential to be considerably improved. This type of training would require stringent competency standards, which would need to be met prior to promotion to the next training level. This approach, which would be based on objective assessment of surgical services, is frequently disorganized, limiting the quantity and quality of such education. Due to the fact that responsibility for instruction is typically unassigned, various team members teach students when convenient. Historically, the educational skills of surgical residents were not considered in their evaluations, even for trainees pursuing academic careers. Residents' development as educators has gotten extensive attention in recent years, and numerous programs have been designed to promote resident maturation.[18]

Structured feedback, on the other hand, has the ability to significantly accelerate the acquisition of skills. Each training module should be built around a comprehensive training and assessment curriculum utilizing a systematic stepwise approach.[2]

Evidence-based medicine should not be merely addressed in lectures; it should be actively taught by faculty and observed and applied in the clinical setting by residents. Residents learn directly from their teaching faculty and gain medical knowledge and experience. Surgical procedures can and have been studied rigorously in order to evaluate nearly every possible component, from preoperative skin preparation and antibiotics to incision techniques and dissection techniques to the incidence of complications and mortality. When new surgical procedures are introduced, the scientific community can study and assess them first. Thus, a safe, successful, and validated surgical procedure can be passed on to surgical trainees after it has been subjected to a thorough review by other physician-scientists.[3]

Skills Lab

The practice of surgery has changed dramatically over the last two decades. Minimally invasive surgical treatments have been widely adopted and applied, and more recently, robotic technologies have been developed.

Table 5: Working hours

System	USA	United Kingdom	India
Week	80 hours	48 hours	No limit
One shift	Up to 24 hours	Up to 13 hours	No limit
Minimum rest	24 hours/week	24 hours/week	None set

Table 6: Operative requirements in the USA

Surgery		Cases
Head and Neck		25
Breast		40
Skin and Soft Tissue		25
Alimentary Tract		
	Esophagus	5
	Stomach	15
	Small Bowel	25
	Large Bowel	40
	Appendix	40
	Anorectal	20
Abdominal		
	Liver	5
	Biliary	85
	Pancreas	5
	Hernia	85
Vascular		50
Endocrine		15
Trauma		
	Operative	10
	Non-operative	40
Thoracic		20
Pediatric		20
Plastic		10
Critical Care		40
Laparoscopic		
	Basic	100
	Complex	75
Endoscopy		85
Total Major Cases		850
	Chief Year	200
	Teaching Assistant	25

Table 7: Evaluation

Evaluation
Resident Evaluation: The faculty must evaluate and document resident performance in a timely manner. The program should • Complete objective assessments of ACGME competencies • Document progressive resident performance improvement appropriate to educational level • Provide each resident with documented semiannual evaluation of performance with feedback • Utilize a formal exam such as the American Board of Surgery in Training Examination (ABSITE) or other cognitive exams to assess the resident's knowledge. Summative evaluation for each resident upon completion of the program, which then becomes part of the resident's permanent record maintained by the institution.
Faculty Evaluation • Should be completed at least annually • Review faculty's ability of clinical teaching, commitment to the educational program, professionalism, clinical knowledge, and scholarly activities • Administer confidential annual evaluations by the residents
Program Evaluation • Completed by the residents and faculty • Must at least annually document formal, systematic evaluation of the curriculum • Monitor graduate performance, including performance of program graduates on the certification examination
Rotation Evaluation • Completed in a timely manner by the residents and faculty
360 Degree Evaluations • Completed by multiple evaluators (e.g., peers, patients, self, and other professional staff like nurses in floor and operating rooms)

Surgical instruments such as electrosurgical dissection tools, mechanical staplers, and laser therapies help surgeons to improve the quality of the operative procedure, resulting in improved patient outcomes.[19]

Training would begin in the skills lab with simulated models and clinical scenarios until predetermined proficiency standards are fulfilled. The trainee will then be able to advance to clinical situations on the ward and operating room. There has been substantial research into the methods for training and testing surgical abilities. According to research, an hour spent in a virtual reality simulator is equivalent to two hours in the operating room. Additionally, randomized experiments have established that abilities acquired in a virtual environment are transferable to the operating room. The pace of skills laboratory sessions is equally important. Multiple distributed sessions have been demonstrated to result in enhanced learning as compared to single skills laboratory sessions.[2]

Laparoscopic cholecystectomy on the same day has become the acknowledged standard of care. With treatment advancements and a better understanding of the science of patient safety, healthcare professionals must improve and perfect their skills to improve patient care. Historically, the skill acquisition "learning curve" was predicated on repetitive, but supervised, "practice" on patients. Therefore, early in the trainees' learning, there were longer operating times and a higher risk of complications. This is no longer a feasible ethical or economic strategy. Despite this, it is crucial for the inexperienced surgeons to learn the necessary knowledge, skills, and attitudes to perform. This is a life-long process because both junior trainees and practicing surgeons must learn new techniques. Now, the majority of the surgery training curriculum can be performed through simulators rather than real patients.[19] Organizing tools, space, learners, and faculty is a significant challenge, the only greater challenging is keeping up to date with the continuously evolving new technology in daily practice, such as telerobotic and natural orifice transendoscopic surgery.[19] As our understanding of this field advances, the implementation of well-designed local and national simulation-based curricula is likely to become more prevalent.[20]

RESEARCH

Scholarly activities include journal clubs, case reports, case series, basic science, and research projects. The next generation of surgical scientists is developed by drawing the top students to surgery and providing them with a structured research curriculum that is appropriately supervised. Academic surgery's future is contingent upon an ongoing influx of young individuals with creative and curious minds who are nurtured and trained to explore innovative frontiers dedicated to the progress of knowledge and science.[21]

Continuous surgery research and innovation over the centuries greatly contributed to scientific and best patient care knowledge. Surgery's future as an academic and professional field may be contingent on how highly it is regarded in surgical practice and education.

Institutions must commit to sustaining the highest standards of research training, ensuring that successful trainees can function independently as scientific investigators following graduation. This requires the institution to provide the necessary facilities, resources, specialized course material and curriculum, and a suitable environment for the development of high-quality work. While mentoring is crucial for the trainee, it involves a significant amount of effort and dedication on the part of the mentor.[21] Appointment of basic scientist (PhD holder) as director of research helps in providing guidance and assistance to residents with their research activities.[22]

After completing their training, trainees should be able to independently formulate meaningful hypotheses, design and perform experiments to test their hypotheses, critically assess their findings, and comprehend the importance and potential applicability of their research findings. It is critical for trainees to be educated to adhere to the highest ethical standards in all aspects of research and patient care, both during and after their research training.[21]

CERTIFICATION

There is a yearly in-training examination conducted nationally by the American Board of Surgery. The scores of this examination are used for assessment of the program, residents and for fellowships selection.[23] Most of the programs conduct annual mock oral examination either on a free standing in-house, or on a consortium basis. Both these examinations help the residents and program by providing an insight into the deficiencies and their remedies.

In the modern era of surgical education, a training program must evaluate a resident's performance against specific core competencies, objectifying and documenting performance against a set of criteria, in order to produce a measure of each resident's effective training.[2] Effective patient communication is a critical skill for surgical trainees when diagnosing and managing clinical problems. This is an area that may be sub-optimally tested.[4]

ADVANCED TRAINING

Based on a survey done in the USA, there is an increasing orientation of surgical trainees toward fellowship training.

Indeed, nearly 75 percent of current trainees' plan to pursue fellowships after general surgery training.[25] Fellowships available post general surgery residency in USA include Bariatric, Breast, Burns, Colorectal, Endoscopy, Hepatopancreatobilliary, Minimally Invasive, Plastic, Surgical Critical Care, Surgical Oncology, Transplant, Trauma, and Vascular Surgery. To help residents decide on future careers and fellowships, specialty rotations are provided in the general surgery residency curriculum (Table 8).

The majority of the institutions training surgical residents in India lack a setting for critical care, vascular surgery, plastics, thoracic surgery, and trauma. As training in these specialties is an integral part of general surgery training, residents should be sent on outside rotations to nearby institutions with such facilities. There is an ever-increasing role of imaging and interventional radiology in surgical management. Residents should complete their training with a rotation in radiology.

SYSTEMIC CHANGES

The traditional time-based approach to surgical education is predicated on the premise that all surgical trainees acquire knowledge at the same rate. A growing body of evidence suggests that this is not the case. The existing time-based model must be replaced by an outcome-based system that awards certification based on demonstrated competence rather than on training duration. Prior to graduation, each resident should be objectively evaluated and demonstrate mastery of all competencies.[2]

Table 8: Specialty rotations

Apart from General Surgery, residents rotate in the following specialties:
Anesthesiology
Burn Care
Cardiac Surgery
Gastroenterology
Gynecology
Neurosurgery
Orthopedic Surgery
Pediatric Surgery
Radiology
Thoracic Surgery
Transplant Surgery
Urology

Surgeons of the future will be expected to fulfill higher standards and perform increasingly sophisticated, demanding surgeries on patients who may have a variety of health-care challenges. Recent pressures appear to imply that these will be to overcome issues difficult using conventional methods. There mast be alternation in the training system; else, risk graduating residents who are less skilled. Therefore, new methods of training, experiment with new models, and most importantly, study our new techniques must be adepted comeptent.

Reforms should be on strong educational research, with government entities held accountable for regulations that are evidence-based. If these reforms are successful, the improvement of surgical education will have a global impact.[5]

REFERENCES

1. Udwadia TE, Sen G. Surgical training in India. World J Surg 2008;32(10):2150-5. PMID: 18679746.
2. Grantcharov TP, Reznick RK. Training tomorrow's surgeons: what are we looking for and how can we achieve it? ANZ J Surg 2009;79(3):104-7. PMID: 19317771.
3. Franzese CB, Stringer SP. The evolution of surgical training: perspectives on educational models from the past to the future. Otolar yngol Clin North Am. 2007;40(6):1227-35, vii. PMID: 18021837.
4. West H. Training of general surgical residents: What model is appropriate? Am J Surg 2008;195(1):136-8. PMID:18070737.
5. Supe A, Burdick WP. Challenges and issues in medical education in India. Acad Med 2006;81(12):1076-80. PMID: 17122473.
6. Bell RH Jr. Graduate education in general surgery and its related specialties and subspecialties in the United States. World J Surg 2008;32(10):2178-84. PMID: 18581168.
7. Longo WE, Seashore J, Duffy A, Udelsman R. Attrition of categoric general surgery residents: results of a 20-year audit. Am J Surg 2009; PMID: 19178898.
8. Mammen JM, Fischer DR, Anderson A, James LE, Nussbaum MS, Bower RH, Pritts TA. Learning styles vary among general surgery residents: analysis of 12 years of data. J Surg Educ 2007;64(6):386- PMID: 18063274.
9. Webb TP, Weigelt JA, Redlich PN, Anderson RC, Brasel KJ, Simpson D. Protected block curriculum enhances learning during general surgery residency training. Arch Surg 2009;144(2):160-6. PMID: 19221328.
10. Srivastava SK. Surgical training in India. Natl Med J India 2003;16(1):48-9. PMID: 12715961.
11. Singh B, Saradananda S. Ethics and surgical training in ancient India-a cue for current practice. SAfr Med J 2008;98(3):218-21. PMID: 18350226.
12. Helft PR, Eckles RE, Torbeck L. Ethics education in surgical residency programs: a review of the literature. J Surg Educ 2009;66(1):35-42. PMID: 19215896.
13. Mittal V, Salem M, Tyburski J, Brocato J, Lloyd L, Silva Y, Silbergleit A, Shanley C, Remine S. Residents' working hours in a consortium- wide surgical education program. Am Surg 2004;70(2):127-31; PMID:15011914.
14. Council directive 93/104/EC. Official J. Eur. Commun 1993; L307: 18–24.

15. Mittal VK, Portenier D. Continuity of care in the 80-hour workweek era?. Curr Surg 2006;63(1):31-4. PMID: 16373157.
16. Grantcharov TP, Reznick RK. Teaching procedural skills. Br. Med. J 2008;336:1129–31.
17. Aggarwal R, Grantcharov TP, Darzi A. Framework for systematic training and assessment of technical skills. J Am Coll Surg 2007; 204:697–705.
18. Jamshidi R. Formalizing teaching responsibilities for junior surgical housestaff encourages educator development. J Surg Educ 2008;65(6):514-7. PMID: 19059187.
19. Aggarwal R, Darzi A. From scalpel to simulator: a surgical journey. Surgery 2009;145(1):1-4. PMID: 19081469.
20. Scott DJ, Cendan JC, Pugh CM, Minter RM, Dunnington GL, Kozar RA. The changing face of surgical education: simulation as the new paradigm. J Surg Res. 2008;147(2):189-93. PMID: 18498868.
21. Suliburk JW, Kao LS, Kozar RA, Mercer DW. Training future surgical scientists: realities and recommendations. Ann Surg 2008;247(5):741-9. PMID: 18438110.
22. Sabir M, Penney DG, ReMine SG, Mittal VK. Scholarly activities— essential to surgical education. Curr Surg 2003;60(4):459-62. PMID:14972241.
23. Schneider JR, Coyle JJ, Ryan ER, Bell RH Jr, DaRosa DA. Implementation and evaluation of a new surgical residency model. J Am Coll Surg 2007;205(3):393-404. PMID: 17765154.
24. Chung R. Evaluating surgical residents the old school way: clues to how surgical training works and why. J Surg Educ 2008;65(6):512-3. PMID: 19059186.
25. Foley PJ, Roses RE, Kelz RR, Resnick AS, Williams NN, Mullen JL, Kaiser LR, Morris JB. The state of general surgery training: a different perspective. J Surg Educ 2008;65(6):494-8. PMID:19059183.

❑❑❑

19

CHAPTER

Global History of Surgery

Lawrence Chen
Austin Lee
Ethan Tabaie
Yavar Abgin
Dinesh Vyas

INTRODUCTION

Today, you can arrive in an emergency room after a car accident, be quickly evaluated and recommended for surgery, and get carted off into the operating room. There, the attending surgeon can employ any number of techniques, from bone setting, exploratory laparotomies, to whole organ transplants; and depending on the severity of the case, the patient might be able to get patched up and go home the next day. Nowadays, there are countless maladies that can be treated or cured via surgical intervention, providing millions of patients with another chance at life or the opportunity for a healthier one. Of course, this was not always the case. Only through numerous innovations and paradigm shifts have we coursed through time to arrive at where we are now. Historical civilizations from all over the world, ranging from Hammurabi in ancient Babylon to Hua To during the Han Dynasty in China, have all made notable contributions to modern surgery. Analyzing and truly understanding the history of how the field of surgery has evolved not only can provide context for your current practice but may even provide a window to see where the future of surgery may possibly go.

Year	Event
1600 BC	Evidence of early surgery in Egypt
600 BC	Shushrita Samhita copies Ayurveda, describing creating flaps for plastic surgery
1505 CE	Royal College of Edinburgh established
1606 CE	Wilhelm Fabricius von Hilden published *Six Hundred Surgical Observations and Treatments,* where he described various surgical treatments
1785 CE	John Hunter performs ligation of superficial femoral artery to treat popliteal arty aneurysm
1846 CE	William T.G. Morton adopted the use of ether as an anesthetic
1881 CE	Theodor Billroth carried out first successful partial gastrectomy for gastric cancer
1901 CE	Georg Kelling conducted the first intra-abdominal laparoscopic surgery using a fiber-optic lens system.
1910 CE	Flexner Report was published allowing lawmakers to enact state licensing laws to ensure the quality of physicians produced
1954 CE	Joseph Murray conducts the first successful kidney transplant

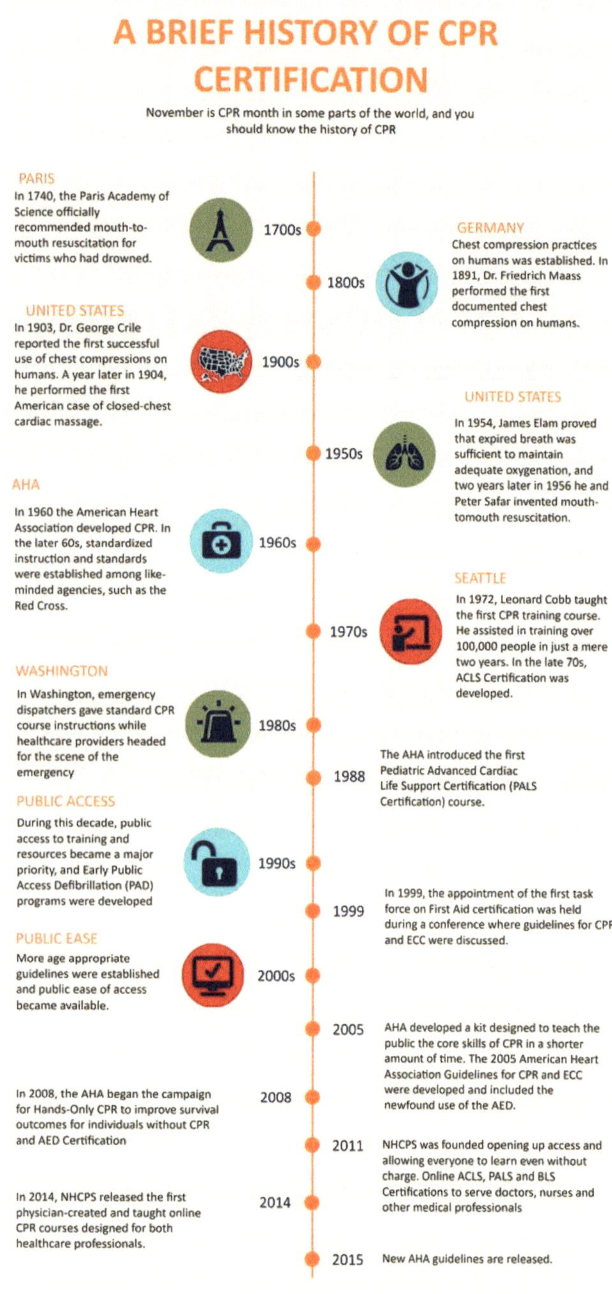

Figure 1. Abridged timeline of major events in the history of surgery.

Before Modern Surgery (1600BCE)

Evidence of primitive surgery being practiced can be found all over the globe, suggesting that separate ancient civilizations developed their own methods of approaching medicine and healing independently. One of the early pieces of evidence of surgery can be found around 1600 BCE in the Edwin Smith Surgical Papyrus. Named after the antiquities dealer who bought the papyrus after it was unearthed from a tomb in Thebes, Egypt, where it had resided for over 3000 years, this document contains descriptions of injuries of the spinal column and spinal cord, as well as diagnostic and therapeutic techniques.[1] Similarly, evidence of surgery can be found in ancient Sumeria. The Code of Hammurabi, perhaps most recognizable by its popularization of *lex talionis* or the concept of "an eye for an eye", even has distinct clauses regarding operating incisions by physicians. Clause 215 of the Harper translation reads "If a physician operate on a man for a severe wound (or make a severe wound upon a man) with a bronze lancet and save the man's life; or if he open an abscess (in the eye) of a man with a bronze lancet and save that man's eye, he shall receive ten shekels of silver (as his fee).[2]"

There is evidence of cranial surgical intervention in 7th century BCE ancient Greece, including a case study of a right occipitoparietal cranium that showed a 14.78 mm by 9.19 mm cerebral opening, indicative of a surgical opening made in order to treat a head wound.[3] This procedure is also found in the Hippocratic corpus, further supporting the claim Hippocrates has as the founder of scientific medicine. His books describe the structure of the vertebrae, the curvature of the spine, and diseases including tuberculous spondylitis, scoliosis, concussion, and dislocation, among others. His treatises *On Fractures* and *On Joints* contain some principles that still hold true today; for this reason, he is regarded by many as the father of Spine Surgery.[4]

Chinese Surgery (1100BCE- 207CE)

Given the large geographic distance and challenging terrain between China and Europe, it was difficult to exchange science and ideas between the two regions. The Silk Road provided an avenue to exchange goods and culture between Europe and China, but it seems throughout China's history, their medical practices progressed separately from Europe. However, around the same time as the first recordings of surgery in Europe, there was evidence of surgery in China in a feat of parallel thinking.

China's written history spans over three thousand years, and descriptions of medical workers such as surgeons who treated infections and trauma were recorded during the Zhou dynasty, which lasted between 1100 and 700BCE.[5] Due to the metaphorical nature of some texts from this period of time, it is difficult to parse mythology from reality; however, the event of recognizing and recording surgical theories should not be understated. One notable example of this situation is the Chinese physician Pien Chueh, also known as Ch'in Yueh-yen, who lived from 407 to 310 BCE and was noted in Lieh-tzu's *Book of Master Lieh* to have prepared a medicinal wine which rendered two patients unconscious and allowed him to open their chests and switch their hearts with each other.[6] This instance showed understanding of general anesthesia and the potential to transplant organs from two different individuals. In reality, surgeons in China at this time dealt with trauma from weapons or fractures, infections, ulcers, and tumors.[5]

China's most famous and regarded surgeon was the "God of Surgery," Hua To, who lived from 141 to 207 CE.[5] His life was well documented in the Chinese classic texts *Wei Shu* in the *San-kuo Chi* (*Record of Wei* in the *Record of the Three Kingdoms*) and *Hua-tuo Chaun* in the *Hua-huan Shu* (*Biography of Hua Tuo* in the *History of the Later Han Dynasty*).[7] In *Wei Shu*, Hua To was noted to have treated a patient's diseased organs where herbs or acupuncture could not help by preparing *ma-fei-san*, a numbing agent, which made the patient unconscious and allowed Hua To to open the abdomen, cleanse and resect the affected parts, and stitch the patient.[6] This concoction is theorized to be composed of a combination of *Papava somniferum* (opium) possibly with or without *Cannabis indica* (hashish), *Rhododendron molle* root, *Jasmina sambac* root, *Angelica sinensis* root, and *Acorus calamus* root.[6] Thus, it appears that this feat may be one of the first recorded events of practical anesthesia and open abdomen surgery recorded in Chinese history.

Ayurveda

India's contribution to surgery began many thousands of years ago around 3,500 BC when the oldest of the four sacred books maintained the knowledge of the culture's medicine.[8] This book is called the Rig Veda and is the oldest of the four VEDAS.[8] The book contains descriptions of lacerated limbs that were sutured, the goal being to walk after surgery.[8] There are four VEDAS, Ayurveda, the science of life is a subdivision of the Atharva Veda.[8] Sushruta Samhita, in 600 BC, known as the original plastic surgeon, copied much of the original information on the Ayurveda where it maintained its significance throughout the generations.[8] Several different procedures are described in this book including the creation of flaps for plastic surgery.[8] These flaps were used in several well-documented procedures such as in rhinoplasties and cleft palate fixtures.[8] Extracapsular surgical technique for cataract extraction and detailed explanations of surgical instruments, incisions, suturing and bandaging techniques, fracture reductions, and techniques for foreign body extraction were recorded in the book.[8] The Ayurveda persisted through the generations and even describes a form of sterile technique for operations.[8] The Ayurveda's maintenance throughout the generations expresses the significance of the book in Indian and global medicine.

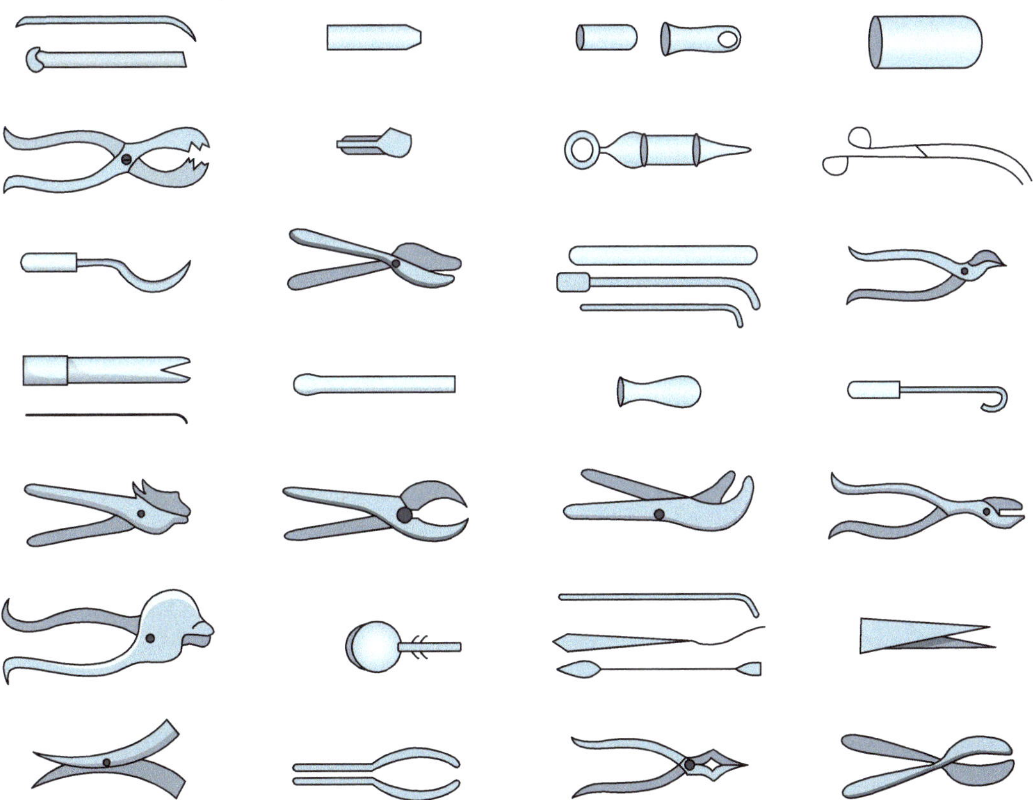

Figure 2. Selection of Blunt Instruments Described by Shusruta Samhita. Strikingly, these instruments resemble many of the modern surgical tools used today.

British Surgery Before Lister (1505CE- 1827CE)

The transition of surgery from the pre-modern era to the modern era is not a definitively marked moment in history. With surgeries being performed and practiced throughout history in pre-modern societies, it is difficult to truly define eras in surgical history, especially when capabilities to disseminate scientific discoveries were limited, and these findings took prolonged time to be accepted into common surgical practice. However, the first tracings of modern surgical societies and their influence on surgery today could be traced back to Britain.

During the Middle Ages throughout Europe and in England, it appeared that the art of surgery was lost with the division of medicine from surgery. Although the root cause of how this dichotomy arose ultimately leading to the loss of knowledge is debated, the fact remains that physicians during the Middle Ages practiced medicine through unproven theories without the extensive knowledge of surgery, anatomy, or chemistry; surgery being reserved for unknowledgeable craftsmen.[9] The rise of British surgery began soon after the fall of Constantinople marked the end of the Middle Ages in 1453.[10]

Medieval trade guilds were originally established to train apprentices and protect one's craft such as butchers and blacksmiths. In 1505, Britain founded one of the oldest surgical organizations in the world. The Edinburgh School of Surgery's roots lie with the Barber Surgeons of Edinburgh who were incorporated with the 'Seal of Cause,' giving the Barber Surgeons the exclusive privilege to practice surgery in the city and surrounding area.[11] The Barber Surgeons of Edinburgh were significant in the progression of British surgery by being one of the first guilds to establish important guidelines and duties to maintain the highest professional standards when practicing surgery. These codes helped lay the foundation of surgical ethics still relevant today such as ensuring surgeons are experts in their craft and masters of the anatomy, nature, and complexion of every human's body.[11]

Despite the significance of the Barber Surgeons of Edinburgh being one of the first surgical craft guilds established, they were not the only ones who were prominent in Britain during the 1500s. Thirty-five years after the Barber Surgeons of Edinburgh were approved and approximately four-hundred miles away in London, the English Company of Barber Surgeons was chartered in 1540.[12] Given the great distance between Edinburgh and London as well as limitations in travel capabilities, the founding of another institution tasked with the training of surgeons in the capital city of England seemed inevitable. The Company of the Barber Surgeons combined the Company of Barbers with the Fellowship of Surgeons, where barbers performed bleeding and abscess lancing while surgeons tried to advance surgical principles.[13] Eventually over the next two centuries, differences grew between the barbers and surgeons as the surgeons slowly improved themselves, and the surgeons eventually separated on May 2, 1745 to later form the Royal College of Surgeons on March 22, 1800 after being granted a Royal Charter by George III.[13] In the Royal College of Surgeons, colleagues established professorships to lecture students.[12]

RICHARD WISEMAN (1621-1676)

Richard Wiseman was an important surgeon during the English Civil War, who served as sergeant surgeon to Charles II.[14] In his book published in 1676, *Severall Chirurgicall Treatises*, Wiseman included comprehensive surgical knowledge, from his extensive experience and knowledge from working many years in the military, navy, and civilian field. This work included the definition, cause, signs, prognostics, and cure to different pathology and became the authoritative body of information on surgery for many years to come.[14] Wiseman's notable discoveries and operations included tuberculous joints, suturing arteries, importance of suturing the abdominal peritoneum to prevent hernia, removing all foreign bodies from wounds during the first dressing, and early reduction of fractures to minimize swelling.[14] Many of these discoveries are now currently accepted practice and have been studied to maximize patient benefit today.

JOHN HUNTER (1728-1793)

John Hunter is generally regarded as the father of modern scientific surgery. Hunter studied surgery with Cheselden at Chelsea Hospital and under Percival Pott at St Bartholomew's; later, he served as a staff-surgeon during the Seven Years War, became a Fellow at the Royal Society, taught anatomy and researched surgery at Earl's Court, and ultimately became Surgeon General and Inspector of Regimental Hospitals in the British Army.[15,16] Hunter practiced and thoroughly applied the concept of examining anatomy and physiology, comparing symptoms and diseases, proposing treatments, testing on animals, and trying on humans.[15] For example, he used this method after studying collateral circulation in a deer's antler to treat a popliteal artery aneurysm through ligating the superficial femoral artery in 1785.[17] Hunter contributed greatly to the advancement of surgery through his meticulous research and use of the scientific method to lay the foundation of questions to be answered by future surgical discoveries.

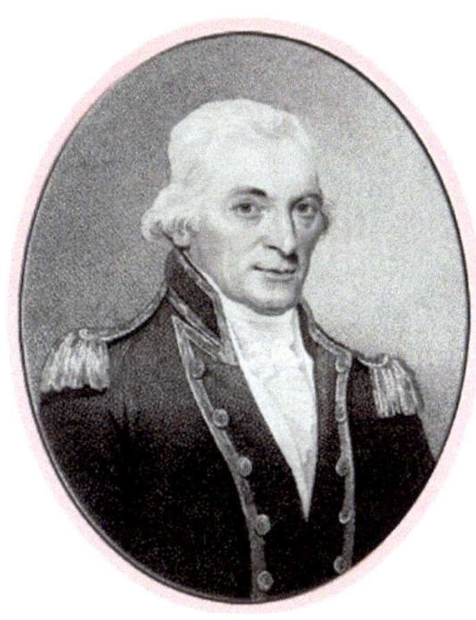

Image 1. Portrait of John Hunter from the Rijksmuseum

German Surgery

Concurrent with the development of Surgery in the British Isles, German Surgical innovations started to gain traction during the late renaissance period. Generally considered the founder of *scientific* German surgery, Wilhelm Fabricius von Hilden (1560-1634) published his surgical treatise *Observationem et cuationem chirurgicam cenuriae sex* (Six Hundred Surgical Observations and Treatments) in 1606, where he described various surgical treatments for nasal polyps, stone bladder, breast cancer, ocular cancer, hydrocele, ascites, and amputation techniques.[18,23]

In the 17th Century, Johannes Scultetus (1595-1645), published his textbook *Armamentarium Chirurgicam* 10 years postmortem, which catalogs his surgical instruments, illustrations of his operations, as well as 100 case reports.[19,23] Furthermore, Scultetus' name, which is sometimes translated as Johann Schulte or Johannes Schultheiss depending on if it appears in German or Latinized, is still used in surgical wards today.[20,21] Born in Ulm, Germany and studied at the University of Padua in Italy, his lasting impact can be seen whenever a scultetus binder is used to provide additional abdominal support.

Lorenz Heister (1683-1758) was an eighteenth-century German surgeon, who published his textbook, *Systems of Surgery*, in 1739. This book became the standard text on the subject, being translated into many languages, and was the first textbook of this subject to be translated into English.[22,23] Further building on from the surgeons that came before him, August Gottlieb Richter (1742-1812) is a German surgeon whose treatise on hernias earned him the eponym for Richter's hernia, a term still used today to describe a non-obstructive strangulation of a herniated anti-mesenteric wall.[23,24]

The next chapter of German Surgery was heavily influenced by Lister's innovation of antiseptic surgical technique, allowing surgeons to operate with much greater control and decreased risk for post-operative infections. Bernhard von Langenbeck (1810-1887) is known not only for the numerous techniques and tools that are named after him, the establishment of a surgical journal, and co-founding the German Surgical Society, but also for teaching an array of students, including but not limited to Theodor Billroth and Emil Theodor Kocher.[25] Theodor Billroth (1829-1894) is generally considered to be the founder of modern abdominal surgery, specifically known for his two gastric reconstruction surgeries.[26] In 1881, Billroth carried out the first successful partial gastrectomy for gastric cancer.[27]

Ernst von Bergmann (1836-1907) further built on Lister's techniques by turning the antiseptic method into an aseptic one. Using carbolic acid spray and heat, Bergmann sterilized the operating room, instruments, and clothes, making surgeries an even safer venture.[11,12]

Anesthetics and Antiseptics

The first demonstrated use of a chemical anesthetic came with the discovery of ether and its use as an anesthetic in 1846. Prior, the prospect of surgery was uncommon and grisly. While ether had been prepared since the 1500s, its use was limited to recreational drug abuse rather than having medical value. In 1846, Dr. William T.G. Morton, a Dentist from Boston, adopted the use of ether as an anesthetic for pain relief after dental procedures. Inspired by a presentation of the anesthetic applications of Nitrous Oxide by Horace Wells, also a dentist, Dr. Morton demonstrated and popularized the use of ether as an inhaled anesthetic. He even conducted several demonstrations at the Harvard Medical School; one of the amphitheaters at Massachusetts General Hospital is now known as the "Ether Dome" after one of his public demonstrations.[36] The use of ethers as a general anesthetic began to wane in the 1960s, when fluorinated hydrocarbons, such as halothane and enflurane, began to replace it. The advent of anesthetics served as a watershed moment in the history of surgery, making the public image of surgical procedures more palatable. However, it was not until anesthetics were combined with antiseptics, that surgery became truly commonplace.

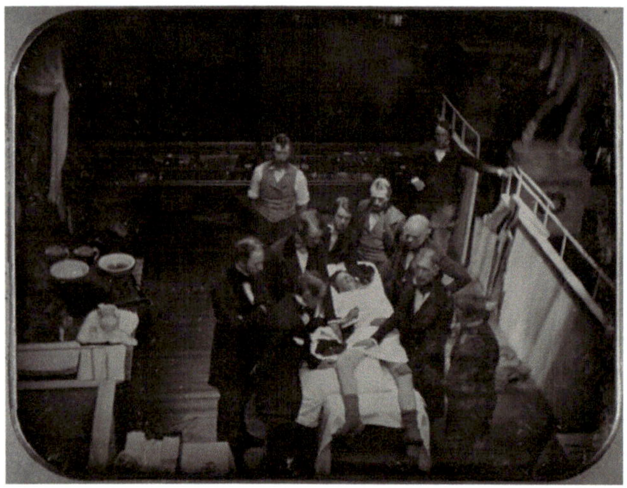

Image 2. Ether Dome Daguerrerotype No. 3, 1847, from Photographs of Early Ether Anesthesia in Boston: The Daguerreotypes of Albert Southworth and Josiah Hawes Rajesh Parsotam Haridas

Pasteur and Lister

The advent of germ theory and antisepsis was pivotal in the progression of surgery and infection control. Joseph Lister (1827-1912) is widely considered to be a pioneer in infection control and antisepsis, who studied the arts at the University College, London before pursuing surgery training in Edinburgh from 1853 to 1860, then working in Glasgow, Edinburgh again, and London again.[30] At this point in history, mortality was extremely large in hospitals, especially with amputations being the treatment of choice for compound fractures with mortality rates ranging anywhere from 24.3% at best up to 46% throughout America, Paris, and Britain.[31] Therefore, the infection and death following amputations was widely prevalent and essentially inevitable, making these operations death sentences for patients. During the wars of this era, infections from wounds essentially killed as many people as bullets fired from guns.[31]

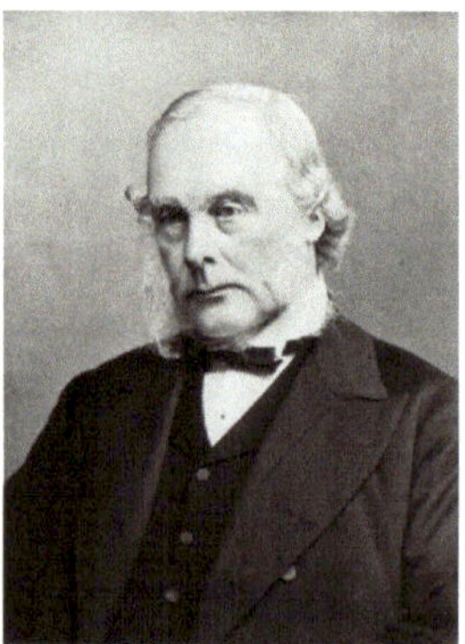

Image 3. Portrait of Joseph Lister, from Weltrundschau zu Reclams Universum 1902

Joseph Lister built his reputation through his work researching blood coagulation in Edinburgh, but his influence from Louis Pasteur cemented Lister in history.[30] Louis Pasteur (1822-1895) was a French scientist who is most famous for his work in disproving spontaneous generation and the development of germ theory.[32] In Pasteur's famous swan neck experiment, he boiled a culture broth and fashioned a swan neck vessel to allow air sterilized from the humidity to enter.[32] When life did not appear within the vessel until the vessel's neck was broken, Pasteur disproved the theory of spontaneous generation and laid the foundation of germ theory.[32] The spontaneous generation experiment showed that decomposition, disease, and suppuration are results of living microorganisms; Lister recognized that killing or preventing these microorganisms from entering living tissue could prevent infection and improve results of surgery.[31] Lister then searched for suitable antiseptic agents that could effectively eliminate microorganisms and save patients. During this time, smoking and salting were used to preserve food, and honey, wax, wine, and vinegar were used before as natural methods of antisepsis.[31]

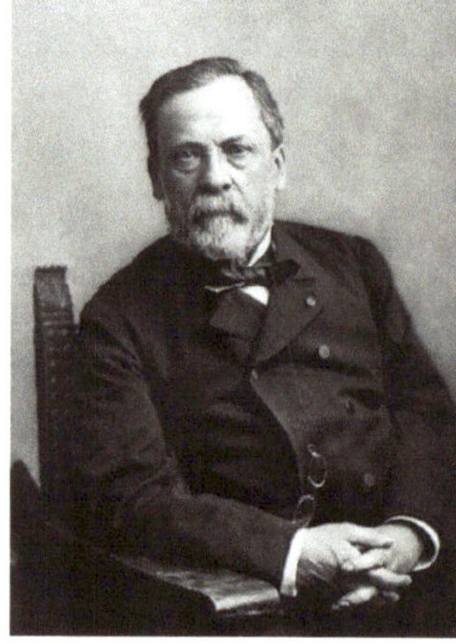

Image 4. Portrait of Louis Pasteur, photo from Paul Nadar.

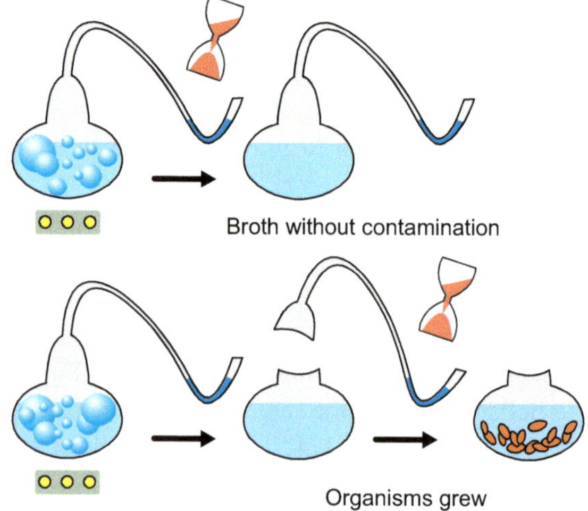

Figure 3. Diagram of the swan-neck flask experiment.

In Lister's seminal publication, *On the Antiseptic Principle in the Practice of Surgery*, Lister settled on a solution of carbolic acid combined with boiled linseed oil as an antisepsis that could kill microorganisms while preserving the human tissue. Lister further discusses that wounds are not naturally purulent, and use of antisepsis could work on various wounds, abscesses, and surgical preparation with overarching effects on the overall cleanliness and general healthiness of the hospital.[33] Examples of case studies where he used his carbolic acid solution showed great promise, and Lister urged the quick adoption of these antiseptic principles to save patient lives.[33]

His work on antisepsis was met with skepticism and great opposition by his British colleagues, but the positive results spoke for themselves through patient outcomes.[34] However, his reputation soared in Germany, who championed Lister's antiseptic technique, and later the United States, France, and finally Britain adopted antiseptic techniques.[34] Today, antisepsis is a commonplace and integral part of surgical preparation in modern medicine, thanks to the work of Joseph Lister and his colleagues in Glasgow.

Modern Surgical History

After the advent of antiseptic technique and anesthesia, post-surgical mortality dropped to a more acceptable level, allowing increased leeway for future surgeons to innovate in the area. In 1901, German Doctor Georg Kelling pioneered the first intra-abdominal laparoscopic surgery using an advanced fiber-optic lens system.[37] This technique was then introduced to the United States when Dr. Bertram M. Bernhein of Johns Hopkins.[38,39]

Also at Johns Hopkins, Dr. Halstead spearheaded a different system of surgical care called the "school of surgery." He introduced this system with a focus on research to demonstrate when and what were the indications for certain procedures. Generally regarded as the father of American Surgery, William Stewart Halstead (1852-1922) modeled the Halstead School of Surgery after the German system, which included a team of assistants, residents, and a chief resident. In his system, he would directly teach his chief resident, who would then go on to teach the residents beneath them, many of which are estimated to have become surgery professors at other medical schools, including Yale and Stanford.[40]

In 1910, Abraham Flexner published the Flexner report, which effectively criticized American Medical education. At the time, medical education was a for-profit business that produced an overabundance of inadequately trained physicians. Taking inspiration from the German system and reading Theodore Billroth's *Medical Education in the German Universities*, Flexner categorically evaluated the clinical facilities, admissions standards, and laboratory equipment, among other aspects, to judge the quality of education offered at each institution. The report rated a majority of medical schools as deficient in numerous areas, claiming that there were of such poor quality that closure was indicated. These claims procured the evidence that allowed lawmakers to enact state licensing laws to ensure the quality of physicians produced by medical schools.[40,41]

After these revolutions in both surgery and surgical education, innovative doctors continued to push the line and began introducing increasingly ambitious procedures. While human organ transplant has been a subject of both study and mythology for thousands of years, innovations in aseptic surgery and basic science elucidation of antigen compatibility allowed the first kidney transplant to successfully occur in 1954. Dr. Joseph Murray was able to bypass the barrier of transplant rejection by using the recipient's identical twin as a donor. While skin grafts between identical twins had occurred for years prior, the first successful organ transplant garnered widespread enthusiasm for prospects in the future.[43,44]

Table 1. Other notable modern surgical advancements.

Year	Achievement
1913	Dr. Alexis Carrell transplanted a kidney and heart in animals[45]
1913	Dr. Daniel H. Williams successfully repaired a pericardial and splenic stab wound[46]
1920	Dr. Ernest Codman started 1st cancer registry for bone sarcoma[47]
1945	Drs. Alfred Blalock and Helen Taussig cured 1st "blue baby" by operation[48]

Surgeon Nobel Laureates for Physiology/Medicine

Table 2. List of surgeons who have won a Nobel prize for physiology/medicine[49,50]

Name	Year	Reason for Nobel Prize
Emil Theodore Kocher	1909	Thyroid physiology, pathology, and surgery
Alvar Gullstrand	1911	Refracted light path through ocular lens
Alexis Carrel	1912	Suturing blood vessels and transplantation methods
Robert Barany	1914	Vestibular apparatus function
Frederick Grant Banting	1923	Insulin extraction and diabetes treatment
Alexander Fleming	1945	Penicillin discovery
Walter Rudolf Hess	1949	Brain mapping for internal bodily function control
Werner Theodor Otto Forssmann	1956	Cardiac catheterization
Charles Brenton Huggins	1966	Prostate cancer hormonal control
Joseph Edward Murray	1990	Organ transplantation
Shinya Yamanaka	2012	Mature cell reprogramming for pluripotency

History of Surgical Specialties

Table 3. Major modern surgical advancements in oncological, pulmonary, cardiac, vascular surgery, and minimally invasive surgery.

Oncological Surgery	Pulmonary, Cardiac and Vascular Surgery	Minimally Invasive Surgery
• 1920: Dr. Ernest Codman of MGH started the 1st cancer registry for bone sarcoma[47] • 1922: The ACS initiated a Committee on Treatment of Malignant Disease. Later it was re-organized as the Commission on Cancer • 1935: Dr. Allen O. Whipple of Columbia University1st performed en-bloc radical duodeno-pancreactomy for cancer of the pancreas. This "Whipple procedure" remains one of the few effective treatments against pancreatic cancer today[51] • 1975: Fischer's randomized clinical research studies showed that radical mastectomy should no longer be a standard treatment for breast cancer[52]	• 1923: Dr. Elliott C. Cutler performed the 1st successful section of the stenosed mitral valve[53] • 1953: Dr. Michael DeBakey performed the 1st successful carotid endarterectomy, establishing the field of surgery for strokes[54] • 1964: Dr. H. Edward Garrett performed the 1st successful coronary artery bypass graft (CABG) procedure using a saphenous vein graft[55] • 1969: Dr. Denton Cooley of Texas 1st successfully implanted an artificial heart in a patient[56]	• 1901: German Dr. Georg Kelling pioneered laparoscopy with advanced fiber-optic lens system[37] • 1985: A robot, using a software developed by Dr. Yik San Kwoh, assisted in performing a brain biopsy[58] • 1992: Dr. Camran Nezhat reported the 1st laparoscopic radical hysterectomy and lymphadenectomy[57] • 1998: Robot 1st assisted in the open-heart coronary artery bypass graft (CAGB) operation[59] • 2006: First "Un-manned Operation": a robot placed a defibrillator in a patient in Milan using logic of thousands of operative data stored in a computer in Boston

WAR AND SURGERY

Overview

The surgeons' work on civilian vs soldier-in-war drastically differs. The quality of tissue damage and contamination does not compare to that which is seen in contemporary practice. Wars throughout history provided the opportunity for and also obliged surgeons to experiment, improvise, and innovate their techniques. Soldiers sustained a myriad of injuries and wounds in emergent settings; thus, surgeons were not constrained by the legalities and ethics that would normally hinder their ability to render aid. Consequently, the evolution of surgery was expedited in war. A number of key features distinguish the history of surgery in war from the practice of surgery outside of war. The epidemiology of wounds is dictated by war on land, at sea, in air, weapons available in war throughout history, and protective armor. The wound pathologies also greatly differed, as bullets, shrapnel, bombs, blasts, and toxic agents produced problems which surgeons outside of war would not routinely treat. War surgery is also emergency surgery - no place for enhanced technique or reconstructions.[60] Throughout history, surgeons entering war fronts were successively better trained to address appropriate demands of trauma. The necessity of rapid care for an imposingly growing number of wounded soldiers led to the development of basic principles in managing war wounds. Bravely, surgeons in wartime worked in hostile and violent environments, and surgeons must be ready to adapt to various unforeseen circumstances. Three main wars were pivotal and fostered a breeding ground for surgical experimentation, improvisation, and innovation - The American Civil War, World War I, and World War II.

United States Civil War

The large patient populations during these wars and the opportunity to save as much life as possible, provided surgeons opportunity to expand their scope of practice. Focusing on the American Civil War, there were a number of advancements in surgery that assisted in reducing the mortality of soldiers in war. Advances in anesthesia, bacterial wound care, and amputation were seen not only through the creation of protocols, but also the advancement and opportunity to use innovative technology created before or during the war.

Many of these innovations came in the use of anesthesia since anesthesia had only been introduced to the United States in the 1840s.[35] Despite anesthesia being recently introduced to the U.S, it was used in over 80,000 cases in the Civil War and solely led to 43 anesthesia-related deaths.[35] Through its use in the Civil War, chloroform became preferred as it was not flammable, had a quick onset of action, and required a small volume to present the desired aesthetical effects.[35] The volume of cases involving anesthesia greatly expanded the field as no civilian use case could ever amount to the experimental knowledge that was obtained from 80,000 cases in a four year span.

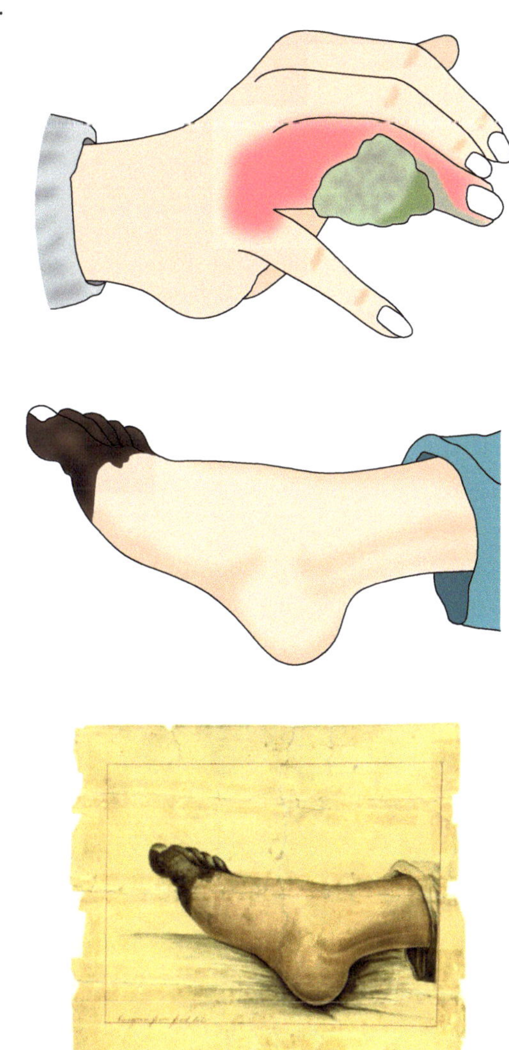

Figure 4: Gangrene often seen in war patients

Bacterial wound care was also greatly expanded upon during the Civil War. During the war, postoperative infections producing a thick, creamy pus were found to have a better prognosis than pus that was thin and bloody.[35] Necrotizing fasciitis was even described and shown to have a 48% mortality rate.[35] As a result, a procedure to dissect away necrotic tissue and inject bromine into the margins while under anesthesia was developed, and since nurses working with these patients developed erysipelas they started washing their hands in chlorinated soda.[35] This innovation in a short time was the result of the massive patient population that war provided and the insatiable desire to improve patient outcomes those wartime doctors expressed.

The largest effect the Civil War had on innovation was through the knowledge of surgical amputation. Out of every four procedures done during the war, three were amputations which resulted in a 26.3% mortality rate.[35] Before and during the war, amputations would last days. However, due to the large-scale necessity for these surgeries, it was learned that survivability improved when amputations lasted less than 24 hours.[35] Public perception also helped guide the future of amputations during the Civil War by not allowing just any physician trained medicine to amputate. Only the most senior physicians were allowed to amputate, and as a result, one in every fifteen physicians were permitted to amputate.[35] This is due to the public backlash that came from the perception the doctors would amputate excessively over the course of the war.[35] Most of this surgical knowledge would have been gained without war. However, war clearly elevated the progression of knowledge for amputation surgery and post operative surgical infections. Therefore, war does allow for the massive boost in innovation that pushes medicine forward years ahead of its original course during peacetime.

WORLD WAR I

World War I became the first conflict where soldiers died predominantly due to traumatic wounds.[60] World War I also became the first conflict where wounds and trauma were caused by automatic weapons, heavy artillery, and weaponized gasses. Thus, the pivotal shift in the quality of patients seen by surgeons in this new-styled warfare exponentially increased the innovation and development of technique within surgery. Nevertheless, infection remained a critical issue surgeons needed to address, as "Trench Foot" - a fungal infection caused by the cold damp soil within the trench fighting grounds - affected more than 75,000 British soldiers before 1917.[65]

Highlighting the new demand of surgically treating the disfigured and severely damaged faces of soldiers comes Herold Delft Gillies. Prior to World War I, reconstructive plastic surgery was a seldom practiced specialty.[62] However, the pioneering surgeon from New Zealand, Herold Delft Gillies, rapidly became the most respected reconstructive plastic surgeon during World War I.[63] He operated on soldiers who had missing or violently damaged jaws or cheeks as a result of peeking over the trenches, or being met with the shrapnel of a rifle or the blast of proximal artillery. To pay homage to the history of surgery, before Dr. Gillies the field of surgery, and particularly reconstructive plastic surgery, became much easier to practice after the improvements of asepsis and anesthetics[63]. Dr. Gillies' focus was more so set in aesthetics, wanting to make his patients resemble their pre-war self. For this task, he developed the tubed pedicle technique. This involved partially releasing tissue from a site near the wound allowing the pedicle to retain blood supply, then transferring the free end of the skin to the site of injury without completely disconnecting the donor tissue from the original site. Maintaining that physical connection increased the chance of the graft being accepted and also reduced the risk of infection.[63] To this day, Dr. Gillies is considered by many to be the father of modern plastic surgery, and many techniques he pioneered during the first world war are still used today. The birth of cosmetic surgery stems from Gillies' work as well, as restoration of enhanced appearance while maintaining functionality permeated society at large.

Injuries sustained by weapons of war did not produce neat single fractures within bone; Rather, soldiers sustained compound fractures or entirely shattered bone, so the established technique of splinting would not have been effective. In 1865, Hugh Owen Thomas, described in his book *Diseases of the Hip, Knee and Ankle Joints with Their Deformities Treated by a New and Efficient Method* how he used The Thomas Splint to immobilize injuries while allowing access for dressing and cleaning. Unfortunately, this new technology was not vastly distributed to armies until 1917. However, when the Thomas Splint was consistently utilized, the innumerable deaths from bleeding or infection as a result of orthopedic injury saw an enormous reduction, from 80% to 15.6%.[66] Overall, war grounds were fertile soil for the revolution of surgical practice and innovation, and many revolutionary ideas were built upon in the coming World War II only several decades later.

WORLD WAR 2

Sulfonamide powders were sprinkled into open wounds to prevent blood poisoning, Penicillin and Streptomycin were both developed and being distributed, soldiers were inoculated with vaccinations for smallpox, typhoid, tetanus, cholera, typhus, and yellow fever. Improvements from better helmets to advanced pharmaceutical, medical, and surgical techniques such as removing dead tissue in order to minimize amputation, allowed for surgeons of World War II to dedicate less of their time on issues that surgeons of the past would have had to treat.[70,71] Instead, surgeons during World War II were able to focus on practices such as "debridement" to preserve tissue and life. Surgeons of World War II learned that simply removing bullets or shrapnel from a wound, sprinkling it with sulfonamides, and stitching it up was not optimal.[70] Understanding that bullets, dirt, and bacteria would penetrate and disperse deep tissues motivated the practice of debridement. The practice consisted of enlarging the entrance and exit of wounds, clearing away all dead tissue, dirt, and other foreign bodies, covering it with antiseptics and a pressure-dressing for about a week, and if the wound remained clean, it was closed.

In conjunction with advancements in the management of traumatic wound healing came improved methods for control of hemorrhage, shock, and vascular surgery at large. Between World War I and World War II, treatment of hemorrhage and shock was a primary concern and grew as a greater concern with the advent of weapons capable of firing more deadly rounds at higher velocity. Although the chances of vascular injury rose, the practice of vascular surgery remained inapt until World War II as the demand for complex vascular surgery was absent in civilian life, and not developed during World War I to be practiced within battlegrounds.[72] Moreover, the lack of competent, specialized, and experienced surgeons for the large number of vascular injuries was addressed during World War II with the development of the Zone of Interior[72] of vascular centers. Here, vascular surgeons, surgeons in training, and patients were housed, and it finally became possible to provide adequate care with a large amount of equipment and focused efforts toward individual patients. Prior to World War II, the scattering of patients, and the thinly spread distribution of resources hindered the ability for this level of care toward vascular injuries. With a central system of care in place, surgeons could keep pre and post operative data on their patients, allowing for the research, study, and advancement of future surgical practice within this specialty.[72]

The brave soldiers who fought in World War I and II granted us physicians the ability to experimentally treat, learn, and develop enhanced surgical practices that have revolutionized medicine and continue to be built upon. Modern medicine thus stands on the shoulders of past giants in order to see further and do better.

Ethics of Surgery and Medical Innovation

Many of the major pushes in medical research and advancement occurred as a direct effect of war and as a result some of the medical practices used to achieve knowledge and practice surgery in the past are not considered ethical. For instance, during the Civil War minimal anesthesia was used during amputations, which would be considered unethical in today's standards. However, some methods to obtain research and perform surgery were still performed, especially during wartime despite their obvious unethicality. During WWII, there were many experiments in the field of gynecology that were practiced on victims of the war such as forced abortions and sterilizations.[64] The experiments may have resulted in novel information but were still clearly unethical even by the standard of the times during wartime.

When looking at the past there were clearly instances of unethical practices performed for surgical knowledge both by the standards of the time they were practiced in and the higher standard of ethics that is maintained today. However, looking towards the future there are several practices in today's surgical practices that may be questioned in the future. The process of supplying organ donations for transplant surgery has been one that involves plenty of ethical dilemmas.[73] In some countries, there is profit to be made from the transaction of organs for transplant surgery allowing wealthier patients to receive expedited surgeries.[73] Despite the existence of organ exchange organizations such as the Euro-transplant, there are still unethical practices that can go unnoticed in the field of transplant surgery especially in countries without proper regulations.[73] In the future, there may be a better method of handling organ donations that negates all unethical practices, and therefore, the process by which we handle organ transplants today may be considered unethical.

One especially common practice in the training of medical students is the use of cadavers for dissection. This practice is commonplace amongst most medical education and is seen as a necessity. In a study conducted in Punjab, 27.9% of doctors thought the most effective method of teaching anatomy was through cadavers, and surgeons were significantly less likely to say the use of cadaveric dissection is unethical over other physicians.[74] In the future, cadavers may be completely replaced by three dimensional models using virtual reality, synthetic tissue, or both. Although the current consensus may be that cadavers are essential for learning anatomy, this may not be the case in the future when technologies are able to imitate the same experience without requiring a human body to gain knowledge.

Culture of Superspecialization and Surgical Deserts

The history of surgery has led us through specialization into days of superspecialization. Although specialization in surgical practice has improved the treatment and care of particular ailments, a culture of superspecialization may be producing a separation between the wants of surgeons and needs of patients. Moreover, excessive specialization may produce net-negative effects on the totality of patient care, the education of rising surgeons, training and establishing a foundation in the skill-set of general surgery as a medical student or resident, and surgical research.[76] Throughout history the general surgeon focused on and developed upon expertise ranging from surgery of the alimentary tract to surgical problems of the vasculature, head, and neck. Advances in endoscopic and laparoscopic surgeries will aid general surgeons in their broad-based surgical expertise. Additionally, the general surgeon will continue to play a major role in leading the future surgeons of the modern era, as well as take on a greater role and responsibility in times of superspecialization.

Superspecialization incentives surgeons to base their practice and focus their attention in areas with voluminous patient populations. As a result, many regions of the United

States remain below the Graduate Medical Education National Accreditation Council (GMENAC) and Solucient standard recommended general surgeons per 100,000 population - 4.7 general surgeons (GMENAC) and 6.01 (Solucient) respectively.[75] Many factors play a role in the general surgeon's decisions toward focusing their expertise in urban areas, such as the uncertainty of generating the cost of running a critical access hospital (CAH).[75] Although surgeons practicing in surgical deserts will receive bonuses and enhanced reimbursements from Medicare and Medicaid, the distribution of surgeons among urban and rural populations remains uneven.

According to 2016 data from AAMC's State Physician Workforce Data Report, the number of active general surgeons per 100,000 population still drastically varies by state.[77] Moreover, 2006 data from AMA Physician Masterfile reports surgeons per 100,000 population with respect to counties across the United States.

Many north-western counties of South Dakoda such Harding, Perkins, and Corson, some of the biggest counties in our country within Nevada such as Nye, Lincoln, and Clark, and large patches of counties across the Midwest as well as a greater majority of Alaska remain at a under 5 general surgeons per 100,000 population.[75] In an age of superspecialization, surgical deserts may likely persist and it will be a responsibility of future surgeons to work toward ameliorating the variance in surgeon representation.

Telesurgery and Its Advancements and Future

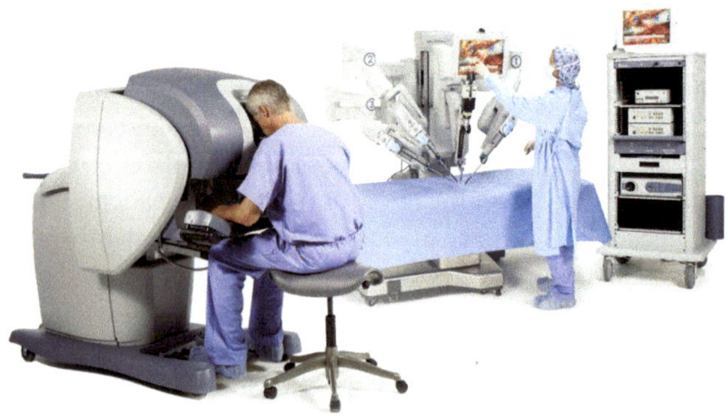

Image 5. Da Vinci Robotic Surgery allows for a minimally invasive surgery approach, image from da Vinci.

The future of medicine will be filled with technological advancements in every subspecialty within surgery. However, focusing on advancements that are more broad and have a potential to impact nearly all surgical specialties, telesurgery might be the most impactful. Telesurgery is the operation of a surgical procedure by a surgeon in a different location from the patient through real-time data transfer that allows a robot to follow the procedure. There are already several examples of telesurgery in practice. In one paper, two cases of vitreoretinal surgery were performed successfully over a 5G cellular network transferring data from one part of Massachusetts to another.[78] Due to the advent of 5G allowing higher speeds of data transfer, there could be the potential to do telesurgical operations where one country with more surgeons and advancements operates over the cellular network in another country with less resources. This has the potential to revolutionize care and expand surgical advancements to more people and populations.

Automation in surgery may be another powerful innovation that dominates the future of surgery. Having many aspects of surgery become automated, could result in improved patient outcomes as less of the cognitive capacity and attention of the surgeon has to be absorbed when performing a demanding operation. One study showed that even a semi-autonomous suction tool can help alleviate the mental workload of a surgeon.[79] When considering the next decade of surgery, it is much more likely that certain aspects of surgery may become automated; however, the full automation of a surgeon seems impossible in the next several decades. Because the human body is immensely variable and complicated, teaching an AI or creating a machine that could take the complete role of a surgeon becomes increasingly difficult.

REFERENCES

1. van Middendorp JJ, Sanchez GM, Burridge AL. The Edwin Smith papyrus: a clinical reappraisal of the oldest known document on spinal injuries. Eur Spine J. 2010 Nov;19(11):1815-23. doi: 10.1007/s00586-010-1523-6. Epub 2010 Aug 10. PMID: 20697750; PMCID: PMC2989268.
2. Hammurabi. The Code of Hammurabi, King of Babylon, about 2250 B.C.: Autographed Text, Transliteration, Translation, Glossary, Index of Subjects, Lists of Proper Names, Signs, Numerals, Corrections and Erasures, with Map, Frontispiece and Photograph of Text. Translated by Robert F. Harper. Chicago, IL: University of Chicago Press, Callaghan, 1904.
3. Agelarakis A. Early Evidence of Cranial Surgical Intervention in Abdera, Greece, a Nexus to On Head Wounds of the Hippocratic Corpus. Mediterranean Archaeology and Archaeometry, Vol.6. 2006 Dec.
4. Marketos SG, Skiadas P. Hippocrates: The Father of Spine Surgery. Spine: July 1, 1999 - Volume 24 - Issue 13 - p 1381.

5. We Y-kai, Cheng Z-fen, Shang T-yu, Wu X-zhong. Surgery in Ancient China Ying-kai Wu, Zhi-fan Cheng, Tian-yu Shang and Xian-zhong Wu. *Chinese Medical Jounal*. 1988;101(02):79-83. doi:10.5555/cmj.0366-6999.101.02.p79.01.
6. Fu L. Surgical history of ancient China: Part 1. ANZ Journal of Surgery. 2009;79(12):879-885. doi:10.1111/j.1445-2197.2009.05138.x.
7. Fu LK. Hua Tuo, the Chinese god of surgery. Journal of Medical Biography. 2002;10(3):160-166. doi:10.1177/096777200201000310.
8. Vyas D, Gupta Nav Y, Mittal V. *Comprehensive Textbook of Surgery*. (Vyas D, ed.). Jaypee Brothers Medical; 2012.
9. Parker G. The early history of surgery in Great Britain: Its organization and development. British Journal of Surgery. 1920;8(31):380-381. doi:10.1002/bjs.1800083121.
10. Şahin K. Constantinople and the end time: The Ottoman conquest as a portent of the last hour. Journal of Early Modern History. 2010;14(4):317-354. doi:10.1163/157006510x512223.
11. MacLaren I. A brief history of the Royal College of Surgeons of Edinburgh. *Res Medica*. 2005;268(2). doi:10.2218/resmedica.v268i2.1030.
12. Miles A. Chapter 1. In: The Edinburgh School of Surgery before Lister. London, England: A. & C. Black; 1918:1-10.
13. Robinson JO. The barber-surgeons of London. Arch Surg. 1984;119(10):1171-1175. doi:10.1001/archsurg.1984.01390220053012.
14. Smith AD. Richard Wiseman: his contributions to English surgery. Bull N Y Acad Med. 1970;46(3):167-182.
15. Guthrie D. John Hunter: Surgeon and Naturalist. Edinb Med J. 1942;49(2):119-135.
16. Stevenson LG. John Hunter, surgeon-general 1790–1793. Journal of the History of Medicine and Allied Sciences. 1964;XIX(3):239-266. doi:10.1093/jhmas/xix.3.239.
17. Murley R. John Hunter, velvet and vascular surgery. Ann R Coll Surg Engl. 1984;66(3):214-218.
18. Laios K. Wilhelm Fabricius von Hilden (1560-1634): The Pioneer of German Surgery. Surg Innov. 2018 Jun;25(3):301-303. doi: 10.1177/1553350618759152. Epub 2018 Feb 23. PMID: 29473453.
19. Schultheiss D, Jonas U. Johannes Scultetus (1595-1645). Urologic aspects in the 'Armamentarium chirurgicum'. Eur Urol. 1998 Dec;34(6):520-5. doi: 10.1159/000019794. PMID: 9831796.
20. Strohl EL. Johannes Scultetus (1595-1645). Arch Surg. 1963;87(3):396–397. doi:10.1001/archsurg.1963.01310150032007.
21. Bahşi İ, Adanır SS. The life and works of Johannes Schultheiss (1595–1645), who was the pioneer surgeon. Childs Nerv Syst 37, 2125–2129 (2021). https://doi.org/10.1007/s00381-019-04110-6.
22. Shklar G, Chernin DA. Lorenz Heister and oral disease with the original text from his papers. J Hist Dent. 2007 Summer-Fall;55(2):68-74. PMID: 17848045.
23. Surgery: Principles and Practice, Third Edition. Moyer, Rhoads, Allen, Harkins. 1965.
24. Rutkow IM. A selective history of hernia surgery in the late eighteenth century: the treatises of Percivall Pott, Jean Louis Petit, D. August Gottlieb Richter, Don Antonio de Gimbernat, and Pieter Camper. Surg Clin North Am. 2003 Oct;83(5):1021-44, v. doi: 10.1016/S0039-6109(03)00131-2. PMID: 14533901.
25. Goldwyn RM. Bernhard Von Langenbeck. His life and legacy. Plast Reconstr Surg. 1969 Sep;44(3):248-54. doi: 10.1097/00006534-196909000-00005. PMID: 4895616.
26. Lin TY, Seal A. Theodor Billroth: Surgeon, Musician, and Composer. Am Surg. 2021 Apr;87(4):507-510. doi: 10.1177/0003134820949520. Epub 2020 Oct 16. PMID: 33064016.
27. Androutsos G. Theodor Billroth (1829-1894) and other protagonists of gastric surgery for cancer. J BUON. 2004 Apr-Jun;9(2):215-20. PMID: 17415819.
28. Nordlander NB. Den moderna kirurgins födelse--en synopsis [The birth of modern surgery]. Sven Med Tidskr. 2007;11(1):89-93. Swedish. PMID: 18548947.
29. Zimmermann M. Leben und Wirken des Chirurgen Ernst von Bergmann (1836-1907). Langjähriger Herausgeber des "Zentralblatt für Chirurgie" [Life and work of the surgeon Ernst von Bergmann (1836-1907), long-term editor of the "Zentralblatt für Chirurgie"]. Zentralbl Chir. 2000;125(6):552-60. German. PMID: 10919251.
30. Newsom SW. Pioneers in infection control-Joseph Lister. J Hosp Infect. 2003;55(4):246-253. doi:10.1016/j.jhin.2003.08.001.

31. Edgar II. Modern surgery and lord Lister. Journal of the History of Medicine and Allied Sciences. 1961;XVI(2):145-160. doi:10.1093/jhmas/xvi.2.145.
32. Bordenave G. Louis Pasteur (1822-1895). Microbes Infect. 2003;5(6):553-560. doi:10.1016/s1286-4579(03)00075-3.
33. Lister J. On the Antiseptic Principle in the Practice of Surgery. Br Med J. 1867;2(351):246-248. doi:10.1136/bmj.2.351.246.
34. Pitt D, Aubin JM. Joseph Lister: father of modern surgery. Can J Surg. 2012;55(5):E8-E9. doi:10.1503/cjs.007112.
35. Reilly RF. Medical and surgical care during the American Civil War, 1861-1865. Proc . 2016;29(2):138-142.
36. Chang CY, Goldstein E, Agarwal N, Swan KG. Ether in the developing world: rethinking an abandoned agent. BMC Anesthesiol. 2015 Oct 16;15:149. doi: 10.1186/s12871-015-0128-3. PMID: 26475128; PMCID: PMC4608178.
37. American College of Surgeons (2012). Remembering Milestones and Achievements in Surgery: Inspiring Quality for a Hundred Years 1913-2012. Tempa, FL: Faircount Media Group.
38. Lee Y. (2016) Historical Development of Modern Surgery in America. Advances in Historical Studies, 5, 168-182. doi: 10.4236/ahs.2016.54015.
39. Williams GM. Bertram M. Bernheim: a southern vascular surgeon. J Vasc Surg. 1992 Sep;16(3):311-8. PMID: 1522632.
40. Tan SY. Uyehara P. William Stewart Halsted (1852-1922): father of American surgery. Singapore Med J. 2010 Jul;51(7):530-1. PMID: 20730390.
41. Flexner A. Medical education in the United States and Canada. From the Carnegie Foundation for the Advancement of Teaching, Bulletin Number Four, 1910. Bull World Health Organ. 2002;80(7):594-602. Epub 2002 Jul 30. PMID: 12163926; PMCID: PMC2567554.
42. Duffy TP. The Flexner Report--100 years later. Yale J Biol Med. 2011 Sep;84(3):269-76. PMID: 21966046; PMCID: PMC3178858.
43. Barker CF, Markmann JF. Historical overview of transplantation. Cold Spring Harb Perspect Med. 2013 Apr 1;3(4):a014977. doi: 10.1101/cshperspect.a014977. PMID: 23545575; PMCID: PMC3684003.
44. Nordham KD, Ninokawa S. The history of organ transplantation. Proc (Bayl Univ Med Cent). 2021 Oct 19;35(1):124-128. doi: 10.1080/08998280.2021.1985889. PMID: 34970061; PMCID: PMC8682823.
45. Vernon G. Alexis Carrel: 'father of transplant surgery' and supporter of eugenics. Br J Gen Pract. 2019 Jul;69(684):352. doi: 10.3399/bjgp19X704441. PMID: 31249090; PMCID: PMC6592355.
46. Britannica, The Editors of Encyclopaedia. "Daniel Hale Williams". Encyclopedia Britannica, 31 Jul. 2022, https://www.britannica.com/biography/Daniel-Hale-Williams. Accessed 22 November 2022.
47. Codman EA. The classic: registry of bone sarcoma: part I.--Twenty-five criteria for establishing the diagnosis of osteogenic sarcoma. part II.--Thirteen registered cases of "five year cures" analyzed according to these criteria. 1926. Clin Orthop Relat Res. 2009 Nov;467(11):2771-82. doi: 10.1007/s11999-009-1049-6. Epub 2009 Aug 19. PMID: 19690927; PMCID: PMC2758960.
48. Blalock A, Taussig HB. Landmark article May 19, 1945: The surgical treatment of malformations of the heart in which there is pulmonary stenosis or pulmonary atresia. By Alfred Blalock and Helen B. Taussig. JAMA. 1984 Apr 27;251(16):2123-38. doi: 10.1001/jama.251.16.2123. PMID: 6368878.
49. Radhakrishnan J, Ezzi M. Nobel Laureate Surgeons. World Journal of Surgery and Surgical Research. 2020;3(1).
50. Toledo-Pereyra LH. Nobel laureate surgeons. Journal of Investigative Surgery. 2006;19(4):211-218. doi:10.1080/08941930600840592.
51. Whipple AO, Parsons WB, Mullins CR. TREATMENT OF CARCINOMA OF THE AMPULLA OF VATER. Ann Surg. 1935 Oct;102(4):763-79. doi: 10.1097/00000658-193510000-00023. PMID: 17856666; PMCID: PMC1391173.
52. Fisher B, Jeong JH, Anderson S, Bryant J, Fisher ER, Wolmark N. Twenty-five-year follow-up of a randomized trial comparing radical mastectomy, total mastectomy, and total mastectomy followed by irradiation. N Engl J Med. 2002 Aug 22;347(8):567-75. doi: 10.1056/NEJMoa020128. PMID: 12192016.
53. Cutler EC, Levine SA. Cardiotomy and Valvulotomy for Mitral Stenosis; Experimental Observations and Clinical Notes Concerning an Operated Case with

Recovery. The New England Journal of Medicine, 188, 1023-1027.

54. DeBakey ME. Successful carotid endarterectomy for cerebrovascular insufficiency. Nineteen-year follow-up. JAMA. 1975 Sep 8;233(10):1083-5. PMID: 1174155.
55. Garret HE, Cartmill TB, Thiele JP, Howell JF, DeBakey ME. Experimental Evaluation of Venous Autografts as Aorta to Left Ventricular Myocardial Shunts in Revascularization of the Heart: A Preliminary Report. Cardiovasc Res Cent Bull. 1964 Jul-Sep;3:15-20. PMID: 14195356.
56. Cooley DA, Bloodwell RD, Hallman GL, Leachman RD, Nora JJ, Rochelle DG, Milam JD. Human cardiac transplantation. Circulation. 1969 May;39(5 Suppl 1):I3-12. doi: 10.1161/01.cir.39.5s1.i-3. PMID: 4893439.
57. Nezhat CR, Burrell MO, Nezhat FR, Benigno BB, Welander CE. Laparoscopic radical hysterectomy with paraaortic and pelvic node dissection. Am J Obstet Gynecol. 1992 Mar;166(3):864-5. doi: 10.1016/0002-9378(92)91351-a. PMID: 1532291.
58. Kwoh YS, Hou J, Jonckheere EA, Hayati S. A robot with improved absolute positioning accuracy for CT guided stereotactic brain surgery. IEEE Trans Biomed Eng. 1988 Feb;35(2):153-60. doi: 10.1109/10.1354. PMID: 3280462.
59. Loulmet D, Carpentier A, d'Attellis N, Berrebi A, Cardon C, Ponzio O, Aupècle B, Relland JY. Endoscopic coronary artery bypass grafting with the aid of robotic assisted instruments. J Thorac Cardiovasc Surg. 1999 Jul;118(1):4-10. doi: 10.1016/S0022-5223(99)70133-9. PMID: 10384177.
60. Giannou C, Baldan M. (2010) International Committee of the Red Cross. Available at: https://www.icrc.org/en/doc/assets/files/other/icrc-002-0973.pdf.
61. Barr J. (2019) From Trench to Bedside: Military Surgery During World War I Upon Its Centennial, Academic.oup.com. Available at: https://academic.oup.com/milmed/article/184/11-12/214/5518569.
62. The birth of plastic surgery (no date) National Army Museum. Available at: https://www.nam.ac.uk/explore/birth-plastic-surgery.
63. Bell L. (2018) Medical developments in World War One, British Library. Available at: https://www.bl.uk/world-war-one/articles/medical-developments-in-world-war-one.
64. Frobenius W, Kinzelbach A, Anthuber C, Dross F. German gynecologic societies investigating their Nazi past. Arch Gynecol Obstet. 2014;290(5):925-928.
65. Atenstaedt RL. Trench foot: the medical response in the first World War 1914-18. Wilderness Environ Med. 2006;17(4):282-289. doi:10.1580/06-weme-lh-027r.1.
66. Gordon P, O'Connor K. (2021) The Thomas Splint - vastly improving mortality rates in World War one, State Library Of Queensland. Available at: https://www.slq.qld.gov.au/blog/thomas-splint-vastly-improving-mortality-rates-world-war-one.
67. Vergun D. (2020) Medical improvements saved many lives during World War II, U.S. Department of Defense. Available at: https://www.defense.gov/News/Feature-Stories/story/Article/2115192/medical-improvements-saved-many-lives-during-world-war-ii/.
68. Adams S. Medical advances behind the line, part 2. Legion Magazine. https://legionmagazine.com/en/medical-advances-behind-the-line-part-2/. Published July 5, 2021.
69. Elkin D, DeBakey M. Surgery In World War II Vascular Surgery. Defense Technical Information Center. https://apps.dtic.mil/sti/pdfs/ADA291756.pdf. Published 1955. Accessed 2022.
70. Vergun, D. (2020) Medical improvements saved many lives during World War II, U.S. Department of Defense. Available at: https://www.defense.gov/News/Feature-Stories/story/Article/2115192/medical-improvements-saved-many-lives-during-world-war-ii/.
71. Adams S. Medical advances behind the line, part 2. Legion Magazine. https://legionmagazine.com/en/medical-advances-behind-the-line-part-2/. Published July 5, 2021.
72. Elkin D, DeBakey M. Surgery In World War II Vascular Surgery. Defense Technical Information Center. https://apps.dtic.mil/sti/pdfs/ADA291756.pdf. Published 1955. Accessed 2022.
73. Cohen B, Persijn GG, Vanrenterghem Y. Commerce in transplantation: how does it affect European legislation? Clin Transplant. 2000;14(1):28-31.
74. Ghazanfar H, Rashid S, Hussain A, Ghazanfar M, Ghazanfar A, Javaid A. Cadaveric Dissection a Thing of the Past? The Insight of Consultants, Fellows, and Residents. Cureus. 2018;10(4):e2418.
75. Belsky D, Ricketts T. Surgical Deserts in the U.S.: Counties without Surgeons. https://www.researchgate.

net/profile/Thomas-Ricketts-3/publication/50934943_Surgical_deserts_in_the_US_counties_without_surgeons/links/02bfe514327e046ee5000000/Surgical-deserts-in-the-US-counties-without-surgeons.pdf. Published 2010.

76. Nambiar RM. General surgery in an era of superspecialisation--what is the future?. Ann Acad Med Singap. 1995;24(1):180-187.
77. 2017 State Physician Workforce Data Report. AAMC.ORG. https://store.aamc.org/downloadable/download/sample/sample_id/30/. Published 2017. Accessed 2022.
78. Lu ES, Reppucci VS, Houston SKS 3rd, Kras AL, Miller JB. Three-dimensional telesurgery and remote proctoring over a 5G network. Digit J Ophthalmol. 2021;27(3):38-43.
79. Yang J, Barragan JA, Farrow JM, Sundaram CP, Wachs JP, Yu D. An adaptive human-robotic interaction architecture for augmenting surgery performance using real-time workload sensing-demonstration of a semi-autonomous suction tool. Hum Factors. Published online November 11, 2022:187208221129940.

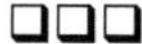

SECTION 2: SKIN AND SOFT TISSUE

20

CHAPTER

Head and Neck Mass

Madan Mohan Reddy Paluru, MD
Binit Katuwal, MD
Vijay K. Mittal, MD

INTRODUCTION

Neck mass or a lump in the neck is a common clinical finding encountered in General Surgery Practice. A neck mass is defined as an abnormal lesion (congenital or acquired) that is visible, palpable, or seen on an imaging study.[1] A neck mass can be seen across all age groups and has a very complex differential diagnosis; therefore, a systematic approach is essential in evaluating and managing a neck mass. The differential diagnosis of a neck mass includes congenital, inflammatory, and neoplastic disease processes and it is helpful to approach the neck mass by broadly dividing it into these three categories.

Table 1: Differential diagnosis of a neck mass

Congenital	Inflammatory	Neoplastic
• Branchial cleft cyst • Thyroglossal duct cyst • Lymphangi oma/heman-gioma • Ectopic thyroid tissue • Pharyngeal diverticulum • Laryngocele • Ranula • Teratoma • Dermoid cyst • Thymic cyst	• Lymphadenopathy • Bacterial • Viral • Granulomatous • Tuberculosis • Cat Scratch disease • Sarcoidosis • Fungal • Sialadenitis • Parotid • Submandibular • Congenital cyst	• Primary benign • Lipoma • Angioma • Carotid body tumor • Primary malignant • Epidermoid carcinoma • Melanoma • Adenocarcinoma • Lymphoma • Thyroid • Salivary • Metastatic • Unknown primary • Epidermoid CA

CONGENITAL NECK MASS

Congenital neck masses are the second most common cause for neck masses in children, after infections. They are usually seen at birth but can present at any age. Understanding embryology and the development of structures in the neck is crucial in identifying and managing these conditions.

BRANCHIAL CLEFT CYST

During the development of the pharyngeal pouches, the endodermal and ectodermal linings separate the arches by coming together. The adjacent arches then fuse as the external cleft and internal pouches are obliterated. Anomalies of the branchial cleft are due to incomplete obliteration of the cleft or pouch during this process. Cysts of the branchial cleft are the second most common congenital neck masses seen in children.[2] They are usually asymptomatic and unrecognized by the patient until a cyst develops from the infection. The cysts are located anterior to the sternocleidomastoid muscle and can present as either cysts, sinuses, or fistulas. Branchial cysts are lined by stratified squamous epithelium and contain keratinous material inside the cyst. They are further divided into four types based on developmental origin.

First Branchial Cleft Cyst: Subclassified into two types (Work classification). Type I cysts are purely ectodermal in origin and present as duplication anomalies of the external auditory canal. They are usually present lateral to the facial nerve and pass through the parotid gland. Type II cysts contain both ectoderm and mesoderm. They are usually located below the angle of the mandible, pass through the parotid gland either medial or lateral to the facial nerve, and pass between branches of the facial nerve.

Second Branchial Cleft Cyst: These are the most common type of branchial cysts, usually located inferior to the angle of the mandible and anteromedial to the sternocleidomastoid muscle. The fistulous tract arising from this cleft travels deep to the platysma and then it goes between the internal and external carotids, running superficial to the glossopharyngeal nerve and the hypoglossal nerve where it then connects to the tonsillar fossa.[3] If bilateral, these second branchial cleft cysts are often associated with branchio-oto-renal syndrome (i.e., second branchial cleft anomalies, deafness, preauricular pits, auricular malformation, renal anomalies).

Third Branchial Cleft Cyst: These are located anterior to sternocleidomastoid muscle, typically in the lower one third of the muscle. The sinus tract passes deep to the platysma, the internal carotid artery, passes between the glossopharyngeal and hypoglossal nerves, and ends in the pyriform sinus in the larynx.

Fourth Branchial Cleft Cyst: These are very rare, and the exact course of the cyst is not well described owing to its rarity. Typically, the sinus tract runs deep to the common carotid and will then either loop around the aortic arch (left-sided anomaly) or the subclavian (right-sided anomaly) and terminate in the pyriform sinus in the larynx.

Clinical Features

Branchial cysts are more common than fistulas and are seen more often in children, while fistulas are usually seen in teenagers. Cysts are often asymptomatic and can get infected secondary to upper airway tract infections. Infected cysts that present with abscess can compress the upper airway causing dysphagia, dyspnea, and stridor. The presentation and the best way to perform a thorough physical examination will depend on the type of the branchial cleft cyst.[4]

A first branchial cleft cyst is between the external auditory canal and submandibular area. It can present with punctum from which fluid may be expressed. The parotid gland and the facial nerve are involved, additionally a connection to the middle or external ear may exist, thus an otologic exam must be performed. A second branchial cleft cyst presents as a punctum of the skin at the sternocleidomastoid's lower anterior border. It may be close to the glossopharyngeal nerve, the hypoglossal nerve, and the carotid vessels. When infected, the cysts may lead to airway compromise. The skin and the pharynx may have mucoid or purulent discharge when an associated sinus tract is present. Third and fourth branchial cleft cysts are rare. These cysts are generally found on the left side of the neck or the suprasternal notch/clavicular area.

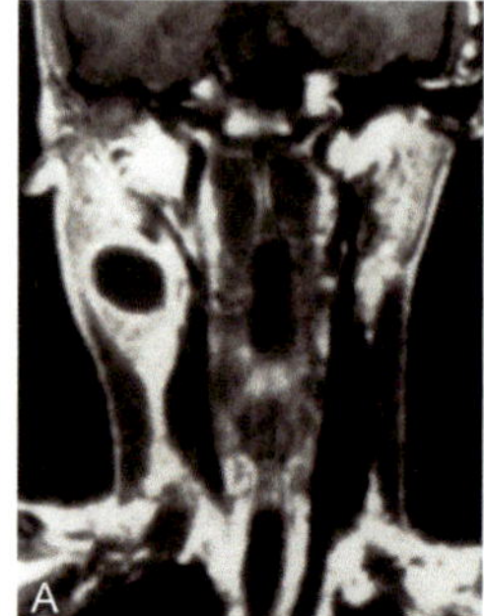

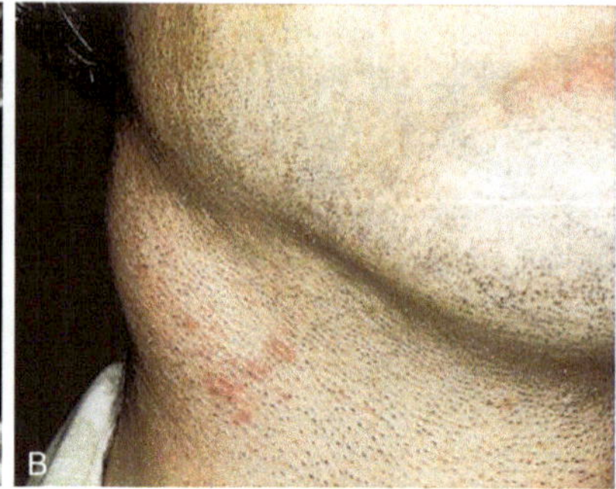

Figure 1: CT demonstrating right branchial cyst and adjacent image showing associated clinical finding

Evaluation

Clinical examination alone is sufficient in establishing a diagnosis of a branchial cleft cyst (Figure 1. A sinogram or a fistulogram can be done to identify the location and course of the tract. CT (Figure 1) and MRI of the neck can delineate the anatomy very well and establish the exact relationship of the cyst or tract its relation to major structures in the neck. Ultrasound is the best modality of imaging in the pediatric population since it avoids radiation exposure. Ultrasound can help determine the relationship of the lesion to the cervical vasculature. It can further help with needle decompression of the infected cyst, while avoiding a formal incision and drainage. Ultrasound can also help image third or fourth arch anomalies that pass near or through the thyroid gland.[5] When the diagnosis is in doubt, FNAC helps rule out malignant diseases that can appear or other differential diagnoses that have a similar presentation to branchial cleft cysts.

Management

Management depends on the acuity of presentation. Patients who present with large abscesses with clinical signs of sepsis or patients who present with airway compromise should undergo emergent surgery. These surgeries often include incision and drainage in addition to IV antibiotics. Non emergent abscess can be dealt with antibiotics and needle aspiration. Definitive management is excision of the cyst.

First branchial cleft cysts, sinuses, and fistulas are excised similarly to a parotid lobectomy.[5] The parotid gland is dissected posteriorly from the sternocleidomastoid and anteriorly from the external auditory canal. Then the posterior belly of the digastric must be identified, followed by the facial nerve trunk as the cyst exits the stylomastoid foramen. To remove the cyst in total, an excision of either part or all of the parotid gland's superficial lobe may be required. Then to ensure complete tract resection, it is dissected to the external auditory canal.

For second branchial cleft cysts incision is made transversely within a natural skin crease of the neck. If a fistula or sinus is present, a lacrimal probe can be dipped into a solution of methylene blue which is then inserted into the tract to make the fistula or sinus easier to identify intraoperatively.[3] The tract is then dissected around carcfully. If thc track is long, then exposure can be made with a second (step-ladder) incision placed within a skin crease proximal to the primary incision. Ethanol ablation can be used in patients who cannot undergo surgery for other reasons. Third and fourth branchial cleft cysts often require thyroid lobectomy with preservation of the recurrent laryngeal nerve to completely excise the tract in the piriform sinus. Direct laryngoscopy should be performed prior to cervical incision to confirm and cannulate the internal opening into the piriform sinus which facilitates dissection during excision. Estimated recurrence rate after surgery is low at around 3%.

THYROGLOSSAL DUCT CYST

Thyroglossal duct cysts are the most common congenital cysts in the neck. The prevalence is around 7%. The usual presentation is a midline neck cyst that is near the hyoid bone. They are seen in patients of all age groups, but the majority are seen in children.

Embryology

The thyroid gland develops during the fourth week of gestation. Initially, the first and second pharyngeal pouches form a ventral diverticulum of foramen cecum (the medial thyroid anlage). The diverticulum is connected to the tongue and descends in the neck midline, usually anterior to the hyoid bone and ends anterior to the first few tracheal rings by the end of week seven. By week ten of gestation, the tract should atrophy and disappear. In 50% of people, the distal portion of the duct differentiates into the thyroid gland's pyramidal lobe. A thyroglossal duct cyst arises from the persistent remnant of the thyroglossal duct tract. Lymphoid tissue within the tract can get hypertrophied due to local infection, thereby occluding the tract with resultant cyst formation.[6]

Clinical Features

Thyroglossal duct cysts are typically mobile midline neck masses near the hyoid bone and elevate during swallowing or torque protrusion (Figure 2). The cyst is usually asymptomatic but can get infected secondary to an upper respiratory tract infection. Once infected, they can become an abscess or a sinus that drains intermittently. The cyst is usually located at or just below the hyoid bone adjacent to the thyrohyoid membrane but can appear at any point along the thyroglossal duct tract, between the foramen cecum at the base of the tongue to the level of the suprasternal notch. Head and neck radiation for treating cancers can acutely enlarge subclinical thyroglossal duct remnants.

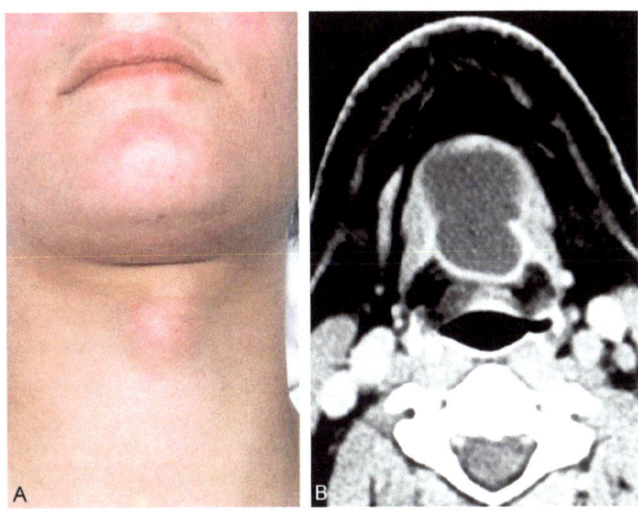

Figure 2: Midline mass in the neck consistent with thyroglossal duct cyst, adjacent image showing CT finding

Evaluation

Thyroid function tests should be performed in all patients who present with thyroglossal duct cysts. Sometimes the only thyroid tissue in these patients is in the thyroglossal cyst. Clinical examination of the thyroid gland in its normal anatomical location should be completed to confirm its presence or absence. Imaging modalities help diagnose the thyroglossal duct cyst and identify healthy thyroid tissue. Ultrasound is the preferred modality in children. The cyst appears as a well-defined, thin-walled, anechoic, or hypoechoic mass with posterior acoustic enhancement in the midline anterior neck. CT of the neck with contrast is the preferred imaging modality in adults (Figure 2). CT and MRI help identify the relationship of the cyst to the hyoid bone and also identifies normal orthotopic thyroid tissue.

Management

Infected thyroglossal duct cysts should initially be treated with antibiotics and then definitive surgery should be done once the infection has resolved. Abscesses that do not respond to antibiotics should be treated with incision and drainage. Recurrence rates generally increase after incision and drainage due to seeding of ductal cells outside the cyst. The usual culprits are the oropharyngeal flora and thus antibiotics are directed towards them.

Sistrunk Operation

Incidentally found cysts on imaging can be monitored closely. All symptomatic thyroglossal duct cysts should be treated surgically unless the patient is not a surgical candidate. Surgery should be avoided during the acute inflammation phase as this can lead to recurrence. Sistrunk operation is the recommended procedure for thyroglossal cysts and involves resection of the cyst along with the midportion of the hyoid bone, and resection of a core of tissue from the hyoid upwards toward the foramen cecum. A transverse cervical incision is made at the midpoint between the hyoid bone and the superior edge of the thyroid cartilage. Next the subplatysmal flap is raised superiorly and care should be taken not to rupture the cyst. Dissection should be performed starting below and moving upwards from the pyramidal lobe (if present) going to the hyoid bone. The cyst is generally adherent to the inferior part of the hyoid bone. The central part of the hyoid bone is sectioned and resected en bloc with the cyst. Next, the Sistrunk maneuver is performed by using the left index finger (for a right-handed surgeon) with the fingertip facing down towards the foramen caecum, which helps guide the dissection. The thyroglossal duct is then ligated at the level of the foramen cecum and transected. Recurrence rates after the sistrunk procedure is 1.5 to 10%.[7] Sclerotherapy using a percutaneous ethanol injection is useful in patients who are not surgical candidates.

Thyroglossal Fistula

Thyroglossal fistulas are an acquired condition that can result from rupture of an infected thyroglossal duct cyst or due to recurrence from an inadequate cyst excision. Management is similar to thyroglossal duct cysts and involves the sistrunk operation after adequate control of the infection.

Thyroglossal Duct Cyst Carcinoma

The incidence of thyroglossal duct cyst carcinomas is less than 1% and is generally seen in adults. Typically, they are diagnosed on final pathology and the sistrunk operation is usually sufficient to treat true thyroglossal duct cyst cancers. The majority of the carcinomas are papillary-type thyroid cancers. If the cyst is found to have thyroid cancer, it should be further evaluated to see if the cancer is arising from within the cyst and is not a cystic metastasis to a midline lymph node from a primary thyroid cancer. If preoperative ultrasound shows a normal thyroid gland, then the sistrunk operation is usually sufficient. Thyroidectomy is done in cases where a primary thyroid malignancy cannot be excluded or when a secondary thyroid malignancy is detected.

CYSTIC HYGROMA

Cystic hygroma is the most common type of lymphangioma. They result from lymph accumulation in the jugular lymphatic sacs due to obstruction of the lymphatic system, most commonly in the fetal neck. Cystic hygroma arises from embryonic lymphatic tissue remnants that can still proliferate and is associated with chromosome aneuploidies, hydrops fetalis, and intrauterine death.

Embryology and Pathophysiology

Embryologically, cystic hygromas originate at the point of lymphatic-venous collection and as a result of this, they are commonly seen in the posterior triangle of the neck. Lymph accumulates when the communication between the lymph and venous pathways fails and subsequently a cystic structure form. They often cross the body's midline and extend into both the axilla and the mediastinum.[8] Rapid growth in a previously stable cystic hygroma should raise concerns of lymph accumulation.

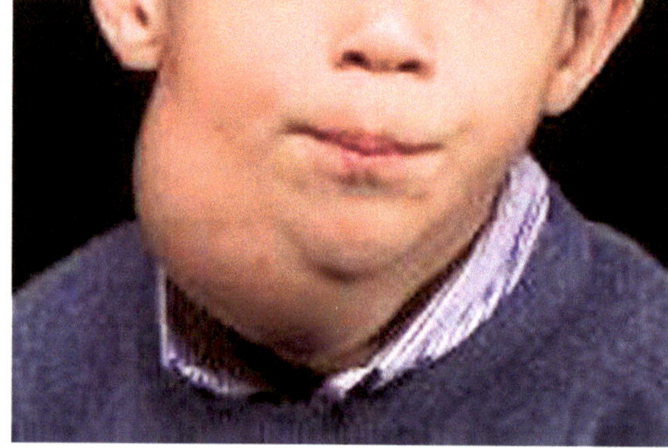

Figure 3: Cystic hygroma seen in right neck

Clinical Features

Cystic hygromas are mostly seen in children less than two years and are extremely rare in adults. Children usually present with a large, diffuse, and painless lump. On physical exam, cystic hygromas are soft, fluctuate, are freely mobile, and transilluminate well (Figure 3). Generally, they are non-pulsatile and become larger with coughing and crying. Symptoms depend on the lump's location and size and include pain, hoarseness, dysphagia, or shortness of breath.

Evaluation

Clinical examination alone is often sufficient to establish the diagnosis of a cystic hygroma. Ultrasonography, CT, and MRI can reveal involvement of and relation to surrounding structures and are useful in delineating the lesion further for planning surgery. Imaging usually shows multicystic lesions with internal septations. Karyotyping can be done if there is suspicion of a chromosomal disorder. Prenatal diagnosis of cystic hygromas can be done in the first trimester, ultrasound shows single or multilocular fluid-filled structure in the nuchal region or extending along the entire length of the fetus. In euploid fetuses, the majority of simple cystic hygromas resolve within four weeks of diagnosis, and septated cystic hygromas often resolve between 15 and 30 weeks of gestation

Management

Asymptomatic cystic hygromas can be monitored without any intervention. Treatment should be started if there is infection, hemorrhage, respiratory distress, dysphagia, or disfigurement. Treatment is individualized and depends on cystic size, anatomical location, and complications. Management is generally surgical, but other options include sclerotherapy, drainage, radio-frequency ablation, or cauterization. Surgical excision rates can be improved by using sclerotic agents as adjuncts. The approved sclerosing agents include OK-432 produced by Streptococcus sp., Bleomycin, and Doxycycline.

HEMANGIOMA

Hemangiomas are caused by endothelial cell proliferation and are the most common benign tumors of infancy. They are congenital if visible at birth or infantile if they arise later in infancy. Infantile hemangiomas have early, rapid growth, and then spontaneously involutes.

Etiology and Pathophysiology

The most accepted hypothesis of the etiology of hemangiomas is that hypoxic stress upregulates GLUT-1 and VEGF expression. This results in the endothelial progenitor cell mobilization. Infantile hemangiomas are more frequently seen amongst Caucasian infants than other racial groups. There is a 5:1 female to male ratio. Other risk factors include premature infants who often have low birth weights or prenatal hypoxia. Additionally, having an older mother increases the risk of an infant with infantile hemangioma. Hemangioma evolution has three phases:

- *Early proliferative or growth phase:* In the first three months of the infant's life, the hemangioma grows rapidly. Then when the infant is five to eight months, it grows gradually.
- *Plateau phase:* When the infant is six to twelve months old, the lesion remains inactive and dormant for a period of months.
- *Involution phase:* From one year old to several years old, the color of hemangioma changes from a bright red to a purple/gray and it becomes softer and more compressible.

Evaluation

Infantile hemangiomas are generally diagnosed clinically (Figure 4). However, if unsure, a skin biopsy can be taken and will stain positive for GLUT 1. Imaging (i.e., ultrasonography, CT, and MRI) are needed for diagnosis confirmation and help determine the extent of deep infantile hemangiomas without superficial changes.

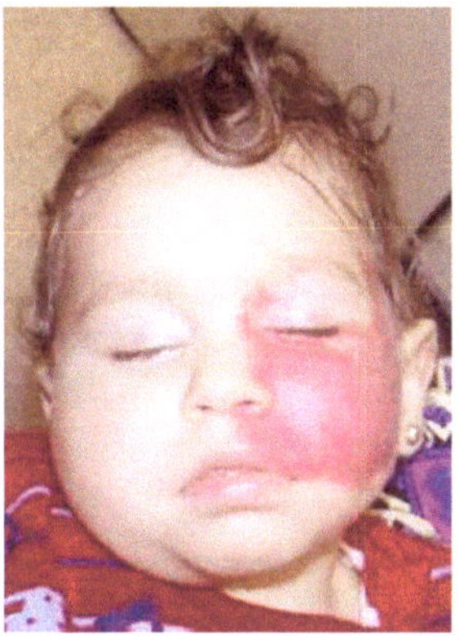

Figure 4: Hemangioma seen in an infant

Management

Most infantile hemangiomas resolve on their own and do not require treatment, so watchful waiting is recommended. Fifty percent of hemangiomas resolve in 5 years, 70% resolve in 7 years, and 90% resolve in 9 years. If complicated, the hemangioma will require treatment with beta blockers (i.e., oral propranolol) and oral prednisone. If the lesion is small and localized, intralesional and topical corticosteroids can be used. If there is concern for complications, surgical excising the residual fibrofatty tissue may be considered.

LARYNGOCELE

A laryngocele is an abnormal cystic dilatation of the laryngeal saccule. It is in communication with the larynx and contains air within the lumen.[9] The laryngeal saccule is a pouch in the upper portion of the laryngeal ventricle of Morgagni. Since there are mucinous glands in the ventricle, there may be mucus in the laryngocele. Obstruction of the laryngocele lumen can result in a laryngo-mucocele and potentially infection, forming a laryngopyocele.

Pathophysiology

Laryngoceles can be congenital or acquired. Raised intraluminal laryngeal pressures for prolonged periods can lead to the formation of laryngoceles. Thus, people at a higher risk of having a laryngocele include glass blowers and trumpet players. Additionally, a laryngeal tumor can obstruct the lumen, increase intralaryngeal pressure, and result in the formation of a laryngocele. Other causes include amyloidosis, chondroma, and scleroderma. They are classified into three types: (1) internal, which is confined within the thyrohyoid membrane, (2) external, which dissects superiorly through the thyrohyoid membrane into the subcutaneous tissues of the neck, and (3) a mixed form containing both parts.

Clinical Features and Evaluation

Common symptoms include hoarseness of voice and neck swelling. It is a clinical diagnosis. AP and lateral plain radiographs of the soft tissue are helpful, especially if the patient does the Valsalva maneuver. CT and MRI help define the laryngocele boundaries and its relation to the thyrohyoid membrane; it is particularly helpful in distinguishing between the internal, external, or mixed components. MRI is important for working up a laryngocele and laryngopyocele because it helps distinguish obstructed mucous and inflammation from neoplastic disease

Management

The treatment of choice is surgical excision. For external and combined laryngoceles, an external approach is indicated. Internal laryngoceles require an endolaryngeal approach.

INFLAMMATORY NECK MASS

Inflammatory neck masses in the neck result from enlarged lymph node groups secondary to an infectious or an inflammatory process.

Viral Lymphadenopathy

Reactive viral lymphadenopathy is the most common cause for cervical lymphadenopathy in children. Adenovirus, rhinovirus, and enterovirus are the most common pathogens that can cause upper respiratory tract infection leading to cervical lymphadenopathy. Enlarged Lymph nodes are usually seen along the jugular chain or in the submandibular region. These lymph nodes measure 1 to 1.5 cm and have preserved vascular hilum with no central hypodensity on imaging. Lymph nodes can be monitored and usually self-resolve in a few weeks. Failure to self-resolve or improve warrants biopsy and workup for other inflammatory disorders. Epstein-Barr virus, which causes infectious mononucleosis, is often associated with neck nodes that are quite large (>2 cm) and enlarged lymph nodes in the posterior triangle.

Bacterial Lymphadenopathy

Staphylococcus aureus and group A Beta-*Streptococcus* are the most common bacteria which can cause cervical lymphadenitis secondary to pharyngitis. Antibiotics alone are usually sufficient in managing these conditions and lymphadenopathy will resolve after treating the primary source. Other bacteria that can cause cervical lymphadenopathy includes *Rochalimaea or Bartonella henselae* (cat scratch disease), *Francisella tularensis* (Tularemia), Brucella (Brucellosis), Actinomycosis, and Mycobacterial infections.

Tuberculous Lymphadenitis (Scrofula)

Tuberculosis (TB) of cervical lymph nodes is the most common extrapulmonary manifestation of pulmonary TB. It is caused by the lymphatic spread or hematogenous dissemination of either reactivated TB or pulmonary TB. Mycobacterium tuberculosis and nontuberculous mycobacteria are the major causes of scrofula in immunocompromised patients.[10]

Pathophysiology

Cervical lymphadenitis due to TB is most often caused by reactivation of latent tuberculosis. Cervical lymph nodes (i.e., mandibular, upper jugular, and tonsillar) are more susceptible to cervical lymphadenitis due recurrent bacterial throat infections lowering nodal resistance. TB infections may also arise in the tonsils and adenoids and result in caseous necrosis and abscess formation underneath the deep fascia (cold abscess). This inflammation and necrosis have a fibrous capsule that prevents spreading of the infection. If this fibrous capsule ruptures, there may be abscess accumulation under the superficial fascia which can have cross fluctuance with deep fascia (collar-stud abscess). This abscess can rupture leading to formation of a sinus tract that drains yellow caseating material.

Clinical Fearures

Clinical manifestations of tuberculous lymphadenitis depend on the site of the lymphadenopathy and the immune status of the patient. Physical examination reveals a firm, discrete mass or matted nodes fixed to surrounding structures; the overlying skin may be indurated, or the lymph nodes can be complicated by ulceration, fistula, or abscess formation. Additional symptoms are those of systemic TB infection such as weight loss, failure to thrive, fever, rigors, and night sweats.

Evaluation

FNAC of the lymph node along with microscopic examination, cytology, and PCR is the initial diagnostic modality of choice.

If FNAC is nondiagnostic, excisional biopsy of the lymph node should be done. Specimens should be submitted for histology, acid-fast stain, culture, and nucleic acid amplification testing. Imaging modalities such as CT help monitor treatment and to differentiate tuberculous lymphadenitis from metastatic cancer or lymphoma. The interferon-gamma (IFN-gamma) Release Assay can detect T-cell IFN-gamma which is released due to stimulation with the highly TB-specific antigen. This assay has a high sensitivity and specificity for tuberculous lymphadenitis. Chest X-ray and Mantoux test are done to evaluate for pulmonary TB.

Management

Treatment for immunocompetent individuals consists of antimycobacterial therapy for six months which includes a two month, four drug regimen (Isoniazid, Rifampicin, Ethambutol, and Pyrazinamide) and followed by a four-month regimen of Isoniazid plus Rifampicin. Immunocompromised patients such as patients with HIV will need a longer duration of therapy. In immunocompetent patients, excision and removal of affected lymph nodes can sufficiently treat scrofula as long as there is not a concomitant pulmonary TB. Cold abscess of the neck can be treated by non-dependent drainage or aspiration and excision of the diseased nodes.

SIALADENITIS AND SIALOLITHIASIS

Inflammation and swelling of a salivary gland are known as sialadenitis. It is usually caused by salivary stasis that leads to retrograde seeding of bacteria from the oral cavity. Acute sialadenitis is rapid in onset and has swelling and pain associated with the salivary gland. Chronic sialadenitis is due to recurrent inflammation and oftentimes obstruction of the salivary duct. Benign, non-inflammatory swelling of the salivary gland is known as sialadenosis, usually associated with metabolic conditions. Parotid gland sialadenitis is more common than submandibular gland sialadenitis.[11]

Etiology

- Infections: bacterial (*Staphylococcus aureus* is most common, *H. Influenza*, anaerobes, tuberculosis), viral (HIV, Mumps)
- Inflammatory: radiation, contrast induced
- Autoimmune and Granulomatous: Sjogren syndrome, Sarcoidosis
- Obstruction: sialolithiasis, stricture, foreign body, external compression
- Others: poor oral hygiene, dehydration, immuno-compromised state, malnutrition, and drugs (diuretics, antihistamines)

SIALOLITHIASIS

Salivary gland stones usually occur in major salivary glands such as the submandibular (most common), parotid, and sublingual glands. Pathogenesis of stone formation is unknown. Elevated salivary calcium concentration and obstruction or stagnation of salivary flow can predispose to stone formation.[12] Salivary stones are mainly composed of calcium phosphate and carbonate. The submandibular gland may be more prone to stone formation because it is a long duct, the flow of saliva is slow and against gravity, and the saliva is more alkaline with a high mucin and calcium content. Additionally, there is hooking of the duct by the lingual nerve during its anatomical course. Submandibular duct stones are more common and the most common location for the stone is at the duct genu (an acute bend over the posterior free border of the mylohyoid muscle). The most common location for a parotid duct stone is at the parotid hilum or the main duct overlying the masseter muscle.

Clinical Features

Acute bacterial sialadenitis presents with a rapid onset of tender swelling over the involved gland. Purulent drainage can be expressed from the affected duct orifice. Viral sialadenitis usually involves multiple salivary glands and presents with generalized symptoms such as fever, headache, malaise, and myalgia in addition to mild pain and swelling over the involved glands. Patients with salivary stones usually present with unilateral salivary gland swelling and an acute onset of pain that worsens with eating or by the anticipation of eating. Stones can also present as painless swelling or may be noted incidentally on physical examination or imaging.

Evaluation

On physical exam, stones are often seen at the opening of the ducts or palpated along the course of the duct. The submandibular gland duct (Wharton's duct) opening is seen at its orifice near the frenulum of the tongue. Opening of the parotid gland duct (Stensen's duct) is adjacent to the second upper molar. Conventional radiographs using occlusal views have largely been replaced by more advanced imaging such as CT, MRI, and Ultrasound. CT and MRI have higher sensitivity and specificity in identifying stones compared to the conventional X-ray. Sialography is done by injecting a radiopaque dye into the duct after duct cannulation, followed by plain films.

Management

- Acute sialadenitis can be managed conservatively with antibiotics, proper hydration, warm compresses, and massage. Pain relief is with analgesics. For empiric and prophylactic antibiotic therapy, use amoxicillin/clavulanate or clindamycin. Antibiotics can be switched later depending on culture and sensitivities.
- Chronic sialadenitis is managed with hydration, oral hygiene, analgesics, and antibiotics in cases with associated infection. In the case of sialolithiasis, salivary gland stone removal should take place. The salivary glands should be excised in cases of recurrent sialadenitis (>3 episodes/year) or in chronic sclerosing sialadenitis.
- Sialendoscopy can be done for salivary stones that do not resolve with conservative management. Sialendoscopy has a working channel through which miniaturized wire baskets and forceps can be passed for extracting stones. Micro drills and laser fibers can be used for fragmenting larger stones. Extracorporeal lithotripsy, laser lithotripsy, and wire basket retrieval under fluoroscopic guidance are other minimally invasive approaches.

Surgical removal is recommended when minimally invasive approaches have failed in removing the salivary stones. Submandibular stones that are palpable within the mouth can be removed via a transoral approach. Transcervical excision of the submandibular gland (sialoadenectomy) is reserved for cases where transoral or minimally invasive approaches have failed, but the procedure carries risks of injury to the lingual and hypoglossal nerves. Parotid stones are usually not approachable through the transoral route. Parotidectomy is reserved for patients who have debilitating symptoms from the stone, but the procedure carries risks of injury to the auriculotemporal nerve and the facial nerve during dissection.

NEOPLASTIC HEAD AND NECK MASSES

CAROTID BODY TUMOR

Carotid body tumors, also known as chemodectomas or non-chromaffin paragangliomas, are a type of paragangliomas that arises from chemoreceptive tissue located at the carotid bifurcation. They typically reside in the adventitia of blood vessels.[13] The normal carotid body is ovoid in shape and measures approximately 5 mm. The carotid body is developed from both neural crest ectoderm and mesodermal tissue from the third branchial arch. The neural crest cells that migrate in close association with autonomic ganglion cells are known as paraganglioma cells. These cells differentiate into two types of cells called glomus cells. Type I glomus cells function as chemoreceptors. Type II glomus cells are formed from mesoderm and support chemoreceptor cells. The carotid body receives its arterial supply from branches of the external carotid artery. Venous drainage is through tributaries of the lingual and laryngopharyngeal veins. Nerve supply is from the carotid sinus nerve or Hering's nerve (branch of the glossopharyngeal nerve).

Pathophysiology

The carotid body acts as a chemoreceptor that transmits signals to the medulla oblongata in the brain, regulating breathing and blood pressure. The carotid body is stimulated primarily by the partial pressure of O_2 and stimulated less by the partial pressure of CO_2 and arterial pH. Stimulated type I glomus cells release neurotransmitters that act on the receptors of afferent nerve fibers. This signal is carried through the glossopharyngeal nerve to the medulla oblongata. A carotid body tumor is the most common type of paraganglioma in the head and neck. They represent neoplastic growths of the chemoreceptive tissue. Most carotid body tumors are benign and rarely are aggressive with local invasion and malignant transformation. They lack a true capsule and are reddish brown, rubbery, and well circumscribed. They are highly vascular, can invade the adventitia of adjacent carotid vessels, and can distort the carotid bifurcation leading to the "lyre sign" (splaying of the internal and external carotid arteries) seen on angiography. The Shamblin classification distributes carotid body tumors into three categories. The classification is based on the relationship between the carotid arteries and the adjoining nerves that surround the tumor. Type I tumors are small, they mildly displace the carotid vessels, and they lie beneath the hypoglossal and superior laryngeal nerves. Type II tumors are larger, more adherent to the adventitia, they partially surround the carotid vessels, and they lie beneath the hypoglossal and superior laryngeal nerves. Type III tumors encase the carotid vessels.

Clinical Features

Carotid body tumors are usually asymptomatic but can present with a mass in the neck or incidentally on imaging studies (i.e., a CT or MRIs scan performed for other reasons). On palpation, the lesions are firm, smooth, lobulated, and are mobile laterally but fixed longitudinally due to its close association with the carotid artery. Carotid pulsation may be transmitted through the mass and an audible bruit can be heard over the tumor. Local compression or invasion can lead to dysphagia, hoarseness, chronic cough, tinnitus, and rarely Horner's syndrome. Carotid body tumors are usually nonfunctional in secreting catecholamines.

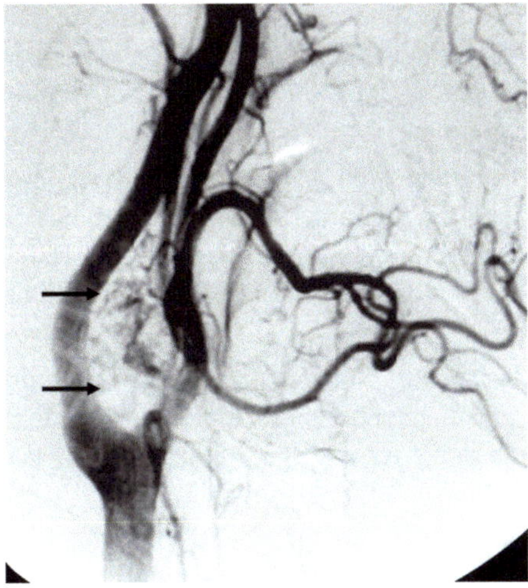

Figure 5: Conventional angiography showing carotid body tumor

Evaluation

Duplex ultrasound is the initial imaging of choice for carotid body tumors. It can provide anatomical details of the tumor, estimate tumor vascularity with color Doppler, and determine tumor size, vessel encasement, and underlying atherosclerotic disease in carotid vessels. Conventional angiography (Figure 5) used to be the gold standard, and can also identify synchronous and contralateral tumors, carotid atherosclerotic or ulcerative disease, and other anatomic variations of carotid vessels. It can also identify intracranial vascular lesions and it provides the opportunity for preoperative embolization if needed. Computed tomography angiography (CTA) and magnetic resonance angiography (MRA) have replaced conventional angiography. These methods are noninvasive and provide high levels of anatomic and vascular detail when compared to duplex ultrasound. Percutaneous biopsy and incisional biopsy are contraindicated due to the highly vascular nature of the tumor.

Management

Carotid body tumors must be resected surgically if the patient is deemed a good operative candidate. Smaller lesions are relatively easier to resect with minimal complications, however if they are allowed to grow, they can invade into the skull or involve cranial nerves, complicating resection. Chemotherapy is ineffective and these tumors are generally not radiosensitive. Patients who are deemed poor operative candidates, and for patients with bulky, unresectable, or recurrent tumors, radiation therapy can offer some benefit; however preoperative radiation can result in fibrosis and makes any subsequent surgery in the neck very difficult.

Preoperative embolization is not routinely performed and there are no guidelines supporting this type of intervention. Further it can lead to inadvertent cerebral embolization and stroke. Surgery is usually done under general anesthesia with cerebral monitoring and protection using EEG or shunting of the internal carotid artery. A longitudinal incision is made through the skin and subcutaneous tissues along the anterior border of the sternocleidomastoid centered over the carotid bifurcation. The sternocleidomastoid muscle is then reflected off the carotid sheath and the carotid sheath is opened along the anterior border of the internal jugular vein. The facial vein is then ligated and divided to expose the carotid bifurcation. Care should be taken to identify and protect the hypoglossal, vagus, and laryngeal nerves. In Type I tumors, the branches of the external carotid artery that supply the tumor can be divided and ligated and the external carotid artery can be preserved. For Type II tumors that are adherent to the external carotid artery, the vessel can be divided at its origin, the proximal stump is oversewn, and the external carotid artery is resected en bloc with the tumor. Type III tumors usually require removal of both external and internal carotid arteries that are involved with the tumor. The external carotid artery is ligated, and the internal carotid artery can be reconstructed with a prosthetic or autologous vein interposition graft.

LYMPHOMAS IN THE NECK

Lymphomas are usually more common in children and young adults. Up to 80% of children with Hodgkin's lymphoma can have a neck mass. Lymphomas arise when there is clonal proliferation of B-cells, T- cells, or natural killer (NK) cells. Lymphomas are generally classified into Hodgkin lymphomas (10%) and Non-Hodgkin lymphomas (90%). Hodgkin lymphomas can be further classified into classical and non-classical types. Non-Hodgkin lymphomas can be further classified into B-cell, T-cell, and NK cell types. Clinically, lymphoma is considered to be aggressive (high grade) and indolent (low grade).[14]

Hodgkin Lymphoma

Hodgkin lymphoma is an uncommon lymphoproliferative malignancy of B-lymphocytes. Presentation is bimodally distributed and has four subgroups: nodular sclerosis, lymphocyte-rich, mixed cellularity, and lymphocyte-depleted. The etiology is unclear, but risk of development is higher among first-degree relatives of patients with Hodgkin lymphoma. Patients usually present with cervical lymphadenopathy (Figure 6) and B symptoms (i.e., unexplained profound weight loss, high fevers, and drenching night sweats). Incisional or excisional biopsy with immunohistochemistry is needed for diagnosis and histology shows scattered large mononuclear Hodgkin and multinucleated cells (Reed-Sternberg) within a mix of non-neoplastic inflammatory cells (Figure 6). Imaging studies such as chest x-ray, chest/abdomen/pelvis CT, and PET-CT scans help stage lymphomas. Management depends on the histologic subtype, stage at diagnosis, and prognostic factors. Treatment consists of various chemotherapy combinations and radiation therapy of the involved site. PET-CT is used to assess the patient's response to the initial therapy and individualize ongoing treatment.

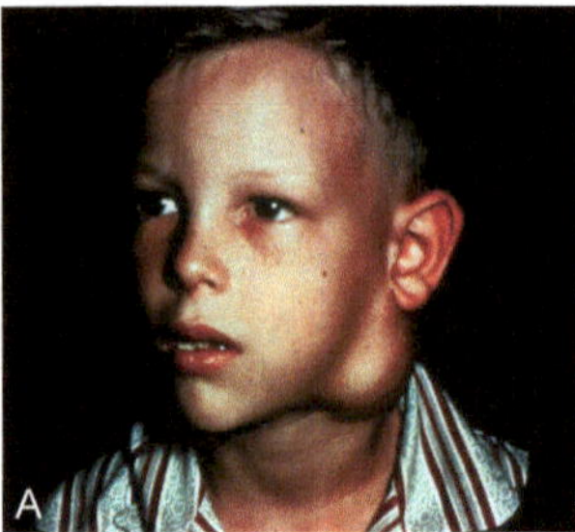

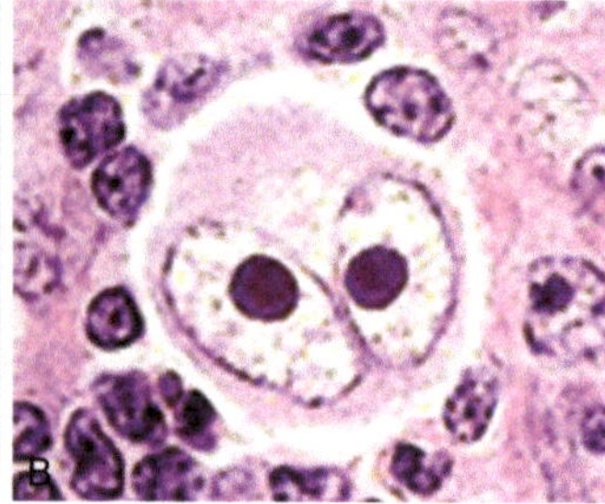

Figure: 6 Lymphoma in the neck, adjacent picture showing Reed-Sternberg cell on microscopy

Non-Hodgkin Lymphoma

The incidence of Non-Hodgkin's Lymphoma (NHL) increases with age; with the majority of patients being above 60 years of age. Diffuse large B-cell lymphoma is the most common subtype and in patients with HIV, NHL is the most common tumor (followed by Kaposi's sarcoma). Factors associated with an increased risk of NHL include immunosuppression, a previous history or family history of lymphoma, and drugs like Methotrexate and TNF-α inhibitors. Patients usually present with lymphadenopathy. Aggressive lymphomas have an acute or subacute presentation with increasing mass size. B symptoms like unexplained weight loss, fever, fatigue, and night sweats are also present. Indolent lymphomas have a chronic course, with asymptomatic lymphadenopathy and slowly progressive cytopenias. Excisional or incisional surgical biopsy with immunophenotyping, immunohistochemistry +/− flow cytometry are usually needed for accurate diagnosis. Rituximab based chemotherapy like R-CHOP (rituximab plus cyclophosphamide, doxorubicin, vincristine, and prednisone) or rituximab along with Bendamustine is currently recommended for the management of NHL.

CERVICAL LYMPH NODES

Lymph nodes in the head and neck are classified into seven levels (Table 2) based upon their anatomical location.

Level I Nodes: These are further divided into two groups. Level Ia (submental nodes) are located in the submental triangle, boundaries include the virtual midline medially, the anterior belly of the digastric muscle laterally, and the hyoid bone inferiorly. Level Ib (submandibular nodes) are located in the submandibular triangle, boundaries include the inferior border of the mandible, and the anterior and posterior bellies of the digastric muscle.

Level II Nodes: This level includes upper jugular nodes and is adjacent to the superior third of the internal jugular vein (IJV) and upper spinal accessory nerve. The boundaries include superiorly the insertion of the posterior belly of the digastric muscle and inferiorly the hyoid bone.

Level III Nodes: This group includes the middle jugular nodal group, adjacent to the middle third of the IJV. It is bounded superiorly by the hyoid bone, and inferiorly by the cricoid cartilage.

Level IV Nodes: This group includes the lower jugular nodal group adjacent to the inferior third of the IJV. It is bounded superiorly by the cricoid cartilage, and inferiorly the level ends at two centimeters superior to the sternoclavicular joint.

Level V Nodes: This group includes lymph nodes in the posterior triangle of the neck. It is bounded anteriorly by the posterior border of the sternocleidomastoid muscle and posteriorly by the anterior border of the trapezius muscle.

Table 2: Levels of Lymph nodes in neck

Level	Nodes	Possible Site of Malignancy
IA	Submental	Lower lip, floor of the mouth, lower jaw
IB	Submandibular	Face, nose, paranasal sinuses, oral cavity, submandibular gland
II	Upper Jugular	Oral cavity, oropharynx, nasopharynx, hypopharynx, supraglottic larynx
III	Middle Jugular	Thyroid, larynx, hypopharynx, cervical esophagus
IV	Lower Jugular	Hypopharynx, larynx, thyroid, cervical esophagus
V	Nodes in Posterior Triangle	Nasopharynx, thyroid, lung, esophagus, breast
VI	Central Compartment nodes	Lower lip, thyroid, oral cavity, glottic and subglottic larynx, apex of pyriform sinus, cervical esophagus
VII	Anterior Superior Mediastinum and Tracheoesophageal groove	Subglottic, thyroid, cervical esophagus

Level VI Nodes: Includes the central or anterior compartment nodes. Boundaries include the hyoid bone superiorly, suprasternal notch inferiorly, and laterally it extends up to the medial borders of both common carotid arteries.

Level VII Nodes: This group includes lymph nodes in the anterior superior mediastinum and the tracheoesophageal grooves, extending from the suprasternal notch to the innominate artery.[15]

Cervical Lymph Node Metastasis

Oral cavity tumors usually spread to the regional lymph node levels I, II, and III. Tumors of the lateral aspect of the oropharynx, hypopharynx, and larynx spread to the deep jugular lymph nodes at levels II, III, and IV. Metastasis from thyroid cancer usually goes to lymph nodes of the peri-thyroid, tracheoesophageal groove, and superior mediastinum. Metastasis from parotid gland tumors goes to preauricular, periparotid, intraparotid regions and the upper deep jugular nodes.

NECK

Evaluation and Management of Occult Primary in the neck

Evaluation should begin with a complete history and physical examination. Flexible fiberoptic laryngoscopy should be done to evaluate the sinonasal cavity, nasopharynx, pharyngeal walls, base of the tongue, larynx, and hypopharynx. Next, FNA of the mass should be done to identify the type of cancer like SCC, adenocarcinoma, lymphoma, melanoma, or cancer from the thyroid gland. CT or MRI with contrast is done to find the primary. If CT or MRI is unable to find the primary, then positron emission tomography (PET) with fluorodeoxyglucose (FDG) or integrated PET/CT should be performed. If the above methods are unable to identify the primary, the patient should undergo panendoscopy or triple endoscopy which includes direct laryngoscopy (i.e., evaluating the oropharynx, larynx, and hypopharynx), nasopharyngoscopy, and upper esophagoscopy. If the primary is found by any of the above methods, then the patient is treated according to specific guidelines for the respective primary. If the primary is not found and pathology is suggestive of adenocarcinoma, then Levels I through III neck dissections with parotidectomy is indicated. For levels IV and V, evaluate for an infraclavicular primary and perform a neck dissection if indicated. For SCC and anaplastic cancers, neck dissection or radiotherapy is preferred for N1 tumors, radiotherapy with concurrent systemic therapy or induction chemotherapy is preferred for N2-N3 tumors.

SALIVARY GLAND TUMORS

Salivary glands include the major glands such as the parotid, submandibular, sublingual, and minor salivary glands. These glands are located throughout the submucosa of the mouth and upper aerodigestive tract. The parotid gland accounts for 80 to 85 percent of salivary gland tumors. Approximately three-fourths of parotid lesions are benign, and approximately 25 percent are malignant.[16] 40 to 45 percent of submandibular gland tumors, 70 to 90 percent of sublingual gland tumors, and 50 to 75 percent of minor salivary gland tumors are malignant. The most common type of benign salivary gland tumor is a pleomorphic adenoma. Other benign salivary gland tumors include Warthin tumor, basal cell adenoma, and canalicular adenoma. The most common malignant salivary gland tumors are mucoepidermoid carcinoma and adenoid cystic carcinoma

Classification of Salivary Gland Tumors

WHO identified 24 different malignant salivary gland cancers and 11 different benign epithelial salivary gland tumors. They can be briefly classified as shown in Table 3.

Table 3: Classification of Salivary Gland Tumors

Benign	Malignant
Pleomorphic adenoma	Mucoepidermoid carcinoma
Warthin tumor	Adenoid cystic carcinoma
Oncocytoma	Malignant mixed tumors
Monomorphic tumors	Acinic cell carcinoma
Sebaceous tumors	Adenocarcinoma
Benign lymphoepithelial tumors	Lymphoma
Papillary ductal adenoma	

Pleomorphic Adenoma

Pleomorphic adenomas are the most common parotid neoplasm (80%). It is due to the proliferation of epithelial and myoepithelial cells of ducts. Most pleomorphic adenomas are encapsulated by podocytes which have irregular peripheral borders and local extensions of fingerlike processes into the capsule, seen on microscopy. They are slow growing tumors and present as a mass in the lateral neck raising the ear lobule (Figure 7). The recurrence rate is 1-5% after excision. Malignant degeneration is seen in 2-10% of tumors. Carcinoma ex pleomorphic adenoma is a malignant neoplasm that arises in association with a pleomorphic adenoma.

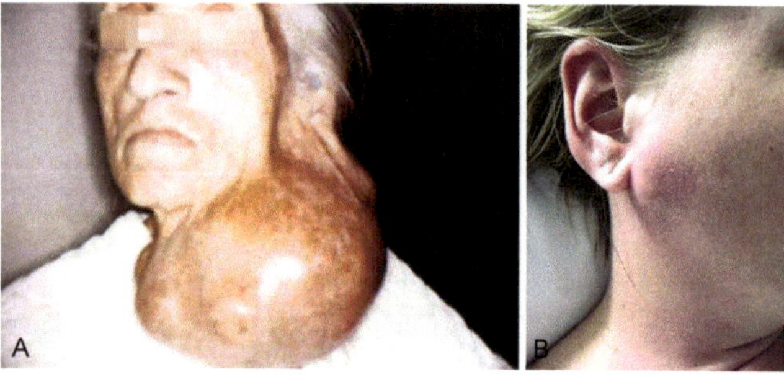

Figure 7: Parotid gland tumors in various stages of presentation

Warthin's Tumor (Papillary Cystadenoma Lymphomatosum)

Warthin's tumor is the second most common benign parotid tumor. It is the most common bilateral benign neoplasm and is seen in 10% of patients. It is more common in males and usually occurs in the 5th decade of life. On microscopy, the tumor is composed of eosinophilic glandular epithelium lined by basaloid cells, it has papillary cystic spaces, and is embedded in dense lymphoid tissue.

Mucoepidermoid Carcinoma

Mucoepidermoid carcinomas are the most common malignant salivary gland tumor. Most are seen in the parotid gland. The tumor shows epidermoid, mucous, and intermediate cells arranged in cystic or glandular structures or in a solid growth pattern on microscopy. The tumor is locally invasive and has low metastatic potential. Local metastasis to lymph nodes is seen. The most important prognostic factor is the histological grade. The 5-year survival rate is 75% for low grade tumors and 5% for high grade tumors respectively.

Adenoid Cystic Carcinoma

Adenoid cystic carcinomas are a slow growing tumor, but they show a high degree of perineural invasion, local invasion, and high recurrence after surgical resection. The tumor shows three main growth patterns: cribriform, tubular, and solid. The tumor is locally invasive to the facial nerve. Grade has no significance on survival rate. Prognosis depends upon the type of growth pattern, where tumors with solid components show worse survival rates. Lymph node metastasis is rare and distant metastasis to the lungs is more common.

Evaluation of Salivary Gland Tumors

CT and MRI are excellent in showing the anatomy of the salivary glands and show their relation to surrounding structures. FNA should be done in all cases with either direct palpation or under image guidance (i.e., ultrasound or CT). FNA can help identify benign versus malignant salivary tumors. Preoperative FNA is helpful in planning the surgery and determining the need for a neck dissection in the case of a malignancy. Intraoperative frozen section is helpful in identifying occult tumors and decreases reoperative and recurrence rates.

TNM Staging of Salivary Gland Tumors

Primary Tumor (T)

TX - Cannot assess the primary tumor

T0 - No evidence of the primary tumor

Tis - Carcinoma in situ

T1 - The greatest dimension of the tumor is ≤2 cm. No extraparenchymal extension

T2 - The greatest dimension of the tumor is 2 to 4 cm. No extraparenchymal extension

T3 - The tumor is >4 cm +/- extraparenchymal extension

T4 - The tumor is moderately or very advanced disease

T4a - The tumor is invasive, reaching the skin, mandible, ear canal +/- the facial nerve. Moderately advanced disease.

T4b - The tumor is invasive, reaching the skull base +/- pterygoid plates +/- encases the carotid artery. Very advanced disease.

Regional Lymph Nodes (N)

NX - Cannot assess the regional lymph nodes

N0 - No evidence of regional lymph node metastasis

N1 - Single, ipsilateral lymph node metastasis. The greatest dimension of the node is ≤3 cm

N2 - Single, ipsilateral lymph node metastasis. The greatest dimension of the node is 3-6 cm

N3 - Metastasis. The greatest dimension of the node is >6 cm

Distant Metastasis (M)

M0 - There is no distant metastasis

M1 - There is distant metastasis

Management

Surgical excision is the mainstay of therapy for all salivary gland tumors. Most pleomorphic adenomas of the parotid gland are seen in the superficial lobe, thus superficial parotidectomy is usually sufficient. For benign tumors lying deep to the plane of the facial nerve, the facial nerve is preserved by carefully removing selected tumors in the inferior portion of the gland. Low grade malignant tumors which are confined to the superficial lobe can be treated with superficial parotidectomy alone. For low grade tumors in the deep lobe and high-grade tumors, total parotidectomy is recommended. The facial nerve and its branches must be preserved unless the tumor grossly involves the nerve.

Benign tumors of the mandibular salivary gland are treated by simple excision of the gland. The marginal mandibular branch of the facial nerve, the hypoglossal nerve, and the lingual nerve should be spared. Malignant tumors of the mandibular salivary gland are removed en bloc with the affected gland. Effort should be made to preserve the marginal mandibular branch of the facial nerve, the lingual nerve, and the hypoglossal nerve, unless they are encased with tumors.

Patients presenting with nodal metastases should be treated with neck dissection of the areas involved and lymph node groups at highest risk should have adjuvant radiation therapy in most cases. For patients with clinically negative nodal metastasis, elective neck dissection is reserved for patients who are at high risk for occult nodal disease: high-grade tumors, large tumors (T3 and T4), and facial nerve paralysis/weakness.

ORAL CANCER

Squamous cell cancer constitutes the majority of cancers found in the oral cavity. The oral cavity extends from the upper lip (skin-vermillion junction) and runs superiorly to the junction of the hard and soft palate and runs inferiorly to the line of circumvallate papillae of the tongue. Laterally anterior tonsillar pillars and glossotonsillar folds serve as the boundaries between the oral cavity and oropharynx. Oral cavity cancer can include the lips, alveolar ridges, hard palate, floor of the mouth, and the anterior two-thirds of the tongue.

Etiology

Risk factors for the development of oral cancer include tobacco use, HPV infection (primarily types 16 and 18), alcohol use, immunocompromised state, prior exposure to radiation, betel nut chewing, and solar radiation.

Clinical Presentation

Oral cancers can present in varied forms of patches, lesions, and growth. Oral leukoplakia is a white patch or plaque that develops in the oral cavity. The condition is potentially malignant and is strongly associated with tobacco use. Erythroplakia is a lesion of the oral mucosa that presents a bright-red velvety plaque. Generalized symptoms of malignancy like weight loss, fatigue and anorexia may be seen. Local invasion into adjacent structures can present with oral ulcers or mass, choking, dyspnea, dysphagia, odynophagia, hoarseness, globus sensation, otalgia, hemoptysis, trismus, neck mass, and pain in the head and neck region.

Evaluation

Initial evaluation of the primary should start with a thorough history and physical examination including inspection and palpation of the oral cavity, indirect mirror examination, or direct flexible laryngoscopy. FNA biopsy is useful in determining the type of primary cancer. CT, MRI, PET, and integrated PET/CT are important for assessing the degree of local infiltration, the involvement of regional lymph nodes, and the presence of distant metastases or of a second primary tumor.

TNM staging

Primary Tumor (T)

TX - Cannot assess the primary tumor

T0 - No evidence of the primary tumor

Tis - Carcinoma in situ

T1 - The tumor is ≤2 cm in size and has a ≤5 mm depth of invasion (DOI)

T2 - The tumor is ≤2 cm, DOI 5-10 mm; or the tumor is >2 cm and DOI 4-10 mm

T3 - The tumor is 2-4 cm, DOI >10 mm; or the tumor is >4 cm, DOI ≤10 mm

T4 - The tumor shows moderately or very advanced disease

T4a - The tumor shows moderately advanced, local disease. The tumor is >4 cm, DOI >10 mm; or the tumor is invasive into only adjacent structures

T4b - The tumor shows very advanced, local disease. The tumor invades the masticator space, pterygoid plates, or skull base +/- encases the internal carotid artery

Regional Lymph Nodes (N)

NX - Cannot assess the regional lymph nodes

N0 - There is no metastasis to the regional lymph node

N1 - Single, ipsilateral lymph node metastasis. The greatest dimension of the node is ≤3 cm

N2 - Single, ipsilateral lymph node metastasis. The greatest dimension of the node is 3-6 cm

N3 - Metastasis. The greatest dimension of the node is >6 cm

Distant Metastasis (M)

M0 - There is no distant metastasis

M1 - There is distant metastasis

Prognostic Stage Groups

Stage 0 - Tis N0 M0

Stage I - T1 N0 M0

Stage II - T2 N0 M0

Stage III - T1, T2 N1 M0, T3 N0, N1 M0

Stage IVA - T1 N2 M0, T2 N2 M0, T3 N2 M0, T4a N0, N1, N2 M0

Stage IVB - Tis to T4b N3 M0, T4b Any N M0

Stage IVC - Tis to T4b N M1

Management

For patients with stage, I or II oral cavity tumors, surgery is recommended over radiotherapy (RT) because it is typically associated with less long-term morbidity than RT and offers more detailed pathologic staging, including depth of invasion (DOI). Definitive RT is reserved for patients who are ineligible for surgery or for whom surgical resection would result in severe functional impairment. R0 resection must be achieved, and re-resection should be done if needed to achieve negative margins. Locoregionally advanced tumors (stage III and localized IV) that are resectable are typically approached by upfront surgery followed by adjuvant radiation and/or chemotherapy. Unresectable patients are typically treated with definitive chemotherapy and radiotherapy. Patients with stage III and IV oral cancer require treatment of the neck. Elective lymph node dissection for clinically N0 tumors should include at least 18 lymph nodes.

CARCINOMA OF LIP

Cancer of the lip is the most common malignant tumor affecting the head and neck. Cancers arising on the inner surface of the lip are considered as oral cavity cancers and cancers of the vermillion. Cancers arising on the external surface of the lip are now classified with skin cancers. SCC is the most common cancer of the lower lip and basal cell cancer is more common cancer of the upper lip. Non-SCCs of the lip are due to tumors arising from minor salivary glands.

Etiology

Carcinoma of the lip is seen in individuals who are associated with chronic sun exposure, alcohol use, and tobacco exposure. Lower lip cancers are more common than upper lip cancers due to increased sun exposure.

Clinical Features

Carcinoma of the lip usually presents as an exophytic, crusted lesion with variable invasion into the underlying muscle (related to the size of the primary tumor (Figure 8. The adjacent lip often shows features of actinic sun damage such as color change, mucosal thinning, and various associated areas of leukoplakia.[17]

Evaluation

Clinical evaluation of carcinomas of the lip includes a wedge biopsy which usually confirms the diagnosis. Advanced tumors of the lip with concerns for local invasion into surrounding structures require CT or MRI to allow for complete staging and treatment planning with regards to resection margins which may include resection of adjacent bone. Oral cavity tumors are almost always staged with cross-sectional imaging including the chest where the demonstration of simultaneous pulmonary parenchymal disease may influence curability.[17]

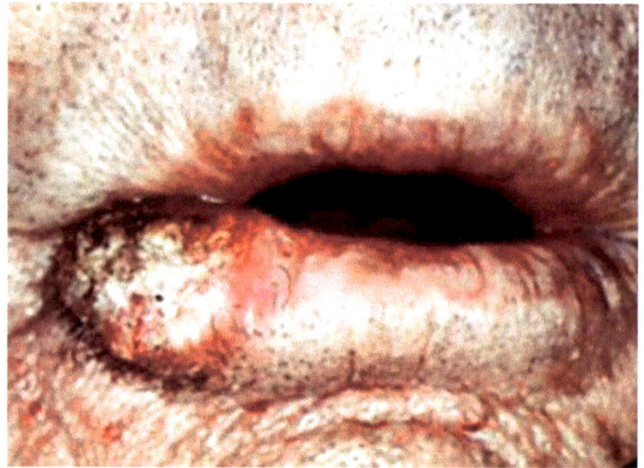

Figure 8: Carcinoma over lower lip

Management

Surgery or radiotherapy is equally effective for early-stage lip cancers (T1 and T2). Superficial lesions affecting the external vermilion of the lip such as leukoplakia or actinic keratosis are best managed via a lip shave and mucosal advancement.[18] Larger lesions of the lip are better treated with excision and reconstruction. To avoid contracture during reconstruction, full thickness skin flaps which consist of skin, muscle, and mucosa are used. If there are no clinically suspicious lymph nodes, neck dissection is often not indicated because greater than 5 percent of patients develop recurrence in the neck. Cervical nodes have a poor prognosis. If the cancer is in the upper lip, they can invade the premaxilla and nasal cavity; thus, treatment of the neck is often performed for prophylactic measures, these include early-stage upper lip SCCs. Neck dissection is often not completed if the cancer is in the lower lip, this is especially true if there is no involvement of the cervical lymph nodes because there are low rates of recurrence.

CARCINOMA OF THE TONGUE

The tongue is divided into two anatomical regions. It consists of an anterior two-thirds of the tongue (part of the oral cavity) and a posterior third (base of tongue). This tongue is a component of the oropharynx. SCC is thc most common type of tongue cancer

Etiology and Pathogenesis

Tongue SCC risk factors include smoking tobacco, alcohol use, betel nut chewing, radiation exposure, immunocompromised states, poor oral hygiene, and HPV infection. Head and neck SCCs generally involve tumor suppressor gene p53 mutations and overexpression of the oncogene epidermal growth factor receptor (EGFR).[19]

Clinical Features

Reported symptoms include localized pain, dysphagia, weight loss, dysarthria, and odynophagia. Patients usually report a history of trauma to the region (Figure 9). Ipsilateral tongue deviation is seen when the hypoglossal nerve is involved. Altered sensation to the tongue is noticed when the lingual nerve is involved. Involvement of the inferior alveolar nerve means the disease is advanced and the patient will have symptoms of numbness in the chin, lower lip, and/or mandibular teeth.[20]

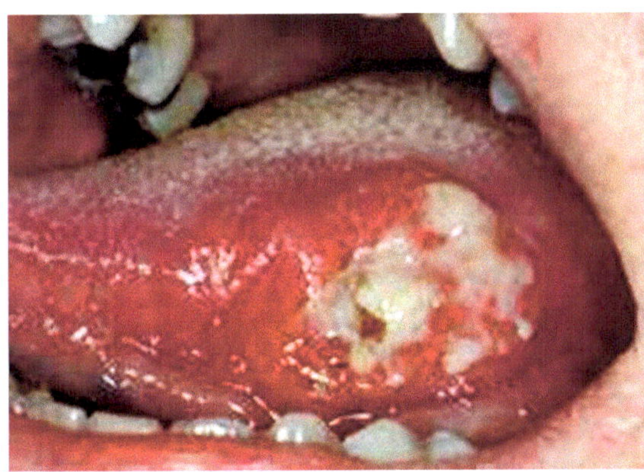

Figure 9: Carcinoma of Tongue

Evaluation

A thorough physical exam with an emphasis on the head and neck exam should be performed. The neck exam includes searching for palpable lymphadenopathy, especially of the submental, submandibular, and jugulodigastric regions. If the patient undergoes an incisional biopsy or punch biopsy, they should be put under local anesthesia. The biopsy can reveal the cancer type. Gross neck lymphadenopathy requires an ultrasound guided FNA biopsy. A head and neck CT can reveal tumor size, location, extension, and radiologic appearance of the draining neck lymph nodes. PET/CT helps reveal distant metastasis.

Management

Similar to carcinoma of the lip, T1 and T2 tumors can be managed with surgery or radiotherapy with similar outcomes. T3 and T4 tumors are managed with surgical excision and postoperative chemoradiation. Resection margin should be at least 1cm when possible. After resection, frozen sections will go to pathology to confirm that the margins are disease-free. For functional deficits, reconstruction with flaps should be done to improve swallow and speech functions. Flaps for tongue reconstruction are generally taken from the radial forearm free flap and anterolateral thigh free flap. When mandibular reconstruction is necessary after resection, a fibular free flap is used. Locoregional pedicled flaps such as a submental island flap, latissimus dorsi pedicle flap, and the pectoralis major myocutaneous flap are used when free flaps fail or if there is a contraindication to use a free flap.

If a patient with tongue cancer has a preoperative or intraoperative palpable neck disease, they should undergo a radical neck dissection on the ipsilateral side. The tongue usually drains to neck levels I to III, which is also the first location of tumor metastasis. The depth of invasion of a tongue tumor is the main determinant when deciding to do a neck dissection for non-palpable disease. Most patients with primary tongue SCC must be offered an elective neck dissection to rule out occult nodal disease by pathology. Also, a selective dissection of levels I to III (supraomohyoid neck dissection) is done.

CARCINOMA OF LARYNX

The larynx is divided into three anatomic regions: the supraglottis, glottis, and subglottis. Glottic, supraglottic, and subglottic cancers represent approximately two-thirds, one-third, and 2 percent of laryngeal cancers. Most laryngeal cancers are SCC.

Etiology

Laryngeal cancer risk factors are smoking, alcohol, advanced age, HPV infection, chronic laryngitis, exposure to paint, asbestos, gasoline fumes and radiation. Also, a diet with little green leafy vegetables, high in fats, and/or high in salt-preserved meat is a risk factor. The peak incidence is in the sixth decade, with 80% of cases detected in males. Approximately 60% of cases present an advanced disease (stages III to IV).

Clinical features

Involvement of the glottis presents with hoarseness of voice. Involvement of the supraglottis and subglottis is usually asymptomatic and can present with late symptoms such as cervical lymphadenopathy, neck or ear pain, discomfort and/or pain during swallowing. In later stages symptoms include hoarseness, dysphagia, and airway obstruction.

Evaluation

Evaluation of a laryngeal mass includes a history, physical examination, and direct larynx visualization (Figure 10) including a sample of the tissue. The patient should have a FNA of any suspicious nodal disease. FNA of a primary mass in the larynx can reveal the type of primary malignancy. CT neck with contrast is the imaging modality of choice. Metastatic workup includes chest CT and PET/CT. If suspicious of invasion of the hypopharynx, an esophagogastroduodenoscopy (EGD) and/or barium swallow is indicated to differentiate the origin of the cancer tissue.

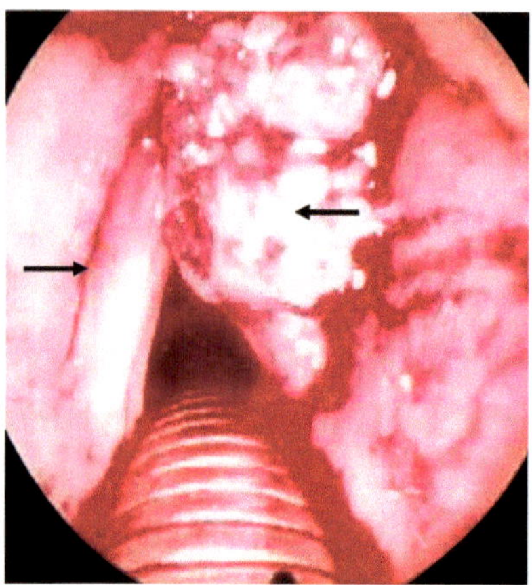

Figure 10: laryngoscopy showing cancer of larynx

Management

Management of early-stage laryngeal cancer is primarily based on the anatomic location of the tumor. For patients with early stage glottic cancer, a larynx-preserving approach with either transoral laser microsurgery or radiation therapy is the treatment of choice. For patients with early stage supraglottic laryngeal cancer, initial therapy with either RT or surgical resection is recommended. For patients with early stage supraglottic laryngeal cancer, initial therapy with either RT or surgical resection is recommended. Advanced-stage patients are treated with concurrent chemotherapy and radiotherapy as initial therapy; salvage laryngectomy is reserved for cases of treatment failure. For unresectable cancers, the treatment consists of definitive chemotherapy and radiotherapy followed by neck dissection. If hypopharyngeal involvement exists, then laryngopharyngectomy with neck dissection and postoperative radiotherapy with or without chemotherapy is required.

REFERENCES

1. Pynnonen MA, Gillespie MB, Roman B, et al. Clinical Practice Guideline: Evaluation of the Neck Mass in Adults. Otolaryngology–Head and Neck Surgery. 2017;157(2_suppl):S1-S30. doi:10.1177/0194599817722550.
2. Fanous A, Morcrette G, Fabre M, Couloigner V, Galmiche-Rolland L. Diagnostic Approach to Congenital Cystic Masses of the Neck from a Clinical and Pathological Perspective. *Dermatopathology (Basel)*. 2021;8(3):342-358. Published 2021 Aug 1. doi:10.3390/dermatopathology8030039.
3. Bajaj Y, Ifeacho S, Tweedie D, Jephson CG, Albert DM, Cochrane LA, Wyatt ME, Jonas N, Hartley BE. Branchial anomalies in children. Int J Pediatr Otorhinolaryngol. 2011 Aug;75(8):1020-3. doi: 10.1016/j.ijporl.2011.05.008. Epub 2011 Jun 15. PMID: 21680029.
4. Coste AH, Lofgren DH, Shermetaro C. Branchial Cleft Cyst. [Updated 2021 Jul 18]. In: StatPearls [Internet]. Treasure Island (FL): StatPearls Publishing; 2021 Jan-. Available from:https://www.ncbi.nlm.nih.gov/books/NBK499914/.
5. Prosser JD, Myer CM 3rd. Branchial cleft anomalies and thymic cysts. Otolaryngol Clin North Am. 2015 Feb;48(1):1-14. doi: 10.1016/j.otc.2014.09.002. PMID: 25442127.
6. Noyek, A M (02/1981). "Thyroglossal duct and ectopic thyroid disorders.". *Otolaryngologic clinics of North America* (0030-6665), 14 (1), p. 187.
7. Righini CA, Hitter A, Reyt E, Atallah I. Thyroglossal duct surgery. Sistrunk procedure. Eur Ann Otorhinolaryngol Head Neck Dis. 2016 Apr;133(2):133-6. doi: 10.1016/j.anorl.2015.11.008. Epub 2015 Dec 22. PMID: 26725753.
8. Bloom DC, Perkins JA, Manning SC. Management of lymphatic malformations. Curr Opin Otolaryngol Head Neck Surg. 2004 Dec;12(6):500-4. doi: 10.1097/01.moo.0000143971.19992.2d. PMID: 15548907.
9. Juneja R, Arora N, Meher R, Mittal P, Passey JC, Saxena A, Bhargava EK. Laryngocele: A Rare Case

Report and Review of Literature. Indian J Otolaryngol Head Neck Surg. 2019 Oct;71(Suppl 1):147-151. doi: 10.1007/s12070-017-1162-x. Epub 2017 Jul 21. PMID: 31741950; PMCID: PMC6848569.

10. Bhandari J, Thada PK. Scrofula. [Updated 2021 Jun 7]. In: StatPearls [Internet]. Treasure Island (FL): StatPearls Publishing; 2021 Jan-. Available from: https://www.ncbi.nlm.nih.gov/books/NBK557700/.
11. Adhikari R, Soni A. Submandibular Sialadenitis and Sialadenosis. [Updated 2021 Aug 14]. In: StatPearls [Internet]. Treasure Island (FL): StatPearls Publishing; 2021 Jan-. Available from: https://www.ncbi.nlm.nih.gov/books/NBK562211/.
12. Williams MF. Sialolithiasis. Otolaryngol Clin North Am. 1999 Oct;32(5):819-34. doi: 10.1016/s0030-6665(05)70175-4. PMID: 10477789.
13. Neumann HP, Pawlu C, Peczkowska M, Bausch B, McWhinney SR, Muresan M, Buchta M, Franke G, Klisch J, Bley TA, Hoegerle S, Boedeker CC, Opocher G, Schipper J, Januszewicz A, Eng C; European-American Paraganglioma Study Group. Distinct clinical features of paraganglioma syndromes associated with SDHB and SDHD gene mutations. JAMA. 2004 Aug 25;292(8):943-51. doi: 10.1001/jama.292.8.943. Erratum in: JAMA. 2004 Oct 13;292(14):1686. PMID: 15328326.
14. Jamil A, Mukkamalla SKR. Lymphoma. [Updated 2021 Jul 21]. In: StatPearls [Internet]. Treasure Island (FL): StatPearls Publishing; 2021 Jan-. Available from: https://www.ncbi.nlm.nih.gov/books/NBK560826/.
15. Shah JP, Patel SG. Head and neck surgery and oncology. 3rd ed. London: Mosby; 2002. p. 355.
16. Spiro, R H (01/1986). "Salivary neoplasms: overview of a 35-year experience with 2,807 patients.". *Head & neck surgery* (0148-6403), 8 (3), p. 177.
17. Wolff KD, Follmann M, Nast A. The diagnosis and treatment of oral cavity cancer. Dtsch Arzteblatt Int. 2012;109:829–35.
18. Kerawala C, Roques T, Jeannon JP, Bisase B. Oral cavity and lip cancer: United Kingdom National Multidisciplinary Guidelines. J Laryngol Otol. 2016 May;130(S2):S83-S89. doi: 10.1017/S0022215116000499. PMID: 27841120; PMCID: PMC4873943.
19. Rivera C. Essentials of oral cancer. Int J Clin Exp Pathol. 2015 Sep 1;8(9):11884-94. PMID: 26617944; PMCID: PMC4637760.
20. Gonzalez M, Riera March A. Tongue Cancer. [Updated 2021 Sep 14]. In: StatPearls [Internet]. Treasure Island (FL): StatPearls Publishing; 2021 Jan-. Available from: https://www.ncbi.nlm.nih.gov/books/NBK562324/.

❑❑❑

21

CHAPTER

Soft Tissue Sarcomas

David Machado-Aranda, MD
Binit Katwal, MD
Vijay K. Mittal, MD

INTRODUCTION

Soft Tissue Sarcomas (STS) represent a group of heterogeneous malignant tumors primarily derived from a wide variety of tissues of mesodermal origin. In the United States, despite the awareness of the generalist and widespread technological capacity for imaging, their incidence and detection is approximately 3 cases per 100,000; constituting less than 1% of all adult malignancies,[1] with a male preponderance, and with a male: female ratio of 1.4:1.[2] An estimated 12,000 new cases are diagnosed in the US each year and approximately 5000 patients die annually, because of advance stage disease.[3] Most soft tissue sarcomas are diagnosed in the extremities (59.5%), followed by the trunk (17.9%).[4] The thigh is the most common site in the body, accounting for 44% of all extremity STS. Adequate surgical resection with negative margin on their initial presentation may be the patient's only hope for cure, supported by advancing multimodal therapies including chemotherapy and radiotherapy. It is extremely important then that a general practitioner recognize a worrisome soft tissue mass and refer them right away for complete oncologic resection.

Epidemiology and Etiology

Because of the rarity of these tumors, no single etiological factor has been identified. Several environmental factors have been associated with a possible increase in incidence in the United States; these are listed in Table 1. However, this increment may be the result of improved detection and registry rather than reflecting a true increase of disease.

How these environmental factors produce sarcoma is poorly understood. It is thought that similar to what happens in epithelial tissues where squamous cell cancer can be the product of chronic irritation, each environmental factor could produce a chronic inflammatory response with the subsequent development of sarcomas.[5] Most chemicals associated with sarcomas have a very long half-life causing prolonged injury. For example, polyvinyl chloride can cause a chronic foreign body reaction with the subsequent development of an angiosarcoma. Overall, there has been an increase in the incidence of soft-tissue sarcomas. This may be due to the increased numbers of Kaposi's sarcoma, which is due to increased numbers of the acquired immunodeficiency syndrome (AIDS) and improved recognition and diagnosis.[6]

In Stewart-Treves syndrome, chronic upper extremity lymphedema after modified radical mastectomy has an increased incidence of lymphangiosarcoma.[7]

Host immunosuppression increases the risk of several types of sarcomas. The association of AIDS and Kaposi Sarcoma (KS) has been well established. KS is an endothelial proliferation produced by the human herpesvirus 8 (HHV8) infection. Leiomyosarcomas induced by the Epstein-Barr virus (EBV) have been seen in pediatric AIDS. [8] The recuperation of the host immune system regresses these tumors. Another group at risk are solid organ transplants recipients.

Radiation has been implied as an important risk factor for sarcomas. The increased use of radiation therapy for the treatment of breast, testes, ovarian, lung, and prostate cancer has shown an increased incidence of sarcomas in surrounding tissues. Typically, these tumors arise on the radiation field margins where the dose may cause mutations but is insufficient to kill these genetically modified cells. [9]

Due to these genetic alterations causing sarcomas, significant progress has been made in identifying an increasing number of modifications in the genome and their consequences in cellular function. These constitute potential targets for further drug development. As an example, Gastrointestinal stromal tumors (GIST) which have a mutation on a cell surface tyrosine receptor (c-KIT) are treated very well with several biological drugs (e.g., Imatinib, Sumatinib). It is possible that soon most of these tumors will be treated with molecular directed therapy.

Table 1: Etiologies and risk factors for development of sarcomas

Risk Factor		Resulting Sarcoma Subtype
Environ-mental pollutant/ chemical	• Ionizing radiation, previous or environmental • Herbicides (e.g., phenoxyacetic acids, chlorophenol) • Vinyl chloride • Dioxins	• Especially osteosarcoma, angiosarcoma • Non-specific • Hepatic angiosarcoma • Non-specific
Infection	• HIV, human herpes virus 8	• Kaposi's sarcoma
Genetic disorder	• Li-Fraumeni syndrome • Neurofibromato-sis type 1 • Rb-mutation (13q14) • Paget disease • Werner syndrome • Bloom syndrome • Gardner syndrome	• Any cancer, (e.g., 30% of sarcomas, osteosarcoma, and several soft-tissue sarcomas • MPNST • Osteosarcoma, if survived retinoblastoma • Osteosarcoma in adults • Osteosarcoma • Osteosarcoma • Fibrosarcoma

Clinical Presentation

Most patients present with an enlarging painless soft tissue mass present either in an extremity or in the trunk. For tumors developing in the retroperitoneum, non-specific GI symptoms are more common, these include abdominal or back pain, early satiety, constipation, and weight loss. Many times, patients perceive these lesions as unresolved hematomas or muscle strains that do not resolve, triggering a visit to the physician. Any perception of enlargement should raise concerns for malignancy. A focused history should include location, duration, changes in size, presence of skin changes and pigmentation, and/or associated symptoms.

Physical examination allows the appreciation of size, mobility, anatomical relationships with fascial planes, and involvement with neighboring organs, nerves, or blood vessels. A comprehensive neurovascular exam should be performed in the affected limb. An abdominal exam can differentiate if a tumor is arising from the retroperitoneum as opposed to the mesentery, GI tract, or a visceromegaly. Table 2 and Table 3 summarize the differential diagnosis of soft tissue masses located in the extremities and retroperitoneum, respectively.

Table 2: Differential diagnosis of soft tissue masses of extremities

Common benign adult soft tissue tumors
• Lipoma • Ganglion cyst • Hemangioma • Fibrous histiocytoma • Giant cell tumor of tendon sheath • Schwannoma • Neurofibroma • Fibromatosis • Ossified myositis
Common adult soft tissue sarcomas
• Malignant fibrous histiocytoma • Liposarcoma • Leiomyosarcoma • Synovial sarcoma • Malignant schwannoma
Others
• Peripheral artery aneurysm • Pseudoaneurysms • Benign cysts • Hematomas

Table 3: Differential diagnosis of retroperitoneal mass

Primary retroperitoneal tumors
• Liposarcoma • Leiomyosarcoma • Hemangiopericytoma • Malignant fibrous histiocytoma
Adrenal tumors
• Biochemical active • Adrenal cancer • Metastatic
Secondary retroperitoneal tumors
• Lymphoma • Germ cell tumor • Metastatic

Renal mass
Aortic abdominal aneurysm
Other • Mesenteric cyst • Hepatomegaly • Splenomegaly

Radiologic evaluation

The use of radiological imaging is a fundamental part in the diagnosis and management of soft tissue sarcomas. Conventional X-rays continue to be used in the evaluation of bone trabecular detail and the characterization of bone sarcomas. Myositis ossificans, a calcified hematoma and hemangioma with phleboliths, while common, is associated with distinct presenting histories. Ultrasound can be used to further characterize the lesion and can also be utilized in image guided biopsies. Adjuncts to ultrasound can be color doppler to determine the vascularity of the tumor. Increased or decreased changes in neovascularization can reflect an absence or presence of a tumor. [10] Cross sectional imaging, especially the Magnetic Resonance Imaging (MRI), has now become the standard of care in newly discovered masses. MRI allows the characterization of a mass based on features such as enhancement pattern, local extent of disease and neurovascular involvement; information that is extremely important in times of operative planning.[11] MRI scans are also important in differentiating benign from malignant tumors. Lipomas have a typical enhanced T1 weighted imaging and are suppressed with fat saturation sequences. Because sarcomas grow in a centripetal fashion, the compression of normal surrounding tissue creates an appearance of encapsulation, pushing away major nerves and vascular structures as opposed to invading them. Dynamic contrast-enhanced MR studies with rapid image acquisition after intravenous bolus administration of Gd-DTPA is very valuable. It can distinguish between benign from malignant soft tissue tumors, monitor patient's response to chemotherapy, guide biopsy procedures, and detect local tumor recurrence early (Figure 1).[12]

Computed tomography (CT) also has its place in the evaluation of soft tissue sarcomas. It can be used where MRI is contraindicated (i.e., the presence of metal foreign bodies, pacemakers, etc.). Thin cut and reconstruction software allow a better spatial resolution and characterization of these tumors, especially in the retroperitoneum. Since the lung is the most common site of metastatic spread, CT thorax is an integral part of the staging workup.[13] (Figure 2 and 3) New modalities include the use of Positron Emission Tomography (PET) scan for full body evaluation of spread. Sarcomas are metabolically active tumors and avidly capture the radionuclide tracer (16-Fluoro-deoxy-glucose). Recent studies have shown that the magnitude of clinical response to Imatinib against metastatic GIST can be followed effectively with PET (Figure 4).[14]

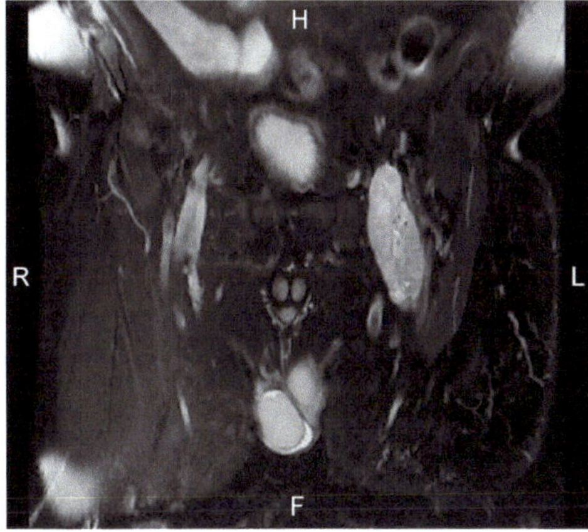

Figure 1: Magnetic Resonance Imaging (MRI) of left groin mass located inside the left common femoral vein. Wide local excision with extensive venous reconstruction was performed afterwards, pathology showing an intraluminal Leiomyosarcoma.

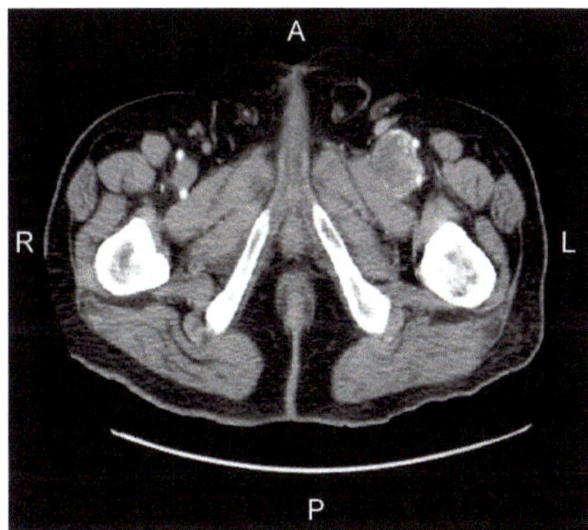

Figure 2: Computed Tomography (CT) of the same tumor showing its anatomical relationships with the rest of the neurovascular bundle.

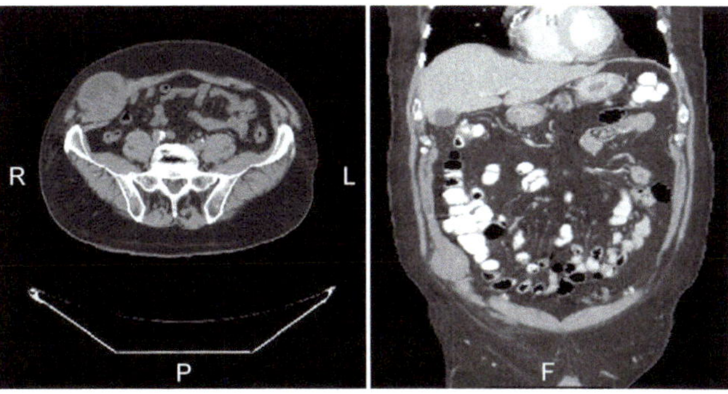

Figure 3: Computed Tomography (CT) of abdominal wall Malignant Fibrous Histiocytoma. The use of fine cuts and software allow the reconstruction in different orthogonal planes which are important in preoperative planning.

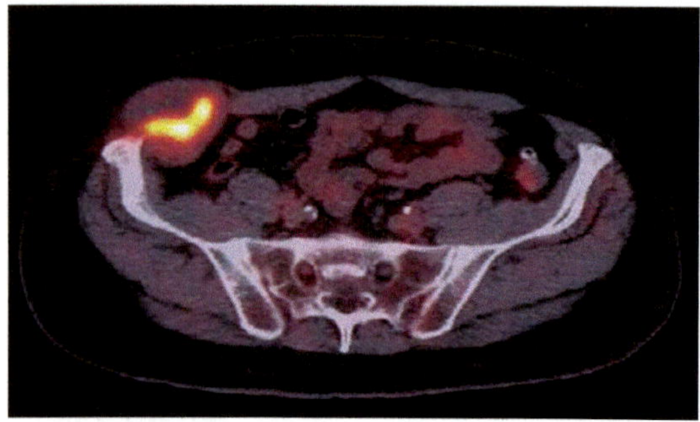

Figure 4: Positron Emission Tomography of the same tumor seen in Figure 3, showing metabolic activity that can be used for further follow up. Whole body tomography did not reveal any other areas of abnormal activity.

Figure 5: Initial evaluation of soft tissue sarcomas

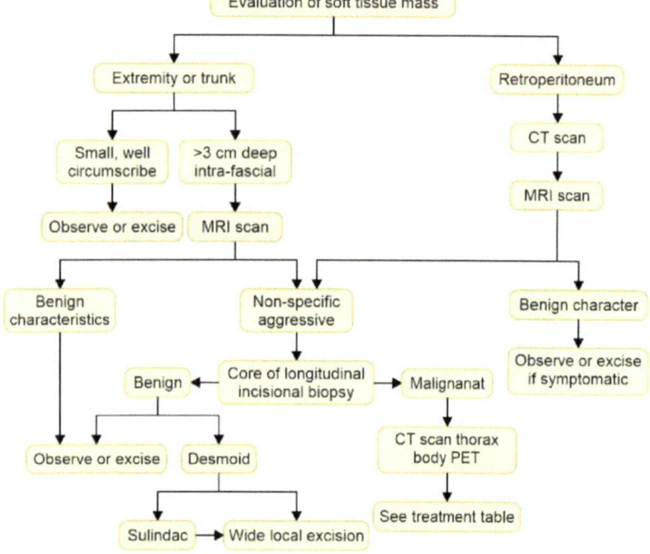

Staging of Soft Tissue Sarcomas

Tissue diagnosis of sarcomas must be achieved in an orderly and systematic fashion and should be made by the surgeon that will attempt its complete resection. Core needle biopsies deliver sufficient tissue for adequate diagnosis. For larger tumors, an incision biopsy can be performed following the long axis of a limb. Importantly this will not compromise subsequent stages, allowing for the incorporation of the resulting scar in the specimen during the definitive resection.

Regardless of the etiologic factors that induce the appearance of soft tissue sarcomas (STS) it is of great importance to determine the lineage of the tumor, as it may have implication for a specific treatment (i.e., gastrointestinal stromal tumors and its susceptibility to imatinib therapy). The World Health Organization (WHO) classification includes over 50 histological subtypes, however the distinction between tumors is not always clear. Table 4. Summarizes the five major subtypes of STS according to the national surveillance database and includes more than two thirds of all diagnosis. Once confirmation of diagnosis has been achieved the health care provider will now perform studies to assess initial staging and incorporate the patient into a multidisciplinary program for multimodal treatment.

Table 4: Surveillance, Epidemiology and End Results (SEER) Database (1978-2001) National Cancer Institute

Histology	Linage	Percentage
Leiomyosarcoma	Smooth muscle cells	23.7%
Malignant fibrous histiocytoma	Fibroblasts	17.1%
Liposarcoma	Adipose cells	11.5%
Dermatofibrosarcoma	Skin fibroblasts	10.5%
Rhabdomyosarcoma	Skeletal muscle cells	4.6%

A simplified version of AJCC (TNM) staging system is as follows.

Primary Tumor (T)

T1 < 5 cm

T2 > 5 cm

T2a superficial

T2b deep

Regional Lymph Nodes (N)

N0 none

N1 present

Distant metastasis

M0 none

M1 present

Histological grade

G1 differentiated well

G2 differentiated moderately

G3 differentiated poorly

G4 differentiated poorly with aggressive features or undifferentiated.

Several differences can be made between sarcomas and other types of cancer. First, of the different categories, grade is the most important prognostic factor in terms of predicting the local recurrence as well as presence of distant metastatic disease, and therefore is an integral part of the staging system.[15] Second, any nodal spread is considered metastatic disease. Figure 6 offers a simplified version of stage grouping. The 5-year survival for extremity sarcoma is 81% for localized disease, 56% for regional spread, and drops down to around 15% for distant metastasis.[16]

Table 5: Simplified Soft Tissue Sarcoma Staging system (modified from Makary 2008)

	T1A	T1B	T2A	T2B
Low Grade	I			
High Grade	II			III
N1	IV			
M1				

Treatment of Soft Tissue Sarcomas

Management is done by an experienced multidisciplinary team of specialists and, from the time of diagnosis, should be the standard of care. This team generally consists of a pathologist, radiologist, radiation and medical oncologist, and surgical and orthopedic oncologist who specialize in sarcoma treatment.[17] The overall treatment of soft tissue sarcomas remains a controversial topic as the anatomic site, histologic subtype, and treatment resources may dictate the need for a referral to a high-volume center to ensure a better patient outcome.[18] However, the principles of treatment remain the same, that is resection with wide margin. Due to the outward growth pattern, sarcomas compress surrounding tissue without infiltration, thus causing a pseudo capsule effect that can be mistaken as the margin of resection.[6] As said above the resection should include unaffected tissue surrounding the tumor for at least 1 cm with the fascia intact.[19] If the margin involves important structures such as vessels and nerves, these structures can be preserved as long as frozen sections are taken to assure no tumor involvement. However, preoperative planning is imperative as it may require a multidisciplinary team to allow oncologic clearance and reconstruction.

Table 6: Treatment table for soft tissue sarcomas

Clinical Scenario	Possible grade	Treatment	Follow up
Small tumor <5cm, low grade	I	Wide local excision with clear margins	Quarterly with annual CT-thorax for next 5 years, then Annual exam with CT-thorax
Large tumor >5cm, low grade	I	Wide local excision with clear margins Postoperative radiation	Quarterly with annual CT-thorax for next 5 years, then Annual exam with CT-thorax
Tumor <10cm, high grade	II	Wide local excision with clear margins Postoperative radiation	Quarterly with annual CT-thorax for next 5 years +/- PET, then Annual exam with CT-thorax
Tumor >10cm, high grade Retroperitoneal tumor or tumor close to vital structures	III	Preoperative radiation Wide local excision with clear margins Postoperative radiation +/- chemotherapy	Quarterly with annual CT-thorax for next 5 years +/- PET, then Annual exam with CT-thorax
Metastatic Disease	IV	Palliative care Palliative radiation with resection	

Alternatively preoperative adjuvant therapy can be used to downstage a locally advanced tumor affecting vital structures or involving the retroperitoneum. This in theory would allow an easier surgery with better outcome. Indications for postoperative radiation include tumors that are >5 cm, high grade, resections with close margins and/or close to vital structures that were not sacrificed.[20]

Despite the use of doxorubicin or ifosfamide-based chemotherapy, resection has not proven a significant impact in survivability for soft tissue sarcomas.[21] However, as we further understand the biology behind sarcomatogenesis new drugs are in development. Imatinib mesylate (STI571) has proven to be very effective as a general inhibitor of c-KIT, platelet growth factor receptor (PDGFR) and Bcr-Abl receptor tyrosine kinases. It has been proven to be an enormous success against both local and metastatic Gastrointestinal Stromal Tumors (GIST) with relatively low toxicity.

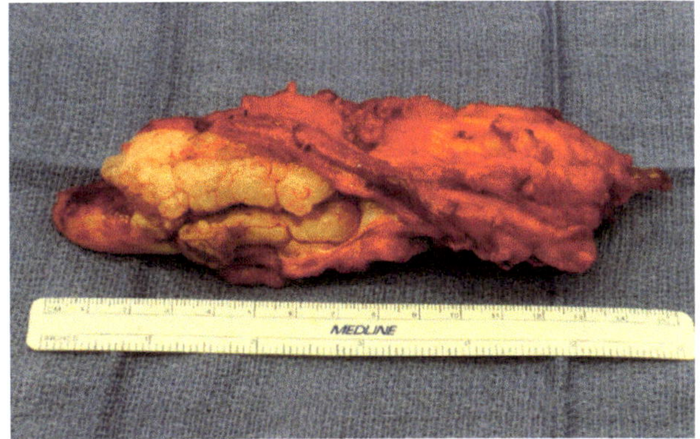

Figure 6: Intraluminal femoral vein leiomyosarcoma tumor resected from patient shown on Figures 1 and 2. Notice that a portion of the Superficial Femoral Artery (SFA) had to be sacrificed to achieve complete oncologic resection. Patient required extensive arterial and venous reconstruction using contralateral saphenous vein graft. His treatment was later completed with post-adjuvant chemotherapy.

New Strategies

After the success of Imatinib against GIST, new insights into the biology of sarcomas have allowed us to identify further therapeutic targets. Vascular Endothelial Growth Factor is a protein that is responsible for tumor angiogenesis and is expressed in both ligand and receptor form in several sarcomas, thus it is thought that the monoclonal antibody Bevacizumab (Avastin) is a suitable target against VEGF, although with poor results.[22] Similarly, thalidomide has immunomodulatory and antiangiogenic effects and has been used against Kaposi's Sarcoma. Sirolimus which can inhibit mTOR (Mammalian target of rapamycin) can regulate several proteins during mitosis and can produce a cell cycle arrest in G1 phase has been used in clinical trials against bone sarcomas, leiomyosarcomas, and liposarcomas.[23] Newer targeted therapies like Pazopanib have been developed and have shown some promise in the treatment of soft tissue sarcomas.[24]

Because of the rarity of these tumors, the difficulty remains in performing a well powered randomized placebo-controlled trial with all the different therapeutic combinations and sequences. The molecular biology study of these tumors has allowed further insight of oncogenesis of all cancers and thus the arrival of a new generation of powerful biological drugs with better clinical responses and a smaller side effect profile. Perhaps these drugs can substitute the way we treat cancer in general.

REFERENCES

1. Dvm AJ, Tiwari RC, Murray T, et al. *Cancer Statistics, 2004*. Vol 54.; 2004. Accessed May 3, 2021. http://caonline.amcancersoc.org.
2. Hui JYC. Epidemiology and Etiology of Sarcomas. *Surg Clin North Am*. 2016;96(5):901-914. doi: 10.1016/j.suc.2016.05.005.
3. Siegel RL, Miller KD, Jemal A. Cancer statistics, 2015. *CA Cancer J Clin*. 2015;65(1):5-29. doi:10.3322/caac.21254.
4. Lawrence W, Donegan WL, Natarajan N, Mettlin C, Beart R, Winchester D. Adult soft tissue sarcomas: A pattern of care survey of the American College of Surgeons. *Ann Surg*. 1987;205(4):349-359. doi:10.1097/00000658-198704000-00003.
5. Radons J. Inflammatory stress and sarcomagenesis: A vicious interplay. *Cell Stress Chaperones*. 2014;19(1):1-13. doi:10.1007/s12192-013-0449-4.
6. Brennan MF, Singer S, Maki RG OB. No Title. In: *Sarcomas of the Soft Tissue and Bone, in DeVita VT (Ed): Cancer: Principles and Practice of Oncology, Ed 7. Philadelphia, PA: Lippincott Williams and Wilkins*. Lippincott Williams and Wilkins; 2005:1581-1637.
7. Huang J, Mackillop WJ. Increased risk of soft tissue sarcoma after radiotherapy in women with breast carcinoma. *Cancer*. 2001;92(1):172-180. doi:10.1002/1097-0142(20010701)92:1<172:AID-CNCR1306>3.0.CO;2-K.
8. McClain KL, Leach CT, Jenson HB, et al. Association of Epstein–Barr Virus with Leiomyosarcomas in Young People with AIDS. *N Engl J Med*. 1995;332(1):12-18. doi:10.1056/nejm199501053320103.
9. Radiation-Induced Sarcoma: Diagnosis, Treatment and Prognosis. Accessed May 3, 2021. http://sarcomahelp.org/radiation-induced-sarcoma.html.
10. Van der Woude HJ, Bloem JL, Van Oostayen JA, et al. Treatment of high-grade bone sarcomas with neoadjuvant chemotherapy: The utility of sequential color Doppler sonography in predicting histopathologic response. *Am J Roentgenol*. 1995;165(1):125-133. doi:10.2214/ajr.165.1.7785571.
11. Elias DA, White LM, Simpson DJ, et al. Osseous invasion by soft-tissue sarcoma: Assessment with MR imaging. *Radiology*. 2003;229(1):145-152. doi:10.1148/radiol.2291020377.
12. Sanders TG, Parsons TW. Radiographic imaging of musculoskeletal neoplasia. *Cancer Control*. 2001;8(3):221-231. doi:10.1177/107327480100800302.
13. Aga P, Singh R, Parihar A, Parashari U. Imaging Spectrum in Soft Tissue Sarcomas. *Indian J Surg Oncol*. 2011;2(4):271-279. doi:10.1007/s13193-011-0095-1.
14. Kumar R, Chauhan A, Vellimana AK, Chawla M. Role of PET/PET-CT in the management of sarcomas. *Expert Rev Anticancer Ther*. 2006;6(8):1241-1250. doi:10.1586/14737140.6.8.1241.
15. Coindre J, Terrier P, Guillou L, et al. Predictive value of grade for metastasis development in the main histologic types of adult soft tissue sarcomas: a study of 1240 patients from the French Federation of Cancer Centers Sarcoma Group. *Cancer Interdiscip Int J Am Cancer Soc*. 2001;91(10):1914-1926.
16. Howlader N, Noone AM, Krapcho M, et al. SEER cancer statistics review, 1975–2017. *Natl Cancer Inst*. Published online 2020.

17. Gamboa AC, Gronchi A, Cardona K. Soft tissue sarcoma in adults: An update on the current state of histiotype specificmanagementinaneraofpersonalized medicine. *CA Cancer J Clin.* 2020;70(3):200-229. doi:10.3322/caac.21605.
18. Maurice MJ, Yih JM, Ammori JB, Abouassaly R. Predictors of surgical quality for retroperitoneal sarcoma: Volume matters. *J Surg Oncol.* 2017;116(6):766-774. doi:10.1002/jso.24710.
19. Geer RJ, Woodruff J, Casper ES, Brennan MF. Management of Small Soft-Tissue Sarcoma of the Extremity in Adults. *Arch Surg.* 1992;127(11):1285-1289. doi:10.1001/archsurg.1992.01420110027007.
20. Haas RLM, Delaney TF, O'Sullivan B, et al. Radiotherapy for management of extremity soft tissue sarcomas: Why, when, and where? *Int J Radiat Oncol Biol Phys.* 2012;84(3):572-580. doi: 10.1016/j.ijrobp.2012.01.062.
21. Verma S, Younus J, Stys-Norman D, Haynes AE, Blackstein M. Ifosfamide-based combination chemotherapy in advanced soft-tissue sarcoma: A practice guideline. *Curr Oncol.* 2007;14(4):144-148. doi:10.3747/co.2007.130.
22. Ray-Coquard IL, Domont J, Tresch-Bruneel E, et al. Paclitaxel given once per week with or without bevacizumab in patients with advanced angiosarcoma: A randomized phase II trial. *J Clin Oncol.* 2015;33(25):2797-2802. doi:10.1200/JCO.2015.60.8505.
23. Demetri GD, Chawla SP, Ray-Coquard I, et al. Results of an International Randomized Phase III Trial of the Mammalian Target of Rapamycin Inhibitor Ridaforolimus Versus Placebo to Control Metastatic Sarcomas in Patients after Benefit from Prior Chemotherapy. In: *Journal of Clinical Oncology.* Vol 31. American Society of Clinical Oncology; 2013:2485-2492. doi:10.1200/JCO.2012.45.5766.
24. Lee ATJ, Jones RL, Huang PH. Pazopanib in advanced soft tissue sarcomas. *Signal Transduct Target Ther.* 2019;4(1):1-10. doi:10.1038/s41392-019-0049-6.

❑❑❑

22

CHAPTER

Benign Breast Diseases

Neelima Rehil, MD
Vijay K. Mittal, MD

INTRODUCTION

Many women will experience benign breast diseases during their lifetime. This makes it essential to properly work-up these patients to differentiate benign and malignant diseases to reduce unnecessary anxiety. Breast has cells of different origin and are responsible for different benign lesion. These lesions have appreances of malignant tissue and proper workup is required to diagnosis. In the following section, we will discuss various types of benign lesions of the breast and the workup required to properly diagnose such lesions.

Screening

Detection of breast masses and abnormalities is essential in the proper diagnosis and treatment of both malignant and benign diseases. Screening is an invaluable tool in identifying breast lesions that allows for the early detection of breast cancer. This is imperative in order to achieve the best outcomes with treatment, as well as early detection and diagnosis of benign lesions. The breast self-examination (BSE) is an examination that should be performed by patients in the comfort of their own home. The exam consists of palpation of the breasts and axillae to detect irregularities. It is recommended that women perform such an exam monthly to assess for any changes in the breast that may occur with their menstrual cycles, as well as any new lesions or abnormalities.

In addition to the breast self-examination, female patients should have an annual breast exam in a clinical setting by their primary care provider. Patients with a known history of breast cancer or other breast lesions, who have undergone lumpectomy or excision should follow-up regularly with their surgeon in the clinical setting for examination. Patients over the age of 40 should also undergo an annual mammogram to evaluate for microcalcifications or other abnormalities.

Imaging

Many imaging modalities have been found useful in identifying both benign and malignant lesions of the breast, including mammography, ultrasound, magnetic resonance imaging and computed tomography. Among these, the most commonly used imaging for both screening and diagnostic purposes are mammography and ultrasound.

Mammography

The only breast imaging modality which has been proven to reduce breast cancer mortality is mammography. Mammography can be used both for screening and diagnostic purposes. Screening mammography is used to detect for early clinically occult lesions in asymptomatic patients. Due to the limitations of screening mammography in younger patients with more dense breast tissue, annual screening is not recommended to begin until the age of 40. In women with a higher risk of breast cancer, such as those with a strong family history, annual screening mammography can be started at an earlier age. Though no upper age limit for screening mammography has been established, patients older than 70 years with comorbidities reducing life expectancy to less than 10 years are no longer recommended to undergo screening.

Diagnostic mammography is used in patients who have a clinical complaint such as a palpable mass, discharge, focal pain, or whose screening mammography was abnormal. Diagnostic mammography for an abnormal screening mammogram is conducted by the radiologist and involves spot and roll views, with or without magnification which help to determine if lesion on the initial exam was present or due to overlapping of normal breast tissue. If lesions are confirmed on diagnostic mammography, they are assigned a Breast Imaging Reporting and Data System (BI-RADS) score which will determine the need for patient follow up and possible surgical intervention shown in Table 1.

Table 1: American College of Breast Imaging Reporting and Data Collections (BI-RADS) classification of diagnostic mammography findings

Category	Assessment	Recommendation
0	Additional imaging required	Additional imaging recommended
1	Negative finding	Routine screening recommended
2	Benign finding	Routine screening recommended
3	Probably benign finding	Short interval follow-up suggested for stability
4	Suspicious abnormality	Probability of malignancy, biopsy should be considered
5	Abnormality highly suggestive of malignancy	High probability of cancer, appropriate action should be taken
6	Biopsy proven malignancy	Appropriate treatment for malignancy

Breast Ultrasound

High frequency ultrasonography is usually used in conjunction with mammography in the diagnosis of breast lesions and serves as a follow-up modality. The main role of ultrasound in breast imaging is to aid in diagnosis after a screening mammogram returns an abnormal result. Breast ultrasound is useful in distinguishing between solid and cystic lesions and in diagnosing breast lesions in younger patients due to limitations of mammography in dense breast tissue.

In solid breast lesions, or patients with BI-RADS scores of 4 or 5, it is important to obtain a tissue sample in order to properly diagnose a lesion. Ultrasound-guided core needle biopsy is a beneficial modality to use when a mass is visualized sonographically, as it is relatively inexpensive and requires no exposure to harmful radiation.

MRI

Magnetic resonance imaging uses strong magnetic fields and peripheral intravenous administration of gadolinium-based contrast to create cross-sectional images to detect breast masses. MRI is useful in detecting both in situ and invasive breast carcinomas, as it is highly sensitive for both. MRI has also been noted to be useful in detecting mammographically occult lesions in the ipsilateral breast.

Due to its sensitivity, MRI was initially thought to be an invaluable tool during initial diagnosis of breast lesions and in identifying recurring lesions. Though MRI is still used in imaging of breast lesions, recent literature has questioned its benefits and costs in comparison to mammography and ultrasound imaging. A study published in the Journal of Clinical Oncology in January 2008, involved 756 patients who were diagnosed with early-stage invasive breast carcinoma or carcinoma in situ and underwent breast conservation therapy. Of the 756 patients, 215 women had an MRI study in addition to mammography and ultrasound. In the 5-year follow-up, no significant difference in failure rate or overall survival in the patients that had an initial MRI and those patients that did not.[11]

The same trends in magnetic resonance imaging have been noted in patients in which recurring lesions were identified and required reoperation. A randomized controlled trial published in February 2010 from the United Kingdom demonstrated that the addition of MRI to conventional imaging such as mammography and ultrasound was not associated with reduced rate of reoperation and was therefore an unnecessary expense.[12] As studies into the efficacy and cost of MRI will continue, magnetic resonance imaging used in addition to conventional mammography and ultrasound still remains an option for breast imaging and is most commonly used at the discretion of the surgeon.

Benign Breast Lesions

Benign breast disease is often classified into non-proliferative, atypical hyperplastic, proliferative, and miscellaneous lesions. These lesions are separated based on the degree of atypia and cellular proliferation of a lesion and its propensity for becoming breast cancer. Non-proliferative lesions are common but does not change the risk of becoming breast cancer. Proliferative lesions without atypia are the most commonly seen benign breast lesion and have a small increase in developing into breast cancer risk. Atypical hyperplasia has a moderate to high risk of becoming breast cancer, especially when patients present with a strong family history of breast cancer.[3] Miscellaneous lesions range from simple lipomas to more complex lesions which can mimic malignancy, but they generally have no association with increased risk of breast cancer.

Non-proliferative Breast Lesions

Non-proliferative breast lesions are epithelial lesions that have very little to no association with the development of breast cancer. Some common non-proliferative lesions include breast cysts, fibrocystic disease, chronic cystic mastitis, and mammary dysplasia.

Breast Cysts

Cysts are the most common type of non-proliferative breast lesion. These lesions are round or ovoid fluid-filled masses noted most commonly during physical exam or as a mammographic anomaly. Cysts occur mostly in patients between 35 and 50 years of age and may cause sudden onset of severe, localized pain if they become acutely enlarged. Generally, breast cysts are divided into three categories: simple cysts, complicated cysts, and complex cysts.

Simple Cysts

Simple breast cysts are non-fixed, round masses, generally non-painful and benign by definition. Cysts are very common in women of all ages and can present as multiple cysts in the ipsilateral or contralateral breast. Diagnosis of simple cysts is usually made by ultrasonography, especially in younger patients. They are easily identified on ultrasound of the breast as anechoic, circumscribed lesions with posterior acoustic enhancement and an absence of solid components (Figure 1).[3]

In patients who have no discomfort or pain caused by the cyst, no intervention is necessary. Symptomatic patients should have resolution of the cyst and symptoms with simple fine needle aspiration. Generally, fluid from simple cysts consists of clear or serous, non-purulent, non-bloody fluid.

In cases where bloody or purulent fluid is obtained, the specimen should be sent for culture and cytology. Simple cysts do recur and a second attempt at aspiration to reduce the cyst can be performed. If the cyst continues to recur, surgical excision is the next option for the patient, and is recommended when the recurrent lesion is associated with pain.

Complicated Cysts

Complicated cysts most commonly present as non-painful lumps or masses in the breast and, like simple cysts, are easily identified on ultrasound of the breast. Complicated cysts are defined by their appearance on breast ultrasound, having homogenous low level internal echoes due to echogenic debris, lacking solid components, thick walls, and vascular flow (Figure 2). Complicated cysts are sometimes visualized on mammography as well as ultrasound.[10]

These lesions are rarely malignant but should be followed up with imaging and clinical examination. A repeat mammogram, ultrasound and clinical exam should be performed every six months for the first two years after diagnosis to establish the stability of the lesion. Aspiration of a complicated cyst for diagnosis is indicated if the lesion resembles differentials including abscess, hematoma, galactocele, or fat necrosis. Fine needle aspiration or biopsy is also indicated if a lesion changes on follow up imaging, including increased size, new and different characteristics or the potential for a solid component cannot be ruled out.

Complex Cysts

Complex cysts are lesions with cystic and solid components as well as thick walls, or septa, measuring greater than 0.5 cm. On ultrasound, they demonstrate both anechoic and echogenic components. Inflamed or ruptured cysts, abscesses, hematomas, and fat necrosis often present as complex cysts, but malignancy cannot be ruled out in complex cysts and biopsy of the lesion is imperative in diagnosis.

Fine needle aspiration can be performed if a lesion is thought to be a simple cyst, however if a lesion has an obvious solid component, core needle biopsy under ultrasound guidance is a safe and accurate technique for diagnosis. A metal clip should be left in the biopsy site as a marker for follow up and potential surgical excision.

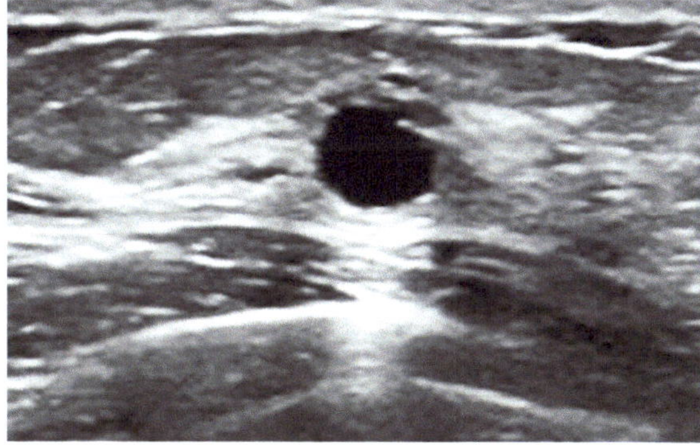

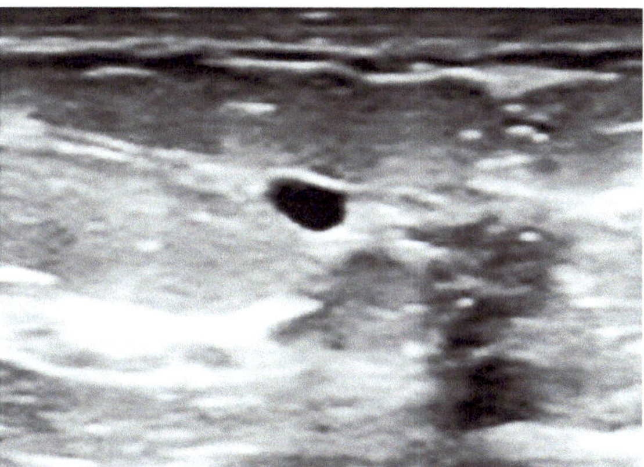

Figure 1: Ultrasound images of simple cysts

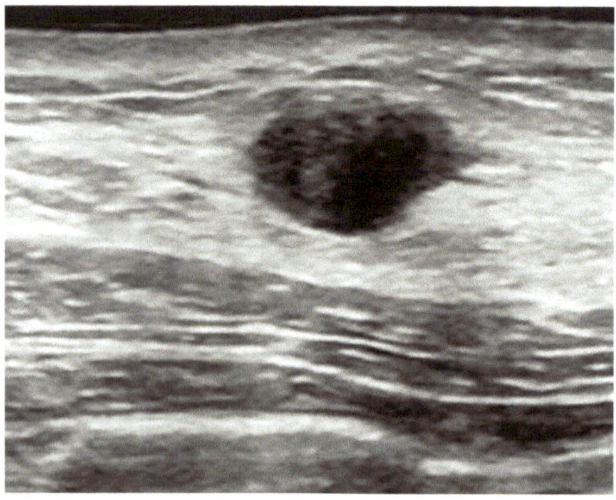

Figure 2: Ultrasound image of a complicated cyst with echogenic debris

Fibrocystic Condition

Fibrocystic disease, more recently referred to as fibrocystic condition, is the most common benign breast lesion. It commonly occurs in women between 30 and 50 years of age but is also known to occur in postmenopausal women taking hormone replacement therapy. Women who drink alcohol, especially those between 18 and 22 years of age also have an increased risk of developing this condition. Estrogen is thought to be a cause of the development of fibrocystic conditions.

Clinically, patients often present with one or more painful, palpable masses found bilaterally. Breast tissue in patients with fibrocystic change are often described as lumpy or having a cobblestone texture. The masses or lumps are smooth with well-defined edges and are most often non- fixed or free moving masses. Masses are most often found in the upper outer quadrant of the breast. Patients with fibrocystic change complain of persistent or intermittent pain that occurs most often in conjunction with their menstrual cycle. However, in some patients the masses may be asymptomatic and are only detected by screening in the office or at home.

Treatment for fibrocystic change is observation. Fibrocystic change in the breast is managed conservatively. Imaging with mammography (women >40 years old) and/or targeted ultrasound of the area of concern is necessary to rule out an underlying pathologic lesion. If both studies are negative or benign, a follow-up clinical exam in 3-6 months is advised. Associated mastodynia or breast pain can be alleviated by a properly fitting and supportive brassiere, cutting caffeine in the diet, a low fat and low salt diet, and NSAID's as necessary. This is a common condition among women and due to the alteration in size of the cysts with hormone fluctuation. The minimal breast cancer risk associated with this condition requires no aggressive treatment.

Proliferative Breast Lesions without Atypia

Fibroadenoma

Fibroadenomas are benign tumors showing evidence of both epithelial proliferation and proliferation of connective tissue. Clinically, they present as well-circumscribed rubbery, mobile, smooth masses. In 10 to 15 percent of patients, fibroadenomas present as multiple masses in the ipsilateral breast or bilaterally. Fibroadenomas are the most common cause of a new palpable breast mass in female patients under the age of 25. These benign tumors are considered an aberration of normal development resulting in hyperplasia or proliferation of a single terminal duct unit. About 10 percent of fibroadenomas spontaneously disappear each year and of those that do not, most only grow to be about 2-3 centimeters large.[8]

Imaging modality depends on patient factors including patient age at presentation. Ultrasonography is useful in diagnosis of fibroadenoma in patients younger than 30 years of age, patients with palpable masses or patients who are pregnant. Breast ultrasound of a fibroadenoma will demonstrate a hypoechoic mass with smooth, partially lobulated margins typical of a fibroadenoma. Mammography is generally useful in patients older than 30 and typically show well-circumscribed round or oval masses with coarse calcifications.[10] Magnetic resonance imaging is also useful in breast tissue to identify fibroadenomas and can be used to distinguish them from carcinomas. MRI reveals smooth masses which have high signal intensity on T2- weighted images and enhance with gadolinium-based contrast.[11]

Treatment of fibroadenomas ranges from conservative to invasive, depending on the certainty of diagnosis on imaging. Monitoring of the lesions with mammography and clinical exam does not expose patients to unnecessary risk, therefore it is common practice. In patients with rapidly growing fibroadenomas, lesions that cannot be distinguished from carcinoma, or suspicion for phyllodes tumor, more invasive treatment becomes necessary. Core needle biopsy can produce a definitive diagnosis and rule out phyllodes tumor, as well as carcinoma. The current recommendations for follow-up of fibroadenomas, whether diagnosed solely by imaging or with tissue biopsy confirmation, includes a clinical breast exam and targeted ultrasound every 6 months for 2 years to confirm stability of the mass.[23] If a presumed or biopsied fibroadenoma increases in size or is symptomatic, then excision is mandated to rule out malignant change and confirm the diagnosis. Enucleation of the fibroadenoma is an adequate initial treatment. Any finding of phyllodes tumor will warrant re-excision of cavity with at least 1 cm margins. Any incidental finding of a malignancy should be treated appropriately.[8]

Cryoablation and percutaneous excision are relatively new treatment modality which is effective and less invasive than open surgical excision. For accurate results, the American Society of Breast Surgeons recommends that the fibroadenomas being treated with either cryoablation or percutaneous excision if it is less than 4 centimeters in diameter, sonographically visible, and confirmed to be fibroadenomas on histology (Figures 3A and B). These procedures are convenient for patients as it takes little time and can be performed in an office setting. For cryoablation, an ultrasound is used to allow for image guided insertion of the cryoablation probe which is inserted through a small 3-millimeter incision. Once inside, the probe reaches extremely cold temperatures of less than 40 degrees Centigrade and destroys the fibroadenoma and a small margin of surrounding tissue. After removing the probe, the skin is dressed, and patients can go home.[9] Cryoablation can be used on multiple fibroadenomas in the same setting with enough allotted time to treat each lesion.

Ultrasound-guided percutaneous vacuum-assisted core biopsy of fibroadenomas has become widely available. The procedure allows the removal of all sonographically imaged tumors with a hand-held, large-bore, vacuum-assisted biopsy device. Initial success rates are reported at 75-100%.[20,21]

Patients undergoing cryoablation or percutaneous excision of a fibroadenoma should have clinical follow up by the treating physician. Treatment for local recurrence of a fibroadenoma is re-excision because of the small risk of a more active tumor. If recurrence is elsewhere in the breast, this mass should be followed up based on the same principles as the original fibroadenoma.[22]

Juvenile Fibroadenoma

Juvenile fibroadenomas are fibroadenomas which occur in a young patient population, usually in females under the age of 18. They tend to grow more aggressively than fibroadenomas in adults and in some cases result in deformity of the breast. Juvenile fibroadenomas are often referred to as giant fibroadenomas or giant juvenile adenomas due to their size and growth and are on occasion mistaken for phyllodes tumors. Histologically, juvenile fibroadenomas are not different from common fibroadenomas. They are composed of stromal and epithelial hyperplastic tissue and lack the leaf-like growth pattern and stromal atypia of phyllodes tumors.[8] Ultrasonogram demonstrates a hypoechoic mass with smooth, partially lobulated margins typical of a fibroadenoma.

Due to the size and rapid growth of juvenile fibroadenomas, surgical excision is the best choice of treatment. Patients are young and deformities of the breast tissue can be easily reduced with resection of the mass. The nature of the juvenile adenoma to mimic phyllodes tumor is also an indication for excision so proper diagnosis can be made in pathology.

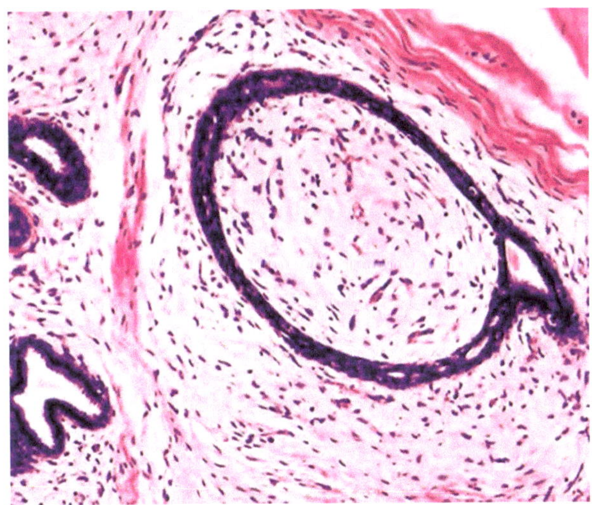

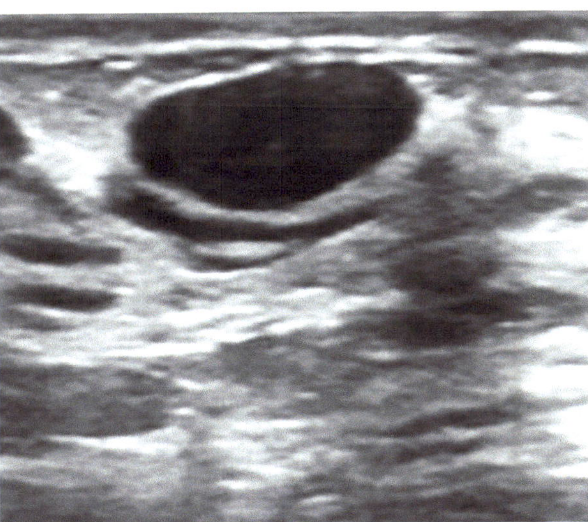

Figure 3: Histological and ultrasonographic appearance of a fibroadenoma

Atypical Hyperplasia

Atypical hyperplasia is usually an incidental finding discovered after biopsy of a radiographic abnormality on mammogram or ultrasound. Hyperplasia can be divided into proliferative lesions affecting the ducts or atypical ductal hyperplasia and lesions affecting the lobules, or atypical lobular hyperplasia. Atypical hyperplasia is associated with an increased risk of developing breast cancer. In most cases where advancement to breast cancer occurs, the ipsilateral breast is involved, however disease has been known to occur in the contralateral breast as well. Once diagnosis is made with core-needle biopsy, areas of atypical hyperplasia in the breast should be surgically excised and examined more closely. Analysis of a larger tissue sample may result in an upgrade of the diagnosis to ductal carcinoma in situ (DCIS) or invasive breast cancer in 10 to 20 percent of cases depending on the gauge of the needle used at percutaneous biopsy and the number of cores procured.[24,25]

Women diagnosed with atypical hyperplasia should be counseled on breast cancer risk reduction strategies. Surveillance with annual mammography and breast exams every 6 months is essential for early detection of abnormal tissues suspicious for breast cancer. Patients with atypical hyperplasia who are taking oral contraceptive pills or other types of hormone therapy should discontinue them immediately. Women with additional factors for developing breast cancer may be candidates for breast cancer risk reduction therapies including tamoxifen and raloxifene.

Miscellaneous Breast Lesions

Phyllodes Tumor

Phyllodes tumor, also known as cystosarcoma phyllodes, a term derived from the Greek for 'leaf-like fleshy tumor' is a predominantly benign breast tumor found in females. Grossly, phyllodes tumors resemble malignant sarcoma, however when it is sectioned it displays a unique leaf-like appearance and histologically consists of epithelial cyst- like spaces (Figure 4). The tumors have a smooth, well- demarcated texture, are freely mobile and tend to recur. Size varies from case to case, with the average tumors being 5 cm or smaller, however due to aggressive growth, some phyllodes tumors have been documented to reach substantially larger sizes of up to 30 cm.

Phyllodes tumor is the most commonly occurring nonepithelial breast tumor but is still a rare tumor as it only makes up 1 percent of all breast tumors. They occur almost exclusively in females, with no predilection for race. Though phyllodes tumors can occur in patients of all ages, they most often occur in the fifth decade of life. Patients present with a firm, well-circumscribed mass. The masses are usually nontender and mobile. Patients will commonly report a history of a small mass that rapidly changed size in a few weeks' time. Phyllodes tumors occur more in the left breast than in the right breast, however, the cause for this is unknown.

Though almost 90 percent of phyllodes tumors are benign, they are grossly indistinguishable from their malignant counterparts. Malignant phyllodes tumors metastasize through hematogenous spread, with the lungs being the most susceptible organ affected. The skeleton, heart, and liver are other organs where malignant phyllodes tumors tend to metastasize. Patients with metastasis of malignant disease present with symptoms of dyspnea, fatigue, and bone pain.

Imaging such as mammogram and ultrasonography is not reliable in the diagnosis of phyllodes tumor due to its propensity to look like malignant sarcoma, therefore, a more invasive approach is required.[5] Although needle biopsy and core needle biopsy are options, they are usually inadequate for diagnosis and a surgical biopsy is required. In small lesions, excisional biopsy with margins is both diagnostic and therapeutic, while in large lesions, incisional biopsy is indicated until the diagnosis is confirmed histologically.[6,13]

Phyllodes tumors have a stromal and fibrous component and can appear similar to fibroadenomas, except for the clefts found in the walls of the tissue. Benign phyllodes tumors will demonstrate a large number of fusiform fibroblasts in the stromal tissue, and occasionally anaplastic cells with myxoid changes. Malignant phyllodes tumors will demonstrate a high degree of cellular atypia with increased mitotic count and increased stromal cellularity.

Treatment for phyllodes tumor is a wide excisional biopsy with margins of normal tissue. Wide local excision entails margins of at least 1 cm to minimize local recurrence. The surgical specimen should be oriented so as to guide subsequent re-excision if necessary. It is important to remove the tumor and its wall without shelling out the lesions, as recurrence is much more likely when components of the phyllodes tumor are left behind. In cases where the breast is markedly distorted, a mastectomy can be performed with reconstruction, however, in most cases of phyllodes tumor, a minimal resection is recommended.[6] Any local recurrence of a phyllodes tumor warrants re-excision with at least 1 cm margins with or without radiation to help avoid the morbidity of yet another recurrence and the need for additional aggressive surgical intervention. Chest imaging to rule out lung metastasis is advised prior to excision, especially in malignant cases.[23]

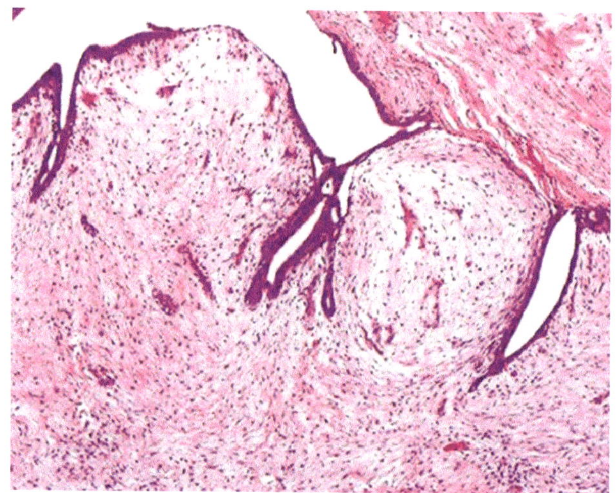

Figure 4: Histological appearance of phyllodes tumor

Breast Abscess

Breast abscesses are painful benign masses with surrounding erythema which arise spontaneously and have a sudden onset.

Breast abscesses often have an area of fluctuance or are found to be draining pus and typically localize to the lower half of the breast. These lesions tend to occur more often in patients who have large breasts, are overweight, or have poor personal hygiene. These patients may have a long history of similar abscesses in the breast, or other areas of the body. Diabetic patients with poor sugar control are also at higher risk for developing abscesses and should be treated aggressively.

Abscesses are caused by bacterial colonization in either in the central breast or in the periphery triggering an inflammatory reaction and collection of neutrophils, white blood cells, and bacteria in a localized area of the breast resulting in a painful mass. Diagnosis of breast abscess is based on the history of the lesion and clinical examination. Patients present with a sudden onset of painful, growing mass that may be associated with fever and drainage of pus. The lesions usually present with a central area of fluctuance with surrounding erythema and induration and may have a history of purulent drainage. Ultrasound confirms the diagnosis. Nipple discharge consisting of pus or blood is concerning and requires a breast ultrasound to evaluate the abscess cavity as well as follow up with a surgeon to further work up the lesion and rule out breast carcinoma as a cause. Once the diagnosis of abscess is made definitively, several options are available for treatment. If the overlying skin is normal and ultrasound confirms simple abscess measuring < 5 cm, then aspiration of the abscess under ultrasound guidance using generous local anesthesia is the preferred method of management. Infiltration and irrigation with local anesthetic reduces pain and the use of epinephrine reduces subsequent bruising.[26] If the overlying skin is compromised or the abscess is > 5 cm, or complex looking on ultrasound, open surgical drainage with local anesthetic will be required.Wound cultures should be taken at the time of incision and followed for culture and sensitivity so the appropriate antibiotic can be administered.[7] If the abscess cavity is small and the patient shows no signs of systemic effect or increase in white blood cell count, empiric antibiotics may be given orally to the patient with instructions to follow up as an outpatient. In cases where the white cell count is elevated above normal limits, if patients are febrile or immunocompromised, or the areas of erythema and cellulitis are extensive, the patient should be admitted for intravenous antibiotics, fluid hydration and pain control.

Mastitis

Postpartum mastitis is a localized cellulitis that is caused by an irritated or fissured nipple resulting in bacterial invasion into the lactiferous sinuses and milk ducts. Patients generally present with a history of abrasion, trauma from breastfeeding, or a dry cracked nipple. Postpartum mastitis occurs in 2 to 3 percent of lactating women and most commonly occurs after the second postpartum week. Milk stasis plays a role in bacterial colonization as nutrients and temperature creates an ideal growth medium for bacteria once introduced. Stasis occurs when one breast is favored for breastfeeding due to positioning or infant preference.

The most common organism involved in postpartum mastitis is Staphylococcus aureus, however Staphylococcus epidermidis and streptococci are occasionally isolated as well. Treatment involves drainage of the affected segment by milking the breast or using a breast pump. Antibiotics that are effective on Staphylococcus species are prescribed as well. Warm compresses can be applied to the affected breast to reduce pain and aid in emptying of breast.[3] Lactating women should be encouraged to alternate breasts when feeding or pumping milk to avoid milk stasis.

Mastitis unassociated with lactation can be divided into peri-areolar lesions and peripheral lesions. Periductal mastitis is a condition in which nondilated subareolar breast ducts become inflamed and occur more commonly than peripheral nonlactating breast abscesses. Peripheral lesions are associated with conditions such as diabetes, rheumatoid arthritis, trauma and in patients who are being treated with steroids.[7] Patients present with localized erythema, warmth, and pain in addition to fever and chills. Ultrasound should be used to rule out an abscess or cystic mass. Treatment involves anti-staphylococcal antibiotics, followed by warm compresses and NSAIDs such as ibuprofen for control of pain and inflammation.[3]

Fat Necrosis

Fat necrosis is a condition of the breast that can easily mimic breast cancer and was first differentiated from breast carcinoma as early as 1924.[1] Fat necrosis of the breast is a result of enzymatic breakdown of the subcutaneous fatty tissue into fatty acids. It usually occurs secondary to trauma to the breast tissue but can occur spontaneously or less often as a result of diagnostic or therapeutic modalities involving the breast. Patients present with a painless, hard, indurated, fixed mass which has evolved over weeks to months after a traumatic event. The hard or firm nature of the mass and the appearance of fixation to the skin is due to the growth of new connective tissue in place of the lost subcutaneous fat. The masses often seem attached to deeper tissues as well, which is likely due to the inflammatory process involved in the necrosis. On occasion, the breakdown of subcutaneous fat can lead to the formation of an oil cyst, or a sac-like collection of greasy fluid composed of triglycerides and fatty acids.

Imaging used to evaluate lesions suspicious for fat necrosis includes ultrasonography (Figure 5) and mammogram. Ultrasonography reveals solid masses which may be complex or cystic with ill-defined or discrete borders, and posterior shadowing. On mammogram, the appearance of fat necrosis ranges from lesions which are radiographically benign to those which are suspicious for malignancy. Radiographically benign lesions present as radiolucent masses with thin, well-defined capsules, while those suspicious for malignancy are complex masses with ill-defined borders.[10]

Fine needle aspiration should be performed for lesions suspicious for carcinoma of the breast if radiological imaging is not definitive for breast necrosis. Histologically these lesions will demonstrate anuclear fat cells, unlike the atypia and increase in mitotic cells found in breast carcinoma. In radiographically benign lesions with areas of fluctuance, or oil cysts, aspiration can be therapeutic. Small masses, when left alone, tend to spontaneously resolve on their own over several months, where large lesions may require surgical excision of the area of necrosis, depending on patient preference and location of the lesion.

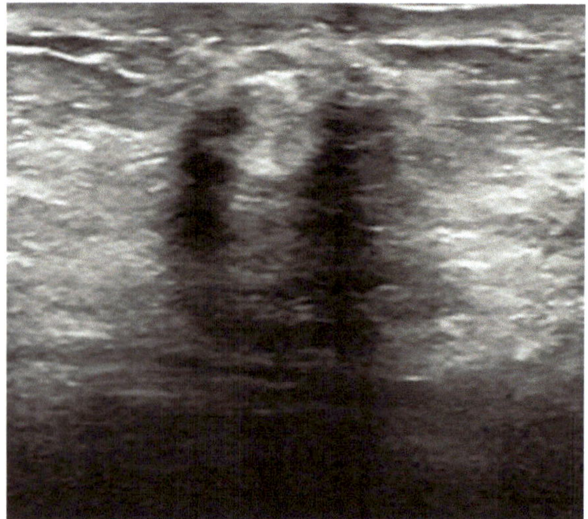

Figure 5: Ultrasound image of fat necrosis

Hamartoma

Breast hamartomas are often referred to as fibroadenolipomas, lipofibroadenomas or adenolipomas. They consist of normal breast parenchyma including glandular tissue, adipose tissue, and fibrous tissue, organized in a haphazard or unorganized fashion. Hamartomas of the breast are commonly discovered as an incidental finding on imaging but can also present in patients as discrete, painless, and encapsulated masses. Though these lesions are benign, coincidental malignancy can occur in the region of growth of a hamartoma, therefore excision is recommended to rule out malignancy on pathological specimens.

Galactocele

Galactoceles, also known as milk retention cysts, are collections of fluid consisting of breast milk which occur secondary to an obstruction of a milk duct. Patients present with a soft, round, mobile cystic mass, and a history of breastfeeding. Galactoceles usually occur when a patient cease breastfeeding or a significant change occurs in breast- feeding pattern and can occur weeks to months after cessation. The masses tend to be located centrally, just behind the nipple. Treatment is needle aspiration which will reveal a thick, creamy material. On occasion the aspirate is tinged brown or green, giving it the appearance of purulence, however this fluid is usually sterile, and aspiration alone is sufficient. In cases where an infection is present, showing signs of erythema, tenderness and possibly an elevated white blood cell count, or when a galactocele cannot be aspirated, excisional biopsy is indicated.

Intraductal Papilloma

Benign duct papillomas occur in 3 main forms: solitary (discrete), multiple, and juvenile. Solitary papillomas are the most common of the three and they usually will be found in a subareolar duct, and usually present as nipple discharge. Multiple papillomas are rare and more peripheral in location and have a greater malignant potential. Juvenile papillomatosis is very rare.[14]

Papillomas can harbor areas of atypia or ductal carcinoma in situ (DCIS). The standard recommendation for management of papillomas on core biopsy is surgical excision although there is some debate in the literature about this recommendation.[15,16]

When the diagnosis of papilloma is confirmed by surgical excision, additional treatment is not warranted. Unless there is associated atypia, there is not an increased risk of breast cancer recurrence.

Radial Scars

Radial scars, also known as complex sclerosing lesions, are diagnosed pathologically and are normally discovered incidentally as a breast mass on physical exam or radiological abnormality is removed or biopsied. Radial scars are characterized microscopically by a fibroelastic core with radiating ducts and lobules.

The recommendation for these lesions is that they be surgically excised since most series show that 8 to 17 percent of surgical specimens at subsequent excision are positive for malignancy.[17,18]

Aside from potentially finding an unrecognized in situ or invasive component, some studies show that radial scars are potentially premalignant lesions, meaning that they can slowly progress from scar to hyperplasia to carcinoma over time.[19]

Radial scars require no additional treatment beyond excision. The risk of subsequent breast cancer after excision is small and chemoprevention is not indicated.

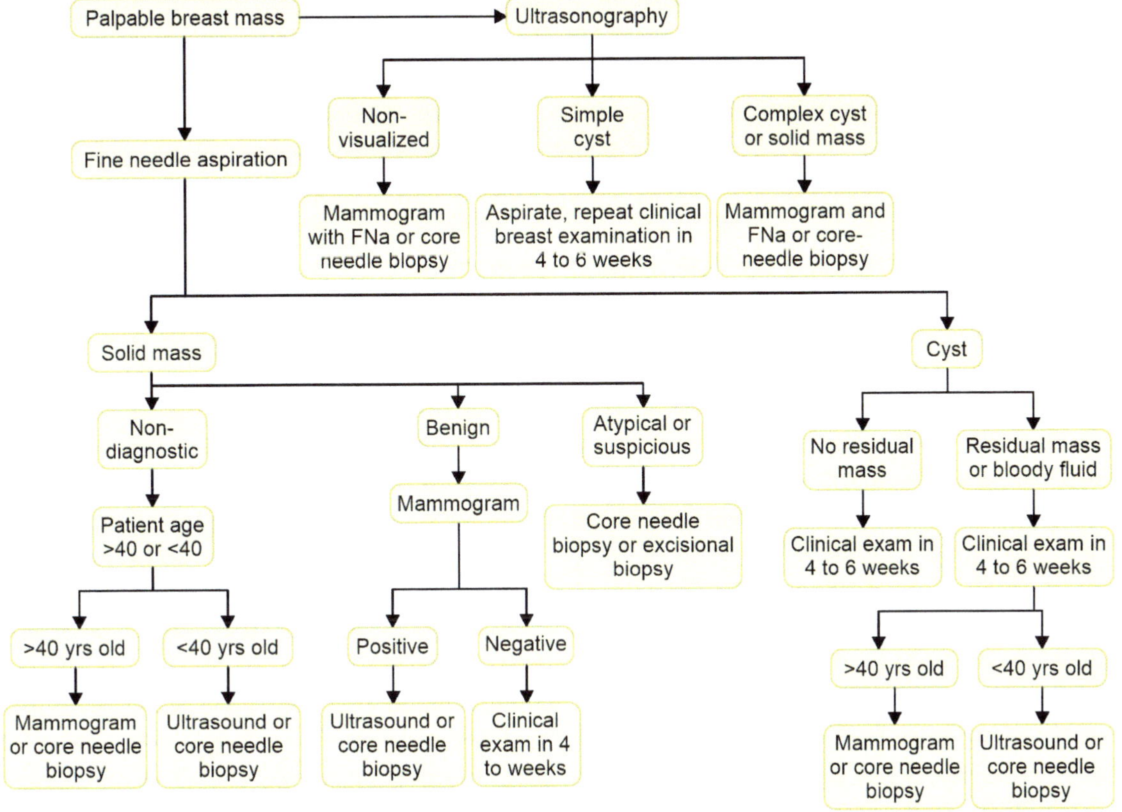

Figure 6: Algorithmic work-up of palpable breast mass

REFERENCES

1. Adair FE, Burton JL. Traumatic fat necrosis of the female breast and its differentiation from carcinoma. Ann Surg 1924;80(5):670–91.
2. American Cancer Society. Breast Cancer Facts and Figures 2007-2008. Available at http://www.cancer.org/downloads/STT/BCFF-Final.pdf.Accessed 06/04/2010.
3. Brennan M, Houssami N, French J. Management of benign breast conditions. Part 3—Other breast problems. Aust Fam Physician 2005;34(5): 353-5.
4. Brooks HL, Priolo S, Waxman. Cystosarcoma phylloides: a case report of an 11-year survival and review of surgical experience. Contemp Surg 1998;53:169-72.
5. Cole-Beuglet C, Soriano R, Kurtz AB. Ultrasound, x-ray mammography, and histopathology of cystosarcoma phylloides. Radiology 1983;146(2):481-6.
6. Chen WH, Cheng SP, Tzen CY, et al. Surgical treatment of phyllodes tumors of the breast: retrospective review of 172 cases. J Surg Oncol 2005;91(3):185-94.
7. Dixon JM. Outpatient treatment of non-lactational breast abscesses. Br J Surg 1992;79(1);56-7.
8. Greenberg R, Skornick Y, Kaplan O. Management of breast fibroadenomas. J Gen Intern Med 1998;13(9): 640-45.
9. Kaufman CS, Littrup PJ, Freeman-Gibb LA. Office-based cryoablation of breast fibroadenomas with long-term follow-up. Breast J 2005;11(5): 344-50.
10. Kerlikowske K, Smith-Bindman R, Ljung BM, et al. Evaluation of abnormal mammography results and palpable breast abnormalities. Ann Intern Med 2003;139(4):274-84.
11. Solin LJ, Orel SG, Hwang WT, Harris EE, Schnall MD. Relationship of breast magnetic resonance imaging to outcome after breast-conservation treatment with radiation for women with early-stage invasive breast carcinoma or ductal carcinoma in situ. Journal of Clinical Oncology 2008;26(3):386-91.
12. Turnbull L, Brown S, Harvey I, Olivier C, et al. Comparative effectiveness of MRI in breast cancer (COMICE) trial; a randomized controlled trial. Lancet 2010;(9714):563-71.

13. Wurdinger S, Herzog AB, Fischer DR. Differentiation of phyllodes breast tumors from fibroadenomas on MRI. AJR Am J Roentgenol 2005;185(5):1317-21.
14. Hughes, Mansel and Webster's Benign Disorders of the Breast 3rd ed. 2009 Elsevier limited. pp 213-216.
15. Lewis JT, Hartmann LC, et al. An analysis of breast cancer risk in women with single, multiple, and atypical papilloma. Am J Surg Pathol. 2006;30(6):665.
16. Valdes EK, Feldman SM, Boolbol SK. Papillary lesions: a review of the literature. Ann Surg Oncol. 2007;14(3):1009.
17. Kennedy M, Masterson AV, Kerin M, Flanagan F. Pathology and clinical relevance of radial scars: a review. J Clin Pathol. 2003;56(10):721
18. Linda A, Zuiani C, Furlan A, Londero V, Girometti R, Machin P, Bazzocchi M. Radial scars without atypia diagnosed at imaging-guided needle biopsy: how often is associated malignancy found at subsequent surgical excision, and do mammography and sonography predict which lesions are malignant? AJR Am J Roentgenol. 2010;194(4):1146.
19. Manfrin E, Remo A, Falsirollo F, Reghellin D, Bonetti F. Risk of neoplastic transformation in asymptomatic radial scar. Analysis of 117 cases. Breast Cancer Res Treat. 2008;107(3):371.
20. Thurley P, Evans A, Hamilton L, et al. Patient satisfaction and efficacy of vacuum-assisted excision biopsy of fibroadenomas. Clin Radiol 2009; 64:381-385.
21. Grady I, Gorsuch H, Wilburn-Bailey S. Long-term outcome of benign fibroadenomas treated by ultrasound-guided percutaneous excision. Breast J 2008; 14:275-278.
22. Mansel, Robert Edward, et al. "Hughes, Mansel & Webster's Benign Disorders and Diseases of the Breast." Amazon, Saunders, 2009, https://www.amazon.com/Hughes-Mansel-Websters-Disorders-Diseases/dp/B01K0S14AG.
23. Soft Tissue Sarcoma, Version 2.2012: Featured Updates to. https://www.unmc.edu/orthosurgery/images/J_Natl_Compr_Canc_Netw2012von_Mehren951_60_1.pdf.
24. Margenthaler JA, Duke D, Monsees BS, Barton PT, Clark C, Dietz. Correlation between core biopsy and excisional biopsy in breast high-risk lesions. Am J Surg. 2006;192(4):534.
25. Degnim AC, Visscher DW, Berman HK, Frost MH, Sellers TA, Vierkant RA, Maloney SD, Pankratz VS, de Groen PC, Lingle WL, Ghosh K, Penheiter L, Tlsty T, Melton LJ. Stratification of breast cancer risk in women with atypia: a Mayo cohort study. 3rd, Reynolds CA, Hartmann. J Clin Oncol. 2007;25(19):2671.
26. Ozseker B, Ozcan UA, Rasa K, Cizmeli OM. Treatment of breast abscesses with ultrasound-guided aspiration and irrigation in the emergency setting. Emerg Radiol. 2008;15(2):105.

❑❑❑

23

CHAPTER

Malignant Breast Diseases

Megan Nelson, MD
Vijay K. Mittal, MD

RISK FACTORS

Factors that increase the duration or quantity of estrogen exposure increase the likelihood of developing breast cancer. Early menarche, late menopause, and nulliparity are all high estrogen states due to a higher number of menstrual periods, which subsequently increases breast cancer risk.[1-2] Additionally obesity, alcohol use, and hormone replacement therapy increase the amount of estrogen exposure. Patients who undergo their first pregnancy after the age of 35 are also at increased risk.[3]

Non-hormonal factors have also been implicated in breast cancer risk. Radiation therapy predisposes women to development of breast cancer. First-degree relatives with breast cancer, a personal history of prior breast cancer, and certain genes substantially increase the risk as well.[4] Additionally, the presence of lobular carcinoma in situ or atypical hyperplasia increases the relative risk of breast cancer development fourfold.[5]

The average U.S. female has a 12% risk of developing breast cancer over the course of her life. As noted above, the risk for each woman is multifactorial. Several risk assessment models have been developed to assess individual risk.[6] The most commonly implemented model is the Gail Model, first developed by Gail and associates in the 1970s. The Claus model is another commonly used risk assessment tool that places heavier emphasis on family history of breast cancer.[7] Neither the Gail nor Claus model take into account specific genetic abnormalities, a risk factor that is gaining significance as further research is undertaken.

Based on the risk assessed, several medical decisions may be affected. Post-menopausal women at high risk for breast cancer may elect to abstain from hormone replacement therapy (HRT) for control of vasomotor symptoms that could otherwise be ameliorated with estrogen replacement. The Women's Health Initiative was a large-scale phase III trial that evaluated the effect of HRT on cardiovascular disease, bone health, and breast cancer. Based on results published in 2002, there were minimal protective cardiovascular effects of HRT, but a concerning three-fold increased risk of breast cancer when taken for greater than 4 years.[8]

Screening mammography is a noninvasive, cost-effective method for breast cancer detection. While recent recommendations have raised the age of screening mammography to 50 years, the American College of Surgeons continues to recommend screening mammography yearly for women greater than 40 years of age. The case for waiting to begin screening after the age of 50 years stems from an increased number of false-positive findings in women younger than 50 years as well as difficulty in reading the studies based on increased breast density in younger women.[9]

Tamoxifen, a selective estrogen receptor modulator, is currently recommended for women with a Gail relative risk greater than 1.70. In the Breast Cancer Prevention Trial (NSABP P-01) that looked at over 13,000 women with a Gail score greater than 1.7, breast cancer development was reduced by 49 percent in those who received Tamoxifen compared to the placebo group. Tamoxifen has been found to increase the risk of endometrial cancer development by 2.5%. Due to this adverse effect, Raloxifene (another selective estrogen receptor modulator) was compared to Tamoxifen with hopes of finding the same preventative effect on breast cancer but with a better side effect profile. In the STAR trial, 19,000 post-menopausal women at high risk for breast cancer were randomly assigned to treatment with Tamoxifen or Raloxifene. Both drugs were found to reduce the risk of breast cancer by half, but Raloxifene was not associated with as high a risk of developing endometrial cancer.[10-12]

Genetic Mutations

Genetic mutations such as BRCA1 and BRCA2 are associated with 5-10% of all breast cancers. These are autosomal dominant mutations that display variable penetrance. Both genes function as tumor suppressors, and loss of both alleles is necessary for cancer development. These genes are involved in transcription, cell-cycle control, and DNA damage repair. BRCA1 gene is found in chromosome 17q21. Mutations have been implicated in 45% of hereditary breast cancers and carry an associated lifetime risk of 40% for ovarian cancer development as well. Breast cancer secondary to BRCA1 mutations is associated with earlier onset, higher propensity for bilateral breast cancer, and the presence of other malignancies such as ovarian, colon, and prostate cancers.[13-16] Two specific mutations of the BRCA1 gene have been found in Jewish populations, specifically Ashkenazi Jews. 1% of Ashkenazi Jews carry the 185delAG mutation, sometimes in conjunction with the 5382insC mutation, and these have been implicated in almost all BRCA1 mutations in this particular population.[17]

BRCA2 is also a DNA damage repair gene found on chromosome arm 13q12.3, made up of 70 kb. It is believed to be co-regulated with BRCA1. Over 250 mutations of BRCA2 have been identified. BRCA2 infers an 85% lifetime risk of breast cancer development and is also associated with ovarian cancer. BRCA2 is of particular importance in male carriers, as it is associated with a 100- fold increase in breast cancer development compared to that of the general male population (6% risk). BRCA2 is associated with a higher incidence of invasive ductal carcinomas. Like BRCA1, carriers of BRCA2 are more likely to develop breast cancer at a young age and develop bilateral breast cancer. It is linked to a greater variety of associated cancers: ovarian, colon, prostate, pancreatic, gallbladder, stomach, and melanoma. It is found with increased incidence in Ashkenazi Jewish and Finnish populations.[13-14]

BRCA mutation testing should be considered in women diagnosed with breast cancer before the age of 45, before age 50 with family history of breast and/or ovarian cancer, with two breast primaries when the first breast cancer diagnosis occurred before age 50, triple negative breast cancer before 60, Ashkenazi Jewish, known BRCA mutation in the family, those who have concurrent breast and ovarian cancer, male breast cancer at any age, and those with a history of hereditary breast and ovarian cancer. Detailed family history should be obtained in all of these patients. In women without breast cancer, genetic testing is advised if there is a known BRCA mutation in the family, if there is suspicion of BRCA mutation in the family based on history and clustering of various cancers, or if she has a personal history of epithelial ovarian carcinoma.

The decision to proceed with genetic testing requires informed consent and must be preceded by appropriate counseling. The affected individual is tested via a panel of mutations, and once the mutation is identified, other family members may be tested specifically for the identified mutation. A positive test is one which finds a BRCA mutation that affects translation or transcription. If no mutation is identified, the woman carries an identical risk for developing breast cancer as that of the general population, and her children need not be tested for the mutation. The possibility of an unidentified genetic mutation remains. The Health Insurance Portability and Accountability Act (HIPAA) made it illegal for genetic information to be taken into account by insurance plans to deny coverage.[18-21]

Once a BRCA mutation has been identified, there are several options for risk management. These include prophylactic mastectomy with reconstruction, prophylactic oophorectomy with HRT, intensive surveillance for breast and ovarian cancer, and chemoprevention. Prophylactic mastectomy greatly reduces the risk for breast cancer, though any remaining breast tissue is still at risk. If intense surveillance is chosen, annual mammography and MRI should begin at age 25 for screening in unaffected women, and post-treatment in women already diagnosed with breast cancer. MRI is more sensitive for identifying masses in dense breast tissue of younger patients, but also leads to more identification of benign masses and subsequent false negatives. Tamoxifen has been suggested but has not been reliably found to decrease incidence of breast cancer with BRCA mutations. Tamoxifen is most effective on estrogen receptor (ER) positive cancers, and most breast cancers associated with BRCA mutations are ER negative.

The American College of Obstetrics and Gynecology recommends that BRCA1 or BRCA2 carriers consider a prophylactic oophorectomy after childbearing or after 35 years of age. In those who defer or delay oophorectomy, the Cancer Genetics Studies Consortium recommends yearly transvaginal ultrasound and annual serum cancer antigen 125 screens beginning at age 25. However, there is no reliable screening modality or test for ovarian cancer. Hereditary breast cancer is also associated with Cowden's disease and Li-Fraumeni syndrome, which are related to TP53 and PTEN gene mutations respectively.[18-22]

EPIDEMIOLOGY

Breast cancer is the most common cancer in women and is the leading cause of cancer death in women aged 20 to 59 years. Overall, it is surpassed only by lung cancer as the most frequent cause of death from cancer in all women. The probability of a woman in the United States developing breast cancer is now 1 in 8, increased from 1 in 13 in the 1970s. While the incidence of overall breast cancer has increased (in part due to greater detection via mammograms), the incidence of local metastasis and mortality from breast cancer has declined. Survival rates in the 1960s for Caucasian and African American women were 63% and 46% respectively, while in the late 1980s they were 85% and 71% respectively.

Breast cancer around the world varies greatly in incidence, from 29.6 per 100,000 in Cyprus to 2.0 per 100,000 in Haiti. The United States sits in the middle with 19.6 per 100,000. The incidence of breast cancer is higher in more industrialized nations. Atypically high incidences are found in the Ashkenazi Jewish population (due to higher incidence of BRCA mutations) and nuns (due to nulliparity and resultant increased estrogen exposure). Though the rates of breast cancer rose throughout the 1990s in the United States, the incidence has since leveled off and declined. The rise was attributed to the increased number of women taking HRT, which has since reduced. The variations in breast cancer incidence stem from cultural reductions in risk factors. In less developed countries, women often begin childbearing at younger ages. However, due to reduced access to mammography, the breast cancer is often more advanced at time of presentation. In the United States, disparity exists based on socioeconomic status. Lack of access to screening leads to delayed diagnosis and presentation in minorities and the poor. Additionally, follow-up systemic treatment and reconstruction are less common in lower socioeconomic groups. Notably, African American women have the highest incidence of breast cancer under the age of 45 years, specifically ER negative breast cancer.[23-26]

PRIMARY BREAST CANCER

Breast cancer begins with fibrosis that involves the stroma and epithelial tissue of the breast. When cancer invades into surrounding tissue, a desmoplastic reaction develops that entraps the Coopers ligaments and results in a classic retraction of the skin. When this spreads to involve the lymph flow, *peau d'orange* develops, a thickened, dimpled skin. This progresses to invasion of the skin, areas of ulceration, and satellite nodules. These features can be seen in Figure 1.

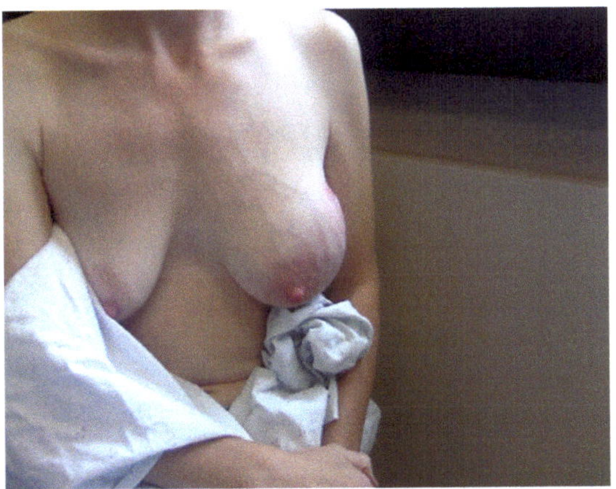

Figure 1a: Large breast mass involving the skin.

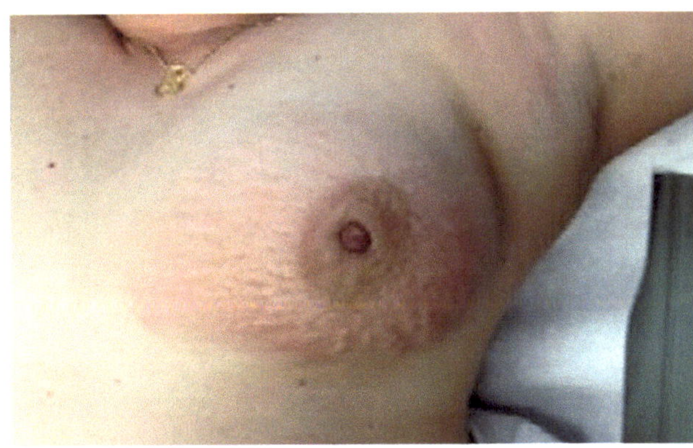

Figure 1b: Breast showing *peau d'orange.*

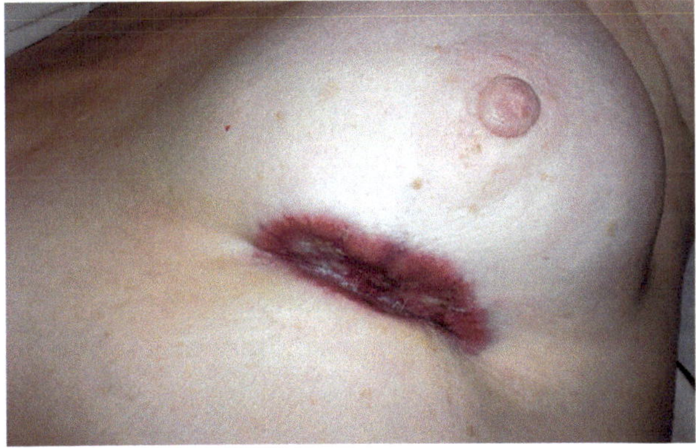

Figure 1c: Breast mass involving the chest wall.

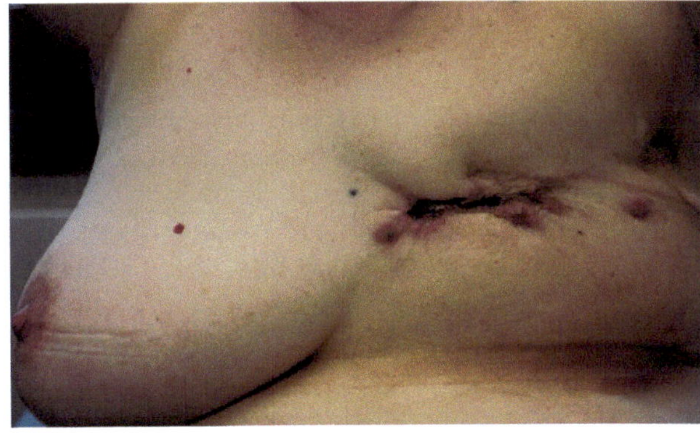

Figure 1d: Tumor recurrence at the surgical site.

The most important prognostic component is axillary metastasis. Breast cancer usually spreads first to the low axillary lymph nodes (Level I: lateral to the pectoralis minor), then to the middle nodes (Level II: posterior to pectoralis minor) and then to the apical nodes (Level III, medial to the pectoralis minor). At first the nodes are soft and mobile but become firm and fixed as the cancer progresses.

Distant metastasis (Figure 2) occurs after breast cancers receive their own blood supply from neovascularization, which occurs after the 20th cell division. Distant metastasis is especially likely to occur after the 27th cell division, at which point the lesion has usually grown to greater than 5 millimeters. Metastasis is the leading cause of cancer-related death for up to 10 years after treatment of the original focus.[27]

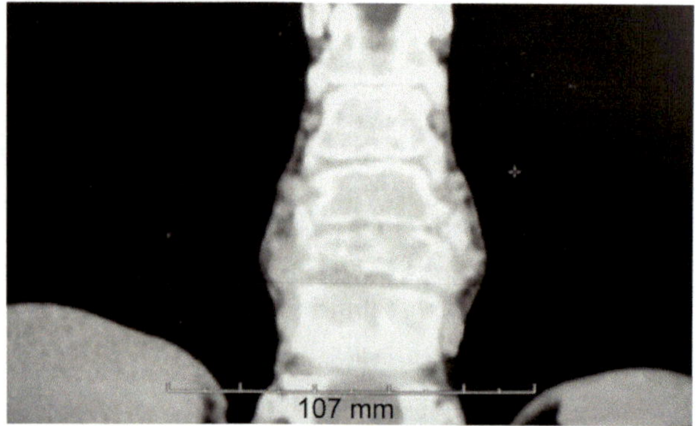

Figure 2: Breast cancer metastasis to L4 lumbar spine.

PATHOLOGY

Breast cancer is first divided into two subtypes: Noninvasive and invasive. A cancer is deemed invasive after it invades through the basement membrane, a characteristic seen on microscopic examination.

Noninvasive Breast Cancer

Noninvasive malignancies include lobular carcinoma in situ (LCIS) and ductal carcinoma in situ (DCIS). While previously considered a separate, malignant neoplasm, LCIS has recently been classified as a risk factor for breast cancer rather than a separate malignant sub-type. LCIS is indistinguishable from normal breast tissue on gross examination- it appears the same as normal anatomic lobular breast tissue.[28] LCIS develops from the terminal duct lobular units. It is characterized by mucoid cytoplasmic globules and may be associated with nearby calcifications.

The average age at diagnosis is 44 years. Five percent of the time, a concurrent invasive breast cancer will be found (in either breast). LCIS is currently regarded as a marker for future development of breast cancer, usually ductal in origin. Prior to the use of screening mammography, LCIS was the most frequently diagnosed *in situ* lesion, but now DCIS is diagnosed more with a ratio of >2:1. LCIS occurs bilaterally in 50-70 percent of cases.[29]

LCIS on core biopsy is managed with surgical excision. (NCCN Guidelines V2012). There may be an upgrade to DCIS or invasive carcinoma in 18-30% of cases after analysis of a larger tissue sample based on observational studies. If only LCIS is diagnosed on an excisional breast biopsy, no further surgery is required. Wide surgical excision with histologically negative margins (i.e., lumpectomy) is not needed since LCIS is often multicentric and is not managed as a precursor lesion. If an invasive carcinoma is detected, appropriate management should be initiated. Patients with LCIS are candidates for breast cancer chemo-preventive therapy (i.e., Tamoxifen). Surveillance alone without medical therapy is also an option.

DCIS is regarded as a malignant lesion. It is present in 5 percent of male breast cancers. It is often classified as intraductal, which carries a higher risk of development into invasive cancer. Papillary growths project into the minor duct lumen on a histological level. Initially they are difficult to distinguish from benign lesions because of their lack of atypia. As the lesion progresses, it fills the lumen and develops pleomorphic and highly mitotic characteristics. DCIS is further subdivided into four histologic types: papillary, cribriform, solid, and comedo. DCIS lesions consist of discrete areas of malignant tissue contained within the basement membrane. Solid and comedo histotypes are more aggressive, progressing more quickly to invasive malignancy than cribriform and papillary lesions. However, more than one sub-type is often found in a single lesion.[28] DCIS is bilateral in less than 20 percent of cases.[30] The presence or history of DCIS places women at a fivefold increased risk for invasive breast cancer, usually in the same quadrant of the same breast.

Calcifications may be the first detectable sign of malignancy, identified on mammograms. The blood supply is from outside the basement membrane and as a result, the lesions develop central necrosis and subsequent central calcification. It is not well understood what causes transformation into invasive cancer, but the lesions usually retain their morphologic structures (papillary DCIS develops into papillary invasive cancer, etc.). Counter-intuitively, histologic grade does not progress when the lesion becomes invasive: high grade DCIS becomes high grade invasive cancer, and likewise for low grade.[28] Multifocal lesions refer to the presence of more than one breast cancer within the same quadrant as the primary. Multicentricity refers to more than one cancer within the same breast, but within different quadrants.

INVASIVE BREAST CANCER

Invasive breast cancers differ from noninvasive primarily due to their lack of basement membrane and, as a result, lack of containment of malignant cells. Like noninvasive breast cancer, invasive is divided into lobular and ductal histologic origin. Lobular malignancies extend in a linear nature, which makes it more difficult to detect until the lesion has grown to be quite large. On the other hand, ductal malignancies invade in a haphazard direction, creating a discrete mass that is picked up earlier on both mammography and physical exam.

Fifty to seventy percent of invasive breast cancer is ductal cancer. Ten to fifteen percent of breast cancer is lobular carcinoma. Invasive ductal cancer often has no specific identifying features and is subsequently known as infiltrating ductal carcinoma, not otherwise specified (NOS). When there is further differentiation, the lesions are named according to their identifying features.[28]

Invasive breast cancer can be divided into special type cancers, which require 90 percent of the histologic features of the lesion to be made up of one defining type or no special type (NST), which carries a worse prognosis. Drs Foote and Stewart proposed the following classifications of special type breast cancer.[31]

- Paget's disease of the nipple
- Invasive ductal carcinoma
- Adenocarcinoma with productive fibrosis, 80 percent
- Medullary carcinoma, 4 percent
- Mucinous (colloid) carcinoma, 2 percent
- Papillary carcinoma, 2 percent
- Tubular carcinoma, 2 percent
- Invasive lobular carcinoma, 10 percent
- Rare cancers, including adenoid cystic, squamous cell, apocrine.

Inflammatory breast cancer

Paget's disease presents as a chronic, scaly eczematous lesion that may progress to ulceration as shown in Figure 3. It is often confused with superficial melanoma and can be distinguished using S-100 antigen immunostaining (positive in melanoma) and carcinoembryonic antigen (CEA, positive in Paget's disease). Paget's disease is diagnosed by a nipple biopsy which reveals Paget's cells: large pale, vacuolated cells. It is often associated with underlying DCIS or invasive breast cancer. Treatment depends on the extent of the underlying lesion and may range from lumpectomy to mastectomy.

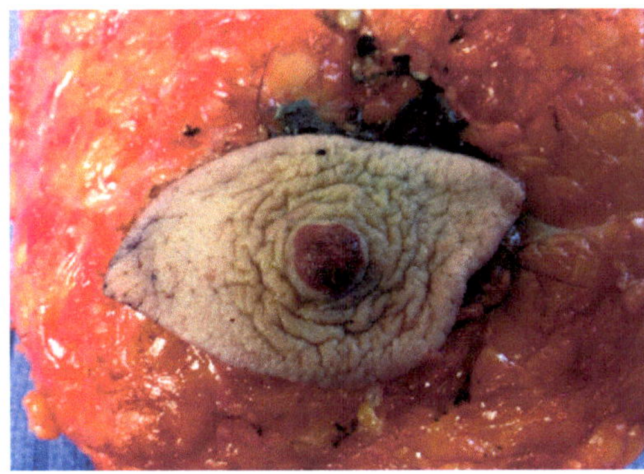

Figure 3: Nipple changes due to Paget's Disease.

Invasive ductal carcinoma with productive fibrosis makes up 80 percent of invasive lesions. In up to two-third of cases, micro- or macroscopic axillary lymph node metastases are present at the time of diagnosis. Invasive ductal carcinoma usually presents in 50 to 60-year-old women as a firm, discrete mass. On mammography it displays stellate calcifications, and often involves several clusters of cancer cells. Within this classification there is a broad variety of cellular and nuclear grades.[31]

Medullary carcinoma is associated with BRCA 1 hereditary breast cancer and presents as a large, soft mass deep in the breast. It is associated with a favorable 5-year survival rate. Necrosis with hemorrhage may occur and result in a rapid increase in size. Histologically, medullary carcinoma has dense lymphoreticular infiltration with lymphocytes and plasma cells, large poorly differentiated pleomorphic nuclei, and a sheet-like growth pattern without ductal differentiation. DCIS is present along the borders of medullary carcinoma lesions in half of these cases. Since medullary breast carcinoma carries with it an intrinsic involvement of lymph nodes that is usually simply benign or hyperplastic, this particular special-type cancer is often clinically staged incorrectly.[32]

Mucinous or colloid carcinoma presents in the elderly as a bulky mass. Extracellular mucin pools surround low- grade cancer cells. On a gross exam the cancer is gelatinous, shiny, and firm. Two-thirds of these cancers carry hormone receptors while one-third have lymphatic involvement. Histologically, these carcinomas require many sections for diagnosis as the mucinous cells displace the few cancer cells.

Papillary carcinoma occurs in non-white females over the age of 70. These are small tumors, less than 3 cm in diameter with papillae that have fibrovascular stromal epithelium. They rarely involve lymph nodes.

Tubular carcinoma occurs usually in perimenopausal women and is found via mammography. It is characterized by a random array of tubular components. One tenth of these women present with level 1 axillary node involvement.

Invasive lobular carcinoma makes up one tenth of all breast cancers. The presentation of this particular type of cancer varies from clinically undetectable to entire breast replacement. It can be multifocal, multi-centric, and/or bilateral at time of presentation. Histologically invasive lobular carcinoma has rounded nuclei with minimal cytoplasm. Using special staining, intracytoplasmic mucin may be identified as signet-ring cells. Invasive lobular carcinoma grows slowly and displays subtle findings on mammography, leading to delayed diagnosis.[32]

Inflammatory Breast Cancer

Occurs in women in their 30-40s and has one of the worst prognoses (Figure 4). Diagnosed with clinical examination followed by biopsy. Histologically, there is involvement of subdermal lymphatics. Treatment with chemoradiation followed with mastectomy.

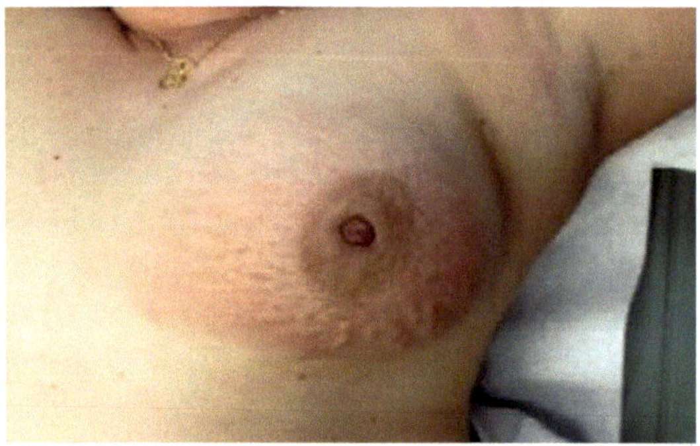

Figure 4: Inflammatory breast cancer.

Diagnosis

Despite the push for breast self-examination, only one third of all breast cancers are first discovered as a palpable mass noted by the woman herself. More frequently, women present with complaints of breast enlargement or asymmetry, changes in the appearance of a nipple or associated discharge, erythema, axillary masses, or pain (rarely).

Physical Exam

First, the woman should be examined with her arms by her side, then with her arms extended upward, then with her hands on her hips. The breast should be visually examined during this time for symmetry, size, edema, nipple retraction, or any skin changes. When the woman leans forward, this should exaggerate any underlying skin retraction. Once proper visual inspection has been performed, the physician should move to physical examination.

With the patient lying supine with her ipsilateral arm raised and her hand underneath her head, all quadrants of the breast should be palpated, from the sternal border medially to the edge of the latissimus dorsi laterally, and from the clavicle superiorly to the inframammary fold inferiorly. The three axillary levels of lymph nodes should then be palpated with the arm held in a relaxed position so the axilla may be palpated deeply. Attention should also be paid to the presence of parasternal nodes.

IMAGING

Mammography

Mammography first came into use in the 1960s but has since gained more frequent use as technology. It is especially useful as a screening tool to detect unexpected lesions. If a palpable mass is felt, two-view chest radiography may be employed. This utilizes a craniocaudal (CC) and a mediolateral oblique (MLO) view. The MLO view is useful for examining the greatest amount of breast tissue. However, the CC view is more efficacious in examining the medial aspect of the breast. Spot compression improves definition and decreases the radiation dose required. Magnification may also be used to better examine microcalcifications.[33] Suspicious findings on mammography include the following: solid masses, especially with stellate characteristics, thickened breast tissues, and areas of microcalcifications. Multiple pinpoint calcifications are highly suspicious and occur in half of non-palpable malignancies. This is particularly important in early cancer detection in young women.

Mammography may be performed as part of routine screening examination or as further investigation of a clinical abnormality. Mammography looks for density abnormalities and microcalcifications as findings suspicious for underlying malignancy. The findings are classified according to the Breast Imaging Reporting and Data System (BI-RADS).[34]

Nonpalpable abnormalities identified on mammography may be density lesions, microcalcifications, or a combination of both. Stellate dense lesions with associated microcalcifications are the most suspicious for breast cancer. All suspicious lesions should undergo biopsy. BI-RADS 1-3 may be monitored with interval mammography (annually for BI-RADS 1-2, Bi-annually for BI-RADS 3) (Table 1). A diagnostic mammogram may be used to further investigate a concerning, palpable lesion. According to two reports, a striking 10 to 22 percent of palpable lesions were not visualized on screening mammography.[35-36] In such cases, a marker may be placed on the area of concern to guide the study to focus on that area.[35] Additionally, ultrasound may be employed as an alternate investigation for those palpable, concerning areas not visualized on mammogram.[36]

Table 1: Breast cancer treatment (PDQ): Health professional version, National Cancer Institute

BI-RADS category	*Description*	*Likelihood of malignancy*	*Recommendation*
0	Need more information	2-10%	Further imaging studies
1	Normal	0.05-0.1%	Routine screening mammography
2	Benign	0.05-0.1%	Routine screening mammography
3	Probably benign	0.3-1.8%	Short-term follow up (6 months)
4	Highly suspicious	10-55%	Biopsy
5	Malignant	60-100%	Biopsy
6	Known cancer	100%	Treat malignancy

Score	Chemotherapy Treatment Benefit
0-15	No benefit
16-20	1.6%
21-25	6.5%
26-100	Great benefit

Ultrasound

Ultrasound is of particular use in breast examination, especially when evaluating palpable breast masses (Figure 5). Two major advantages are its non-invasiveness and its availability: most breast surgeons have this easily on-hand at their offices. Ultrasound is useful in examining cystic masses as well as further investigating echogenic qualities of abnormalities. Qualities that are suspicious for malignancy are ill-defined, irregular borders, stellate shapes, and strong internal echoes. Ultrasound can be used to guide needle aspiration and core biopsy. Ultrasound is of limited use in lesions less than one centimeter in diameter.[22,33,37] Ultrasound used in conjunction with mammography increases sensitivity and accuracy and has a higher negative predictive value. However, the efficacy of ultrasound imaging is operator-dependent and relies on an experienced technician to achieve the highest sensitivity and specificity as possible. Additionally, ultrasound may be more helpful in younger women as the density of their breasts makes mammography more difficult.[5]

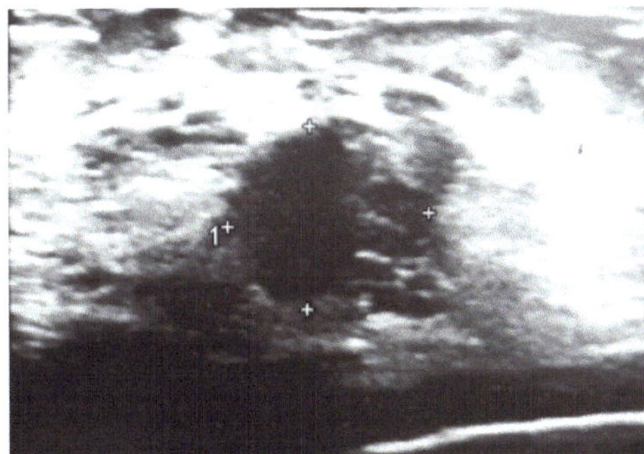

Figure 5: Breast ultrasound: tumor with hemorrhage

MRI

Magnetic resonance imaging (MRI) is rapidly gaining utility in breast cancer work-up. It is even more sensitive than mammography and can be used to further examine abnormalities found on mammography. In a study of 426 women with known cancer, MRI identified additional abnormalities in one quarter of these patients. Almost 2/3 of those sampled were found to have additional occult cancer foci.[38] This study has been used in arguments that suggest these patients would benefit from mastectomy instead of breast conserving therapy, though there have been no studies further evaluating outcomes of women with additional malignancy identified on MRI treated with BCT versus mastectomy. NCCN has released guidelines for using breast MRI together with mammography as a screening modality. The guidelines include women with a higher risk of developing breast cancer, namely those with the BRCA mutation, those with a first-degree relative with the mutation, and those who have a >20% risk of developing breast cancer in their lifetime based on the BRCAPRO model and other risk assessment models dependent on family history. MRI for screening is also recommended, although the evidence is not as strong, in those who have had chest radiation in their childhood (i.e., history of lymphoma) and in those who have personal or family history of Li-Fraumeni and Cowden syndromes. Due to the presence of naturally dense breast tissue in younger women, mammography is often less effective in identifying small lesions (Figure 6). MRI potentially has an advantage in early detection in these young patients.[22,33,37] Downsides to the utilization of MRI include high cost, lack of standard procedure, increase in number of biopsies performed due to false positive MRI findings, delay in treatment, and difficulty in biopsying lesions identified on MRI.[5] MRI has also been suggested to be of use in identifying ruptured implants, locating primaries in women presenting with axillary adenopathy in multifocal or multicentric breast cancers, as well as in assessing tumor response to neoadjuvant chemotherapy (Figure 6)

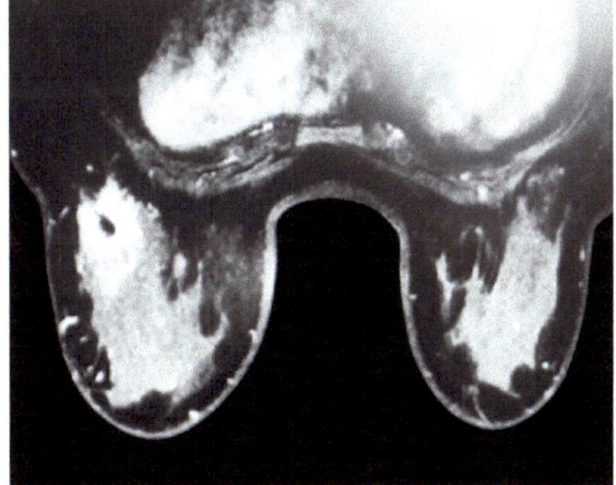

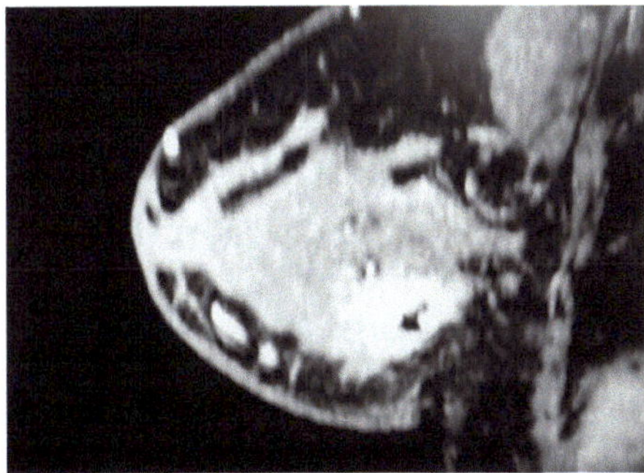

Figure 6a: MRI of Dense Breast of young female with BRCA, tumor not seen on mammogram

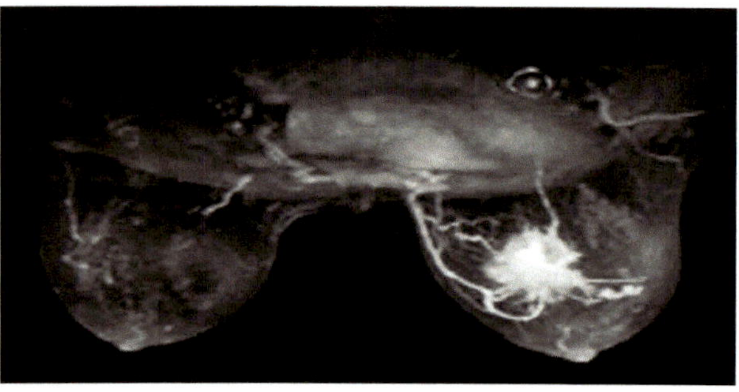

Figure 6b: MRI showing normal and abnormal breast mass.

Ductography

If nipple discharge (Figure 7) is the presenting symptom, a ductogram can be performed. This involves dilation of the suspicious duct with subsequent injection of radio-opaque dye while the patient is in the supine position. CC and MLO views are then obtained, and the duct is outlined with the dye. It is examined for areas of obstruction or filling defects, which are suggestive of tumoral involvement.

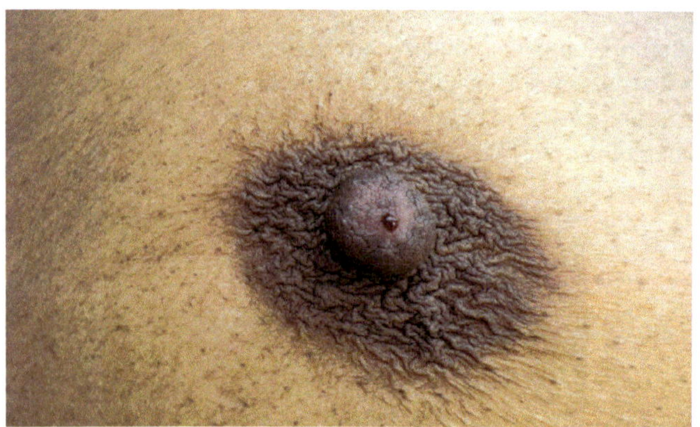

Figure 7: Bloody nipple discharge.

BIOPSY

While ultrasound can be used to guide biopsies in palpable lesions, stereotactic techniques must be utilized when the lesions are non-palpable, such as in the case of microcalcifications. The combination of diagnostic mammography, ultrasound or stereotactic localization, and subsequent fine-needle aspiration is almost 100 percent accurate in successfully diagnosing breast cancer via cytology. Open breast biopsy must be undertaken to analyze breast tissue architecture and grade. For non-palpable lesions, core biopsy as an initial step is preferred not only because of cosmesis, but because it allows definitive surgery to be achieved with a single, better-planned surgery. This has the added benefit of lower overall cost to the patient as well.

For palpable lesions, intra-office fine-needle aspiration (FNA) is ideal. Under ultrasound guidance a 1.5- inch 22-gauge needle is advanced into the lesion. The needle is gently moved within the breast to create cellular debris. Once this is performed the cells are aspirated and then deposited on microscope slides. The slides are fixed and then sent for analysis. In palpable breast masses, the sensitivity and specificity of FNA is almost 100 percent. Core needle biopsy using a 14-gauge Tru-Cut needle is an alternative diagnostic modality. The downside to fine needle biopsy is that a specimen that does not show malignant cells cannot completely rule out breast cancer.[28] Additionally, an experienced cytopathologist is necessary for accurate assessment of the specimen. Small, fibrotic tumors, or those with histology consistent with infiltrating lobular, tubular, and cribriform are associated with higher false-negative results.[5] As always, if radiologic findings are suspicious despite a negative core biopsy or FNA, open biopsy should be undertaken.

BREAST CANCER STAGING AND BIOMARKERS

Although there are multiple ways of staging breast cancer, the most frequently used is TNM (Tumor, Node, Metastasis) created by The American Joint Committee on Cancer. While there is correlation between tumor size, axillary lymph node metastasis and disease-free survival, the single greatest predictor of 10 and 20-year survival is the presence and extent of axillary lymph node metastasis.

PROGNOSIS

The five-year survival for stage I breast cancer is 94 percent for stage IIA and 85 percent for stage IIB 70 percent. Once a stage III cancer is diagnosed, the survival at five years is significantly impacted, dropping to 52 percent for stage IIIA and 48 percent for stage IIIB. Stage IV breast cancer has a dismal 18 percent five-year survival rate. However, breast cancer survival rates continue to increase as early detection improves and treatment modalities are advanced.

CHEMOPREVENTION

For estrogen- receptor (ER) positive breast cancers, tamoxifen (an estrogen antagonist) given for at least 5 years has been found to reduce breast cancer risk and decrease the risk of contralateral breast cancer development. The Early Breast Cancer Trialists' Collaborative Group (EBCTCG) found a 47% reduction of contralateral breast cancer development in women treated with Tamoxifen. This was met with mixed results in four subsequent studies, though definite improvement was demonstrated by the National Surgical Adjuvant Breast and Bowel Project (NSABP) in women with LCIS or atypia.[28]

The ATAC trial (Arimidex, Tamoxifen, Alone or in Combination trial) has also proven that an aromatase inhibitor achieves equal if not better results in breast cancer treatment and prevention in postmenopausal women with ER positive breast cancer. There was a 5-year study of 9366 postmenopausal women who had localized breast cancer, comparing the drugs anastrozole, an aromatase inhibitor, with tamoxifen. After follow-up at a median of 68 months, anastrozole greatly prolonged disease-free survival and time-to-recurrence, and reduced distant metastases.

SURGICAL TECHNIQUES

Lumpectomy With or Without Needle/Wire Localization

The complete removal of a breast malignancy with cancer-free margins is referred to as a lumpectomy. The possibility of mastectomy should be discussed with all patients prior to the operation for the possibility of worse- than-expected findings. Subareolar and centrally located lesions should be approached via circum-areolar incisions, which result in excellent scars. For lesions located outside the nipple-areolar complex, curvilinear incisions along Langer's lines should be utilized. For the inferior quadrants, radial incisions result in the best outcomes. Once excised, the lesion is marked for orientation for the pathologists using silk suture (for example, long tails for lateral margin, short tails for superior margin, air-knot for anterior margin) or by painting the 6 margins with a pre-specified legend. Hemostasis is obtained using electrocautery. While not usually necessary to approximate the subcutaneous tissue, some approximation using absorbable suture may help prevent dimpling if a large lesion was removed. A running subcuticular stitch is used to close the skin and a surgical bra is applied to prevent seroma formation. This approach is the same for stereotactic or ultrasound-guided/needle localized lesions. A J-shaped wire is placed using mammographic or ultrasound guidance. The surgeon then excises a core of tissue around the length of the wire. Before the skin is closed, intra-operative radiography of the surgical specimen is performed to ensure full excision of the lesion and achievement of biopsy clip.

Sentinel Lymph Node Dissection

Sentinel lymph node dissection (SLND) is used to assess the lymph node status in women with early breast cancer and no detectable nodes on clinical exam. SLND is only useful in early breast cancer – by stage III and IV, full axillary lymph node dissection should be undertaken. It should also not be used in cases of palpable nodes or prior axillary surgery. Additionally, SNLD can be used in pregnancy, but only the technetium-99 radioisotope is safe for use. Use of blue dye is contraindicated. In cases of DCIS, SLND should be done when performing a mastectomy and is recommended for palpable DCIS lesions, those with comedo necrosis (both have a higher incidence of underlying invasive or microinvasive disease), and when the lesion is in the upper outer quadrant of the breast (might make subsequent SLND technically more difficult).

SLND can be performed using several techniques. Studies have shown that a combination of intraoperative gamma probe detection of radio-labeled colloid and methylene or lymphazurin blue for sentinel lymph node detection yields the best results. On the morning of surgery, the area around the prior biopsy site, known lesion location, and/or retro-areolar location is injected with 0.5 mCi of 0.2 Technetium (Tc) 99m-labeled sulfur colloid. Immediately prior to the operation, 3-5 mL of methylene blue dye is injected in the sub-areola and peri-tumor areas and massaged gently. Women should be notified that the methylene or lymphazurin blue may change the color of their urine to blue as well for 24-48 hours. Anaphylactic reactions are rare, though there is a slightly higher risk associated with lymphazurin blue over methylene blue. Total radiation exposure is minimal with this technique.

Intraoperatively, a hand-held gamma probe is used to transcutaneously detect the lymph node with the highest concentration of colloid. A 3 cm transverse incision along the axillary hairline should be made and dissection carefully undertaken. Attention should be paid to identifying areas of blue dye concentration. If delicate lymphatic channels can be identified and preserved, this results in cleaner dissection, less edema, and less spilling of dye onto non- nodal tissue (creating less distraction during dissection). The node with the highest gamma-probe signal (and hopefully concurrent greatest concentration of blue dye) should be removed. Ex-vivo, the node undergoes a ten-second radioactive count, which is recorded.

The remainder of the axilla is then checked for areas with a radioactive count greater than 10 percent of that of the highest count. Any node with greater than 10 percent should be excised and sent for pathology. Additionally, any node with a high concentration of blue dye should be excised. Any grossly palpable, suspicious lymph node should also be excised.

The overall success rate in identifying the sentinel node is 97.2 percent. The false-negative rate is 9.8 percent. This was found to be associated with tumors located near the axillary tail, as peri-tumor injections may lead to false results. The fewer lymph nodes removed, the less diagnostic the dissection. According to the NSABP B-32 trial, there was a 7.7 percent reduction in false negative rates when three lymph nodes were removed compared to two (10 percent versus 17.7 percent). Additionally, prior excisional biopsy contributes to disruption of normal lymphatics, and for this reason core biopsy is recommended prior to surgery to aid in better pre-surgical planning and the possibility of a single, definitive surgery. Of note, a peritumoral injection may help identify SNL outside of the usual expected level I and II nodes.

Complications of sentinel lymph node biopsy were as follows: wound infection 1 percent, seroma, or hematoma 1.4 percent, axillary paresthesias 8.6 percent, and lymphedema in 2 percent. These numbers are greatly reduced compared to those found in patients undergoing SLND with completion of axillary lymph node dissection.[39]

Management of positive SLN's has evolved in the past year or so after the release of the results of the ACOSOG Z-11 trial. In this randomized, controlled trial, 813 patients with clinical T1-2 node-negative tumors who also had 1-2 hematoxylin and eosin (H&E)-positive SLNs were randomized into ALND compared to no additional axillary surgery. All patients in the study had a lumpectomy with clear margins, had whole breast radiation, and most had some sort of systemic adjuvant treatment. At follow-up after 6.3 years, the study found no differences between the 2 groups in regard to the rates of axillary recurrence (0.5% vs 0.9%), in-breast recurrence (3.6% vs 1.9%), or overall locoregional recurrence (4.1% vs 2.8%, P = 0.53). Both overall and disease-free survival were alike (82.2% vs 83.8% and 91.9% vs 92.5%) between the groups as well. This trial suggests that ALND can be omitted in selected patients with 1 or 2 positive SLNs.

Conservation Therapy

Patients may opt for breast conservation therapy, which involves resection of the primary breast lesion with assessment of regional lymph node status and radiation therapy. The surgical therapy may involve wide local excision, lumpectomy, partial mastectomy, or segmental mastectomy with a minimum of 1-2 mm margins. This is particularly ideal for stage I or II breast cancer because results are equivalent to those after total mastectomy with the added benefit of preservation of the breast. Six randomized trials showed equivalent disease-free survival rates with breast conserving therapy (BCT) as compared to mastectomy. BCT also is often preferred in terms of cosmesis and quality of life. It offers additional protection of sensation preservation and less psychological adjustment for women as opposed to those undergoing total mastectomy. BCT is the current standard of care for DCIS, stage 0, I and II breast cancer with post- operative radiation treatment.

SLND is the preferred staging procedure if there are no clinically positive nodes. This should be performed prior to the excision of the primary tumor. Local recurrence in BCT is primarily determined by the adequacy of surgical margins during the primary operation. If clear margins are not able to be obtained during re-excision, the decision should be made to proceed with mastectomy.

Oncoplastic surgery may be considered at the time of segmental mastectomy. This should be considered only in situations where re-excision is not a possibility. Oncoplastic surgery should be considered when large amounts of breast tissue are removed, when there is an expected unfavorable cosmetic outcome, and when there is concern for mal positioning of the nipple.

Mastectomy

A skin-sparing mastectomy removes all breast tissue including the nipple-areolar complex and prior biopsy scars. A total mastectomy removes the aforementioned tissue with the additional removal of overlying skin. An extended simple mastectomy removes all that of a total mastectomy as well as level I axillary nodes. A modified radical mastectomy adds the removal of level II nodes. The Halsted, or radical mastectomy, requires removal of the pectoralis major and minor muscles, as well as all III lymph node levels. With the improvement of chemotherapy, radiation therapy, and hormonal therapy, radical mastectomies are rarely required. Some women who would be good candidates for BCT may elect to proceed with mastectomy. This may be due to preferred single-stage treatment, economic reasons, genetic predisposition, or lack of access to follow-up care with chemotherapy or radiation. As always, the patient should be evaluated from a complete medical and psychosocial standpoint to yield the best personal results.

Prophylactic Mastectomy

Prophylactic mastectomy is also known as preventative mastectomy. It is performed on one or both breasts to reduce the risk of developing breast cancer in either the ipsilateral or contralateral breast. It is indicated in patients who have the BRCA1 or the BRCA2 gene mutation because it can decrease the chance of developing breast carcinoma in 90 to 95% of cases, as reported by the National Cancer Institute.

This procedure can be advocated in patients with a family history of breast carcinoma and the BRCA1 or BRCA2 mutation. Additionally, patients who have breast carcinoma on one side can opt for prophylactic mastectomy of the other breast.

Women of Ashkenazi Jewish descent have an increased incidence of the BRCA mutation. Patients who have multiple generations with breast carcinoma, have the BRCA mutation, or had breast carcinoma at a younger age (<50 years old) are also considered for prophylactic mastectomy.

Overall, the prophylactic mastectomy is becoming more popular in patients who have a breast mutation and patients with unilateral breast carcinoma and patients with a family history (e.g., mother, sister, or daughter with breast carcinoma at an age <50 years old). Patients who had radiation therapy to the chest for other conditions have also benefited from the prophylactic mastectomy because radiation therapy at a young age increases the incidence of breast carcinoma. Patients with recurrent breast carcinoma are also considered for preventative mastectomy. The prophylactic mastectomy is getting more and more adapted in the younger patient. The indications mentioned above can reduce the chance of developing breast carcinoma in 90 to 95% of the patients.

Reconstruction

There are a variety of reconstruction options once all chemotherapy and radiation have been finished. Depending on the remaining breast tissue, a pedicled flap, such as a latissimus dorsi flap or a transverse rectus abdominus flap may be utilized. Some women may elect to undergo immediate reconstruction after mastectomy with tissue expander and subsequent implants. Free flaps (free TRAM's, gluteus flaps, etc.) are also being used for reconstruction. Expertise in microvascular surgery is required to be able to perform these types of reconstruction. Proper preoperative planning and discussion helps to expedite reconstruction via early involvement of all necessary specialists.

Radiation Therapy

Radiation therapy is utilized in all patients undergoing BCT to prevent local recurrence. Radiation should also be used in patients who had positive margins after undergoing mastectomy. Women with axillary involvement of 4 or more nodes or those pre-menopausal women with 1-3 positive nodes should also be considered for adjuvant radiation therapy. For stage IIIB and IV, neoadjuvant chemotherapy with segmental mastectomy should be followed by radiation of the supraclavicular lymph nodes and chest wall. Partial breast radiation via brachytherapy or external beam radiation using three-dimensional conformal radiation is increasingly being used in low-risk populations as part of prospective trials.

Adjuvant Chemotherapy

Adjuvant chemotherapy is recommended for women with blood vessel or lymphatic invasion, high nuclear grade, high histologic grade, and HER-2/neu over-expression.[40-45] A large meta-analysis that looked at the major prospective, randomized trials of chemotherapy was performed by the Early Breast Cancer Trialists Collaborative Group. It found that adjuvant chemotherapy reduced the risk of death equally in patients with node positive as well as node negative disease. Doxorubicin was found to have a slightly increased benefit over other chemotherapy. Adjuvant chemotherapy reduced the odds of death by 8 percent in women ages 60- 69 years, and a staggering 27 percent in women under the age of 40 years.[46] The addition of a taxane to doxorubicin slightly increases the benefit to women with node-positive disease. Recently, the use of Herceptin, an antibody to c- HER2-neu protein, and vinorelbine, have been the focus of new avenues of adjuvant therapy.[46] Tamoxifen acts as a selective estrogen receptor modulator (SERM). It acts against estrogen in the breast via competitive blockade of estrogen receptors. It has the added benefit of preserving bone density and lowering cholesterol as an estrogen agonist. Unfortunately, tamoxifen also acts to increase the incidence of endometrial carcinoma. In patients who have tumors that are ER positive, PR positive, or both, tamoxifen has been found to reduce the annual odds of recurrence by 47 percent and annual odds of death by 26 percent. These results have been replicated in over 63 trials. Another avenue of interest has been aromatase inhibitors such as Anastrozole, which prevent the peripheral conversion of androgens to estrogen. In a large randomized clinical trial, Anastrozole has shown to be slightly more effective than tamoxifen alone or when used in combination, with a more favorable side-effect profile.[47]

In metanalysis of randomized, controlled trials, the combination of chemotherapy and tamoxifen is beneficial in all groups of women, though the side-effects in post-menopausal women must be considered. The proportional reduction in mortality must be evaluated in terms of absolute reduction to calculate the benefit for the individual patient.[48-49]

The development of prognostic profiles has been particularly useful in guiding decision-making about adjuvant systemic therapy. The 21-gene recurrence score (RS, Oncotype Dx) is among the best-validated and most widely used prognostic assays, has some value in predicting chemotherapy response, and is relatively unique in that it can be used in fixed tissue. This test analyzes a panel of 21 genes within a tumor specimen to determine a Recurrence Score (RS). This Recurrence Score is a number between 0 and 100 that corresponds to a specific likelihood of breast cancer recurrence within 10 years of the initial diagnosis when the patient receives / abides to 5 years of Tamoxifen or an aromatase inhibitor (prognostic benefit). The RS has also been validated to predict response and benefit to chemotherapy. A low RS score will have minimal benefit, while a high RS has substantial benefit with use of chemotherapy (predictive benefit). It is recommended by the American Society of Clinical Oncology (ASCO) for women who have node-negative, estrogen receptor (ER)-positive breast cancer. Other molecular gene profiling assays used in breast cancer include the Amsterdam 70-gene prognostic profile (Mammaprint) and the Rotterdam/Veridex 76-gene prognostic signature.

Neoadjuvant Chemotherapy

Neoadjuvant chemotherapy is given to patients before their primary course of either surgery or radiation treatment. The aim of neoadjuvant chemotherapy is to shrink the tumor by using chemotherapy drugs prior to their primary treatment (Figure 8). This therapy is indicated for very large tumors or is used to kill tumor cells that are not visible on routine imaging (occult tumor). Response to the neoadjuvant chemotherapy is seen based on the tumor size, the tumor type, the cancer progression, and the symptoms of the patient. The effectiveness of this therapy is determined by the decrease in size, the progression free survival, the easing of symptoms, and the slowing of growth.

Neoadjuvant therapy also provides the benefit of having an easier surgical removal of the tumor, making non-operable tumors into operable case, and decreasing the need for mastectomies in up to 43% of the cases.

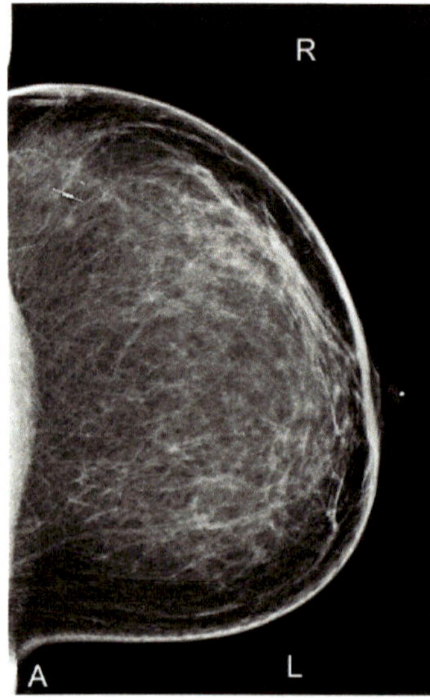

Figure 8a: Pre-Neoadjuvate MRI

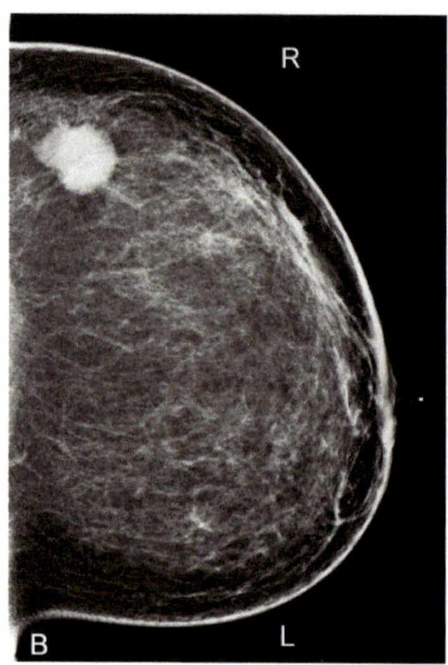

Figure 8b: Post-Neoadjuvant MRI

Immunotherapy and Targeted Therapy for Breast Cancer

In a certain select group of patients with breast carcinoma, a certain hormone receptor status and gene expression as determined on the histological specimen may provide useful clinical prognostic information. Recently, various clinical trials have validated and have been the approach in treating breast cancer as a targeted therapy with multiple new drugs.

At present, there are multiple gene expression tests available (e.g., a 21-Gene-expression) which provide supporting evidence that tests will be a useful platform for evaluating patients for further treatment. It also provides the highest level of evidence supporting the clinical validity and usefulness of these new biomarkers. There is also a 70-Gene expression assay available with the same validity in clinical trials.

The targeted therapy or immunotherapy is considered for (1) certain hormone receptor statuses and (2) the stage of the disease. These therapies are implied before and after surgical procedures for stage two carcinoma, recurrent carcinoma locally, and metastatic breast carcinoma in other parts of the body.

There are multiple newer drugs available against certain genes. The archival histological specimen of the patient is tested on these genes and the treatment is based on the positivity of those gene receptors. The various agents commonly used and available at this time include Ipilimumab (Verboy), Pebrolizumab (Keytruda), Livolumab (Opdivo), and Atezolizumab (Tecentriq). The various groups of medication currently available for PD-L1/PD-1 inhibitors, Kinase inhibitors, CDK 4/6 inhibitors, M-Tor inhibitors, P-13

K inhibitors, and BRCA gene mutation medications are detailed in Table 2. All these immunotherapy agents are targeted therapy agents and can be used individually or in combinations. Currently there are multiple clinical on-going trials to see the benefit of these therapy in terms of progression-free survival, disease-free survival, and overall survival.

Table 2: Targeted therapies and immunotherapy options for breast cancer

Immunotherapy types for metastatic breast cancer		Mechanisms of action
Immune checkpoint PD-1	Nivolumab (Opdivo) Pembrolizumab (Keytruda) Atezolizumab (Tecentriq) Durvalumab (Imfinzi)	Nivolumab: PD-1 on T cells/PDL1 interaction is blocked, T cell activation Pembrolizumab: Blocks PD-1 receptors, immune system targets cancer cells Atezolizumab: Blocks interaction of PD-I and CD80 receptors Durvalumab: Blocks PD-1/PDL1 interaction
CDK4/6 inhibitors	Abemaciclib (Verzenio) Palbociclib (Ibrance) Ribociclib (Kisqali)	CDK4/CDK6 inhibition, prevents cell cycle progressing to S phase, induce apoptosis
Her2Neu	Trastuzumab (Herceptin) Trastuzumab-emtansine (Kadcyla)	Cell surface HER2/neu receptors, inhibits the receptors, arrest of G1 phase of growth cycle, inhibition of downward MAPK signaling pathway
PARP inhibitors	Olaparib (Lynparza) Niraparib (Zejula)	PARP(Poly ADP ribose polymerase) used by cancer cells for DNA repair, PARP inhibitors affect this process of DNA repair by cancer cells
PI3K/AKT	Eganelisib Ipatasertib	Phosphatidylinositol-3 kinase inhibitor, disrupts PI3/AKT/mTOR signaling pathway
MAPK/ERK (MEK inhibitor)	Cobimetinib (Cotellic)	Inhibits MEK1/MEK2, ultimately affects the MAPK/ERK pathway Also used in Vemurafenib resistant malignant melanoma
ADC	Sacitizumab (Trodelvy) SGN-LIV1A/Ladiratuzumab	Sacituzumab is conjugate of anti-Trop2 monoclonal antibody with SN-38, a metabolite of irinotecan, inhibits Topoisomerase (works in DNA)
PIK3CA activating mutation	Alpelisib (Piqray)	PIK3CA mutation breast cancer
NTRK fusion	Larotrectinib (Vitrakvi) Entrectinib (Rozyltrek)	NTRK genes abnormally fuses with other genes causing TRF fusion protein that leads to growth and survival of cancer cells This group of drugs inhibit this interaction
mTOR inhibitors	Everlimus (Afinitor)	mTOR inhibition: late blockage of G1/S phase of cell growth cycle, leads to apoptosis
Tyrosine kinase inhibitors	Neratinib (Enhertu)	Dual inhibitor of HER2 and EGFR kinases

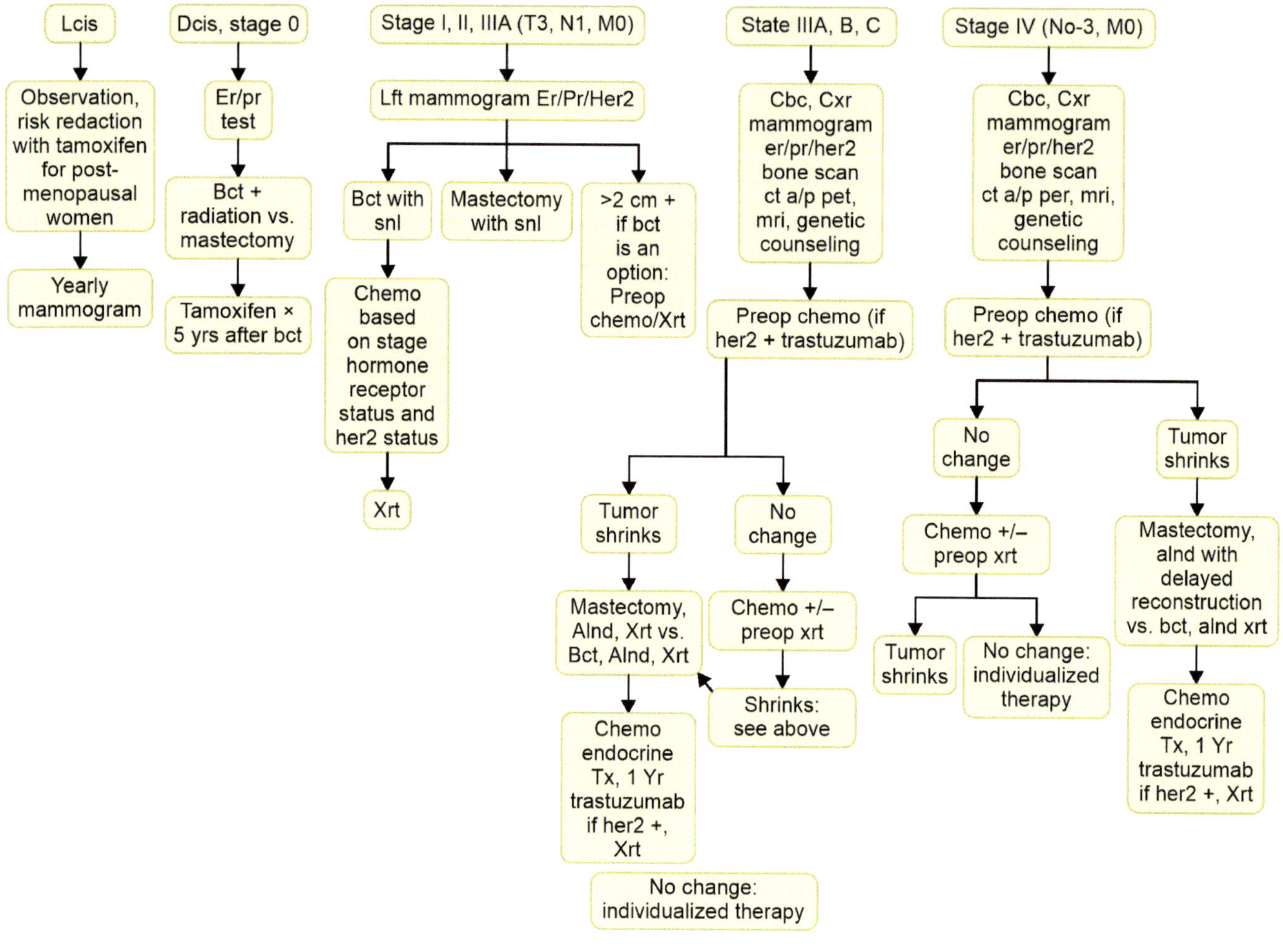

Figure 9: An algorithm for management of breast cancer.

REFERENCES

1. Singletary SE. Rating the risk factors for breast cancer. Ann Surg 2003;237:474.
2. Hulka BS. Epidemiologic analysis of breast and gynecologic cancers. Prog Clin Biol Res 1997;396:17.
3. Pujol P, Galtier-Dereure F, Bringer J. Obesity and breast cancer risk. Hum Reprod 1997;1:12 Suppl: 116.
4. Goss PE, Sierra S. Current perspectives on radiation-induced breast cancer. J Clin Oncol 1998;16:338.
5. Mulholland M, et al. Greenfield's Surgery: Scientific Principles and Practice. Breast Disease, 4th edn. 2005.
6. Wynder EL, et al. Breast cancer: Weighing the evidence for a promoting role of dietary fat. J Natl Cancer Inst 1997;89:766.
7. Gail MH, et al. Projecting individualized absolute invasive breast cancer risk in African American women. J Natl Cancer Inst 2007;99:1782.
8. Edwards BK, et al. Annual report to the nation on the status of cancer, 1975-2002, featuring population-based trends in cancer treatment. J Natl Cancer Inst 2005;97:1407.
9. Kerlikowske K, et al. Efficacy of screening mammography. A meta- analysis. JAMA 1995;273:149.
10. Fisher B, et al. Tamoxifen for prevention of breast cancer: Report of the National Surgical Adjuvant Breast and Bowel Project P-1 Study. J Natl Cancer Inst 1998;90:1371.
11. Grodstein F, et al. Postmenopausal hormone therapy and mortality. N Engl J Med 336:1769, 1997.52. Har tmann LC, et al: Efficacy of bilateral prophylactic mastectomy in women with a family history of breast cancer. N Engl J Med 1999;340:77.
12. Wu K, Brown P. Is low-dose tamoxifen useful for the treatment and prevention of breast cancer? J Natl Cancer Inst 2003;95:766.

13. Martin AM, Weber BL. Genetic and hormonal risk factors in breast cancer. J Natl Cancer Inst 2000;92:1126.
14. Ford D, et al. Genetic heterogeneity and penetrance analysis of the BRCA1 and BRCA2 genes in breast cancer families. The Breast Cancer Linkage Consortium. Am J Hum Genet 1998;62:676.
15. Gowen LC, et al. BRCA1 required for transcription-coupled repair of oxidative DNA damage. Science 1998;281:1009.
16. Wooster R, Weber BL. Breast and ovarian cancer. N Engl J Med 2003;348:2339.
17. Oddoux C, et al. The carrier frequency of the BRCA2 6174delT mutation among Ashkenazi Jewish individuals is approximately 1%. Nat Genet 1996;14:188.
18. Haffty BG. Molecular and genetic markers in the local-regional management of breast cancer. Semin Radiat Oncol 2002;12:329.
19. Morabito A, et al. Prognostic and predictive indicators in operable breast cancer. Clin Breast Cancer 2003;3:381.
20. Rogers CE, et al. Molecular prognostic indicators in breast cancer. Eur J Surg Oncol 2002;28:467.
21. Esteva FJ, et al. Molecular prognostic factors for breast cancer metastasis and survival. Semin Radiat Oncol 2002;12:319.
22. Schnall MD. Breast MR imaging. Radiol Clin North Am 2003;41:43.
23. American Cancer Society: Cancer Facts and Figures 2008. Atlanta: American Cancer Society, 2008. Available at http:// www.cancer.org/downloads/STT/2008CAFFfinalsecured.pdf [accessed January 29, 2009].
24. Clarke CA, et al. Recent declines in hormone therapy utilization and breast cancer incidence: Clinical and population-based evidence. J Clin Oncol 2006;24:e49.
25. Ferlay J, et al. Globocan 2002: Cancer Incidence, Mortality and Prevalence Worldwide. Lyon, France: IARC Press, 2004. IARC Cancer Base No. 5, Version 2.0.
26. Ries LAG, et al. SEER Cancer Statistics Review, 1975-2002, National Cancer Institute. Bethesda, MD, http://seer.cancer.gov/ csr/1975_2002/ [accessed January 29, 2009].
27. Khan SA, Stewart AK, Morrow M. Does aggressive local therapy improve survival in metastatic breast cancer? Surgery 2002;132:620; discussion 626.
28. Townsend CM, et al. Sabiston Textbook of Surgery: Expert Consult. Breast Disease. (18th edn) Nov 2007.
29. Gallager HS, Martin JE. The study of mammary carcinoma by mammography and whole organ sectioning. Early observations. Cancer 1969;23:855.
30. Consensus conference on the classification of ductal carcinoma in situ. Hum Pathol 1997;28:1221.
31. Foote FWJ, Stewart FW. Lobular carcinoma in situ: A rare form of mammary carcinoma. Am J Pathol 1941;17:491.
32. McDivitt RW, et al. Tubular carcinoma of the breast: Clinical and pathological obser vations concerning 135 cases. Am J Surg Pathol 1982;6:401.
33. Bassett LW. Breast imaging: Bland KI, Copeland EM III (eds): The Breast: Comprehensive Management of Benign and Malignant Diseases. Philadelphia: WB Saunders, 1998;648.
34. Birads: bestpractice.bmj.com. Accessed 7/21/10.
35. Shelty MK, Shah YP, Sharman RS. Prospective evaluation of the value of combined mammographic and sonographic assessment in patients with palpable abnormalities of the breast. J Ultrasound Med 2003;22:263–8.
36. Morrow M, Schmidt RA, Bucci C. Breast conser vation for mammographically occult carcinoma. Ann Surg 1998;227:502–
37. Fletcher SW, Elmore JG. Clinical practice. Mammographic screening for breast cancer. N Engl J Med 2003;348:1672.
38. Holland R, Veling SH, Mravunac M, et al. Histologic multifocality of Tis, T1-2 breast carcinomas. Implications for clinical trials of breast-conserving surgery. Cancer 1985;56:979–90.
39. Hunt KK, et al. The Breast A Brief History of Breast Cancer Therapy. Schwartz's Principles of Surgery (9th edn) 2010.
40. Tamoxifen for early breast cancer: An overview of the randomised trials. Early Breast Cancer Trialists' Collaborative Group. Lancet 1998;351:1451.
41. Polychemotherapy for early breast cancer: An overview of the randomised trials. Early Breast Cancer Trialists' Collaborative Group. Lancet 1998;352:930.
42. Fisher B, et al. Two months of doxorubicin-cyclophosphamide with and without interval reinduction therapy compared with 6 months of cyclophosphamide, methotrexate, and fluorouracil in positive-node breast cancer patients with tamoxifen-nonresponsive tumors: Results from the National Surgical Adjuvant Breast and Bowel Project B-15. J Clin Oncol 1990;8:1483.
43. Kelleher M, Miles D. 21. The adjuvant treatment of breast cancer. Int J Clin Pract 2003;57:195.
44. Loprinzi CL, Thome SD. Understanding the utility of adjuvant systemic therapy for primary breast cancer. J Clin Oncol 2001;19:972.

45. Wood WC, et al. Dose and dose intensity of adjuvant chemotherapy for stage II, node-positive breast carcinoma. N Engl J Med 1994;330:1253.
46. Early Breast Cancer Trialists' Collaborative Group. Polychemo- therapy for early breast cancer: an overview of the randomized trials. Lancet 1998;352:930–42.
47. Baum M, Buzdar A, Cuzick J, et al. Anastrozole alone or in combination with tamoxifen versus tamoxifen alone for adjuvant treatment of postmenopausal women with early-stage breast cancer: results of the ATAC (arimidex, tamoxifen alone or in combination) trial efficacy and safety update analyses. Cancer 2003;98:1802–10.
48. Schneiderman M, Axtell LM. Deaths among female patients with carcinoma of the breast treated by surgical procedure alone. Surg Gynecol Obstet 1979;148:193–6.
49. Early Breast Cancer Trialists' Collaborative Group. Tamoxifen for early breast cancer: an overview of the randomized trials. Lancet 1998;351:1451–67.

24

CHAPTER

Melanoma

Richard Englehadt, MD
Manu Kaushik, MD
Vijay K. Mittal, MD

INTRODUCTION

Among all the cancers, melanoma has the highest increase in incidence. There are many possible causes for this rapid rise in cases. The dominant contributing factor is an increased exposure to ultraviolet radiation from sunlight. Other risk factors for melanoma include a family history, freckles, red or blonde colored hair, fair skin pigmentation, a history of at least one blistering sunburn, and the presence of multiple nevi, particularly any dysplastic nevi.

From 2003-2007, the median age of melanoma diagnosis in the United States was 60 years old. Table 1 displays the age distribution of melanoma diagnosis. The age-adjusted incidence rate was 20.1 per 100,000 persons per year (Table 2).[1] Additionally, the median age of death due to melanoma was 68 years old. Table 3 displays the age distribution of deaths due to melanoma. The age-adjusted death rate was 2.7 per 100,000 persons per year (Table 4).[1]

Table 1: Age Distribution of Melanoma Diagnosis

Age Range of Melanoma Diagnosis	Percent of Melanoma Cases
<20 years old	0.8%
20 to 34 years old	7.5%
35 to 44 years old	11.8%
45 to 54 years old	18.7%
55 to 64 years old	20.4%
65 to 74 years old	17.8%
75 to 84 years old	17.0%
> 85 years old	6.0%

Table 2: Incidence of melanoma based on race and gender

Race/Ethnicity	Male	Female
All Races	25.6 per 100,000 men	16.2 per 100,000 women
White	29.7 per 100,000 men	19.1 per 100,000 women
Black	1.1 per 100,000 men	1.0 per 100,000 women
Asian/Pacific Islander	1.6 per 100,000 men	1.3 per 100,000 women
American Indian/Alaska Native	4.1 per 100,000 men	3.7 per 100,000 women
Hispanic	4.4 per 100,000 men	4.7 per 100,000 women

Table 3: Age Distribution of Deaths due to Melanoma

Age Range of Death	Percent of Melanoma Deaths
<20 years old	0.1%
20 to 34 years old	2.7%
35 to 44 years old	6.3%
45 to 54 years old	14.3%
55 to 64 years old	19.6%
65 to 74 years old	20.9%
75 to 84 years old	24.1%
> 85 years old	11.9%

Table 4: Mortality secondary to melanoma as distributed by race and gender

Race/Ethnicity	Male	Female
All Races	4.0 per 100,000 men	1.7 per 100,000 women
White	4.5 per 100,000 men	2.0 per 100,000 women
Black	0.5 per 100,000 men	0.4 per 100,000 women
Asian/Pacific Islander	0.4 per 100,000 men	0.3 per 100,000 women
American Indian/Alaska Native	1.6 per 100,000 men	0.8 per 100,000 women
Hispanic	1.0 per 100,000 men	0.6 per 100,000 women

Suspicious lesions for melanoma include those that are asymmetric, have an irregular border, or have multiple or unusual colors such as gray, white, red, blue, or dark black. Lesions with a diameter >5 mm or have undergone any new changes should also be regarded as suspicious.[2]

Melanomas are further classified into different categories based on their patterns of growth. These classes include superficial spreading, acral lentiginous melanoma, nodular melanoma, and lentigo maligna.

Superficial spreading melanoma (Figure 1) is the most common presentation of melanoma, comprising more than 70% of all melanomas. These generally arise from pre-existing nevi in sun-exposed areas of the body. Growth generally occurs in a superficial pattern initially, with later development of a vertical growth phase.[3,4]

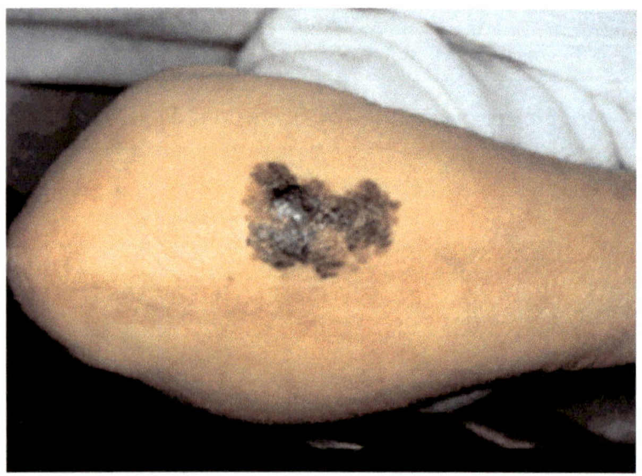

Figure 1: Superficial spreading melanoma characteristically demonstrates asymmetry and color variability.

Acral lentiginous melanoma accounts for approximately 5% of all melanomas in the Caucasian population. In contrast, it makes up between 30 and 60% of all cases of melanoma among African American, Asian, and Hispanic races. As opposed to the superficial spreading melanomas, acral lentiginous lesions are more commonly found in non-sun-exposed areas such as the nail beds, soles of the feet or palms, and the perineum. These lesions develop quickly and are often very aggressive. They tend to be very large, with an average diameter of 2.5-3 cm. Acral lentiginous melanomas are notable for their irregular borders, ulceration, and unusual color patterns.[3,4]

Nodular melanoma (Figure 2) makes up 15 to 25% of the melanomas found in the Caucasian population. Nodular lesions are generally more pronounced, dome-like lesions with well-defined borders. They are more commonly found in the elderly, and are often located around the head, neck, and trunk. Nodular melanomas are notable for having an aggressive vertical growth phase, and as a result often are diagnosed as deep, invasive lesions.[3,4]

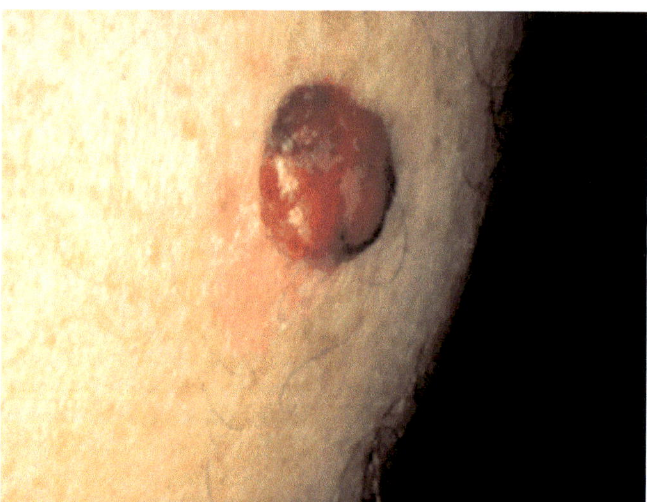

Figure 2: Nodular melanoma common present as discrete nodules with dark pigmentation.

Lentigo maligna melanoma (Figure 3) accounts for roughly 4 to 10% of all melanomas. While lentigo maligna lesions tend to be locally advanced with high recurrence rates following excision, they also have the lowest propensity for metastatic spread compared to other subtypes. Lentigo maligna is generally found in sun-exposed areas and is noted for having irregular borders and a more horizontal growth pattern.[3]

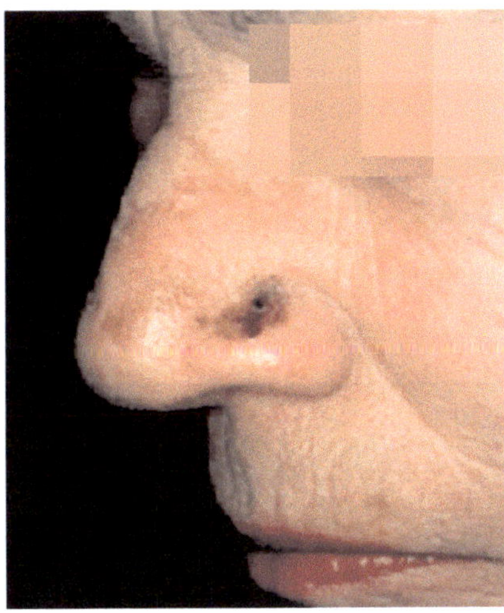

Figure 3: Lentigo maligna melanoma. This melanoma most often arises in sun-exposed parts of the skin, especially the head and neck.

GENETICS AND MELANOMA

Melanoma is most often associated with the familial gene CDKN2A/p16 (cyclin-dependent kinase inhibitor 2A), located on chromosome 9p21. This gene acts through the cyclin D1/cyclin-dependent kinase 4 complex, an upstream regulator of the retinoblastoma gene pathway. By acting through this complex, the CDKN2A/p16 gene controls the passage of cells through the cell cycle by stopping damaged cells at the G1/S checkpoint and repairing any DNA damage prior to continuing the cycle. This mutation accounts for 35 to 40% of familial melanomas. In one large case series, CDKN2A mutations were present in all of families with seven to ten individuals affected, 60 to 71% of families with four to six cases, and 14% of families with two cases. Other genetic markers associated with increased risk of melanoma include mutations to the CDK4 and CDK6 genes. These mutations cause disruption along a similar signaling pathway as the CDKN2A gene. Germline CDK4 mutations are very rare while germline mutations in CDK6 have not been identified in any melanoma families.[5]

Germline mutations in CDKN2A are identified by clinical testing. Current practices regarding testing for this mutation follow two different schools of thought. Some believe that identifying a potential cause of disease is beneficial for the individual due to the reassurance of a negative test. However, a negative test result is uninformative in cases of unknown familial mutations and a genetic cause of disease must still be identified for these families. Additionally, it is important to remember that even if an individual does not carry the mutation that runs in their family, they remain at an increased risk of melanoma. Currently, clinical management does not change for individuals with that identified CDKN2A mutation. Close dermatologic follow-up is indicated, regardless of genetic testing result. Any genetic testing performed in this population should be accompanied by genetic counseling in order to clarify the role of the testing.[6]

STAGING OF MELANOMA

The stage of development of the primary tumor is one of the most important prognostic factors associated with melanoma. The current micro-staging method, which is now the standard for classification, was originally described by Breslow. In this method the primary tumor is classified according to its thickness in millimeters as measured from the top of the granular layer to the base of the tumor.[7] There are many studies which demonstrate an inverse correlation between the thickness of the tumor and patient survival. The ulceration status and mitotic rate have also been used as independent factors that aid in the micro-staging of the lesion.[6]

Prior to the use of the Breslow system for micro-staging, melanomas were staged using the Clark's level classification system. Clark's system stages lesions according to the level of invasion into the histologic layers of the skin. It separates the degree of invasion into five levels, with level 1 consisting of in situ involvement only and level 5 extending to the subcutaneous tissue. Several studies have subsequently confirmed that the Breslow staging based on thickness conveys a more accurate prognostic evaluation than Clark's system.[8,9]

Clark Classification System of Micro-staging
Level I: Confined to the epidermis (in situ)
Level II: Invasion into the papillary dermis
Level III: Penetration to the papillary-reticular interface
Level IV: Invasion into the reticular dermis
Level V: Penetration into subcutaneous fa

Presence of regional lymph node metastasis is associated with a worse prognosis in melanoma lesions. The degree to which the lymph node is involved (microscopic versus macroscopic disease) has demonstrated an inverse correlation with long-term survival. The use of sentinel lymph node biopsy has been instrumental in identifying a subgroup of patients with micro-metastatic nodal disease who have been found to have a more favorable prognosis than those with macroscopic nodal involvement. This difference in prognosis has led to the incorporation of the type of nodal involvement into the staging system.[10,11]

DIAGNOSIS OF MELANOMA

Examination of nodal metastases by H and E alone often leads to either overdiagnosis or underdiagnosis of metastatic disease due to hypercellularity of the lymph node and similar staining of the cells. Several antigens have been identified on melanoma cells, with associated monoclonal antibodies generated and used for diagnostic immunohistochemistry. Frequently used markers include S-100 protein, HMB-45, Melan-A, Mitf, and Tyrosinase.[12] Comparison of the sensitivities and specificities of the various markers is shown in Table 5.

Table 5: Comparison of the sensitivity, specificity, positive and negative predictive values and likelihood ratio of S-100, HMB-45, Mitf, Melan-A, and Tyrosinase as markers for diagnosing melanomas

	Sensitivity	Specificity	Positive Predictive Value	Negative Predictive Value	Likelihood Ratio
S-100	88	70	78	82	26
HMB-45	92	97	97	92	69
Mitf	100	97	97	100	90
Melan-A	95	97	97	94	75
Tyrosinase	98	84	89	96	59
S-100 and HMB-45	80	100	100	80	59
Mitf and Melan-A	95	100	100	94	84

TREATMENT OF MELANOMA

Any lesion thought to be suspicious for melanoma should be biopsied. The goal of any biopsy is to provide the pathologist with sufficient tissue to allow for a complete evaluation of the lesion. In order to accomplish this, the melanoma must be biopsied at its deepest portion so that the Breslow depth can be determined. Excision or punch biopsies are the preferred methods of biopsy. When possible, complete excisional biopsies are preferred; however, if the lesion is large and in an anatomic location (face, scalp, or hands) which would make complete excision disfiguring, a punch biopsy may be performed. Shave biopsies or curette biopsies should be avoided if melanoma is suspected.

Once confirmed via biopsy, complete treatment of a primary melanoma tumor consists of complete excision with a margin of tissue determined by the depth of invasion. Previously, 5 cm margins were used for all melanomas. Multiple studies and trials have shown that narrower margins can be used without increasing the risk of local recurrence or overall survival. The narrower margins also allow for less morbidity and decreased need for skin grafting. The current standard of practice determines the width of margins based on the depth of invasion of the lesion.[5,8,9]

Melanoma in situ can safely be excised with 5 mm margins. Melanoma with invasion less than 1 mm in thickness can be excised with 1 cm margins. Lesions between 1 to 4 mm in thickness should ideally be excised with 2 cm margins. In locations where a 2 cm margin cannot be obtained, a 1 cm margin is acceptable. Melanomas with a thickness greater than 4 mm should undergo resection with 2 cm margins (Table 6). If tissue allows for a 3 cm margin around these lesions, a wider margin should be considered.[5,8,9]

Table 6: Recommended clinical excision margins for melanoma based on thickness[5]

Tumor Thickness	Recommended Margins
In situ	0.5 cm
<1 mm	1 cm
1-4 mm	2 cm
>4 mm	2 cm

In addition to obtaining adequate horizontal margins, resection should be carried down to the underlying fascia, although the fascia itself does not need to be excised. A number of reconstructive options exist following wide excision. A simple local advancement flap is most commonly used, often by performing the resection in an elliptical fashion. Ideally a length-to-width ratio of 3:1 should be observed in order to allow for ideal tissue closure. Rotational flaps, Z-plasty closures, V-Y flaps, as well as pedicled or free flaps can be used in difficult situations; however, they are not often necessary.

Skin grafting in general provides good closure in situations where closure by an advancement flap is not possible. Full thickness skin grafting should be used for the face, scalp, and hands. Split-thickness grafts can be used to cover larger areas such as the chest, back, or proximal extremities.

SITE-SPECIFIC CONSIDERATIONS

There are general recommendations indicating the extent of surgical resection that are applicable to most of the body.

However, some anatomic sites do not follow such rigid surgical criteria. Situations which require special surgical considerations include subungual melanomas and lesions involving the digits, face, and sole of the foot.

More than 75% of subungual melanomas involve either the great toe or the thumb. Melanoma on a digit or under the nail is usually removed via a partial digital amputation. Amputations of the finger are often performed at the middle interphalangeal joint. Amputations of the thumb are often performed proximal to the interphalangeal joint. Amputations that are more proximal are not shown to have improved survival and are rarely indicated. For melanoma located on a toe, the entire digit is amputated at the metatarsal-phalangeal joint, except for the great toe, where the amputation is often proximal to the interphalangeal joint.[14]

When the melanoma is excised on the foot plantar surface, a significant weight-bearing area defect is made and thus a plantar flap is often placed to provide well-vascularized local tissue. Staged closure of some plantar melanomas have been performed with the initial use of a negative pressure wound vacuum to stimulate granulation tissue formation which is then followed by skin graft application.[14]

When working with facial lesions, more than a 1 cm margin cannot be excised due to adjacent vital structures; in these cases, it is important to consider the tumor's diameter, thickness, and exact location on the face when margin width is planned. Mohs surgery using repeated microscopic analysis to obtain negative margins has been used with some success for facial lesions. Best results have been reported for melanoma in situ; however, it has also been used successfully for select deeper lesions.

EVALUATION OF LYMPHATIC INVOLVEMENT

Melanomas generally metastasize through lymphatic spread using a predictable route. The most likely site of initial spread of melanoma disease is to the regional lymph nodes. Any palpable lymph node should be considered highly suspicious for metastatic disease. Presence of metastatic disease can be confirmed with fine needle aspiration biopsy. Patients with clinical evidence of nodal metastasis at the time of their initial operation should undergo lymph node dissection at the time of the initial surgery. However, In the majority of cases the status of the regional lymph nodes is not known beforehand.[4,10,11]

The use of lymphatic mapping and sentinel lymph node biopsy allows for identification of occult lymphatic metastasis without subjecting patients to an initial morbid procedure like lymphadenectomy (Figure 4). Sentinel lymph node biopsy is indicated in all patients whose melanomas are 1 mm or greater in thickness. Sentinel node biopsy should be selectively used in patients with tumor thickness between 0.75 mm and 1 mm when other worrisome features such as ulceration, a high mitotic rate, young age, or a Clarks stage IV or greater are present. Patients who are found to be node negative on sentinel lymph node exam are more than 6 times more likely to survive than patients who have a positive sentinel lymph node. Thus, the predictive value of a sentinel lymph node biopsy is one of the most valuable prognostic factors. Additional evidence suggests that early removal of micro-metastatic disease from the lymph node basins may improve overall survival as opposed to waiting for regional recurrence before performing a lymphadenectomy.[4,10,11]

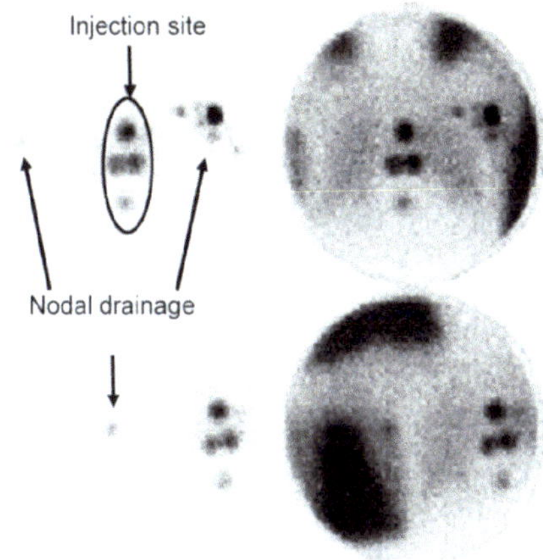

Figure 4: Mapping the area of radioactivity during a sentinel node imaging procedure. Images derived from the use of the gamma camera to detect foci of radioactive uptake after injection of radiocolloid. The images on the left show the tracer activity in the injection sites and nodes. The corresponding images on the right are obtained by waving a sheet source of radioactivity behind the patient to produce a body (and lung) outline for reference.

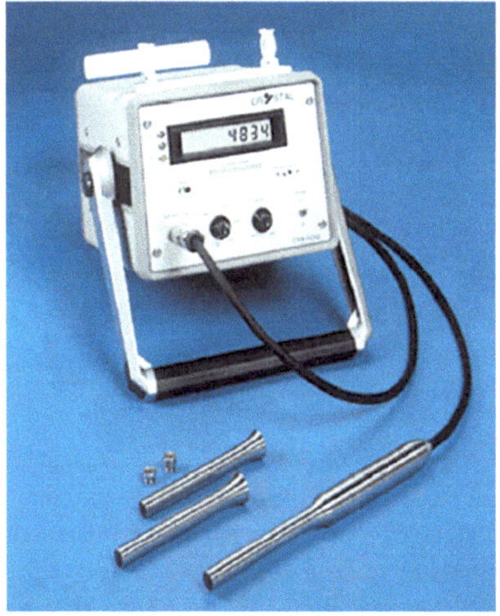

Figure 5: Gamma detector for SLN biopsy. Hand-held gamma probe that is used intraoperatively to detect a sentinel lymph node (SLN) after local injection of radioactive colloid around the primary tumor.

The sentinel lymph node is defined as the first lymph node to receive lymphatic drainage from the primary tumor site. In order to identify the sentinel node, a radiocolloid such as technetium–sulfur colloid, a blue dye such as lymphazurin or isosulfan blue dye, or a combination of both dye and radiocolloid are used. Preoperative lymphoscintigraphy is performed to identify all possible draining lymphatic basins. The site of the sentinel node can then be marked on the patient. In the operating room, before preparing the operative site, the blue dye is injected at the biopsy site as a second aid in identifying the sentinel node. The injection should be intradermal to allow for maximal passage of dye within the lymphatics. Approximately 1-2 ml of dye should be used. Sentinel lymph node dissection should be performed prior to excision of the primary melanoma.[4]

A gamma probe is used intraoperatively to confirm the location of the sentinel node prior to making an incision as well as intermittently following incision to localize the site of the sentinel node. The sentinel node can be identified by color or high radioactivity measured with the gamma probe. More than one sentinel node may be present, so the nodal basin should be re-examined after removal of the first sentinel node to ensure no significant radioactivity remains. Nodes that measure within 10 percent of the highest measured lymph node should be excised.[3]

In patients with nodal metastasis, a complete lymphadenectomy is the standard of care. A complete lymph node dissection is significantly more invasive that a sentinel lymph node biopsy and carries a much higher rate of morbidity, particularly with regard to lymphedema.[3]

CHEMOTHERAPY AND RADIOTHERAPY

Traditional chemotherapeutic regimens have generally been shown to be ineffective in the treatment of melanoma. The cytokine IFN alfa-2b has been shown to improve overall survival and lengthen the disease-free period in patients without evidence of systemic metastasis. IFN alfa-2b therapy generally requires a 12-month treatment plan and is notable for having substantial toxic side effects. Despite this, IFN alfa-2b is currently the only approved adjuvant therapy of melanoma, and all patients with high-risk melanoma should be informed of the option as well as its risks and benefits.[15]

Melanoma is traditionally thought of as a radioresistant cancer. Despite this, there is some evidence to suggest that the use of radiotherapy may decrease the risk of recurrence in lymph node dissection basins in cases where multiple lymph nodes are involved or there is gross extracapsular extension. The use of radiotherapy is not without significant risks. There is an increased risk of lymphedema following radiation therapy. In lymphatic basins such as the cervical region where there is a higher incidence of nodal recurrence, the risks of radiotherapy may outweigh the possible benefits.[13]

TREATMENT OF LOCAL RECURRENCE AND IN-TRANSIT METASTASIS

Isolated local recurrence is rare when appropriate surgical practices are followed during the initial operation. Local recurrence can be treated with a repeat wide local excision with 2 cm margins.[5] 2-3 percent of patients who have had a primary melanoma removed will develop in-transit metastatic disease. This disease pattern is peculiar to melanoma, and results from foci of tumor cells that spread via lymphatics without reaching the lymph nodes. They present as dermal or subcutaneous lesions.

Management of in-transit metastasis is dictated by the number and size of the lesions. In cases where there are a small number of lesions, the metastases may be excised with a small negative pathologic margin. More commonly however, the extent of the disease prohibits local excision and leads to common disease recurrence. Hyperthermic isolated limb perfusion is one treatment strategy for in-transit metastasis in an extremity that allows for chemotherapeutic administration. The concentration is 15-25 times higher than is possible with systemic chemotherapy and without the systemic side effects. Hyperthermic isolated limb perfusion uses the drug Melphalan as the standard chemotherapeutic agent due to its efficacy and low regional toxicity. Use of isolated limb perfusion has not been shown to significantly improve survival; however, it has been shown to provide substantial palliation of local and regional symptoms when other options have been exhausted.[16]

Some centers have employed the use of local immunotherapy in patients with in-transit disease. This involves injection of Bacilli Calmette-Guerin (BCG), or interferon-alpha combined with topical application of imiquimod cream. This results in local inflammation and toxicities such as erythema, ulceration, and edema. Some centers report a regression of approximately 80 percent of injected lesions, particularly among the smaller lesions.[4]

METASTATIC DISEASE

Distant metastatic disease has traditionally been seen as a contraindication for surgery. In a carefully selected subset of patients however, resection may be appropriate. Recent studies have shown that while systemic therapy has never shown an improved survival, postoperative adjuvant vaccine therapy following resection of distant metastatic disease has demonstrated a nearly 40 percent 5-year survival rate. Isolated small bowel metastases appear to have a particularly favorable prognosis.[14] Preoperative staging and careful selection of appropriate patients for resection is crucial. Workup should include CT (Figure 6 and 7) of the chest, abdomen, and pelvis, as well as PET scan and MRI of the brain. So long as all lesions can be resected, the number of metastases does not have a major impact on the overall outcome.[8]

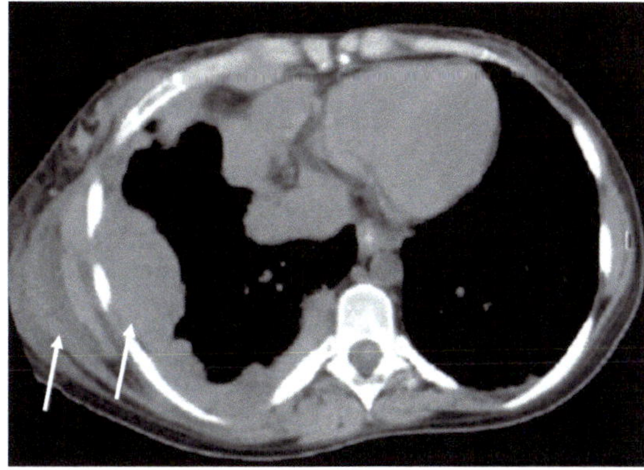

Figure 6: Thoracic metastases from melanoma. Axial CT shows extensive pleural metastases due to melanoma. There is an associated soft tissue mass in the right chest wall.

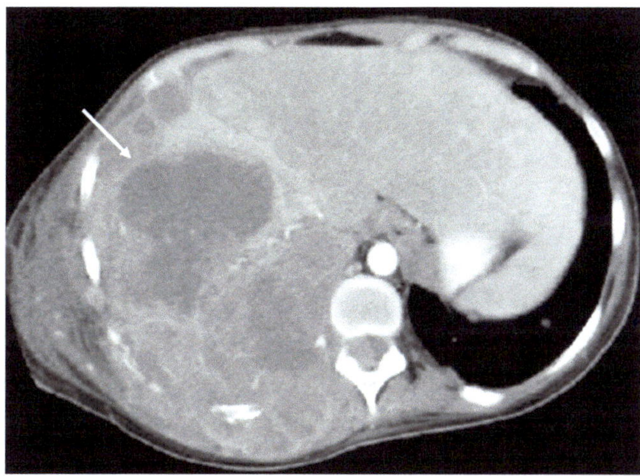

Figure 7: Necrotic metastases from melanoma. Large hepatic metastasis with central necrosis due to metastatic melanoma.

REFERENCES

1. Altekruse SF, Kosary CL, Krapcho M, et al (Eds). SEER Cancer Statistics Review, 1975-2007, National Cancer Institute. Bethesda, MD, http://seer.cancer.gov/csr/1975_2007/, based on November 2009 SEER data submission, posted to the SEER web site, 2010.
2. Harmful effects of ultraviolet radiation. Council on Scientific Affairs. JAMA 1989;262(3):380-4.
3. Sabel MS. Oncology. In: Doherty G (Ed). Current Diagnosis and Treatment: Surgery, (13th edn). New York: McGraw Hill 2010;1225-7.
4. Farles MB, Morton DL. Cutaneous melanoma. In: Cameron JL (ed). Current Surgical Therapy. (9th edn). Philadelphia: Mosby 2008;1096-1100.
5. Goldsmith L, Koh HK, Bewerse B, et al. Proceedings from the national conference to develop a national skin cancer agenda. American Academy of Dermatology and Centers for Disease Control and Prevention, April 8-10, 1995. J Am Acad Dermatol 1996;34(5 Pt 1): 822-3.
6. Balch CM, Soong SJ, Gershenwald JE, et al. Prognostic factors analysis of 17, 600 melanoma patients: validation of the American Joint Committee on Cancer melanoma staging system. J Clin Oncol 2001;19:3622-34.
7. Breslow A. Tumor thickness, level of invasion and node dissection in stage I cutaneous melanoma. Ann Surg 1975;182:572-5.
8. Balch CM, Buzaid AC, Soong S, et al. Final version of the American Joint Committee on Cancer staging system for cutaneous melanoma. J Clin Oncol 2001;19:3635-48.
9. Edge SB, et al. AJCC Cancer Staging Handbook, (7th edn). Springer Publishing, 2010.
10. Morton DL, et al. Sentinel node biopsy or nodal observation in melanoma. N Engl J Med 2006; 355:1307.
11. Vaquerano J, Kraybill WG, Driscoll DL, et al. American Joint Committee on Cancer clinical stage as a selection criterion for sentinel lymph node biopsy in thin melanoma. Ann Surg Oncol 2006;13:198-204.
12. Sheffield MV, Yee H, Dorvault CC, et al. Comparison of five antibodies as markers in the diagnosis of melanoma in cytologic preparations. Am J Clin Pathol 2002;118:930-6.
13. Balch CM, et al. Cutaneous Melanoma (4th edn). Quality Medical Publishing, 2003.
14. Gershenwald JE, Hwu P. Melanoma. Holland-Frei Cancer Medicine, (8th edn). In: Hong WK, Bast RC, et al (eds). Peoples Medical Publishing House, 2010.
15. Sabel MS, Sondak VK. Pros and cons of adjuvant interferon in the treatment of melanoma. Oncologist 2003;8:451.
16. Blazer DG, Sondak VK, Sabel MS. Surgical therapy of cutaneous melanoma. Semin Oncol 2007;34:270.

❑❑❑

SECTION 3: GASTROINTESTINAL

25. Acute Abdomen
26. Femoral and Inguinal Hernia, and Testicular Diseases
27. Esophagus
28. Stomach
29. Liver
30. Gallbladder and Biliary System
31. Pancreas
32. Spleen
33. Appendix
34. Bariatric and Metabolic Surgery
35. Small Bowel Neoplasms
36. Large Bowel Tumors
37. Anorectal Diseases

25

CHAPTER

Acute Abdomen

Melissa Wong, MD
Yogendra Patel, MD

INTRODUCTION

BACKGROUND/HISTORICAL PERSPECTIVE

Acute abdominal pain is sudden-onset, non-traumatic abdominal pain, lasting fewer than 7 days (most common 1-2 days) in duration, where there is an urgent need to determine if surgery is necessary or not. Acute abdominal pain accounts for about 5-10% of all emergency room visits. In addition, 2-3% of patients presenting to their primary care physicians' office report abdominal pain, including Internal Medicine, Family Practice, Pediatrics, and Obstetrics/Gynecology. Therefore, a thorough knowledge of the differential diagnosis of acute abdominal pain is important not only for surgeons, but also for non-surgical specialists to enable early diagnosis and prompt referral to a surgeon, if necessary. However, approximately two thirds of patients who present with acute onset of abdominal pain will not need surgical intervention. Pain lasting more than 6 hours in duration, but fewer than 48 hours is most characteristic of surgical etiologies. Beyond this timeframe, non-surgical causes are more likely.[1,2] In a survey of 10,320 patients with abdominal pain, the most common diagnosis was idiopathic abdominal pain; no cause for pain was identified in 34% of patients. In this series, the four most common surgical diagnoses were acute appendicitis (28.1%), acute cholecystitis (9.7%), small bowel obstruction (4.1%), and acute gynecologic disease (4.0%).[3] Furthermore, the most common diagnoses differed by patient age (Table 1). However, in children, the most common cause of abdominal pain was nonspecific (62%), followed by acute appendicitis (32%).

Table 1a: Incidence of Most Common Diagnoses in Adults with Acute Abdominal Pain in the World Organization of Gastroenterology (OMGE) Study, by Patient Age[4]

	Frequency (% of Patients)	
Diagnosis	**Age <50 years old (N = 6,317)**	**Age ≥50 years old (N = 2,406)**
Abdominal pain is nonspecific	39.5	15.7
Appendicitis	32.0	15.2
Cholecystitis	6.3	20.9
Obstruction	2.5	12.3
Pancreatitis	1.6	7.3
Diverticular disease	< 0.1	5.5
Cancer	< 0.1	4.1
Hernia	< 0.1	3.1
Vascular disease	< 0.1	2.3

Table 1b: Examples of common causes of acute abdominal pain arising from various abdominal organs are listed below.

Organ	Disease
Stomach & duodenum	Perforated Peptic Ulcer Perforated gastric cancer Acute Alcoholic gastritis Food Poisoning
Small Intestine	Obstruction Incarcerated hernias Inflammatory bowel disease Intussusception Mesenteric arterial or venous occlusion

Organ	Disease
Colon	Acute diverticulitis Sigmoid volvulus
Appendix	Acute appendicitis
Liver	Acute hepatitis Congestive hepatomegaly
Gallbladder	Acute cholecystitis Acute Cholangitis Obstructive jaundice
Spleen	Acute splenomegaly Splenic infarct Spontaneous rupture of pathological splenomegaly
Pancreas	Acute / chronic Pancreatitis
Kidney	Acute pyelonephritis Pyonephrosis Renal stones
Female Pelvic Organs	Pelvic Inflammatory Disease Ectopic pregnancy Torsion of ovary or fibroid Ruptured ovarian cyst
Retroperitoneal	Ruptured aortic aneurysm Aortic dissection

The subject of acute abdomen, and this chapter, owe much to Zachary Cope's *Early Diagnosis of the Acute Abdomen*. He was driven by the principle of "earlier diagnosis means better prognosis.[5]" In 1921, when his book was first published, Cope's primary tools were his understanding of anatomy and physiology, which he applied to the patient's history and physical examination. Notwithstanding the technological advances of the past century, anatomy and physiology remain the keys to deciphering the acute abdomen.

ANATOMY AND PATHOPHYSIOLOGY

ANATOMY

The abdominal cavity is lined by the peritoneal membrane, a layer of simple squamous mesothelium. The total surface area of the peritoneum is approximately 1.4 m^2.[6] Parietal peritoneum covers the anterior, lateral, and posterior abdominal walls. Visceral peritoneum, also called the serosal layer of the gastrointestinal tract, envelops the intra-abdominal organs. These peritoneal coverings tend to stick together in intra-peritoneal infections as the body's response to localize the infection.

The peritoneal fluid that is secreted into the peritoneal cavity by the peritoneum enables the mobile viscera to glide easily on one another. Since there is constant movement of the diaphragm, abdominal muscles, and peristaltic movements of the intestinal tract, peritoneal fluid is not static and has a direction of flow moving towards the subphrenic spaces. Further, the peritoneal cavity contains about 50 mL of normal physiologic fluid.

The peritoneal cavity is divided into greater and lesser sacs. Both sacs communicate through the omental foramen, or Foramen of Winslow. The lesser sac is bordered by the stomach, liver, transverse colon, gastrocolic ligament (greater omentum), and lesser omentum. The greater sac or main peritoneal cavity is divided by the transverse mesocolon into the supra-colic and infra-colic regions. The infra-colic region is divided by the mesentery of the small intestine into right upper and left lower halves. Below the sacral promontory is the lesser pelvis, which contains the Pouch of Douglas. Aside from these main divisions, there exist other smaller recesses: the right and left subphrenic spaces, the hepato-renal space, also known as Morrison's pouch (the most dependent portion in supine position aside from the pelvic cavity), and the right and left paracolic gutters, lateral to the ascending and descending colons, respectively. Fluid, blood, or pus can collect in these various spaces.

The omentum, the "fatty apron" hanging from the greater curvature of the stomach and from the transverse colon, is a vascular double layer of peritoneum containing focal concentrations of macrophages. It is constantly on the move and may adhere to other peritoneal surfaces around a focus of infection. The omentum plays a vital role in localizing inflammation and infection, and sealing off viscus perforations, leading to its nickname "the policeman of the abdomen."

The retroperitoneum contains the bare area of the liver, the second and third portions of the duodenum, the pancreas, the kidneys and ureters, and variable portions of the posterior walls of the ascending and descending colons and retrocecal appendix.

SOURCES AND MECHANISMS OF ABDOMINAL PAIN

There are three main types of abdominal pain: visceral, parietal, and referred pains.

VISCERAL PAIN

Visceral peritoneum covers the abdominal solid organs and intestines. It is innervated by the autonomic nervous system, mediated by afferent C fibers running in a bilateral distribution. This makes visceral pain vaguely localized, usually midline. The axial location of visceral pain follows the embryologic origin of the viscera. Pain from all foregut-derived structures is perceived in the upper abdomen, in the epigastric region, and both upper quadrants. Pain arising from midgut-derived structures is perceived in the mid-abdomen or periumbilical area. Pain from hindgut-derived structures is perceived in the lower abdomen which includes the hypogastric area and both lower quadrants.

Visceral pain is triggered by inflammation, ischemia, distension, and obstruction. Except for the latter, the pain caused by these stimuli will be steady and aching in nature. If the pain is due to obstructive pathology of any hollow viscus, with resulting distension, it will be colicky in nature.

Inflammation: Whether the underlying etiology is bacterial infection, chemical irritation, or ischemia, mediators of the inflammatory response (e.g., prostaglandins, histamine, bradykinin, and serotonin) stimulate afferent nerve endings and produce visceral abdominal pain.

Ischemia: When tissues without adequate blood supply become ischemic, metabolites and other wastes build up and stimulate pain receptors. As the ischemia persists, the accumulated toxins build up and the pain intensifies.

Distension: Afferent nerve endings are also directly stimulated by distension of the capsule in solid organs, and of the wall in hollow viscus organs, which can result from mechanical obstruction, pseudo-obstruction, or ileus (Figure 1), or edema linked to bacterial, chemical, or viral inflammation. The rate of distension of the visceral peritoneum, whether rapid (as in the case of dilated small bowel loops in mechanical obstruction) or more gradual (as in distension of Glissen's capsule in acute hepatitis), leads to severe or mild visceral pain, respectively.

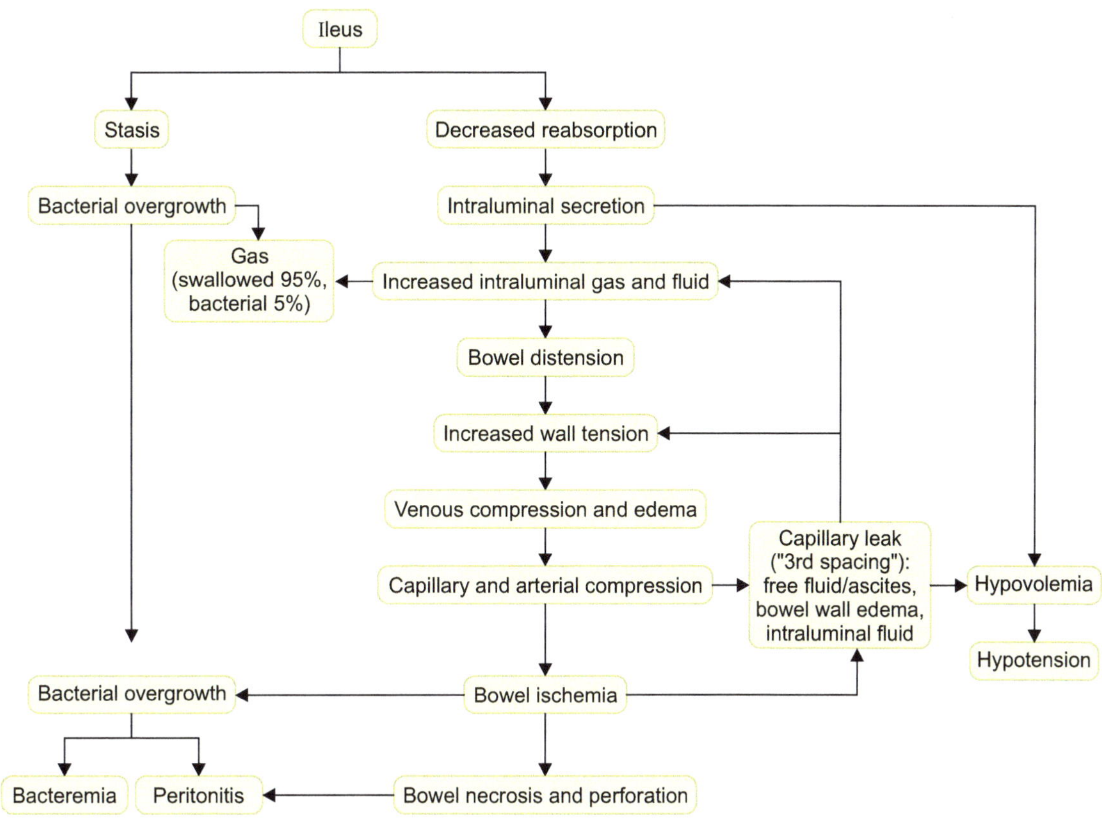

Figure 1: Pathophysiology of ileus

PARIETAL PAIN

Parietal peritoneum covers the anterior, lateral, and retroperitoneal walls of the abdominal cavity. It is innervated by somatic nerves with unilateral distribution, making parietal pain sensations more precisely localized to the anatomical location of the underlying pathology. Unlike visceral pain, parietal pain is more acute, localized, and severe. Visceral pain being replaced by parietal pain generally indicates that the condition has progressed and is potentially worsening. It may be due to painful stimuli including inflammation due to infection or chemical irritation by various body fluids (e.g., blood, pus).

It is worth noting that parietal peritonitis can induce spasm in the overlying muscles of the abdominal wall, giving rise to rigidity or voluntary guarding, as well as to abdominal wall tenderness. This fact forms the basis of many physical examination findings in acute abdominal conditions (e.g., psoas sign and obturator sign).

REFERRED PAIN

Referred pain is perceived by patients at a location that is embryologically related to, but anatomically remote from, the source of pathology. For example, pain from diaphragmatic irritation, either superior or inferior surface, is felt in the ipsilateral shoulder. Thus, left shoulder pain may indicate irritation of the inferior left diaphragm from splenic rupture (Kehr's sign), ruptured ectopic pregnancy (Danforth sign), pancreatitis (tail), or splenic flexure inflammation. Irritation of the right hemidiaphragm from an inflamed gallbladder may produce referred pain to the right shoulder. Irritation of the pleural surface of the diaphragm (e.g., pleurisy, empyema, or basilar pneumonia) can also cause referred pain in the ipsilateral shoulder and/or corresponding upper quadrant. Inferior wall myocardial infarctions may produce referred pain to the upper abdomen and epigastrium. Conditions involving retroperitoneal structures, such as the pancreas, aorta, and duodenum, may produce referred pain to the back. Testicular pain can be referred to the upper abdomen due to its embryonic origin from the abdomen. Referred pain from the gastrointestinal tract also follows a definite relationship between the embryonic origin of the viscera and location of pain as the nerves follow the blood vessels (Table 2).

Table 2a: Embryologic Basis for Referred Pain from the Intestines

Embryonic Structure	Blood Supply	Organs Derived	Location Of Pain
Foregut	Celiac Artery	Esophagus, Stomach, Duodenum, Pancreas, Liver, Gallbladder, common bile duct, Spleen	Upper Abdomen Epigastric Right or left upper quadrants
Border Landmark	Ligament of Treitz (Embryologic border is second part of duodenum)		
Midgut	Superior Mesenteric Artery	Small intestine, appendix, Meckel's diverticulum, cecum, ascending colon & proximal 2/3 of transverse colon	Mid-abdomen Periumbilical
Border Landmark	Junction of proximal 2/3 with distal 1/3 transverse colon		
Hind Gut	Inferior Mesenteric artery	Splenic flexure, descending colon, rectosigmoid colon	Lower abdomen Hypogastric area Right or left lower quadrants

Table 2b: Embryologic basis for referred pain - Miscellaneous

Source	Embryological relationship	Location of pain
Diaphragm, gallbladder, pancreas	Phrenic nerve C3-5	Shoulder Pain
Kidney	Metanephros, Wolffian ducts, gonadal ridge	Testis

Extra-Abdominal Sources of Abdominal Pain

While most cases of acute abdomen will be traceable to an intra-abdominal pathology, there are many extra-abdominal conditions that present with sudden-onset, severe abdominal pain similar to that associated with parietal peritonitis. This is commonly interpreted by patients as abdominal pains, making them part of the differential diagnosis of the acute abdomen. Some originate from near the abdomen, such as the abdominal wall (e.g., rectus sheath hematoma), retroperitoneum or back (e.g., retroperitoneal hemorrhage, psoas abscess, osteomyelitis of spine), genitourinary system (e.g., pyelonephritis, pyonephrosis, acute cystitis, prostatitis, epididymo-orchitis, testicular torsion, perinephric abscess, ureteral stones), and thoracolumbar nerve root pain (e.g., disc disease, herpes zoster, spinal cord tumor, multiple sclerosis). Some of these are cases of referred pain, as discussed above (e.g., pneumonia, pleurisy, empyema, inferior wall myocardial infarct). Others are related to metabolic derangements (e.g., diabetic ketoacidosis, Familial Mediterranean fever, hypercalcemic crisis), toxic syndromes (e.g., tetany, Black Widow spider bite, drug withdrawals, or arsenic or mercury poisoning), or autoimmune disorders, (e.g., systemic sclerosis, polyarteritis nodosa, systemic lupus erythematosus, Henoch-Schoenlein Purpura).

Two rare neurologic syndromes of paroxysmal abdominal pain (usually associated with nausea and vomiting) are worth mentioning. The first, abdominal migraine, is not initially associated with a headache component but patients tend to develop traditional migraine headaches later in life. Consensus diagnostic criteria exist for pediatric patients, but this condition is increasingly suspected to occur in adults as well. It demonstrates the same familial clustering, female predominance, and trigger-responsiveness as traditional migraines, and responds to migraine treatments such as triptans and propranolol.[7] Abdominal epilepsy is a rare syndrome of seizure activity manifesting primarily as abdominal pain, accompanied by neurologic symptoms. It is more common in the pediatric than adult population and is treated with anti-seizure medication.[8]

INITIAL PRESENTATION AND EVALUATION

HISTORY

An accurate history of the acute abdomen often accurately indicates the diagnosis. Three cardinal symptoms in any history of the acute abdomen are abdominal pain, fever, and vomiting. Understanding the pathogenesis of these symptoms helps predict the underlying pathology.

PAIN

Pain is a primary and often the most severe feature in cases of acute abdomen. The three major types of abdominal pain, described above, are visceral, parietal, and referred. While it is usually possible to distinguish among these once a complete description of the pain has been elicited, cases of true acute abdomen often present with more than one of these types of pain. A complete description of the pain includes its location, quality (e.g., sharp versus aching, intermittent versus constant), onset (e.g., sudden versus gradual), duration, progression (e.g., worsening versus improving), and alleviating or aggravating factors (e.g., position, fatty foods) (Table 3).

Table 3: Typical pain patterns

RUQ pain radiating to the back, scapular region, or shoulder. Associated with fatty food intolerance	Acute Cholecystitis
Epigastric or periumbilical colicky pain that shifts to RLQ steady aching pain	Acute Appendicitis
Epigastric pain exacerbated by lying down and relieved by sitting up	Acute Pancreatitis
Postprandial pain 30-60 minutes after food intake	Mesenteric Ischemia (Intestinal Angina)
Pain relieved by eating or antacids	Peptic Ulcer Disease

Table 4: Common causes of acute abdominal pain by pathophysiology

Inflammation/Infection	Obstruction	Ischemia	Hemorrhage
• Spontaneous bacterial peritonitis	• Int. Obstruction due to adhesion, Incarcerated Hernia,	• Mesenteric occlusion	• Blunt & penetrating trauma
• Perforated viscus	• Volvulus, Gallstone	• Splenic infarct	• Ectopic pregnancy
• Ruptured ovarian cyst	• Ileus, Intussusception,	• Strangulated Hernia	• Ruptured aortic or visceral artery aneurysm
• Mittelschmerz	• Foreign bodies, bezoars & parasites	• Torsion of ovarian cyst	• Ruptured ovarian cyst
• Acute gastritis	• Gastric outlet obstruction,	• Torsion of fibroid	• Endometriosis
• Acute gastroenteritis	• Colonic obstruction due to volvulus, tumor, diverticulitis	• Omental Torsion	• Aortic dissection
• Acute viral hepatitis		• Necrotic fibroids	
• Acute cholecystitis			
• Acute suppurative cholangitis			
• Acute pancreatitis			
• Inflammatory Bowel Disease			
• Meckel's Diverticulitis			
• Acute Appendicitis			
• Acute Diverticulitis			
• Bacterial Colitis			
• Amoebic dysentery			
• Ulcerative colitis			
• Intraperitoneal abscesses			
• Mesenteric adenitis[9]			
• Epiploic Appendagitis			
• Salpingo-oophoritis			
• Tubo-ovarian abscess			
• Endometritis			
• Ruptured Pyonephrosis			

COLIC

Colicky pain, a type of visceral pain caused by smooth muscle contraction of a hollow viscus against an obstruction, is worth particular mention. Colic is typically paroxysmal, with sudden severe episodes between intervening periods of partial or full relief. Patients may grimace and assume a fetal position for relief or be writhing in bed trying to find a comfortable position. The severity of the colic is proportional to the force of peristaltic activity present in the organ. It is important to realize that many acute abdominal conditions start with obstruction of a hollow organ (Table 5).

Table 5: Obstruction of a hollow organ leading to acute abdomen

Site and cause of obstruction	Resulting pathology
Appendix, by fecalith or lymphoid hyperplasia	Acute appendicitis
Cystic duct, by gallstone	Acute cholecystitis
Colonic diverticulum, by fecalith	Acute diverticulitis
Pancreatic or common bile duct, by gallstone	Acute pancreatitis
Common bile duct, by gallstone	Acute suppurative cholangitis

Different organs produce colics of different quality:

- Esophageal and gastric obstruction do not produce typical colicky type pain. Gastric outlet obstruction manifests as vague epigastric discomfort associated with projectile vomiting due to reverse peristalsis.
- Biliary colic, from cystic or common bile duct obstruction by a gallstone, is felt in the epigastric and/or right upper quadrant and may radiate toward the back, at the angle of the right scapula. Unlike other colics, it tends not to be spasmodic because the gallbladder and bile ducts are sparsely muscular. Instead, the pain is primarily due to distention and will feel constant, dull, and aching.
- Intestinal and appendicular colics are classic non-radiating, paroxysmal pains. Pain in the periumbilical or mid-abdominal regions originates from the small intestine, Meckel's diverticulum, appendix, and right colon. Whereas colic from the left colon is felt in the hypogastric region. In small bowel obstruction, the pain is more severe with distal rather than proximal obstruction.
- Ureteral colic radiates from the loin to the groin, may radiate to scrotum or labia, and is usually associated with micro- or macroscopic hematuria. Pain due to obstruction at the uretero-pelvic junction is constant and not colicky as there is no peristaltic activity in the renal pelvis and calyces.
- Uterine colic can present as menstrual cramps (spasmodic dysmenorrhea) or as labor pains in the gravid uterus. It is colicky pain localized in the lower abdomen and in the lower back.

The most severe colicky pain is ureteral, followed in descending order by intestinal, biliary, and colonic pain. Colonic obstructive pain is more likely to be due to distension rather than strong peristaltic contractions.

ANOREXIA, NAUSEA AND VOMITING

This triad represents the same symptoms on a continuum of increasing severity. They are all caused by either peritoneal irritation or by distension of a hollow viscus (Figure 2). They represent nature's protective reflex to decompress the gastrointestinal tract. In contrast to gastroenteritis, where vomiting generally precedes pain, most cases of acute abdomen are associated with vomiting that follows the onset of pain.

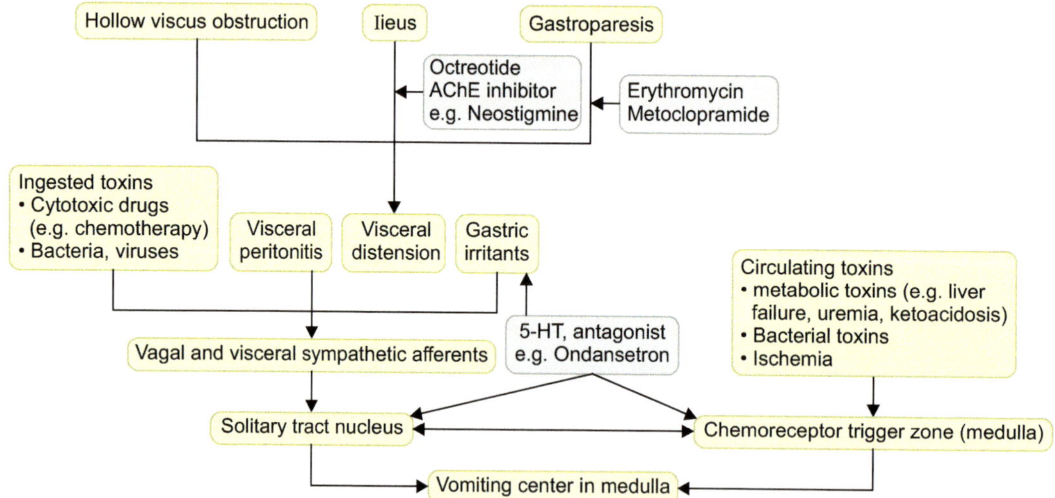

Figure 2: Vomiting in the acute abdomen[10]

The severity and frequency of vomiting varies by the location of the pathology. In an upper intestinal obstruction, vomiting starts early, is copious, and more frequent. In a distal small bowel obstruction, vomiting tends to start later. In colonic obstruction, vomiting occurs late and only if the ileocecal valve is incompetent.

The quality of vomitus can also shed light on the location or type of intestinal pathology. For example, feculent vomitus results from the bacterial proliferation and fermentation in a distal small bowel obstruction. Hematemesis or rectal bleeding associated with abdominal pain is highly suggestive of intestinal ischemia and hence is in urgent need for surgical evaluation.

It is important to remember that the absence of anorexia, nausea, or vomiting does not rule out severe intra-abdominal pathology. In several studies of patients with proven acute appendicitis, about one third of patients have a normal appetite.[11-13]

FEVER

The presence of fever indicates an infectious or inflammatory etiology. In the early stages of acute abdomen, the patient may be afebrile or may have low grade fever. A septic patient may exhibit hypothermia. On the other extreme, high fever at the beginning of the presentation of acute abdomen is more likely to be from pneumonia, acute pyelonephritis, or acute suppurative cholangitis. Fever with chills may indicate bacteremia. Patients who are immunocompromised, elderly, or taking steroids may not mount a febrile response (Figure 3).

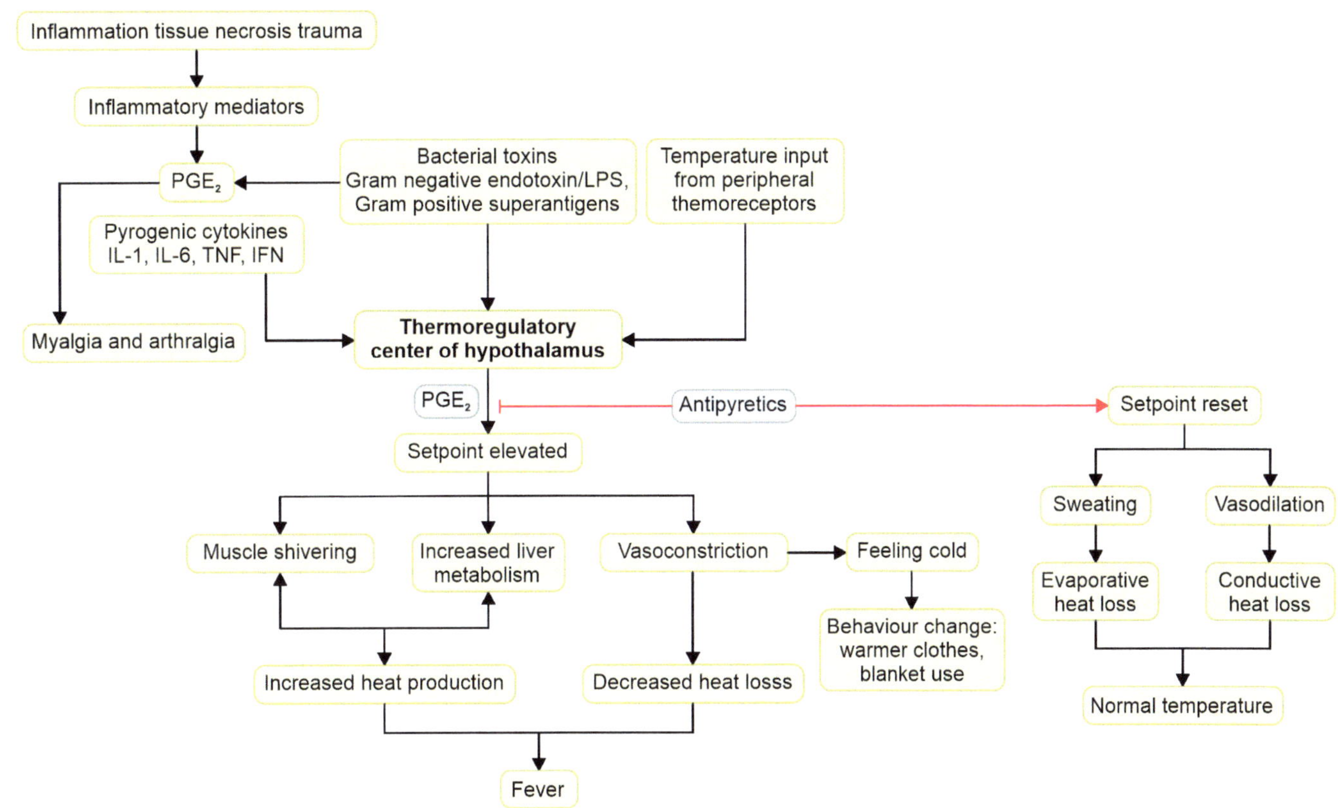

Figure 3: Pathogenesis of fever in the acute abdomen

OTHER SYMPTOMS

Symptoms associated with the presentation of abdominal pain often give important clues. Abdominal pain and distension with constipation and obstipation suggest a complete obstruction, whereas the same pain and distension with diarrhea suggest partial obstruction, intra-abdominal abscess (especially pelvic abscess) (Figure 4), or other pathology. A general review of systems may also elicit other relevant symptoms, such as urinary frequency or a new cough which the patient may not remember to mention or recognize as being related. As with any description of accompanying symptoms (e.g., jaundice, hematuria, hematemesis, vaginal discharge), it is important to note whether it started before or after the onset of pain, and whether it is improving, worsening, or stable.

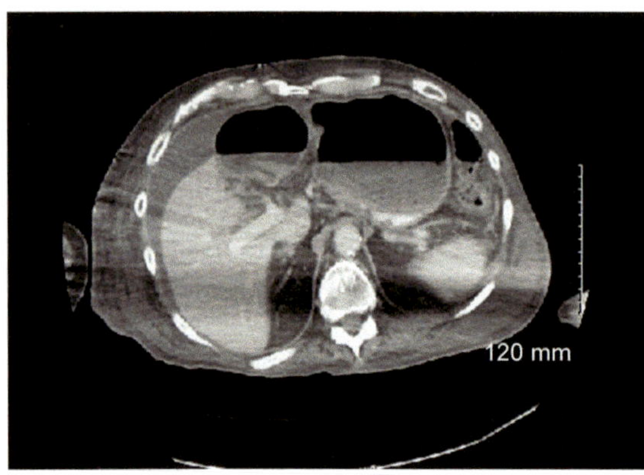

Figure 4: Intraabdominal collection

PAST MEDICAL HISTORY

It is important to understand the patient's past medical history because (1) this may alter the presentation of their illness (e.g., atypical pain presentation of acute MI in diabetics), and in the case of a patient who requires urgent or emergent surgery, (2) may add significant perioperative risk (e.g., risk of perioperative tachyarrhythmias or MI in patients with significant cardiac history), and (3) increase their risk of postoperative complications (e.g., poor wound healing among diabetics). If these conditions are known ahead of time, the proactive surgeon can anticipate and preempt likely complications (e.g., frequent blood glucose measurements and early initiation of insulin drip for patients developing diabetic ketoacidosis). Further, beware of the patient who reports no medical problems, particularly among the elderly and obese. The stress of the illness itself, or of operative intervention, may uncover undiagnosed medical problems.

In addition to a general medical history, pay attention to these specific areas:

Screenings: Compliance with appropriate screenings is particularly important among higher risk patients, particularly older or obese patients and those with significant medical history. For example, it may be judicious to ascertain when patients had their last colonoscopy, including the colonoscopy results.

Medications: Review the patient's medication regimen as medication history is integral to their baseline physiology. Are they on immunosuppressive medication? If so, be vigilant for subtle signs of clinical deterioration because they may not mount a fever or leukocytosis. Are they on daily beta-blocker therapy? If so, make sure to continue the medications perioperatively as tolerated, to minimize the risk of perioperative tachyarrhythmias. Are they on daily aspirin, or other antiplatelet or anticoagulation medications? If so, prepare to address coagulopathy and blood loss in the operating room and post-operatively.

Exposures: A history of certain exposures can help make some diagnoses, particularly esoteric ones. Ask about travel, trauma, occupational and social histories. Has the patient traveled to areas endemic for typhoid fever, malaria, or amoebic dysentery? If so, suspect possible ileal perforation, ruptured malarial spleen, or liver abscess, respectively. Trivial trauma can lead to rupture and bleeding from a pathologically enlarged spleen (e.g., malaria, infectious mononucleosis, malignant liver mass). Occupational exposures can alert you to toxic syndromes that are associated with acute abdomen. A history of intravenous drug use or unprotected sex may alert acute hepatitis, undiagnosed HIV, or hepatitis C.

Family History: A patient's family history can be an important clue when determining the cause of acute abdominal pain. For example, most patients with Familial Mediterranean Fever have a first abdominal attack at some point, with fever and acute abdomen, often similar to the presentation of acute appendicitis. An inability to distinguish these conditions may lead to unnecessary surgery.

Gynecologic History: Time of last menstrual period is helpful in the diagnosis of ectopic pregnancy. Duration of the period and amount of bleeding are important to differentiate a normal period from breakthrough spotting experienced in early pregnancy. Abnormal vaginal discharge may be present in pelvic inflammatory disease (PID). History of intrauterine contraceptive device usage, previous tubal surgery, or ectopic pregnancy are risk factors for ectopic pregnancy.

Surgical History: A history of prior abdominal surgery increases a patient's risk for specific post-surgical complications which may present as acute abdomen. In a patient with intestinal obstruction, a history of prior abdominal operation makes post-surgical adhesions, or perhaps incisional hernias, the most likely causes, whereas an occult malignancy is the more likely cause if no such history exists. Patients who have had an aortic graft surgery may develop an aorto-enteric fistula.

PHYSICAL EXAM

When evaluating a patient with acute abdomen, a surgeon seeks to answer a few basic questions: What is the underlying pathology? Does the patient need surgery urgently or emergently? And if so, what approach would be most effective? A surgeon can often obtain the decisive information from a focused physical exam. A systematic approach to the physical exam enables it to be focused without being cursory.

VITAL SIGNS

Vital signs can reveal a lot about a patient if used appropriately. They are quick to obtain and should be followed serially. Interpret initial vital signs in the context of the patient's presenting history and co-morbidities. For example, intractable vomiting will often result in tachycardia and hypotension from dehydration. A normal-appearing blood pressure may be an early sign of relative hypotension in a hypertensive patient. Similarly, a normal-appearing heart rate is falsely reassuring when the patient is taking a beta-blocker.

Orthostatic vital signs, particularly an increase in heart rate with position, are more sensitive to intravascular volume than ordinary blood pressure readings. Orthostatic hypotension is an early indication of hypovolemia due to dehydration or bleeding. An increase in the heart rate of 30 bpm or greater may signify a substantial volume loss.

A fall in cardiac output will cause systolic blood pressure to decrease, while an increase in systemic vascular resistance (SVR) will cause diastolic blood pressure to increase or be maintained. This produces a narrowed pulse pressure (the difference between the systolic and diastolic blood pressures), which is a sign of hypovolemia.

ABDOMINAL EXAM

Most causes of acute abdomen manifest as visceral and/or parietal peritonitis. Once recognized, the presence of peritonitis focuses the diagnosis of acute abdomen (Figure 5).

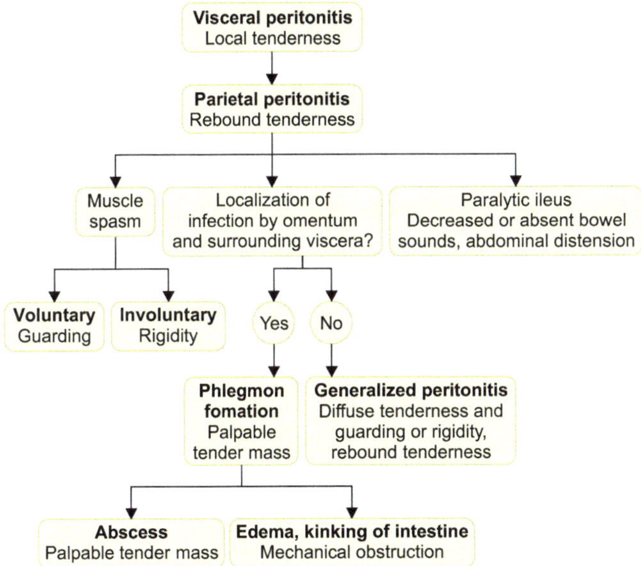

Figure 5: Evolution of peritonitis and associated physical exam findings

Abdominal examination should be done in a systematic manner in the following order:

1. **Inspection:** Much can be learnt from observing a patient's general appearance and demeanor. Does the patient appear well, or toxic? Is he jaundiced? Notice the pallor and cold sweat of a bleeding patient. Notice the apprehension and total stillness of a patient with peritonitis. Mark the restlessness of a colicky patient. Notice the subtle confusion or dullness of a septic, older patient. A dyspneic patient with cough may have pneumonia, whereas a patient with intractable hiccups may have obstruction or ileus, or subphrenic irritation due to abscess, bile, or blood. The presence of old scars suggests a patient's surgical history, even if the patient does not remember and thus, they potentially have intestinal obstruction from adhesions.
2. **Auscultation:** Auscultation of the abdomen is traditionally done in four quadrants to listen for bowel sounds. High-pitched, hyperactive sounds suggest a mechanical obstruction. A total lack of bowel sounds suggests paralytic ileus, which could be due to underlying peritonitis. However, the presence of bowel sounds does not rule out acute abdomen.
3. **Percussion:** Percuss the liver span to see if the patient has hepatomegaly, acute stretching of Glisson's capsule may be due to hepatitis. Gentle percussion which produces disproportionate pain, indicates rebound tenderness and peritonitis. The presence of tympany suggests either bowel obstruction or ileus.
4. **Palpation:** In children and apprehensive adults, voluntary guarding may be present and may not signify underlying peritonitis. Examining with warm hands and asking the patient to flex their hips and knees can help reduce voluntary guarding.

Prior to palpation of the abdomen, ask the patient to point with one finger to where the pain is greatest, and start with gentle palpation away from this area. As you move towards this area, take note of the patient's reaction to help determine whether the pain is localized or diffuse. Is there involuntary guarding or rigidity, or rebound tenderness, indicating peritonitis? Shake the stretcher and watch the patient's reaction to test for peritonitis. Palpate to localize and quantify the patient's pain, if they do not need surgery, this gives you a baseline to compare to when you reexamine the patient later. If they need surgery, this can help you decide what incision to make, and how to prioritize your intra-operative approach.

Pay attention to any masses or lymphadenopathy. A pulsatile abdominal mass, signifying an abdominal aortic aneurysm, may become apparent on deep palpation. A pelvic mass may be a gravid uterus or distended bladder. Periumbilical lymph nodes, also called Sister Mary Joseph nodes, may clue an undiagnosed gastric cancer.

In cases of pelvic inflammatory disease (PID), pelvic appendicitis, or perforated diverticulitis with pelvic abscess, a patient may present with only suprapubic tenderness. When peritonitis is confined to the lesser pelvis, the usual signs of rebound tenderness, abdominal wall guarding, and rigidity may be absent. Only subtle clues of pelvic peritonitis may be apparent, such as evidence of a local bladder or rectosigmoid irritation by history (e.g., dysuria, urinary frequency, abnormal urinalysis diarrhea, tenesmus), digital rectal examination (see pelvis and rectal examinations), or laboratory tests (pyuria).

All possible locations for hernia defects need to be carefully examined by inspection and palpation to avoid missing a small incarcerated or strangulated abdominal wall hernia, particularly in obese patients. If the swelling is not overtly visible, it can easily be missed by the patient.

PELVIC AND RECTAL EXAMINATIONS

Digital rectal exam (DRE) is sometimes eschewed out of consideration for the patient's comfort or sensibilities, but it carries virtually no morbidity and can yield important information. A rectal mass and occult intestinal bleeding suggest an undiagnosed malignancy, whereas a rectal or pelvic mass and tenderness suggest an abscess. A lateral mass palpable on a rectal exam in a patient presenting with small bowel obstruction may indicate an incarcerated obturator hernia. Fullness in the pouch of Douglas indicates pelvic fluid or abscess.

DRE is diagnostic and therapeutic for elderly patients with fecal impaction. In a patient with pelvic peritonitis and abscess due to perforated diverticulitis, salpingitis, tubo-ovarian abscess, or acute appendicitis in a pelvic-lying appendix, DRE reveals the presence of a mass or of pelvic wall tenderness. This is especially true for appendicitis in children. In a study of 181 American children with acute appendicitis, up to 25% had a rectally palpable mass.[14] Overall sensitivity of DRE for acute appendicitis was 41% and specificity 77%.[13] If the underlying pathology is outside the lesser pelvis, DRE is less likely to provide any diagnostic clues of clinical significance.

In female patients, a pelvic exam is an important addition to the physical exam. Pelvic inflammatory disease (PID), pelvic appendicitis, and perforated diverticulitis may cause secondary pelvic abscess or pelvic peritonitis. The patient may present with suprapubic tenderness, but abdominal wall guarding, and rigidity may be absent. A pelvic exam, in combination with a digital rectal exam, will reveal pelvic tenderness, a pelvic mass, cervical motion tenderness, or a feeling of fullness in Douglas's pouch if any fluid or abscess is present. Pelvic peritonitis should be suspected in the presence of any signs and symptoms of bladder irritation (e.g., dysuria, frequency, and abnormal urinalysis) or rectosigmoid irritation (e.g., diarrhea and tenesmus).

Table 6: Clinical significance of history and physical exam findings

Physical Exam Finding	Clinical Significance
Pallor	Signs of shock, hemorrhage, or dehydration
Cyanosis	Primary respiratory problem or secondary to abdominal distension
Scleral icterus, Jaundice	Biliary disease (e.g., cholangitis) or hepatitis
Rales, rhonchi, wheezing	Pneumonia
Hematemesis	Mallory-Weiss syndrome, Boerhaave Syndrome, ischemia
Hematuria	Ureteral colic, acute cystitis, severe UTI
Diarrhea	Gastroenteritis, *Clostridium difficile* colitis
Blood in stool	Ulcerative or granulomatous colitis, dysentery, intestinal ischemia
History	**Clinical Condition**
Timing in menstrual cycle	Mittelschmerz
Relation of pain to menstrual cycle	Endometriosis
Vaginal discharge	PID
Prior STD	PID, Ectopic pregnancy
Breakthrough bleeding	Ectopic pregnancy
Steroid use	Perforation, mask signs of inflammation
Crack cocaine	Duodenal perforation[15]
Anticoagulants (e.g., clopidogrel, warfarin, etc.)	Retroperitoneal hematoma, rectus sheath hematoma, duodenal hematoma

LABORATORY

Laboratory studies are useful adjuncts in the evaluation of patients with acute abdomen but should be interpreted with caution (Table 7). While the decision to operate can be informed by lab values, beware of the false comfort of unremarkable lab values in patients who warrant an operation by clinical exam.

When acute abdomen is suspected, a complete blood count (CBC), basic metabolic panel (BMP), and urinalysis are useful baseline tests to guide diagnosis and management. A urine pregnancy test should be checked in all menstruating female patients. Blood type and screen should be sent for patients for whom an urgent or emergent surgery with blood transfusion is likely to be needed. In addition, liver function tests, amylase and lipase levels are useful for patients with the appropriate presentation (e.g., epigastric, or right upper quadrant abdominal pain, jaundice, etc.).

In any potentially septic patient, samples for culture (including blood, urine, sputum, CSF if applicable, and stool if applicable) should be sent prior to antibiotic administration if possible. Each culture, particularly blood cultures, should be collected in a sterile fashion and sent in duplicate sets. Suspected central lines should be removed if possible, and the tip should be sent for culture.

Table 7: Laboratory tests useful in the work up of acute abdomen

Blood Test	Values	Clinical significance
CBC	Elevated hemoglobin or hematocrit	Dehydration, third space losses
	Decreased hemoglobin or hematocrit	Acute Hemorrhage (e.g., esophageal varices, peptic ulcer, diverticular disease, ruptured ectopic pregnancy, ruptured abdominal aortic aneurysm) Chronic blood loss (e.g., G.I. malignancy, anemia of chronic disease)
	Leukocytosis	Infection or inflammation present
	Leukopenia	Viral disease or sequestration of WBC at site of infection
	Neutrophil predominance, Increased immature, or band cells ("Left shift")	Infection
	Thrombocytosis	Infection or inflammation (acute phase reactant)
Serum Electrolytes	Electrolyte derangements (Na, K, Mg, Ca, Cl, Phos)	Dehydration (secondary to diarrhea, vomiting, etc.), inappropriate diuretic use
	Increased bicarbonate	Metabolic alkalosis (secondary to vomiting)
	Decreased bicarbonate	Metabolic acidosis (secondary to lactic acidosis, diabetic ketoacidosis, etc.)
	Elevated BUN and/or Cr	Dehydration, acute kidney injury, severe third space losses
	Glucose	Diabetic ketoacidosis
Liver Function Tests	Elevated bilirubin	Acute cholecystitis, obstructive jaundice suppurative Cholangitis, acute hepatitis
	Elevated alkaline phosphatase	Obstructive jaundice, liver metastases, cholangitis
	Elevated AST, ALT	Severe in acute hepatitis, mild in acute cholecystitis
Amylase and lipase	Markedly elevated	Acute pancreatitis
	Mild elevation	Perforated peptic ulcer, intestinal infarct or obstruction, inflammation of salivary glands
Serum Lactate	Elevated	Intestinal ischemia
PT, PTT, INR	Coagulopathy	Liver failure (acute or chronic), pharmacologic anticoagulation, disseminated intravascular coagulation
Troponins	Elevated	Acute Coronary Syndrome, demand ischemia
C-Reactive Protein (CRP)	Elevated	Inflammation, infection
Urine test		
Urinalysis	Pyuria, bacteriuria, nitrites, leukocyte esterase	UTI, possible cystitis or pyelonephritis
Urine Pregnancy test	Positive	Ectopic pregnancy, choriocarcinoma

RADIOLOGY

Acute abdominal pain may be caused by a myriad of diagnoses. Imaging improves the diagnostic accuracy of clinical evaluation and plays an important role in the management of patients with acute abdomen. Conventional plain abdominal X-rays, once the initial imaging study of choice, is now primarily useful in the setting of bowel obstruction or suspected visceral perforations. It has been superseded by ultrasound (US) and computed tomography (CT), which offer better diagnostic accuracy.

X-RAY

The classic X-ray series for evaluating the acute abdomen includes three views: upright and supine abdominal films, and an upright chest X-ray. A normal abdominal X-ray will show a variable gastric air bubble and air in the colon. The small intestine does not normally contain air, although this finding can be benign in a patient with aerophagia (Table 8). The upright chest X-ray is useful to screen for intrathoracic diseases that can mimic abdominal emergencies such as pneumonia, pleural effusion, pulmonary infarction, or esophageal disease.

Table 8: Difference between small intestine and colonic gas pattern

Small Intestine	Colon
Presence of valvulae conniventes extends across full width of intestine (stacked coin appearance)	Haustral markings. Extends only partially into lumen, indentation of colonic wall
Absence of fecal gas pattern	Fecal gas pattern present
Central location	Peripheral distribution

X-ray is useful primarily in cases of intestinal ileus, obstruction, or perforation. Air in distended small bowel loops usually indicates ileus or mechanical obstruction. Air-fluid levels on the upright abdominal view were traditionally interpreted as evidence of mechanical obstruction instead of ileus, but in fact they appear in both conditions and are relatively nonspecific.[16] Similarly, air in the rectum was thought to indicate ileus instead of mechanical obstruction but is also nonspecific.[17] Extraluminal air in the abdomen suggests perforated viscus or abscess. This is commonly seen as hyperlucent air on both sides of an intestinal wall (Rigler's sign), or under the diaphragm, especially above the liver. The appearance of free air on plain X-ray should be interpreted with caution since it is present in only 70-80% of perforated peptic ulcer cases. Conversely, it can be mimicked by other conditions including basal curvilinear atelectasis, subdiaphragmatic abscess, or Chilaiditi's syndrome, where the colon is interposed between the liver and the anterior abdominal wall. The latter can be distinguished by the presence of haustral markings within a subdiaphragmatic hyperlucency.

Certain X-ray findings may accompany pathologies other than the three discussed above (Table 9) but are not meaningful when absent. For example, radio-opaque stones in a suggestive location can be diagnostic in certain cases of nephrolithiasis, or acute appendicitis with fecalith. Pneumobilia, especially alongside dilated bowel loops and, rarely, a radiopaque stone overlying the right lower quadrant, can indicate gallstone ileus. The psoas margins and flank stripes may become asymmetrically blurred by an overlying mass or edema. A plain radiograph, as a rapid screening tool in cases of suspected foreign body ingestion, shows metal and glass best, but may be able to detect other radiopaque items.[18] None of these conditions, however, can be confidently ruled out with a normal X-ray finding and further imaging is often necessary.

Table 9: Interpretation of radiographic findings

Radiographic finding	Pathology or Clinical Significance
Distended small bowel loops, multiple air-fluid levels	Paralytic ileus (i.e., usually secondary to peritonitis, gastroenteritis, abscess, etc.), mechanical obstruction, aerophagia
Sentinel loop (localized air-filled bowel): • Of small intestine in RLQ • Of transverse colon	 • Acute appendicitis • Acute pancreatitis
String of pearls (chain of small air bubbles trapped between valvulae conniventes)	Intestinal obstruction
Thickened bowel wall	Wall edema secondary to bowel obstruction or ischemia
Thumbprinting of bowel wall	Submucosal edema or hemorrhage due to bowel ischemia
Generalized distension of colon	Colonic ileus (i.e., secondary to toxic megacolon, Ogilvie's pseudo-obstruction, etc.)
Massively dilated loop of colon extending from LLQ to RUQ, with characteristic central stripe	Sigmoid volvulus

Radiographic finding	Pathology or Clinical Significance
Distended cecum in LUQ (or RUQ) with absence of cecal shadow in RLQ, collapsed left colon, and distended small intestine	Cecal volvulus (or bascule)
Calcifications: RUQ RLQ RLQ or pelvis (in the setting of dilated bowel loops and pneumobilia) Punctate pancreatic calcifications Along distribution of ureter Overlying renal shadow	 Cholelithiasis (15%) Appendicular fecalith Gallstone ileus Chronic pancreatitis Ureteral stone (85%) Staghorn calculus
Intraperitoneal air under diaphragm, between loops of bowel (Rigler's sign)	Perforated viscus
Pneumobilia (central air overlying biliary tree, close to hilum)	Cholecysto-enteric fistula, gallstone ileus
Portal venous air (peripheral location)	Abdominal sepsis or ischemia
Pneumatosis intestinalis (linear gas pattern or small bubbles of gas in thickened bowel wall, especially in dependent portion of intestine)	Ischemic necrosis of bowel Idiopathic
Extraluminal gas in speckled pattern, retroperitoneal or intraperitoneal	Ruptured duodenum, abscess
Pleural effusion: Left-sided, unilateral Right-sided, unilateral Bilateral	 Acute pancreatitis Acute cholecystitis, subdiaphragmatic abscess Systemic disease (e.g., CHF)
Obliteration of psoas shadows and/or flank preperitoneal fat lines	Retroperitoneal mass, hemorrhage, abscess Acute appendicitis (right side) Acute diverticulitis (left side)

Some authors have advocated reducing or eliminating the use of plain X-ray for the evaluation of the acute abdomen because its results seldom change management. One study found pathologic findings on only 20% of abdominal X-rays and 13% of chest X-rays. Moreover, the supine abdominal view and upright chest X-rays together diagnosed normality or abnormality in 98% of study patients.[19] By eliminating the upright abdominal X-ray from the classic 'acute abdominal series', or even bypassing plain X-rays altogether in favor of CT and US when indicated, radiation exposure could be decreased, radiology staff and budget used more efficiently, and finally useable information can be gained for making management decisions and planning an operative strategy.[20,21]

ULTRASOUND

Abdominal sonography is highly operator-dependent, but in the best hands is a fast, accurate, non-invasive, and portable imaging modality that avoids ionizing radiation. US is the imaging modality of choice for a patient suspected to have biliary disease, or gynecologic pathologies like ectopic pregnancy, pelvic inflammatory disease, or ovarian cysts and its complications (e.g., rupture, torsion) (Figure 6). It is helpful in the diagnosis of abdominal aortic aneurysms. In children and pregnant patients, it is the first test of choice in the diagnosis of acute appendicitis.

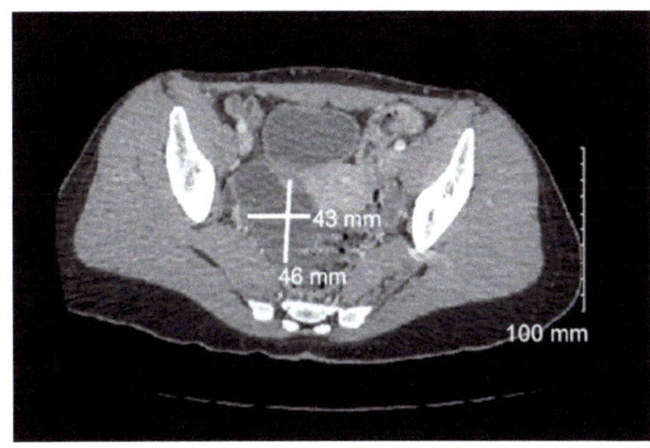

Figure 6: Ovarian cyst presenting as acute abdomen

COMPUTED TOMOGRAPHY

Abdominal CT is a detailed, accurate, reproducible, and relatively quick imaging modality that frequently increases diagnostic certainty and helps form the initial treatment plan, particularly in urgent conditions.[22] Non-contrast studies are obtained when renal colic secondary to nephrolithiasis is suspected. More often, the scan is performed with intravenous (IV) contrast to delineate vascular and solid organ pathologies, as well as highlight abscesses and inflammatory changes. Impaired renal function, a common consequence of severe cases of acute abdomen, and a history of prior allergic reaction are relative contraindications to the use of IV contrast. Nonetheless, when weighed against the risks of delayed or missed diagnosis and inappropriate treatment, judicious use of IV contrast may be warranted in select cases. Common measures used to mitigate the risk of IV contrast in at-risk patients include (1) premedication with steroids (oral is preferred to IV) and an H1 antihistamine (diphenhydramine) against allergic reactions and (2) pre-hydration with isotonic crystalloids (possibly with the addition of sodium bicarbonate and/or N-acetylcysteine, although neither have demonstrated consistent benefit despite numerous studies) against contrast-induced nephropathy.[23] Oral contrast is useful when ileus or obstruction are suspected, or to locate a perforation or fistula. Rectal contrast differs from oral contrast in that the rectum and part of the colon distend with contrast under some pressure. This is most commonly helpful in two situations: (1) suspected appendicitis, where distending the cecum with enteric contrast can help identify the appendix or (2) rectal or rectosigmoid perforation, where contrast is more likely to extravasate from a perforation when under the pressure of the rectally administered contrast enema.

In general, CT findings provide anatomic information, and clues of physiologic processes, which must be interpreted in a clinical context to be fully understood. Fat stranding, the increased attenuation of fat due to edema or lymphatic engorgement, indicates inflammation, infection, or sometimes malignancy. Bowel wall thickening may be seen in many neoplastic, infiltrative, or inflammatory processes; details about its specific appearance (whether homogeneous or heterogeneous, localized, or diffuse, contrast-enhancing or not) help distinguish which underlying pathology is present. Free extraluminal fluid and air are easy to identify but must be interpreted with extreme care. A small amount of free fluid is a physiologic finding in a female patient of reproductive age but may be an ominous sign of capillary leak and third-spacing of fluid in a male patient. Free intra-abdominal air is suspicious for perforated viscus, although within the first week after an abdominal operation it may be an expected, benign finding. Optimal CT interpretation combines anatomic detail, abnormal findings, and pertinent negative or normal findings with clinical context (Table 10).

Table 10: Specific visceral findings on CT Scan

Organ	CT findings	Interpretation
Adrenal	Contrast-enhancing, normal size	Hypovolemia & shock
	Bilateral hemorrhage	Addisonian crisis
Kidney	Patchy enhancement, especially in excretory phase	Acute pyelonephritis
	Hypodense lesion with wall enhancement	Abscess vs cystic carcinoma
	Gas within renal parenchyma	Emphysematous pyelonephritis
	Air fluid level in renal pelvis	Pyonephrosis
Peritoneal cavity	Pneumoperitoneum, loculated gas and fluid, focal omental or mesenteric infiltration, focal enhancement of parietal peritoneum	Perforated viscus
	Low-attenuation center with enhancing rim, air-fluid levels or gas bubbles, displacement of adjacent structures, thickening of continuous fascial planes and mesenteric or omental fat	Intra-abdominal abscess
Omentum	Well-circumscribed region of inflamed omental fat with areas of haziness and streak-like inflammatory stranding; normal appearing adjacent small bowel, appendix, and colon	Omental infarction
Gallbladder	Distension, wall enhancement and thickening >3 mm, pericholecystic fluid, haziness of pericholecystic fat, increased attenuation of the gallbladder bile	Acute cholecystitis
	Intraluminal or intramural gas	Perforation, gangrene, emphysematous cholecystitis
Pancreas	Diffusely enlarged gland with shaggy contour, edema of gland and surrounding fat, peripancreatic fat stranding, thickened fascial planes	Acute pancreatitis
	Diminished or absent parenchymal enhancement, high attenuation peripancreatic exudates which obliterate the surrounding fat and fascial planes	Necrotizing pancreatitis
	Splenic artery pseudoaneurysm, splenic or portal vein thrombosis	Vascular complications of pancreatitis

Organ	CT findings	Interpretation
Small Intestine	Dilated loops of small bowel, a discrete transition point, distal collapsed loops of bowel containing little or no air, fluid, or contrast	High-grade obstruction
	Above findings, with the transition point at a hernia defect (inguinal, abdominal wall, obturator foramen, etc.)	Incarcerated hernia
	Above findings, with thickened and poorly enhancing bowel walls, engorgement of mesenteric vessels	Strangulated hernia
	U- or C-shaped loop of bowel, with radial fanning and haziness of associated mesentery, swirling of mesenteric vessels	Closed-loop obstruction Volvulus
	Edematous bowel walls, which appear in concentric layers in cross-section ("target sign")	Intussusception
	Dilated small bowel loops (usually colon is collapsed), air within biliary tree, stone may be located near terminal ileum	Gallstone ileus
	Filling defect within proximal mesenteric vessels (most commonly SMA) with lack of distal enhancement, bowel wall edema and pneumatosis intestinalis, air within the mesenteric veins and portal venous system	Mesenteric ischemia
Colon	Mural stratification (i.e., mucosa, submucosa and muscularis propria appear as distinct layers) indicating submucosal edema	Colitis, any type
	Above findings, with wall thickening, diverticula, and pericolonic fat stranding	Acute diverticulitis
	Above findings, with extraluminal air (may be localized or diffuse)	Perforated diverticulitis
	Above findings, with air in bladder or uterus, or phlegmon or abscess formation	Complications of diverticulitis (colovesical or colovaginal fistula, peri-colonic or pelvic abscess, etc.)
	Segmental wall thickening with scalloped irregular edges ("thumbprinting sign"), caused by submucosal edema	Ischemic colitis
	Wall thickening and layering ("target" or "halo" pattern of submucosal edema), accordion-like pattern of luminal contrast caused by deep ulcerations between thickened haustra (or lumen may be completely effaced), ascites and pericolonic inflammatory changes	Pseudomembranous colitis
Appendix	Dilated >6 mm diameter (although up to 10 mm is increasingly considered the upper limit of normal),[26] fluid-filled, with wall enhancement and stranding of surrounding fat, and sometimes a calcified appendicolith	Acute Appendicitis
	Phlegmon or abscess, pelvic free fluid, secondary wall thickening of the adjacent terminal ileum and cecum	Perforated appendicitis
Aorta	Aneurysm with retroperitoneal hematoma or frank extravasation of IV contrast material, surrounding fat stranding	Ruptured aneurysm
	Intimal flap, false lumen	Aortic dissection

Apart from the exceptions discussed above under US, CT is increasingly considered the primary imaging technique for the diagnosis of acute abdominal pain. CT alters the management in more than half of patients with acute abdominopelvic pain, most notably in averting unnecessary laparotomy.[27] Studies have demonstrated that abdominal CT is a reliable and cost-effective test for diagnosing acute appendicitis among female patients of reproductive age who present with right lower quadrant abdominal pain.[28] In cases of perforated viscus, CT is the most sensitive way to detect free intraperitoneal air and may be valuable in determining the cause of the perforation. Imaging studies generally have poor sensitivity for bowel ischemia, although there are some highly specific signs on CT which, if found, are virtually diagnostic. Thus, CT is the preferred initial imaging modality for most patients presenting with acute abdomen, except in patients clinically suspected of having acute cholecystitis. When cost and exposure to ionizing radiation are primary concerns, US may be performed initially in all patients with acute abdominal pain, followed by a CT scan in those patients where US was nondiagnostic.

MAGNETIC RESONANCE IMAGING AND CHOLANGIO-PANCREATOGRAPHY

The benefit of MRI over CT is avoiding exposure to ionizing radiation, and for this reason, it is still preferred in the workup of acute abdomen in the pregnant patient after an inconclusive US. However, there are few studies on the role of MRI in evaluating the acute abdomen outside of pregnancy, and the wider use of MRI has also been hindered by cost, availability, duration of the study, and relative difficulty in interpretation compared to CT.[29] Magnetic resonance cholangiopancreatography (MRCP) is used to evaluate the biliary tree in patients with suspected choledocholithiasis, biliary obstruction, or acute pancreatitis.

HEPATOBILIARY IMINODIACETIC ACID SCAN

Although the hepatobiliary iminodiacetic acid (HIDA) scan is the gold standard for the diagnosis of acute cholecystitis, it is seldom performed because it is not always available and not usually necessary if the US is diagnostic. In patients with suspected acute cholecystitis, if the US study is equivocal, a HIDA scan can be used to establish or rule out the diagnosis of acute cholecystitis.

DIAGNOSTIC LAPAROSCOPY

Although not an imaging modality in the strict sense, diagnostic laparoscopy is being considered earlier in the work-up of acute abdominal pain. It is particularly valuable in female patients with lower abdominal pain to differentiate between pelvic inflammatory disease and acute appendicitis. Laparoscopy carries the additional benefit of allowing therapeutic intervention if a treatable surgical cause is found.

IMPORTANCE OF EARLY DIAGNOSIS

Early diagnosis is very critical as many conditions are due to infection, ischemia, or hemorrhage which, if left untreated due to delay in diagnosis, can progress to sepsis, septic shock, and even death. For this reason, patients require prompt evaluations (i.e., clinical, laboratory, and radiologic).

All physicians should be familiar with the clinical presentations of the most common acute abdominal conditions. However, there are many causes of abdominal pain, and approximately one third of patients do not present with a typical textbook description. For this reason, the common approach to the diagnosis of a disease by pattern recognition is fraught with the twin dangers of missing a diagnosis or making a wrong diagnosis. A pathophysiology-based approach to analyzing symptoms and physical findings is more likely to improve diagnostic accuracy. An understanding of the pathophysiologic mechanisms of pain, tenderness, and other abdominal physical findings is critical, as is a knowledge of the natural history of abdominal pathologies and of the progression of peritonitis.

When applying the pain classifications to a clinical situation and helping clarify how understanding the information can help one recognize acute abdominal conditions, take the case of acute appendicitis. The process usually starts as an obstruction of the appendicular lumen, either by a fecalith or by lymphoid hyperplasia. This leads to colicky visceral pain, which is felt in the periumbilical region due to its origin from the embryonic midgut. As a result of trapped secretions, bacterial proliferation, and ischemia due to distension occur, which causes inflammation of the appendix. At this time, the colicky pain subsides and shifts to the right lower quadrant. The nature of pain here is steady due to the presence of inflammation. As this visceral peritonitis spreads to the abdominal wall, causing parietal peritonitis, the character of the pain changes. It becomes sharper, more intense, constant, and localized to the right lower quadrant. Physical examination at this point would reveal localized tenderness and rebound tenderness at McBurney's point. This change from visceral peritonitis (clinically seen as localized direct tenderness) to parietal peritonitis (clinically manifested as rebound tenderness, and a positive Rovsing's sign) indicates progression or worsening of the underlying inflammatory condition. Despite recent advances in sonography, CT scan and laparoscopy, they cannot take the place of detailed history taking and a thorough physical examination, and the analytical interpretation of physical findings.

DIFFERENTIAL DIAGNOSIS

A presentation of acute abdomen may be caused by many different pathologies, not all of which are intra-abdominal, and not all requiring a surgeon. Therefore, keep a broad differential diagnosis in view and systematically address each possibility with evidence. Referred pain from myocardial infarction, radiculopathies, basal pulmonary pathologies like pneumonia and pleuritis, and testicular torsion may present with severe abdominal pain. Metabolic, congenital, and autoimmune disorders such as sickle cell crisis, acute porphyria, diabetic ketoacidosis, aspirin overdose, and connective tissue diseases with abdominal crises,[30] can present with acute abdomen in a patient in distress.

Non-acute abdominal pathologies causing abdominal pain include rectus sheath hematoma and abscess. Even among intra-abdominal pathologies, many causes can lead to a similar presentation. A classic example is right lower quadrant pain with nausea and vomiting, which may represent appendicitis, nephrolithiasis, ovarian torsion, tubo-ovarian abscess, or perforated peptic ulcer, among others.

At times, despite your best efforts, it will not be possible to make a definitive diagnosis. Anatomic variation, past surgical adventure, delay in presentation, and many other factors will add to the complexity and uncertainty of a case. In these circumstances, it is best to narrow the differential as much as possible (two or three most likely), and then proceed with treatment. Avoid delay in treatment solely out of diagnostic uncertainty.

Cases of acute abdomen highlight the challenges of clinical decision-making: the surgeon is confronted with a high degree of uncertainty and given a limited window of opportunity for diagnosis and treatment. The disease process relentlessly imposes a cost on the patient for any delays in treatment. Each new test result or therapeutic outcome shapes the next choices available to the patient, for better or for worse. Surgeons who deal with these scenarios efficiently and accurately can achieve safe outcomes for their patients, save time and resources, and minimize errors. How, then, can effective clinical decision-making be developed?

Clinical decision-making has been characterized by several cognitive strategies, described below.[31] It is notable, however, that these same approaches are considered cognitive biases when they result in error. The reality is that decisions are often reached by a method that combines, and yet is not fully described by, these strategies. This good clinical intuition or acumen is primarily developed through experience but can also be learned. Defining these cognitive strategies and recognizing their contribution in clinical decisions is the first step towards becoming better clinical decision-makers.

Pattern Recognition: Groupings of relevant data ("bottom-up") resemble prior experiences, with the clinician's expectations shaping further data collection and/or interpretation ("top-down"). Weaknesses of this approach are (1) initial misinterpretation of the data as a pattern that it is not present ("anchoring bias") and (2) vulnerability to a clinician's experience or pet beliefs in discerning the initial pattern or subsequently selecting data to support the initial impression ("confirmation bias"). Please keep in mind that a mental template of disease that fits a typical patient may not fit all.

Rule Out Worst-Case Scenario: The greatest perceived risk to the patient is identified through a pattern recognition, and a focus on must-not-miss scenarios regardless of the probability ("value-induced bias"). The discussion below about abdominal pain associated with hypotension exemplifies this scenario.

Availability Bias: A clinician's past experiences, especially recent ones, make certain diagnoses seem more common than they are. The weakness of this approach is that it trades excessive use of resources for incremental safety. It also becomes narrow focused, and one is likely to miss less common diagnoses.

Shotgun Approach: Indiscriminate, formulaic search through all data for an answer. This approach does not depend on clinical judgment or experience, and thus is often used where uncertainty is high (e.g., among inexperienced clinicians, or in unfamiliar situations). The weakness of this approach is that it requires more time and resources.

Hypothetico-Deductive Method: Initial information about the patient's clinical presentation is used to generate a short-list of potential diagnoses or actions, which is then the focus of efforts to narrow down the list further. This approach also combines bottom-up with top-down methods: data is the basis for generating the initial hypothesis list, which then serves as the framework for subsequent maneuvers. This method is vulnerable to premature diagnostic closure.

Heuristics: "Rules of thumb" can be developed for clinical decision-making through experience. These short-cuts are often practical, efficient, and effective for most cases.[31]

TREATMENT

PAIN CONTROL IN ACUTE ABDOMEN

The old adage that pain medications should not be given to a patient with acute abdominal pain, so as not to mask vital symptoms and physical findings, dates back many decades. The suffering patient is made to wait for a long period while the initial evaluation by a nurse and a physician is completed and while the patient is getting various laboratory and radiologic studies performed. However, it is cruel and inhumane to do so. Many studies have demonstrated that a judicious use of analgesics, for example morphine, does not mask physical findings or interfere with making the correct diagnosis.[32,33] The United States Agency for Healthcare Research and Quality recommended adequate analgesia in the acute abdomen patient after a review of the literature.[34] A prospective study by Thomas et al. found that administering up to 15 mg of morphine did not affect diagnostic accuracy in patients with acute abdominal pain.[32] Another study in children with acute abdominal pain showed similar safety with analgesic use.[35]

OPERATIVE APPROACH

As we have already seen, acute abdomen represents the gamut of pathologies. Those that require an urgent or emergent surgical treatment share this in common: a specific, localized source exists which is surgically correctable. While the reality is often much more complicated than this, we have found a few guidelines helpful in virtually any case.

Prepare the skin widely and plan the incision carefully: A classic example of this principle is the trauma laparotomy, where the patient is prepped from chin to knees, table to table, and the operation can later proceed into the chest or groins as needed. Even in less extreme situations, a wide prep is one way to prepare for intraoperative surprises. The incision itself is a separate plan and warrants forethought, particularly in patients where the pre-operative diagnosis is uncertain, or who have had prior abdominal surgeries. Will reopening an old scar present a manageable challenge, or many enterotomies? Choose an incision that offers you the best chance of addressing your pathology and allows you to extend or improve upon it if the exposure is poor.

If an urgent or emergent surgery is indicated, patients will be in some degree of extremis. Therefore, look for the source of the pathology, address it, and finish up. The temptation to lyse stray adhesions, resect some redundant omentum, or address some similar incidental finding, is strong but should be resisted. Each additional unnecessary maneuver prolongs the patient's physiologic stress, is an unnecessary delay to post-operative resuscitation and stabilization and may burn a bridge that you miss later on.

In the operating room, surgeons and anesthesiologists are tackling the same problem from different sides. Communicate your findings and plan across the drapes to recruit the anesthesiologists to your team. Does the patient need an urgent transfusion before you proceed? Will your patient be ready to be transferred to the ICU within the hour? The anesthesia team can accomplish these tasks while you suture. Listen to and ask for anesthesia updates. You may be able to curtail your operative plan in a patient who is becoming acidotic or oliguric or hemodynamically unstable. You may decide to leave the abdomen open if you hear that his peak pressures are high. The best operative team includes an anesthesiologist.

While open approaches are still more common, the use of laparoscopy in abdominal emergencies is growing. Studies among groups skilled in laparoscopy have shown low complication rates and low conversion rates.[36]

NON-OPERATIVE MANAGEMENT: WATCHFUL OBSERVATION AND THE THRESHOLD FOR SURGERY

Depending on the clinical scenario, a trial of observation and non-operative management may be indicated. In some respects, this approach is more active than a plan to operate. The safety of non-operative management depends on two parts: a method and a threshold. The method involves a serial clinical examination of the patient every 1-2 hours (by the same surgeon, if possible), supplemented by serial laboratory testing and imaging studies when appropriate. The threshold for operative management should be chosen at the outset of the observation period. This gives the team some objective standard by which to assess the patient. Often, this threshold may be a length of time to watch for improvement, beyond which some action will be taken. An increase in temperature, pulse rate, abdominal pain, or tenderness on examination, white blood cell count, lack of symptom resolution, or failure to respond appropriately to treatment suggest a progression of the underlying pathologic process and the need for possible surgery.

SPECIAL CONSIDERATIONS

ACUTE ABDOMEN ASSOCIATED WITH HYPOTENSION

When early-onset hypotension accompanies a presentation of acute abdomen, the differential diagnosis should include the following possible etiologies:

1. Ruptured abdominal aortic aneurysm
2. Ruptured ectopic pregnancy
3. Acute mesenteric ischemia
4. Esophageal perforation
5. Acute suppurative cholangitis
6. Inferior wall myocardial infarction
7. Acute pancreatitis

The importance of ruling out these etiologies in a methodical, efficient, and safe manner cannot be overemphasized. Although a CT scan with IV contrast would be diagnostic for most of these pathologies, the clinical reality of an unstable patient necessitates a more resourceful approach. There is often a relevant history (e.g., drop attack, tearing back pain, missed period, food fear, etc.) which the patient in extremis may be unable to supply. Thus, the initial workup should include a broad laboratory screen, including complete blood count, chemistry, liver function tests, amylase and lipase, lactate, troponin, and pregnancy test; an upright portable chest X-ray; and a 12-lead electrocardiogram. Bedside US is an invaluable adjunct in these cases, as the patient can be examined for most of the above conditions without interrupting monitoring and initial resuscitation.

ACUTE ABDOMEN IN PREGNANCY

The non-obstetric causes of acute abdomen during pregnancy are similar to those among the general population (Table 11), the exception being ovarian torsion which is more common in pregnant patients than non-pregnant. However, diagnostic workup and treatment of these conditions are significantly influenced by the physiologic changes of pregnancy and concern for the wellbeing of the fetus.[37] The stakes for delayed or missed diagnosis can be high. In one study, the rate of fetal loss in nonperforated appendicitis was 1.5% but increased to 36% once perforated.[38]

Table 11: Incidence of non-obstetric diagnosis causing acute abdomen in pregnancy[38]

Diagnosis	Incidence
Acute appendicitis	1: 1500
Acute cholecystitis	1: 1 600 to 10000
Pancreatitis	1: 1 000 to 10000
Ovarian torsion	1: 2 000 to 5000
Bowel obstruction	1: 2 500 to 3500

Laboratory values of a pregnant patient must be interpreted in the context of the normal physiologic changes during pregnancy. A pregnant woman's intravascular volume increases by 30-50%, primarily due to expanded plasma volume, and results in physiologic anemia where normal hematocrits may be 30-35%. The physiologic leukocytosis in pregnancy may be as high as 16,000 cells/mm^3, and even higher during labor. Alkaline phosphatase, normally useful as a marker of biliary obstruction, is physiologically elevated by high estrogen levels during pregnancy. During the first 2 trimesters, both amylase and lipase are also normally elevated in pregnancy up to 1,000 U/L and 2,000 U/L, respectively.[39]

Diagnostic imaging starts with graded compression US and MRI, which are both considered safe during pregnancy. CT is sometimes used when the need for more diagnostic certainty outweighs the risk of ionizing radiation to the fetus. The impact of ionizing radiation on fetal development and on the risk of childhood cancer, particularly leukemia, depends on gestational age at exposure and dose. Protocols for focused scans with helical CT, which uses less radiation than conventional CT, have been developed to limit radiation exposure to pregnant patients. Selected use of diagnostic laparoscopy appears to be safe.

The classic non-obstetric operation in pregnancy was open appendectomy, performed through a muscle-splitting incision over the point of maximal tenderness. Care was taken to position the patient on a leftward tilt with a hip roll to keep the gravid uterus from impeding venous return in the IVC. While these pearls are still relevant today, operative management for acute abdomen in pregnant patients is changing. Opinion on intraoperative fetal heart rate monitoring is divided, some groups recommend using it routinely while others cite the lack of evidence that it detects intraoperative fetal distress and only recommend using it pre- and post-operatively. Laparoscopy in pregnancy was initially considered dangerous, particularly in the 3rd trimester; insufflation was thought to decrease blood supply to the uterus, and extrapolation from animal studies suggested a risk of hypercarbic acidosis to the fetus. However studies have found no increased risk to the fetus in the short term, and laparoscopy is now being used more frequently, particularly for laparoscopic cholecystectomy and diagnostic laparoscopy.[40] Indeed, biliary disease during pregnancy, traditionally managed non-operatively, is a growing indication for laparoscopic cholecystectomy based on evidence of high rates of recurrence during the same pregnancy (58% of patients with acute cholecystitis, and 50% of those with pancreatitis), and lower risk of spontaneous abortion in the 1st trimester and preterm labor in the 3rd trimester after laparoscopic cholecystectomy.[38,41] Many current guidelines are based on expert opinion and more research on long-term outcomes is needed.

ACUTE ABDOMEN IN IMMUNOSUPPRESSED PATIENTS

Immunosuppressed patients presenting with abdominal pain should be evaluated with caution because they are not able to mount an appropriate immune response to infection. Thus, their presentation may appear misleadingly benign: afebrile, unremarkable abdominal exam without peritoneal signs, and normal white blood cell count. They are also brittle, and more likely to succumb to a lesser insult. Any patient on chronic steroid therapy, chemotherapy, or immunosuppression (e.g., transplant patients), as well as HIV/AIDs patients are at risk.

Classic examples in specific populations are worth mentioning. Patients on chemotherapy presenting with abdominal pain who also have neutropenia may have neutropenic enterocolitis, an acute inflammatory and necrotizing process that affects the terminal ileum, cecum, and appendix. Complications such as colonic perforation, pneumatosis intestinalis, or intractability despite medical management, are indications for surgery. Acute graft-vs-host disease may manifest as acute abdominal pain in transplant patients. HIV/AIDS patients are at an increased risk for infections such as cytomegalovirus, tuberculosis, and fungal infections. Barring evidence of intestinal extremis (e.g., severe bleeding, peritonitis, or perforation), these opportunistic infections are initially managed medically with antiviral, anti-tubercular, and antifungal medications, in addition to HIV treatment with antiretroviral therapy as appropriate.

ACUTE ADBOMEN IN THE POSTOPERATIVE PATIENT

Tertiary peritonitis as a result of laparotomy and gastrointestinal surgery is the most common cause of pain in post-operative patients and usually improves steadily with supportive care. Other etiologies to consider if improvement does not occur, or if other symptoms develop, include non-occlusive mesenteric ischemia (NOMI) from a low-flow state, segmental inferior mesenteric artery ischemia after abdominal aortic surgery, acalculous cholecystitis, and Clostridium difficile colitis. The index of suspicion for post-operative complications is based on patient symptoms and time course from the initial operation. For example, pain or peritonitis on postoperative day (POD) 4-9 may be the result of anastomotic leak, whereas pain or peritonitis on POD 7-10 with an associated fever may be from an abscess.[42] Prolonged or persistent ileus may also provide a clue to the intra-abdominal septic process.

ACUTE ABDOMEN IN PARAPLEGIC PATIENTS

Delayed diagnosis is very common in this group of patients as typical signs like tenderness and guarding are not reliable due to loss of sensation and paralysis. However, referred pain to the shoulder from phrenic nerve irritation is intact. Nausea, vomiting, and abdominal distension due to ileus are not affected either and provide a clue to the diagnosis.[43]

ACUTE ABDOMEN IN THE TROPICS

A presentation of acute abdomen in the tropics, or in a patient who has visited the tropics, carries two important implications: high burden of infectious disease and delayed presentation. Indeed, these challenges stem as much from socioeconomic and political factors (e.g., lack of access to health care, underdeveloped public health and healthcare systems, and poor sanitation and hygiene) as from climate-related factors (e.g., ecological habitat of mosquito vectors, excessive heat). Specific countries and regions carry different patterns of endemic disease, both infectious and otherwise. Clinicians should apply knowledge of these patterns in forming their differential diagnosis.

Remembering that regional variation exists, the most common surgical cause of acute abdomen in the tropics is acute appendicitis. A prospective series of 3,114 patients in Ghana admitted with acute abdominal pain found that other common causes included typhoid ileal perforation, acute intestinal obstruction, and gastroduodenal perforation.[44] Most of the latter were related to ulcer disease, notable because this region has a higher prevalence of *H. pylori* and lower use of H2-blockers or proton pump inhibitors than populations in temperate climates. Half a century ago, intestinal obstruction was the most common cause of emergency surgical admissions in many parts of Africa. Not only has its incidence declined, but its etiologies are shifting too. Causes such as adhesions and colorectal cancer are increasing, whereas ascariasis is decreasing.[45] Recent series of acute intestinal obstruction in Nigeria found that the most common causes were external hernias, especially inguinal, intussusception, and sigmoid volvulus.[46,47]

Excessive hot weather in the tropics can lead to heat stroke or severe acute dehydration and electrolyte depletion. This may cause abdominal pain and muscle spasm which can be confused with peritonitis.

Infectious causes of acute abdomen can manifest in a myriad of ways, from obstruction to perforation to abscess and more. A careful history may yield valuable clues, but the physical exam is often nonspecific. Initial work-up should always include eosinophil count and stool studies.[48] We briefly describe the common infectious etiologies of acute abdomen below and refer the reader to a textbook on tropical diseases for more detail.

- Typhoid fever is the most common cause of ileal perforation.
- Ascariasis (roundworm) can also lead to intestinal obstruction or perforation, typically of the ileum. Infestation leading to obstruction of the appendix or biliary tree manifests as acute appendicitis or cholangitis, respectively.
- Filariasis may cause retroperitoneal lymphadenitis and abdominal pain.
- Tuberculosis, endemic in much of the tropics, usually manifests as a chronic abdominal peritonitis, which feels dough-like to palpation except in the uncommon case of intestinal perforation. Patients usually complain of heaviness rather than pain, and the onset of symptoms is gradual. There may be free fluid in the abdomen. CT scan will reveal a thickened omentum and peritoneal granulomas.
- Malaria can produce severe splenomegaly with left upper quadrant pain, and risks rupture with minor trauma. Other causes of an enlarged spleen in the tropics include sickle cell trait, schistosomiasis, leishmaniasis, etc.
- Acute cholera infection presents with severe abdominal pain, rice water-like profuse diarrhea, and signs of severe dehydration.
- Amoebiasis can present as amoebic colitis or dysentery, amoebic hepatitis, or amoebic liver abscess that can rupture and cause peritonitis.

AGE CONSIDERATIONS

ACUTE ABDOMEN IN CHILDREN

In the two extremes of ages, presentation of acute abdomen is extremely variable. In children, the inability to accurately communicate their symptoms poses the first diagnostic challenge. Even their response to the physical examination, overshadowed by anxiety, fear, and crying makes the interpretation of real pain and tenderness difficult. The challenge in this age group is to differentiate between self-limited, non-surgical conditions that cause abdominal pain, which are the majority of cases, and the less common surgical conditions which are potentially life threatening. Sometimes there may be tell-tale signs of surgical pathology, such as bilious vomiting in an infant to indicate midgut volvulus or malrotation. However no specific diagnosis is made in 50%

of children with abdominal pain. In addition, many non-abdominal conditions can cause non-specific abdominal pain, including sickle cell disease, lower lobe pneumonia, hepatitis, lead poisoning, acute porphyria, and Henoch-Schoenlein purpura.

Among pediatric patients, age influences the differential diagnosis significantly. Congenital pathologies like intestinal atresia or stenosis, necrotizing enterocolitis, and Hirschsprung's disease present in newborns and young infants. Among children up to 2 years of age, the possibilities of malrotation, midgut volvulus (Figure 7), intussusceptions, and inguinal hernias are most likely. In children of 2-5 years of age, acute appendicitis is the most common etiology, although other possible causes include Meckel's diverticulitis and incarcerated inguinal hernias. In children over 5 years of age, acute appendicitis, Meckel's diverticulitis, testicular torsion, and, among teenage girls, pelvic inflammatory disease and other tubo-ovarian pathologies should be considered.

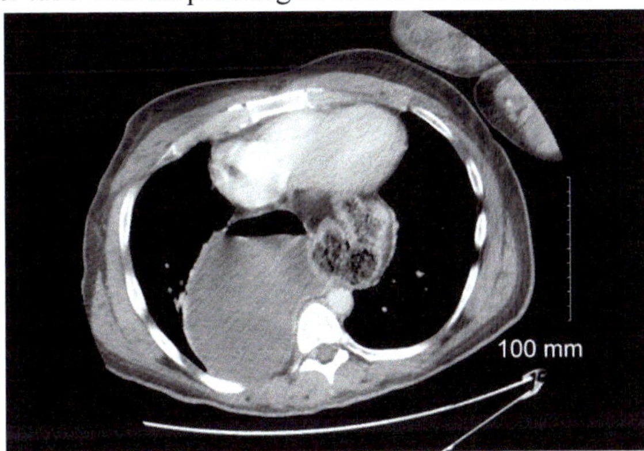

Figure 7: CT abdomen showing hiatal hernia with gastric and transverse colonic volvulus

ACUTE ABDOMEN IN THE ELDERLY

In a series of 472 patients, over 70 years of age in the United States, the most common cause for emergency operation was biliary disease. Other prevalent causes include appendicitis and intestinal obstruction.[49] Men required surgery more often than women. Further, malignant disease is encountered more often among elderly patients than in younger adults.

Among elderly patients presenting with acute abdomen, three factors increase mortality: comorbidities, need for emergency operation, and delay in diagnosis and treatment.[50] The latter is modifiable but requires the clinician to look for subtle signs and to approach elderly patients with a high index of suspicion. In the older patient, the available history can be inaccurate or incomplete, and is sometimes compounded by dementia. Clinical symptoms and physical signs may reflect a blunted response to physiologic stimuli. For example, elderly patients may exhibit a reduced ability to develop fever, with only a modest rise in temperature in the face of severe infection.[51] Finally, they often present later, among adult patients with appendicitis, older patients are more likely to perforate.[52]

SUMMARY

There are many possible etiologies of acute abdominal pain, and only a few that are addressed surgically. Early evaluation by a surgeon, early diagnosis where possible, and early intervention improve patients' outcomes. Understanding the anatomy and pathophysiology of the abdominal solid organs and gastrointestinal tract is the key to making a diagnosis. It is the basis for interpreting any history or physical exam findings elicited from the patient; for choosing the appropriate labs and imaging studies to order and interpret; for formulating a treatment plan, operative or otherwise; and for adapting to special patient circumstances, such as pregnancy or immunocompetency.

REFERENCES

1. Brewer BJ, Golden GT, Hitch DC, Rudolf LE, Wangensteen SL. Abdominal pain. An analysis of 1,000 consecutive cases in a University Hospital emergency room. *Am J Surg* 1976 Feb;131(2):219-23.
2. Staniland JR, Ditchburn J, De Dombal FT. Clinical presentation of acute abdomen: study of 600 patients. *Br Med J* 1972 Aug 12;3(5823):393-8.
3. de Dombal FT. The OMGE acute abdominal pain survey. Progress report, 1986. *Scand J Gastroenterol Suppl* 1988;144:35-42.
4. Nagle A. Gastrointestinal Tract and Abdomen: Acute Abdominal Pain. In: *ACS Surgery: Principles & Practice*. Hamilton, Ontario & Philadelphia, PA: Decker Publishing Inc.; 2013. STAT!Ref Online Electronic Medical Library. http://online.statref.com/Document.aspx?fxId=61&docId=780. Accessed October 15, 2013.
5. Silen W. *Cope's Early Diagnosis of the Acute Abdomen* (22nd ed.) New York: Oxford University Press; 2010:ix.
6. Albanese AM, Albanese EF, Miño JH, Gómez E, Gómez M, Zandomeni M, Merlo AB. Peritoneal surface area: measurements of 40 structures covered by peritoneum: correlation between total peritoneal surface area and the surface calculated by formulas. *Surg Radiol Anat* 2009 Jun;31(5):369-77.
7. Roberts JE, deShazo RD. Abdominal Migraine, Another Cause of Abdominal Pain in Adults. *Am J Med* 2012 Nov;125(11):1135-1139.
8. Zinkin NT, Peppercorn MA. Abdominal epilepsy. *Best Pract Res Clin Gastroenterol* 2005 Apr;19(2):263-74.

9. Macari M, Hines J, Balthazar E, Megibow A. Mesenteric adenitis: CT diagnosis of primary versus secondary causes, incidence, and clinical significance in pediatric and adult patients. *Am J Roentgenol* 2002 Apr;178(4):853-8.
10. Hasler WL. Chapter 39. Nausea, Vomiting, and Indigestion. In: Longo DL, Fauci AS, Kasper DL, Hauser SL, Jameson JL, Loscalzo J, eds. *Harrison's Principles of Internal Medicine* (18th ed.) New York: McGraw-Hill; 2012. http://www.accessmedicine.com/content.aspx?aID=9112783. Accessed October 14, 2013.
11. Rothrock SG, Green SM, Dobson M, Colucciello SA, Simmons CM. Misdiagnosis of appendicitis in nonpregnant women of childbearing age. *J Emerg Med* 1995 Jan-Feb;13(1):1-8.
12. Alvarado A. A practical score for the early diagnosis of acute appendicitis. *Ann Emerg Med* 1986 May;15(5):557-64.
13. Wagner JM, McKinney WP, Carpenter JL. Does this patient have appendicitis? *JAMA* 1996 Nov 20;276(19):1589-94.
14. Rothrock SG, Skeoch G, Rush JJ, Johnson NE. Clinical features of misdiagnosed appendicitis in children. *Ann Emerg Med* 1991 Jan;20(1):45-50.
15. Abramson DL, Gertler JP, Lewis T, Kral JG. Crack-related perforated gastropyloric ulcer. *J Clin Gastroenterol* 1991 Feb;13(1):17-9.
16. Lappas JC, Reyes BL, Maglinte DD. Abdominal radiography findings in small-bowel obstruction: relevance to triage for additional diagnostic imaging. *AJR Am J Roentgenol* 2001 Jan;176(1):167-74.
17. Simpson A, Sandeman D, Nixon SJ, Goulbourne IA, Grieve DC, Macintyre IM. The value of an erect abdominal radiograph in the diagnosis of intestinal obstruction. *Clin Radiol* 1985 Jan;36(1):41-2.
18. Halverson M, Servaes S. Foreign bodies: radiopaque compared to what? *Pediatr Radiol* 2013 Sep;43(9):1103-7.
19. Mirvis SE, Young JW, Keramati B, McCrea ES, Tarr R. Plain film evaluation of patients with abdominal pain: are three radiographs necessary? *AJR Am J Roentgenol* 1986 Sep;147(3):501-3.
20. Kellow ZS, MacInnes M, Kurzencwyg D, Rawal S, Jaffer R, Kovacina B, Stein LA. The role of abdominal radiography in the evaluation of the nontrauma emergency patient. *Radiology* 2008 Sep;248(3):887-93.
21. Gans SL, Stoker J, Boermeester MA. Plain abdominal radiography in acute abdominal pain; past, present, and future. *Int J Gen Med* 2012;5:525-33.
22. Tsushima Y, Yamada S, Aoki J, Motojima T, Endo K. Effect of contrast-enhanced computed tomography on diagnosis and management of acute abdomen in adults. *Clin Radiol* 2002 Jun;57(6):507-13.
23. American College of Radiology Committee on Drugs and Contrast Media. ACR Manual on Contrast Media, Version 9. 2013. Available from http://www.acr.org/Quality-Safety/Resources/Contrast-Manual. Accessed December 15, 2013.
24. Curry CA, Urban BA, Fishman EK. CT of the acute abdomen: GI manifestations. *Appl Rad* 1999 Dec;28(12):23-31.
25. Gore RM, Miller FH, Pereles FS, Yaghmai V, Berlin JW. Helical CT in the evaluation of the acute abdomen. *AJR Am J Roentgenol* 2000 Apr;174(4):901-13.
26. Daily R, Danton G, Munera F. ER radiology evaluation of appendicitis and alternative diagnoses of the right lower quadrant: Emphasis on multidetector CT. *Appl Rad* 2011 Jul;40(7):14-24.
27. Chambers A, Halligan S, Goh V, Dhillon S, Hassan A. Therapeutic impact of abdominopelvic computed tomography in patients with acute abdominal symptoms. *Acta Radiol* 2004 May;45(3):248-53.
28. Morse BC, Roettger RH, Kalbaugh CA, Blackhurst DW, Hines WB Jr. Abdominal CT scanning in reproductive-age women with right lower quadrant abdominal pain: does its use reduce negative appendectomy rates and healthcare costs? *Am Surg* 2007 Jun;73(6):580-4; discussion 584.
29. Stoker J, van Randen A, Laméris W, Boermeester MA. Imaging patients with acute abdominal pain. *Radiology* 2009 Oct;253(1):31-46.
30. Coughlin LM, Sparks DA, Chase DM. Scleroderma Mimicking the Acute Abdomen. *Am Surg* 2012 Dec;78(12):E536-7.
31. Croskerry P. Achieving Quality in Clinical Decision Making: Cognitive Strategies and Detection of Bias. *Acad Emerg Med* 2002 Nov;9(11):1184-1204.
32. Thomas SH, Silen W, Cheema F, Reisner A, Aman S, Goldstein JN, Kumar AM, Stair TO. Effects of morphine analgesia on diagnostic accuracy in Emergency Department patients with abdominal pain: a prospective, randomized trial. *J Am Coll Surg* 2003 Jan;196(1):18-31.
33. Manterola C, Vial M, Moraga J, Astudillo P. Analgesia in patients with acute abdominal pain. *Cochrane Database Syst Rev* 2011 Jan 19;(1):CD005660.
34. Brownfield E. Pain management. Use of analgesics in the acute abdomen. In: *Making Health Care Safer: a*

critical analysis of patient safety practices. Evidence Report/Technology Assessment, No 43. AHRQ Publication No 01-E058. Rockville: Agency for Healthcare Research and Quality; 2001. pp. 396–400. Available from: http://www.ahrq.gov/clinic/ptsafety/. Accessed February 26, 2011.

35. Kim MK, Strait RT, Sato TT, Hennes HM. A randomized clinical trial of analgesia in children with acute abdominal pain. *Acad Emerg Med* 2002 Apr;9(4):281-7.
36. Agresta F, Mazzarolo G, Ciardo LF, Bedin N. The laparascopic approach in abdominal emergencies: has the attitude changed?: A single-center review of a 15-year experience. *Surg Endosc* 2008 May;22(5):1255-62.
37. Tarraza HM, Moore RD. Gynecologic causes of the acute abdomen and the acute abdomen in pregnancy. *Surg Clin North Am* 1997 Dec;77(6):1371-94.
38. Sharp, HT. The Acute Abdomen During Pregnancy. *Clin Obstet Gynecol* 2002 Jun;45(2):405-413.
39. Stone, K. Acute Abdominal Emergencies Associated with Pregnancy. *Clin Obstet Gynecol* 2002 Jun;45(2):553-561.
40. Society of American Gastrointestinal and Endoscopic Surgeons. Guidelines for Diagnosis, Treatment, and Use of Laparoscopy for Surgical Problems during Pregnancy. Apr 2011. Available from http://www.sages.org/publications/guidelines. Accessed October 13, 2013.
41. Kilpatrick CC, Orejuela FJ. Management of the acute abdomen in pregnancy: a review. *Curr Opin Obstet Gynecol* 2008 Dec;20(6):534-9.
42. Silen W. The postoperative abdomen. In: *Cope's Early Diagnosis of the Acute Abdomen* (20th ed.) New York: Oxford University Press; 2000. pp 255-9.
43. Bar-On Z, Ohry A. The acute abdomen in spinal cord injury individuals. *Paraplegia* 1995 Dec;33(12):704-6.
44. Ohene-Yeboah M. Acute surgical admissions for abdominal pain in adults in Kumasi, Ghana. *ANZ J Surg* 2006;76:898-903.
45. Ajao OG. Abdominal emergencies in a tropic African population. *Br J Surg* 1981 May;68(5):345-7.
46. Adesunkanmi AR, Agbakwuru EA. Changing pattern of acute intestinal obstruction in a tropical African population. *East Afr Med J* 1996 Nov;73(11):727-31.
47. Otu AA. Tropical surgical abdominal emergencies: acute intestinal obstruction. *Afr J Med Med Sci* 1991 Jun;20(2):83-8.
48. Hoffman SH. Tropical medicine and the acute abdomen. *Emerg Med Clin North Am* 1989 Aug;7(3):591-609.
49. Reiss R, Deutsch AA. Emergency abdominal procedures in patients above 70. *J Gerontol* 1985 May;40(2):154-8.
50. Vogt DP. The acute abdomen in the geriatric patient. *Cleve Clin J Med* 1990 Mar-Apr;57(2):125-30.
51. Marco CA, Schoenfeld CN, Keyl PM, Menkes ED, Doehring MC. Abdominal pain in geriatric emergency patients: variables associated with adverse outcomes. *Acad Emerg Med* 1998 Dec;5(12):1163-8.
52. Kraemer M, Franke C, Ohmann C, Yang Q. Acute Abdominal Pain Study Group. Acute appendicitis in late adulthood: incidence, presentation, and outcome. Results of a prospective multicenter acute abdominal pain study and a review of the literature. *Langenbecks Arch Surg* 2000 Nov;385(7):470-81.

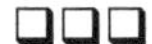

26

CHAPTER

Femoral and Inguinal Hernia, and Testicular Diseases

Dinesh Vyas, MD

Testicular Disease

Scrotal pathology requires urgent workup and treatment as persistence can result in poor outcomes (e.g., testicular torsion, testicular cancer) nercsotic bovel. The testicular examination helps to evaluate the tunica vaginalis and the epididymis. The spermatic cord consists of the testicular vessels and the vas deferens, another essential anatomical structure easily palpated on a routine exam. The examiner must appreciate changes from normal anatomy to help diagnose the pathological condition.

History

A focused history and examination helps in diagnosis and includes following key points:

- Details of pain - onset and severity
- Common etiologies - testicular torsion, torsion of testicular or epididymal appendages, and epididymitis
- Trauma
- Change in testicular or scrotal size
- Flank pain or hematuria
- Sexually active
- Onset of change, diurnal variation, variation with position or Valsalva maneuver
- Varicocele or hydrocele with and without hernia

Physical

The examination should be preceded by a brief discussion with the patient regarding the procedure. An upright patient is the best position for the physical exam, while the examiner is either sitting or standing. During an examination, the patient should be facing sideways so that the hernia is at the physician's eye level. For a small hernia, the physician should examine the hernia while the patient is coughing, straining, or performing a Valsalva maneuver.

The physical exam includes evaluation of the abdomen, inguinal region, and genitalia (e.g., testes, epididymis, spermatic cord, penis, scrotal skin). Herniography is not very sensitive, ultrasound is still not commonly used, and MRI, though an option, has a high cost which prevents its everyday use.

Genital examination

Inspection - Inspect the penis and the groin area while the patient is standing. In addition, notice the position and orientation of the testicles, the left testicle is lower than the right testicle. A varicocele will be obvious in the standing position after evaluation in both the standing and supine positions.

Palpation - Palpate the testis and epididymis for induration and abnormalities.

Cremasteric reflex - This has limited clinical use. It is present in boys between the ages of 2 to 12 years old but is almost always absent in patients with testicular torsion.

Prehn sign - This involves elevating the scrotal contents for symptomatic pain reduction in patients with epididymitis but has no effect on the pain in patients with testicular torsion. However, this is not a reliable test to clinically differentiate between testicular torsion, epididymitis, and other testicular conditions.

Painful Testicular Conditions

- Workup is done for the following differential diagnosis:
  - Testicular torsion - the abrupt onset of severe pain
  - Always perform urgent doppler ultrasonography - this is a surgical emergency

- Operative scrotal exploration for a confirmed torsion or an equivocal imaging study
- Incarcerated inguinal hernia
- Torsion of the appendix testis also has an abrupt onset of pain, but the severity is less than in testicular torsion and is localized to the region of the appendix testis
- Epididymitis - subacute pain with swelling of the epididymis only
- Scrotal trauma
- Another surgical emergency - Fournier's gangrene (necrotizing fasciitis of the perineum)

Painless Testicular Conditions

Hydrocele - cystic scrotal fluid collection that transilluminates and are either communicating or non-communicating. They are differentiated by a change in size over the day's progression. Communicating hydroceles increase in size as the day progresses.

Varicoceles - the spermatic cord feels like a bag of worms.

Testicular Cancer - painless mass and approximately 20% of cancers in males 15 to 35 years old. Common risk factors include cryptorchidism, a family history of testicular cancer, and cancer of the other testicle.

Management of Testicular Conditions

The management of common testicular conditions are:

1. **Testicular torsion:** A medical emergency and needs immediate surgical untwist of the affected testicle as delaying treatment may result in infertility.
2. **Testicular cancer:** Treatment typically involves surgery to remove the affected testicle, followed by chemotherapy or radiation therapy. In some cases, surveillance may be an option for low-risk tumors.
3. **Epididymitis:** This is typically treated with antibiotics to clear the infection, along with pain management medications and scrotal support.
4. **Varicocele:** Treatment may not be necessary if there are no symptoms or fertility concerns. If treatment is desired, options include surgical repair or embolization, which involves blocking the abnormal veins.
5. **Hydrocele:** Treatment may not be necessary if there are no symptoms or concerns about fertility. If treatment is desired, options include surgery to remove the fluid-filled sac or draining the fluid with a needle.

Pathophysiology

The inguinal canal is a fibromuscular tunnel of the abdominal wall through which the spermatic cord/round ligament passes from the abdomen. It is imperative to understand the anatomy of the tunnel, as it is helpful in the treatment of hernias. The tunnel is formed by the aponeurosis of the external oblique muscle (anteriorly), transversus abdominus muscle, and the transversalis fascia (posteriorly).

Floor weakness increases the risk for direct hernias through the zone known as Hesselbach's triangle (Figure 2): bounded by the inferior epigastric vessels, the inguinal ligament, and the rectus sheath. The canal is barely present in infants, increasing the incidence of indirect hernias. Additional risk factors (e.g., collagen disease type I and III, smoking, and steroid use) may contribute to the weakening of the collagen fiber. Ventral hernias are seen in patients with an aortic aneurysm which are often seen in patients with a metalloproteinase or elastase genetic disorder.

It is important to discuss anatomical landmarks for hernias.

- The external inguinal ring defect in the external oblique muscle - superior and lateral to the pubic tubercle
- The internal inguinal ring - defect in the transversalis fascia with a muscular shutter of the transversus abdominus and internal oblique muscles
- Indirect inguinal hernias - lateral to the deep epigastric vessels, the hernia contents reside and travel through the inguinal canal
- Direct inguinal hernias - are medial and inferior to the deep epigastric vessels and the hernia contents do not traverse the inguinal canal
- Femoral hernias - are below the inguinal ligament and medial to the femoral artery

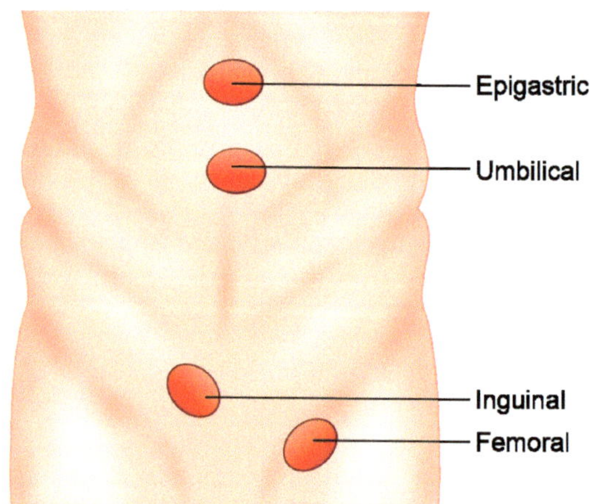

Figure 1: Common locations of hernias

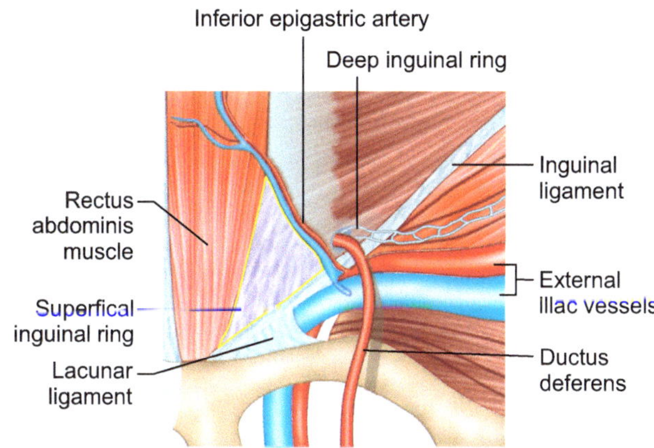

Figure 2: Hesselbach's Triangle

Diagnosis of Inguinal and Femoral Hernias

Repairing a hernia is one of the most routine surgical procedures. More than 95% of groin hernias are inguinal and occurs nine times more frequently in males.[1] The lifetime risk of an inguinal hernia is 25-30%. There is an ongoing debate over the indications for inguinal hernia surgery, but all femoral hernias require surgery.

Indirect inguinal hernias - the most common groin hernia in men and women. Its origin is lateral to the inferior epigastric artery, in contrast to direct hernias which arise medial to the inferior epigastric vessels.

Direct inguinal hernias - a defect in Hesselbach's triangle which can be due to a congenital defect, a weakness in the muscle fibers with age, or both.

Femoral hernias - an uncommon hernia, more often seen in elderly females, is due to decreased muscle mass and post-pregnancy anatomical changes. Approximately 40% of cases are emergencies from the incarceration or strangulation of bowel in the empty space at the medial aspect of the femoral canal.[2] Femoral hernias are difficult to differentiate from inguinal hernias, and at times, imaging studies like CT scans and MRIs can be useful in identifying anatomy. There is some financial cost attached to it; hence in most cases, clinical history and examination assist in making a diagnosis, and then the definitive diagnosis is made intra-operatively. Of all the hernias, the femoral hernia has a higher percentage of bowel symptoms.

The clinical presentation of hernias can be a slight bulge or bubonocele, incarceration, strangulation with bowel gangrene and peritonitis. Pain out of proportions is a sign of incarceration or strangulation, and it follows a sequence of venous and lymphatic congestion, leading to incarceration and subsequent arterial blockage, leading to gangrene. Patients may also have obstructive symptoms before incarceration, which can be relieved with gentle reduction (taxis). There are also situations where pre-peritoneal fat or omentum gets involved, and patients have pain from the ischemia or necrosis of fat. These patients have a non-obstructive abdominal presentation with fever and localized redness. Patients with an incarcerated hernia should be treated with emergency surgery to rescue the bowel. Once the hernia is reduced, the patient must be observed in the hospital to ensure the reduced bowel is not gangrenous. Patient with concern for gangrene needs emergency surgery. Patients with emergency surgery may not get definitive hernia repair with mesh to prevent infection.

Inguinal Hernia

One to five percent of all newborns and 9-11% of those born prematurely have an inguinal hernia. Thirty-three percent of kids with a birth weight of less than 1000g have a hernia. Newborns with an inguinal hernia should undergo operation urgently. The management of an inguinal hernia is surgical repair only. Clinical studies have shown that patients with light-duty work can delay surgery for a small reducible hernia as long as they have close monitoring by a surgeon.

Incarcerated hernias are a surgical emergency and must be reduced immediately using sedation, Trendelenburg position, ice packing, and, most importantly, manual reduction (taxis) to avoid strangulation of the contents of the hernia sac. Manual reduction is the treatment if the patient appears healthy but contraindicated with peritonitis or when septic from gangrenous bowel. Emergency surgery has more complications; hence, a manual reduction is opted for, with a fairly large number of patients doing well. Manual pressure can take up to half an hour for reduction. The technique for reduction is highly specific and one must learn it from an experienced surgeon.

There are differences in the surgical repair of children compared to adults.

Hernia in Children

Even though hernias are less common in female children, it requires a thorough evaluation as the reproductive structure can be inadvertently ligated and excised. In the pediatric population, high ligation is the procedure of choice and laparoscopic herniorrhaphy can be advised in recurring cases. Another strong indication for laparoscopic repair is a proven or suspected bilateral hernia. Once the incarcerated hernia is reduced, a delay of 5-10 days generally enables a more successful surgery. This duration gives tissue swelling an opportunity to normalize, allowing a better repair and a low recurrence.

Premature infants should undergo operation sooner, as there is a higher likelihood of incarceration. Hernias diagnosed in one-year-old children must be offered surgery as soon as possible, even if they do not have any incarceration, as the chances of incarceration are high. Pre-term infants with low birth weights have a 33% chance of having a hernia, and surgery should be done before discharge, once the infant is stable. Female infants with incarcerated hernias require emergency surgery even after reduction, as there is a risk of ovarian torsion and gangrene. The chances of salvaging the ovary are good if surgery is performed in 2 hours.

There is an increasing trend to not operate on the contralateral side for an inguinal hernia if it is non-clinical. It is more likely that the patent processus vaginalis will obliterate if left alone. Post-surgery, patients can have a seroma and hydrocele, which may take 3 weeks to 3 months for swelling to resolve. Patients have a 1% risk of infection. There is a 5-10% chance of testicular atrophy and vas injury.

Hernia Repair

Inguinal hernioplasty has seen changes in the philosophy of the technique, with the intention of reducing hernia recurrences. The main principles of hernia repair were aimed at strengthening the floor of the inguinal canal and tightening the external inguinal ring. Then came the focus of tension-free repair to reduce recurrences. There are various techniques of tension-free repair which include releasing or relaxing the incision of rectus, placement of mesh, and laparoscopic repair. As of 2023, the community has not come to a consensus on the superiority of open mesh and laparoscopic hernia repair. Each technique has its strengths and weaknesses, as discussed in the latter part of this chapter.

It is imperative to learn the old-time tested non-mesh techniques, tissue approximation repairs such as the Bassini or McVay repairs, as they are still the techniques used in infected and gangrenous hernias. The use of mesh is absolutely contraindicated in these situations.

The open approaches are the Lichtenstein repair, a plug and patch, and an open preperitoneal approach. They have recurrence rates from 1-5%, depending on the patient's comorbaitiesand the surgeon's experience. It is the duty of a surgeon to discuss the risks and benefits of surgery with their patients. All potential complications must be addressed in light of the benefits.

Lichtenstein Repair

The Lichenstein repair (Figure 3) is the most common technique and is currently the gold standard open surgery technique to treat inguinal hernias.[3] All patients are administered pre-operative antibiotics, and selected patients receive subcutaneous heparin (i.e., patients over 40 with other medical comorbidities). Surgery can be performed with different anesthesia (i.e., local, spinal, or general) depending on the patient's requirements and the surgeon's expertise. A nerve block of the ilioinguinal and iliohypogastric nerves helps surgery with minor tissue swelling. Another important aspect is that polypropylene or synthetic mesh covers the inguinal area. The medial edge of the mesh should be at least an inch medial to the pubic tubercle. Its medial border is sewn to the shelving edge of the inguinal ligament. The upper border of the mesh is sewn to the rectus sheath and internal oblique muscle. Finally, a keyhole defect in the mesh is used to pass the cord structure and helps prevent future recurrences.

The mesh-induced scarring prevents long-term hernia recurrence, and tension during mesh placement is the common cause of hernia recurrence. It is important to always secure mesh tension free.

Nerve pain is the most common and dreaded complication of the procedure nerve entrapment should be avoided during the procedure.

The Lichtenstein repair does not help in the femoral hernia. If there is difficulty finding an inguinal hernia during repair, explore the femoral hernia by opening the transversalis fascia.

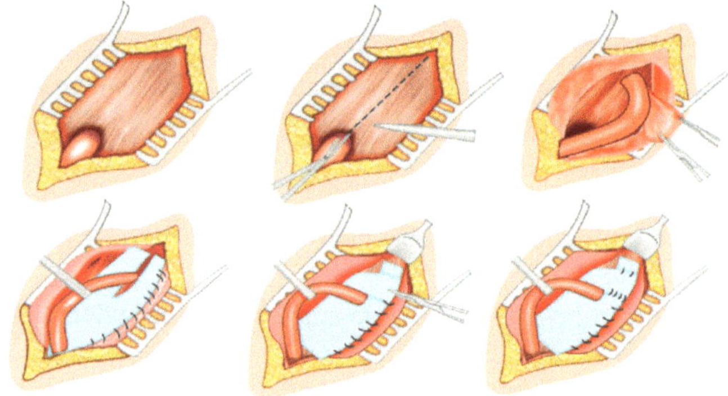

Figure 3: Lichtenstein Hernia Repair

Other Repair Techniques

Shouldice repair - this is a non-mesh technique developed by Shouldice Institute, Canada. The institute makes tissue approximation in layers and has a long post-op rehabilitation path. It claims a recurrence rate of 1%, which has not been achieved by any study using any technique thus far.

Bassini repair (Figure 4) - this technique approximates the conjoined tendon to the inguinal ligament from the pubic tubercle medially to the area of the internal ring laterally, using suture and closing the hernia defect. The use of this procedure is still advocated in an infected situation where the prosthetic mesh is contraindicated. This technique is only used for inguinal hernias, not femoral hernias.

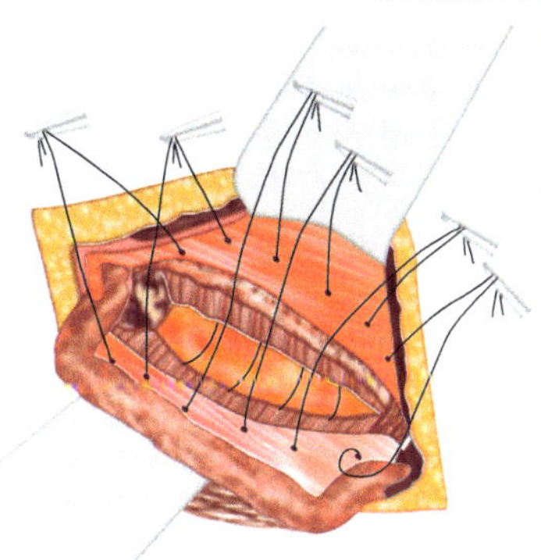

Figure 4: Bassini Repair

McVay repair (Figure 5) - is used for the repair of femoral and inguinal hernias. It is the most challenging inguinal surgery to understand, as the anatomical landmarks require meticulous dissection. The repair creates tension and requires a relaxing incision. A quick review of the steps includes dividing the transversalis fascia (Hesselbach's triangle) and delineating the pectineal ligament (Cooper's ligament, an extension of the lacunar ligament on the pectineal line) in the pre-peritoneal space. Subsequently suturing the conjoined tendon to Cooper's ligament from the pubic tubercle medially to the femoral vein laterally. Here on, place a suture including the conjoined tendon, Cooper's ligament, and the inguinal ligament. The remaining repair is done by approximating the conjoint tendon to the inguinal ligament lateral to the internal ring. The relaxing incision involves exposing the rectus sheath. It is critical to remember to spare the external oblique aponeurosis in a relaxing incision. Almost two to three inches of relaxation incision is required. This procedure has a painful postoperative course.

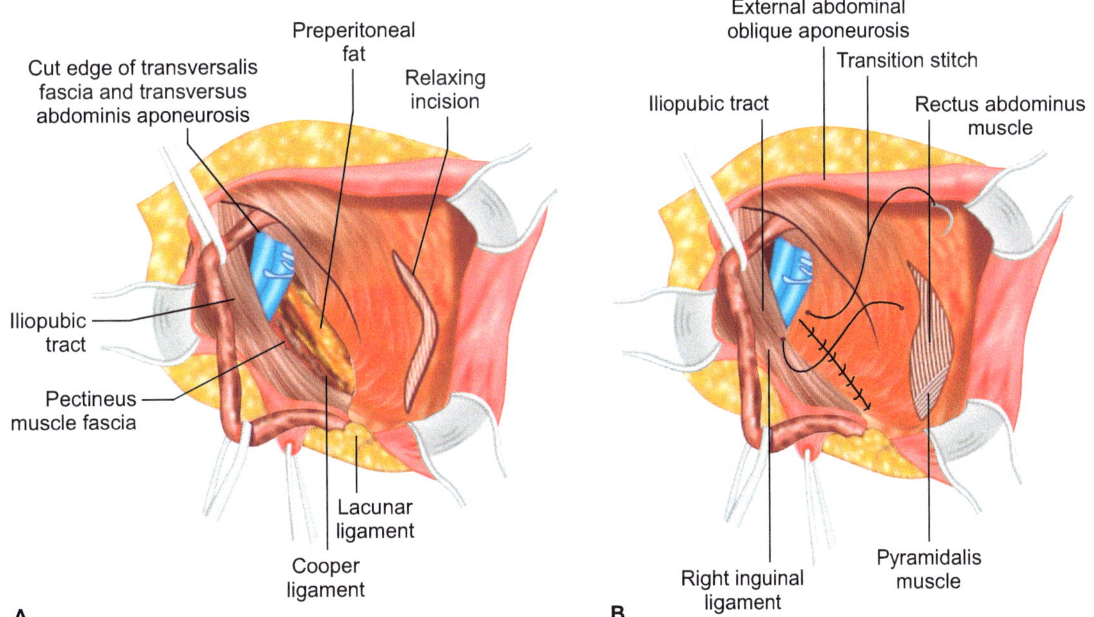

Figure 5: McVay Repair

A femoral hernia must be suspected when exploration of the inguinal hernia reveals no sac with cord, or it is in Hesselbach's triangle. This is achieved by opening the fascia transversalis and opening pre-peritoneal space.

Special Considerations

Incarcerated femoral hernias have some challenges. In complex cases, the lacunar ligament is incised to enlarge the femoral ring. In another challenging situation, the inguinal ligament is divided above the defect. If gangrenous bowel needs to be resected, and if there is difficulty delivering bowel, a lower midline incision can also be used.

Laparoscopic Repair

The objective of laparoscopic surgery is to have tension-free placement of mesh, both TEP (total extraperitoneal) and TAPP (transabdominal pre-peritoneal repair) (Figure 6).

The totally extraperitoneal (TEP) repair is performed in the pre-peritoneal space. The peritoneum is not violated. Three ports are placed in the midline from the umbilicus down, and the space is developed. This is the most common of all three repairs.

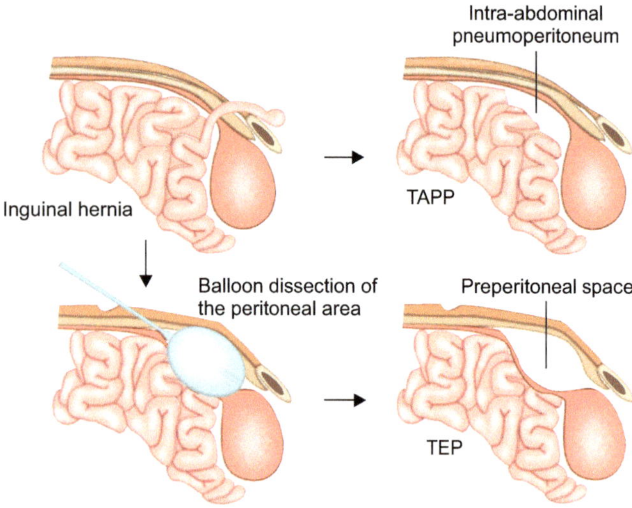

Figure 6: Laparoscopic inguinal hernia repair TAPP and TEP

The following is a quick overview of surgical steps:

1. Pre-peritoneal repair - the transversalis fascia over Hesselbach's triangle is opened in the same direction as the inguinal incision.
2. The fascia is opened from the pubic tubercle to the deep epigastric vessels.
3. Subsequently, the preperitoneal space is dissected, and the peritoneum and preperitoneal fat is freed from the muscles above.
4. The extension of dissection is from the linea alba medially and the anterior superior iliac spine laterally.
5. The extent of exposure posteriorly is to the symphysis pubis, Cooper's ligament, femoral ring, cord structures, psoas muscle, and external iliac vessels.

The transabdominal pro-peritoneal patch (TAPP) repair, as the name suggests, involves entering and reducing the hernia from the abdominal side and then placing the mesh and covering it with peritoneum to prevent adhesions. This technique raises the peritoneum flap, and the hernia sac is reduced after identifying the anatomy. Then mesh is used to cover all direct, indirect, and femoral defects. TAPP can visualize all the defects in view, and the same mesh covers all three openings. Mesh is mainly secured to the pubic bone.

In the intraabdominal pro-peritoneal onlay mesh (IPOM) repair, the mesh is placed from the peritoneal side to cover the defect exposing the mesh to the bowels.

Considerations

There are a few technical considerations in laparoscopic repairs. TEP is technically challenging in female patients due to dense scar between the sac and round ligament. Females are more likely to have obstetric or gynecological procedures, making laparoscopic procedures more challenging. Pre-peritoneal repair makes any future anterior prostate surgery challenging in male patients, so patients with questionable prostate issues are better off with the Lichtenstein repair.

Laparoscopic Surgery Advantages and Disadvantages

Significant benefits of laparoscopic surgery include reduced postoperative pain, examination of all hernia defects especially if there is the possibility of another hernia, visualization and repair of a bilateral hernia, simultaneous repair of a bilateral hernia, and evaluation of other intra-abdominal conditions. However, severe complications with laparoscopic surgery have also been reported, including significant vascular injury, bowel obstruction, bladder injury, and nerve injury.

Many in the surgical community are still not convinced of the advantages of laparoscopic repair. The surgeon's preference and competence in repair and fixation can be good, as long as the surgeon has expertise in his technique. Laparoscopic repair enables heavy manual labor to work quicker. Open repair helps an older and debilitated patient, as the surgery is done under local anesthesia.

Robotic Surgery

Robotic inguinal hernia repair is a new and revolving technique. It has equivocal result in postoperative pain, recovery, and outcomes compared to laparoscopic hernia repair. More studies will fully evaluate the long-term outcomes and its known its not cost-effective.

Other Repairing Techniques

The Bassini repair has a relaxing incision for incarcerated and strangulated inguinal hernias. The McVay repair is indicated for incarcerated and strangulated femoral hernias.

Another challenging area in hernia surgery is recurrence. The chances of failure increase with each surgery. The rule of thumb is as follows:

1. Recurrence after open surgery - laparoscopic repair is a better option, depending on the expertise of the surgeon
2. Recurrence after laparoscopic surgery - open repair is a better option
3. The most common area of recurrence after the repair is next to the pubic tubercle
4. Hernia recurrence in standard hands is less than 5%, with a target of 2%. Common reasons for recurrence are technical failure and failure in identifying the anatomy

Complications

The postoperative complications include mesh infection, chronic testicular pain, and testicular ischemia. The most common and bothersome complication to the patient is groin pain. Thirty percent of patients may complain of pins and needles for one month and close to 5-10% for three months or more. Seroma is a common finding after surgery and not a complication unless infected. Infected wounds generally end up in the removal of mesh and primary repair.

REFERENCES

1. Oberg S, Andresen K, Rosenberg J. Etiology of Inguinal Hernias: A Comprehensive Review. Front Surg. 2017 Sep 22;4:52. doi:10.3389/fsurg.2017.00052. PMID:29018803; PMCID:PMC5614933.
2. Nilsson H, Stylianidis G. Haapamaki M, Nilsson E, Nordin P. Mortality after groin hernia surgery. Ann Surg. 2007 Apr;245(4):656-60. doi:10.1097/01.sla.0000251364.32698.4b.
3. Samaali I, Zenaidi HH, Dougaz W, Khalfallah M, Jarraya H, Nouira R, Bouasker I, Dziri C. Treatment of inguinal hernia by Lichtenstein technique: an open prospective study. Tunis Med. 2016 Dec; 94(12):872. PMID: 28994888.

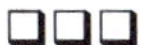

27

CHAPTER

Esophagus

Richard Berri, MD

ANATOMY

Surgeons who plan to treat esophageal disorders must have detailed knowledge of esophageal anatomy and its relationships. This is vital to performing safe surgeries as well as to understanding the meaning of abnormalities detected on specific diagnostic studies. By recognizing early pathological changes and being able to interpret tests of esophageal function, the surgeon can optimize the care provided to patients with esophageal diseases.

Embryology of the esophagus is vital to understanding the normal anatomy and its variants, as well as congenital malformations. The embryonic esophagus forms during the fourth week of development when a diverticulum forms on the ventral surface of the foregut. This tracheobronchial diverticulum has two paired grooves on each side that form the tracheoesophageal septum via medial growth. This septum later separates the foregut into the trachea ventrally, and the esophagus dorsally. The esophagus elongates rapidly with cranial growth of the embryonic body and reaches its final length by week seven of development. Subsequently, blood vessels enter the submucosa, and the endoderm rapidly proliferates nearly occluding the esophageal lumen. By week ten the lumen recanalizes leaving a superficial layer of ciliated epithelial cells, which are later replaced by squamous epithelium. Caudal branchial arches give rise to the striated muscle of the upper esophagus which is innervated by the vagus nerve. The smooth muscle of the lower esophagus derives from splanchnic mesenchyme and is supplied by a visceral nerve plexus.

The adult esophagus begins at the pharyngoesophageal junction and ends at the gastroesophageal junction, ranging from 18 to 26 cm in length.[1] The cervical esophagus begins at C6, ends at T1 and is approximately 5 cm in length. As it descends it makes a slight curve to the left, and is surrounded by the carotid sheaths laterally, the trachea anteriorly, and the retroesophageal space and vertebral column posteriorly.

The thoracic esophagus superiorly is intimately related to the trachea, passing just posterior to the tracheal wall and coursing to the right of the descending aorta. At the level of the tracheal bifurcation, approximately T8, the esophagus turns left and passes behind the left mainstem bronchus and descends to the diaphragm. At the level of T10, the esophagus passes through the hiatus of the diaphragm and enters the stomach. The esophageal hiatus is formed by the left and right crura, which arise from the first four lumbar vertebrae and anterior longitudinal ligaments. The crura are joined together caudally by the median arcuate ligament at the level of the celiac axis.

The abdominal esophagus varies from 0.5 to 2.5 cm in length.[2] At this level the esophagus is surrounded by a fibroelastic membrane, the phrenoesophageal ligament. The phrenoesophageal ligament is derived from subdiaphragmatic fascia and inserts into the circumference of the esophagus above and below the diaphragm.[3,4] At the lower limit of the phrenoesophageal ligament there is a large fat pad that corresponds to the gastroesophageal junction.

The esophagus has three areas of anatomic narrowing. The cervical constriction at the level of the cricopharyngeal sphincter is the narrowest point of the gastrointestinal tract. The bronchoaortic constriction is located behind the tracheal bifurcation where the left main bronchus and aortic arch about the esophagus. The diaphragmatic constriction occurs where the esophagus enters the diaphragm.

Numerous segmental arteries contribute to the extensive capillary network that supplies the esophagus. The inferior thyroid artery provides the majority of the blood supply to the cervical esophagus, with some contribution from the superior thyroid artery and other collaterals as well. The major blood supply to the thoracic aorta is from the right intercostal and bronchial arteries proximally, and branches directly from the aorta distally. The abdominal esophagus receives its blood supply from branches of the left gastric, short gastric, and left inferior phrenic arteries. The venous drainage is also extensive and includes the inferior thyroid vein proximally, bronchial, azygous, or hemiazygos veins in the thorax, and the left gastric vein in the abdominal portion of the esophagus.

The esophagus contains a dense network of lymph vessels that drain into nodes in the periesophageal connective tissue. The flow of lymphatics in the upper two thirds of the esophagus is cephalad, whereas in the distal third it is in both directions. In the cervical region, lymphatic drainage is towards the internal jugular and upper tracheal nodes. Dorsally, the thoracic esophagus drains into posterior mediastinal nodes. Drainage from the anterior thoracic esophagus is to tracheal nodes superiorly, and paraoesophageal and subcarinal nodes inferiorly. The lymphatics from the abdominal esophagus drain into cardiac and celiac nodes, which may drain into the thoracic duct or cisterna chyli. Unlike the arterial supply, the lymphatic drainage is not segmental, and all lymphatics intercommunicate. This accounts for the frequent and wide intramural and mediastinal lymphatic metastases of esophageal carcinomas.

The esophagus has parasympathetic and sympathetic innervation. The vagus nerve supplies only parasympathetics to the esophagus, but below the neck the vagus nerve holds a mixture of parasympathetic and sympathetic fibers. The superior laryngeal nerves arise from the vagus nerve in the neck, dividing into external and internal branches. The internal branch is the sensory nerve of the pharyngeal surface of the larynx and base of the tongue. The external branch innervates the cricothyroid muscle and partly the inferior pharyngeal constrictor muscle. The recurrent laryngeal nerve provides parasympathetic innervation to the cervical esophagus and upper esophageal sphincter. Branches of both vagus nerves and the left recurrent laryngeal nerve innervate the upper thoracic esophagus. Left and right vagus nerves entwine with fibers from the thoracic sympathetic chain to form the esophageal plexus. This plexus is on the anterior and posterior wall of the esophagus and innervates the lower portion of the esophagus. Distal to the esophageal plexus, each vagus trunk contains fibers from both the left and right original vagus nerves. The left vagus trunk (under the diaphragm) splits into a hepatic branch and gastric branches (anterior). In contrast, the right vagus trunk gives off a branch to the celiac plexus as well as the gastric branches (posterior). The superior cervical ganglion, celiac ganglion, thoracic aortic plexus, major splanchnic nerve, and sympathetic chain contribute to overall sympathetic innervation.

PHYSIOLOGY

The esophagus serves to transport swallowed material from the pharynx into the stomach. Once initiated, swallowing is entirely a reflex. Oropharyngeal swallowing begins with an oral phase followed by a pharyngeal phase. The oral phase is largely voluntary and varies depending on factors such as taste, hunger, and motivation. The pharyngeal phase of swallowing is a complex event referred to as the *swallow response* and is regulated by afferent sensory nerves of the pharynx.

When food is taken into the mouth, it is broken up and lubricated with saliva to prepare for swallowing. Once the food is ready, swallowing can be initiated voluntarily, or as a reflex due to stimulation of areas in the mouth and pharynx, particularly the posterior lateral walls of the hypopharynx, or anterior and posterior tonsillar pillars. Afferent sensory fibers of the pharynx derive from the glossopharyngeal nerve and superior laryngeal branches of the vagus nerve. These sensory fibers converge and terminate in the medullary swallow center. The swallow center coordinates the act of swallowing via signals to cranial nerves 5,7, 10-12, and motor neurons of C1-C3. The overall swallow response can be divided into several coordinated actions:[5] elevation and retraction of the soft palate to close the nasopharynx, upper esophageal sphincter (UES) opening, laryngeal closure by the epiglottis, tongue loading, tongue pulsion, and pharyngeal clearance. The whole pharyngeal part of swallowing occurs within 1.5 seconds.[6]

Pressure in the hypopharynx rises quickly during swallowing. This is attributed to the backward movement of the tongue and contraction of posterior pharyngeal constrictors. The pharyngeal constrictors contract to push the food forward into the thoracic esophagus, and the UES contracts and closes upon initiation of the swallow. Closure of the UES creates increased intraluminal pressure, and when combined with peristaltic waves, prevents food from refluxing back into the pharynx.

The esophageal phase of swallowing is initiated by pharyngeal activity. This phase represents work done by the esophagus to move food from the negative pressure of the intrathoracic cavity to the positive pressure of the abdominal cavity. Three types of contractions are seen in the body of the esophagus: primary peristalsis, secondary peristalsis, and tertiary contractions. Primary peristalsis is triggered by voluntary swallowing and is progressive in nature. Secondary peristalsis is triggered by distention or irritation, rather than voluntary swallowing. Secondary peristalsis begins in the smooth muscle of the esophagus and is progressive, continuing until retained intraesophageal contents empty into the stomach. Tertiary contractions are simultaneous contractions that occur spontaneously between swallows or after voluntary swallowing. These contractions represent uncoordinated smooth muscle contractions throughout the esophagus and are often responsible for esophageal spasm.

When a swallowed bolus enters the esophagus, a primary peristaltic wave is activated. Primary waves move down the esophagus at 2 to 4 cms per second and reach the distal esophagus about 9 seconds after swallowing is initiated.[6] Peristaltic pressures range from 20 to 100 mm Hg with contractions lasting 2 to 4 seconds.[7] If the entire bolus does not empty into the esophagus, secondary peristaltic waves are initiated.

The lower esophageal sphincter (LES), although not a distinct anatomic structure, serves as a resting pressure barrier between the stomach and esophagus. The LES is more accurately referred to as the *LES mechanism* and represents a functional sphincter. The sphincter remains closed at a resting pressure of 10 to 20 mm Hg to prevent reflux of gastric contents into the esophagus and relaxes to open during a pharyngeal swallow. LES pressure returns to resting level after the peristaltic wave passes through the esophagus.

MOTILITY DISORDERS

The physiological and anatomic divide between oropharynx and gut is provided by the esophagus. The oropharynx which consists of striated muscle is controlled by the medulla and is capable of precise tactile sensation. The distal esophagus is made of smooth muscle, capable of imprecise sensation, and is regulated by the enteric nervous system. Due to this structure, motility disorders of the esophagus can be categorized as pharyngeal or esophageal. Pharyngeal dysphagia includes physiological abnormalities of the UES and proximal esophagus, whereas esophageal dysphagia involves purely esophageal motor disorders. Pharyngeal dysphagia differs from esophageal dysphagia in several aspects. Pharyngeal dysphagia most commonly arises from neurogenic or myogenic diseases or structural anomalies, while esophageal dysphagia results almost entirely from primary disease of the esophagus. Secondly, because airway protection plays a significant role in the oropharyngeal swallowing mechanism, pharyngeal dysphagia has a high risk of aspiration. Additionally, unlike esophageal dysphagia, pharyngeal dysphagia frequently requires a multidisciplinary approach to management involving radiologists, gastroenterologists, neurologists, speech-language pathologists, otolaryngologists, and dieticians.[8]

Pharyngeal Dysphagia

Pharyngeal dysphagia is estimated to range between 16% and 22% in persons older than age 50, is associated with high morbidity, mortality, and cost.[9,10] Most cases of pharyngeal dysphagia are structural or functional in nature, with stroke being the most common cause overall. The dysphagia is localized between the thyroid cartilage and the suprasternal notch. Symptoms often include feeling a lump in the throat, occasional pain radiating to the jaw and ears, hoarseness, expectoration of excessive saliva, and symptoms associated with gastroesophageal reflux. Sequelae of pharyngeal dysphagia are severe including dehydration, malnutrition, choking, aspiration, pneumonia and death. Video-fluoroscopic Swallowing Study is the study of choice for evaluating pharyngeal dysphagia, although manometry and video-endoscopy may be used as adjuncts.

Structural Causes of Pharyngeal Dysphagia

Structural anomalies frequently associated with pharyngeal dysphagia include pharyngeal diverticula and cricopharyngeal bars. Lesions such as webs, strictures, or tumors can cause obstructive dysphagia. Additionally, because of the close opposition of the posterior pharynx to the anterior cervical vertebrae, cervical osteophytes can also cause obstructive dysphagia.

Pharyngeal diverticula are classified according to anatomical site, either lateral or posterior. The most frequent site is in the posterior midline between the oblique fibers of the inferior pharyngeal constrictor and cricopharyngeus muscle (Killian's dehiscence).[11] This is the location for Zenker's diverticulum. Lateral diverticula protrude from the lateral wall of the mid pharynx and may be congenital or more commonly acquired. The common theme of these locations is that they are sites of potential weakness of the muscular lining of the hypopharynx. These diverticula rarely cause symptoms until they are large enough to store a significant amount of food or liquid. In addition to dysphagia, symptoms can include halitosis, regurgitation, aspiration of material from the diverticula, and recurrent chest infections.

Zenker's Diverticulum is the most common of the esophageal diverticula. It is a pulsion diverticulum, in which the herniation of the pouch is due to incomplete opening of the UES.[12] This restricted opening of the UES is thought to be the result of intrinsic disease of the cricopharyngeus muscle, where muscle fiber degenerates and is replaced by fibroadipose tissue.[13] A barium swallow establishes the diagnosis, although occasionally an air fluid level can be seen on a plain film. Treatment of Zenker's diverticulum can be done surgically or endoscopically. Surgical treatment involves doing a cricopharyngeal myotomy, and resection of the diverticulum or diverticulopexy. Resection of the diverticulum is usually preferred for diverticulum larger than 3 cm. Alternatively, myotomy may be done via the endoscopic approach. Through a rigid esophagoscope, the septum between the posterior wall of the cricopharyngeus muscle and anterior wall of the Zenker's diverticulum is incised. This incision can be done using a needle-knife papillotome and monopolar cautery, laser, or stapler.

Cricopharyngeal bar is a common incidental radiologic finding that rarely causes symptoms. It is visualized on barium swallow as a characteristic prominent projection on the posterior wall of the pharyngoesophageal junction. The Valsalva maneuver, and upper GI studies (performed on patients without dysphagia) can result in transient cricopharyngeal bar.[14] dermatomyositis, or inclusion body myositis can lead to persistent cricopharyngeal bar.[14] These lesions turn up in the investigation of many patients with dysphagia, but rarely cause dysphagia. Additional esophageal or pharyngeal abnormalities should be ruled out by radiologic, manometric and endoscopic studies. When considered symptomatic, these lesions are treated by either cricopharyngeal myotomy or dilatation.

Esophageal webs are thin transverse membranes comprised of mucosa and submucosa. They usually occur in the proximal few centimeters of the esophagus and are usually eccentric, but sometimes are circumferential. These lesions are visible transiently on barium swallow, and better visualized on video-fluoroscopy. Webs have been associated with iron deficiency anemia, as part of Plummer-Vinson or Patterson-Kelly syndrome.[15] Patients with these syndromes have been shown to have increased risk of squamous carcinoma.[16] Some webs are asymptomatic but most typically present with intermittent dysphagia for solids. When symptomatic, these lesions are best treated with bougienage.[5]

Functional Causes of Pharyngeal Dysphagia

Functional causes of pharyngeal dysphagia are often neurogenic or myogenic. Neurogenic disorders such as stroke, Parkinson's Disease, motor neuron disease, poliomyelitis, and tumors of the medulla are associated with dysphagia. Stroke is the most common cause of pharyngeal dysphagia. Typical findings seen on video-fluoroscopy include difficulty initiating the swallow, absent or delayed pharyngeal swallow response, pharyngeal weakness with poor pharyngeal clearance, post-swallow pooling in vallecula and pyriform sinuses, and aspiration.[8] Brainstem strokes to the medulla can result in failure of UES relaxation which is detectable by manometry.[17]

Myogenic diseases causing dysphagia include inflammatory myopathies such as polymyositis, dermatomyositis and inclusion body cyst myositis,[18] myasthenia gravis, myopathy of thyrotoxicosis, oculopharyngeal dystrophy and myotonic dystrophy. Video-fluoroscopic features may vary based on the causative disease. Management of dysphagia aims at specifically treating the underlying disease.

Esophageal Dysphagia

A basic characteristic of esophageal motility disorders is failure in preserving esophageal emptiness. This can manifest as retained material within the esophagus or excessive entry of material into the esophagus. Dysphagia of this nature is categorized as disorders of peristalsis or sphincter competence. Patients typically present with odynophagia, esophagopharyngeal regurgitation, heartburn, chest pain, and intermittent esophageal obstruction. Patients with primary esophageal motility disorders will also experience dysphagia with both solids and liquids, as opposed to just solids as seen in disorders of mechanical obstruction.

Disorders of peristalsis causing esophageal dysphagia

Achalasia

Achalasia is a motor disorder of the esophagus characterized by loss of peristalsis, failure of the LES to completely relax with swallowing, and increased LES resting pressure, all of which are seen on manometry. It is thought to result from loss of ganglionic cells in the intermyenteric (Auerbach's) plexus. The cause of ganglion cell loss is unknown but there is increasing evidence consistent with an immune related response.[5] An additional cause is Chagas' disease, a parasitic infection characterized by destruction of the smooth muscle ganglion cells of the Auerbach plexus, with resulting motor dysfunction of the esophagus, colon, ureters and other viscera. Injury to Auerbach's plexus by cold, heat, chemicals, or excision can also lead to characteristic manometric signs of achalasia.[19]

Patients with achalasia classically present with dysphagia, regurgitation, and weight loss. Some patients also suffer from bronchopulmonary complications as the result of regurgitation such as aspiration, pneumonia, lung abscess, bronchiectasis, hemoptysis, or bronchospasm. The characteristic appearance on chest X-ray shows an air-fluid level in a dilated esophagus. Barium swallow shows esophageal dilation with tapering of the LES, giving the distal esophagus a beak-like appearance. Pseudoachalasia, caused by tumor at or near the gastroesophageal junction, can be differentiated from true achalasia by endoscopy. Retention esophagitis is also seen on endoscopy in advanced achalasia.

Treatment of achalasia aims at relieving the obstruction caused by the nonrelaxing LES. In early stages of the disease, smooth muscle relaxing agents given before or during meals such as sublingual nitroglycerin, nitrates, or calcium channel blocking agents may offer some relief. Botulinum toxin injection into the LES has been shown to decrease LES pressure and improve dysphagia. Dilation with an endoscope or bougies provides temporary relief for several days to weeks but is not a long-term solution. Definitive treatment involves destruction of the circular layer of smooth muscle within the LES. This can be done by forceful pneumatic dilation, or esophageal myotomy. During pneumatic dilation, a long cylindrical balloon is positioned across the LES using fluoroscopy or an endoscope and inflated using a handheld manometer. The balloon is usually inflated to a pressure of 300 mm Hg for 15 seconds.[19] Surgical myotomy involves incising enough muscle to relieve dysphagia, but not cause gastroesophageal reflux. The circular muscle of the lower end of the esophagus is divided via an open or video-assisted thoracoscopic approach, but most surgeons prefer a laparoscopic transabdominal approach. Adding an antireflux procedure can prevent reflux, but dysphagia may recur with a tight wrap.

Diffuse Esophageal Spasm

Diffuse esophageal spasm (DES) is a hypermotility disorder seen in patients with unexplained chest pain or dysphagia associated with disordered peristalsis and tertiary contractions. The cause of DES is unknown, but studies suggest that it is a result of a hypersensitive smooth muscle response to cholinergic and hormonal stimulation. Most commonly patients complain of recurrent chest pain similar to angina, and intermittent dysphagia. Symptoms appear more prominent during periods of emotional stress or anxiety.

There are no uniform radiographic or manometric findings for DES. Since the abnormal events are intermittent, many examinations may be normal if the patient is not experiencing a spasm at the time of the study. Radiographic findings may include classic curling, "corkscrew esophagus", "rosary bead esophagus", or pseudodiverticula. Classic manometric criteria are high amplitude, non-peristaltic, prolonged contractions that occur in the smooth muscle after a swallow and spontaneously. However, these radiographic and manometric criteria can be seen in asymptomatic patients. The key to diagnosing DES is the correlation of these results with the patients' subjective complaints of pain and dysphagia.

Treatment for DES is ill defined. Calcium channel blockers, antispasmodics, nitrates and hydralazine have been shown to be helpful occasionally. Esophageal dilation may be therapeutic for chest pain and dysphagia. If symptoms of reflux are present, anti-reflux therapy should be initiated to help with esophageal pain. Behavioral modifications such as avoiding stress during meals and biofeedback have also been shown to successfully manage symptoms. Esophageal myotomy for symptomatic relief of DES only has a success rate of 50-60%, so this option should be reserved for patients incapacitated by chest pain or dysphagia, or in the presence of an intrathoracic esophageal pulsion diverticulum.[19]

Other abnormalities of peristalsis

Nutcracker esophagus is a hypermotility disorder where the manometric abnormality is defined as average distal esophageal peristaltic pressures greater than two standard deviations above normal in a symptomatic patient.[20] These high amplitude contractions are progressive and prolonged, and patients often complain of chest pain, odynophagia and dysphagia. Treatment is similar to that for DES.

Esophageal dysmotility is well characterized with collagen vascular diseases such as lupus erythematosus, dermatomyositis, polymyositis, and particularly scleroderma. Scleroderma is recognized by normal proximal esophageal peristalsis, with weak to absent distal peristalsis, and weak or absent LES pressure on manometry.[21] Patients with esophageal scleroderma mainly present with dysphagia and heartburn. Although there is no specific treatment for scleroderma of the esophagus, gastroesophageal reflux should be identified and treated according to its severity. Combined Collis gastroplasty-fundoplication may be beneficial in patients with esophageal scleroderma complicated by severe esophagitis, stricture formation, fibrinoid degeneration and atrophy of distal esophageal smooth muscle, all of which may compromise success of traditional operations.[19]

Other nonspecific esophageal motility disorders are seen in patients with chest pain, dysphagia and gastroesophageal reflux. These disorders are recognized as manometric abnormalities of peristalsis, but with patterns inconsistent with previously described diseases. Abnormal findings include frequent non-transmitted contractions, retrograde contractions, repetitive contractions, low-amplitude contractions, prolonged contractions, high amplitude contractions, spontaneous contractions and incomplete LES relaxation.

Disorders of sphincter competence causing esophageal dysphagia

Hypertensive lower esophageal sphincter (HLES) is a manometric abnormality of unknown etiology defined as resting LES pressure two standard deviations above normal, with normal residual pressures associated with normal peristalsis.[8] It is typically seen in patients being evaluated for nonspecific chest pain, and dysphagia is a common presenting symptom. Since most radiographic and nuclear emptying studies are normal, the mechanism of dysphagia or chest pain is unknown. HLES is relatively uncommon, whereas the major dysfunction of sphincter competence occurs with gastroesophageal reflux disease.

GASTROESOPHAGEAL REFLUX DISEASE

Gastroesophageal reflux is the effortless retrograde movement of gastric contents into the esophagus. It is a normal physiologic process that occurs multiple times a day especially after large meals. It occurs in almost everyone without producing signs or symptoms of mucosal damage. In contrast, gastroesophageal reflux disease (GERD) is a chronic disorder that produces a spectrum of symptoms with or without mucosa damage.

Pathologic reflux results when the acidity and volume of gastroduodenal contents overcomes the defensive factors protecting the esophagus (esophageal acid clearance, tissue resistance, antireflux barriers). The antireflux barrier is an anatomic region consisting of the LES, diaphragmatic crura, the intra-abdominal location of the LES, the phrenoesophageal ligaments, and the acute angle of His.[5] The main component of the antireflux barrier is the LES, and dysfunction of this muscular segment is the major cause of GERD. Patterns of LES dysfunction are hypotensive LES pressure, transient LES relaxations, and swallow-induced LES relaxations. Hypotensive LES pressure is the main cause of GERD in patients with severe reflux disease such as in patients with scleroderma. Transient LES relaxation accounts for the reflux of gasses during belching and is the most common mechanism for reflux episodes in healthy persons and those with mild GERD. Refluxes during swallow-induced LES relaxation is often associated with a hiatal hernia due to pooling of gastric contents in the hernia, and loss of diaphragmatic support normally present during LES relaxation.[22] Presence of a hiatal hernia also displaces the LES into the chest, which reduces basal LES pressure, and leads to loss of the intra-abdominal segment of the LES. Certain foods, medications, and lifestyle behaviors can also lead to decreased LES pressure and contribute to the onset of GERD.

Typical presentation of patients with GERD is a long-standing heartburn with a shorter history of regurgitation. Extraesophageal symptoms include respiratory, ear, nose, and throat manifestations as well as non-cardiac chest pain. "Alarm" signs include dysphagia, odynophagia, weight loss, advanced age, anemia, gastrointestinal (GI) bleeding, and a family history of upper GI cancer. Complications from long-standing GERD include esophageal ulcers, esophagitis, bleeding from esophageal erosions or ulcerations, strictures, perforation, Barrett's esophagus, and esophageal carcinoma.

GERD is first diagnosed clinically by taking a history of the patient's history. It is then confirmed by the patient's response to treatment with proton pump inhibitors (PPI). If a patient is not responsive to medical treatment, 24-hour pH monitoring may be helpful. The pH monitoring will confirm the diagnosis of GERD, or if the patient requires more medical or surgical treatment. Esophageal pH monitoring is useful in patients who have atypical GERD symptoms (i.e., chronic cough) and who have not responded to PPI therapy. For patients with suspected GERD or extraesophageal symptoms of GERD and negative pH testing, esophageal impedance testing is helpful to establish diagnosis. This test is helpful in detecting antegrade and retrograde movement of liquid and gas, enabling the differentiation between acid and non-acid reflux. "Alarm" signs necessitate further evaluation with an upper endoscopy or imaging such as barium esophagram or upper GI series.

Goals of therapy for GERD are to relieve acid-related symptoms, prevent symptomatic relapses and complications of GERD, and heal esophagitis if present. Lifestyle changes should be part of initial management of all patients. These include avoiding foods and beverages that exacerbate reflux, refraining from lying down for three hours after meals, avoiding evening snacks before bedtime, head of bed elevation, weight loss, smoking cessation, alcohol restriction, and avoidance of tight-fitting clothing. Additionally, drugs that act to lower LES pressure or drugs that cause localized esophagitis should be avoided.

Medical management includes antacid and antisecretory agents. Antacids that are from over-the-counter help treat mild heartburn by buffering the gastric acid that is in the esophagus and stomach. Antisecretory agents include Histamine-2 (H_2) receptor blockers which reduce gastric acid secretion by acting on gastric parietal cells and competitively blocking H_2 receptors. They mostly control reflux symptoms associated with nocturnal acid secretion in patients who have mild to moderate GERD[23].

PPIs inhibit acid secretion by blocking the H+/K+ ATPase pump on parietal cells. They inhibit acid secretion better than H2 blockers at all times of the day.[24] PPIs should be administered when fasting and 30 minutes prior to meals. They are the initial therapy for moderate to severe GERD and in patients who have complications including strictures and bleeding.

Surgical antireflux therapy can be used in patients with persistent symptoms despite medical therapy, patients who have atypical GERD but still respond to PPIs, or patients with PPI controlled GERD but who discontinue medications due to affordability of the drug, have poor compliance, or fear the side effects of the drug. The goal of surgery is to prevent GER by reducing the diameter of the esophageal lumen. The most popular procedure is the Nissen fundoplication, followed by the Toupet partial fundoplication. Additionally, if hiatal hernia is present, surgery aims at increasing basal LES pressure by reducing the hernia back into the abdomen to restore proper length of intra-abdominal LES and reconstructing the hiatus.

BARRETT'S ESOPHAGUS

In some patients, chronic GERD becomes esophagitis and metaplastic changes, also may exhibit known as Barrett's esophagus. Barrett's esophagus is when the distal esophagus is changed from squamous epithelium to specialized intestinal columnar epithelium with goblet cells. This is thought to be a protective mechanism against further injury to the esophagus by gastric contents.

Barrett's esophagus is more prevalent in patients with GERD versus healthy individuals, and this is due to longer periods of acid reflux resulting in greater acid exposure. The acid and bile salts contained in the refluxed gastric contents have been shown to induce certain homeobox (ffox) genes which regulate cell differentiation, and this is believed to result in metaplasia.[14] Although this metaplasia may be protective, it also increases the patient's risk for esophageal cancer.

Barrett's esophagus is suspected at endoscopy and confirmed by biopsies. Normally the columnar epithelium of the reddish pink gastric mucosa meets the glossy white squamous mucosa of the esophagus at the squamocolumnar junction (SCJ) or Z-line. This corresponds to the GE junction and endoscopically is seen at the top of the gastric folds. If the SCJ is displaced proximally into the tubular esophagus, then metaplasia is likely present, and biopsies should be taken. Strictures and esophagitis can also be seen at the new SCJ.

There are three main types of Barrett's esophagus: Long-segment, short segment, and intestinal metaplasia. With regards to characteristics, 3 cm of columnar epithelium must be identified for long segments, and less than 3 cm for short segments. The latter are biopsy findings under the microscope; however, they are not visible during an endoscopy.[25]

Characteristically, histology of Barrett's esophagus will show the presence of glandular epithelium with mucin-type cells, additionally there will be goblet cells. Biopsy specimens are classified as (1) dysplasia is not present, (2) dysplasia is indefinite, (3) dysplasia is low-grade, or (4) dysplasia is high-grade. Dysplasia is diagnosed based on lesions with nuclear atypia on mucosal surfaces. In indefinite-grade dysplasia, nuclear enlargement, crowding, hyperchromatism and prominence of nucleoli with mild stratification is confined to the lower gland. The upper gland has either fewer abnormalities or is normal. Low-grade dysplasia is when the mucosal cells have large, hyperchromatic nuclei with irregular contours in the basal cell layer of the esophagus. Additionally, there is little to no stratification. High grade dysplasia is when there is marked distortion of glandular structure, with epithelium on the mucosal surface, and nuclear polarity abnormalities.

Patients with Barrett's esophagus have an increased risk of developing esophageal cancer compared with the general population, specifically adenocarcinoma. Dysplasia is a major risk factor for progression of the cells to an adenocarcinoma. Patients with short-segment Barrett's esophagus have 6-8% incidence of dysplasia versus 15-24% in long-segment Barrett's esophagus.[14] Subsequently the risk of adenocarcinoma is estimated to be 2-15 times higher with long-segment Barrett's esophagus compared to short-segment Barrett's esophagus.[14]

Treatment for Barrett's esophagus varies based on presence and extent of dysplasia. However, it is recommended for all patients with Barrett's esophagus to be placed on PPIs due to data showing lower rate dysplasia becoming adenocarcinoma in patients taking PPIs than patients not taking PPIs.[14] This should be done whether symptoms of GERD are present or not. If biopsy specimens show indefinite-grade dysplasia, the patient should be started on an aggressive antisecretory therapy and have repeat surveillance biopsies every 3 months. Initial diagnosis of low-grade dysplasia should prompt repeat EGD and biopsies within 3-6 months. Low-grade dysplasia may regress to nondysplastic Barrett's esophagus on subsequent biopsies, but as long as low-grade dysplasia persists on histology, biopsies should be done annually. For high-grade dysplasia that is "focal" (involving 5 or fewer crypts) on a single biopsy, endoscopic surveillance is reasonable, and more invasive treatment reserved for patients who progress to adenocarcinoma. For patients with high grade dysplasia in a nodule or discrete lesion, options for treatment include endoscopic mucosal resection, photodynamic therapy or endoscopic ablative techniques using radiofrequency, focal thermal, or cryoablation.

NEOPLASMS

Benign Neoplasms

Benign neoplasms of the esophagus are rarely seen. They may be classified based on location between those within the muscular wall and those within the lumen of the esophagus.[27] Leiomyomas are the most common benign neoplasm. Polyps are also uncommon but may be encountered at specialty centers.

Leiomyomas are the most common of the benign esophageal neoplasms, representing two thirds of these.[26] They are mesenchymal in origin and intramural, occurring mainly in the lower two thirds of the esophagus.[27] They are generally found as single lesions but may be multiples. Leiomyomas are slow growing tumors with a minimal risk of malignant degeneration.

Most leiomyomas are asymptomatic. When symptoms are present, they consist of dysphagia and retrosternal pain. Diagnostic work-up entails barium swallow and endoscopy. Barium swallow provides the characteristic image of a smooth non-circumferential well-demarcated mass. Endoscopy reveals a freely movable mass invading the esophageal lumen. Biopsy should not be undertaken as it augments the chances of mucosal perforation at the time of resection.[27] Endoscopic ultrasound may also be utilized to further evaluate the tumor.

Treatment of leiomyomas is controversial. There is a consensus that symptomatic lesions and those larger than 5cm require surgical excision.[19] Asymptomatic and smaller lesions may be observed or surgically removed. These lesions are removed with simple enucleation, where the tumor location determines the surgical approach. Right thoracotomy is employed for tumors in the proximal and middle esophagus, and left thoracotomy is utilized for those of the distal esophagus.[27] The outer longitudinal muscle is repaired after tumor removal. Esophageal resection may be required for larger lesions and those involving the gastroesophageal junction.[27] Minimally invasive techniques have also been employed for tumor removal.

Polyps are uncommon benign lesions of the esophagus. They are intraluminal and cervical in location. Their presenting symptoms include dysphagia and potentially asphyxiation, if a larger polyp drops into the airway. Polyps usually have a stalk allowing them to be easily removed endoscopically. Cervical esophagomyotomy, and potentially a right thoracotomy is necessary for larger polyp removal.[26]

Malignant Neoplasms

Adenocarcinoma and squamous cell carcinoma remain the most common of the malignant neoplasms of the esophagus. Worldwide, squamous cell carcinoma is the most prevalent.[27] Its incidence varies based on geographical location, with the highest rates in the Mid-East and Asia. Local diet may serve as a risk factor and account for this trend, with food containing nitrosamines and nitrosyl compounds, such as smoked meats, and mineral deficiencies.[27] Tobacco and alcohol use remain strong risk factors in addition to medical conditions such as achalasia, strictures, human papillomavirus, Plummer-Vinson syndrome, and tylosis.[26] Squamous cell carcinoma is generally located in the proximal and middle two-thirds of the esophagus.

Adenocarcinoma is rapidly becoming the most common of the malignant esophageal neoplasms.[26] In recent decades, its incidence has grown more than any other cancer in the Western world. This change is largely due to its strong association to gastroesophageal reflux disease and Barrett's esophagus. Diagnoses are therefore becoming more common in younger patients with earlier stages being identified.

Clinical presentation varies for esophageal carcinoma. Early cancers are usually asymptomatic, but patients may present with dysphagia and stridor from invasion of the tracheobronchial tree. Aspiration pneumonia may result from a tracheoesophageal fistula that develops later in the course of disease. Weight loss may be present and is indicative of a poor prognosis. Local and systemic invasion may lead to severe bleeding, vocal cord paralysis, jaundice, and bone pain. A palpable left supraclavicular lymph node or Virchow's node represents metastatic disease.

Thorough diagnostic work-up entails the use of multiple modalities, including the main techniques of barium swallow and endoscopy. Barium swallow is utilized to delineate intraluminal and intramural lesions, and intrinsic and extrinsic compression. This may also reveal the characteristic apple core lesion present with some esophageal carcinomas. Endoscopy is utilized to further characterize the lesion by identifying its location and consistency and provides an opportunity for biopsy and endoscopic mucosal resection for biopsy.[28] Endoscopic ultrasound will identify the involvement of regional lymph nodes and adjacent structures. Other ancillary tests include computed tomography, CT scan, positron emission tomography, PET scan, and magnetic resonance imaging, MRI, which provide additional anatomic characterization, lymph node involvement, and distant spread of the disease. Minimally invasive techniques, such as bronchoscopy, thoracoscopy, mediastinoscopy, and laparoscopy provide means to biopsy local nodes and aid in staging.

Staging is essential in characterizing the patient's disease and in dictating its treatment strategy (Table 1). Chest X-ray, CT scan, and PET scan may be utilized initially to evaluate for lymph node involvement, invasion into adjacent structures, and distal metastasis. Endoscopic ultrasound, thoracoscopy, and laparoscopy provide additional information on lymph node involvement and supplement the staging process. Through these treatment modalities, important prognostic factors are identified, including lymph node metastasis and esophageal wall penetration. Metastasis of five or less lymph nodes indicate a more favorable prognosis.[27]

Table 1a: AJCC Prognostic Stage Groups for Squamous Cell Carcinoma

Clinical Staging (cTNM)			
	cTumor	cNode	Metastasis
Stage 0	Tumor is	Node 0	Metastasis 0
Stage I	Tumor 1	Node 0 to 1	Metastasis 0
Stage II	Tumor 2	Node 0 to 1	Metastasis 0
	Tumor 3	Node 0	Metastasis 0
Stage III	Tumor 3	Node 1	Metastasis 0
	Tumor 1 to 3	Node 2	Metastasis 0
Stage IVA	Tumor 4	Node 0 to 2	Metastasis 0
	Tumor 1 to 4	Node 3	Metastasis 0
Stave IVB	Tumor 1 to 4	Node 1 to 3	Metastasis 1

Table 1b: Pathological TNM

Pathological (pTNM)					
	pTumor	pNode	Metastasis	Grade	Location
Stage 0	Tumor is	Node 0	Metastasis 0	Not Applicable	Anywhere
Stage 1A	Tumor 1a	Node 0	Metastasis 0	G1	Anywhere
	Tumor 1a	Node 0	Metastasis 0	GX	Anywhere
Stage 1B	Tumor 1a	Node 0	Metastasis 0	G2 to G3	Anywhere
	Tumor 1b	Node 0	Metastasis 0	G1 to G3	Anywhere
	Tumor 1b	Node 0	Metastasis 0	GX	Anywhere
	Tumor 2	Node 0	Metastasis 0	G1	Anywhere
Stage IIA	Tumor 2	Node 0	Metastasis 0	G2 to G3	Anywhere
	Tumor 2	Node 0	Metastasis 0	GX	Anywhere
	Tumor 3	Node 0	Metastasis 0	G1 to G3	Lower
	Tumor 3	Node 0	Metastasis 0	G1	Upper or Middle
Stage IIB	Tumor 3	Node 0	Metastasis 0	G2 to G3	Upper or Middle
	Tumor 3	Node 0	Metastasis 0	GX	Lower or Upper or Middle
	Tumor 3	Node 0	Metastasis 0	Any Grade	Location X
	Tumor 1	Node 1	Metastasis 0	Any Grade	Anywhere
Stage IIIA	Tumor 1	Node 2	Metastasis 0	Any Grade	Anywhere
	Tumor 2	Node 1	Metastasis 0	Any Grade	Anywhere
Stage IIIB	Tumor 2	Node 2	Metastasis 0	Any Grade	Anywhere
	Tumor 3	Node 1 to 2	Metastasis 0	Any Grade	Anywhere
	Tumor 4a	Node 0 to 1	Metastasis 0	Any Grade	Anywhere
Stage IVA	Tumor 4a	Node 2	Metastasis 0	Any Grade	Anywhere
	Tumor 4b	Node 0 to 2	Metastasis 0	Any Grade	Anywhere
	Tumor 1a to 4b	Node 3	Metastasis 0	Any Grade	Anywhere

Table 1c: Post Neoadjuvant Therapy (ypTNM)

Post Neoadjuvant Therapy (ypTNM)			
	ypT	ypN	Metastasis
Stage I	Tumor 0 to 2	Node 0	Metastasis 0
Stage II	Tumor 3	Node 0	Metastasis 0
Stage IIIA	Tumor 0 to 2	Node 1	Metastasis 0
Stage IIIB	Tumor 3	Node 1	Metastasis 0
	Tumor 0 to 3	Node 2	Metastasis 0
	Tumor 4a	Node 0	Metastasis 0
Stave IVA	Tumor 4a	Node 1 to 2	Metastasis 0
	Tumor 4a	Node X	Metastasis 0
	Tumor 4b	Node 0 to 2	Metastasis 0
	Tumor 0 to 4b	Node 3	Metastasis 0
Stage IVB	Tumor 0 to 4b	Node 0 to 3	Metastasis 1

The treatment of esophageal carcinoma begins by determining the type of surgical resection. The stage and location of the tumor in addition to the patient's overall health are evaluated to determine whether the carcinoma is amenable to curative or palliative treatment. Palliative treatment is appropriate when the patient is too debilitated to undergo surgery or has a tumor that is unresectable, and when there is recurrence of resected or irradiated tumor, and/or metastases. Options for palliation include esophageal dilatation/stenting, radiation, photodynamic therapy, and laser ablation. Cervical tumors represent about 8% of esophageal carcinomas and are generally unresectable secondary to their rapid regional spread.[27] Esophagolaryngectomy may be employed but is met with a multitude of complications. Chemotherapy and radiation are the most effective treatment strategy for cervical tumors.[27]

If there is no metastatic disease, patients with resectable tumors can undergo an esophagectomy. A gastric pull-up is the preferred technique for reconstruction unless precluded by extensive tumor involvement or poor anatomy or blood supply. Four different esophagectomies have been described:

enbloc, transhiatal, transthoracic and video-assisted.[19] Enbloc esophagectomy entails complete resection of the thoracic esophagus with a two- or three-field lymph node dissection, using a midline laparotomy, right thoracotomy and a cervical incision for the proximal anastomosis of the stomach to the cervical esophageal remnant. Transhiatal esophagectomy requires a cervical incision to mobilize the esophagus and perform the proximal anastomosis, and a midline laparotomy to mobilize the stomach and esophagus. Transthoracic esophagectomy involves a midline laparotomy for mobilization of the stomach and a right thoracotomy for proximal esophageal lesions, or a left thoracotomy for distal lesions. In the video-assisted esophagectomy technique, many approaches are employed to mobilize different areas: VATS for esophagus, and laparoscopy for the stomach, VATS to mobilize the esophagus, and a cervical incision for anastomosis of the stomach and cervical esophageal remnant. No certain technique has been shown to have a relative survival advantage. Additionally, despite improvements in surgical outcomes and increasing 5-year survival rates for esophagectomy patients, the esophageal carcinoma survival rate has not changed significantly.[19]

TRAUMA

Esophageal Perforation

Esophageal perforation is an emergency. Survival is dependent upon early identification and repair. Survival rates dramatically decrease with intervention after the initial twenty-four hours. Perforation results from a variety of causes, including iatrogenic injury, Boerhaave's syndrome, trauma, and foreign bodies. Boerhaave's syndrome is esophageal perforation resulting from vigorous vomiting (Figure 1). This recurrent forceful vomiting increases intrathoracic esophageal pressure, leading to perforation as the vomiting reflex and trigger for sphincter relaxation are disrupted.[28] The most common cause of esophageal perforation is that of iatrogenic injury, namely endoscopy and its associated procedures.

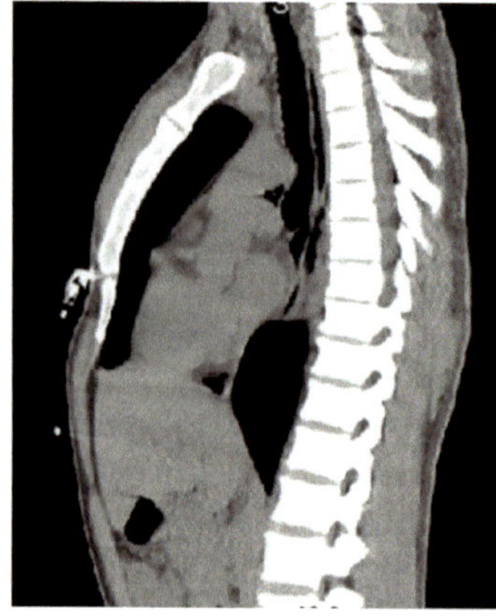

Figure 1: Pneumomediastinum secondary to esophageal perforation

Thorough symptomatology and history should be elicited when esophageal perforation is suspected. Intense and persistent pain in the neck or thorax is a common presenting symptom. Dysphagia and nausea and vomiting may be present. Shortness of breath and abdominal pain may occur from perforation in the thoracic esophagus and abdominal region, respectively. Signs initially include tachypnea, tachycardia, and fever and may progress to hemodynamic compromise and shock. Subcutaneous emphysema in areas of the cervical or thoracic esophagus strongly supports esophageal perforation. A detailed history should also be taken to identify risk factors of recent endoscopy, vomiting, foreign body ingestion, and trauma.

Diagnostic work-up mainly entails X-ray and swallow studies. Chest X-ray is the initial study and may demonstrate a hydropneumothorax. Mediastinal air and widening will present on X-ray as contamination progresses. A barium swallow then follows, eliciting a leak and extravasation of contrast. As most esophageal perforations occur on the left and superior to the gastroesophageal junction, the patient must be in the lateral decubitus position to best demonstrate the perforation.[28] Additionally, a chest CT may supplement the work-up and demonstrate free air and fluid in the mediastinum. Endoscopy may also be performed to confirm or negate a perforation, preoperatively delineate the perforation, or identify a mucosal injury.

Treatment is most successful when performed early. Primary anastomosis in the initial twenty-four hours is ideal.[27] Inflammation would be minimal at this point, allowing repair by primary anastomosis. The surgery includes dissecting away the stomach, gastroesophageal fat pad removal, and debridement and closure of the area of injury. Reinforcement of the repair may be achieved with a pleural patch or Nissen fundoplication. Otherwise, if the diagnosis and repair are after the initial twenty-four hours or if the patient is unstable, resection of the esophageal injury is necessary. The esophageal remnant is then utilized for an end cervical esophagostomy, and a drain and feeding jejunostomy are placed. After adequate time for recovery is allowed, final reconstruction of the esophagus is completed with substernal colon interposition.[27] Other conditions not amenable to primary repair and anastomosis include carcinoma, megaesophagus, caustic injury, and peptic strictures as these conditions are prone to narrowing and obstruction.[28]

The injury location dictates the surgical approach. An ipsilateral neck incision is utilized for cervical perforations. For thoracic injuries, a right thoracotomy is utilized for the proximal two-thirds of the esophagus and a left thoracotomy for the distal third.[28] A left thoracotomy or abdominal approach is utilized for abdominal esophageal injuries, depending on the degree of contamination, as more contamination necessitates an abdominal approach.

Treatment options also include non-operative management. Injuries from endoscopic dilation may be treated in this manner. Also, injuries that are contained within the mediastinum and hence result in mild symptomatology, and low concern for sepsis may be treated with conservative management of antibiotics, H2-receptor blockers, parenteral nutrition, and/or stent placement.[27] The patient is followed clinically, radiographically, and endoscopically to determine when the perforation has healed and when it is safe to resume oral feeding. Failure of conservative therapy will require surgical treatment.

Acquired Fistulas

Traumatic fistulas may be created between the trachea and bronchus, and the esophagus. Tracheoesophageal fistulas are likely to be created secondary to their close location. Esophageal fistulas may also be due to surrounding carcinoma and diverticula, and their inherent inflammation. The mechanisms of injury that create traumatic fistulas include penetrating trauma, iatrogenic means such as intubation and tracheostomy cuffs, and caustic injury.[27]

Fistulas present with readily apparent symptoms. Patients typically have recurrent coughing attacks after meals and frequent respiratory infections. Fevers and bile-stained mucous may present later with advanced disease and contamination.[28]

Diagnosis of esophageal fistulas is achieved with endoscopy, bronchoscopy, and barium swallow. These modalities delineate the anatomy, location, size, and characteristics of the fistula.

Treatment for acquired fistulas is varied and depends upon the cause of the fistula. Initially, the patient is not allowed oral intake, and receives parenteral or a source of enteral nutrition in addition to antibiotics to combat any existing pulmonary infection. A stent may also be placed for large fistulas. Next, the fistula is ablated either by surgery or endoscopy. Surgical intervention is generally required and entails dividing the fistula, resecting the injured pulmonary area, and repairing the esophagus utilizing a pleural flap.[27] Malignant fistulas are mainly treated with palliation of an endoprosthesis and rarely, diversion and feeding jejunostomy.[27]

Mallory-Weiss Syndrome

Mallory-Weiss Syndrome is when an increase in intra-abdominal pressure, most likely from forceful vomiting, results in mucosal tearing at the gastroesophageal junction, leading to upper gastrointestinal bleeding. It causes about 15% of all upper gastrointestinal bleeding, and the bleeds are generally arterial in nature.[27] Coughing, and seizures may also lead to a large enough rise in intra-abdominal pressure to create an esophageal tear. Endoscopy is utilized for diagnosis by showing bleeding longitudinal fissures in the stomach mucosa. Treatment is generally non-operative and involves blood transfusions, stomach decompression, and anti-emetics.[27] During endoscopic diagnosis, epinephrine injections may be administered to control bleeding. Rarely, surgical intervention is required and entails a laparotomy, high gastrotomy, and oversewing of the injury.[27] Prognosis is usually good as mortality and recurrence are rarely seen.

REFERENCES

1. Meyer GW, Austin RM, Brady CE, et al. Muscle anatomy of the human esophagus. J Clin Gastroenterol 1986;8:131.
2. Harrington SW. Esophageal hiatal diaphragmatic hernia. Surg Gynecol Obstet 1955;100:277.
3. Peters PM. Closure mechanisms at the cardia with special reference to the diaphragmatic oesophageal elastic ligament. Thorax 1955;10:27.
4. Bombeck CT, Dillard DH, Nyhus LM. Muscular anatomy of the gastroesophageal junction and role of phrenoesophageal ligament. Autopsy study of sphincter mechanism. Ann Surg 1966;164:643.
5. Yamada T, Alpers DH, Kaplowitz N, et al. Textbook of Gastroenterology Volume One 2003.
6. Mulholland MW, Lillemoe KD, Doherty GM, et al. Greenfield's Surgery Scientific Principles and practice Fifth Edition 2011.
7. Duranceau AC, Devroede G, LaFontaine E, et al. Esophageal motility in asymptomatic volunteers. Surg Clin North Am 1983;63:777-786.
8. Castell DO, Richter JE. The Esophagus Third Edition 1999.
9. Bloem BR, Lagaay AM, Van Beck W, et al. Prevalence of subjective dysphagia in community residents over 87. BMJ 1990;300:721.
10. Lindgren S, Janzon L. Prevalence of swallowing complaints and clinical findings among 50-70 year old men and women in an urban population. Dysphagia 1991;6:187.
11. Wilson CP. Diverticula of the pharynx. J R Coll Surg 1959;4:236.
12. Koufman JA. The otolaryngologic manifestations of gastroesophageal reflux disease (GERD): A clinical investigation of 225 patients using ambulatory 24-hour PH monitoring and an experimental investigation of the role of acid and pepsin in the development of laryngeal injury. Laryngoscope 1991;101:78.

13. Cook IJ, Blumberg P, Cash K, Jamieson GG, Shearman DJ. Structural abnormalities of the cricopharyngeus muscle in patients with pharyngeal (Zenker's) diverticulum. J Gastroenterol Hepatol 1992;7:556.
14. Greenberger NJ, Blumberg R, Burakoff R. Current Diagnosis and Treatment: Gastroenterology, Hepatology and Endoscopy Second Edition 2012;13:168.
15. Waldenstrom J, Kjellberg S. Roentgenologic diagnosis of sideropenic dysphagia (Plummer-Vinson syndrome). Acta Radiol 1939;20:618.
16. Chisolm M. The association between webs, iron, and post-cricoid carcinoma. Postgrad Med 1974;50:215.
17. Cook IJ, Wallace KL, Zagami AS, Enis JM. Mechanisms of pharyngeal dysphagia in lateral medullary syndrome (LMS). Gastroenterology 1996;110:A650.
18. Dalakas MC. Polymyositis, dermatomyositis and inclusion body myositis. N Engl J Med 1991;325:1487.
19. Townsend CM, Beauchamp RD, Evers BM, Mattox KL. Sabiston Textbook of Surgery The Biological Basis of Modern Surgical Practice 17th Edition 2004.
20. Richter JE, et al. Esophageal manometry in 95 healthy adult volunteers. Dig Dis Sci 1987:32:583.
21. Turner R, Lipshutz W, Miller W, et al. Esophageal dysfunction if collagen disease. Am J med Sci 1973;265:191.
22. Mittal RK, Lange RC, McCallum RW. Identification and mechanism of delayed esophageal acid clearance in subjects with hiatus hernia. Gastroenterology 1987;92:130.
23. Lipsy RJ, Fennerty B, Fagan TC. Clinical review of histamine-2 receptor antagonists. Arch Intern Med 1990;150:745.
24. Klinkenberg-Knol EC, Festen HPM, Meuwissen SGM. Pharmacological management of gastro-esophageal reflux disease. Drugs 1995;49:697.
25. Spechler SJ, Goyal RK. The columnar-lined esophagus, intestinal metaplasia, and Norman Barrett. Gastroenterology 1996;110:614.
26. Mulholland MW, Lillemoe KD, Doherty GM, Maier RV, Upchurch GR. *Greenfield's Surgery: Scientific Principles & Practice, Fourth Edition.* Philadelphia: Lippincott Williams & Wilkins, 2006.
27. Brunicardi F, Andersen D, Billiar T, Dunn D, Hunter J, Matthews J, Pollock R. *Schwartz's Principles of Surgery, Ninth Edition.* 2010.
28. Townsend. *Sabiston Textbook of Surgery, 19th Edition.* St Louis: W.B. Saunders, 2012.

28

CHAPTER

Stomach

Jasneet Singh Bhullar, MD
Ravi Kapadia, MD
Vijay K. Mittal, MD
Simranjit Singh, MD

NTRODUCTION

The stomach is an extraordinary organ with vital digestive, nutritional and endocrine functions. The primary function of the stomach is to store food, facilitate digestion, regulate appetite, and aid in absorption of nutrients. Stomach diseases are common. In order to provide patients with accurate diagnosis and treatment options, surgeons must be familiar and have a profound understanding of stomach anatomy, pathophysiology, benign & malignant diseases, and its implications in clinical practice.

ANATOMY

The stomach is a pear-shaped, asymmetrical, organ in the digestive tract.[1] It originates as the tubular embryonic foregut dilation during the fifth week of gestation. By the seventh week, it rotates, dilates, and descends with elongation of the greater curvature into its normal anatomic shape and position.[1] After birth, this becomes the most proximal organ of the alimentary tract. The stomach resides in the left upper quadrant of the abdomen. The majority of the amount of the anterior portion of the stomach is covered by the left lateral segment of the liver. Inferiorly, the stomach is attached to the spleen, transverse colon, and caudate lobe of the liver. The hepatogastric ligament, sometimes referred to as pars flacida or the lesser omentum, is bound to the lesser curvature. The gastrosplenic ligament attaches to the spleen to the proximal greater curvature. The cardia is the most proximal region of the stomach and is attached to the esophagus, and the lower esophageal sphincter (LES) is located just proximal to the cardia. The superior most portion of the stomach is fundus that is floppy and distensible, bounded laterally by the spleen and superiorly by the diaphragm. The angle of his is the intersection of the left side of the gastroesophageal (GE) junction. The inferior part of the fundus lies in the horizontal plane of the GE junction and serves as the transition point to the body (corpus) of the stomach. Although the parietal (oxyntic) cells are mostly in the body of the stomach, they are also present in the cardia and fundus. The body of the stomach is bounded on the right by the lesser curvature, which is relatively straight, and the more elongated portion of the greater curvature on the left. The body of the stomach ends where the lesser curvature abruptly angles to the right at the angularis incisura, marking the anatomic beginning of the antrum.

The antrum comprises nearly 30% of the distal stomach. Inferiorly, the antrum is connected to the proximal duodenum through the pylorus. The stomach is fixed at the GE junction and pylorus but is quite mobile at its large midportion.[2]

Arterial and Venous Blood Supply

The stomach is a highly vascularized organ that gets most of its blood supply from the celiac axis.[2] Four main arteries supply the stomach: the left and right gastric arteries supply the lesser curvature of the stomach, while the left and right gastroepiploic arteries form an arcade around the greater curvature of the stomach (Figure 1). The left gastric artery is the largest artery that supplies the stomach and arises directly off the celiac trunk. In 15-20% of patients, an aberrant left hepatic artery originates from the left gastric artery.[2] Rarely, is the left hepatic artery the only source of arterial supply to the liver, but inadvertent ligation may result in left sided acute hepatic ischemia.

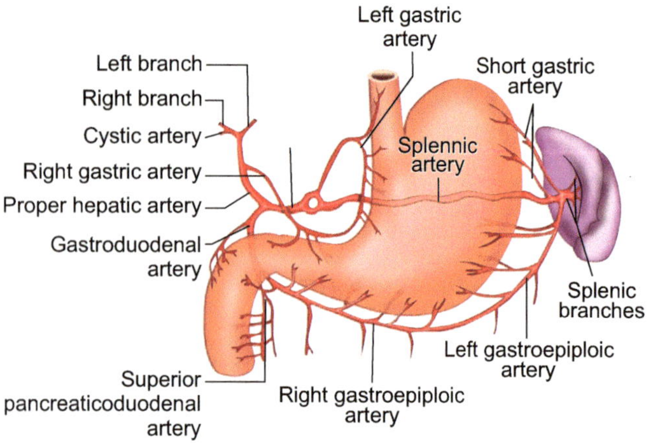

Figure 1: Arterial Blood Supply to the Stomach.

The right gastric artery arises from the hepatic artery and courses along the most inferior portion of the stomach. Behind the first portion of the duodenum, the right gastroepiploic artery arises from the gastroduodenal artery. The right gastroepiploic artery is the main supply to the gastric conduit after esophagectomy. The left gastroepiploic artery originates from the splenic artery and forms an anastomotic arcade with the right gastroepiploic artery to supply the greater curvature. The fundus receives blood from the short gastric arteries that arise as branches from the splenic artery (Figure 1).

The venous drainage of the stomach usually parallels the arteries. The left gastric (coronary vein) and right gastric veins drain into the portal vein. Occasionally, the coronary vein drains into the splenic vein.[2] The left gastroepiploic vein drains into the splenic vein, while the right gastroepiploic vein drains into the superior mesenteric vein.

Lymphatic Drainage

Generally, the lymphatics parallel the blood vessels. Four zones of lymph nodes have been identified that provide drainage.[3] The superior gastric group provides drainage for the antrum along the lesser curvature into the right suprapancreatic nodes. The pancreaticolienal nodes drain lymph high on the greater curvature into the left gastroepiploic and splenic nodes. The inferior gastric and subpyloric group of nodes drains lymph along the right gastroepiploic vessels.[3] Due to its rich lymphatic plexus, the gastric wall can have microscopic evidence of malignant cells several centimeters away from the primary tumor. This is the reason that surgeons perform an extensive lymphadenectomy for gastric cancer.

Innervation

The stomach has an extensive extrinsic and intrinsic nerve supply. As represented in Figure 2, the vagus nerve provides extrinsic parasympathetic innervation to the stomach, while the celiac plexus provides sympathetic innervation. The vagus nerve originates in the vagal nucleus, which is located in the floor of the fourth ventricle and travels via the carotid sheath to the mediastinum.[2] In the mediastinum, the recurrent laryngeal nerve originates from the vagus and divides into several branches around the esophagus. At the esophageal hiatus, these branches combine to produce the right and left vagus nerves. The left vagus nerve runs anteriorly, and the right vagus nerve runs posteriorly at the GE junction; this can be remembered using the mnemonic LARP (Left Anterior, Right Posterior).[2] The anterior branch gives off another branch that goes to the liver. It is contained in the gastrohepatic ligament and then runs along the lesser curvature of the stomach where it is called the anterior nerve of Latarjet. The nerves of Latarjet transmit segmental branches to the body of the stomach and terminate in the angularis incisura, forming the crow's feet (Figure 2). The criminal nerve of Grassi, the first branch off the posterior vagus, innervates the posterior fundus. If the nerve of Grassi is not divided, it may act as a causative factor for recurring ulcers.[2] By dividing the crow's feet to the proximal stomach and retaining innervation to the antrum and pylorus, a highly selective vagotomy can be accomplished. Truncal vagotomies are performed by ligating the vagus above the celiac and hepatic branches.

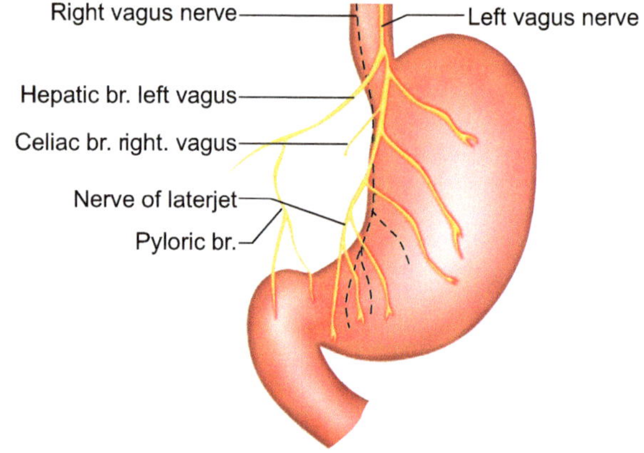

Figure 2: Innervation of the stomach.

Sympathetic nerve fibers originate at spinal levels T5–T10 and go to the celiac ganglion via the splanchnic nerves. Postganglionic fibers then move along the arterial system to innervate the stomach.

Two nerve plexuses, Auerbach and Meissner's, provide enteric or intrinsic innervation of the stomach. This region consists of a dense collection of serotoninergic, cholinergic, and peptidergic neurons. Although the exact function of these neurons remains unknown, various neuropeptides associated with these neurons have been identified.[2] They include substance P, calcitonin gene-related peptide (CGRP), bombesin, acetylcholine, serotonin, cholecystokinin (CCK) and somatostatin.

Certainly, assuming that the stomach contains exclusively parasympathetic input from the vagus and sympathetic input from the adrenergic system is an oversimplification. Acetylcholine is a vital neurotransmitter that mediates vagal function and epinephrine in sympathetics, however, some interplay between the two systems does co-exist.[2]

Histology

The gastric wall is made up of four distinct layers: serosa, muscularis propria, submucosa and mucosa.[4] The mucosa, which is the innermost layer, is lined with columnar glandular epithelial cells; the mucosa is composed of three layers: the epithelium, the lamina propria, and the muscularis mucosa. The lamina propria is a layer of connective tissue, blood vessels, nerve fibers, and inflammatory cells that lies beneath the basement membrane. Depending on their location, gastric glands are lined with different epithelial cells. Endocrine cells such as somatostatin (D) cells and gastrin (G) cells are also present in gastric glands. Mucous secreting surface epithelial cells (SECs) are present throughout the stomach, which secrete bicarbonate and form a protective barrier against injury from pepsin, acid, and ingested irritants. Except for endocrine cells, all epithelial cells in the stomach have the ability to produce bicarbonate.[4]

The glands of the stomach vary in morphology, according to location. For example, the glands in the cardia tend to be more branched with shorter pits and secrete higher concentrations of bicarbonate than acid. The glands in the fundus and body are more tubular with deeper pits. In the body of the stomach, glands are lined with mostly parietal and chief cells. In the intracellular space, parietal cells release acid, intrinsic factor, and bicarbonate. Pepsinogen is secreted by chief cells (also known as zymogenic cells) and activated at a pH of 2.5.

Gastric glands in the antrum are more branching and are more shallow, containing G cells that secrete gastrin and D cells that secrete somatostatin. Parietal cells, however, are rare in the antrum. The antrum, in general, produces more gastrin than acid, whereas the proximal stomach produces acid rather than gastrin. Parietal cells make up 13% of epithelial cells in the stomach, according to histologic studies. Chief cells account for 44%, mucous cells for 40%, and endocrine cells about 3%.[4]

Blood arteries, lymphatics, nerve fibers, inflammatory cells, and Meissner's submucosal plexus are all abundant in the submucosa of the stomach. The submucosa and the mucosa give the stomach its characteristic grossly appearing rugal folds.[4]

Beneath the submucosa lies the muscularis propria also called the muscularis externa. It is composed of two muscular layers, an inner oblique layer, a complete middle circular layer and a complete outer longitudinal layer. This layer contains a rich collection of nerves and autonomic ganglia, which also comprises Auerbach's myenteric plexus. This layer also contains the interstitial cells of Cajal (ICC).[4]

The outermost layer, the serosa is also referred to as the visceral peritoneum. This layer provides significant tensile strength, particularly for anastomoses.[4] Microscopic or gross peritoneal metastases are common when tumors that originate in the mucosa penetrate and breach the serosa, presumably due to shedding of tumor cells that only occurs due to the penetration of the serosa. Thus, the serosa might be thought of as the stomach's outer envelope. Microscopic and gross metastases from primary tumors into the stomach are common as a result of penetrating the mucosa and serosa. This would not have occurred in the absence of a penetration of the serosa. In this regard, the serosa can be viewed as an exterior layer that acts as a barrier against tumor infiltration.[4]

PHYSIOLOGY

General Considerations

The stomach's primary function is twofold: it acts as a storage vessel for food, and it assists the small intestine in digestion and nutrient absorption. The stomach's function is influenced by a variety of neurological and hormonal mediators. Acid production is specific to the stomach and is a central component of the stomach's function during the digestion process.

A phenomenon known as receptive relaxation allows the stomach to function as a storage compartment. The proximal region of the stomach relaxes in anticipation of food during normal oral intake.[5] As a result, liquids move from the stomach and into the small intestine with ease. Solid components settle along the greater curvature of the fundus until they are tiny enough to be released into the small intestine by coordinated antrum propulsions. While the food bolus is being stored in the stomach, it is bathed in acid, which aids in its digestion. Ulceration is prevented by an intact defense mechanism against mucosal damage caused by the stomach›s acidic fluids.[5]

Acid Secretion

Food consumption acts as a stimulant for acid secretion. The stomach's response to food is categorized into three phases: cephalic, gastric, and intestinal.[5] The cephalic phase of digestion begins at the thought, sight, smell, or taste of food. This activates a neurohormonal signal via the vagus nerve. Enter-Chromoffim Like (ECL) cell ECL and parietal cells. This phase is often referred to as the vagal phase and accounts for nearly 30% of total meal stimulated acid secretion.[5]

When food enters the stomach, the gastric phase of acid secretion begins and terminates when the stomach is empty. It accounts for nearly 60% of meal stimulated acid secretion.[5] Gastric distention serves as an additional signal for acid secretion via a vasovagal reflex. Acetylcholine stimulates the production of gastrin, which then stimulates the release of histamine from ECL cells. It can be said that acetylcholine coupled with the actions of gastrin and histamine potentiate the effects of the parietal cell's acid secretion capability.

The exact mechanism of the intestinal phase is not completely understood. This phase begins with food entering the small intestine from the stomach and remains active until nutrients remain in the proximal small bowel.[5]

Gastric Peptides

Gastrin

The G cells located in the antrum of the stomach produce gastrin. It is secreted as a propeptide that undergoes cleavage to its active form. Lab studies have isolated various molecular forms of gastrin, such as big gastrin which consists of 34 amino acids (G-34), little gastrin (G-17) and mini gastrin (G-14). A majority of the gastrin produced by the antrum is secreted with the 17 amino acid sequence, or G-17.[6]

Gastrin has a fundamental role in regulating the gastric phase of acid release in response to food.[7] Its secretion is stimulated by histamine; therefore, it makes sense that H2-antagonists serve as potent inhibitors of acid secretion. Gastrin also exerts a significant trophic impact on parietal and ECL cells. This is why prolonged hypergastrinemia caused by pernicious anemia or long-term use of acid suppressants is related to mucosal hyperplasia and increased ECL cell numbers.

Somatostatin

Somatostatin is synthesized by D cells in the body and antrum and is present as a 14- or 28-amino acid peptide; the main form in humans is the 14-peptide sequence, somatostatin-14. Its effect is mediated in a paracrine fashion; the secretion is stimulated by acidification of the antrum. In addition to inhibiting acid secretion from the parietal cells and gastrin release from the G cells, somatostatin also has a role in reducing histamine release from the ECL cells.[7]

Gastrin-Releasing Peptide

Gastrin releasing peptide (GRP) is the mammalian analogue of bombesin, which was identified in 1970 in an extract of the amphibian Bombinabombina's skin.[8] By attaching to receptors on G and D cells in the antrum, GRP induces the release of gastrin and somatostatin. Immunohistochemistry staining for GRP is abundant in nerves terminating in the body and antrum of the stomach. Additionally, it is prevalent in the circular muscle layer.

Animal studies have demonstrated that peripheral administration of GRP increases acid secretion but decreases acid secretion when given centrally in the ventricles. This inhibitory pathway is unaffected after vagotomy and does not seem to be due to humoral factors, but rather due to a pathway mediated by the sympathetic nervous system.

Leptin

Leptin is a polypeptide synthesized in adipocytes and chief cells in the stomach. In animal studies, leptin has demonstrated decreased food intake.[8] It functions as a satiety signal hormone and is thought to function via a vagal mediated pathway.

Ghrelin

Ghrelin, discovered in 1999, is a short peptide generated by the endocrine cells of the stomach's oxyntic mucosa.[8] Ghrelin has a strong growth hormone releasing action via activation of growth hormone receptor type 1a.[8] Exogenous administration of ghrelin in humans demonstrates a dose-dependent release of growth hormone. In addition, exogenous administration also triggers release of prolactin, ACTH, cortisol and aldosterone. Recent studies have also demonstrated a potential role of ghrelin regulating glycemic control, after decreased levels of insulin were noted following exogenous ghrelin administration.[9]

In humans, ghrelin administration enhances appetite, leading to increased food intake. Plasma ghrelin levels are often reduced in patients who have undergone gastric bypass or sleeve gastrectomy. Appetite control is a complex mediated function, with distinct overlapping orexigenic and anorexigenic signals. This indicates that ghrelin could be critical in the treatment and prevention of obesity.[9]

Gastric Motility

The stomach plays a critical role in digestion and serves as a significant processing center of ingested food and delivery of chyme to the duodenum. Gastric motility is a complex process with an extensive integration of neural and hormonal inputs. Gastric motility disorders can present with a wide variety of symptoms ranging from minor discomfort to debilitating and potentially fatal symptoms. Symptomatic patients are managed conservatively, and surgery is reserved for those whose symptomatology is severe and medically refractory. Surgeons who operate in the foregut must be aware of current diagnostic and therapeutic approaches for abnormalities of gastric motility.

Normal Gastric Motility

The activity of the smooth muscle of the stomach is regulated by myogenic, neuronal, and hormonal factors. The intrinsic myogenic contraction is the underlying mechanism of stomach motility, which occurs independently of external inputs. The intrinsic myenteric plexus regulates the nervous system, with extrinsic vagal and splanchnic input. The *interstitial cells of Cajal (ICC)* are specialized cells found in the muscularis propria, which serve as a modulator of motility.[10] Gastric peristalsis occurs in the distal stomach and is governed by a slow wave, which is a depolarization of the smooth muscle cell membrane at a rate of 3 cycles per minute. The ICC regulates the speed of these slow waves.

Fasting Gastric Motility

During fasting, the stomach's electrical activity follows a cyclical pattern composed of electrical spikes and slow waves, known as the myoelectric migrating complex (MMC).[10] The proximal stomach contracts tonically, whereas the gastric slow wave controls the distal stomach's coordinated peristalsis. The MMC is approximately 90-120 minutes in duration with four unique phases.

Phase I is the quiescent phase lasting between 40-60 minutes. Slow waves exist without action potentials; therefore, an increase in gastric tone is seen without gastric contractions. Phase II is characterized by a progressive, irregular increase in the size of the peristaltic wave over a course of 30 to 50 minutes. Regular contractions with a large amplitude occur at a rate of 3 cycles per minute during phase III. During this phase the stomach clears the maximal food content. The pylorus remains open during this phase to allow for complete emptying. Phase IV is defined by a brief period of recovery followed by a return to baseline before the following MMC cycle.

Postprandial Gastric Motility

The MMC gives way to the fed state of stomach muscle activity five to ten minutes after food administration. The proximal stomach expands to accommodate a meal's contents and to enable the mixing of gastric contents with pepsin and hydrochloric acid to commence digestion.[11] Receptive relaxation of the proximal stomach occurs in response to swallowing and expansion of the proximal stomach, termed gastric accommodation. These processes occur by stimulatory vagal input and by intrinsic and vasovagal reflexes in response to stretch. The rate of gastric motility and emptying can be influenced by systemic factors such as fear, anxiety, depression, and exercise.

Generally speaking, liquids empty faster than solids. Liquids at ambient temperatures have a tendency to empty at a faster rate than those at extreme temperatures (hot or cold). The enteric nervous system regulates these responses.

In the proximal small bowel, osmoreceptors and pH-sensitive receptors exhibit negative feedback on gastric emptying.[11] CCK, vasoactive intestinal peptide, glucagon, and gastric inhibitory peptide are said to exhibit an inhibitory role in gastric emptying.

Gastric Motility Disorders

Nausea, fullness, early satiety, stomach pain, and discomfort are all symptoms of abnormal gastric motility. In clinical practice, the most often seen gastric motility disorders are dysmotility following vagotomy, delayed gastric emptying due to uncontrolled diabetes mellitus, and dysmotility secondary to H. Pylori infection. Vagotomy results in loss of receptive relaxation and gastric accommodation, resulting in early satiety, postprandial bloating, and accelerated emptying of solids.[12] Diabetic gastropathy can occur in diabetes mellitus that is insulin dependent or insulin independent, and its clinical presentation resembles that of post-vagotomy gastroparesis. Hyperglycemia impairs the antrum's contractility, increases pyloric contraction, and inhibits the MMC's phase III activity.[12] *H. pylori* infection has been shown to impair gastric emptying due to a reduction in gastric compliance.

Treatment for gastroparesis involves prokinetic agents such as metoclopramide and erythromycin. Surgical management is indicated for patients who are refractory to medical management. Multiple options are available, ranging from percutaneous gastrostomy to near complete gastrectomy. Unfortunately, these therapies provide minimal symptomatic improvement and are linked with a high rate of recurrence and morbidity.[13]

Gastric Emptying Studies

The complex symptoms of delayed gastric emptying (DGE) require confirmatory imaging to establish a definitive diagnosis. The gold standard test for diagnosis is a 4-hour radionucleotide colloid scintigraphy gastric emptying study (GES).[14] The test is conducted with the aid of a radiolabeled liquid or meal. It is preferable to utilize an isotope labeled as a low-fat meal because liquid-based scans may be normal in advanced diseases. The diagnosis of DGE is confirmed if there is greater than 60% retention at 2 hours, or greater than 10% retention at 4 hours.[15]

Any diagnosis suggestive of gastric outlet obstruction should be ruled out with an endoscopic evaluation. Retained stomach contents, particularly phyto-bezoars, suggest a significant likelihood of DGE. Upper GI barium series can help rule out mechanical obstruction. However, there are some limitations for this test in terms of successfully diagnosing DGE. Rarely, a diagnostic laparotomy may be required to differentiate between a partial distal small bowel obstruction and a small bowel pseudo-obstruction with DGE in order to diagnose the condition.

PEPTIC ULCER DISEASE

Peptic ulcer disease (PUD) continues to be one of the most common disorders, with an annual incidence of 1.8% or approximately 500,000 cases per year.[16] The rate for elective admissions and surgery has steadily decreased over the last three decades. Approximately 3-4 million patients seek medical care by a physician for the purposes of diagnosing and treating PUD annually. Interestingly, the rate of hospitalization for duodenal ulcers has dropped, whereas the rate for gastric ulcers has remained consistent. While this decrease in hospitalization for duodenal ulcers may reflect a true decrease in incidence, it is more likely the result of a decrease in elective admissions.

Stomach ulcers, on the other hand, are more common in older individuals, and hospitalizations for bleeding gastric ulcers have grown over the past several years. Hemorrhage associated with gastric ulcers tends to be secondary to NSAID use.

The discovery of *H. pylori* has revolutionized our understanding of PUD and convinced many clinicians that PUD is an infectious condition. Human gastric bacteria were found in the early 1900's, and urease was believed to have a protective function in the 1920's. It was not until the 1970's that it was discovered that gastric bacteria were connected with inflammation. In 1982, Marshall and Warren successfully cultured the organism and named it Campylobacter pyloridis. It was discovered in 1987 that eradicating the organism reduced duodenal ulcer recurrence. In 1989, the pathogen was reclassified as *H. pylori*, and the National Institutes of Health (NIH) published guidelines for the care of *H. pylori*-associated peptic ulcer disease.[16] Due to its strong association with PUD, physicians must take *H. pylori* into account when discussing medical and surgical treatment options.

Pathogenesis of Peptic Ulcer Disease

Helioobaoter pylori Infection

The pathophysiology of peptic ulcer disease is due to an imbalance between the antagonistic forces of pepsin and gastric acid and the mucosal defense mechanism of the stomach and duodenum. Nearly 90% of duodenal ulcers and 75% of gastric ulcers are currently believed to be caused by *H. pylori*. Ulcer recurrence is extremely rare once H. Pylori is eradicated.[17]

H. pylori is a helical gram-negative rod that resides in gastric type epithelium beneath the mucus layer, making it resistant to antibiotics and acid. It is a potent producer of urease, which splits urea into ammonia and bicarbonate. *H. pylori* is microaerophilic, preferring temperatures between 35 and 37 degrees centigrade for isolation. Interestingly, *H. pylori* can only survive in the stomach epithelium because it expresses unique adherence receptors in vivo that the organism can recognize. It is, however, also present in heterotopic gastric mucosa.

Patients with active *H. pylori* infections have significantly increased levels of basal and stimulated gastrin levels. This is thought to be due to a reduction in antral D cells.

Additionally, peptic ulcers are significantly linked to gastritis of the antrum. A number of studies performed prior to the discovery of *H. pylori* indicated that patients with PUD had histological evidence of antral gastritis. This is because H. pylori has an inhibiting effect on the somatostatin secreting D cells, which inhibit antral gastrin production. Acid hypersecretion and antral gastritis can lead to antral metaplasia of the duodenum, which allows for *H. pylori* colonization.

There is overwhelming evidence that *H. pylori* plays a critical role in the pathogenesis of PUD. Patients with *H. pylori* infection and antral gastritis are 3 times more likely to develop PUD than patients without *H. pylori* infection. Additional factors contributing to the causation of PUD must be considered when a patient is evaluated, because not every case of PUD is due to *H. pylori*. Interestingly, only 10-15% of patients with *H. pylori* colonization will develop PUD during their life. Notably, *H. pylori* is also associated with gastric cancer and lymphoma.[18]

Nonsteroidal Anti-Inflammatory Drugs

Ingestion of NSAIDs is the most common cause of PUD after *H. pylori* infection. Peptic ulcers occur at a rate of 15-20% per year in patients with rheumatoid arthritis and osteoarthritis who take NSAIDs, and at a rate of 25% in chronic NSAID users.[19] Hemorrhage and perforation of peptic ulcers is much more common in patients taking NSAIDs. Unfortunately, many patients are asymptomatic until unforeseen complications of PUD occur. In the United States, over 20 million individuals take NSAIDs on a regular basis.[19] Consequently, this subset of patients has a higher hospitalization rate for GI complications than those who do not take NSAIDs. Age >60 years, a prior

GI incident, a high NSAID dose, concurrent steroid use, and systemic anticoagulation all predispose patients to NSAID-induced GI complications.

Duodenal Ulcers

Duodenal ulcers are due to multiple etiologies. There is a substantial association between the number of parietal cells and Monoamine Oxidase (MAO), and patients with duodenal ulcers have an increase in parietal cell number.

The presentation of patients with duodenal ulcers is variable. The most common symptom is well-localized mid-epigastric abdominal pain, which is relieved with food. The pain is usually episodic but may also be seasonal and aggravated during times of stress. For these reasons, many people wait years before seeking medical attention. Referred pain to the back indicates penetration to the pancreas, and generalized peritoneal irritation suggests perforation.

Approximately in 5% of cases, peritonitis occurs when an ulcer penetrates the duodenum and enters the peritoneal cavity.[20] In the event of perforation, the patient is usually able to recollect the precise time of onset of abdominal pain. It is usually accompanied by tachycardia, fever, dehydration and ileus. On physical examination the patient will be exquisitely tender, with distention and rebound tenderness. A hallmark sign of perforation will be free air under the diaphragm on an upright acute abdominal radiograph (Figure 3). This represents a surgical emergency, and the patient must be taken to the operating room for repair of the perforation with adequate fluid resuscitation.

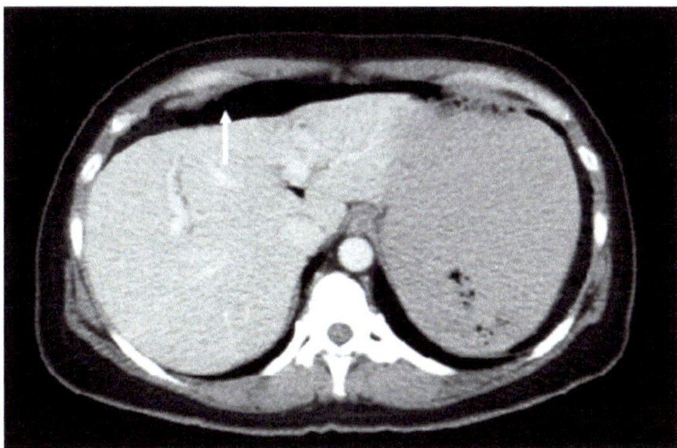

Figure 3: Free air on axial CT scan (red arrow) with perforated peptic ulcer.

The leading cause of death among patients with PUD is hemorrhage. The gastroduodenal artery lies posterior to the duodenal bulb, and most cases of massive hemorrhage are due to ulcer penetration of the gastroduodenal artery. Fortunately, most duodenal ulcers are superficial, and not adjacent to the gastroduodenal artery. Bleeding duodenal ulcers account for 25% of upper GI bleeding.[21]

Gastric Ulcers

Gastric ulcers present a difficulty because they are frequently difficult to differentiate from gastric carcinoma. Patients complain of recurrent cycles of latency and pain. Hemorrhage occurs approximately 35-40% of the time and is more common with type II and type III ulcers (Figure 4).[22] Bleeding is more prevalent in the elderly and is less likely to tamponade.

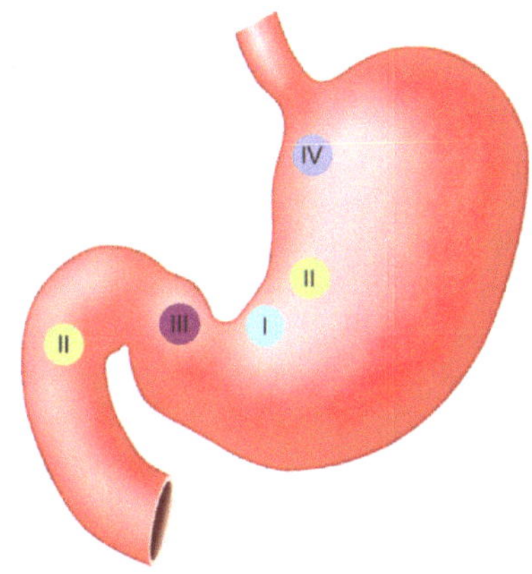

Figure 4: Gastric ulcers according to the modified Johnson classification. Type I: lesser curvature, incisura. Type II: body of stomach, incisura, duodenal ulcer. Type III: prepyloric. Type IV: proximal lesser curvature near GE junction.

The most frequent complication however is perforation, which commonly occurs alongside the lesser curvature's anterior aspect. Older patients have an increased rate of perforation. In addition, larger ulcers carry a significantly higher morbidity and mortality.

Diagnostic Workup

The workup for a patient with suspected PUD includes routine laboratory testing such as a CBC, liver function panel, and serum calcium and creatinine levels (Figure 5). Serum gastrin levels should be determined in patients who are unresponsive to medical therapy or those requiring surgery. To rule out perforation, an upright abdominal radiograph should be taken. The definitive diagnosis of PUD is made through an upper GI endoscopy and/or radiography. Endoscopy affords the ability to take direct biopsies and brushings of suspicious lesions. The probability of diagnosing a malignancy is greater than 90%.

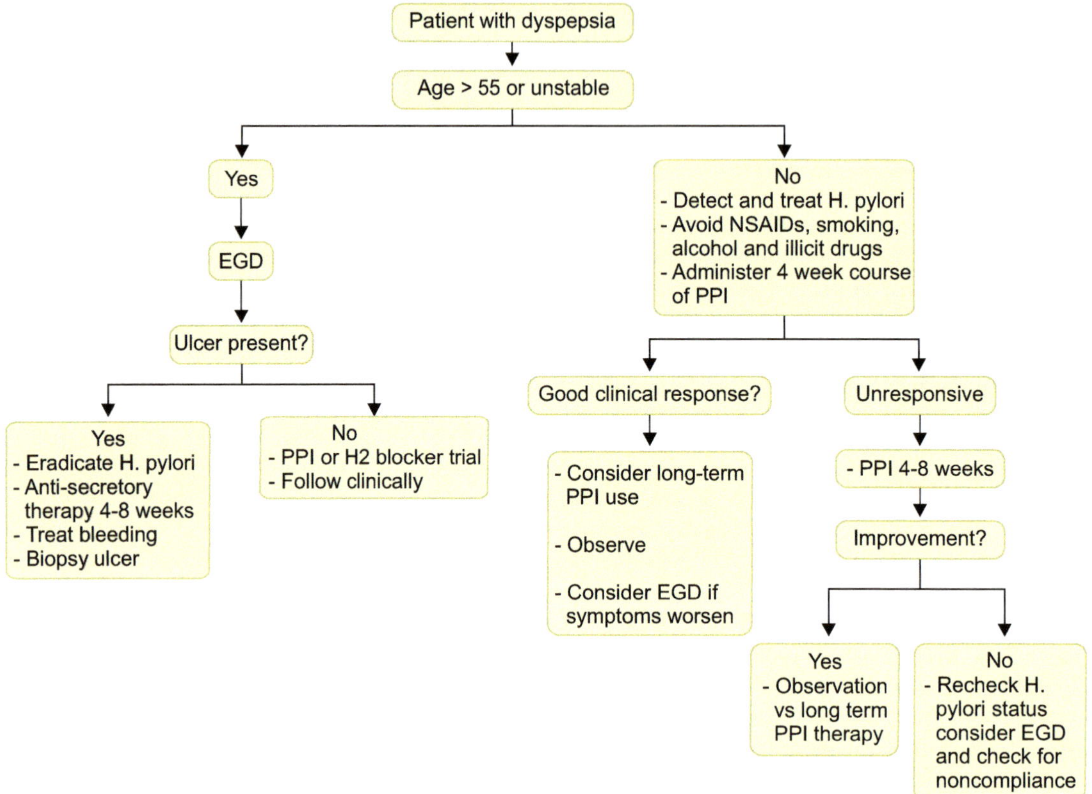

Figure 5: Management algorithm for patients with suspected peptic ulcer disease.

Contrast upper GI radiographs are more cost effective, less invasive and have a 90% diagnostic accuracy. Single contrast radiographs can miss up to 50% of duodenal ulcers. On the other hand, double contrast radiographs can detect between 80-90% ulcer craters (Figure 6). However, a skilled radiologist is required to detect ulcers on radiographs. It is imperative that all patients with symptoms suspicious of PUD be tested for *H. pylori*.

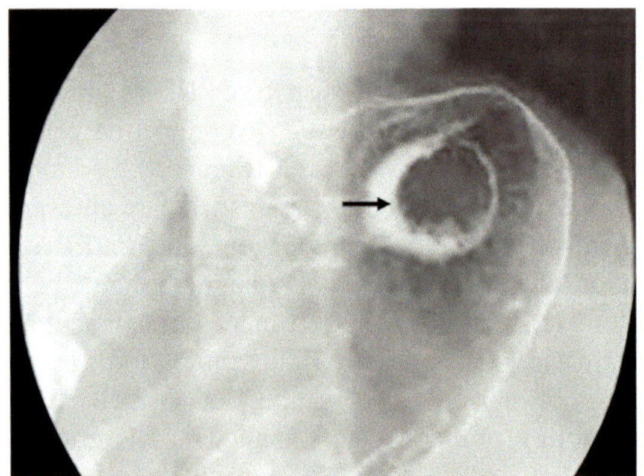

Figure 6: Double contrast conventional barium study demonstrating a focal projecting mass along the gastric fundus.

H. pylori testing

Serological testing (ELISA) is the preferred diagnostic test when endoscopy is not recommended. Serology testing for *H. pylori* has a sensitivity and specificity of 90%.[22] However, antibody titers can remain increased for more than a year. Therefore, serology is not the best test to confirm eradication after treatment.

The urease breath test is another diagnostic tool that is based on *H. pylori's* capacity to hydrolyze urea. It has a greater than 95% sensitivity and specificity.[22] The patient is given a carbon isotope along with radiolabeled urea for this test. If *H. pylori* is present, urea will be converted to ammonia and bicarbonate following consumption of the isotope. The radiolabeled bicarbonate will be expelled as labeled carbon dioxide in the breath. The urea breath test is cost effective and is the best method to confirm eradication after treatment.

If endoscopy must be performed, a rapid urease breath test may be employed, which is based on *H. pylori's* ability to hydrolyze urea. During the procedure the gastric mucosa is biopsied, and samples are placed in a urea-containing medium. Specificity is 98% and sensitivity is 90%. Within hours, results are available.

Treatment

Antacids used to be the most common treatment of PUD. Antacids exert their effect by reducing gastric acidity and inhibiting the actions of pepsin and hydrochloric acid on the mucosal lining of the stomach. Their optimal benefits are achieved if ingested one hour following a meal. When consumed on an empty stomach, they have a transient buffering effect and are emptied from the stomach more rapidly. Magnesium based antacids provide the best buffering action but also acts as a cathartic causing a significant amount of diarrhea.

H2 receptor antagonists share structural similarities to histamine. The liver metabolizes and the kidney excretes all H2 blockers. Famotidine is the most effective H2 blocker, whereas cimetidine is the least effective. Continuous infusions are more efficacious at acid reduction than intermittent infusions.

Proton pump inhibitors (PPIs) exert their effect by forming a covalent connection with the proton pump's alpha subunit and inhibiting acid secretion. Proton pump inhibitors provide better acid inhibition than H2 blockers. PPIs have an 85% healing rate after four weeks and a 96% healing rate after eight weeks.[23] For PPIs to become active and bind to the proton pump, an acidic environment is required.

Sucralfate is a sulfated sucrose aluminum salt that is structurally similar to heparin but has no anticoagulation effects. Studies have proven sucralfate to be effective in treating peptic ulcer disease. 1 gram 4 times daily is comparable to H2-receptor blockers and is superior to placebo.

For *H. pylori*, multiple triple therapy treatment options exist. Treatment involves a PPI with antibiotics such as metronidazole, clarithromycin, or amoxicillin. It involves a two-week course, with the advantage of not taking bismuth with twice daily dosing. Eradication rate with triple therapy is 90%[23] thereby decreasing recurrence rates of both duodenal and gastric ulcers. In patients resistant to metronidazole, quadruple therapy with bismuth is recommended.

Surgical Treatment Options

Despite advances in non-operative management, and newer therapies for *H. pylori* eradication, surgery remains important in the management for some patients. The primary goal of surgery for bleeding peptic ulcers is to control and minimize blood loss. The preferred operation well depends on the ulcer's location.

Bleeding Gastric Ulcers

Bleeding gastric ulcers are best treated by excising the ulcer and repairing the defect. Ulcers should be sent for biopsy, as nearly 5% of grossly benign appearing ulcers are malignant.[24] Ulcers located along the greater curvature of the stomach, antrum or body is best treated with a wedge excision and defect closure. Distally located ulcers along the lesser curvature around incisura are best treated with a distal gastrectomy and Billroth I type anastomosis (Figure 7).

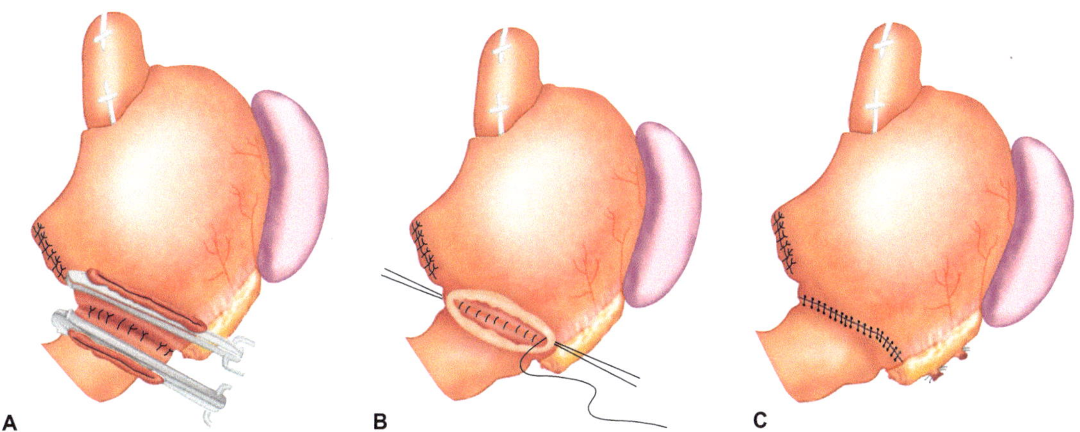

Figure 7: Billroth I Gastroduodenostomy

Type I gastric ulcers (Figure 4) are best treated with distal gastrectomy with Billroth I anastomosis. Vagotomy is not necessary for Type I gastric ulcers. There is always a concern of malignancy in patients presenting with non-healing gastric ulcers without *H. pylori* infection. If malignancy is discovered, treatment consists of either a subtotal gastrectomy with a Billroth II anastomosis (Figure 8) or a Roux-en-Y gastrojejunostomy (Figure 9).

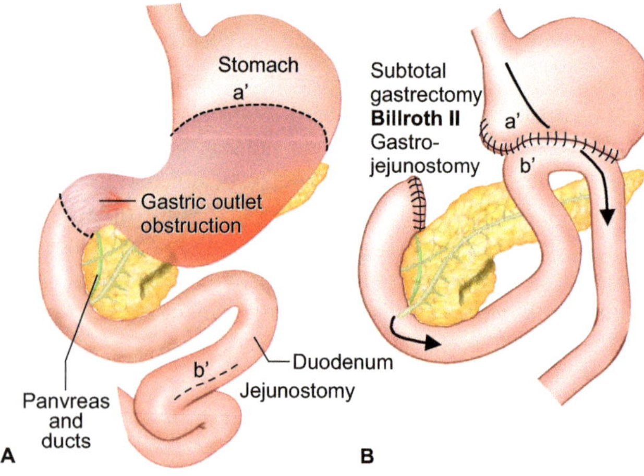

Figure 8: Billroth II Gastrojejunostomy

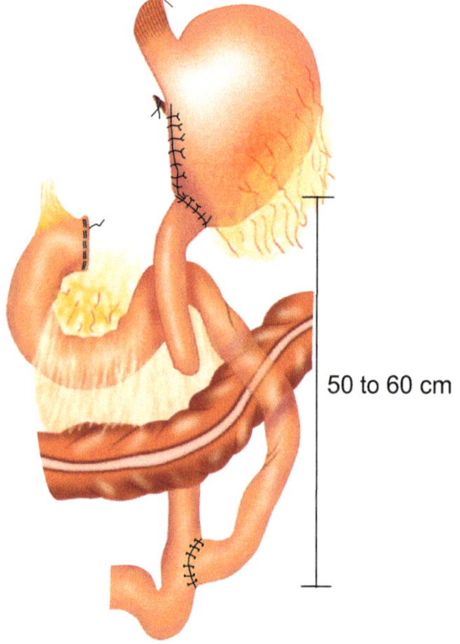

Figure 9: Roux-en-Y Gastrojejunostomy

For Type II gastric ulcers (Figure 4), a distal gastrectomy with truncal vagotomy should be performed once the ulcer has healed sufficiently and the *H. pylori* infection has been cleared. Studies have revealed that individuals getting highly selective vagotomy for Type II or III gastric ulcers had poorer outcomes.

Type IV gastric ulcers (Figure 4) presents a challenge. Surgical treatment is determined by the size of the ulcer, its proximity to the GE junction, and the degree of surrounding inflammation. Ulcers should be excised whenever possible. The most aggressive surgical approach involves a gastrectomy followed by a Roux-en-Y esophagogastrojejunostomy. For type IV ulcers located 2-5cm from the GE junction, the Pauchet procedure should be performed. This involves a distal gastrectomy with the resection to include the lesser curvature with the ulcer. The Sendes procedure may be useful in stable patients or the Kelling-Madlener in unstable patients (Figure 10).

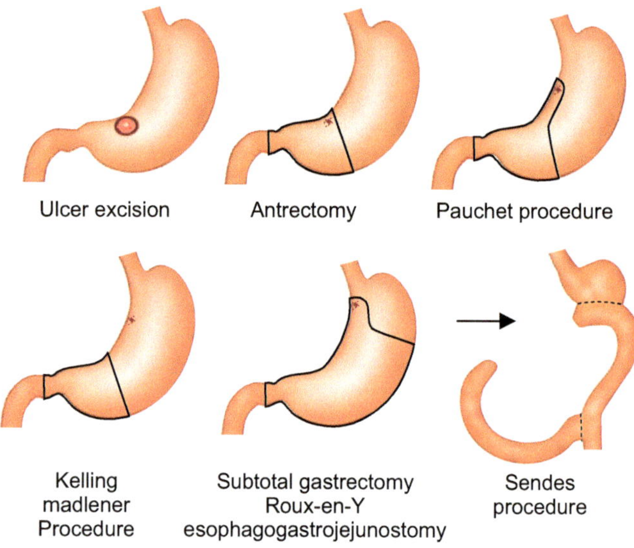

Figure 10: Operative approaches for bleeding gastric ulcers.

Bleeding Duodenal Ulcers

To treat bleeding duodenal ulcers, the standard surgical method is to conduct an anterior longitudinal duodenotomy extending across the pylorus. Bleeding vessels are ligated in the ulcer with 8 sutures at the superior and inferior portion of the ulcer crater to achieve proximal and distal control. The pylorus is repaired in a Heinke-Mikulicz fashion, closing the transverse incision vertically to maintain adequate flow through the conduit (Figure 11). A truncal vagotomy is traditionally performed to lessen the risk of recurrent ulcers. Recurrence rates after truncal vagotomy is between 0-2%.[25] However, the role of vagotomy in bleeding duodenal ulcers remains unclear. According to our current understanding, treating *H pylori* and discontinuing NSAID use should eliminate the underlying risk of ulcer development. Level I data in the literature supports that *H. pylori* eradication eliminates the need for ulcer surgery in perforated duodenal ulcers. However clinical trials with regards to bleeding duodenal ulcers do not exist. According to a survey of surgeons in the UK and US, the majority of surgeons do not conduct a vagotomy as part of an operation to treat a bleeding duodenal ulcer.

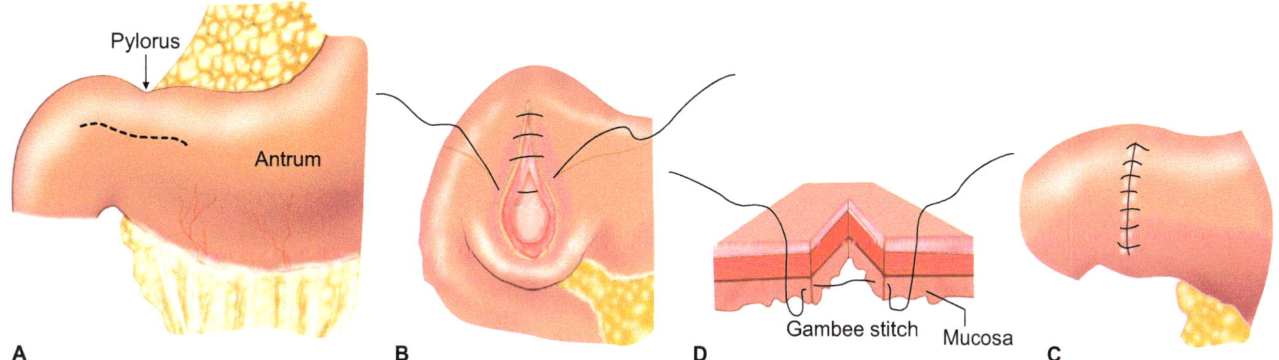

Figure 11: Heineke-Mikulicz pyloroplasty. A transverse incision is made (A) and the defect is then closed longitudinally with a Gambee stitch (C & D).

Perforated Peptic Ulcers

Simple patch closure with parietal cell vagotomy or patch closure with truncal vagotomy are surgical options for perforated duodenal ulcers. Simple patching of the perforation is recommended for patients who are hemodynamically unstable or with exudative peritonitis. Duodenal patch closure can be performed laparoscopically or open. If treated within six hours of perforation, the prognosis is excellent; however, delaying treatment beyond 12 hours is associated with increased morbidity and mortality.[26] Once again, patients should be evaluated for *H. pylori* infection with a urea breath test.

GASTRIC NEOPLASMS

Benign Tumors

Gastric Polyps

Gastric polyps are usually discovered as an incidental finding during endoscopy. Nearly 47% of gastric polyps are located in the fundus and have no malignant potential. They are usually seen as multiple sessile lesions in the body and fundus measuring between 2- to 3-mm. However, gastric polyps can occur in over 50% patients with Gardner's syndrome or familial adenomatous polyposis.[27]

Hyperplastic polyps account for almost 75% of all gastric polyps.[27] These polyps are often less than 1.5cm and are seen in conjunction with atrophic gastritis nearly 75% of the time. Chronic atrophic gastritis usually occurs as a result of *H. pylori* infection. Eradication of *H. pylori* usually results in regression of the polyp. Adenocarcinoma is detected in nearly 2% of all hyperplastic polyps.[27] Therefore, endoscopic polypectomy is indicated for all hyperplastic polyps.

Adenomatous polyps account for nearly 10% of all gastric polyps and pose a risk of malignancy.[27] These polyps are usually encountered in the antrum and are sessile solitary lesions. They can be tubular, tubular-villous or villous. Polyps greater than 4cm, as well as villous adenomas carry the highest malignant potential for gastric adenocarcinoma. Presence of gastric adenomas indicates an increased risk of developing adenocarcinoma in another area of the stomach. Treatment involves complete endoscopic polypectomy. Operative excision is indicated for sessile lesions greater than 2cm, polyps found in areas of an invasive tumor, or those that are secondary to bleeding or pain. Patients should have endoscopic surveillance since these polyps do harbor a malignant potential.

Ectopic Pancreas

The incidence of ectopic pancreatic tissue is rare, with 1-2% being found on autopsy. The stomach, duodenum, and jejunum account for over 70% of these instances.[28] The majority of people are asymptomatic, but others may exhibit symptoms consistent with PUD. Although the tumor can be observed during upper GI endoscopy, diagnosis can be challenging due to its location. Pancreatic rests that cause symptoms can be excised surgically.

Malignant Tumors

The incidence of gastric cancer has declined since the 1930's but remains the second leading cause of cancer death.[29] Gastric cancer incidence varies significantly by geographic region, with the greatest rates occurring in Japan. The lowest rates are found in North America. Gastric cancer affects more males than females. Despite the fact that gastric cancer encompasses a wide range of malignancies, adenocarcinoma is the most common form which accounts for more than 90% of all gastric malignancies.[29]

Gastric Adenocarcinoma

Gastric adenocarcinomas are histologically divided into two groups: diffuse gastric adenocarcinoma (DGCA) and intestinal gastric adenocarcinomas (IGCA). DGCA has a higher incidence in younger patients, with males and females equally affected. Peritoneal metastasis is common via direct tumor extension. Infiltrative growth into the submucosa can occur resulting in Linitis Plastica giving the stomach a thickened, leather bottle type appearance.

IGCA, on the other hand, affects older patients and is linked to environmental factors like atrophic gastritis. It spreads hematogenously, resulting in liver metastases. *H. pylori* does seem to be a risk factor associated with progression to IGCA.[30]

Nearly 1-3% of gastric cancers have a familial preponderance.[31] Hereditary diffuse gastric cancer (HDGC) is the most prevalent kind. HDGC is inherited in an autosomal dominant manner. There is no definitive age at which patients with a CDH1 gene mutation should undergo surgical resection. Total gastrectomy, however, is suggested for CDH1 mutants. For patients who elect out of prophylactic gastrectomy, annual endoscopic surveillance is suggested. A multidisciplinary team approach must be employed when dealing with young patients requiring radical operative management.

Clinical Manifestations

Most patients present with advanced disease, and their symptoms are frequently nonspecific. However, the most common symptom is weight loss secondary to loss of appetite and vague abdominal pain. The patient's symptoms can vary based on their location. Dysphagia is common in tumors involving the gastroesophageal junction. Tumors of antrum frequently produce nausea and vomiting and are associated with an increased risk of gastric outlet obstruction. Iron deficiency anemia with heme positive stools is also common. Frank hematemesis however is rare.

Diagnosis and Staging

A history and physical examination should be performed as part of the initial assessment for gastric cancer. Basic laboratory investigations include a complete blood count to assess for anemia. Certain tumor markers are associated with a poor prognosis and aggressive disease. CEA, AFP, and CA 19-9 elevations are linked with depth of tumor invasion, vascular invasion, pathologic stage, and liver and lymph node metastases.

Flexible upper endoscopy remains the diagnostic test of choice when suspecting gastric cancer. Routine screening is justified for high-risk patient groups and those residing in high incidence areas. Although double contrast barium upper GI radiography is 90% accurate in diagnosis, the inability to distinguish benign from malignant lesions makes endoscopy the preferred method.[32] Multiple biopsy samples should be obtained during endoscopy.

The computed tomography (CT) scan remains the preferred staging modality. CT scans have a sensitivity of 50–95% and a specificity of 40–99% for determining nodal status.[33] Although MRI is somewhat inferior to CT scan, it affords a higher detection of metastatic disease. The best test to assess for tumor depth is endoscopic ultrasound (EUS) to determine T staging.[34]

The AJCC TNM staging classification for gastric adenocarcinoma remains the best prognostic system. There has been extensive discussion in the literature on the number of nodes to be sampled for accurate staging. The latest edition of the AJCC staging manual, the seventh edition, recommends sampling a minimum of seven nodes.[35]

The Japanese Research Society for Gastric Cancer (JRSGC) has developed an alternative method of assessing nodal metastases. The JRSGC system categorizes and organizes lymph node basins based on the primary tumor site's location. A D1 resection removes group 1 lymph nodes, a D2 resection includes both groups 1 and 2, and a D3 resection comprises a D2 resection plus excision of the para-aortic lymph nodes.[36]

Treatment

Nearly 20-30% of gastric cancers are diagnosed at stage IV.[37] Palliative care and quality of life must be considered prior to proceeding with radical surgical intervention. Unfortunately, individuals with stage IV disease are frequently marginal surgical candidates.

However, surgical resection remains the only curative treatment for stomach cancer. The primary goal is to perform an R0 resection, removing gross and microscopic evidence of tumor. Simple gastric decompression helps patients with advanced disease relieve obstructive symptoms (Figure 12).

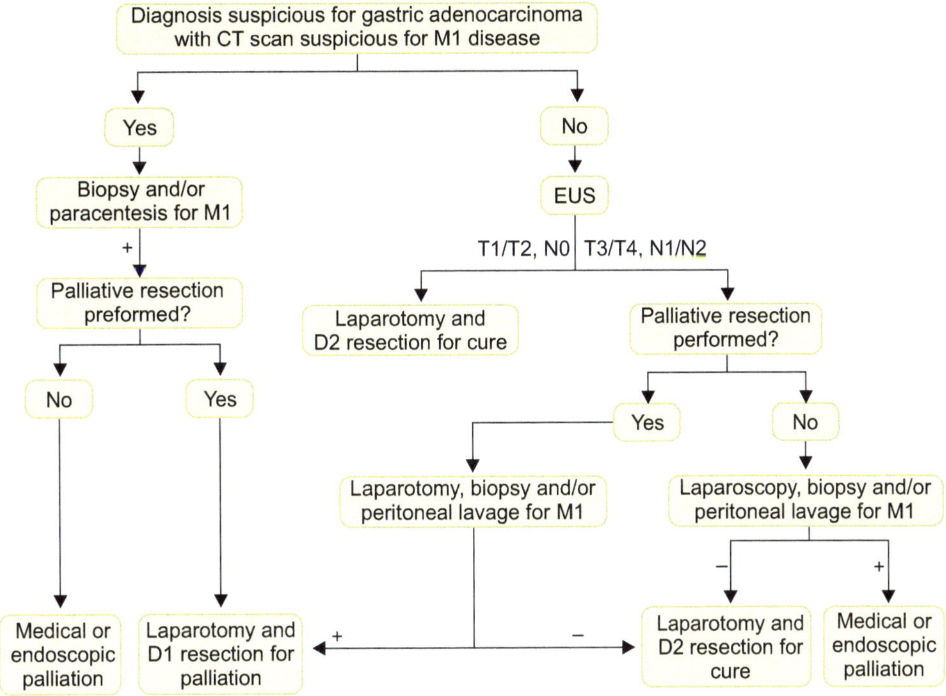

Figure 12: Management algorithm for Gastric Adenocarcinoma.

Chemotherapy and Radiation

Chemotherapy can be used to treat micro-metastatic lesions and downstage illness prior to surgical resection. Recently, MAGIC trial demonstrated improvement in disease free and overall survival in patients treated with preoperative or postoperative chemotherapy. Recently, the NCCN guidelines recommended adjuvant chemoradiation with 5-FU based regimen following complete surgical resection for patients with T3, T4 or node positive results.[38] Patients with microscopically positive resection margins should also have adjuvant therapy.

Numerous trials have been conducted to determine the efficacy of adjuvant chemotherapy alone in patients with resected cancer, with mixed findings.[38]

Gastric Lymphoma

The stomach remains the most common site of lymphomas. However, a primary lymphoma in the stomach is uncommon. Typically, patients come with vague symptoms such as epigastric pain, early satiety and fatigue, with more than half the patients present with anemia. Affected patients tend to be older, in their sixth or seventh decade of life and are more common in men than women. Majority of the tumors occur in the antrum.

It is important to determine the stage and subtype of lymphoma. Multiple classification systems exist. Diffuse large B cell lymphoma is the most prevalent kind of gastric lymphoma, followed by extranodal marginal cell lymphoma (MALToma).[39] Less common lymphomas include mantle cell lymphoma, Burkitt's lymphoma, and follicular lymphoma. *H. pylori* infection and immunodeficiencies are risk factors for primary diffuse large B cell lymphoma development.

Endoscopy typically shows ulcerations or nonspecific gastritis. Mass lesions tend to be uncommon. The use of endoscopic ultrasonography to determine the depth of stomach wall invasion is useful. All patients must be tested for *H. pylori.*

In lymphomas, the role of gastric resection is still controversial. Chemoradiation alone is now being used to treat a large number of patients. The most common chemotherapeutic regimen is CHOP (cyclophosphamide, doxorubicin, vincristine, and prednisolone).[40] Radiation therapy has limited usefulness in larger tumors.

Gastrointestinal Stromal Tumors

Epidemiology

Gastrointestinal Stromal Tumors (GISTs) are the most common gastrointestinal tract mesenchymal tumors, accounting for around 1% to 2% of all gastrointestinal malignancies.[41] They most frequently occur in the stomach and present after the fourth decade of life.[41] The mean age of presentation is 60 years old, with a little male predominance. At the time of presentation, the most common symptoms are bleeding, dyspepsia, abdominal pain, and early satiety. GISTs are usually incidental findings on radiologic imaging, endoscopy and surgery. These tumors are thought to arise from the interstitial cells of Cajal (ICC), the pacemaker cells of the stomach. More than 95% of GISTs express KIT (CD117) protein.[42] The majority are composed of spindle cells, a minority of which are composed of epithelioid cells, and the remainder are composed of a mixture of spindle and epithelioid cells.

Diagnosis

GISTs are frequently discovered following the excision of an unknown mass. The mass appears well confined and primarily extraluminal on CT imaging (Figure 13). A characteristic feature of GISTs is a necrotic center surrounded by a heterogeneously enhancing soft tissue rim.[41] Endoscopic ultrasonography (EUS) can help diagnose these subepithelial lesions.[43] Percutaneous biopsy is not recommended as risk of rupture and seeding into the peritoneal cavity may occur. A tissue diagnosis is only required if neoadjuvant imatinib is to be utilized due to unresectability or if lymphoma is in the differential diagnosis.

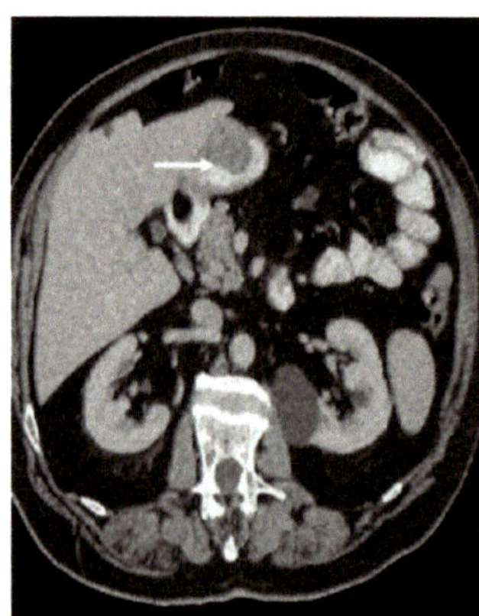

Figure 13: CT scan demonstrating a gastrointestinal stromal tumor (arrow).

Staging

No standardized approach to histopathologic evaluation for GISTs exists. Several factors, however, are associated with clinical behavior. Tumors with a low mitotic rate (5 or fewer mitoses per 50 high power fields) are typically benign. Tumors with a frequency of greater than 5 per 50 HPF are categorized as malignant, and those with a frequency of greater than 50 per 50 HPF as high grade malignant.

Tumors larger than 5cm in diameter, necrosis, cellular atypia, or local invasion are also associated with malignancy. C-kit mutations are found in malignant GISTs, and their presence indicates a bad prognosis.[44] Current studies demonstrate the essential need for a standardized staging approach for GIST specimen reporting in order to improve risk classification and treatment recommendations.

Treatment

The objective of treatment is to perform a gross and microscopic negative resection, as well as an en bloc resection of any implicated neighboring organs. GISTs are friable, soft tumors, and rupture should be avoided to avoid seeding in peritoneum and recurrence. Extended lymphadenectomy is not recommended since lymph node metastases are rare and do not have any added benefit. Tumors less than 10cm in diameter without local invasion have a low morbidity. Wedge resection is indicated for GISTs found in the proximal stomach, particularly along the greater curvature of the stomach. After primary resection, 5-year survival rates are 96% for low-risk patients, 54% for intermediate-risk patients, and 20% for high-risk patients.[45]

With a 50% 5-year recurrence, and ineffective chemotherapy, the 1998 discovery of a mutation in the i-KIT gene and the subsequent development of Imatinib has revolutionized the treatment of GIST.[46] Marketed as Gleevec, Imatinib is a competitive inhibitor of specific tyrosine kinases. Imatinib remains the mainstay treatment for recurrent or metastatic GIST tumors (Figure 14).

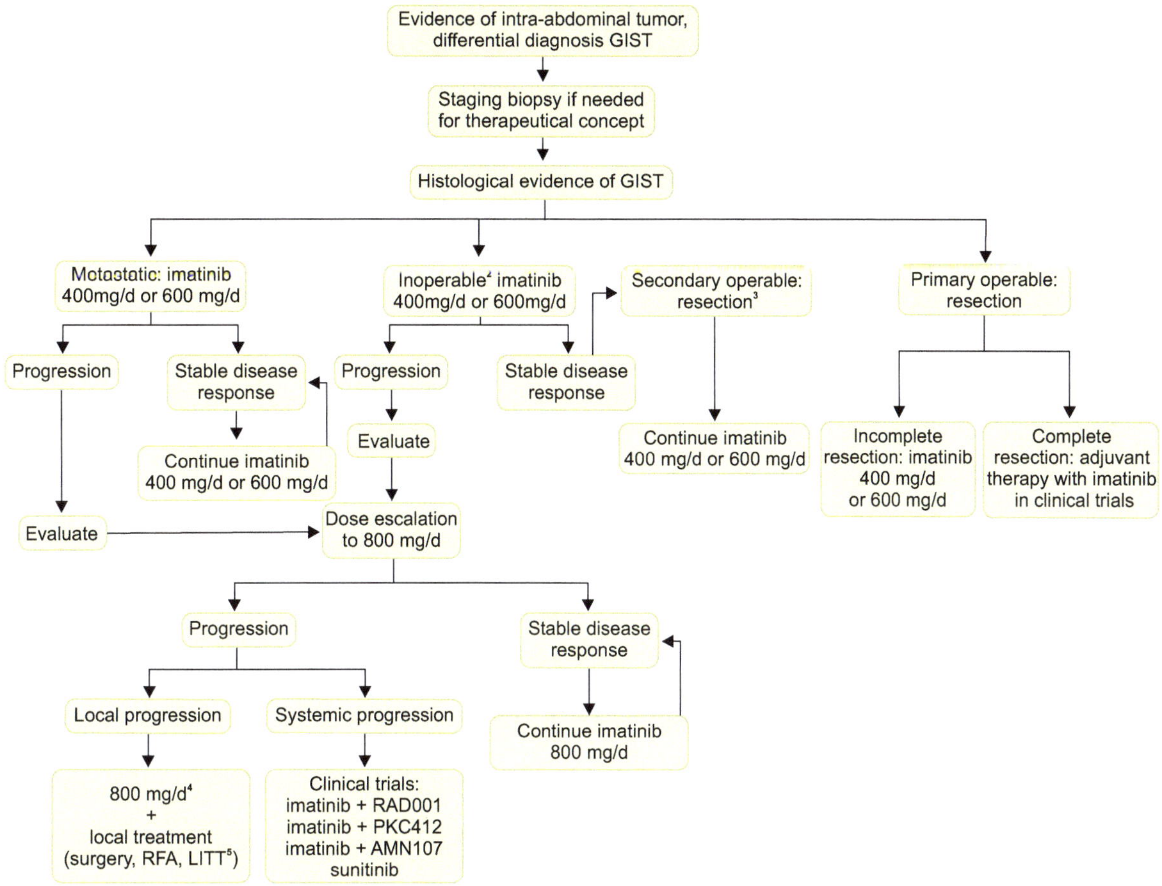

Evidence of intra-abdominal tumor, differential diagnosis GIST

Staging biopsy if needed for therapeutical concept

Histological evidence of GIST

Metastatic: imatinib 400mg/d or 600 mg/d

Progression

Evaluate

Stable disease response

Continue imatinib 400 mg/d or 600 mg/d

Inoperable[4] imatinib 400mg/d or 600mg/d

Progression

Evaluate

Stable disease response

Dose escalation to 800 mg/d

Progression

Local progression

800 mg/d[4] + local treatment (surgery, RFA, LITT[5])

Systemic progression

Clinical trials: imatinib + RAD001 imatinib + PKC412 imatinib + AMN107 sunitinib

Stable disease response

Continue imatinib 800 mg/d

Secondary operable: resection[3]

Continue imatinib 400 mg/d or 600 mg/d

Primary operable: resection

Incomplete resection: imatinib 400 mg/d or 600 mg/d

Complete resection: adjuvant therapy with imatinib in clinical trials

Figure 14: Management algorithm for gastrointestinal stromal tumors.

GASTRIC VOLVULUS

Gastric volvulus is an uncommon disorder. Torsion can occur in two ways, along the stomach's longitudinal axis, organoaxial or along the stomach's vertical axis, mesenteroaxial (Figure 15). Organoaxial torsion is more common than mesenteroaxial torsion, occurring in nearly two thirds and one third of cases, respectively.

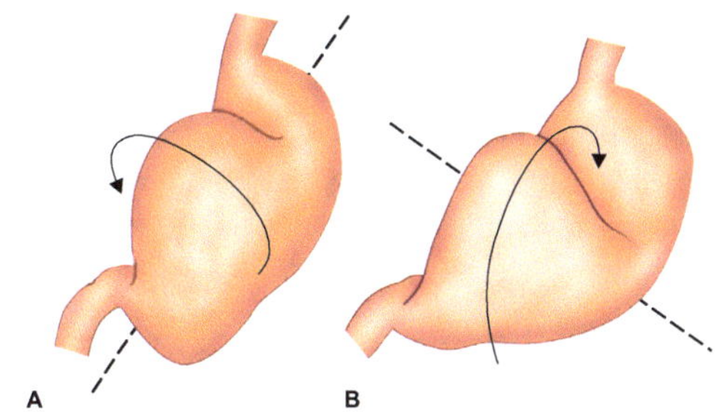

Figure 15: A. Organoaxial volvulus, which is the stomach's rotary torsion along its longitudinal or cardio-pyloric axis. B. Mesenteroaxial volvulus, which is a rotary torsion around the short axis of the stomach, which runs from the center of the greater curvature to the porta hepatis.

In contrast to organoaxial torsion, which develops acutely and is related to a diaphragmatic defect, mesenteroaxial volvulus is a recurrent disorder and is not linked with a diaphragmatic defect. Diaphragmatic defects are caused by trauma or paraesophageal hernias in adults. Congenital anomalies, such as eventration or foramen of Bochdalek are frequent causes of diaphragmatic deformities in children.

Most patients present with abdominal pain that is acute in onset, vomiting, distention, and upper GI hemorrhage. The classic triad of symptoms of gastric volvulus, first described by Bochardt in 1904 consists of severe epigastric pain, retching without vomiting, and inability to pass a nasogastric tube.

Abdominal plain film radiography will reveal a gas-filled viscus in the chest or upper abdomen. A barium contrast or upper GI endoscopy can be used to confirm the diagnosis.

Acute volvulus is a surgical emergency, and the stomach is reduced and uncoiled through a transabdominal approach. In the rare event that the stomach is strangulated, the compromised portion of the stomach is resected. Without a diaphragmatic defect, spontaneous volvulus can be managed by detorsion and fixation with gastropexy or tube gastrostomy.

REFERENCES

1. Zuiderma G. Shackelford's Surgery of the Alimentary Tract, 4th ed. Philadelphia, WB Saunders, 1995.
2. Mulholland MW. Gastric anatomy and physiology. In: Mulholland MW, editor. Greenfield's surgery: scientific principles and practice. 4th edition. Philadelphia: Lippincott Williams and Wilkins; 2006. p 712-20.
3. Bonenkamp JJ, Hermans J, Sasako M, van de Velde CJ. Extended lymph-node dissection for gastric cancer. Dutch Gastric Cancer Group. N Engl J Med 1999; 340:908-14.
4. Owen DA. Normal Histology of the Stomach. The Am J of Pathology. 1986; 10(1):48-61.
5. Mercer DW, Liu TH, Castaneda A. Anatomy and physiology of the stomach. In: Yeo CJ, editor. Ahackelford's surgery of the alimentary tract. 5th edition. Elsevier; 2002. p 3.
6. Verkijk M, Gielkens HA, Lamers CB, et al. Effect of gastrin on antroduodenal motility: role of intraluminal acidity. Gastrointestin and Liver Physiol. Am J Physiol 1998; 275(5):1209.
7. Saffouri B, Weir GC, Bitar KN, et al. Gastrin and somatostatin secretion by perfused rat stomach: Functional linkage of antral peptides. Am J Physiol 238: G495-501, 1980.
8. Cummings DE, Overduin J. Gastrointestinal regulation of food intake. J Clin Invest 117:13, 2007.
9. Murray CD, Kamm MA, Bloom SR, et al. Ghrelin for the gastroenterologist: History and potential. Gastroenterology 125: 1492, 2003.
10. Wood JD. Neurogastroenterology and motility. In: Rhoades R, Bell DR, editors. Medical physiology: principles for clinical medicine. 3rd edition. Baltimore (MD): Lipincott Williams & Wilkins; 2008. p 438-8.
11. Huerta Franco R, Vargas-Luna M, Hernandez E, Capaccione K, Cordova. Use of short-term bioimpedance for gastric motility assessment. Med Eng Phys. 2009; Sep:31(7)770-4.
12. Khoo J, Rayner CK, Feinle-Bisset C, et al. Gastrointestinal hormonal dysfunction in gastroparesis and functional dyspepsia. NeurogastroenterolMotil 2010;22(12):1270-8.
13. Rees WD, Malagelada JR, Miller LJ, et al. Human interdigestive and postprandial gastrointestinal motor and gastrointestinal hormone patterns. Dig Dis Sci 1982;27(4):321-9.
14. Killmar O, Moussavian MR, Richter S, et al. Prophylactic octreotide and delayed gastric emptying after pancreaticoduodenectomy: results of a prospective randomized double-blinded placebo-controlled trial. Eur J SurgOncol 2008; 34(8):868-75.
15. Khayyam U, Sachdeva P, Gomez J, et al. Assessment of symptoms during gastric emptying scintigraphy to correlate symptoms to delayed gastric emptying. NeurogastroenterolMotil 2010;22(5):539-45.
16. Kurata JH. Ulcer epidemiology: An overview and proposed research framework. Gastroenterology 1989; 96:569-580.
17. NIH Consensus Conference. *Helicobacter pylori* in peptic ulcer disease. NIH Consensus Development Panel on *Helicobacter pylori* in peptic ulcer disease. JAMA 1994;272(1):65-9.
18. Dooley CP, Cohen H, Fitzgibbons PL, et al. Prevalence *Helicobacter pylori* infection and histologic gastritis in asymptomatic persons. N Engl J Med 321:1562-1566, 1989.
19. Huang JQ, Sridhar S, Hunt RH. Role of *Helicobacter pylori* infection and non-steroidal anti-inflammatory drugs in peptic ulcer disease: a meta-analysis. Lancet 202;359(9300):14-22.
20. Groenen MJ, Kuipers EJ, Hansen BE, et al. Incidence of duodenal ulcers and gastric ulcers in a Western population: back to where it started. Can J Gastroenterol 2009;23(9): 604-8.
21. Dallal HJ, Palmer KR. Clinical review: Upper gastrointestinal hemorrhage. *BMJ* 323: 1115, 2001.
22. Graham DY, Lew GM, Klein PD, et al. Effect of treatment of *Helicobacter pylori* infection on the long-term recurrence of gastric or duodenal ulcer: A randomized controlled study. Ann Inter Med 116:705, 1992.
23. Mossner J, Caca K. Developments in the inhibition of gastric acid secretion. Eur J Clin Invest 35: 469, 2005.
24. Poxon VA, Keighley MR, Dykes PW, et al. Comparison of minimal and conventional surgery in patients with bleeding peptic ulcer: a multicenter trial. Br J Surg 1991;78(11): 1344-5.
25. Millat B, Hay JM, Valleur P, et al. Emergency surgical treatment for bleeding duodenal ulcer: oversewing plus vagotomy versus gastric resection, a controlled randomized trial. French Associations for Surgical Research. World J Surg 1993; 17(5):568-73.
26. Bertleff MJ, Lange JF. Laparoscopic correction of perforated peptic ulcer: first choice? A review of literature. SurgEndosc 2010;24(6):1231-9.
27. Oberhuber G, Stolte M. Gastric polyps: An update of their pathology and biological significance. Virchows Arch 437:581-590, 2000.

28. Lee YT, Lin H, Guo JC, Yan SL, Hou HJ, Lai YS, Liu YH, Wu HS, Hwang MH. Laparoscopy assisted billroth I gastrectomy for ectopic pancreas in the prepyloric region. Case Rep Gastroenterol. 2012 Sep;6(3):712-9.
29. Parkin DM, Bray F, Ferlay J, et al. Global cancer statistics, 2002. CA Cancer J Clin 2005;55(2):74-108.
30. Figueiredo C, Machado JC, Pharoah P, et al. *Helicobacter pylori* and interlukin 1 genotyping: An opportunity to identify high-risk individuals for gastric carcinoma. J Natl Cancer Inst 94: 1680-1687, 2002.
31. Carneiro F, Oliveira C, Seruca R. Pathology and genetics of familial gastric cancer. Int J SurgPathol 2010; 18:33-6.
32. Sarela AI, Lefkowitz R, Brennan MF, et al. Selection of patients with gastric adenocarcinoma for laparoscopic staging. Am J Surg 191:134-8, 2006.
33. Mani NB, Suri S, Gupta S, et al. Two-phase dynamic contrast-enhanced computed tomography with water-filling method of staging of gastric carcinoma. Clin Imaging 25:38-43, 2001.
34. Ganpathi IS, So JB, Ho KY. Endoscopic ultrasonography for gastric cancer: does it influence treatment? SurgEndosc 2006;20(4):559-62.
35. Schwarz RE, Smith DD. Clinical impact of lymphadenectomy extent in resectable gastric cancer of advanced stage. Ann SurgOncol 2007,14(2):317-28.
36. Japanese Gastric Cancer A. Japanese classification of gastric carcinoma – 2nd English edition. Gastric Cancer 1998; 1(1): 10-24.
37. Saidi RF, ReMine SG, Dudrick PS, et al. Is there a role for palliative gastrectomy in patients with stage IV gastric cancer? World J Surg 30:21, 2006.
38. Lowy A, Mansfield P, Leach S, et al. Response to neoadjuvant chemotherapy best predicts survival after curative resection of gastric cancer. Ann Surg 1999; 229:303-8.
39. Isaacson P, Wright DH. Malignant lymphoma of mucosa associated lymphoid tissue. A distinctive type of B-cell lymphoma. Cancer 52:1410-1416, 1983.
40. Koniaris LG, Drugas G, Katzman PJ, et al. Management of gastrointestinal lymphoma. J Am CollSurg 197:127-141, 2003.
41. Burkhill GJ, Badran M, Al-Muderis O, et al. Malignant gastrointestinal stromal tumor: distribution, imaging features, and pattern of metastatic spread. Radiology 2003; 226:527-32.
42. Antonescu CR, Viale A, Sarran L, et al. Gene expression in gastrointestinal stromal is distinguished by KIT genotype and anatomic site. Clin Cancer Res 2004;10: 3282-90.
43. Shah P, Gao F, Edmundowicz SA, et al. Predicting malignant potential of gastrointestinal stromal tumors using endoscopic ultrasound. Dig Dis Sci 2009; 54:1265-9.
44. Dematteo RP, Gold JS, Saran L, et al. Tumor mitotic rate, size, and location independently predict recurrence after resection of primary gastrointestinal stromal tumor (GIST). Cancer 2008; 112:608-15.
45. Otani Y, Furukawa T, Yoshida M, et al. Operative indications for relatively small gastrointestinal stromal tumor of the stomach based on analysis of 60 operated cases. Surgery 2006; 139:484-92.
46. Blay JY. A decade of tyrosine kinase inhibitor therapy: historical and current perspectives on targeted therapy for GIST. Cancer Treat Rev 2011;37(5):373-84.

❑❑❑

29

CHAPTER

Liver

Manjunath Haridas, MD, FACS
Sachin Patil, M.D, FACS
Michael Jacobs, MD, FACS, FICS
Rakhi Goswami, BS
Srinivas Kavuturu, MD, FACS
Dinesh Vyas, MD, FACS
Vijay Mittal, MD, FAIS (Hon), FICS, FICA, FACS

Anatomy

The average liver can weigh approximately 1,200 to 1,600 grams. The liver is located in the right upper quadrant of the abdomen, embedded in the peritoneum, which forms the liver capsule (Glission's capsule). The lateral peritoneal reflections from liver onto the diaphragm form the suspensory ligaments of the liver, including left and right triangular ligaments (coronary ligaments). The falciform ligament extends anteriorly as a thin membrane from the center of the coronary ligament, onto the diaphragm and abdominal wall, extending up to umbilicus. Historically, the falciform ligament marked the division between the right and left hemilivers. The ligamentum teres (obliterated umbilical vein) runs along the inferior edge of the falciform ligament. The umbilical fissure is on the inferior surface of the left liver and contains the left portal triad. At the hilum, the hepatic arterial and portal venous blood enters the liver.

Segmental Anatomy

The portal and hepatic vein branches divide the liver into the two hemilivers, four sectors and eight sections/segments. The portal fissure, or Cantlie's line, is a vertical plane that stretches from the gallbladder to the left border of the inferior vena cava (IVC), dividing the organ into the left and right hemilivers. The right liver is divided into anterior and posterior sectors. The left liver is divided into a medial (quadrate lobe) and lateral sectors. The medial sector of left liver lies to the right of the falciform ligament and umbilical fissure, and the lateral sector lie to the left. The right scissura contains the right hepatic vein, dividing the right liver into an anterior (segments V and VIII) and posterior (segments VI and VII) sections, respectively. Furthermore, the right portal pedicle comprises the right hepatic artery, portal vein, and bile duct, and is split into the right anterior and posterior pedicles which supply the anterior and posterior sectors, respectively. The left portal pedicle splits into an anterior (segments III and IV) and posterior (segment II-the only sector comprised of a single segment) pedicles. The caudate lobe (segment I) posteriorly abuts the IVC, inferiorly lies posterior to the left portal triad, and superiorly the left and middle hepatic veins. Most of the caudate lobe lies to the left of the IVC, but inferiorly, it traverses between the IVC and left portal triad to fuse to the right liver (segments VI and VII), called the right portion of the caudate process. The left portion of the caudate lobe is in the lesser omental bursa and the anterior portion is covered by the lesser omentum (gastrohepatic ligament) that separates it from segments II and III anteriorly (Figure 1).

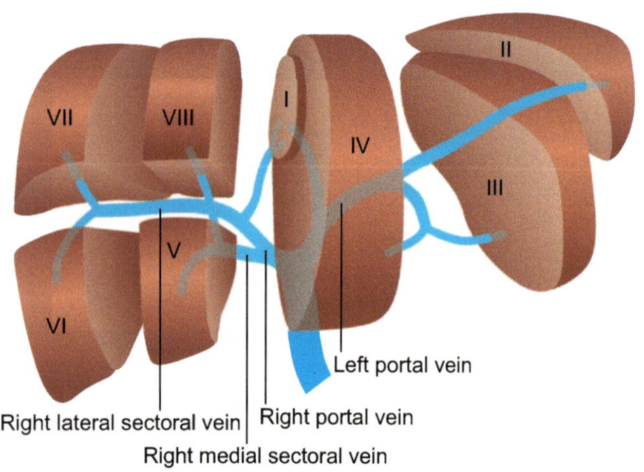

Figure 1: Liver Segmental Anatomy

Blood Supply

Approximately 75 percent (%) of hepatic blood flow is supplied by the portal vein. Due to the lack of valves in the portal venous system, there is low resistance, allowing the accommodation of high flow blood supply, at low pressures. Absence of valves allows for the portal venous pressure to be measured throughout the system. The portal vein forms directly behind the neck of pancreas by the convergence of the splenic and superior mesenteric veins, at the level of second lumbar vertebra, which further bifurcates into left and right branches at the hilum of liver. The length of main portal vein ranges between 5.5 to 8 centimeters (cm), with a diameter of about 1 centimeter (cm).

The hepatic artery supplies high flow oxygenated systemic arterial blood flow to the liver, gallbladder, pancreas, duodenum, and pylorus of the stomach (Figure 2). It supplies about 25 percent (%) of the hepatic blood flow and contributes to 30 to 50% of hepatic oxygenation. The liver also receives blood supply from many small perihepatic arteries, which come from the inferior phrenic and gastroduodenal arteries. The small vessels are essential for maintaining collateral blood flow, in case occlusion of the main hepatic artery occurs. If ligation of the left or right hepatic artery were to occur, then the intrahepatic collaterals would reinforce nutrient blood flow. Arterial flow to the liver and biliary tree only occurs about 60% of the time. The celiac trunk, a short vessel arising from the aorta, below the aortic diaphragmatic hiatus, gives off three major branches: the splenic, left gastric, and common hepatic arteries.

The common hepatic artery runs forward and to the right, along the pancreas' superior border. From there, it moves up towards the hepatic hilum, left of the bile duct, and anterior to the portal vein. The branches of the common hepatic artery are first the gastroduodenal artery then the supraduodenal artery, and then the right gastric artery before entering the hepatic hilum. After the gastroduodenal artery branches, the common hepatic artery becomes the proper hepatic artery and then divides into left and right branches at the hilum. The left hepatic artery runs vertically toward the umbilical fissure, suppling segments I, II, and III. Usually, the left hepatic artery also has a middle hepatic artery branch that runs toward the right side of the umbilical fissure, supplying segment IV. The right hepatic artery usually moves posterior to the common hepatic duct and enters Calot's triangle (liver edge, cystic duct, common hepatic duct. In the Calot's triangle right hepatic artery offers the cystic artery branch, which supplies the gallbladder, and continues towards the right lobe. An accessory vessel adds to the normal branch patterns, while a replaced vessel will substitute or replace normal branches. Commonly, the hepatic artery will come from the celiac trunk. However, different branches or even the entire hepatic arterial system may originate from the superior mesenteric artery. In such cases, the replaced or accessory right hepatic artery will traverse posterior to the head of the pancreas and portal vein and then, to the right of the portal vein.

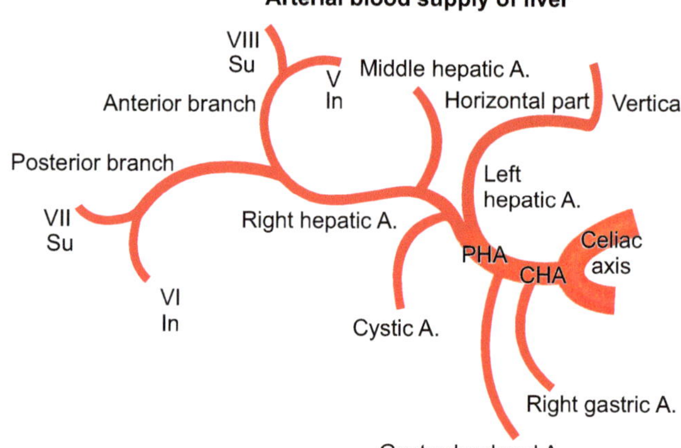

Figure 2. Hepatic Arterial Supply

There are three major hepatic veins draining from the superior and posterior liver surfaces, directly into the inferior vena cava. The right hepatic vein drains most of the right liver to the right of the IVC, after a one centimeter (cm) extrahepatic course. The left and middle hepatic veins connect intrahepatic and form a single vessel and enter to the left of the IVC. The middle and left hepatic veins may occasionally drain separately into the IVC. There are additional hepatic veins providing venous drainage to liver. The umbilical vein runs below the falciform ligament, in between the middle and left hepatic veins, to drain into the left hepatic vein. The various small venous branches posteriorly drain into the IVC, and an inferior accessory right hepatic vein is commonly seen and can be of substantial size. The caudate lobe drains directly into IVC through various smaller hepatic veins, and an additional large tributary drains superiorly into the left hepatic vein (Figure 3).

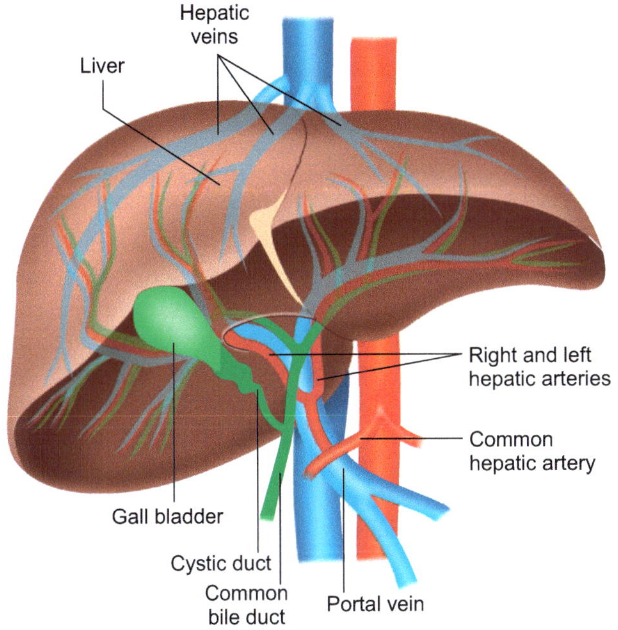

Figure 3. Hepatic Venous Drainage

Hepatocytes

The hepatocytes are complex and multifunctional cells in the liver that accounts for 60 percent (%) of the cellular mass and 80 percent (%) of the cytoplasmic mass. Hepatocytes, polyhedral with centrally located spherical nuclei, arrange themselves in single cell layered plates, and are lined with blood-filled sinusoids. All hepatocytes are in contact with adjacent hepatocytes. The biliary space, or bile canaliculus, as well as the sinusoidal space allow the cells to carry on various functions. Some of these essential functions may include, but are not limited to the uptake, storage, and release of nutrients. Additionally, hepatocytes synthesize multiple plasma proteins, glucose, fatty acids, and lipids; produce and secrete bile, and thus digest dietary fats; and degrade and detoxify toxins.

Biliary System

The biliary tree is a system of ducts that emerges from the bile canaliculi within the liver and acts as conduit to bile and pancreatic secretions. The bile canaliculi are lined by specialized hepatocytes membrane which coalesces to form hepatic lobular ductules, which in turn coalesce to form large segmental bile ducts which drain each hepatic segment. Both anterior and posterior right sectoral ducts join to form the main right hepatic duct. The ducts that drain the segments II, III, and IV constitute the left hepatic duct, which also has a longer extrahepatic course, as compared to the right. Segment I, or the caudate lobe, drains into the left hepatic duct. Supplemental smaller ducts drain into the right hepatic ducts, or into the hepatic duct confluence, whereas the major lobar ducts unite to form the common hepatic duct. The common hepatic duct plunges into the hepatoduodenal ligament for a discernible interval to unite the cystic duct of the gallbladder to form the common bile duct.

Anatomical variations of the biliary duct have been observed in about 30% of patients, commonly involving the right hepatic duct. In about a quarter of patients, the right posterior sectoral duct independently connects to the common or left hepatic duct.

Lymphatics

The liver produces and contributes the most lymph in the human body, accounting for 25 to 50% of lymph that flows through the thoracic duct. Lymphatics that drain the superficial lobules take sub-capsular course and drain into the lymphatics along the diaphragm, the suspensory ligaments, and the posterior mediastinum. The remaining lymphatics will join the porta hepatis. Lymphatics that arise from the deeper lobules of the liver will either travel along the vena cava with the hepatic veins, or into the porta hepatis with the portal veins. A majority of the liver's lymphatic system drains into the hepatoduodenal ligament.

DIAGNOSIS

Ultrasonography

Ultrasonography, commonly recognized as an ultrasound, translates high-frequency sound waves into images that may be used in the evaluation of abdominal symptoms. Ultrasounds are widely accessible, inexpensive, well-tolerated, and do not risk exposure to radiation. Therefore, ultrasounds of the liver are excellent for obtaining initial images for the diagnosis of biliary pathology and focal hepatic lesions. In trauma cases, the focused abdominal sonography for trauma (FAST) examination, expedites the detection of liver injury. Doppler augmented ultrasound may be used to detect blood vessels and the direction and velocity of blood flow. However, ultrasound imaging of the liver has limitations. Ultrasound has a limited role in the assessment of deep-seated lesions near the diaphragm, and the quality is compromised in morbidly obese patients and the presence of ileus or bowel obstruction. In such cases, further evaluation with CT scan or an MRI is routinely required to arrive at proper diagnosis. Having said that, intra-operative ultrasound is a valuable adjunct in liver surgery, with 20% to 30% increase in the detection of liver lesions during surgery. The utility of intra-operative ultrasound is broad, including helps in obtaining adequate resection margins, in tumor staging, visualizing intrahepatic vasculature, and guidance of the resection plane by assessing mass to vessel relationships, obtaining biopsy and tumor ablation.

The advancement of contrast-enhanced ultrasound technology has greatly impacted the capability to distinguish between malignant and benign hepatic lesions. The contrast medium consists of micro-bubble agents (size < 10 microns) are injected in the peripheral vein prior to imaging; minimize noise while maximizing echo energy. By identifying high-powered magnification patterns and the vascular anatomy of the liver lesions, contrast-enhanced ultrasounds may allow for clear depiction of liver lesions.

Computerized Tomography

Computerized tomography (CT) scans are a large digital series of *x*-ray images produced in slices and stacked together to form cross-sectional images of the human body. Compared to the earlier conventional axial CT techniques, the advancement of helical, or spiral, CT scans allows for clearer, detailed images, especially of the liver. With a combination of continuous table motion and spiral rotation of the CT machine, the helical CT scanners are able to obtain up to 60 centimeters of adequate volumetric data acquisition, as the patient holds a single breath. Due to the high scanning speed, the helical CT technique eliminates the presence of motion artifacts from movement or breathing, while producing optimal contrast delivery.

Triple phase contrast CT scan, which captures images in arterial phase, portal venous phase and delayed phase helps to differentiate tumors due to the differences in blood supply.

The arterial phase scan is obtained thirty to forty seconds, portal venous phase scan is obtained sixty to seventy seconds and delayed scans are obtained two to five minutes after contrast injection, respectively. Most hepatic tumors are well delineated in the arterial phase as they obtain most of their blood supply from the hepatic artery or other hypervascular lesions in their presence. The liver parenchyma obtains a majority of its blood supply from the portal vein; therefore, the portal phase provides the ability to detect hypovascular lesions. Hypovascular lesions in the CT scans will appear to be hypo-attenuated, when compared to the bright normal liver parenchyma in the portal venous phase.

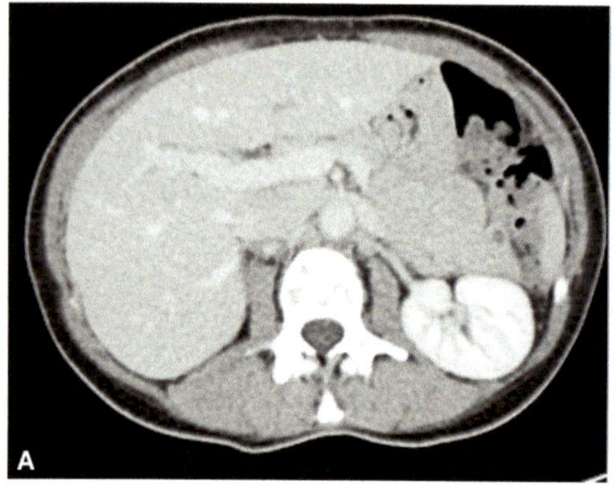

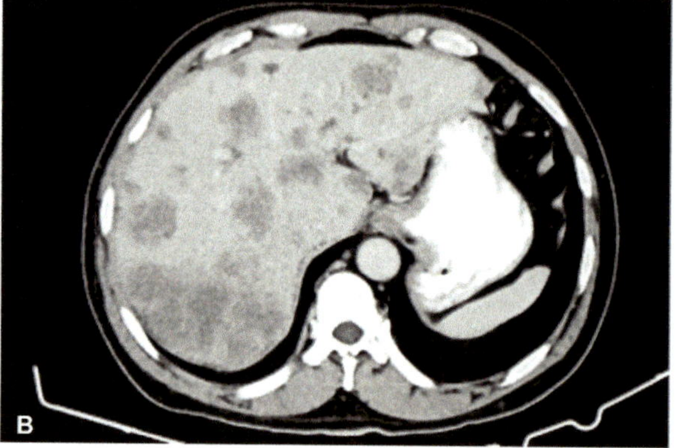

Figure 4: (A) Normal CT scan of Liver, isodense liver and (B) abnormal CT scan of liver, several hypodense lesions indicating metastatic disease

Magnetic Resonance Imaging

Magnetic resonance imaging (MRI) is an imaging technique that uses the magnetic field and computer-generated radio waves to produce images of organs and structures in the human body. The large MRI scanner generates a strong magnetic field to align tissue/fluid protons in the direction of the magnetic field. Radio waves delivered during MRI alter the alignment and move the protons from their original position. The protons will return to their original position after the radio waves are turned off, during this process they release electromagnetic energy, which is captured and converted into real-time image. The T1 and T2 relaxation times may be used to differentiate between tissues. T1 phase measures the rate at which a tissue is magnetized, while T2 phase measures the rate at which the tissue loses magnetization. Similar to the advancements in CT technology, MRI may also be performed as T1-weighted imaging within a single breath hold and T2-weighted imaging triggered by respirations. Imaging technologies with the ability to perform MRI within breath hold time have diminished the motion artifacts and increased the sensitivity of MRI Advancements in the contrast agents for MRI have helped to increase signal intensity and hence help to differentiate various liver lesions. Similar to the iodine-based contrast used for CT scan, gadopentetate dimeglumine is the contrast agent used for MRI. This agent is a salt of the gadolinium complex of diethylenetriamine penta-acetic acid. Some contrast agents used during MRI may be liver-specific, and therefore depend upon excretion from Kupffer cells or secretion in bile by hepatocytes, which helps to improve the sensitivity and specificity.

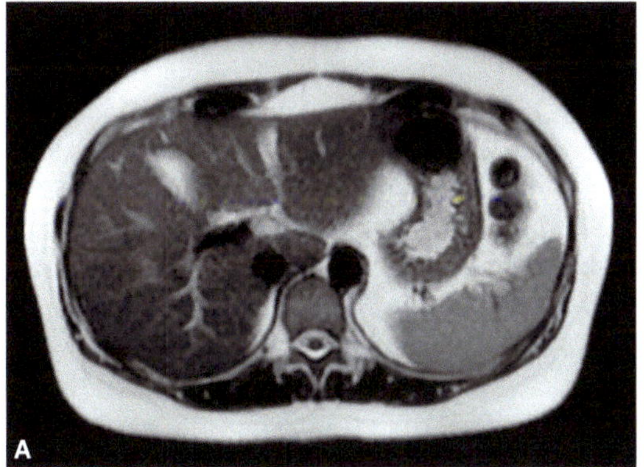

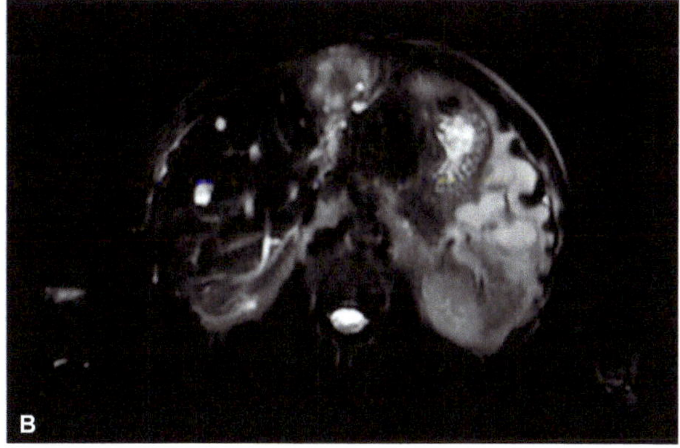

Figure 5: (A) Normal T2 weighted MRI of liver, isointense appearance and (B) Abnormal T2 weighted MRI of liver homogeneous hyperintensity indicating simple liver cyst (small arrow) and heterogeneous hyperintensity indicating colorectal liver metastases (large arrow)

Positron Emission Tomography

Positron emission tomography (PET) is an imaging technique that uses nuclear medicine technology to produce images of tissues based on their metabolic activity. In these techniques, a radioisotope is tagged with glucose, which is absorbed by metabolically active tissue, or a tumor and the gamma rays emitted by the radioisotope are captured by a gamma camera. The most prevalent active metabolic molecule utilized for PET scans is ^{18}fluorodeoxyglucose. Unlike the traditional imaging techniques previously described, PET scans provide functional images of tissues that are experiencing high metabolic activity, as well as most tumors and metastatic deposits. PET scans are a valuable tool, with higher sensitivity and specificity to assess the disease burden. Expanded access to integrated PET and CT scans will result in increased diagnostic accuracy, compared to the sole use of standard PET and CT scans.

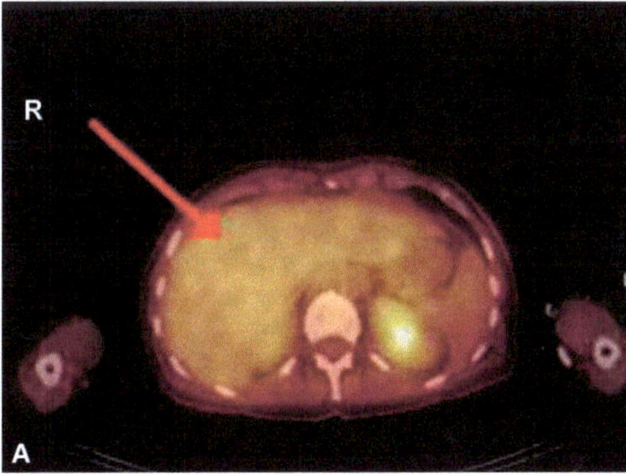

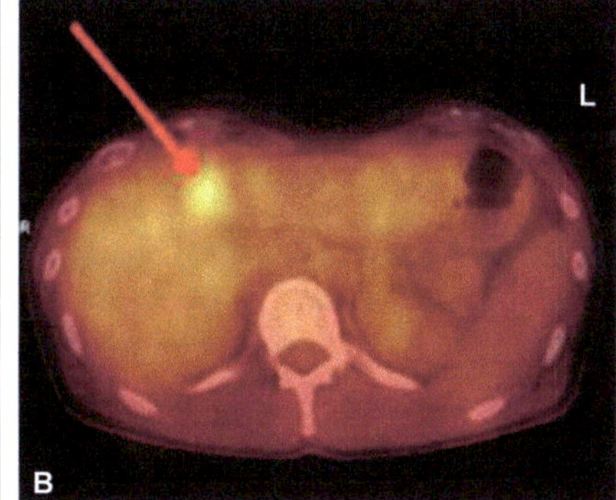

Figure 6: (A) Normal PET scan of liver, homogeneous uptake of radiotracer (arrow). (B) Abnormal PET scan of liver demonstrating increased focal uptake of radiotracer (arrow), indicating colorectal liver metastases

Infectious Diseases

Pyogenic Abscess

Incidence and Etiopathology

Pyogenic liver abscess was once a surgical disease, but now with newer antibiotics and minimally invasive techniques, most do not require such surgical procedures. The incidence of liver abscess has varied over the past two decades as better and improved imaging techniques. Pyogenic liver abscess was most commonly seen as a complication of acute appendicitis; recently it is commonly associated with acute diverticulitis. It is commonly seen in 6th and 7th decade of life with a male to female ratio of 1.5: 1.[1] The liver receives most of the blood supply via the portal system. When the bacterial load exceeds the liver's ability to clear it, a hepatic abscess is formed. This is a result of tissue invasion and neutrophil infiltration leading to formation of an organized abscess. The routes of exposure include (1) biliary tree, (2) portal vein, (3) hepatic artery, (4) direct extension of a nearby focus of infection, and (5) trauma.[2] Ascending pyogenic liver abscess secondary to cholangitis is the most common form. In Asia, intrahepatic stones and cholangitis are common. Previous biliary-enteric anastomosis is also a risk factor for hepatic abscess formation. The most common causes of infection via the portal vein include pancreatitis, appendicitis, diverticulitis, inflammatory bowel disease, perforated viscus, pelvic inflammatory disease, or omphalitis in the newborn.[3] Hepatic abscess can also be associated with malignancy. Systemic infection like endocarditis, pneumonia, and osteomyelitis can also result in liver infection. Immunocompromised patients including children are susceptible. Other routes of infection are iatrogenic hepatic necrosis, such as hepatic artery embolization, and thermal ablative procedures which may complicated by liver abscess. Cryptogenic abscess is when a possible etiology cannot be found after proper examination and imaging studies.

Majority of hepatic abscesses involve the right lobe of the liver, half of which are solitary. Liver abscess arising from portal pyemia or ascending cholangitis are polymicrobial, mainly gram-negative rods. Blood borne liver abscess is commonly due to a single organism. The most common organisms causing liver abscess include Escherichia coli and Klebsiella pneumoniae. Other organisms include Staphylococcus aureus, Enterococcus species, Streptococcus viridans, and Bacteroides species. Klebsiella is frequently associated with gas-forming abscesses. Enterococcus sp. and S. viridans are generally found in polymicrobial abscesses, whereas staphylococci in monomicrobial abscess. In 50 to 60% of cases, blood culture will be positive. In immunosuppressed patients, usually undergoing chemotherapy, fungal and mycobacterial hepatic abscesses may occur, but are otherwise rare.

Clinical Presentation

Majority of patients present with right upper abdominal pain and fever with chills and very few patients will have associated jaundice. The triad of symptoms is seen in <10% of patients. Nonspecific symptoms may include malaise, nausea, and vomiting.[4] Presentation could be acute (days) or chronic (weeks to months). Acute presentation is associated with identifiable inra-abdominal pathology, whereas a chronic presentation typical for cryptogenic liver abscess. Jaundice is seen in about 25% of patients and is often secondary to underlying biliary disease. Hepatomegaly is also commonly noted and present in about half of cases. Ascites, splenomegaly, and severe sepsis are possible presentations.

Diagnosis

Leukocytosis is common along with mild transaminitis. Severe liver function abnormalities are almost always associated with underlying biliary disease. Hypoalbuminemia or mild elevations of the prothrombin time can be present and reflect a degree of chronicity. Tumor markers like alpha fetoprotein, CEA and CA 19-9 will be elevated in abscess related to tumor necrosis. Ultrasonography and CT scan are critical for diagnosing hepatic abscess. Chest radiographs will show abnormal findings related to subdiaphragmatic pathology, including elevated right hemidiaphragm, right pleural effusion, or atelectasis. Ultrasonography will help to differentiate between solid and cystic lesions. Ultrasound has 80-95% sensitivity rate for diagnosing hepatic abscesses. On ultrasound abscess cavity will appear as hypoechoic round or oval shaped area. CT scan has 95-100% sensitivity rate for diagnosing hepatic abscess. Liver abscess will appear as hypottenuating lesions with peripheral ring enhancement on contrast enhanced CT scan (Figure 7). High-quality CT scans may help to identify very small abscesses. Ultrasounds and CT scans are both highly useful for diagnosing other intra-abdominal pathology, such as biliary disease or inflammatory disorders such as appendicitis or diverticulitis. MRI scans don't have any distinct advantages when compared to CT scans, but they are extremely useful in suspected liver abscess related to malignancy.

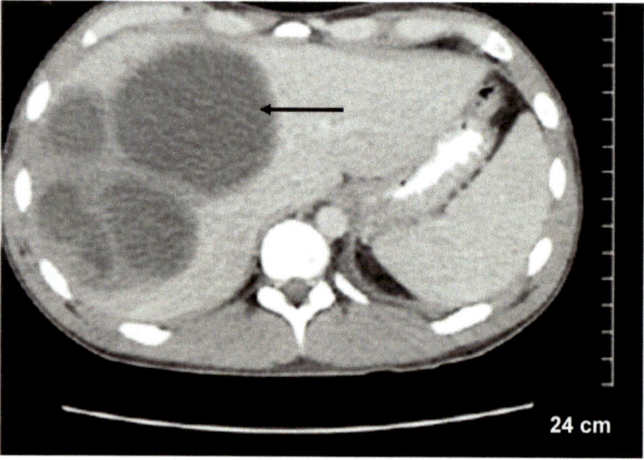

Figure 7. CT scan demonstrating pyogenic liver abscess

Management

Broad-spectrum IV antibiotics should be initiated to cover coliform bacteria and streptococcal species, as soon as possible. Blood and aspirates from the abscess should be sent for aerobic and anaerobic cultures, and where necessary mycobacterial and fungal cultures may be included. In suspected amebic infections, amebic blood serologic studies may be obtained. If diagnostic aspiration of the abscess is not feasible, antibiotic therapy should not be delayed. A combination of beta lactimase inhibitor penicillin, or an aminoglycoside, with metronidazole or a third-generation cephalosporin with metronidazole are appropriate. Parenteral antibiotics are continued for two-three weeks or till the resolution of systemic signs of infection such as fever, chills, or leukocytosis. Beyond this, additional two to four weeks of oral antibiotics are recommended based on culture and sensitivity results. Percutaneous drainage of the abscess larger than 5cm should be attempted where facilities are available. Success rates range from 69% to 90%.[5] Percutaneous drainage of multiple abscess usually has a lower success rate. Surgery should be reserved for patients who require surgical intervention for primary pathologic process (e.g., appendicitis, diverticulitis) or for those who have failed percutaneous techniques. Laparoscopic drainage procedures have been reported. Hepatic abscesses may occasionally require hepatic resection, especially for infected hepatic malignancies, hepatolithiasis, or intrahepatic biliary structures.[6]

AMEBIC ABSCESS

Incidence and Etiopathology

Amebic liver abscesses are the most prevalent extraintestinal manifestations of the parasitic protozoan Entamoeba histolytica. Amebiasis is a widely spread parasitic disease affecting both developing and developed countries. The disease is most common in residents of tropical and underdeveloped countries with suboptimal public health, sanitation, and personal hygiene. Amebic liver abscess is common among immigrant populations between 20 and 40 years of age. The disease is more common in men than in women with a male to female ratio of 10:1.[7] Risk factors include impaired immunity, malnutrition, pregnancy, steroid use, and chronic infections such as tuberculosis or syphilis.

Amebiasis occurs via fecal-oral route of transmission, where E. histolytica parasitic cysts are transmitted by consuming contaminated food, or water. Patients with chronic amebiasis or asymptomatic carriers are the major source of infection. The ingested E. Histolytica cysts pass through the stomach and into the small intestines, where excystation and multiplication of trophozoites by binary fission takes place. Amebiasis in most patients will result in asymptomatic colonization of the gastrointestinal tract; however, in some patients the parasite will invade the colon. Lesions on the colon are typically described as being flask-shaped ulceration extending through the mucosa and muscularis mucosa into the submucosa. Amebic liver abscess occurs when E. histolytica invades mesenteric venules and lymphatics, and travels to the liver via the portal vein. The trophozoites aggregate in the liver parenchyma where, through a process of acute inflammation, granuloma formation, and progressive tissue necrosis (hence the name histolytica), an amebic liver abscess is formed. The contents of the amebic abscess, classically described as "anchovy paste," is acellular, proteinaceous debris and blood, surrounded by an outer rim of Entamoebae that invade healthy hepatic tissue.

Clinical Presentation

The symptoms are similar to those of a pyogenic liver abscess as shown in Table 1. History of travel to endemic area is extremely crucial for diagnosis. Symptomatic patients developed fever, chills, anorexia, right upper quadrant pain and tenderness, and hepatomegaly over a few days to several weeks. Some reportedly experienced gastrointestinal symptoms, including nausea, vomiting, abdominal cramping or distention, diarrhea, or constipation. Rupture of the abscess is not uncommon. Intra-abdominal rupture may result in peritonitis, intrapericardial rupture may result in cardiac tamponade and failure, and pleural rupture may result in pleuritis and decreased breath sounds.[8]

Table1: Amebic vs. Pyogenic Hepatic Abscess

Clinical Features	Amebic Abscess	Pyogenic Abscess
Age (years)	20 to 40	Greater than 50
Male to female Ratio	Less than 10 to 1	1.5 to 1
Solitary vs. multiple	Solitary greater than or equal to 80%	Solitary 50%
Location	Typically in right lobe	Typically in right lobe
Travel to endemic area	Yes	No
Diabetic	Uncommon (≈2%)	More common (≈27%)
Alcohol Abuse	Yes	Yes
Jaundice	Rare	Common
↑ bilirubin	Uncommon	Common
↑ alkaline phosphatase	Common	Common
Blood culture positive	Negative	Common
Amebic serology positive	Positive	Negative

Diagnosis

Mild abnormalities of LFTs are common. Enzyme immunoassays (EIA) with a reported sensitivity of 99% and specificity greater than 90% for serum antibodies, is commonly used serological test. Ultrasound findings include a rounded non-homogeneous hypoechoic lesion abutting the liver capsule without significant rim echoes .[9] CT scan has greater sensitivity, as compared to ultrasound and is useful in differentiating between amebic and pyogenic hepatic abscesses. Amebic liver abscess share most of the CT scan characterstics of pyogenic abscess, however an incomplete rim of edema is characteristic to the former (Figure 8). CT scans may also aid in the identification of simple cysts and necrotic tumors. MRI of the liver has no distinct advantages over CT or ultrasound in typical cases, but it may be helpful in differentiating atypical lesions. Nuclear medicine studies, such as gallium scanning or technetium-99 liver scans, may also be useful in the differential between pyogenic and amebic abscesses, where the former will appear as hot lesion due to the presence of WBC and the later as cold lesion.

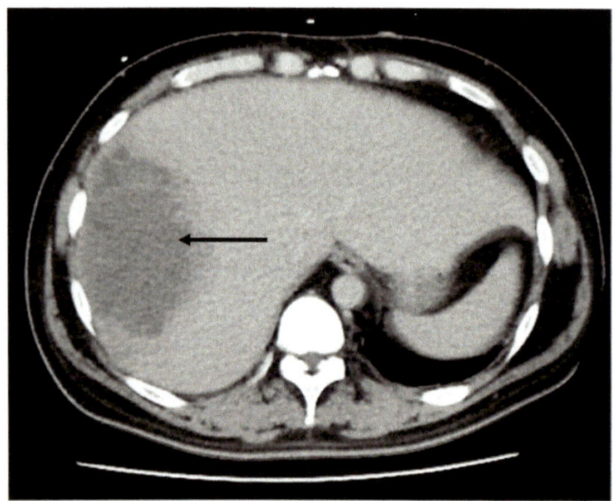

Figure 8 CT scan demonstrating amebic liver abscess

Management

Minor amebic liver abscesses may be treated with the sole use of amoebicidal drugs. Select patients may benefit from additional therapeutic options including simple aspiration, percutaneous drainage, and open surgical drainage. Metronidazole is preferred drug for treating amebic liver abscesses including for both systemic and intestinal amebiasis. A majority of patients experience rapid clinical improvement within 72 hours, and more than 90% are cured with metronidazole given at 750 milligrams orally three times a day for 10 days. In patients who are intolerant to metronidazole, or failing to respond to metronidazole within 5 days of prescription, chloroquine may be used as a substitute or addition to the metronidazole therapy.[10] All patients who have been treated for amebic liver abscess should have additional treatment with a luminal agent such as iodoquinol, paromomycin, or diloxanide furoate to eradicate the asymptomatic colonization state. In some patients, aspiration should be considered such as those with (1) abscesses larger than five centimeters due of the increased risk of rupture, (2) abscesses located in the left hepatic lobe because of the increased risks of peritoneal leakage or rupture into the pericardium and increased mortality, (3) failure to respond to drug therapy, and (4) amebic abscess with suspected secondary bacterial infection.

HYDATID CYST

Incidence and Etiopathology

Hydatid disease or echinococcosis is a zoonosis that occurs primarily in sheep-grazing areas of the world. Dogs are the definitive hosts. Transmission is from dogs to humans.[11] Echinococcosis is endemic in Mediterranean countries, the Far East, the Middle East, East Africa, South America, Australia, and New Zealand. Different species responsible include E. granulosus, E. multilocularis, and E. oligartus. Men and women are equally affected, commonly in 4th decade of life. Humans are the accidental intermediate host, due to consumption of contaminated food and water contaminated by the fecal matter of an infected dog, where the parasite enters its end stage. It most commonly reaches the liver, especially the right lobe, and then the lungs, where the parasite is in its larval stage known as the hydatid cyst. Then the parasite incubates for about three weeks and emerges as daughter cysts which are true replicas of the mother cyst. Hydatid cysts can die via degeneration of the membranes, which leads to development of cystic vacuoles, and calcification of the wall.

Clinical Presentation

Hydatid cysts are incidentally detected as large and asymptomatic liver cysts, until complications arise. The most common presenting symptoms are abdominal pain, dyspepsia, and vomiting. The most frequent sign is hepatomegaly. Jaundice and fever are less common. Hydatid cyst infections are similar to pyogenic abscesses. Rupture of the cyst into the biliary tree or bronchial tree; or free rupture into the peritoneal, pleural, or pericardial cavities have also been reported. Free ruptures risk the circulation of hydatid disease and potential fatal anaphylactic reactions.

Diagnosis

Eosinophilia is present in one fourth of the cases, however it is only suggestive. Enzyme-linked immunosorbent assay

(ELISA) and hydatid antigen immunobinding assays yield a sensitivity and specificity up to 95% and 90%, respectively. The accuracy of these serological assays varies.[12] Ultrasound is most commonly used for imaging and confirming diagnosis. Various classification systems have evolved, one shown in Table 2. Ultrasound demonstrates a well circumscribed, simple hydatid cyst that contains free-floating echogenic hydatid sand will display budding signs on the cystic membrane. In the presence of daughter cysts, a rosette appearance may be observed.

The cyst may be filled with an amorphous mass which may potentially be diagnostically misleading. Calcifications in the wall of the cyst are highly suggestive of hydatid disease and can be helpful in the diagnosis. Similar findings are seen on CT or MRI (Figure 9).[13] These studies can also assess extrahepatic disease and display explicit hepatic anatomical relations with the cyst. In some patients ERCP is indicated to rule out communication to the biliary tree.

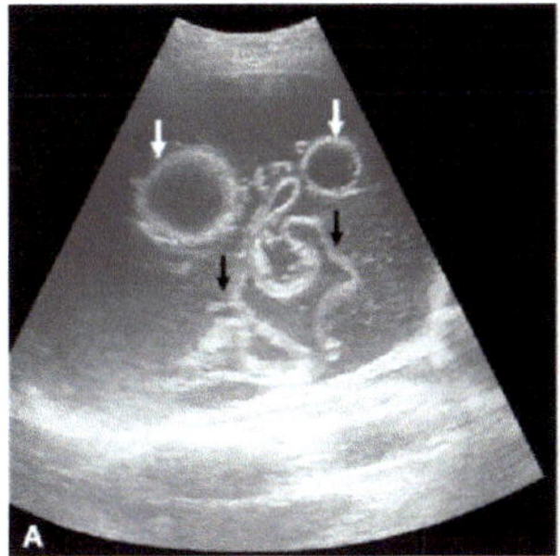

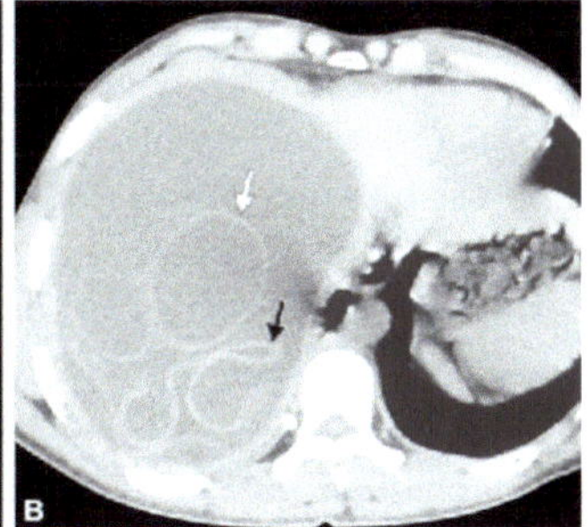

Figure 9. Ultrasound and CT Scan findings of hydatid liver disease

Table 2. Classification of hydatid cyst based on ultrasound features.

CL	Unilocular lesion with no cyst wall visible
CE1	Unilocular lesion with cyst wall visible, hydatid sand, "snowflake" sign
CE2	Multivesicular lesion, multiseptated, honeycomb sign, daughter cysts visible
CE3	Unilocular lesion, detached laminated membrane inside cyst, "water lily" sign
CE4	Heterogeneous hypoechoic or hyperechoic lesion, no daughter cysts, degenerative contents
CE5	Thick calcified lesion, calcification partial to complete, cone-shaped shadow

Management

Hepatic hydatid cysts most commonly require treatment by using surgical interventions. In generally a majority of hepatic hydatid cysts need some kind of intervention. However, elderly patients with small, asymptomatic, and calcified hepatic hydatid cysts, require no treatment. In preparation for an operation, preoperative corticosteroids have been recommended but are not universally used. Anaphylaxis and diffuse seeding are risks associated with ruptures. To avoid the risk of seeding during surgery, packing of the abdominal cavity is essential. If the cyst is large initial aspiration through a closed suction system and injection of scolicidal agents, or hypertonic saline into the cyst may be performed. Smaller cysts may be carefully unroofed and evacuated, then pericystectomy, marsupialization with omentoplasty or even liver resection may be performed[14] Alternatively a total pericystectomy may be performed without entering the cyst. Communication with biliary system should be carefully ruled out during surgery, in case of biliary communication, therapeutic interventions including simple suture repair or roux-en-y reconstruction may be needed. Laparoscopic techniques to drain and un-roof the cysts have been reported in a number of cases with positive results.

The rate of recurrence following surgical treatments ranges from 1 to 20%, but typically occurs in <5% of patients at experienced centers.[15] In the past, aspiration of hydatid cysts was contraindicated due to the risk of rupture and uncontrolled spillage. However, short term follow-up with cyst aspiration and injection of scolicidal agents has shown success rates of approximately 70%.[16]

Fungal Abscess

Approximately 10% of hepatic abscesses are fungal. Candida albicans and other candida species contribute to 80% of these cases, whereas Cryptococcus, Aspergillus, and other mixed fungal infections are less common. Fungal hepatic abscesses are usually multiple and usually prevalent in immunosupressed patients with leukemia undergoing chemotherapy, or those infected with human immunodeficiency virus (HIV) typically have monomicrobial fungal infections. Patients with biliary malignancies, indwelling stents, or those requiring frequent antibiotic therapy typically develop polymicrobial fungal and bacterial abscess. Treatment of fungal liver abscesses includes systemic antifungal therapy, simple aspiration, percutaneous drainage, or even open surgical drainage. Amphotericin B is the first-line drug of choice for systemic antifungal therapy because of its broad fungal efficacy. Patients experiencing mixed fungal and bacterial abscesses should be prescribed the appropriate systemic antibiotic therapy based on the results of culture and sensitivity. Voriconazole or Caspofungin may be used to treat patients who are not responding to Amphotericin B, or those who have aggressive infections caused by other fungal species.

Neoplasms

Liver lesions are commonly encountered in clinical practice. These can be either primary or secondary. It is essential for a general surgeon to be familiar with the clinical presentation, radiographic characteristics, and management of these lesions. Various imaging techniques used to evaluate these lesions include ultrasound, computed tomography and magnetic resonance imaging. Based on the radiographic features, benign lesions can be differentiated from malignant ones. When necessary, serum tumor markers (AFP, CEA, CA 19-9, and CA-125) are also valuable. Liver lesions can be classified as either solid or cystic. These are further classified into either benign or malignant. Primary liver tumors are classified based on cell of origin (hepatocellular, cholangiocellular or mesenchymal). The primary goal in evaluation of a liver lesion is to determine whether surgical resection is possible. A broad classification of liver lesions is shown in Table 3. Various other classifications exist, but for the sake of simplicity, the above-mentioned classification is followed in this chapter.

Table 3: Classification of Liver Neoplasm

Solid	Solid Benign Neoplasm	Hemangioma Focal Nodular hyperplasia Hepatic adenoma Miscellaneous Adenomatous hyperplasia Nodular regenerative hyperplasia Mesenchymal hamartomas Fatty tumors of the liver Benign fibrous tumors and others
	Solid Malignant Neoplasm	Hepatocellular Carcinoma Cholangiocarcinoma Metastatic colorectal cancer Metastatic neuroendocrine Metastatic non-colorectal non-neuroendocrine
Cystic	Cystic Benign Neoplasm	Simple cyst Cystadenoma Adult Polycystic liver disease Bile duct cyst
	Cystic Malignant Neoplasm	Cystadenocarcinoma

Solid Benign Tumors

Benign liver lesions are present in nearly 9% of the population. These are twice more common than malignant lesions. The most common benign liver neoplasm is a hemangioma. Benign neoplasms are commonly found incidentally. Surgical intervention is usually not indicated as majority of benign liver neoplasms tend to have an indolent course. However few lesions lead to complications or become malignant. Hence solid benign tumors will require pathological evaluation and a resection may need to be planned. Commonly seen solid benign tumors may include hemangiomas, hepatic adenomas, and focal nodular hyperplasia, among many others.

HEMANGIOMA

Incidence and Etiopathology

Hemangiomas are the most prevalent benign tumors seen in the liver. They arise from the endothelial lining of the blood vessels. Incidence is reported anywhere from 2% to 20%. These tumors are more prevalent in women with a female to male ratio as high as 6:1.[17] Common ages at presentation varies between 30 to 70 years. It is also commonly found in infants and children. Risk factors include exposure to high estrogen levels during puberty, pregnancy, oral contraceptive use, and androgen treatment. Grossly, the tumor is well circumscribed, compressible, and dark colored. Microscopically, the tumor is composed of various large vascular channels that are lined with a single layer of endothelial cells supported by collagenous walls that branch off the hepatic artery.

Adult hemangiomas vary from a few millimeters to up to twenty centimeters in size and are most prevalent in the right liver, in a subcapsular location. Small, capillary hemangiomas are insignificant compared to large, cavernous lesions. Lesions larger than 5 cm are called as giant hemangiomas and are commonly associated with focal nodular hyperplasia. Some lesions can undergo involution or thrombosis leading to a dense fibrotic mass which can be difficult to distinguish from malignant lesions. Pediatric hemangiomas are typically multifocal and produce pressure effect on surrounding organs. Larger lesions may lead to congestive heart failure due to hyperdynamic circulation. Large symptomatic hemangiomas are treated by either angiographic embolization or surgical resection.[18] However, most pediatric hemangiomas that are asymptomatic often regress and do not require intervention.

Clinical Presentation

Most lesions that are smaller than 5 cm are asymptomatic. Symptoms vary based on the size and location. Patients with giant, subcapsular lesions present with vague abdominal pain due to stretching of the Glisson's capsule. Rapid expansion or acute thrombosis leads to clinical presentation of acute abdomen. Kasabach-Merritt, a syndrome of thrombocytopenia and consumptive coagulopathy, is rare, but well-documented. Spontaneous rupture of liver hemangiomas leading to hemodynamic instability is exceedingly rare.

Diagnosis

LFTs and tumor markers are relatively normal. Radiographic imaging using ultrasound and CT scan can be reliably used to make the diagnosis. Lesions that are a few centimeters in size may need contrast enhanced CT and MRI for making diagnosis. Characteristic features on the contrast enhanced CT include peripheral nodular enhancement and progressive centripetal flow. Areas with contrast pooling can also be visualized as seen in Figure 10. MRI with contrast appears as hypointense on T1 weighted and hyperintense on T2 weighted images. When in doubt, a technetium-99 labeled red blood cell scan can be helpful. Percutaneous biopsy is rarely needed and may potentially lead to bleeding complications.

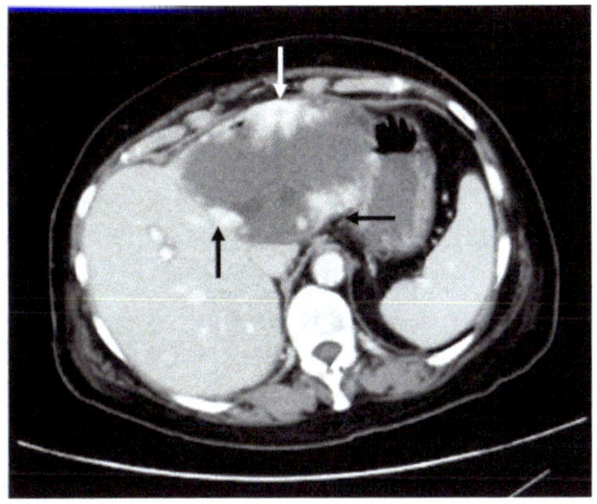
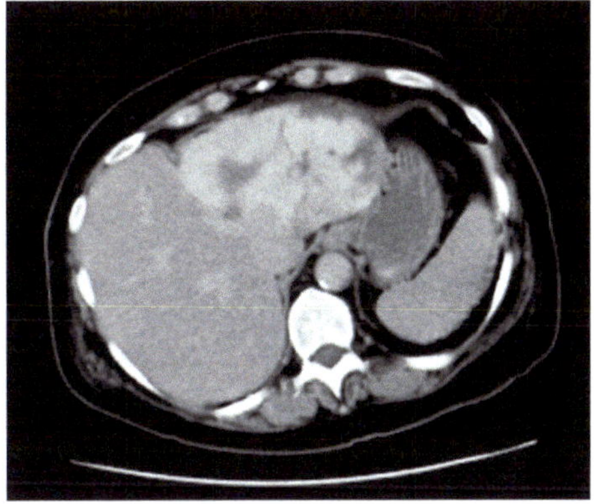

Figure 10. (A) CT Scan demonstrating liver hemangioma, peripheral nodular enhancement and (B) contrast pooling

Management

As most of these lesions are asymptomatic and small, hemangiomas never require resection. Large and symptomatic lesions and lesions that are difficult to differentiate will require resection. For small and peripherally located lesions, simple enucleation or wedge resection can be performed. These lesions can be approached laparoscopically when facilities are available. Lesions that are large and centrally located may require anatomic resection, with vascular inflow control during surgery and preoperative angio-embolization to decrease intraoperative blood loss. Various energy devices including argon beam coagulator and hydro-jet dissector are important adjuncts. For large lesions that are technically unresectable, transplantation is an option.

Outcome

Resection of hemangioma is associated with overall low morbidity and mortality. Lesions that are deemed benign based on radiographic features can be followed up with serial imaging. There are no guidelines as to how closely they need to be followed up. Lesions that are rapidly expanding, and those that do not have characteristic features of hemangiomas should undergo further imaging to rule out other processes including malignancy.

FOCAL NODULAR HYPERPLASIA

Incidence and Etiopathology

Focal nodular hyperplasia (FNH) is the second most prevalent benign hepatic neoplasm. They are considered to be a non-neoplastic hyperplastic response to congenital vascular malformation. Etiology is unknown. They are present in 3% of general population. As with hemangiomas, women are more commonly affected than men with a female-to-male ratio between 6:1 and 8:1. The mean age of presentation is during the fourth decade of life. Risk factors include oral contraceptive use which causes the tumors to grow rapidly. However, contraceptive pills do not predispose to FNH, unlike in hepatic adenoma.[19]

Grossly, FNH are well-circumscribed, non-encapsulated, lobulated tumors. Both lobes of the liver are equally involved. Microscopically, they consist of benign-appearing hepatocytes with cords of fibrous septae radiating from a central scar. The central scar consists of a large artery branching into many smaller arteries in a "spoke wheel" pattern, as shown in Figures 2 and 3. The central scar can often be visualized on imaging studies. In 15% of the cases, this central scar may be absent.

Clinical Presentation

Most patients are asymptomatic. FNHs are usually small nodular masses, less than five centimeters in size, and are found near the hepatic surface. Most common symptoms include vague abdominal pain which is often in the epigastric or right upper quadrant. Occasionally patients report resolution of their symptoms with stopping the use of oral contraceptive pills. Rarely does rupture, bleeding, or infarction occur. Malignant degeneration of FNH has not yet been reported.

Diagnosis

Biochemical tests may be normal. Mild liver function abnormalities have been reported. The serum tumor markers AFP and CEA are not elevated. On ultrasound, FNH appears as a well-demarcated homogenous lesion with a hyperechoic band. Contrast enhanced CT and MRI can diagnose with great accuracy due to the characteristic central stellate scar and "spoke wheel pattern" (Figure 11). As mentioned earlier these features may be absent in some cases. FNH lesions must be differentiated from other lesions because management varies, especially when treating the malignant ones. Nuclear imaging can sometimes be helpful to distinguish FNH from hepatic adenoma because sulfa-colloid is taken up by Kupffer cells that are present in FNH, which are usually absent in adenoma. Further, on angiography, FNH displays a characteristic "spoke-wheel" pattern.[20] Percutaneous biopsy is not often recommended. Surgical resection is recommended for definitive diagnosis.

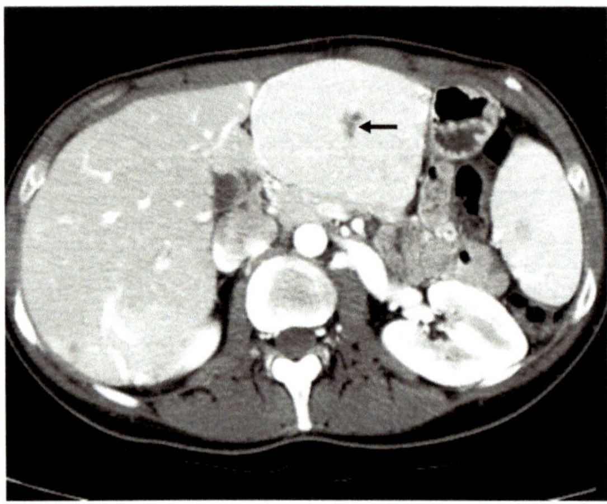

Figure 11. CT scan demonstrating FNH with central stellate scar

Management

Patients with definitive diagnosis and who are asymptomatic do not require further treatment. These patients are followed with routine radiological surveillance every one to two years. Surveillance is stopped after two years if there is no change in size or character of the lesion. In symptomatic patients or in cases of diagnostic uncernity, open or laparoscopic surgical resection is indicated.[21] Transarterial embolization can also be used as an alternative when resection is not possible. For FNH patients who use oral contraceptives, it is controversial whether to recommend discontinuation of the oral contraceptive pills.

Outcome

Lesions that have been diagnosed as FNH can be followed serially with imaging or observed. Lesions that cause symptoms, show evidence of growth, and/or with diagnosis dilemma should be resected for pathological evaluation.

HEPATIC ADENOMA

Incidence and Etiopathology

Hepatic adenoma is a rare proliferation of benign hepatocytes. Its incidence varies between 1 per 100,000 in the general population compared to 3 to 4 per 100,000 populations in those who use oral contraceptives. Again, it is more commonly found in women with a female to male ratio of 11:1. It commonly occurs in women who are 20 to 40 years of age. 70-80% of hepatic adenomas are solitary in nature but benign adenomatosis (ten or more lesions) have also been reported. Risk factors include long term high estrogen use, androgen steroid use, diabetes mellitus, type III glycogen storage disease, type I von Gierke's disease (50%).[22]

Grossly hepatic adenomas are well circumscribed, round, and unencapsulated. A pseudo-capsule is often present. Lesions usually measure 5 to 20 centimeters in size. Intramural fat, necrosis, and hemorrhage are often observed. Microscopically these are hyper-vascular tumors characterized by benign proliferation of bile-producing hepatocytes, but no bile ducts. Hepatocytes may contain fat, glycogen, and occasional calcifications. The liver's normal architecture is lost.

Clinical Presentation

Nearly 75% of patients with hepatic adenoma have symptomatic presentation. Symptoms could be non-specific vague upper abdominal pain, discomfort and fullness, or acute severe abdominal pain due to hemorrhage related to intra-tumoral bleeding or tumor rupture. Intraperitoneal rupture with bleeding, especially with tumors >5cm in size, is more common than intra-tumoral bleeding, leads to presentation with hemodynamic instability in women of childbearing age. These patients may need emergent operation. Angio-embolization, where available, is usually the first step to temporize the bleeding, in a hemodynamically stable patient.

In patients with hypovolemic shock secondary to bleeding, resuscitation will blood transfusion and laparatomy is performed to resect the tumor. These lesions carry a higher risk of rupture during pregnancy and thus should be resected prior to any pregnancy. Women who are on oral contraceptives can also present with vague abdominal pain or discomfort. Occasionally there is complete resolution of the symptoms is noted after discontinuation of oral contraceptive pills. Unlike FNH, hepatic adenoma lesions are at risk of malignant transformation. The true risk remains unknown and may be related to the size.

Diagnosis

LFTs and serum tumor markers are not elevated unless there is malignant transformation. Hepatic adenomas on ultrasound have variable characteristics from hypoechoic to mixed echoic patterns. All lesions appear hyper-vascular. CT characteristics are heterogeneous. On contrast enhanced CT, tumor appears hyperintense on arterial phase and peripheral enhancement with centripetal progression on delayed venous phase (Figure 12). On T1 and T2 weighted MRIs, these often appear as hyperintense.

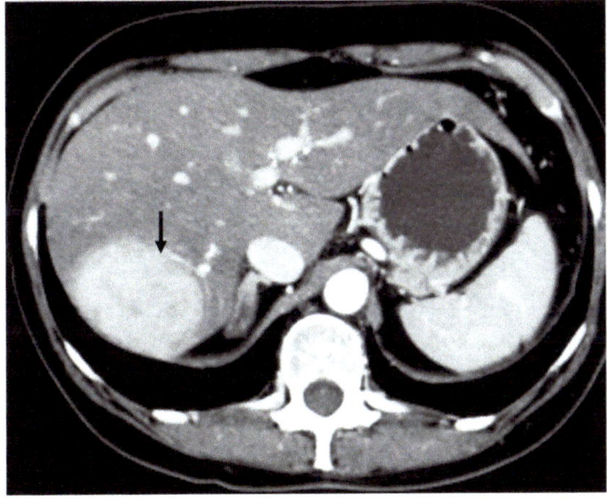

Figure 12. CT Scan demonstrating hepatic adenoma

Management

Generally, hepatic adenomas require resection due to their increased risk of spontaneous rupture, malignant transformation, and indistinguishable from well-differentiated hepatocellular carcinoma. However, in small, asymptomatic hepatic adenomas (<3cm), discontinuation of estrogen, follow-up with surveillance imaging, and serial alpha-fetoprotein measurements can also be considered for management. Surgical treatment options range from enucleation, resection, hepatic artery embolization, and transplantation.[23] Non-anatomic resection is an effective treatment modality and surgeons should aim for 1 cm margin. Anatomic resection is also satisfactory. For tumors with active hemorrhage, hepatic artery embolization should be undertaken as acute treatment. After a period of recovery, the patient may be taken back for formal resection.

Outcome

In small lesions, or those influenced by patient factors, serial imaging and tumor markers should be used. Patients who are of childbearing age should have the lesion resected prior to pregnancy. Adenomatosis are more likely to be diffuse and carry a higher risk of malignant transformation. These are better approached with multi-modality treatments.

Miscellaneous Benign Solid Neoplasms

Patients with existing chronic liver disease may develop adenomatous hyperplasia, a single or multiple, well circumscribed, surface nodule(s). These lesions have very few distinguishing factors from HCC and vary in malignant potential.

Nodular regenerative hyperplasia (NRH) is a rare, diffuse micronodular condition, linked to portal hypertension and chronic systemic diseases. NRH is typically smaller than 1.5 cm in size, with no malignant potential and not related to liver cirrhosis. In doubtful cases percutaneous biopsy is indicated to rule out malignancy.

Mesenchymal hamartoma of the liver (MHL) is a large cystic hepatic tumor that occurs in children. These tumors are rare and only account for approximately 5% of pediatric hepatic tumors. Surgical resection is offered for large lesions are causing significant local pressure effects.

Fatty liver tumors are rare and include primary lipomas, myelolipoma (a lipoma that contains hematopoietic tissue), angiolipoma (a lipoma that contains blood vessels), and angiomyolipoma (a lipoma that contains smooth muscle).

Benign fibrous tumors of the liver must be resected as they grow and become symptomatic. Inflammatory pseudotumors are localized, unregulated mass of inflammatory cells which mimicking neoplastic lesions. Leiomyomas, myxomas, schwannomas, lymphangiomas, and teratomas, are a few other uncommon benign hepatic tumors. Intrahepatic biliary cystadenomas, also referred to as bile duct adenomas, although extremely rare have been reported to cause biliary symptoms in some patients. During an abdominal exploratory surgery, biliary hamartomas or biliary hyperplasia will commonly appear as tiny white surface lesions mimicking smaller metastatic tumors. Ectopic pancreatic tissue and adrenal rest tumors are also prevalent.

Solid Malignant Neoplasms

Malignant neoplasms of the liver are classified as primary or secondary. Primary neoplasms arise from the liver and the bile ducts, whereas secondary neoplasms are metastatic in origin. Primary neoplasms include hepatocellular carcinoma, cholangiocarcinoma (intrahepatic), and other rare tumors. The most common secondary neoplasms are colorectal and neuroendocrine in origin. Tumors that are non-colorectal and non-neuroendocrine in origin are not uncommon.

HEPATOCELLULAR CARCINOMA

Incidence and Etiopathology

Hepatocellular Carcinoma (HCC) is the most common primary liver malignancy. The incidence of HCC is strongly related to the incidence of hepatitis C infection. There is a rapid increase in HCC with an increase in hepatitis C infections. Epidemiological studies have also shown a strong association with environmental factors. Thus, the incidence is greater in Southeast Asian countries. There has been a significant increase in HCC in the United States with both the higher incidence of hepatitis C infections and increased number of immigrants. More than 16,000 people in the United States are expected to die from HCC yearly. HCC occurs commonly in 6th and 7th decade of life and is more common in males compared to females. Risk factors include hepatitis B and C infections, cirrhosis, smoking, alcohol, and certain genetic diseases.[24] The risk of HCC is higher in chronic carriers of hepatitis B and C virus.

HCC is a complex multifactorial disease. HBV infected individuals have an increased risk of developing HCC. The HBV infection leads to chronic inflammation, cirrhosis, and then HCC. The longer the duration of exposure to HBV, the higher the risk of developing HCC. HCV related HCC is most likely due to chronic inflammation and cirrhosis. Increased DNA replication rates are correlated to HCC development. Patients that chronically abuse alcohol and smoke also have an increased the likelihood of developing HCC. Alcohol causes cirrhosis acting as a cocarcinogen. Aflatoxin is a hepatotoxin, which arises from the Aspergillus fungi species. Chronic carcinogenic exposure to aflatoxin, further increases the risk of developing HCC.[25] Other chemicals that have been implicated as carcinogens related to HCC include nitrites, hydrocarbons, solvents, pesticides, and vinyl chloride. Wilson's disease, α1-antitrypsin deficiency, glycogen storage disease, porphyria cutanea tarda and hereditary hemochromatosis are additional hereditary metabolic liver diseases associated with HCC.

Clinical Presentation

Most common clinical presentation is vague right upper abdominal pain associated with weight loss. Some patients may present with a palpable abdominal mass. In advanced cases constitutional symptoms such as anorexia, nausea, lethargy, and weight loss are common. Patients with cirrhosis may develop hepatic decompensation. Rarely these can rupture leading to hemodynamic instability. Both the hepatic vein and portal vein thrombosis can add complexity to the clinical presentation.

Diagnosis

Imaging is extremely important in diagnosis, staging, and assessment of the tumors for resectability. Care must be taken in assessment of the residual liver function if resection is planned. Contrast enhanced CT and MRI supplement each other in diagnosis and staging. HCC shows characteristic arterial enhancement on contrast imaging; thus, biopsy of these lesions is usually not necessary (Figure 13). In preoperative planning, it is critical to evaluate the extent of the lesion, other associated lesions, peritoneal metastases, nodal metastases, and extent of vascular and biliary involvement. Serum tumor marker alpha fetoprotein (AFP) is elevated in more than half of the patients and it is also useful in monitoring for recurrence. Liver biopsy for diagnosis is not required in patients with HCC risk factors and radiology features characteristic of HCC, regardless of AFP levels, and are potential candidates for curative surgery.[26] After a diagnosis has been made based on the CT, MRI, and AFP, every effort should be made to stage the tumor. Various HCC staging systems have been developed, but none have demonstrated superiority or effectiveness over others. The TNM and Okuda staging systems are as shown in Table 4.

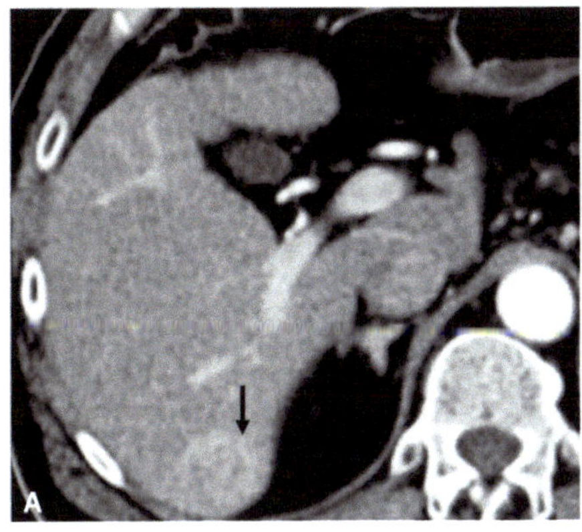

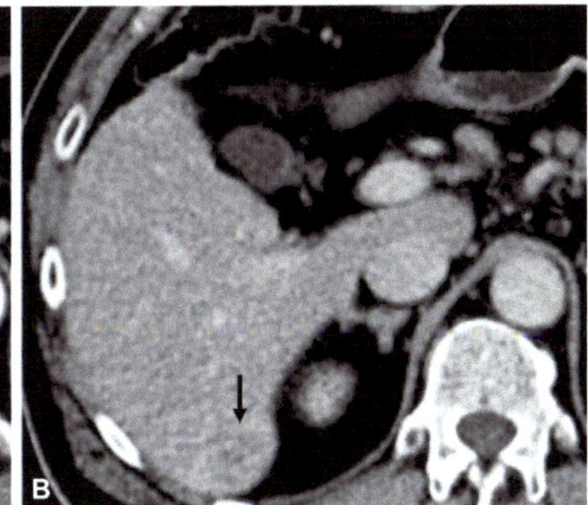

Figure 13. CT scan demonstrating HCC, enhancement in arterial phase (A), washout delayed phase (B)

Table 4: TNM Classification 8th Edition 2017

Primary Tumor (T)

TX	Cannot assess primary tumor
T0	Primary tumor not evident
T1	Solitary tumor, no vascular invasion
T2	Multiple tumors all <5 cm, solitary tumor with positive vascular invasion
T3a	Multiple tumors >5 cm
T3b	Involvement of a major portal vein branch or hepatic vein, can be single or multiple tumors of any size
T4	Tumor(s) directly invading adjacent organs not including the gallbladder, or with perforation of visceral peritoneum

Regional Lymph Nodes (N)

NX	Unable to assess regional lymph nodes
N0	No metastasis to regional lymph node
N1	Metastasis to regional lymph node

Distant Metastasis (M)

M0	No distant metastasis
M1	Presence of distant metastasis

Staging

Stage	T	N	M
I	1	0	0
II	2	0	0
IIIA	3a	0	0
IIIB	3b	0	0
IIIC	4	0	0
IVA	Any	1	0
IVB	Any	Any	1

Management

Patients with HCC have various options for treatment, as listed in Table 5. Various treatment strategies are available in the management of HCC allowing clinicians to tailor the therapy based on individual patient, including surgical resection, tumor ablation, intra-arterial chemo-radiotherapy, and immunotherapy to improve survival.

Surgical resection with negative margins offers highest survival benefits. Patients with unresectable tumors or those at high risk for surgery may benefit from liver transplant. However, only 10-20% of the patients with HCC are candidates for curative resection. Liver resection should be considered after careful assessment of future liver remnant (FLR) or functional liver reserve. In a normal healthy individual major liver resection is safe if FLR is at least 20%, however in post chemotherapy patients or patients with hepatitis or steatohepatitis the FLR has to be at least 30-60% and up to 40%-70% in patients with cirrhosis. Partial hepatectomy mortality rates range between 1-20%. Recent surgical advancements have developed techniques for limited segmental resections, in eligible patients. Overall survival rates for HCC patients after curative resection are as follows, 58-100% at one year, 11-75% at five years, and 19-26% at ten years. Various prognostic factors, as shown in Table 6, are assessed in predicting post-resection survival rates. The most frequently reported negative prognostic factors are cirrhosis, tumor size >5cm, vascular invasion, infiltrative growth pattern, multifocal tumors, intrahepatic metastases, lymph nose metastases, margins less than 1 centimeter, and infiltration of liver capsule. The most effective treatment of HCC would be a liver transplant, which would help maintain liver function, as well as significantly decrease the recurrence rate of HCC. Milan criteria are universally followed to select patients for liver transplantation. Patients qualifying for liver transplant should have a solitary tumor <5cm or 2-3 tumor lesions each less <3cm and Child-Pugh class B or Child-

Pugh class C liver cirrhosis. Both the requirement of chronic immunosuppression and scarce number of organ donors limit transplantation. In addressing the scarcity of organ donors, an increasing recent interest of performing partial hepatectomy from live donors, while controversial, could decrease the gap of supply and demand. Recent studies have shown long-term survival rates of 25-75% following liver transplant for HCC.

Table 5: Treatment Options in Patients with HCC

Surgical Interventions
• Hepatic Resection
• Orthotropic Liver Transplant
Liver Ablation
• Percutaneous Ethanol Injection (PEI)
• Percutaneous Injection of Acetic acid
• Thermal Ablation (cryotherapy, radiofrequency ablation, microwave)
Trans Arterial
• Chemoembolization
• Embolization
Radiotherapy
Combination of Trans Arterial and Ablative Therapies
External Beam Radiation Therapy (EBRT)
Systemic Immunotherapy

Table 6: Prognostic factors in patients with hepatocellular carcinoma

Alpha fetoprotein (AFP)
Fibrosis score
Hepatitis serology
Creatinine (part of the Model for End Stage Liver Disease (MELD) score)
Bilirubin (part of MELD score)
Prothrombin time international normalized ratio (INR) (part of the MELD score)

Nonsurgical local ablative therapy involves percutaneous ethanol injection (PEI), a technique that rapidly dehydrates smaller sized tumors. By combining techniques of cellular dehydration, coagulative necrosis, and vascular thrombosis, complete tumor necrosis may be achieved. A single PEI treatment is capable of ablating tumors smaller than 2cms, however larger tumors would need multiple PEI treatments. For tumors smaller than five centimeters, PEI treatments have shown to have long-term survival rates ranging from 24-40%. Another technique similar to PEI is percutaneous injection of acetic acid. This technique has exceptional necrotizing capabilities and is preferred for ablating septated tumors. Recently, such thermal ablative techniques with freezing or heating abilities are becoming increasingly preferred for ablating tumors. Cryotherapy is a laparoscopic procedure, sometimes using percutaneous techniques, in which a specialized cryoprobe is used to freeze and thaw tumors and their neighboring tissues, causing necrosis.[27] The ball of ice that forms by cryotherapy may easily be monitored using an ultrasound. However, cryotherapy induces a "heat-sink" effect, which limits freezing near major blood vessels, and has a higher complication rate, ranging from 8-14%.

Radiofrequency ablation (RFA) is a minimally invasive and low-risk technique that heats a probe using high frequency alternating currents, to temperatures above 60°C, resulting in immediate cell death. This procedure was initially used for only small tumors. However, technological advancements have allowed RFA probes to ablate tumors up to seven centimeters in size. RFA may be performed percutaneously under image guidance for anterior tumors or laparoscopic/ open technique under intra-operative ultrasound guidance for tumors at a difficult location that are not accessible percutaneously. RFA does not ablate tumors close to blood vessels due to heat sink effect.[28]

Trans-arterial therapy for HCC is an effective form of therapy for unresectable HCC, since tumors derive majority of blood supply from hepatic artery and tumors are hypervascular compared to surrounding liver parenchyma. This therapy is based in three main principles, infusing chemotherapy directly into hepatic artery, injecting drug eluding beads, injecting bland beads, and injecting radiation beads. There have been few studies on hepatic arterial infusion chemotherapy that use 5-fluorouracil–based compounds, doxorubicin, and cisplatin. Trans-arterial chemotherapy is delivered via hepatic arterial infusion pump, which is placed by performing laparotomy The response rate with this approach is 25-60%. The risk of hepatotoxicity during the implantation of the pump limits the use of trans-arterial therapy as a common treatment option. Trans-arterial chemoembolization involves injecting drug eluding beads into the hepatic artery, cisplatin and doxorubicin are the commonly used drugs. The hepatic artery is accessed via a peripheral artery. With this approach the effect is twofold, chemotherapeutic agents provide anti-neoplastic effect and the beads will produce ischemic necrosis. Selective oils absorbable by HCC, such as Lipiodol, ethiodized oil, are also under study. Studies that combine intra-arterial injections of I-131 with either Lipiodol injections or Yttrium-90 (Y-90) in glass microspheres have shown impressive response rates, because they allow for localized radiation to HCC. Trans-arterial radiotherapy has promising potential as a primary or adjuvant therapy for HCC.[29]

External beam radiation therapy (EBRT) delivers high-energy radiation doses to the malignant cells. This form of therapy for HCC, however, risks damaging the normal liver parenchyma and other organs surrounding the liver. Dramatic responses may occasionally occur. Due to technological advancements, scientists have developed conformal radiotherapy and breath-gated techniques to improve the response of EBRT.

Systemic chemotherapy uses various anti-cancer agents to target the entire human body. This treatment, however, has shown to be ineffective in treating HCC, with low response rates of less than 20%, over a short duration. Systemic immunotherapy is new line of treatment for advanced HCC patients with well-compensated liver function, who are not amenable to local therapy. Two oral multikinase inhibitors, sorafenib and lenvatinib, are approved by U.S. Food and Drug Administration (FDA) as a first-line treatment. Regorafenib and cabozantinib are approved for second-line treatment in these patients who have progressed on sorafenib.

HCC Variants

Fibrolamellar HCC (FHCC) is a rare HCC variant with significant differences in the clinical and histological features compared to conventional HCC. These tumors typically affect young adult patients lacking history of cirrhosis. FHCC tumors have well-demarcated margins and dense fibrotic bands that form a central scar resembling FNH. FHCC is made up of large polygonal tumor cells that are embedded in laminated fibrous stroma layers. Tumor marker neurotensin levels may be elevated in FHCC patients, however AFP levels are always normal in these patients. Overall, compared to HCC, FHCC has a better prognosis. This may be because FHCC is much more resectable than HCC and lacks chronic liver disease (CLD). Following complete resection, 50% of FHCC patients are expected to have long-term survival outcomes.[30]

Although rare, HCC may occur as a mixed/combined hepatocellular cholangiocarcinoma (cHCC-CC) It is unknown whether the cHCC-CC is result of two separate primary tumors co-exhisting and infiltrating into each other, mixed differentiation of single primary tumor. Compared to the standard HCC, mixed tumors are more likely to have worse prognoses. HCC has a clear cell variant in which the cells consist of a clear cytoplasm, and has better prognosis compared to standard HCC. Another reported variant of HCC is pleomorphic, also known as a giant cell variant, which consists of large polymorphic, multinucleate cells which may have originated from primary hepatic cells. HCC variants showing sarcomatoid differentiation, also known as sarcomatoid HCC or carcinosarcomas, do not produce AFP and present with a higher incidence of metastases. HCC in children accounts for approximately one-fourth of pediatric hepatic tumors.

INTRA-HEPATIC CHOLANGIOCARCINOMA (PERIPHERAL CHOLANGIOCARCINOMA, PCC)

Incidence and Etiopathology

Cholangiocarcinoma is a rare tumor accounting for <2% of all human malignancies. Despite its rarity, cholangiocarcinoma is the most common malignant tumor arising from the epithelium of the biliary tract, accounting for 15% of all primary liver malignancies. It is classified into three broad categories: 1) Peripheral cholangiocarcinoma (intrahepatic tumors) arising from the intrahepatic bile ducts (PCC), 2) Hilar cholangiocarcinoma (Klatskin tumors) arising at the confluence of right and left hepatic ducts and 3) Extrahepatic or Distal cholangiocarcinoma arising from the common bile duct. The majority of cholangiocarcinoma are sporadic, however there are several identifiable risk factors known to predispose to this neoplasm (Table 7). Cholangiocarcinoma follows, hyperplasia-dysplasia-carcinoma sequence.

Table 7. Risk factors associated with the development of Cholangiocarcinoma

General risk factors	Advanced age (>65 yrs) Smoking Obesity Diabetes
Infections	Liver flukes (Opisthorchis viverini, Clonorchis sinensis)[I] Viral infection (human immunodeficiency virus, hepatitis B virus, hepatitis C virus, Epstein-Barr virus)
Toxin exposure	Thoroium oxide (contrast dye) Dioxin Nitrosamines Asbestos Polyvinyl chloride Heavy alcohol consumption
Chronic inflammatory diseases	Primary sclerosing cholangitis (PSC)[II] Hepatolithiasis (Oriental Cholangiohepatitis, recurrent pyogenic cholangitis)[I] Liver cirrhosis
Congenital liver anomalies	Fibrocystic liver diseases (eg. Caroli's disease) Anomalous pancreaticobiliary junction Choledochal cyst
Post-surgical	Biliary-enteric anastomosis

Clinical Presentation

Abdominal pain is the most common symptom with jaundice being the second most common, however most patients present with nonspecific symptoms such as abdominal pain, jaundice, fever, malaise, and weight loss. Patients in endemic regions typically present in the 4th decade of life, whereas patients in non-endemic regions present in the 7th decade of life. PCC is more common in (1.7:1) and is nearly always clinically silent until late stages of disease making early diagnosis difficult.

Diagnosis

There no specific laboratory test for PCC, however patients may have abnormal LFTs, elevated tumor markers like CEA and CA 19-9. Ultrasound (US) is the most common initial radiologic investigation there are no specific sonographic features to distinguish PCC from other solid intrahepatic mass lesions. Commonly, PPC appears as solitary or multiple mass lesions, but they may also appear as diffuse abnormal liver echotexture displaying hypo, hyper or mixed echogenicity. On the CT scan PCC appears as hypointense irregular large mass, slight contrast enhancement at the periphery, and focal intrahepatic bile ductal dilatation. PCC have a characteristic delayed enhancement from the periphery to center, on dynamic CT scan. On MR imaging PCC appears as irregular large mass with low intensity on T1-weighted images and high intensity on T2-weighted images, with minimal to moderate tumor rim enhancement of the tumors. On dynamic MR imaging the tumor shows progressive and concentric filling with contrast material. Flurodeoxyglucose positron emission tomography (FDG-PET) is a valuable tool to identify satellite nodules, lymph node and systemic metastases, especially when combined with CT scan images by fusion techniques.

Management

Surgical resection with negative margins offers highest survival benefit. The extent of resection depends on the location of the tumor, vascular involvement, and lymph node status. To achieve tumor free margins, hepatic resections are tailored according to local tumor burden. The resectability rate for PCC varies between 50 to 100% and likely reflects selection and treatment bias. Ideal candidates for curative resection are those with: 1) solitary lesion, 2) no evidence of lymph node metastases and 3) those in whom > 1 cm tumor free margin is deemed achievable. There is no role for neo-adjuvant therapy in patients who resectable disease, however adjuvant chemotherapy with Gemcitabine with Oxaliplatin or Capecitabine has shown improved survival following surgical resection with negative margins or microscopically positive margins. Similarly, there is no role for external beam radiation therapy in PCC. Liver directed therapies like trans-arterial chemoembolization, trans-arterial radioembolization are reserved for patients with unresectable tumors. With multimodality treatment approaches PCC patients have a 5-year survival of up to 100% with Stages I and II disease and 46.9% for patients with stage III disease. Stage IV disease carries a poor prognosis with 1-year and 3-year survival of 24% and 6%, respectively. Regardless of stage, survival of patients with PCC who are not candidates for curative interventions is poor with a median survival of 5 to 14 months and a 1-year survival in the range of 11.8% to 36.1%.[36]

Other Primary Malignant Neoplasms

Hepatoblastoma is the most prevalent malignant hepatic tumors in children, with fifty to seventy new cases reported annually in the U.S. Most cases of hepatoblastoma occur before three years of age, with a median age of eighteen months. Hepatoblastomas have been associated with familial polyposis syndrome. These hepatic tumors originate from fetal or embryonic hepatocytes and commonly consist of mesenchymal elements. These hepatic tumors will commonly disguise themselves to appear as an asymptomatic mass. Children with hepatoblastoma tumors may have mild anemia or thrombocytosis. Serum AFP elevation is an effective marker of progressing treatment. Surgical resection with negative margins offers highest survival benefits, in resectable tumors. In unresectable tumors neo-adjuvant chemotherapy is given to downstage the tumor and facilitate surgical resection to improve survival. Adjuvant radiation may have a role in patients with positive resection margins. Patients without existing metastatic diseases or anaplastic variants have 60 to 70% long-term survival rates following complete resection. Around half of the patients diagnosed with pulmonary metastases may be cured with surgical resection of the hepatic tumor and/or pulmonary metastases, and chemotherapy treatments. Trans-arterial chemoembilization and radioembolization have been used to either downstage the tumor for to increase chances or resectability or as a primary modality of treatment in unresectable tumors. Liver transplant is a viable option in unresectable pediatric hepatoblastoma patients with 70% to 80% post-transplant survival rates.

Angiosarcomas are primary hepatic sarcomas presenting in children as numerous hepatic masses and are associated with vinyl chloride or Thorotrast exposure. Primary hepatic angiosarcomas have very low long-term survival rates. Various other sarcomas contribute to primary hepatic malignancy in pediatric patients, including embryonic sarcomas, leiomyosarcomas, primary hepatic rhabdoid tumors, and malignant fibrous histiocytomas. Primary hepatic rhabdoid tumors and embryonic sarcomas are most prevalent in pediatrics. Non-Hodgkin's lymphoma, another rare primary hepatic lymphoma, may occur in the liver regardless of existing extrahepatic diseases. Hepatic non-Hodgkin's lymphoma is amenable to systemic chemotherapy and surgical resection is reserved for unresectable tumors

Primary hepatic neuroendocrine tumors are difficult to distinguish from metastatic lesions most likely due to both the liver being prone to metastases and the extrahepatic primary tumors being radiologically occult. Malignant germ cell tumors, such as choriocarcinomas, teratomas, and yolk sac tumors primarily occur in pediatrics, but are extremely rare. Another rare malignant vascular tumor of the liver is epithelioid hemangioendothelioma, which presents itself in the form of multiple bilateral hepatic masses. These tumors are prevalent in approximately one-fourth of patients and have unpredictable clinical behaviors. A majority of epithelioid hemangioendotheliomas cases led to liver failure and death, however, liver transplants have been reported as successful forms of treatment for these tumors.

METASTATIC TUMORS

Colorectal

Only twenty percent of patients with colorectal metastasis are eligible for a potentially curative liver resection (Figure 14). Upon diagnosis, patients with synchronous metastatic disease of the primary colorectal cancer on preoperative imaging or at laparotomy may also undergo simultaneous resection with curative intent. Elevated LFTs including ALP, GGT, and lactate dehydrogenase (LDH) are seen. Combining contrast-enhanced CT scans with triphasic techniques has been reported to produce the most sensitive study. On contrast CT scan these lesions show enhancement in arterial phase (Figure 15). MRI scans have highest sensitivity and specificity in identifying metastatic lesions. On MRI these lesions appear hypointense on T1-weighted images and hyperintense on T2-weighted images, with arterial enhancement on contrast images. Patients with hepatic colorectal metastasis who are eligible for surgical resection benefit from contrast MRI of the abdomen to identify all the metastatic lesions. If the last screening exam was performed over a year ago, a colonoscopy is also required to ensure the absence of metachronous lesions or local recurrence.[31] Additionally, complete metastatic workup includes contrast CT chest, abdominal and pelvis. For hepatic colorectal metastases, solely using systemic chemotherapy would be largely ineffective, as median survival rate by this approach is approximately twelve months, with a 20-30% partial response rate. Recent advancements in chemotherapeutic agents, such as irinotecan (CPT-11) and oxaliplatin, have shown significantly impressive response rates. These chemotherapeutic agents have gained recent approval as treatment for metastatic colorectal cancers. However, they do not largely impact the survival rates for patients. Memorial Sloan-Kettering Cancer Center (MSKCC) performed a series of 1001 hepatic resections. This multivariate analysis helped to pinpoint the five most influential factors, including the size of the tumors being greater than five centimeters, disease-free interval of less than one-year, multiple tumors, lymph nose-positive primary lesions, and a CEA greater than 200 ng/mL. Metastatic colorectal cancers have a high chance of recurrence, which results in death for most patients. Around 50% of recurrent cases are solely hepatic. Only five percent of recurrent patients are eligible for a second hepatic resection, with a 30-40% five-year survival rate. Following hepatic resection, patients who are candidates for advanced therapeutic interventions must undergo serial CEA and imaging studies which detect early and potentially treatable recurrence. Hepatic arterial infusion (HAI) is form of adjuvant therapy offered in conjunction with systemic chemotherapy at highly specialized centers. Centers offering HAI have demonstrated durable response rates because hepatic tumors obtain most of their blood supply from the hepatic artery. By regionally infusing chemotherapy agents, such as fluorodeoxyuridine (FUDR), the hepatic extraction rate increases by approximately 90 percent. HAI deliver high concentrations of chemotherapeutic agents, while maintaining minimum systemic toxicity. When compared to traditional systemic therapies, HAI therapies have a significantly higher response rate. MSKCC performed a trial which compared systemic chemotherapy, HAI therapy, and systemic chemotherapy using 5-fluorouracil with and without leucovorin only. This trial showed recurrence rates of 9% and 36%, which are significantly low, along with a two-year survival rate of 86%, versus 72%. Thermal ablative techniques, like cryoablation or RFA are used to expand hepatic resection limitations. Combining hepatic resection, cryoablation, and preserved hepatic parenchyma may eradicate numerous bilobar tumors. Sufficient long-term data collection using this approach remains in progress.

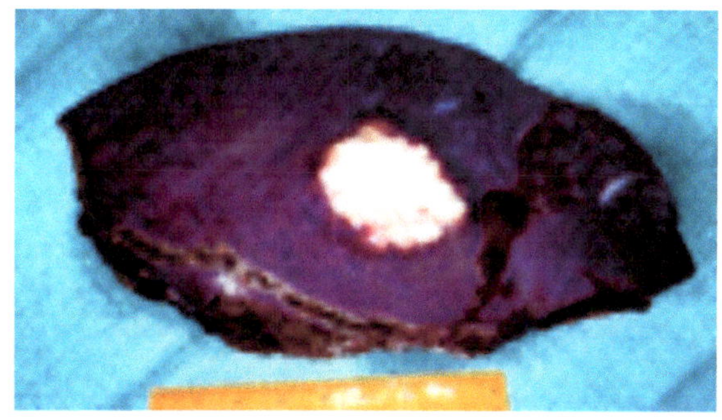

Figure 14. Resected colorectal metastasis

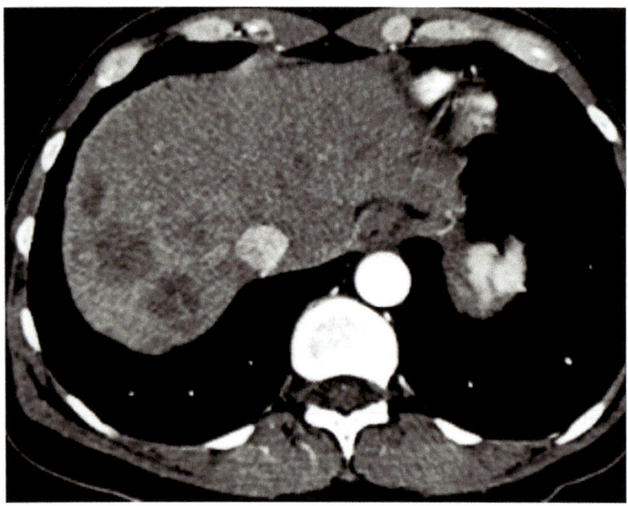

Figure 15. CT scan demonstrating colorectal liver metastases

Neuroendocrine

Tumors with high tendencies of metastasizing to the liver are glucagonomas, somatostatinomas, gastrinomas, and nonfunctional neuroendocrine tumors. Carcinoid tumors and insulinomas have lower tendencies of metastasizing to the liver. Most of these tumors are slow-growing and indolent. Oftentimes, the goal of treatment is to improve quality of life rather than to improve survival. These indolent tumors can only withstand therapies with minimal mortality, which may be achieved in experienced hepatobiliary units. For patients who have with recalcitrant symptoms of hormonal excess after having undergone failed therapy, surgery is a more promising form of treatment. Cytoreductive surgery is shown to improve long-term survival in selected patients, if 90% of the tumor burden is removed without increase in the peri-operative morbidity. Neuroendocrine tumors do not require formal resections with wide margins. Enucleations or wedge resections, as well as thermo-ablative treatments, which include cryoablation and radiofrequency ablation, are also adequate treatment options.[32] Sufficient long-term data collection using laparoscopic RFA remains in progress.

Non-colorectal and Non-neuroendocrine

Metastasis from primary tumors include breast, lung, melanoma, soft tissue sarcoma, Wilms' tumor, ocular melanoma, gastric, pancreas, esophagus, gallbladder, adrenocortical, urologic tumors, and gynecologic tumors (uterine, cervix, and ovarian). When treating these tumors, general principles should be followed in the comparison of isolated liver metastases to metastatic colorectal cancer. In patients with extrahepatic systemic metastasis and short disease-free intervals, a poor prognosis can be expected. Treating genitourinary tumors with hepatic resections in select patients has improved outcomes. Other rare tumors with isolated liver metastasesinclude sarcomas, melanomas, and breast cancers. Liver resection is a viable option in cases where there is a disease-free interval and stability period, while on chemotherapeutic agents, over an extensive period of time. In metastatic non-colorectal, non-neuroendocrine tumors, hepatic cytoreductive resection must be considered only in highly selective patients. .[33] In the case that a symptomatic patient, with a reasonable life expectancy, is not a candidate for any of the existing therapies, then liver resection is an effective treatment option.

CYSTIC NEOPLASMS

Simple Cyst

Simple cysts are spherical or ovoid-shaped, solitary cysts containing serous fluid. Simple cysts lack septations and communication with the biliary tree, and can grow up to approximately twenty centimeters., which risks compression of the liver and induces regional atrophy and hypertrophy. On a histological level, simple cysts are lined with a single layer of cuboidal or columnar cells that lack atypia. These cysts are prevalent in adults and are often incidentally found in asymptomatic patients by radiologists. Large simple cysts will occasionally cause symptoms. As shown in Figure 16, CT scans show anatomical correlation, however, ultrasounds are the preferred methods of imaging technology for confirming thin-walled simple cysts. Additionally, cystadenoma, hydatid disease, and metastatic neuroendocrine tumor are critical differential diagnoses to take into consideration. Intracystic hemorrhage is often a common complication to be aware of, but other complications will rarely occur. Only symptomatic simple hepatic cysts require action of treatments, except for the presence of diagnostic uncertainty. As a majority of simple cysts are asymptomatic, prior to associating the symptoms to the cyst, the etiology of the symptoms must be assessed meticulously. Some nonsurgical treatment options include injecting a sclerosing agent and aspiration. Surgical intervention involves fenestration or unroofing the extrahepatic part of the cyst, either by minimally invasive techniques or as an open procedure.[34]

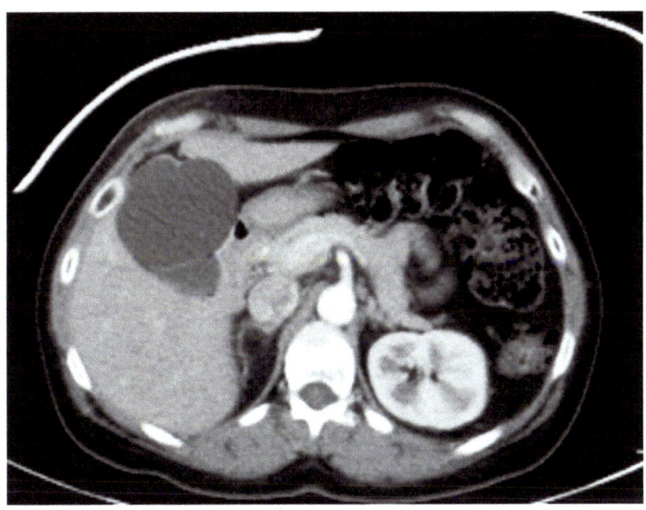

Figure 16. CT scan demonstrating a Simple Cyst

Cystadenoma and Cystadenocarcinoma

Cystadenoma, commonly presented as a large cystic mass, is a rare neoplasm that may reach the size of ten to twenty centimeters. The large cyst has a globular external surface with multiple protruding cysts and locules of varying sizes. These cysts typically contain mucinous fluid. Histologically, the cysts are lined with atypical cuboidal or columnar cells that rest on a basement membrane. Polypoid or papillary projections are commonly made from the epithelium. Hepatic cystadenomas are commonly seen in 5th decade of life with higher incidence in females. Most hepatic cystadenomas are asymptomatic. Symptomatic hepatic cystadenomas may be accompanied by nausea, abdominal pain or distention, and anorexia. If suspected, cross-sectional CT or MRI imaging modalities will assist in differential diagnosis. On ultrasonography, cyst wall thickness, nodularity, septations, and fluid-filled locules may be identified. Contrast enhanced CT scan will show the intensification of the cystic wall and septa. The primary differential diagnosis should include hydatid liver disease. Cystadenomas have a slow growth rate, but they have malignant potential and may transform into cystadenocarcinoma. The presence of large projections and strikingly thick wall indicates malignant degeneration. The complete excision of cystadenoma or cystadenocarcinoma is shown in Figure 17. Any remaining traces of cystadenoma or cystadenocarcinoma will result in recurrence or further development.

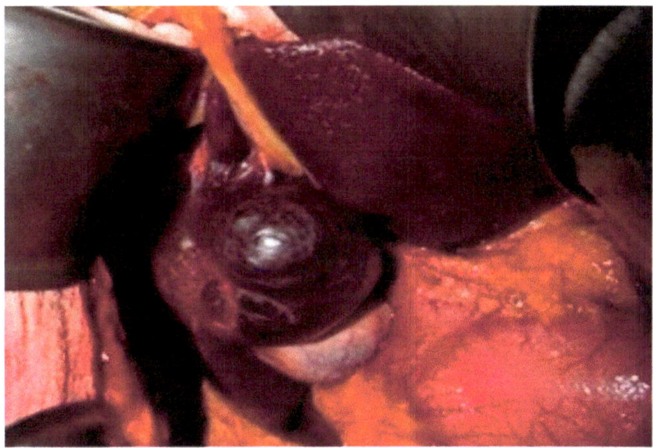

Figure 17. Liver Cyst Intraoperative View

Polycystic Liver Disease (PLD)

Hepatic cysts are most prevalent in patients with autosomal dominant inherited adult polycystic kidney disease. Hepatic cysts resemble simple cysts (as seen above) in appearance, but the number of cysts that occur differentiates the two. In adults with polycystic kidney disease, liver cysts always occur in multiples. Typically, numerous microscopic hepatic and grossly visible macro-cysts can be seen. However, hepatic parenchyma and function are preserved, regardless of the large numbers of liver cysts. Kidney cysts will always precede liver cysts. The prevalence of hepatic cyst in patients with polycystic kidney disease increases with age. Patients below twenty years of age have a 0 percent (%) chance of liver cysts. Patients above the age of 60 years are at a higher risk of liver cysts, at 80 percent (%). Generally, adults with polycystic kidney disease will have asymptomatic liver cysts. Some patients who have cysts numerous cysts larger in size may experience abdominal pain or distention. LFT results will almost always appear normal. Infection or intra-cystic bleeding, although rare, are complications to be aware of. Multiple simple cysts can be seen by ultrasound and CT, throughout the liver and kidneys (Figure 18). Typically, treatments for PLD are reserved for patients experiencing the occurrence of large cysts and complications. Treatments include percutaneous aspiration, with or without sclerotherapy, fenestration by laparotomy or laparoscopy, hepatic resection, or orthotopic liver transplant. Transplants are only performed in patients suffering from progressive diseasing following fenestration or resection, in addition to renal and liver dysfunction. In cases of renal failure, combining kidney and liver transplants could be the most suitable surgical interventions.

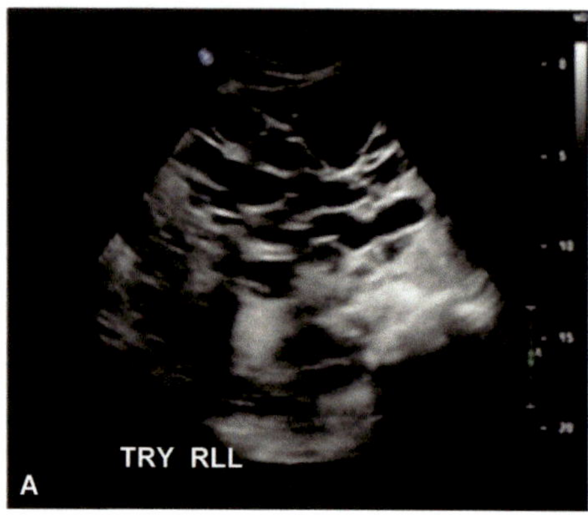

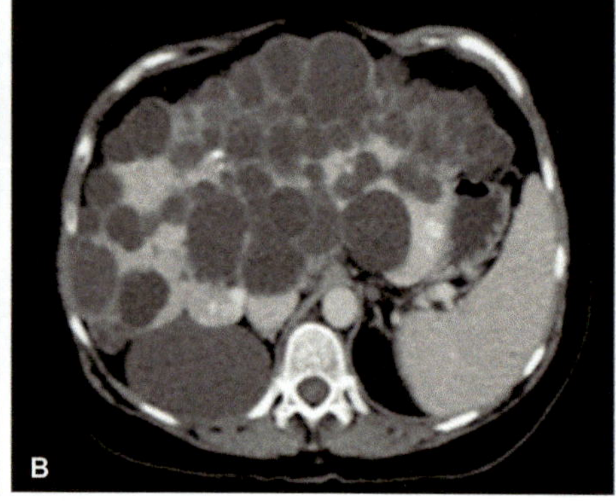

Figure 18. Ultrasound(A) and CT scan(B) demonstrating polycystic liver disease

HAEMOBILIA

Incidence and Etiopathogenesis

Haemobilia is rare condition in which the liver bleeds into the biliary tree due to miscommunication between a blood vessel and the bile duct. There are very limited factors that assist in distinguishing between the haemobilia and gastrointestinal hemorrhage. Haemobilia is most commonly caused by the occurrence of iatrogenic or accidental traumas, cholecystitis, tumors, and inflammatory or vascular disorders. In recent years, iatrogenic trauma has been the most common cause of hemobilia and is usually related to interventional radiologic procedures. Occurrences of hemobilia, following a cholecystectomy, have been reported. Haemobilia, following accidental trauma is more prevalent with blunt traumas, rather than penetrating abdominal traumas. Some risk factors for the development of haemobilia following accidental traumas include central hepatic rupture with a cavity, packing, and inadequate drainage. Primary vascular pathology such as aneurysm, angiodysplasia, and hemangiomas are rare causes of haemobilia. Malignant tumors of the liver, biliary tree, gallbladder, and pancreas; parasitic infection; hepatic abscess; and cholangitis are uncommon causes of hemobilia.[35]

Clinical Presentation

Patients reportedly experience upper abdominal pain, upper gastrointestinal hemorrhage, and jaundice, which are considered to be a classic triad of indications of haemobilia. In 90% of cases of major haemobilia, patients will have melena stool. In major haemobilia, 60% of patients will have hematemesis, 70% will have biliary colic, and 60% will have jaundice. In conjunction to the biliary symptoms, patients with upper gastrointestinal bleeding should raise suspicion of haemobilia. Clots in the biliary tree can cause cholangitis, pancreatitis, and cholecystitis.

Diagnosis

If the occurrence of haemobilia is suspected, the initial assessment should include an upper gastrointestinal endoscopy, to rule-out hemorrhages, and visualize bleeding from the ampulla of Vater. Arterial angiography is the preferred test to rapidly locate the source of bleeding in approximately 90% of haemobilia cases (Figure 19).

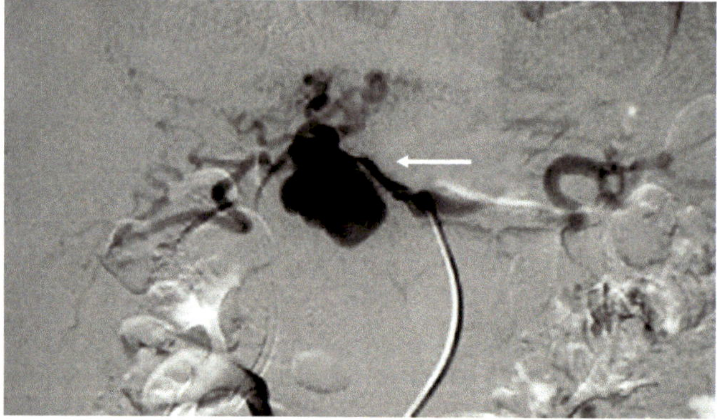

Figure 19. Hepatic angiogram demonstrating hemobilia

Management

Trans-arterial embolization (TAE) is the primary method of treatment for major hemobilia, with reported success rates of 80 to 100%. Angiography with TAE is indicated for major hemobilia requiring blood transfusion. If conservative therapy and TAE are failing, surgical intervention is required. In cases of a mandated laparotomy, TAE therapy should still be the first line of treatment for hemobilia, due to its low morbidity rate. Surgical intervention may include ligating bleeding blood vessels, clipping aneurysms, or nonselective ligation a main hepatic artery. In failed arterial ligations, severe traumas, or tumors, hepatic resection may also be required. In cases of a hemorrhaging gallbladder or hemorrhagic cholecystitis, cholecystectomies are the primary mode of intervention.

Bilhemia

Bilhemia, although extremely rare, occurs when bile invades the bloodstream either by the hepatic vein or portal vein branch. This flow occurs in the context of elevated intra-biliary pressure that exceeds the pressure of the venous system. The etiology can include the erosion of gallstones into the portal vein, or accidental or iatrogenic traumas. In the occurrence of embolization of large amounts of bile into the lungs, bilhemia may be fatal. It commonly presents with direct hyperbilirubinemia without elevating hepatocellular enzyme rates and septicemia. The best test to make this diagnosis is ERCP. Treatment of bilhemia aims to lower intra-biliary pressures with the use of stents or a sphincterotomy.

PRINCIPLES OF HEPATIC RESECTION

Hepatic Resection

The most common indicators of hepatic resections are malignant primary and secondary tumors, and symptomatic benign tumors. Traumatic injuries, infections or abscesses, and transplantations are fewer common indicators of liver resections. Approximately, 80% of the normal liver may be removed with the expectation of the remaining liver regenerating adequately, for survival. Such an extensive resection should be considered only for patients who have normal hepatic function. Patients with cirrhotic livers, steatosis, or significant fibrosis, are much less likely to tolerate or survive from major liver resections. Following an extensive liver resection, patients will experience reduced liver function for several weeks. New functioning hepatocytes will form by the regenerative capacity of the liver. Within the initial 24-hours following a partial resection, cell replication will activate to regenerate new hepatic tissue, until the original capacity is restored. A substantial amount of the liver will be regenerated within the first ten days and completed by the fourth or fifth week. Portions of the liver that have undergone excision will not be re-formed. Instead, new lobules will form, and the residual lobules will expand. Hepatic regeneration is thought to be stimulated by tumor growth factor (TGF), hepatocyte growth factor, hepatopoietin B, heparin-binding growth factor, and disinhibition by TGF. The disinhibition by the tumor growth factor includes decreased inhibitor hepatic growth levels.

Preoperative Evaluation

Prior to hepatic resection, disease and patient-related factors require evaluation, including Child Score and MELD Score. The most important preoperative assessment is that of the liver's functional status. Patients with cirrhosis and high Child score are not good candidates for major hepatic resection. Residual cirrhotic livers have limited reserves, unfit for metabolic demands. In patients with hepatocellular carcinoma, commonly arising along with chronic hepatic parenchymal disease, cirrhosis is concerning. Similarly, patients with hepatic colorectal metastases who have undergone chemotherapy treatments, will have existing hepatic injury impairing the remaining liver to regenerate.

Various tests may be performed to assess hepatic function before surgery, but no test has been deemed perfect. The Child-Pugh Classification, as shown below in Table 7, is the most dependable and widely employed assessment used to arrange hepatic function based on specific factors. The Child-Pugh classification was originally created to assess portosystemic shunt-related mortality and has now evolved to also predict the rate of mortality for patients with cirrhosis, following hepatic resections. According to this classification, cirrhotic patients with Child-Pugh A and highly selected Child-Pugh B may qualify for hepatic resection.

Table 7: Child-Pugh Classification

	Number of Points		
Factor	1	2	3
Bilirubin (mg/dL)	<2	02/03/12	>3
Albumin (g/dL)	>3.5	2.8-3.5	<2.8
Prothrombin time (increased seconds)	1-3	4-6	>6
Ascites	None	Slight	Moderate
Encephalopathy	None	Minimal	Advanced
Grade A 5-6 points, Grade B 7-9 points, Grade C 10-15 points			

Extent of Hepatic Resection

Hepatic resections may be either anatomical or non-anatomical. Anatomic hepatic resection follows the segmental liver anatomy. Some non-anatomical hepatic resections include wedge resections, resection debridement of necrotic tissue, and enucleations. Generally, anatomical hepatic resections are most elected due to their lowered rate of blood loss and lower incidence rate of positive resection margins in malignant cases. Hepatectomies (right, left, or extended) are commonly performed major liver resections and must follow the segmental anatomy. The liver's segmental anatomy allows for minor or bilateral resections as deemed appropriate, as shown in Figure 14. In select cases, the central (V and VIII) or posterior (VI and VII) segments can be resected, as opposed to resecting the entire right lobe. Parenchymal-sparing resections entails removal of a lobe or segment with its afferent and efferent vessels, while avoiding injury to the vessels and bile ducts supplying the residual tissue. As a general rule, in a healthy person 20% future liver remnant is sufficient to provide adequate hepatic function. This would include two adjacent liver segments with intact blood supply, venous drainage, and bile drainage. The amount of future liver remnant varies depending on underlaying liver pathology, as mentioned above.

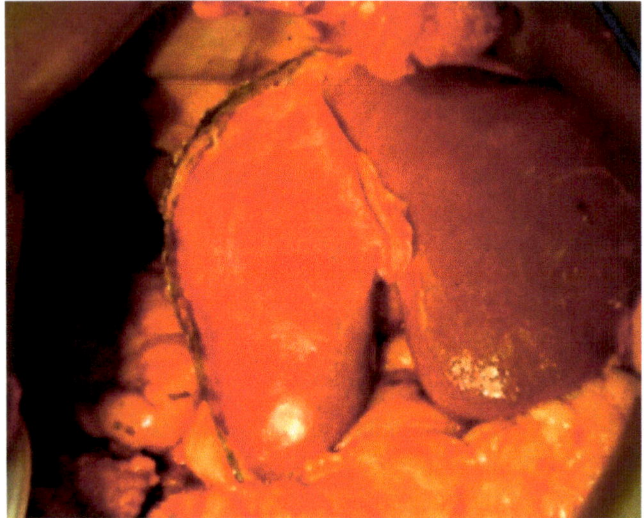

Figure 20: Intraoperative Image of Right Segmental Hepatectomy

As shown in Figure 20, a majority of elective hepatic resections may be performed using an abdominal incision. In select cases, such as large right-lobe tumors, thoracoabdominal incisions are most appropriate. Open hepatectomy are the most common and standard surgical approaches, however surgeons are evolving from the traditional techniques to laparoscopic or robotic approaches. The most effective technique to minimize blood loss during liver resection involves the following steps, a) maintain low central venous pressure by the method of permissive hypotension, b) to obtain vascular inflow control before parenchymal transaction by placing a pringle manure, c) clipping and diving the visible segmental and subsegmental blood vessels during parenchymal transection Pringle maneuver is a procedure in which the portal inflow pedicle is occluded using a Rummel clamp/tourniquet in a sequential manner. The clamp is applied for 15min and removed for 5min. This sequence is continued till the completion of the planned liver resection. is clamped for 15-minute periods, is another operative technique commonly used in minimizing blood loss from the intrahepatic arterial and portal venous branches. The pringle manure is not effective in minimizing hepatic venous bleeding.

Preoperative Portal Vein Embolization

The goal of Preoperative portal vein embolization (PVE) is to increase future liver remnant, by inducing hypertrophy in the contralateral lobe, and potentially prevent or decrease the probability of postoperative liver failure in patients undergoing major resections. This procedure is performed by interventional radiologist under image guidance, to embolize the portal vein branch on the side of the liver that is being resected. For example, if a patient has large tumor in the right liver and requires extended right hepatectomy, it is customary to obtain embolization of right portal vein to achieve atrophy of right lobe and hypertrophy of left lobe, especially in patients with underlying liver disease.

Postoperative Course

Patient who've undergone major hepatic resections must be placed under close observation for several days following the surgery. In most cases, prolonged ICU stays are unnecessary. In this period, post-operative bleeding is the main concern, but most cases don't require reoperation. Most symptoms will normalize in a few days following surgery. For example, non-cirrhotic patients commonly reported to experiencing metabolic changes, consistent to mild hepatic insufficiency. Most postoperative patients may be discharged by the seventh or eighth day of their hospital stay. Complications impairing the postoperative hepatic function may arise, such as consequential hepatic parenchymal diseases, which include the occurrences of fibrosis, steatosis, cirrhosis, or sepsis.

Comparing and assessing postoperative hepatic function to normal hepatic function helps in predicting potential complications or abnormalities. Commonly following major hepatic resections, serum bilirubin levels will increase, but eventually return to normal with regeneration. If serum bilirubin levels are persistently rising, perihepatic fluid collection or hepatic failure is suspected, particularly, when accompanied by additional deteriorating signs or functions. Typically, serum albumin will decrease, and prothrombin time will increase. Fresh frozen plasma (FFP) is only required if the international normalized ratio (INR) is significantly elevated, above 2.0. Ascites may be treated with diuresis. Following a major partial hepatectomy, hepatic glycogen storages are depleted, but hypoglycemia is typically not a postoperative concern. Normoglycemia is achieved using 5% dextrose solution. Acute hypoglycemia is an indication for potential hepatic failure. Serum magnesium, phosphate, and potassium levels also decrease in the initial postoperative days, requiring replacement. Meanwhile, aspartate aminotransferase (AST) and alanine aminotransferase (ALT) hepatic enzymes will increase in the initial postoperative days, but eventually normalize. Compared to AST and ALT levels, alkaline phosphatase (ALP) levels will appear as normal immediately following surgery but become elevated for several postoperative days or even weeks.

Complications

In patients who've had major liver resections of three or more segments, approximately 40% of them have reported to experience complications. Some patients experience relatively minor complications, with most cases being controlled or resolved without long-term ramifications. Complications related to the liver are most prevalent. About 10 to 15% of patients require drainage of perihepatic fluid, which may consist of accumulated blood, bile, chyle, urine, ascites, or pancreatic fluid. Along with regeneration, common cases of hepatic insufficiency, which includes ascites, hyperbilirubinemia, and coagulopathy will resolve, but hepatic failure specifically, is rare in high-volume centers. Pulmonary complications have been reported along with hepatic resection, requiring postoperative pulmonary toilet to assist in clearing the airway of mucus and secretions. Atelectasis or symptomatic pleural effusion are the most prevalent pulmonary complications to occur, with pneumonia rarely occurring. Major liver resections have low mortality rates of 1 to 3%, regardless of the potential complications. Minor liver resections of less than three liver segments have even lower morbidity and mortality rates.

ALTERNATIVE LIVER DIRECTED THERAPIES

Radiofrequency Ablation

Surgical resection, when feasible, offers highest survival benefit, however radiofrequency ablation has its role in the management of unresectable tumors, multiple small tumors in both the lobes, or in patients who are high risk candidates for surgical resection. The technique involves the transfer of electric energy to induce thermal injury within the tissue. The heat formed desiccates the surrounding tissue, leading to coagulation necrosis. The minimum temperature threshold is approximately 50°C, with an optimal temperature of 80° to 100°C. The zone of thermal ablation is based on the size and shape of the electrode used and based on strategies involving novel probe designs such as internally cooled and multi-tined expandable electrodes. A 5 cm sphere of thermal ablation is the approximate limit for a single electrode used to treat tumors no larger than 3 cm in its longest dimension; this ensures that a 1 cm margin around the entire tumor is obtained. Larger tumors can be treated by the use of multiple overlapping applications. Large vessels such as the hepatic veins act as heat sinks by removing the thermal energy in the blood. This effectively protects the vessel wall from thermal injury but may also limit the ablation efficacy (Figure 21).

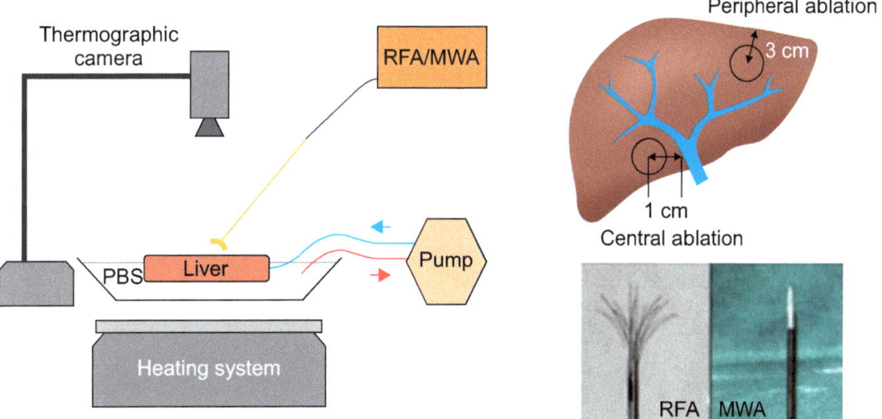

Figure 21. Pictorial demonstration of radiofrequency ablation technique

The indications for RFA continue to evolve, but in general RFA is offered to patients with unresectable tumor due to poor general health, cirrhosis, tumor location, or distribution. In addition, RFA may be used as an adjuvant to hepatic resection to ablate small tumors during major resection, as treatment for the tumors not amenable for surgical resection or used as an alternative to repeated resection in patients with recurrence. A limited life expectancy of less than 6 months, severe cirrhosis, or portal vein thrombosis are considered contraindications to RFA. As the number of lesions increase, the potential for complications increases and the theoretical benefit decreases; therefore, many centers prefer to treat patients with four or fewer lesions. Prospective studies of colorectal metastases comparing surgical resection alone, surgical resection plus RFA, and RFA alone demonstrate that overall and recurrence-free survival is superior with surgery. The data shows a 4-year survival of 65% for surgery compared to 36% for combined and 22% for RFA alone. However, all groups had better survival than patients treated with chemotherapy alone. This suggests that patients who can undergo local treatment of isolated hepatic tumors with RFA improves survival. For patients who were not candidates for surgery, such as those with HCC and decompensated cirrhosis, RFA used as the primary therapy resulted in a 5-year survival of 48% with a recurrence rate of 81% for new tumors and 10% for local tumor progression. Major complications occur in approximately 6% after RFA and include hepatic abscess, bile leak, intrahepatic hematoma or hemoperitoneum, pneumothorax and pleural effusion, intestinal perforation when using the percutaneous technique only, hepatic failure, and death. The results with RFA and indications for its use will continue to expand as our experience and understanding of this technique evolve.

Microwave Ablation

Microwave coagulation causes molecular vibration of dipoles, such as water, producing frictional heat and thermal coagulation, similar to RFA. The coagulative necrosis produced around the microwave needle is rapid, resulting in the formation of a tissue coagulum that prevents further dissipation of heat into the surrounding tissue and thus limiting the area of necrosis. The microwave needle must therefore be advanced 5 to 10 mm through the tumor and surrounding tissue, or multiple needles are required. Studies with microwave coagulation have demonstrated efficacy with both HCC and colorectal metastases with a low local recurrence rate of less than 10%, but survival appears to be inferior to hepatic resection. The results with RFA and microwave coagulation, and the indications for their use will continue to expand as our experience and understanding of these techniques evolve.

REFERENCES

1. Pope IM, Poston GJ, Blumgart, LH, Fong YBW. Pyogenic liver abscess. In eds Surgery of the Liver and Biliary Tract London pp 2000,1135-1145.
2. Johannsen EC, Sifri CD, Madoff LC. Pyogenic liver abscesses. Infectious disease clinics of North America 2000, 14 (3), 547-63, vii.
3. Branum GD, Tyson GS, Branum MA, Meyers WC. Hepatic abscess. Changes in etiology, diagnosis, and management. Annals of surgery 1990, 212 (6), 655-62.
4. Seeto RK, Rockey DC. Pyogenic liver abscess. Changes in etiology, management, and outcome. Medicine 1996, 75 (2), 99-113.
5. Huang CJ, Pitt HA, Lipsett PA. Pyogenic hepatic abscess: changing trends over 42 years. Ann.
6. McDonald MI, Corey GR, Gallis HA, Durack DT. Single and multiple pyogenic liver abscesses. Natural history, diagnosis and treatment, with emphasis on percutaneous drainage. Medicine 1984, 63 (5), 291-302.
7. Hughes MA, Petri WA. Amebic liver abscess. Infectious disease clinics of North America 2000, 14 (3), 565-82, viii.
8. Thomas PG, Ravindra KV, Blumgart LH, Fong YBW. Amebiasis and biliary infection. In eds Surgery of the Liver and Biliary Tract London pp 2000, 1147-1166.
9. Seeto RK, Rocky DC. Amebic liver abscess: epidemiology, clinical features, and outcome. The Western journal of medicine 1999, 170 (2), 104-9.
10. Shandera WX, Bollam P, Hashmey RH, Athey PA, Greenberg SB, White AC. Hepatic amebiasis among patients in a public teaching hospital. Southern medical journal 1998, 91 (9), 829-37.
11. Bouree PJ. Hydatidosis: Dynamics of transmission. World 2001, 25, 4-9.
12. Biava MF, Dao A, Fortier B. Laboratory diagnosis of cystic hydatic disease. World journal of surgery 2001, 25 (1), 10-4.
13. Pedrosa I, Saíz A, Arrazola J, Ferreirós J, Pedrosa CS. Hydatid disease: radiologic and pathologic features and complications. Radiographics: a review publication of the Radiological Society of North America, Inc 2000, 20 (3), 795-817.
14. Zaouche A, Haouet K, Jouini M, El Hachaichi A, Dziri C. Management of liver hydatid cysts with a large biliocystic fistula: multicenter retrospective study. Tunisian Surgical Association. World journal of surgery 2001, 25 (1), 28-39.
15. Ertem M, Uras C, Karahasanoglu T, Erguney S, Alemdaroglu K. Laparoscopic approach to hepatic hydatid disease. Digestive surgery 1998, 15 (4), 333-6.
16. Akhan O, Ozmen MN. Percutaneous treatment of liver hydatid cysts. European journal of radiology 1999, 32 (1), 76-85.
17. Hugh TJ, Poston GJ, Blumgart LH, Fong YBW. Benign liver tumors and masses. In eds Surgery of the Liver and Biliary Tract London pp 2000, 1397-1422.
18. Charny CK, Jarnagin WR, Schwartz LH, Frommeyer HS, DeMatteo RP, Fong YBW, Blumgart LH. Management of 155 patients with benign liver tumours. The British journal of surgery 2001, 88 (6), 808-13.
19. Edmondson HA, Henderson, B, Benton B. Liver-cell adenomas associated with use of oral contraceptives. The New England journal of medicine 1976, 294 (9), 470-2.

20. Fulcher AS, Sterling RK. Hepatic neoplasms: computed tomography and magnetic resonance features. Journal of clinical gastroenterology 2002, 34 (4), 463-71.
21. Nagorney DM. Benign hepatic tumors: focal nodular hyperplasia and hepatocellular adenoma. World journal of surgery 1995, 19 (1), 13-8.
22. Zimmerman A, Blumgart LH, Fong YBW. Tumors of the liver—pathologic aspects. In eds Surgery of the Liver and Biliary Tract London pp 2000, 1343-1396.
23. LaQuaglia MP, Blumgart, LH, Fong YBW. Liver tumors in children. In eds Surgery of the Liver and Biliary Tract London pp 2000, 1397-1422.
24. Lau WY, Blumgart LH, Fong YBW. Primary hepatocellular carcinoma. In eds Surgery of the Liver and Biliary Tract London pp 2000, 1423-1450.
25. Beasley RP, Hwang LY, Vyas GH, Dienstag JL, Hoofnagle JH. Epidemiology of hepatocellular carcinoma. In eds Viral Hepatitis and Liver Disease New York Grune Stratton pp 1984, 209-224.
26. Fong Y, Sun RL, Jarnagin W, Blumgart LH. An analysis of 412 cases of hepatocellular carcinoma at a Western center. Annals of surgery 1999, 229 (6), 790-9; discussion 799.
27. Poon RTP, Fan ST, Tsang FHF, Wong J. Locoregional therapies for hepatocellular carcinoma: a critical review from the surgeon's perspective. Annals of surgery 2002, 235 (4), 466-86.
28. Seidenfeld J, Korn A, Aronso N. Radiofrequency ablation of unresectable liver metastases. Journal of the American College of Surgeons 2002, 195 (3), 378-86.
29. Bruix J, Llovet JM, Castells A, Montañá X, Brú C, Ayuso MC, Vilana R, Rodés J. Transarterial embolization versus symptomatic treatment in patients with advanced hepatocellular carcinoma: results of a randomized, controlled trial in a single institution. Hepatology (Baltimore, Md.) 1998, 27 (6), 1578-83.
30. Craig JR, Okuda K, Tabor E, Churchill Y. Fibrolamellar carcinoma: Clinical and pathological features. In eds Liver Cancer New pp 1997, 255-262.
31. Blumgart LH, Fong Y. Surgical options in the treatment of hepatic metastasis from colorectal cancer. Current problems in surgery 1995, 32 (5), 333-421.
32. Chamberlain RS, Canes D, Brown KT, Saltz L, Jarnagin W, Fong Y, Blumgart LH. Hepatic neuroendocrine metastases: does intervention alter outcomes? Journal of the American College of Surgeons 2000, 190 (4), 432-45.
33. Harrison LE, Brennan MF, Newman E, Fortner JG, Picardo A, Blumgart LH, Fong Y. Hepatic resection for noncolorectal, nonneuroendocrine metastases: a fifteen-year experience with ninety-six patients. Surgery 1997, 121 (6), 625-32.
34. Farges O, Menu Y, Benhamou JP, Blumgart LH, Fong YBW. Non-parasitic cystic diseases of the liver and intrahepatic biliary tree. In eds Surgery of the Liver and Biliary Tract London pp 2000, 1245-1260.
35. Sandblom JP, Blumgart LH, Fong YBW. Hemobilia and bilhemia. In eds Surgery of the Liver and Biliary Tract London pp 1572 2000, 1319-1342.
36. Online article. Bile Duct Cancer (Cholangiocarcinoma) Treatment (PDQ®)–Health Professional Version was originally published by the National Cancer Institute https://www.cancer.gov/types/liver/hp/bile-duct-treatment-pdq. Accessed 09/30/2022

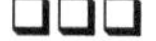

30
CHAPTER

Gallbladder and Biliary System

Manjunath Haridas, MD
Dinesh Vyas, MD

ANATOMY

The gallbladder is a pear-shaped reservoir that is continuous with the common hepatic and common bile duct. The average capacity of the gallbladder is fifty milliliters (mL). It is on the inferior surface of the liver and is partially enveloped in a peritoneal layer. The gallbladder is divided into the fundus, body, infundibulum, and neck. Compared to the gastrointestinal tract it lacks both muscularis mucosa and submucosa and consists mainly of smooth muscles. Both the gallbladder, the neck, and the cystic duct contain spirally oriented mucosal folds known as the valves of Heister. The gallbladder empties into the cystic duct. The cystic duct varies in length from 1 to 4 centimeters (cm) usually joining the common hepatic duct at an acute angle. The area bound by the cystic duct are the common hepatic duct and the liver margin, forming the 'Triangle of Calot'. This relationship is of surgical importance. The extrahepatic biliary tract consists of the left and right hepatic duct bifurcation, the common hepatic duct, common bile duct, cystic duct, and gallbladder. The common hepatic duct is anterior to the hepatoduodenal ligament. It then joins the cystic duct, forming the common bile duct. The common bile duct then extends from the cystic-common hepatic duct junction and is inferior to the papilla of Vater (9 cm in length) where it empties into the duodenum.

Arterial supply of the gallbladder is from the cystic artery, which is often a branch of the right hepatic artery. In anatomical variations, the cystic artery is a branch of the left hepatic, common hepatic, gastroduodenal, or superior mesenteric arteries. In most cases, the cystic artery runs parallel and is medial to the cystic duct, however, there is also variation in the course the artery follows. The arterial supply to the extrahepatic biliary tree begins distally from the gastroduodenal, retro-duodenal, and posterior-superior pancreaticoduodenal arteries. It originates proximally from the right hepatic and cystic arteries. These arteries have branches that run parallel to the duct in the 3 and 9 o'clock positions that supply the common bile and common hepatic ducts.

Bile and Composition

On an average 500 to 1500 mL of bile is produced. The variation in bile composition is shown in Table 1. Between meals bile is stored in the gallbladder where it is concentrated up to 20%. Three factors regulate bile secretion: hepatic secretion, gallbladder contraction, and choledochal sphincter resistance. Ninety percent of bile is made up of bile salts, lecithin, and cholesterol. Bile undergoes enterohepatic circulation where more than 90% of the bile salts are reabsorbed in the jejunum and enter portal circulation. This results in the loss of only about 10% of bile salts via stool. Bile secretion is stimulated by cholecystokinin (CCK). Motilin stimulates partial gallbladder emptying during the interdigestive phase. Amino acids and polypeptides are weak stimuli whereas carbohydrates are not.

Table 1: Composition of bile: Hepatic and Gallbladder

Composition	Levels in Liver (mmol/2)	Levels in Gallbladder
Sodium	160	270
Potassium	5	10
Chlorine	90	15
Bicarbonate	45	10
Calcium	4	25
Magnesium	2	-
Bilirubin	1.5	15
Protein	150	-
Bile acids	50	150

Composition	Levels in Liver (mmol/2)	Levels in Gallbladder
Phospholipids	8	40
Cholesterol	4	18
Total solids	-	125
pH	7.8	7.2

Diagnostic Evaluation

Various diagnostic tools are available for evaluation of the gallbladder and the biliary tree. Among these tools, the most common and widely used are ultrasound, computed tomography (CT), magnetic resonance cholangiopancreatography (MRCP).[1]

Ultrasound

If extrahepatic biliary disease and obstruction is suspected, ultrasound is often the first screening test.[2] The sensitivity and specificity to diagnose biliary tract disease is more than 90%. Ultrasound helps identify gallstones, liver metastases, and occasionally masses of the liver and pancreas. Dilation of the extrahepatic (>10 millimeters (mm)) or intrahepatic (>4 mm) bile ducts, suggestive of biliary obstruction, can also be diagnosed based on ultrasound. It is further used to assess for acute cholecystitis which would show signs of gallbladder wall thickening, pericholecystic fluid, and Murphy's sign. Additionally, ultrasound can be used to assess tumor invasion and flow in portal vein.[3] It can also be used to perform guided biopsy and fine needle aspiration of masses and fluid collections.

Biliary Radio-Nucleotide Scan

Biliary scintigraphy is a noninvasive way to evaluate anatomic and functional aspects of the liver, gallbladder, bile ducts, and duodenum. 99mTechnetium-labeled derivatives of dimethyl iminodiacetic acid (HIDA) are intravenously injected into the patient, cleared by liver Kupffer cells, and excreted in the bile. Biliary scintigraphy is most commonly used for the diagnosis of acute cholecystitis. Biliary scintigraphy can identify cystic duct obstruction which is highly diagnostic for acute cholecystitis, having a 95% sensitivity and specificity. Biliary leaks, a complication of gallbladder or biliary tree surgery, can be confirmed and frequently localized by biliary scintigraphy.[4]

Computed Tomography

Computed Tomography (CT) is an extremely sensitive test at identifying biliary dilation. CT is less sensitive than ultrasound when trying to detect gallstones, but it is more accurate when trying to identify the location and cause of extrahepatic biliary obstruction. When suspecting biliary obstruction from gallstones, ultrasound is the preferred first test. CT or ultrasound is used to evaluate patients when suspecting a malignancy of the gallbladder, the extrahepatic biliary system, or other nearby organs, especially the pancreatic head. CT is particularly helpful in providing staging information, such as vascular involvement in patients who have periampullary tumors.[5]

Other Imaging Modalities

Magnetic Resonance Cholangiopancreatography (MRCP) is important in delineating the site and cause of biliary obstruction, caused either by a benign or malignant process. MRCP is noninvasive and provides great anatomic detail.[6] Both endoscopic retrograde cholangiopancreatography (ERCP) and percutaneous transhepatic cholangiography (PTC) are invasive procedures and have a risk of complications, however both offer a therapeutic intervention opportunity (see later). ERCP is helping in imaging periampullary tumors and choledocholithiasis.[7] Occasionally, ERCP is not possible when a patient has an altered gastroduodenal anatomy. PTC is preferred when there is proximal biliary obstruction or when it is not possible technically.

Biliary Interventions

Endoscopic Procedures

During endoscopic cholangiography, several conditions that cause jaundice can be treated at the same time. Stones can be cleared from the common bile duct with the use of endoscopically passed balloon catheters or baskets after a sphincterotomy. This has a high success of 85% to 90%. Endoscopically placed stents are also used to treat malignant biliary strictures involving the mid or distal common bile duct (e.g., polyurethane, and expandable metallic stents), internally decompressing the biliary tract and relieving jaundice. Metallic stents are patent longer; but are harder to exchange once they occlude.

Endoscopic Ultrasound

When using an endoscopic ultrasound, a special endoscope with an ultrasound transducer at the tip is required. Results are operator dependent; however, it is noninvasive imaging of the bile ducts and adjacent structures. Ultrasound is particularly valuable when evaluating tumors and their resectability. The ultrasound endoscope contains a biopsy channel which enables ultrasound guided needle biopsies of a tumor. Additionally, endoscopic ultrasound is a less invasive technique to identify bile duct stones, however with less sensitivity than ERCP.

Percutaneous Management

The biliary tract can be accessed percutaneously and is a route used to treat obstructive jaundice. This approach is preferred when the obstruction is located more proximally in the bile duct or hepatic duct bifurcation. Polyurethane or metallic stents placed percutaneously can often be passed across an obstructing biliary lesion and into the duodenum, thus allowing internal biliary drainage. Serial dilation of the stent tract enables insertion of a flexible choledochoscope into the biliary tree, thus enabling direct visualization, biopsy, or management of an obstruction.

Gallstones

Incidence and Etiopathology

Gallstone disease is one of the most common pathologies encountered by a general surgeon. Only 1/3 of patients who have gallstones present with symptoms. Complications due to gallstones result in symptoms like cholangitis, common bile duct stone, and acute pancreatitis. Cholelithiasis is present in approximately 10% of adults. More than 20 million people are affected by gallbladder disease in the United States alone.[8] There is marked differences in incidence among various other races and ethnic groups. In general women who are overweight and of childbearing age have a higher incidence. Males seem to be less likely to be affected among all ethnic groups. A majority, more than 98%, of male patients remain asymptomatic. With the new and better resolution imaging techniques, there is increased incidence in this subgroup.

Gallstones are formed due to failure to maintain biliary solutes in their solubilized state. The most common form of gallstones are cholesterol stones (70% to 80%) and pigment stones. The main etiology for gallstone formation is biliary sludge. This is a mixture of cholesterol crystals, calcium bilirubinate, and mucin gel. Formation of cholesterol stones involves cholesterol supersaturation, crystal nucleation, and stone growth. In pigment stones, calcium bilirubinate and calcium palmitate are the major components. These are further classified as either brown or black. Brown pigment stones contain more cholesterol and are commonly associated with infection. These also occur more commonly as primary duct stones. Black pigment stones are frequently associated with conditions associated with hemolysis and cirrhosis.[9] Most patients with gallstones remain asymptomatic. Only about 4% of the population develop symptoms and complications attributable to gallstones. Of those who remain asymptomatic, 10% progress to develop symptoms in 5 years. Less than one fourth will develop symptoms at 20 years. Irrespective of etiology, a symptomatic gallstone will require cholecystectomy either laparoscopic or open. Gallstone disease is classified under various groups for discussion as shown in Table 2.

Table 2: Classification of benign gallbladder disease

Benign calculous disease	Symptomatic Gallstones • Chronic cholecystitis • Acute cholecystitis Asymptomatic Gallstones Acute cholangitis
Benign non-calculous disease	Acalculous cholecystitis Biliary Dyskinesia Sphincter of Oddi dysfunction Intrahepatic stones Polypoid lesions of the Gallbladder Biliary strictures Primary sclerosing cholangitis Biliary cysts

Chronic Cholecystitis

Chronic Cholecystitis is defined as recurrent inflammation involving the gallbladder. Intermittent to complete obstruction of the cystic duct may be seen. In the majority of patients, gallstones are the leading cause. In developing countries infectious causes have also been implicated as an etiology. In symptomatic patients, the pathology varies from minimal inflammation of the wall to thickening and scarring. Microscopically there is a mononuclear cell infiltrate associated with subserosal and subepithelial fibrosis. The mucosa is initially normal and later undergoes atrophy where it protrudes into the muscle layer leading into sinuses known as Aschoff-Rokitansky sinuses.

Clinical Presentation

Symptoms vary from mild abdominal pain to classic right upper quadrant pain associated with fatty food intake. Pain caused by the gallbladder is often called biliary colic. Patients usually have intermittent right upper quadrant pain associated with dyspepsia. In some patients, this pain is so severe that emergency room visits are not uncommon. Cystic duct obstruction results in increased gallbladder wall tension, manifesting as constant pain. This pain can radiate to the right upper back and right scapula. Episodes also consist of nausea and vomiting in 60% to 70% of cases and bloating and belching in 50% of patients. By the time a patient is seen by a general surgeon for symptoms, they would have had an ultrasound or CT documenting gallstones. It is absolutely necessary to correlate the signs and symptoms to the radiographic finding. Findings of a gallstone on a routine or non-focused examination in an otherwise healthy individual without symptoms does not require cholecystectomy. A careful history and examination is the key.

Diagnosis

Cholelithiasis or chronic cholecystitis diagnosis includes biliary colic abdominal pain and the presence of gallstones. Laboratory studies show normal levels of serum bilirubin, transaminases, and alkaline phosphatase in uncomplicated gallstones. In patients with less classic symptoms, other causes including gastroesophageal reflux disease, acute pancreatitis, peptic ulcer disease, or irritable bowel syndrome should first be excluded. Ultrasound is a 95-98% sensitive imaging study for presence of gallstones, and it provides anatomic information including the polyps, the diameter of the common bile duct, or hepatic parenchymal abnormalities.[10] Gallbladder wall thickening and the presence of pericholecystic fluid help in excluding acute cholecystitis as a diagnosis. Gallstones can sometimes be seen on abdominal radiographs (15%) or CT scans (50%). Most of these findings are usually confirmed on ultrasound. In less than 2% of the population where no gallstone has been found and that have a negative scan; ERCP is required to evaluate the cause for biliary obstruction.[11]

Management

Laparoscopic cholecystectomy is preferred treatment for patients who have symptomatic gallstones. The mortality rate is less than 0.1%. Conversion from laparoscopic cholecystectomy to an open cholecystectomy is necessary in less than 5% of patients. The technique and major pitfalls are further expanded below. Conversion rates are increased in the elderly,[12] male, evidence of gallbladder wall thickening, and unclear anatomy.[13] The results of laparoscopic cholecystectomies are excellent. More than 90% of patients are symptom free. Some may develop atypical symptoms of dyspepsia (fatty food intolerance, flatulence, belching, or bloating) and some may complain of increased bowel symptoms. These tend to resolve over time.

Outcome

No further follow-up is required for patients who have undergone an uncomplicated laparoscopic cholecystectomy and had no issues on the first postoperative visit. Review of the pathology should be performed during this visit.

Acute Calculus Cholecystitis

The majority, greater than 90% of acute cholecystitis cases are related to gallstones. Cystic duct obstruction is the primary or the initial event leading to acute cholecystitis. This further leads to inflammation and edema of the gallbladder. When the cystic duct is obstructed without evidence of inflammation, it will eventually lead to hydrops of the gallbladder. However, acute cholecystitis is an inflammatory process in more than half of patients who have positive bile cultures. In some, cystic duct obstruction can be resolve leading to resolution of symtoms.[14]

Clinical Presentation

Symptoms of right upper quadrant abdominal pain, nausea, vomiting, and fever are common. Pain is usually preceded by several days of mild intermittent abdominal pain. In some severe cases, sepsis may be the only initial presentation. On examination, patients may have tachycardia, localized abdominal tenderness, and guarding. A mass can be palpable, and Murphy's sign can be elicited.

Diagnosis

There may be a mild elevation in leukocytes. Mild elevations in serum bilirubin, alkaline phosphatase and transaminases may be present. Jaundice is not a clinical feature of acute cholecystitis. When serum bilirubin is elevated, a common duct stone should be ruled out. Very rare cases of jaundice in acute cholecystitis have been reported as Mirizzi syndrome (Figure 1). Ultrasound remains the key in diagnosis. On ultrasound, acute calculus cholecystitis shows evidence of gallbladder wall thickening, presence of peri-cholecystectomy fluid, and normal common duct. CT images can sometimes be helpful, but care should be taken with interpretation because any inflammation of the liver and transverse colon can also present with similar changes around the gallbladder. In cases with a normal gallbladder, a nuclear medicine scan can be performed.

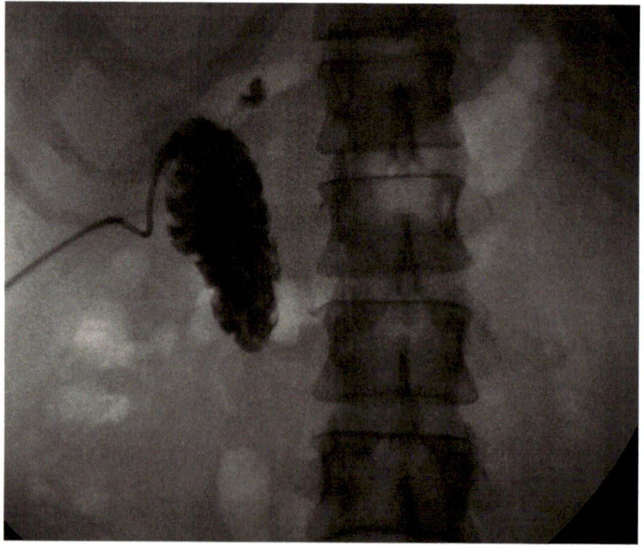

Figure 1: Tubogram showing cholecystoduodenal fistula

Management

Having made a diagnosis of acute cholecystitis, patients should be hospitalized. They should be placed on a restricted diet and started on broad spectrum antibiotics. Escherichia coli, Klebsiella, Enterobacter, Enterococcus, Streptococcus, Bacteroides, and Clostridium are the most common organisms. A second-generation cephalosporin or a fluoroquinolone is sufficient. Cholecystectomy is the definitive treatment of acute cholecystitis. The role of a surgeon in managing acute cholecystitis is quite challenging because the time of decision to intervene will ultimately influence outcome. Early intervention within a week of symptom onset decreases the duration of hospitalization, allowing patients to return to work sooner.[15] Early intervention should be planned in at-risk patients who are elderly, diabetic, cirrhotic, and immunocompromised. At most institutions, patients with acute cholecystitis are operated within the first 24 to 48 hours of hospitalization.

Outcome

Associated complications include empyema of the gallbladder, emphysematous cholecystitis, or perforation of the gallbladder even with the use of antibiotic therapy. Patients with empyema may become septic with fever and leukocytosis. To treat such patients, laparoscopic cholecystectomy can be used, but there is a high rate of conversions to open procedures. Emphysematous cholecystitis is more common in men and patients with a diagnosis of diabetes mellitus. Perforation of the gallbladder, especially the gallbladder fundus, is a sequela of ischemia and gangrene of the gallbladder wall. The perforation is most frequently contained within the subhepatic region. The gallbladder rarely perforates into adjacent viscus (duodenum or colon) or peritoneum. The preferred treatment of gallbladder perforation is intravenous fluids, antibiotics, and emergency cholecystectomy.

Cholecystectomies can be performed in most cases and is the treatment of choice in complicated acute cholecystitis. Sometimes, inflammation can obscure the triangle of Calot, making dissection or ligation of the cystic duct unsafe. Thus, partial cholecystectomy, cauterization of the remaining gallbladder mucosa, and drainage should be performed instead. All measures should be taken to avoid common duct injury. Patients considered too unstable for laparotomy can drain the gallbladder. Such patients include those with concurrent medical comorbidities and percutaneous transhepatic cholecystostomy. Interval laparoscopic or open cholecystectomy should be performed 3 to 4 months later, this provides time for patient recovery and resolution of the acute inflammation.[16]

Asymptomatic Gallstone

Gallstones are found incidentally, and most are asymptomatic. Few studies have been able to identify factors that predict progression of symptoms or complications. The reposed criteria for prophylactic cholecystectomy is shown in Table 3. Patients who have heart transplantation have a greater than 50% incidence of silent gallstones. There is a higher incidence of complications from gallstones, hence prophylactic cholecystectomy is recommended. Similarly in patients suffering from hemoglobinopathies, it is recommended that they undergo prophylactic cholecystectomy if gallstones are present or concomitant cholecystectomy if splenectomy is planned. Expectant management can be followed in patients who are compliant. The risks and benefits of nonoperative management outweigh the risks of doing the procedure.

Table 3: Prophylactic cholecystectomy criteria

Patient has a life expectancy of >20 years
Calculi have a diameter of >2 cm
Calculi are <3 mm and patent cystic duct
Radiopaque calculi
Gallbladder polyps
Calcified or nonfunctioning gallbladder
Women who are <60 years old
Patient living in an area where gallbladder cancer prevalence is high

Acute Acalculous Cholecystitis

Acute acalculous cholecystitis most often occurs in patients who are critically ill. Such critically ill patients include prolonged hospitalization following trauma, burns, long-term parenteral nutrition, and major non-biliary operations (i.e., abdominal aneurysm repair or cardiopulmonary bypass).[17] Acute acalculous cholecystitis has an unclear etiology, but suggested causative factors include gallbladder stasis and ischemia. Acute acalculous cholecystitis presents with decreased arteriolar and capillary filling, which distinguished it from acute calculus cholecystitis which presents with dilation of these vessels.[18]

Clinical signs and symptoms of acute acalculous cholecystitis are similar to those of acute calculous cholecystitis. Patients may have right upper quadrant pain and tenderness, fever, and leukocytosis. Some critically ill patients can have fever of unknown origin. Ultrasound and CT remain the cornerstone to diagnosis. Nuclear medicine scans show absent gallbladder filling.

Emergency cholecystectomy should be performed after diagnosis or if there is high suspicion of acute acalculous cholecystitis because the patient is at high risk for gangrene, perforation, and empyema. Open cholecystectomy is often necessary in emergencies. There remains a high mortality rate for acute acalculous cholecystitis, but this is more often due to the concomitant illnesses.

Acute Cholangitis

Acute cholangitis is an infection of the biliary tract. Risk factors include those that cause biliary obstruction. It is commonly seen in the age group of 50 to 60 years old. The most common etiology for biliary obstruction is a common duct stone. Other non-iatrogenic causes that can lead to biliary stasis and obstruction include primary and secondary choledocholithiasis, pancreatitis (chronic/acute), pseudocyst, papillary, stenosis, Mirizzi's syndrome, choledochal cysts (type V, Caroli's disease), primary sclerosing cholangitis, pancreatic cancer, cholangiocarcinoma, and porta hepatis tumor/metastasis. Iatrogenic causes include obstructed biliary endoprosthesis, iatrogenic biliary stricture, direct surgical trauma, ischemia-induced stricture, and anastomotic stricture (biliobiliary/bilioenteric anastomosis). The most commonly identified bacteria are gram-negative, including Escherichia coli, Klebsiella, and Enterobacter species. Gram positive bacteria are also identified which include Enterococcus species. Certain other pathogens such as helminths, fungi, and viruses have also been reported.

Clinical Presentation

Clinical presentation varies from mild disease to multiorgan failure and septic shock. Fever, jaundice, and abdominal pain is commonly referred to as Charcot's triad. Reynold's pentad includes the presence of mental status derangements and hypotension,

Diagnosis

Acute cholangitis is a clinical diagnosis based on the presence of certain clinical features. The differential diagnosis includes cholecystitis, liver abscesses, and hepatitis all of which can show symptoms of right upper quadrant abdominal pain, jaundice, or fever. Laboratory test findings often include leukocytosis with neutrophilia and liver function test abnormalities (e.g., increased serum alkaline phosphatase, gamma-glutamyl transpeptidase, and conjugated bilirubin concentrations). Increased serum aminotransferase concentrations can occur with acute liver injury resulting from cholangitis-induced hepatic microabscess formation. Serum amylase concentration is elevated in up to 30% of patients with acute cholangitis. If a patient is believed to have cholangitis, blood cultures must be performed. Additionally, one should obtain cultures of bile aspirated from percutaneous biliary catheters, cultures obtained during endoscopic retrograde cholangiopancreatography (ERCP), and cultures of any removed indwelling biliary prostheses. Treatment should be initiated before culture results return and can be modified to a specific antibiotic therapy once results become available.

Ultrasound is the best initial imaging study and should be followed by endoscopic ERCP. Prompt percutaneous transhepatic cholangiography (PTC) should be performed if ERCP is unavailable or if it fails. Patients with indwelling biliary catheters (e.g., T-tubes or U-tubes) can have a cholangiography, using the tubes to instill the contrast if they are externally accessible. CT, MRCP, and EUS do not offer therapeutic capability. ERCP should not be delayed while obtaining these imaging studies.

Management

The main components of management include resuscitation, antibiotics, and biliary drainage. High-risk patients with significant comorbidities should be monitored in a dedicated intensive care unit to ensure invasive monitoring and inotropic support can be provided. Empiric broad-spectrum antibiotic administration should commence when considering a diagnosis of acute cholangitis. In most cases, ERCP should be used first for establishing biliary drainage, while PTC is reserved for patients in whom ERCP failed or is unavailable. If a patient has an external biliary drain, the drain should be placed to gravity drainage once considering a diagnosis of acute cholangitis. Because of the high efficacy rates associated with ERCP and PTC, surgical biliary decompression should only be used in the acute setting if neither of these non-operative procedures succeed in biliary drainage nor are available.

Biliary Dyskinesia

Patients with typical symptoms of biliary colic and who do not show signs of gallstones on ultrasound require further investigation. This is often to rule out diseases that can cause upper abdominal pain. The work-up often includes a CT scan, esophagogastroduodenoscopy, or even an ERCP. Additionally, biliary dyskinesia should be a differential consideration in these patients. In these patients, the CCK-Tc-HIDA scan can be useful in diagnosing biliary dyskinesia. First, the gallbladder must be filled with 99 Tc-labeled radionuclides, then CCK can be infused intravenously. Twenty minutes after administration, a gallbladder ejection fraction can be calculated, with an ejection fraction <35% being abnormal. Patients with biliary dyskinesia should be managed with laparoscopic cholecystectomy.

Sphincter of Oddi Dysfunction

The sphincter of Oddi is a complex muscular structure surrounding the distal common bile duct, pancreatic duct, and ampulla of Vater. Patients present with pain similar to biliary colic and recurrent episodes of pancreatitis. Fibrosis of the sphincter from a gallstone, operative or endoscopic trauma, pancreatitis, or other nonspecific inflammatory processes can result in elevated sphincter pressures. Consider a sphincter of Oddi dysfunction when a patient presents with typical episodic biliary-type pain, but no obvious organic cause. Potential laboratory studies include an elevated serum amylase or transaminases. Ultrasound in these patients reveal a dilated (>12 mm) common bile duct (Figure 2). There can also be an increase in common bile duct diameter in response to CCK. Endoscopic retrograde cholangiopancreatography (ERCP) shows abnormal sphincter function and elevated basal sphincter pressure (>40 mmHg). Both endoscopic sphincterotomy and trans-duodenal sphincteroplasty with trans-ampullary septectomy have been used to manage these patients.

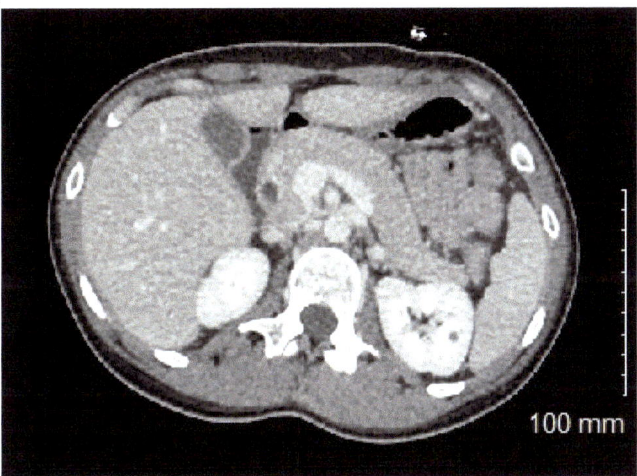

Figure 2: Dilated common bile duct

Gallstone Ileus

Gallstone ileus is mechanical obstruction (small bowel obstruction) from a large gallstone. It most commonly occurs as the stone passes through a biliary-enteric fistula. Other rare causes include fistulous communication between the gallbladder and colon or stomach, or between the common bile duct and duodenum. Gallstone ileus most commonly occurs in older individuals. Patients usually present with signs and symptoms of small bowel obstruction. The symptoms may be episodic as the stone passes through the gastrointestinal tract. Complete obstruction is seen when the stone is impacted at the terminal ileum or occasionally the sigmoid colon. Abdominal films will demonstrate small bowel distension with air-fluid levels and pneumobilia or a calcified gallstone distant from the gallbladder. The goal in management is removal of the gallstone through an enterotomy. Removal of the biliary-enteric fistula and cholecystectomy is warranted because recurrent cholecystitis and cholangitis are common. However, if a patient has a lot of inflammatory process in the right upper quadrant or is too unstable to tolerate a long operative procedure, a second laparotomy can address the fistula.

Intrahepatic Stones

Intrahepatic stones or hepatolithiasis is more prevalent in Asian population. Most cases of hepatolithiasis are associated with common biliary tract conditions such as benign biliary strictures, primary sclerosing cholangitis, choledochal cyst, and biliary tract tumors. Risk factors include bile stasis, bacterial infection, and biliary mucin. The majority of intrahepatic stones are brown pigment stones. Clinical presentation includes right upper quadrant pain and cholangitis in more than half of the patients. Some may also present with jaundice and pruritus. Intrahepatic stones are usually present in both hepatic ducts. These are diagnosed using ERCP or MRCP. Surgical therapy includes cholecystectomy; resection of the extrahepatic biliary tree to include any strictures, tumors, or choledochal cyst; and then choledochoscopy and extraction of any intrahepatic stones. Biliary-enteric continuity is reestablished with a Roux-en-Y hepaticojejunostomy. Partial hepatic resection may be necessary.

Laparoscopic Cholecystectomy

Some of the few indications where laparoscopic surgery is the gold standard is cholecystectomy for benign gallbladder disease. With advancement in laparoscopic techniques and increased comfort and experience of surgeons, this can be expanded to other indications including but not limited to intraoperative cholangiogram common duct stone exploration and extraction of a small group of gallbladder cancers.

The steps involved in the operation are similar to any open cholecystectomy. Variation exists in the dissection of the triangle of Calot. Preoperative preparation should always include the relatively low risk of conversion (5%). Preoperative antibiotics are usually not indicated unless operating on a high-risk patient (e.g., diabetic). Open Hassan technique is used to gain access into the abdomen. After the pneumo-peritoneum is established, the abdomen is carefully visualized for adhesions, inflammation, and any secondary pathology. Next, a second incision is made 5 mm, up to 10 mm, at the subxiphoid, and two additional 5 mm incisions are placed at the right subcostal along the midclavicular and anterior midaxillary lines. The gallbladder infundibulum is grasped and retracted laterally exposing the triangle of Calot.

With blunt and sharp dissection using the two medial 5 mm trocars, the Calot triangle is dissected. This exposes two structures, the cystic artery and cystic duct, which enter the gallbladder. The next step is the division of the cystic artery and the cystic duct between clips. The gallbladder is then dissected off the liver bed. At the end of the operation, the liver bed and the clips at the cystic artery and cystic duct are once again visualized.

Some may perform routine cholangiograms before dividing the cystic duct. During this situation, the cystic duct is identified and a proximal clip towards the gallbladder is placed. An incision is placed on the cystic duct and a cholangio-catheter is advanced laparoscopically. A cholangiogram is obtained, and the anatomy is identified. When the cystic duct is confirmed, the duct is then clipped and divided. In some situations where the anatomy is not identified, an anterograde or "top-down dissection" can be performed.

During pregnancy, laparoscopic procedures can be safely performed in the second trimester. Patients who are pregnant do not present with classical signs and symptoms of cholecystitis. Mild cholecystitis can be safely managed with conservative treatment. Care should be taken when encountering a patient in the first and third trimester because there is higher risk of fetal loss. When acute cholecystitis is encountered during the second trimester, laparoscopic cholecystectomy can be performed safely with lower risk to the fetus. Intra and postoperative fetal monitoring should always be considered.

Complications

The complication rates are low, less than 5%. Some of the complications can be quite disabling to patients because some may need a second operation. In general, patients complaining of pain out of proportion after a laparoscopic procedure should be thoroughly evaluated for complications. The major complications after a laparoscopic cholecystectomy are shown in Table 4. Intraoperative complications include bleeding. These can be from the trocar site, injury to the liver during the trocar placement, and cystic artery stump bleeding. Most conversions are due to bleeding or unclear anatomy. Bleeding from the trocar site can be easily controlled using an energy device, or when a visible vessel is identified, laparoscopic closure of the incision will securely ligate the vessel. Liver injuries that are not actively bleeding will settle down. Some may require the use of an energy device and others will only need simple pressure. There is no role of coagulation factors unless patients had previously low coagulation factors. Bleeding from the cystic artery can be quite difficult to control. The goal of controlling the bleeding is not to lose visualization. Blindly grasping structures or clipping can lead to inadvertent injury to the common duct and other major vascular structures. The suction device itself may be helpful in clearing the field of any blood and identifying the bleeding vessel. A second 5 mm trocar may help control the hemorrhage. When controlling bleeding-time is of essence, care should be taken because major bleeding cannot be managed using minimally invasive techniques and the best option is to convert to an open technique.

Table 4: Complications of laparoscopic cholecystectomy

Intraoperative	Bleeding Bile duct injury Spilled stones
Early postoperative	Retained common duct stone Bile leak Bile duct injury Bowel injury Incidental gallbladder cancer

Spilled stones occur in up to 1/3 of cholecystectomies. There is concern that retained intraperitoneal gallstones can cause abscess formation. The incidence of complications related to retained stones is very low. Care should be taken to suction-irrigate all the stones that are spilled. Spilled stones in the presence of infected bile can lead to abscess formation These may require image guided drainage and antibiotics. All patients should be informed that spilled stones are a potential complication.

When identified, intraoperative bile duct injury will need a cholangiogram. Depending on the skills of the operating surgeon, this can be performed laparoscopically. The biliary anatomy should be identified and injury to the bile duct should be delineated. With an injured common duct, the anatomy should be clearly defined and drainage of the common duct with a T-tube should be performed. Where facilities are not available, these patients should be transferred to a tertiary care center. Late presentation of these patients is not uncommon.

Bile leaks present clinically with recurrent abdominal pain, and imaging will reveal postoperative fluid collections. These are results of bile duct injury or cystic duct stump leakage and require prompt attention. Prompt drainage of intra-abdominal bile and control of sepsis is key. Following drainage and appropriate antibiotics, the next step is to delineate the anatomy. Successful management of patients with biliary injuries following laparoscopic cholecystectomy includes: (1) completely defining the nature of the injury, which may require obtaining a cholangiography from above (a percutaneous transhepatic approach) and below (an endoscopic approach), (2) percutaneously draining the biliary system, (3) treating sepsis and periportal inflammation with antibiotics and drainage of collections, and (4) appropriate timing of expert, definitive repair.

The incidence of retained common bile duct stones is close to 3%. The majority of retained common duct stones can be managed nonoperatively with endoscopic sphincterotomy and stone extraction. Some patients require operative treatment, including those with multiple or large stones and those with prior surgical therapy (e.g., Roux-en-Y gastric bypass or gastric resection with Billroth II anastomosis) that prevents endoscopic access to the ampulla.

Cystic duct leaks are usually treated with endoscopic trans-ampullary stenting percutaneous drainage of localized bile collections. There is about a 90% success rate with nonoperative management of an isolated cystic duct stump leak. Open surgical drainage or closure of cystic duct leaks are rarely necessary.

Bowel Injury with perforation is rare. Small bowel, especially the duodenum, is the most common. The majority of bowel injuries go unnoticed at the time of injury. Electrocautery accounts for nearly half the injuries. All bowel injuries recognized at the time of operation should be repaired primarily. Missed bowel injuries during cholecystectomy present with abdominal pain, fever, and distention. CT may or may not show extravasation and fluid collection. Any fluid collection that is enteric should alert the surgeon for the need of exploration.

Gallbladder cancer is rare. The majority of these cancers are early-stage lesions detected by pathology. When suspicious intraoperatively, it is prudent to convert to open surgery and perform an oncologic resection.

Polypoid Lesions of the Gallbladder

Polypoid lesions of the gallbladder (PLGs) are present in nearly 7% of the population. These are classified as benign pseudotumors (cholesterol polyps, adenomyomatosis), benign (adenoma), and malignant (adenocarcinoma) neoplasms. Cholesterol polyps are the most common and are usually less than 10 mm in size. These have a characteristic echogenic pedunculated appearance on ultrasound and are often multiple in number. Adenomyomatosis appears as a greater than 10 mm sessile polyp with characteristic microcysts on ultrasound. Adenoma and adenocarcinoma may be sessile or pedunculated and are also usually larger than 10 mm. Risk factors for malignancy include age older than 60 years, coexistence of gallstones, and size greater than 10 mm.

Ultrasound is the most effective diagnostic method for detecting polyps. When large lesions of greater than 1 cm are found on ultrasound, CT should be performed to assess for possible gallbladder cancer. All patients with symptomatic PLGs should undergo laparoscopic cholecystectomy. Patients should undergo cholecystectomy if they are asymptomatic PLGs and have one or more risk factors. It is safe to observe PLGs if they are asymptomatic, less than 10 mm, show no ultrasound features of neoplasia, and have interval ultrasound documents showing no change in size.

Benign Stricture/Bile Duct Injury

Benign biliary strictures are associated with many different conditions. The most common cause is during laparoscopic cholecystectomy. Unrecognized or poorly managed biliary strictures lead to recurrent cholangitis, secondary biliary cirrhosis, and portal hypertension.[19] The rate of bile duct injury with laparoscopic cholecystectomy is greater than that observed with open cholecystectomy. The incidence of major bile duct injuries is around 0.55%, and the incidence of bile leaks or minor injuries is 0.3%.

Risk factors for bile duct injuries include chronic inflammation, obesity, fat in the periportal region, poor exposure, and bleeding that obscures the operative field. Generally, older patients, male patients, patients symptomatic for an extended period prior to cholecystectomy, and number of attacks have more difficulty during the procedure. Aberrant biliary anatomy is often encountered during the operation. The most common is an aberrant right hepatic duct that travels through the triangle of Calot and enters the common hepatic duct. Occasionally, the cystic duct enters a small aberrant right hepatic duct, which is mistaken for the cystic duct and is ligated and/or divided. Another intraoperative situation is when the common bile duct is mistaken for the cystic duct; this can lead to the isolation, clipping, and division of the duct which ultimately leads to excessive traction on the cystic duct. If there is a lot of traction on the cystic duct a clip on the common bile duct may be necessary, the clip may dissect into the liver parenchyma too deeply, the clip may be poorly placed on the cystic duct, or injudicious use of cautery may be required.[20] Routine use of intraoperative cholangiogram has shown to reduce the rate of bile duct injury. Other procedures that can lead to bile duct strictures include those that involve the biliary system and the surrounding structures such as common bile duct exploration, gastrectomy with division of the proximal duodenum, and biliary enteric anastomosis.

Clinical Presentation

Some injuries are recognized intraoperatively, and others are present early in the postoperative period. Pain, fever, and/or mild hyperbilirubinemia (2.5 mg/dL) are common. Jaundice with or without abdominal pain is common in injuries that involve the common duct. Other less common symptoms include cholangitis or cirrhosis.

Diagnosis

If a bile leak is suspected, abdominal CT scan or ultrasound can be used to identify peritoneal fluid, abscess, or biloma.

This perihepatic fluid or other intra-abdominal fluid collections should be drained.[21] A sinogram can be helpful in determining the biliary anatomy in patients with a surgical drain or percutaneously placed catheter. PTC and placement of a transhepatic stent decompresses the biliary tree, relieves the jaundice, and defines the proximal extent of the injury.

Management

Cystic duct bile leaks are often managed with percutaneous drainage of any intraabdominal fluid collection, followed by biliary stent placement. If there is a lateral bile duct (partial transection) injury during cholecystectomy, a T-tube should be placed. The T-tube can be placed at the site of injury if it is similar in size to a choledochotomy. If the biliary stent is more extensive, the injury is repaired and stented with a T-tube placed through a proximal or distal choledochotomy. Isolated hepatic ducts <3 mm, or those draining a single hepatic segment can be safely ligated. Ducts >3 mm will probably drain several segments or an entire lobe and will require reimplantation. Major bile duct injuries including transections of the common bile duct or common hepatic duct should be repaired if recognized at the time of cholecystectomy. Injuries diagnosed after the early postoperative period should be managed initially with transhepatic catheters for biliary decompression, followed by operative exploration and repair in 6 to 8 weeks after the acute inflammation has resolved. The goal of surgical repair is to create a duct enteric anastomosis. An end-to-side Roux-en-Y choledochojejunostomy or, more commonly, a Roux-en-Y hepaticojejunostomy should be performed in these patients.

Primary Sclerosing Cholangitis

Primary sclerosing cholangitis is characterized by fibrotic strictures that involve both the intrahepatic and extrahepatic biliary system. The disease is more common in certain HLA haplotypes including B8/DR3 autoimmune diseases, insulin dependent diabetes mellitus, Graves' disease, Sjögren's syndrome, and myasthenia gravis. Primary sclerosing cholangitis is associated with several diseases, the strongest being ulcerative colitis with a 70% association.

Sclerosing cholangitis has a variable presentation in different patients, including some patients being asymptomatic for years, while others present with rapidly progressive obliterative biliary tract changes. The mean age at presentation ranges from 40 to 45 years. Patients can present with cholestatic liver disease (jaundice, pruritus, fatigue), abnormal serum liver function tests, or advanced liver disease. They are also at increased risk of developing cholangiocarcinoma. Primary sclerosing cholangitis diagnosis is made by ERCP which displays diffuse multifocal strictures, often in both the intrahepatic and extrahepatic bile ducts. A liver biopsy is required to determine the degree of hepatic fibrosis or the presence of cirrhosis.

Medical therapy for the disease does not yield good results. Non-operative measures such as stenting and dilatation only result in short-term improvement in symptoms. Patients who are symptomatic and who present with jaundice can undergo surgical therapy. Extrahepatic biliary tree resection with bilateral hepaticojejunostomies have demonstrated to have short-term results in patients with significant extrahepatic or bifurcation strictures. Surgical resection is contraindicated in patients with cirrhosis or significant hepatic fibrosis on liver biopsy. Additionally, exploration is required in patients where a cholangiocarcinoma cannot be excluded. Overall noncirrhotic patients with primary sclerosing cholangitis who are managed with surgical resection have a significantly longer survival relative to patients managed nonoperatively. This is also true for patients needing a liver transplant, where patients managed with surgical resection did not require a transplant for longer than patients managed nonoperatively.[22] This is a progressive disease that can eventually result in biliary cirrhosis. Liver transplantation has demonstrated great results as a treatment with a 5-year actuarial patient survival as high as 85%, and a 5-year graft survival of 72%. Reported recurrent disease has been seen in up to 10% of patients who may require re-transplantation.

Biliary Cysts

Choledochal cyst is a rare congenital condition where there is dilation of the extrahepatic and/or intrahepatic biliary tract. The incidence is only between 1 in 100,000 and 1 in 150,000, with a higher incidence in Asian populations. Females are more commonly affected. The current classification is as shown in Table 5. The clinical triad of choledochal cysts includes right upper quadrant pain, jaundice, and an abdominal mass. The clinical presentation differs among children and adults. Laboratory studies show mild liver function abnormalities. Diagnosis is made on ultrasound or CT, but biliary cysts are often overlooked when not considering it as a diagnosis. Cholangiography (endoscopic, transhepatic, or MR) must be completed to identify the type of choledochal cyst and for making the operative treatment plan. Types I and II choledochal cysts require cholecystectomy, resection of the extrahepatic biliary tract including the choledochal cyst, and Roux-en-Y hepaticojejunostomy. The risk of cholangiocarcinoma is high; hence this supports the role of resection in management. Type IV cysts also potentially require resection of the extrahepatic biliary tract. If the intrahepatic cysts are confined to one lobe, a hepatic lobectomy is considered. Bilobar intrahepatic cysts have an increased risk of intrahepatic stones, thus long-term transhepatic stenting for management is required to have intrahepatic biliary tree access for stone retrieval.

Table 5: Classification of biliary cyst

Type I	Extrahepatic biliary tract is fusiform or has cystic dilations	50%	
Type II	Extrahepatic bile duct is a saccular diverticulum	2-3%	
Type III	Bile duct dilation within the duodenal wall (Choledococele)	<10%	
Type IV	Intrahepatic and extrahepatic biliary tract cystic dilation	35%	
Type V	Intrahepatic cysts (Caroli's disease)	<10%	

Malignant Biliary Disease

Gallbladder Cancer

Incidence and Etiopathology

Gallbladder cancer is a rare cancer and most present in an advanced and unresectable form. It is the most common cancer of the biliary tract. Incidence is 2.5 per 100,000 population. There is a higher incidence in countries where there is a high incidence of gallstones. Mean age of presentation is during the seventh decade of life. Females are more commonly affected than males. Risk factors include gallstones greater than 3 cm, adenomatous polyps, calcification of the gallbladder wall ("porcelain gallbladder"), and anomalous pancreaticobiliary duct junctions. Dysplasia and carcinoma in-situ are found in more than 90% of the gallbladder cancer specimens. Chronic inflammation from stones or other processes is postulated to be the inciting event. Most gallbladder cancers are adenocarcinomas of a papillary, tubular, mucinous, or signet-cell type. Other pathologies include anaplastic carcinomas, squamous cell carcinomas, or adenosquamous cell carcinomas.

The tumor spreads through direct invasion, lymphatics, hematogenous spread, and the peritoneum.

Staging

The most recent (8th) edition of the American Joint Commission on Cancer Staging Manual is shown in Table 6.

Table 6: AJCC classification of gallbladder cancer[23]

Primary Tumor (T)

TX	The primary tumor(s) cannot be assessed.
T0	There is no evidence of a primary tumor.
Tis	Carcinoma in situ.
T1	The tumor invades the lamina propria or muscular layer.
T1a	The tumor invades the lamina propria.
T1b	The tumor invades the muscular layer.
T2	The tumor invades the perimuscular connective tissue and there is no extension past the serosa or into the liver.
T3	The tumor perforates the serosa and/or The tumor directly invades the liver and/or The tumor invades one other adjacent organ or structure.
T4	Tumor invades the hepatic artery or main portal vein or invades at least two extrahepatic organs or structures.

Regional Lymph Nodes (N)a

NX	Cannot assess the regional lymph nodes.
N0	There is no metastasis to regional lymph nodes.
N1	There are metastases to the nodes along the common bile duct, cystic duct, hepatic artery, and/or portal vein.
N2	There are metastases to the pericaval, periaortic, superior mesenteric artery, and/or celiac artery lymph nodes.

Distant Metastasis (M)a

M0	There is no distant metastasis.
M1	There is distant metastasis.

Stage/Prognostic Groups

Stage 0	Tis N0 M0
Stage I	T1 N0 M0
Stage II	T2 N0 M0
Stage IIIA	T3 N0 M0
Stage IIIB	T1 to 3 N1 M0
Stage IVA	T4 N0 to 1 M0
Stage IVB	Any T N2 M0

Clinical Presentation

Gallbladder cancer can present either as an incidental finding post-cholecystectomy or symptomatically with pain or jaundice. Occasionally a mass is found on diagnostic imaging. Constitutional symptoms such as nausea, vomiting, anorexia, and weight loss are also common.

Diagnosis

Ultrasound remains the initial evaluation tool for symptoms related to the gallbladder. This can reveal gallstones, bile duct obstruction, porta hepatis, lymphadenopathy, direct liver extension of a tumor, or even hepatic metastases. In patients with suspected gallbladder cancer, CT or MRI should be performed. Both CT and MRI can demonstrate invasion of a tumor into the hepatoduodenal ligament or the adjacent liver. They can also demonstrate lymph node involvement or encasement of the portal vein or hepatic artery. The extent of adjacent liver involvement is particularly important in planning the extent of liver resection. The finding of paraaortic or peripancreatic nodal disease beyond the head of the pancreas on imaging precludes curative resection. Positron emission tomography (PET) is the most sensitive modality for determining distant metastasis and can reduce surgical explorations for unresectable disease. In patients with advanced disease, and for whom nonsurgical treatment is planned, biopsy guided by ultrasound or CT is a highly sensitive tool to confirm diagnosis. The role of serum tumor markers and other biochemical tests are not helpful.

Management

Surgery is the only potentially curative treatment for gallbladder cancer. Treatment is based primarily on the T-stage of the tumor. Contraindications to surgical therapy are shown in Table 7.

Table 7: Contraindications to surgery in gallbladder cancer

Liver metastases
Malignant ascites
Peritoneal metastases
Distant disease
Extensive involvement of hepatoduodenal ligament
Encasement or occlusion of major vessels
Para-aortic lymph node involvement
Poor performance status

Tis and T1a

For Tis or T1a stage cancers, simple cholecystectomy is the treatment of choice. The cure rate is 85% to 100% as long as the cystic duct margin is negative. If the margin is involved, re-exploration should be performed with common bile duct excision and biliary reconstruction.

T1b and T2 Tumors

T1b tumors have a 15% rate of lymph node metastasis. In T2 tumors, regional lymph node metastasis is found in more than half of cases. Lymphadenectomy and extended resection or radical cholecystectomy resection of the gallbladder fossa with a minimum of 2 cm hepatic parenchymal margin are performed. In patients who are jaundiced, extrahepatic bile duct resection should be performed with reconstruction.

T3 and T4 Tumors

Patients with locally advanced T3 and T4 cancers may benefit from resection if there is no evidence of distant or peritoneal disease and if a resection is technically feasible. There is no survival benefit if the tumor is not completely resected; therefore, debulking operations have no role. For locally advanced T3 or T4 tumors, diagnostic laparoscopy should be strongly considered before exploratory laparotomy. Lesions that have minimal extension into the liver can usually be approached with a simple wedge or a segment 4b and 5 resections. As the lesion size increases or the vascular structures are affected, more extensive resections are required. An aggressive surgical approach with extended liver resection to achieve R0 resection can improve overall survival in T4 tumors with no distant metastasis. The most important factor for survival is resection of the tumor with negative margins, preferably greater than 2 cm.

Stage IV and unresectable disease

Patients who present with locally unresectable or metastatic disease have an overall poor prognosis, often with a survival of less than one year. Unfortunately, there is no effective adjuvant treatment for gallbladder cancers. The majority of patients require palliation for pain, jaundice, and possibly intestinal obstruction. If unresectable disease is encountered during an exploratory laparotomy, choledochojejunostomy and gastrojejunostomy can be performed. Biliary obstruction can be successfully treated with endoscopic or percutaneous drainage. Chemotherapy and radiotherapy have been largely unsuccessful in treating this disease. Modest results have been reported with 5-fluorouracil (5-FU), gemcitabine, or capecitabine based single-agent and multi-agent regimens. Response rates are low, but an occasional disease stabilization can be achieved for a few months. Recurrent disease often occurs locally in the liver and presents with jaundice. Patients who present with peritoneal or distant disease can be offered supportive care or palliative chemotherapy.

Cholangiocarcinoma

Cholangiocarcinoma is more commonly diagnosed than other biliary tract cancers. It represents around 3% of all malignancies. Risk factors include primary sclerosing cholangitis, choledochal cysts, and Asian descent. Males are more commonly affected than females. Microscopically, cholangiocarcinoma is most commonly tubular adenocarcinoma, but papillary adenocarcinoma, signet-cell carcinoma, mucoepidermoid carcinoma, and other histological variants of cholangiocarcinoma have been observed. Bismuth-Corlette classification system is shown in Table 8.

Table 8: AJCC classification of Cholangiocarcinoma

Staging	Stage	Tumor	Node	Metastasis
AJCC TNM Intrahepatic	I	T1, solitary tumor, no vascular invasion	N0	M0
	II	T2, solitary tumor with vascular invasion or multiple <5 cm tumors	N0	M0
	IIIA	T3, major vascular involvement or multiple >5 cm tumors	N0	M0
	IIIB	T4, direct invasion of adjacent organ (not including the gallbladder) or perforation of visceral peritoneum	N0	M0
	IIIC	Any T	N1	M0
	IV	Any T	Any N	M1
AJCC TNM Extrahepatic	0	Tis, carcinoma in situ	N0	M0
	IA	T1, only in bile duct	N0	M0
	IB	T2, past bile duct	N0	M0
	IIA	T3, invades adjacent organs including the liver, gallbladder, pancreas, or unilateral HA or PV	N0	M0
	IIB	T1 or T3	N1	M0
	III	T4, invades other adjacent organs or main HA or PV	Any N	M0
	IV	Any T	Any N	M1
N1, regional lymph node metastasis M1, distant metastasis				

Clinical jaundice is more commonly seen in perihilar and distal lesions. Patients with intrahepatic lesions initially present with pain. Nonspecific symptoms such as anorexia, weight loss, night sweats, malaise, and fatigue are also common. The tumor markers CEA and CA 19-9 are elevated. The biliary anatomy can be imaged using MRCP. Other modalities include ERCP and PTC. CT and MRA are also helpful in evaluation of the vascular structures and tumor extension. Biopsy is usually not required for diagnosis unless the disease is metastatic or unresectable. The most recent (7th) edition of the American Joint Commission on Cancer Staging Manual is shown in Table 8.

Surgery is potentially curative in resectable disease. Contraindications to resection include those as shown in Table 9. Intrahepatic cholangiocarcinoma can be resected using anatomic and nonanatomic (large wedge resection) techniques. Intraoperative ultrasound is used for evaluation of any metastasis. Perihilar cholangiocarcinoma is near the porta hepatis. Preoperative portal vein embolization of the liver portion that is to be resected to stimulate growth of the future liver remnant is not uncommon. Extrahepatic biliary tree and bile duct bifurcation are removed, extensive hilar lymphadenectomy is performed, and biliary-enteric tract reconstruction is performed using a Roux-en-Y limb of jejunum. Distal cholangiocarcinoma is resected with a pancreaticoduodenectomy. The main criteria for resectability includes the absence of metastatic disease and lack of involvement of the portal vein, superior mesenteric vein, hepatic artery, and superior mesenteric artery.

Table 9: Contraindication to resection is cholangiocarcinoma

Hepatic duct involvement. No further than the secondary biliary radicals bilaterally
Encasement/occlusion of the main portal vein. The occlusion is proximal to the main portal vein bifurcation
Atrophy of one hepatic lobe with contralateral encasement of the portal vein branch or involvement of secondary biliary radicals
Unilateral tumor extension to secondary biliary radicles and if there is contralateral vein branch encasement or occlusion

Adjuvant therapy is not well established. Some small studies have provided evidence of modest improvement in survival of cholangiocarcinoma after treatment with external beam radiation treatment. Other studies have evaluated the role of liver transplantation in the treatment of cholangiocarcinoma, with varied success. The primary aim of palliative treatment is to provide biliary drainage with long-term symptomatic relief. Endoscopic placement of biliary stents has low complication rates and high rates of symptomatic relief for patients with biliary obstruction caused by an unresectable tumor. Percutaneous biliary drainage is an acceptable alternative. Surgical bypass can be performed if necessary but is not the first treatment of choice.

Metastatic and Other Tumors

Hepatocellular carcinoma, colorectal carcinoma, and pancreatic carcinoma are the most common primary sites associated with biliary tract obstruction from lymph node metastases. Nodal metastases are also seen in breast and ovarian cancer. Lymphoma can also result in biliary obstruction and mimic either pancreatic cancer or perihilar cholangiocarcinoma.

REFERENCES

1. Ahrendt SA. Biliary tract surgery. Current gastroenterology reports 1999, 1 (2), 107-15.
2. Lee HJ, Choi BI, Han JK, Kim AY, Kim KW, Park SH, Jeong JY, Kang JW. Three-dimensional ultrasonography using the minimum transparent mode in obstructive biliary diseases: early experience. Journal of ultrasound in medicine: official journal of the American Institute of Ultrasound in Medicine 2002, 21 (4), 443-53.
3. Ralls PW, Jeffrey RB Jr, Kane RA, Robbin<. Ultrasonography. Gastroenterol Clin North Am 2002, 31 (3), 801-25, vii.
4. Wexler RS, Greene GS, Scott M. Left hepatic and common hepatic ductal bile leaks demonstrated by Tc-99m HIDA scan and percutaneous transhepatic cholangiogram. Clinical nuclear medicine 1994, 19 (1), 59-60.
5. Breen DJ, Nicholson AA. The clinical utility of spiral CT cholangiography. Clinical radiology 2000, 55 (10), 733-9.
6. Magnuson TH, Bender JS, Duncan MD, Ahrendt SA, Harmon JW, Regan F. Utility of magnetic resonance cholangiography in the evaluation of biliary obstruction. J Am Coll Surg 1999, 189 (1), 63-71; discussion 71-2.
7. Tischendorf JJ, Kruger M, Trautwein C, Duckstein N, Schneider A, Manns MP, Meier PN. Cholangioscopic characterization of dominant bile duct stenoses in patients with primary sclerosing cholangitis. Endoscopy 2006, 38 (7), 665-9.
8. Everhart JE, Khare M, Hill M, Maurer KR. Prevalence and ethnic differences in gallbladder disease in the United States. Gastroenterology 1999, 117 (3), 632-9.
9. Stewart L, Oesterle AL, Erdan I, Griffiss JM, Way LW. Pathogenesis of pigment gallstones in Western societies: the central role of bacteria. J Gastrointest Surg 2002, 6 (6), 891-903; discussion 903-4.
10. Trowbridge RL, Rutkowski NK, Shojania KG. Does this patient have acute cholecystitis? JAMA: the journal of the American Medical Association 2003, 289 (1), 80-6.
11. Binmoeller, K. F.; Schafer, T. W., Endoscopic management of bile duct stones. J Clin Gastroenterol 2001, 32 (2), 106-18.
12. Weber DM. Laparoscopic surgery: an excellent approach in elderly patients. Arch Surg 2003, 138 (10), 1083-8.
13. Lipman JM, Claridge JA, Haridas M, Martin MD, Yao DC, Grimes KL, Malangoni MA. Preoperative findings predict conversion from laparoscopic to open cholecystectomy. Surgery 2007, 142 (4), 556-63; discussion 563-5.
14. Strasberg SM. Cholelithiasis and acute cholecystitis. Bailliere's clinical gastroenterology 1997, 11 (4), 643-61.
15. Shikata S, Noguchi Y, Fukui T. Early versus delayed cholecystectomy for acute cholecystitis: a meta-analysis of randomized controlled trials. Surgery today 2005, 35 (7), 553-60.
16. Patel M, Miedema BW, James MA, Marshall JB. Percutaneous cholecystostomy is an effective treatment for high-risk patients with acute cholecystitis. The American surgeon 2000, 66 (1), 33-7.
17. Ryu JK, Ryu KH, Kim KH. Clinical features of acute

acalculous cholecystitis. J Clin Gastroenterol 2003, 36 (2), 166-9.

18. Pelinka LE, Schmidhammer R, Hamid L, Mauritz W, Redl H. Acute acalculous cholecystitis after trauma: a prospective study. The Journal of trauma 2003, 55 (2), 323-9.
19. Fletcher DR, Hobbs MS, Tan P, Valinsky LJ, Hockey RL, Pikora TJ. Knuiman, M. W.; Sheiner, H. J.; Edis, A., Complications of cholecystectomy: risks of the laparoscopic approach and protective effects of operative cholangiography: a population-based study. Ann Surg 1999, 229 (4), 449-57.
20. Strasberg SM, Hertl, M, Soper NJ. An analysis of the problem of biliary injury during laparoscopic cholecystectomy. J Am Coll Surg 1995, 180 (1), 101-25.
21. Lee CM, Stewart L, Way LW. Postcholecystectomy abdominal bile collections. Arch Surg 2000, 135 (5), 538-42; discussion 542-4.
22. Ahrendt SA, Pitt HA, Kalloo AN, et al. Primary sclerosing cholangitis: resect, dilate, or transplant? Ann Surg 1998, 227 (3), 412-23.
23. Edge SB, Byrd DR, Compton CC, et al. AJCC: Gallbladder. eds.: AJCC Cancer Staging Manual. 7th ed. New York, NY: Springer, 2010, pp 211-7.

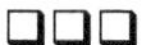

31

CHAPTER

Pancreas

Vijay K. Mittal, MD
Sumeet Virmani, MD

SURGICAL EMBRYOLOGY AND ANATOMY

The pancreas develops during the fourth week of fetal life from dorsal and ventral outgrowths of endoderm that arise from the caudal portion of the foregut. In the seventh week, the ventral and dorsal buds fuse as the duodenum rotates to the right. The dorsal and ventral pancreatic ducts join to form the main pancreatic duct, also known as the duct of Wirsung, and then this duct merges with the common bile duct (CBD). However, a small part remains as an accessory duct, also known as the duct of Santorini, which drains directly into the duodenum. In 5-10% of people, this fusion of the ventral and dorsal pancreatic ducts does not occur, resulting in most of the pancreas needing to be drained through the duct of Santorini and the minor papilla orifice. Failed fusion of pancreatic ducts (pancreatic divisum: Figure 1) may result in pancreatitis arising from the stenosis of the duct of Santorini. Another embryonic anomaly may occur if the second part of duodenum gets trapped in the pancreatic band leading to annular pancreas.

The pancreas is a retroperitoneal organ located in the upper part of the abdomen and weighs 70-100 mg in an adult. The pancreas can be divided into following regions: head (including uncinate process), neck, body, and tail. The head is located between the L1-L2 vertebra in the C-loop of duodenum. The blood supply originates from branches of both the celiac and superior mesenteric arteries (SMA). The pancreatic head is supplied from superior and inferior pancreaticoduodenal arteries. The body is supplied by great, inferior, and caudal pancreatic arteries (all branches from the splenic artery) and the tail is supplied from branches of splenic, gastroepiploic, and dorsal pancreatic arteries. Venous drainage is via the portal system. Lymphatic drains into the celiac and SMA nodes.

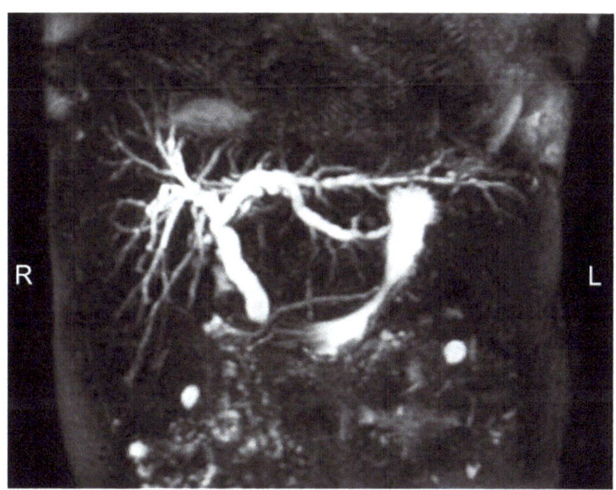

Figure 1: MRI (3D reconstruction) of abdomen showing moderate intra- and extra-biliary ductal dilatation. Pancreatic duct draining the tail, body and anterior aspect of pancreas drains directly into the duodenum. Posterior aspect of pancreatic head mass drains through a second orifice consistent with pancreatic divisum

PHYSIOLOGY

The exocrine pancreas secretes about 1-2 liters/day of clear, alkaline (pH 7-8.5) solution rich in digestive enzymes. Secretin, cholecystokinin (CCK) and parasympathetic vagal discharge stimulate the pancreatic exocrine secretion, whereas somatostatin and pancreatic polypeptide inhibit their release. Ductal cells contain carbonic anhydrase and secrete HCO3, while acinar cells secrete Cl- and digestive enzymes. Digestive enzymes include amylase, lipase, trypsinogen, chymotrypsinogen, carboxypeptidase and HCO3. Amylase is the only pancreatic enzyme secreted in its active form.

Endocrine pancreas secretes glucagon from alpha cells, insulin from beta cells, somatostatin from delta cells, pancreatic polypeptide from F cells, and vasoactive intestinal polypeptide (VIP), serotonin and neuropeptide Y from islet cells.

ACUTE PANCREATITIS

Introduction

Acute pancreatitis is an acute inflammatory process of the pancreas with severity ranging from mild self-limiting disease to one with high morbidity and mortality. It is important to differentiate "acute" from "chronic" pancreatitis which is based on the functional and structural integrity of the gland before and after the attack rather than duration of the disease. Mild cases of acute pancreatitis are often successfully treated conservatively while severe cases may require urgent ICU admission. The incidence is higher in male population as compared to females. Overall mortality from the disease is approximately 5% but may reach 20 to 30% in the presence of multiorgan failure.[1] Acute pancreatitis is a challenging disease to manage, with a significant morbidity, mortality, and financial costs.

Etiology

In developed countries, the leading cause of acute pancreatitis is due to gallstones (i.e., microlithiasis), with alcohol abuse as a close second. Together they account for 80% of the cases. Endoscopic retrograde cholangio-pancreatography (ERCP) induced pancreatitis is responsible for another 5%. Major and less common causes of acute pancreatitis have been summarized in Table 1. In children, acute pancreatitis can be associated with abdominal trauma, hemolytic uremic syndrome, Kawasaki disease, mumps, Reye's syndrome, and viral illnesses.

The exact mechanism causing pancreatitis is not known. However, the disease process is said to start with pancreatic acinar cell injury. Pancreatic enzymes are normally secreted in an inactive form and then become activated when inside the pancreas, at which time they start to digest pancreatic tissue. Subsequently trypsin activates the complement, kallikrein-kinin, coagulation, and fibrinolysis cascades leading to acinar cell injury. This process termed "auto digestion" activates the inflammatory response and in severe cases ultimately leads to necrosis of pancreatic parenchyma. Lipase activation produces the necrosis of fat tissue in pancreatic interstitial and peripancreatic spaces. With further progression of the disease a systemic inflammatory response syndrome (SIRS) is triggered leading to acute respiratory distress syndrome (ARDS), shock, metabolic disturbances, and renal failure. Phospholipase A2 causes injury to alveolar membranes of the lungs. Enzyme rich peri-pancreatic fluid collection often occurs in about 40% of the patients. Fifty percent of these resolve spontaneously while others become infected or form pseudocysts.

Fifty percent of deaths due to acute pancreatitis occur within 2 weeks of symptom onset; most often due to SIRS-induced multisystem organ failure. The remaining causes of death, often 2 to 3 weeks after symptom onset, are due to complications of pancreatic necrosis, in particular infection.

Table 1: Major and less common causes of acute pancreatitis

Major causes	Less common causes
• Gallstones including microlithiasis • Alcohol abuse • ERCP • Infection: Mumps, Epstein-Barr virus, cytomegalovirus, rubella, hepatitis A/B/non-A/non-B, coxsackie B, mycoplasma pneumonia, campylobacter • Drug induced: estrogens, corticosteroids, thiazide diuretics, isoniazid, tetracycline, and azathioprine • Hypercalcemia • Traumatic injury • Pancreatic surgical procedures • Ascaris species • Vasculitis • Idiopathic	• Autoimmune pancreatitis • Abnormalities of bile and pancreatic ducts (e.g., long common duct) • Genetic factors (hereditary pancreatitis) • Pancreatic divisum • Fatty necrosis • Pregnancy • Cystic fibrosis • Pancreatic cancer • Sphincter of Oddi dysfunction

Clinical Findings

The signs and symptoms are variable, depending upon the attack's severity. Acute pancreatitis usually begins after a large meal or alcohol consumption and is associated with abdominal pain radiating to the back, nausea, vomiting and anorexia. Pain often reduces by sitting upright and leaning forward or lying on the side with knees flexed. Some patients complain of pale, foul-smelling and oily stools (steatorrhea). Dehydration, tachycardia, and hypotension, resulting from intravascular hypovolemia, are often seen in patients requiring hospitalization. On abdominal examination, there may be epigastric tenderness with guarding or rigidity depending upon the severity of attack. Bowel sounds are usually decreased or absent. An abdominal mass on palpation may indicate a phlegmon, pseudocyst or an abscess. Low grade fever is secondary to pancreatic inflammation while high-grade fevers are indicative of intra- or extra-pancreatic infection. Diaphragmatic irritation may cause shallow respirations and dyspnea may occur in patients with associated pleural effusion. If there is cholangitis, the patient may present with jaundice. Bluish discoloration in the flank (Grey Turner's sign), periumbilical area (Cullen's sign), or inguinal region (Fox's sign), indicate retroperitoneal hemorrhage. Other less frequently seen findings include subcutaneous nodular fat necrosis known as panniculitis (due to circulating lipases), thrombophlebitis in the legs, and polyarthritis.

Differential Diagnosis

Biliary colic, cholecystitis, small bowel obstruction, severe gastritis, acute mesenteric ischemia, perforation, and ruptured aortic aneurysm need to be considered while evaluating a patient presenting with acute upper abdominal pain. However, blood investigations and imaging tests are often very useful in excluding other causes of acute abdomen.

Laboratory Findings

Complete blood count (CBC) with differential count, liver function test (LFT), blood urea nitrogen (BUN), serum creatinine, serum amylase and lipase are often the initial tests ordered. Acute pancreatitis results in significant loss in the third space and may result in hemoconcentration and an increased hematocrit. WBC count is increased because of pancreatic inflammation. Serum amylase level increases within 6 to 12 hours of attack and then returns to normal (half-life is 10 hours) over next 3 to 5 days in an uncomplicated attack. However, hyperamylasemia is nonspecific and occurs in several other conditions (e.g., acute cholecystitis, parotitis, trauma, radiation, acidosis, or ketoacidosis, macroamylasemia, anorexia nervosa/bulimia, renal failure, and malignancy with ectopic amylase production). Measurement of P-isoamylase (amylase of pancreatic origin) improves diagnostic accuracy.

Serum lipase diagnostic studies have a sensitivity of 85 to 100%. However, like amylase, lipase is also not specific to the pancreas and can be elevated in diseases of salivary glands, perforated viscus, and ischemic bowel disease. Other enzymes like phospholipase A, trypsin, carboxyl ester lipase, carboxypeptidase A, and co-lipase may also be elevated. Levels of pancreatitis-associated protein (PAP), a heat shock protein, are also markedly increased in acute pancreatitis, but this test has not proven to be more sensitive for acute pancreatitis than the other more conventional tests.

Patients with recurrent idiopathic pancreatitis are now screened for mutations in different genes such as cationic trypsinogen (PRSS1), pancreatic secretory trypsin inhibitor (PSTI or SPINK1), and cystic fibrosis transmembrane conductance regulator (CFTR) gene.

Imaging

An abdominal X-ray may show localized ileus of a small intestine segment ("sentinel loop") or the "colon cutoff sign." Chest X-ray (CXR) may reveal pleural effusions, basal atelectasis, and pulmonary infiltrates, especially on the left side. Abdominal ultrasound may reveal gallstones. On ultrasound, acute pancreatitis shows a diffusely enlarged, hypoechoic pancreas. However, about 1/4th of patients have bowel gas thus making the study inconclusive.

CT scan is often not necessary during initial hospital admission, unless considering other diagnoses. However, it is always the first radiological investigation and is indicated in patients with severe acute pancreatitis (Figure 2). A dynamic spiral CT scanning is helpful in identifying the presence and extent of necrosis in the pancreas. The patients are given oral and intravenous contrast (if normal renal function), to identify unenhanced areas which indicate pancreatic necrosis (Figure 3). Diffuse glandular enlargement is the most common finding. Abdominal CT scans are helpful with prognosis based on Balthazar's grading scale (Table 2).

MRI and MRCP are being used more frequently in diagnosing suspected biliary or pancreatic duct obstruction when a patient has pancreatitis. The advantages include (a) the MRI can categorize fluid collection as either acute fluid collections, necrosis, abscess, hemorrhage, or pseudocyst, and (b) the MRI is more sensitive in detecting mild acute pancreatitis compared to the CT. ERCP is normally contraindicated during an acute attack, unless the pancreatitis is due to an impacted common bile duct stone. Under those conditions, sphincterotomy and stone retrieval result in significant reduction in morbidity and mortality.

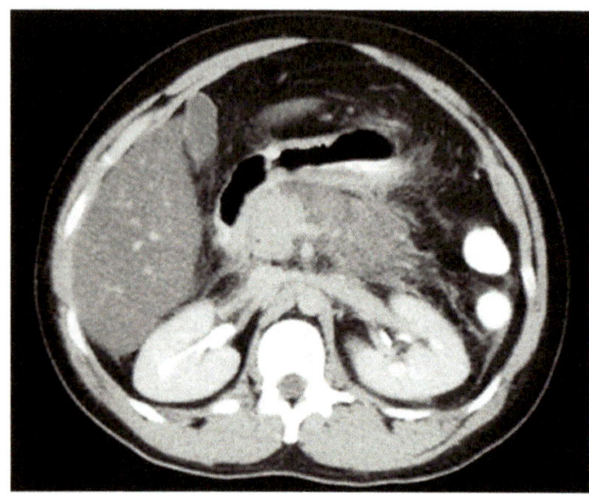

Figure 2: CT scan of the abdomen with contrast showing peripancreatic fluid consistent with acute pancreatitis

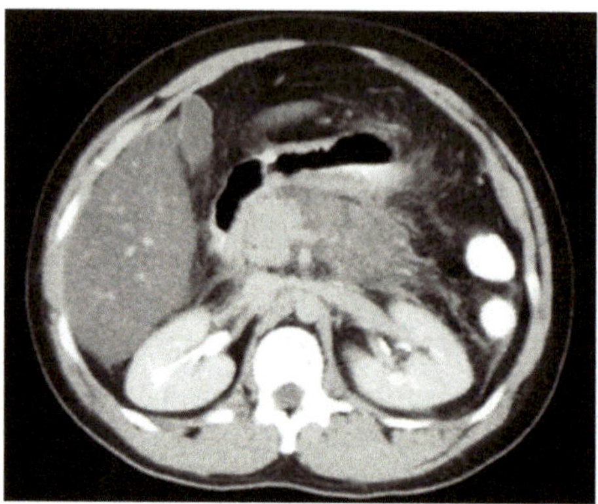

Figure 3: CT scan of the abdomen with contrast showing fluid around the pancreas consistent with pancreatitis. Some hypo-enhancement of the body of the pancreas is also seen suggestive of pancreatic necrosis or impending necrosis

Table 2: CT scan-based Balthazar grading system for acute pancreatitis, CT scan severity index (points for grade of acute pancreatitis) + (points for degree of pancreatic necrosis). Interpretation: minimum score 0, maximum score 10

Criteria	CT Finding	Points
Grade of acute pancreatitis	Normal	0
	Gland enlargement	1
	Peripancreatic inflammation	2
	Single extrapancreatic fluid collection	3
	Extensive extrapancreatic fluid collection, pancreatic abscess	4
Degree of pancreatic necrosis	No necrosis	0
	Necrosis of ⅓ of the pancreas	2
	Necrosis of ½ of the pancreas	4
	Necrosis of >½ of the pancreas	6

Endoscopic ultrasonography (EUS) is used to visualize the pancreas and biliary tract. It is an endoscopic procedure where a high-frequency ultrasound transducer is inserted into the gastrointestinal tract. EUS is often helpful in evaluating the cause of severe pancreatitis, particularly microlithiasis and biliary sludge. It can help to identify periampullary lesions better than any other imaging modalities. A secretin stimulated EUS study is helpful in identifying resistance to ductal outflow at the papilla.

PREDICTORS OF SEVERITY OF ACUTE PANCREATITIS

Clinical, laboratory, and radiologic risk factors cannot be used to predict severity of acute pancreatitis. Acute pancreatitis is divided into two categories by the Atlanta classification. These categories include mild (edematous and interstitial) acute pancreatitis and severe (necrotizing) acute pancreatitis. Severe acute pancreatitis consists of a Ranson's score (Table 3) of 3 or more and/or an Acute Physiology and Chronic Health Evaluation-II (APACHE II) score of 8 or more within the first 48 hours, organ failure (respiratory, circulatory, renal, and/or gastrointestinal bleeding), and/or local complications (pancreatic necrosis, abscess, or pseudocyst). Those with actual or predicted severe disease and those with other severe comorbid conditions should be considered for triage to an intensive care or intermediate medical care unit.

Serum markers of immune activation IL-6, IL-8, IL-10, TNF, PMN elastase, and C-reactive protein, predict an unfavorable outcome of acute pancreatitis. Levels of C-reactive protein above 150 mg/dL at 48 hours discriminate severely from mild disease. C-reactive protein at 48 hours have a sensitivity and specificity of 80 and 76% respectively, using a cutoff of 150 mg/L. Organ failure that begins early and persists is a reliable indicator of a prolonged hospital stay and increased mortality.

Table 3: Ranson's criteria for predicting the severity of acute pancreatitis

At Admission	At 48 Hours
• Age in years >55 years • WBC count >16,000 cells/mm3 • Blood glucose >200 mg/dL (>11 mmol/L) • Serum SGOT (AST) >250 IU/L • Serum LDH >350 IU/L	• Serum calcium <2.0 mmol/L (<8.0 mg/dL) • PO2 <60 mmHg • Hematocrit fall >10% • BUN increased by 5 or more mg/dL (1.8 or more mmol/L) after IV fluid hydration • Base deficit (negative base excess) >4 mEq/L (>4 mmol/L) • Fluids sequestration >6 L

TREATMENT OF ACUTE PANCREATITIS

Treatment of acute pancreatitis is aimed at alleviating the symptoms of nausea, vomiting and pain; hemodynamic stabilization; adequate nutrition; limiting the severity of attack; and management of acute organ failure. Attempts should be made to correct any underlying predisposing factors which may include (a) hypercalcemia reversal, (b) stopping potential causative drugs, (c) administering insulin if a patient is a poorly controlled diabetic usually associated with significant hypertriglyceridemia and (d) an early ERCP if a patient has gallstone pancreatitis (Figure 4) and also have obstructive jaundice or biliary sepsis.[2] If a patient has mild pancreatitis, they will be treated for several days with supportive care. This includes pain control, aggressive fluid repletion, and nothing given by mouth. The algorithm for managing the patients with acute pancreatitis has been outlined in Figure 5.

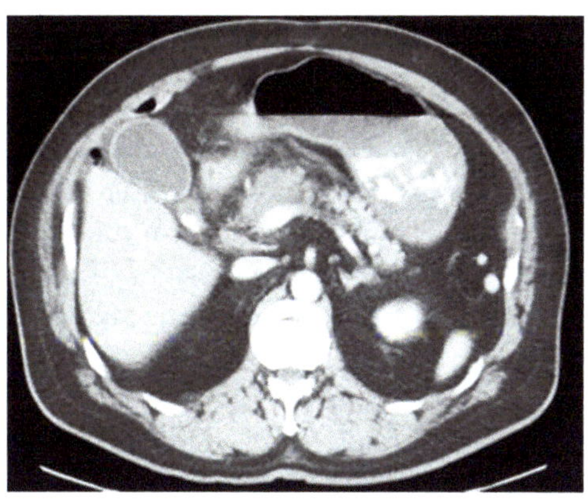

Figure 4: CT scan of the abdomen with contrast showing significant peripancreatic fat stranding and ascites. There is hypoattenuation of the proximal pancreatic body suspicious for pancreatic necrosis. Also seen are innumerable tiny gall-stones highly suspicious for causing the gallstone pancreatitis

History and physical
Abdominal pain radiating to back
Nausea, vomiting, anorexia
Gall stones
Alcohol
Jaundice +/–
Fever, tachycardia, tachypnea

Labs
CBC, LFT, BUN, creatinine, base deficit,
Calcium
Imaging
Abd X-ray, USG

→ Acute pancreatitis → Calculate severity index

Mild → USG
- Gallstones → ERCP
- Normal pancreas → Observe
- Pancreatic mass → Pseudocyst / Cancer

Severe → CT/MRI → Abscess
- No sepsis → Conservative management
- Sepsis → CT/USG guided FNA and culture
  - Infected necrosis → Surgical debridement
  - Sterile necrosis → Continue conservative management → Deterioration / Recovery

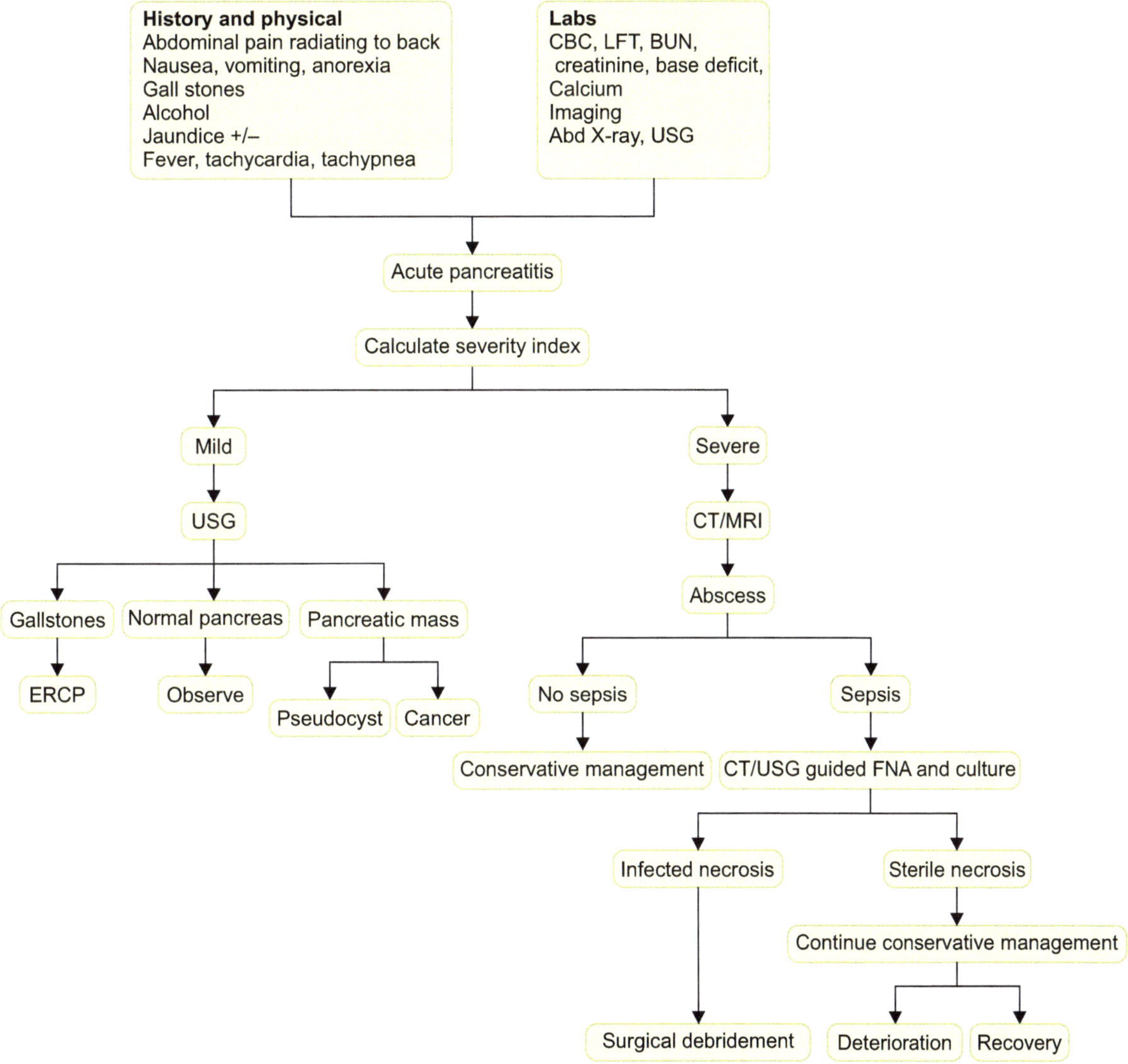

Figure 5: Algorithm summarizing the management of acute pancreatitis

Supportive Treatment

A multidisciplinary approach holds the key to successful management of this disease.[3] In severe pancreatitis, a patient will often be in the intensive care unit so that they can be monitored, and pulmonary, renal, circulatory, and hepatobiliary function can be supported, with the goal of minimizing systemic sequelae. In particular, fluid resuscitation is important, especially if the patient has necrotizing pancreatitis, because these patients can accumulate a lot of fluid in the injured pancreatic bed. At least 250 to 300 cc of intravenous fluids per hour are required for the initial 48 hours (guided by CVP). On the other hand, low urine output often reflects a patient who has already developed acute tubular necrosis, rather than persistent volume depletion. Arterial oxygen saturation should be maintained >95%.

Pain Management

Abdominal pain is often the dominant symptom. Intravenous opiates, usually in the form of a patient-controlled analgesia (PCA) pump are preferred. Morphine causes an increase in sphincter of Oddi pressure, and hence should be avoided; instead, meperidine can be used.

Antibiotics

About one-third of patients who have pancreatic necrosis also develop infected necrosis. It is important to restrict the use of antibiotics to patients with proven infection, unless a patient is decompensating, where infection is suspected, but not quite proven yet. The important organisms causing infection in necrotizing pancreatitis are usually from the intestine including but not limited to Escherichia coli, Pseudomonas, Klebsiella, and Enterococcus species. The majority of infections (75%) are monomicrobial. Imipenem, third generation cephalosporins, piperacillin, mezlocillin, fluoroquinolones, and metronidazole are the antibiotics of choice because of higher penetration in pancreatic tissue. Gut decontamination also helps to decrease the incidence of pancreatic associated infection.

Nutrition

In patients with mild pancreatitis, management can mostly be intravenous fluids, and in patients with severe pancreatitis, nutritional support is also required.[4] Acute pancreatitis creates a state of catabolic stress, promoting a systemic inflammatory response and nutritional deterioration. Oral alimentation is the preferred route, and it can be resumed once the pain and abdominal tenderness subside. Enteral feeding is safe, less expensive, well tolerated and as effective as total parenteral nutrition (TPN). Additionally, it can help maintain mucosal function and decrease endotoxin and cytokine absorption from the gut. Pancreatic stimulation can be avoided by placing the eternal feeding tube distal to the ligament of Treitz. However, if after five days enteral feeding is still not being tolerated, TPN should also be used to meet the patient's caloric and protein requirements.

INDICATIONS FOR SURGERY

With acute pancreatitis, there are several indications for operative intervention. Such indications include patients with an unclear diagnosis to their acute abdomen or patients who develop a complication (e.g., hemorrhage, bowel infarction, or perforation). However, there should be a focus in identifying patients with infected pancreatic necrosis.[5,6] CT guided fine needle aspiration (FNA) is safe and reliable in looking for areas of necrosis/pus and remains the gold standard. A gram stain and culture of the aspirate will diagnose infection, with a positive and negative predictive value of around 90%. Safely delaying any intervention helps with having better demarcation and liquefaction of pancreatic necrosis, which results in a higher success rate for any pancreatic intervention.

CHRONIC PANCREATITIS

Introduction

"Chronic pancreatitis" as the name suggests refers to "progressive inflammation" of the pancreas. It results in permanent structural damage eventually leading to impairment or loss of exocrine and endocrine function. Clinically it presents as a syndrome of persistent/recurrent abdominal pain, steatorrhea, diabetes and/or pancreatic calcification.[7]

Etiology

Chronic pancreatitis is often caused by chronic alcohol abuse (>150 mg/day for 6 to 12 years). Other frequent causes include gallstone-associated pancreatitis, chronic steroid or anti-inflammatory drug use, hereditary, and autoimmune pancreatitis. Tropical pancreatitis is a form of idiopathic pancreatitis occurring in young non-alcoholic individuals. This entity is seen in countries like India, Indonesia and Africa and has been linked to genetic mutations such as the SPINK1 gene mutation and various environmental factors.[8] In children cystic fibrosis and severe protein-energy malnutrition are the most common causes of chronic pancreatitis.

Clinical Presentation

The two main clinical manifestations of chronic pancreatitis are (a) recurrent episodes of acute pancreatitis in a chronically damaged pancreas and/or (b) persistent pain with or without malabsorption. Initially the pain may occur in discrete attacks located deep in the epigastric region often radiating to the back. However, as the condition progresses, the pain becomes more continuous and often increases in severity. The pain in chronic pancreatitis is thought to be caused by inflammation in the pancreatic tissue and perineural sheath. Another hypothesis relates to the increased pressure within the pancreatic duct and parenchyma.

Many patients with chronic pancreatitis do not show any clinically significant protein or fat deficiencies until over 90% of pancreatic function is lost. Pancreatic insufficiency leads to maldigestion and malabsorption of nutrients. A common complication is diabetes due to chronic pancreatic damage. These patients require insulin treatment. Many patients also experience considerable weight loss due to malabsorption. The patient may also have abdominal pain associated with food intake, especially with high fat and protein meals. Pancreatic insufficiency affects fat absorption more, as compared to protein or carbohydrate digestion. This is because protein is also digested by gastric pepsin and carbohydrates are also digested by salivary and intestinal amylase. Patients may also have deficiencies in fat-soluble vitamins (vitamins A, D, E and K), magnesium, calcium, and essential fatty acids, however this may occur later in the disease and are directly related to fat malabsorption. Apart from chronic pancreatitis other causes of exocrine pancreatic insufficiency include cystic fibrosis and Shwachman-Diamond syndrome.

Diagnosis

Chronic pancreatitis diagnosis is usually based on pancreatic structure and pancreatic function tests. Direct biopsy of the pancreas is not done routinely due to the increased risks. Serum amylase and lipase levels are rarely elevated except in cases of acute on chronic episodes. An elevated serum bilirubin and alkaline phosphatase indicate common bile duct stricturing which can be due to edema, fibrosis, or cancer. Elevations in ESR, IgG4, rheumatoid factor, ANA and anti-smooth muscle antibody may suggest an autoimmune process.

The gold standard functional test to diagnose chronic pancreatitis is a secretin-cholecystokinin stimulation test because it has a 95% sensitivity rate in early stages of disease. Pancreatic enzyme activity as well as bicarbonate levels are measured in duodenal juice after stimulation with secretin and cholecystokinin. Pancreatic fluid with bicarbonate concentration of <80 mEq/L and bicarbonate output below 15 mEq/30 min indicates pancreatic insufficiency. Pancreolauryl test, PABA excretion test and fecal fat balance test is also used to evaluate pancreatic exocrine function. Fecal elastase (ELISA test) is the most sensitive and specific test, where <200 ug/g is an indicator of pancreatic insufficiency.

Imaging

Radiological investigations are now commonly used to make a diagnosis of chronic pancreatitis and include abdominal X-rays, ultrasound, EUS, CT scan, MRI, ERCP and MRCP. Pancreatic calcification can often be seen on plain abdominal X-rays. CT scan may show pancreatic atrophy, calcifications (Figure 6), ductal dilatation, pseudocysts, splenic artery pseudoaneurysm, and/or biliary obstruction. ERCP is a highly sensitive radiographic test to detect chronic pancreatitis with a sensitivity and specificity of more than 90%. With the availability of safer and less invasive techniques the role of ERCP in the diagnosis of pancreatic cancer has decreased. However, it can be both diagnostic as well as therapeutic. Sensitivity of MRCP varies between 70 and 92% with ERCP considered as the gold standard. Heavy T2 weighted images allow better visualization of fluid, filled structures, and hence, pancreatic duct.

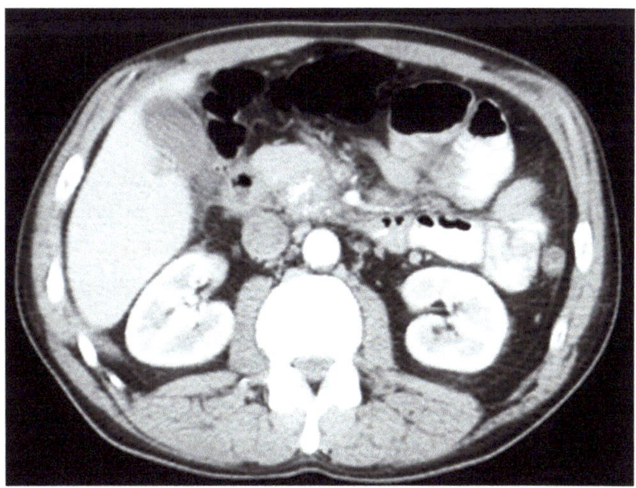

Figure 6: CT scan of the abdomen with contrast showing pancreatic calcification in the head of pancreas suggestive of chronic pancreatitis. Also seen is the fluid located on the medial and superior to the pancreas with peripancreatic inflammatory change

Treatment

Chronic pancreatitis can be treated with medical measures, therapeutic endoscopy, and surgery (summarized in Figure 7). Treatment aims to fix the underlying cause, relieve pain and malabsorption, correct glucose levels, and manage complications. Patients with chronic alcohol use are counseled against taking any alcohol. Although the damage to pancreas is irreversible, abstinence from alcohol often results in reduction of both chronic and acute abdominal pain in more than half of cases. If a patient develops diabetes, they can be treated with long term insulin therapy. Abdominal pain can be severe and may require high dose analgesics, which are often given prior to meals because there is maximal pain postprandially. Finally, chronic pancreatitis can often result in disability and mood problems, thus it is important to diagnose early and provide support.

Pancreatic Enzyme Supplementation

Replacing pancreatic enzymes can help treat malabsorption and steatorrhea. It is indicated if a patient loses >10% body weight or excretes >15 gm/day of fat in stools. Treatment with these enzymes is usually lifelong. Pancreatic enzyme supplements may also relieve pain in some patients. Patients with idiopathic pancreatitis and those without involvement of large ducts benefit from enzyme supplementation, but patients with alcoholic pancreatitis do not respond as well. Pancreatic enzyme products (PEPs) such as pancrelipase are supplemented with diet.[9] They help in the breakdown of fats (lipases), proteins (proteases) and carbohydrates (amylases) into units that can be digested by patients with exocrine pancreatic insufficiency.

Pain Management

Abdominal pain remains the most important symptom in patients with chronic pancreatitis and is the one that is difficult to control. For best results, a stepwise approach starting with some general measures is recommended. Abstinence from alcohol, small frequent meals (low in fat), and pancreatic enzymatic supplementation along with judicious use of analgesics improves the pain in the vast majority of patients. Pancreatic enzyme supplementation reduces pain in some patients.

Short course of opiates along with a low dose of amitriptyline and NSAIDs will break the pain cycle. Admission to the hospital and keeping the patient nil orally on IV fluid supplementation decreases the pancreatic stimulation and hence, the abdominal pain. Chronic opioid use is only recommended in patients with severe chronic pain. Use of long-acting agents such as morphine sulfate and fentanyl patch are usually advised later in the course of disease progression. Benefits from octreotide, and antioxidant[10] therapies have been reported in some studies.

Patients with severe pain refractory to medical management benefit from celiac nerve block, endoscopic stenting of pancreatic duct/pancreatic sphincterotomy, extracorporeal short-wave lithotripsy.[11]

Surgery

Surgery for chronic pancreatitis can be resectional or drainage procedures depending on the extent of pancreatic disease (diffuse vs. localized) and/or dilated on nondilated duct (Figure 7). Timing of surgery is controversial. Early surgery may prevent progression of disease and its complications but at the same time complications of major surgery cannot be ignored.[7,12,13] Many patients choose surgery as the last option. Surgical procedures that have been described are: (a) Decompression/ drainage procedures; (b) Pancreatic resections; (c) Denervation procedures.[14]

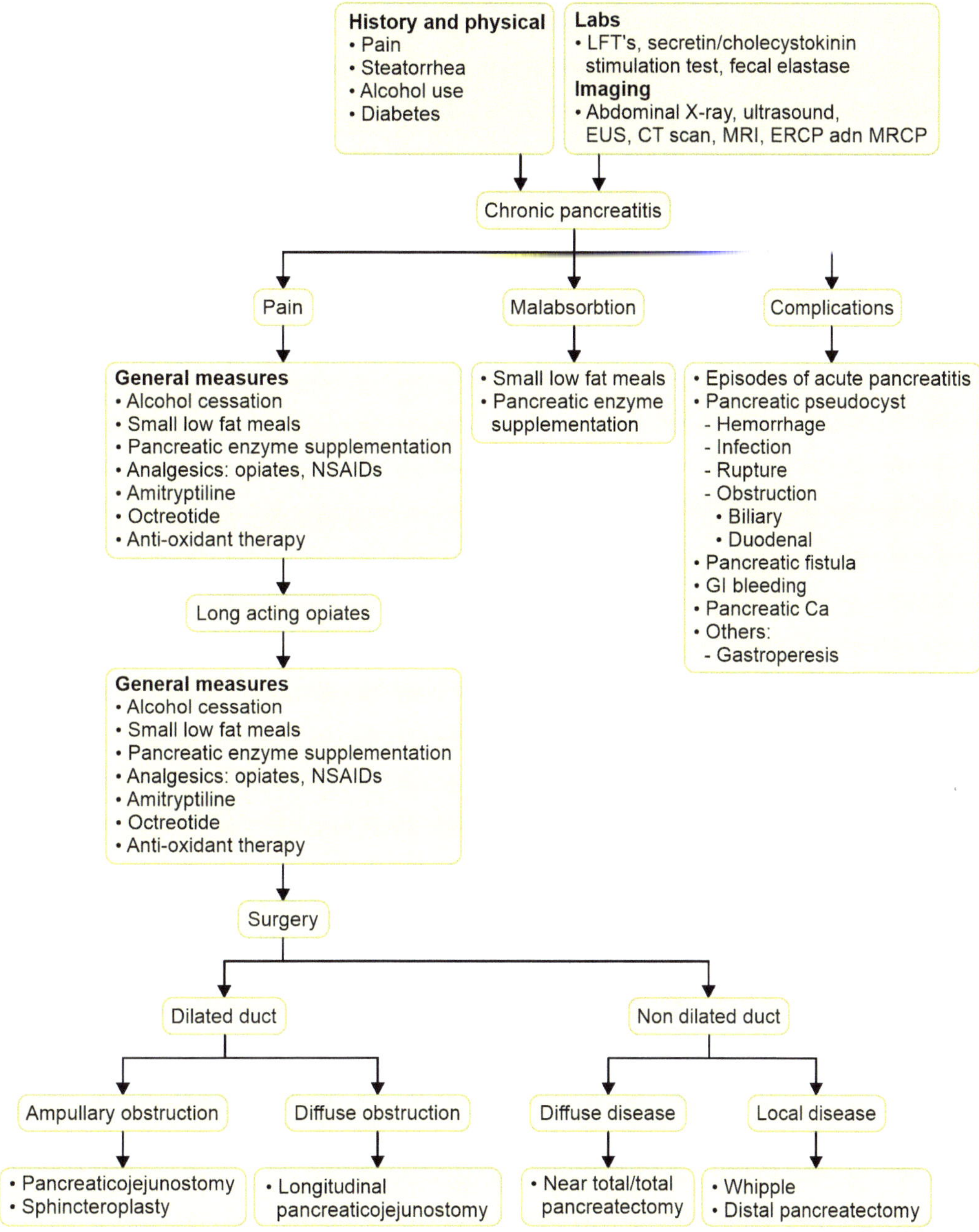

Figure 7: Management of chronic pancreatitis

PANCREATIC PSEUDOCYST

A pancreatic pseudocyst is a collection of fluid in the lesser sac. The fluid collection is usually the pancreatic fluid that has leaked out of a damaged pancreatic duct as a result of acute or chronic pancreatitis but may occur after trauma. Unlike true cysts, which are lined by epithelium; pseudocysts are lined with granulation tissue. In acute pancreatitis, ductal disruption is due to partial pancreatic necrosis with subsequent duct leakage. However, these patients may have increased pancreatic duct pressures due to strictures, ductal calculi, or other causes, and thus resulting in a small ductal disruption, and pseudocyst formation.

Patients usually present with abdominal pain, fever, weight loss or even with features of bowel obstruction from compression. Abdominal USG, CT or MRI helps in the diagnosis of pancreatic pseudocyst. Treatment (Figure 8) is dependent on the pseudocyst size and whether it is causing symptoms. Many self-resolve. Those lasting greater than 6 weeks and have a diameter of >5 cm and/or are symptomatic and continuously increasing in size may require surgery. Patients with symptomatic or growing pseudocyst need MRCP or ERCP to check for duct involvement.[15] CT guided percutaneous drainage of cyst may be done if duct is not involved. In case, a duct involvement is suspected, endoscopic drainage through the gastric or duodenal wall with placements of stents or surgical drainage into an adjacent hollow viscus (e.g., cystojejunostomy or cystogastrostomy, is preferred). Resection of the pseudocyst along with some pancreatic parenchyma may be done if the pseudocyst is located in the tail of the pancreas.

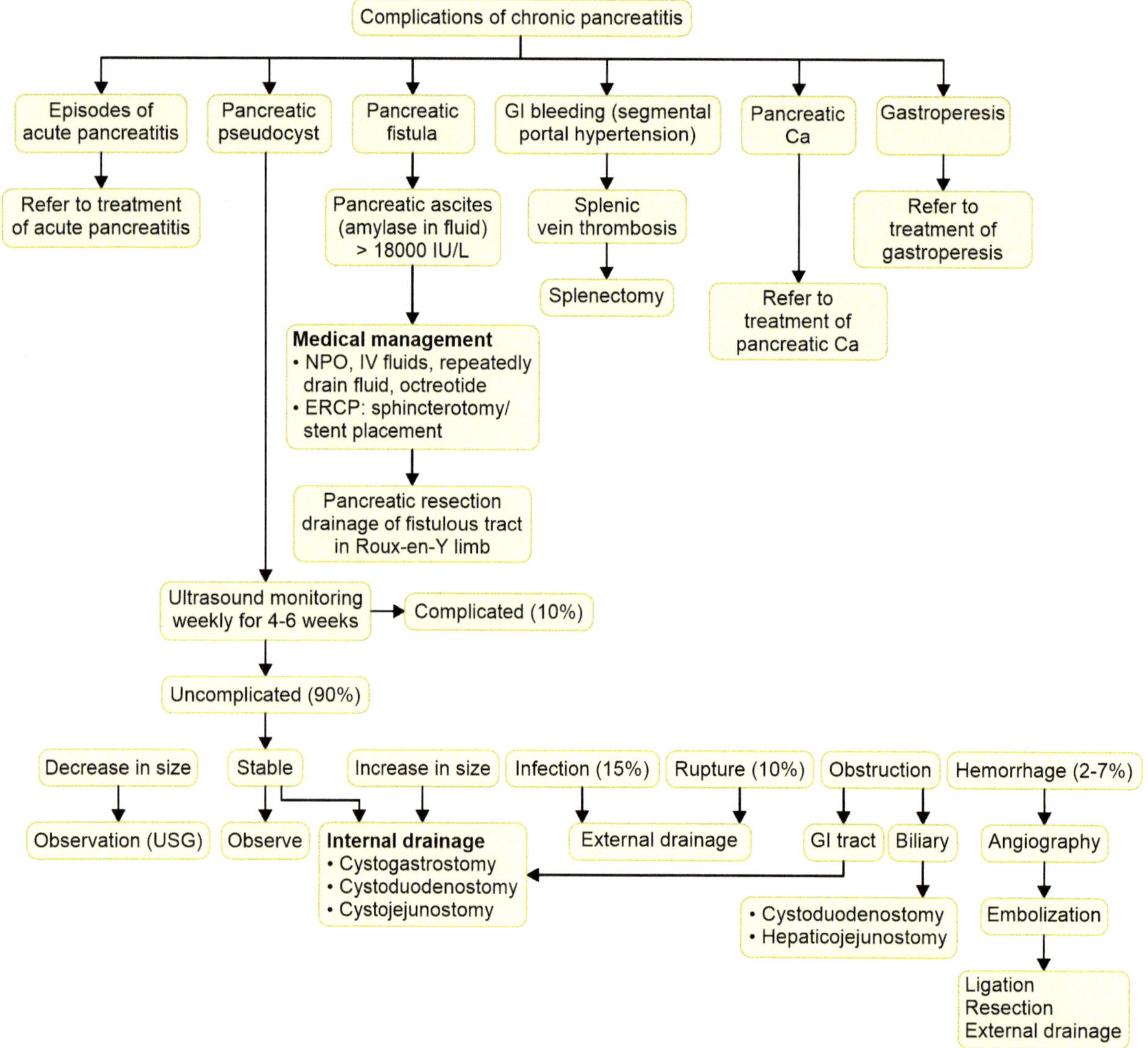

Figure 8: Algorithm summarizing the management for the complications of chronic pancreatitis

PANCREATIC FISTULAS

Disruption of the pancreatic duct or rupture of a pseudocyst usually leads to a leakage of pancreatic secretions and may result in either an external or internal pancreatic fistula. Pancreatic fistulas can be caused by pancreatic disease, trauma, or surgery. Pancreatic cutaneous fistula results in the loss of bicarbonate-rich pancreatic fluid leading to hyperchloremic or normal anion gap metabolic acidosis. An internal pancreatic fistula develops in patients with chronic pancreatitis with the development of pancreatic ascites. Patients usually complain of abdominal distension or dyspnea. Amylase level in fluid is usually elevated (>18,000 IU/L). Most pancreatic fistulas respond to medical management (Figure 8) which includes, nil orally, use of TPN, repeated fluid drainage and octreotide to decrease pancreatic secretions. Patients with failed medical management may benefit from ERCP, sphincterotomy and pancreatic stent placement.[16] Surgery is reserved for patients who fail medical and endoscopic therapy and may include connecting the fistulous tract with a Roux-en-Y loop or rarely pancreatectomy.

PANCREATIC CANCER

Incidence and Epidemiology

Pancreatic cancer is the fifth leading cause of cancer-related deaths in the US. It is more common in men and 80% of cases are above 60 years in age. Risk factors include: (a) High-protein and high-fat diet; (b) Cigarette smoking (doubles the risk); (c) Exposure to industrial carcinogens; (d) Family history of pancreatic cancer; (e) Hereditary or chronic pancreatitis; and (f) Alcohol abuse.

Molecular Biology

Ninety percent of patients with pancreatic cancers demonstrate codon 12 mutations of the KRAS oncogene. Mutations of the p53 tumor suppressor gene (75% of pancreatic cancers) along with other tumor suppressor genes, like p16, SMAD-4/DPC, and DCC have also been reported. Growth factors like epidermal growth factor (EGF) receptor, insulin-like growth factor receptor (IGFR), platelet derived growth factor receptor (PDGFR) and transforming growth factor beta receptor are also up-regulated. KRAS mutations and HER2/neu overexpression are the earliest changes to occur. Alterations in p16 are found primarily in PanIN-2 and PanIN-3.

The incidence of pancreatic cancer is increased in families with hereditary nonpolyposis colon cancer (HNPCC), familial breast cancer (BRCA2 mutation), Peutz-Jeghers syndrome, ataxia-telangiectasia, and familial atypical multiple mole melanoma (FAMMM) syndrome.[17] Patients with hereditary pancreatitis are also at increased risk for developing pancreatic cancer.

Pathology

Solid Epithelial Tumors

Ductal adenocarcinoma and its variants account for 80 to 90% of all pancreatic neoplasms and for an even greater fraction of the malignant tumors. Approximately 70% of ductal cancers arise in the pancreatic head or uncinate process. In more than 80% of the patients at the time of diagnosis, tumor ≤12 is >3 cm in diameter, with both nodal involvement and distant metastases. Perineural growth of the tumor is highly characteristic of this cancer ultimately invading the neighboring neural plexuses resulting in severe upper abdominal and back pain.

Much like colon cancers, pancreatic tumors can progress from benign precursor lesions to malignant lesions. These precursor lesions are known as pancreatic intraepithelial neoplasia (PanIN). PanIN have different stages and grades, PanIN-1A is a proliferative lesion with no significant nuclear abnormality and PanIN-1B is a proliferative lesion with a flat and papillary architecture. PanIN-3 has severe architectural and cytonuclear abnormalities (loss of nuclear polarity, dystrophic goblet cells, mitosis, nuclear irregularities, and prominent nucleoli), but there is no invasion through the basement membrane. True cribriforming, budding off small clusters of epithelial cells into the lumen and luminal necrosis also suggests the diagnosis of PanIN-3. PanIN-2 is an intermediate category and has moderate architectural abnormalities (mucinous epithelial lesions that are flat or papillary) and cytonuclear abnormality (some loss of polarity, nuclear crowding, enlarged nuclei, pseudo-stratification, and hyperchromatism).[18]

Adenosquamous carcinomas are a rare variant of ductal adenocarcinoma with both glandular and squamous differentiation and occur in patients with a previous history of chemoradiation. One percent of pancreatic exocrine tumors are acinar cell carcinomas. These tumors are more common in males and are generally larger than ductal adenocarcinomas, >10 cm. Giant cell carcinomas account for less than 5% of non-endocrine pancreatic tumors, often with average diameters more than 15 cm. Histologically they show pleomorphic cells and have a poor prognosis. Pancreatoblastoma is a rare form of pancreatic cancer that usually presents in young children and contains both epithelial and mesenchymal elements. Nonepithelial cancers of all types, including leiomyosarcomas, liposarcomas, plasmacytomas, and lymphomas, can also develop within the pancreas, however, are quite rare

Cystic Epithelial Tumors

Cystic neoplasms of the exocrine pancreas are less frequent than ductal adenocarcinomas and occur more commonly in females. Almost 70% of the cystic lesions in pancreas are pseudocyst. However, it is important to differentiate these from cystic neoplasms (Figure 9) because of their malignant potential.[19,20]

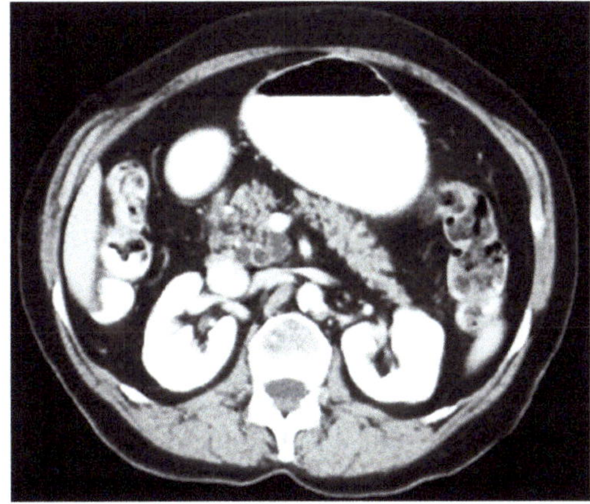

Figure 9: CT scan of the abdomen with contrast showing 2 cm multiloculated cystic mass located in the uncinate process of pancreatic head with mildly prominent duct

Also known as serous cystadenomas, serous cystic neoplasm (SCN) is lined by simple, glycogen-rich cuboidal epithelium and occurs more commonly in females. SCN can have macroscopic variations and is subdivided into either serous microcystic or serous oligocystic adenomas. On CT scan SCN show a honeycomb micro-lacuna, which consists of thin septa that separate the different segments. Additionally, these tumors can have central calcification that has a sunburst pattern. Although benign, with very low malignant potential, symptomatic lesions, or those >4 cm in size, or those that cannot be differentiated from other potentially malignant cysts should be considered for surgical resection.

Mucinous cystic neoplasms (MCN) are composed of mucus-producing cells and are associated with ovarian-like stroma. All MCN are considered potentially malignant and should undergo surgical resection.

Intraductal papillary-mucinous neoplasms (IPMNs) are intra ductal mucin producing neoplasms composed of tall, columnar, mucin-containing epithelium with or without papillary projections. IPMNs are divided into two groups: (a) main-duct type; and (b) branch-duct type which is determined based on pancreatic duct involvement. IPMNs are usually found in elderly patients 60 to 80 years in age and are more often seen in the pancreatic head, neck, and uncinate process, but can occur throughout the gland. CT scan often reveals a cystic mass located in the pancreatic head and has a pancreatic duct communication. ERCP confirms the communication with the pancreatic duct along with mucin oozing out from ampulla of Vater. Main-duct type IPMN have high malignancy potential and thus should be resected. However, branch-duct type IPMN generally show favorable features including a smaller size of <3 cm size and the absence of mural nodules and thus can be managed more conservatively.[21]

Solid and cystic papillary neoplasms (Hamoudi tumors) occurring females in their 4th-5th decade of life. These tumors show solid, cystic, and papillary components and range from 5 to 15 cm in diameter.

Signs and Symptoms

Signs and symptoms usually develop late and depend on the site of the tumor. Eighty percent of patients have metastasis before clinical symptoms arise. Tumors located in the pancreatic head may cause biliary, pancreatic, or duodenal obstruction. Symptoms include unexplained episodes of pancreatitis, painless jaundice, nausea, vomiting, steatorrhea, and unexplained weight loss (>10% of original body weight or 1-2 kg/month). Unlike the pancreatic head tumors, tumors in the pancreatic neck, body, or tail show symptoms of jaundice or gastric outlet obstruction. Symptoms are general including unexplained weight loss and vague upper abdominal pain until the tumor has grown much larger and metastasized. These patients may later develop epigastric pain/back pain when peripancreatic nerve plexuses are involved. Initial metastasis is to the regional lymph nodes followed by hematogenous metastasis to liver (80%) and lungs (50%). Cancers in the body or tail may cause splenic vein obstruction, splenomegaly, gastric/esophageal varices, and GI hemorrhage. The initial symptoms of occult pancreatic cancer are sometimes new-onset diabetes mellitus.[22]

Unexplained migratory thrombophlebitis (Trousseau's syndrome), metastatic sub-umbilical (Sister Mary Joseph node), pelvic peritoneal (Blumer's shelf) deposits, and left supraclavicular lymphadenopathy (Virchow's node) are all indications of distant metastases. Another potential presentation is malignant ascites, caused by peritoneal carcinomatosis.

Periampullary tumors originate from the head of the pancreas, ampulla of Vater, distal common bile duct and the duodenum. They constitute 30% of malignant tumors arising from the pancreatic head region. Gallbladder distention can be due to the tumor causing a distal common bile duct obstruction. Thus, for a patient with painless jaundice (i.e., Courvoisier's sign) and a distended gallbladder which can be examined on palpation, it is important to consider the presence of a periampullary neoplasm.

Blood Tests

Patients with pancreatic head lesions or with liver metastasis frequently have increased serum total bilirubin, alkaline phosphatase and gamma-glutamyl transferase levels. Transaminases can be increased, but it is not normally as great an increase as alkaline phosphatase. Patients who have localized cancer of the pancreatic body and tail, often show normal laboratory values. Nutritional deficiencies of the disease lead to normochromic anemia and hypoalbuminemia. Patients presenting with jaundice can have an abnormally prolonged prothrombin time, often indicating biliary obstruction. Obstruction results in bile being unable to enter the gastrointestinal tract and thus malabsorption of fat-soluble vitamins and less vitamin K-dependent clotting factors being produced in the liver. Laboratory levels of serum amylase and lipase are often normal in pancreatic cancer patients. More than 25% of patients with pancreatic cancer may present with increased glucose levels or worsening of pre-existing diabetes. This has been related to secretion of an anti-insulin hormone "Islet amyloid polypeptide" (IAPP).

CEA and the Lewis blood group carbohydrate antigen CA 19-9 (both tumor markers for pancreatic cancer) are frequently elevated and are often used to monitor the disease. With a normal upper limit of 37 U/mL, CA 19-9 only has an 80% accuracy in identifying pancreatic adenocarcinoma. Increasing the upper limit value to 200 U/mL improves the accuracy to 95%. CA 19-9 levels are correlated with prognosis and tumor recurrence with higher levels prior to surgery indicating a primary tumor of increased size and often correlates well with unresectability. They are also used for monitoring neoadjuvant and adjuvant chemoradiation therapy efficacy. Postoperative increase in CA 19-9 indicates recurrence or progression of disease, whereas decreasing levels indicate a better prognosis.

Imaging Studies

Radiological imaging plays a key role in diagnosis and staging of pancreatic cancer. Abdominal ultrasound due to its wide availability, low cost and non-invasiveness is considered as the screening test for most abdominal conditions. It is considered to be operator-dependent but can demonstrate pancreatic masses (solid or cystic) (Figure 10); dilated intrahepatic and extrahepatic bile ducts, liver metastases, ascites, and enlarged peripancreatic lymph nodes. Its sensitivity ranges from 60 to 100% and specificity from 44 to 99%. Contrast-enhanced CT scan with a dual-phase intravenous contrast study is currently the preferred noninvasive imaging test. Recent advances in this imaging modality have contributed to early tumor detection and thus higher resectability rate. It usually demonstrates hypodense mass (Figures 11 and 12) with poorly demarcated edges with invasion into local structures or metastatic disease if present. Sensitivity depends on the size of the tumor, exceeding 95% for tumors larger than 2 cm in diameter. Positron emission tomography (PET) may be of value in diagnosing small pancreatic tumors that escape CT or MRI detection. It uses the increased glucose metabolism of cancer cells and effectively differentiates benign from malignant lesions.

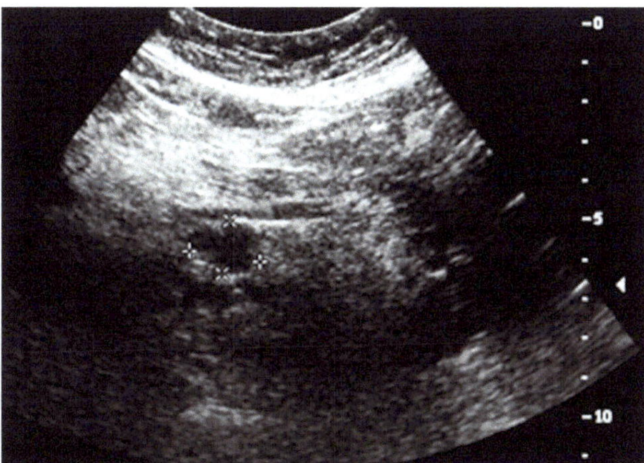

Figure 10: Abdominal ultrasound showing a 1.5 cm hypo- echoic cystic lesion in the head of pancreas

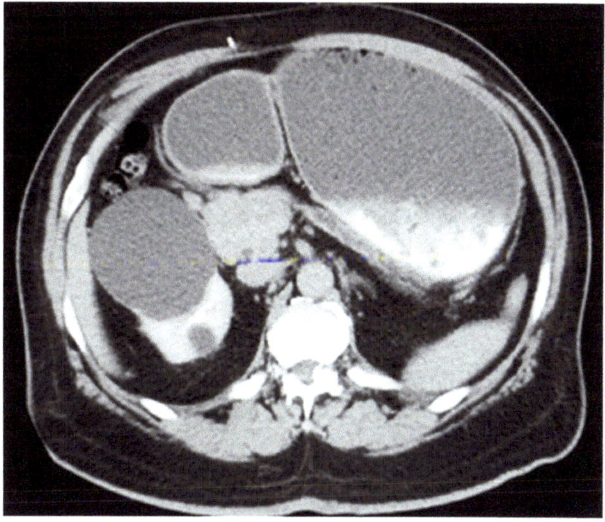

Figure 11: CT scan of the abdomen with contrast showing a3 cm hypodense pancreatic head mass resulting in bowel obstruction at the level of second part of duodenum with marked gastric distension

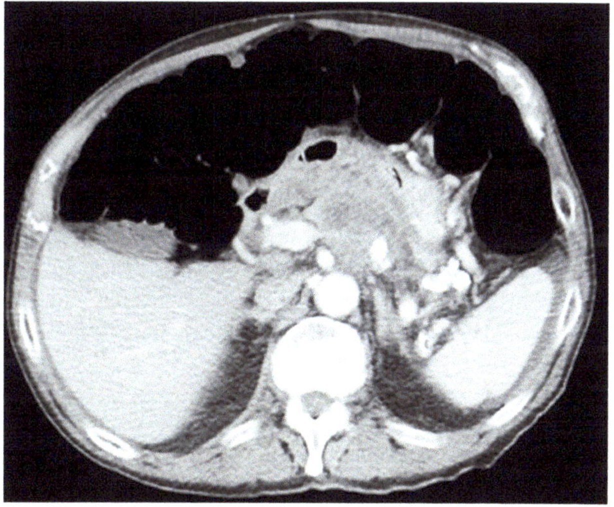

Figure 12: CT scan of the abdomen with contrast showing a 7.4 cm × 6.5 cm mass in the body of pancreas with subtle enhancement and encasement of left renal vein and splenic artery with splenic vein thrombosis and gastric varices

ERCP is a particularly helpful tool in evaluating for obstructive jaundice when CT or MRI fail to display a detectable mass. Pancreatic cancer will look like a long, irregular stricture in an otherwise normal pancreatic duct. It helps in: (a) identifying stones or other nonmalignant sources of obstructive jaundice, (b) locate the bile duct obstruction, (c) identify ampullary and periampullary lesions, and (d) to diagnose IPMN if there is mucus extruding through a fish-mouth papillary opening. Diagnostic ERCP should only be performed in patients where pancreatic cancer is of high suspicion, with or without jaundice with negative imaging studies. Role of EUS is very limited and was developed to eliminate the interface with bowel gas. EUS is operator dependent and its applicability to preoperative staging is dependent on the locally available expertise.[23] Its role is justified in patients with uncertain diagnosis. EUS helps to detect and localize the smaller lesions (<3 cm) better (high resolution) and at the same time gives an opportunity to obtain tissue samples for histological confirmation.

Staging of Pancreatic Cancer

The goal of preoperative staging is to identify unresectable or metastatic disease and to select the patients who qualify for and will benefit from surgical resection. The TNM staging of pancreatic cancer takes into account the size of the tumor (T), lymph node involvement (N), and the distant metastasis (M). The American Joint Committee for Cancer (AJCC) system is the most commonly used classification system. Absence of extra pancreatic disease, a patent superior mesenteric vein (SMV)-portal vein confluence, no evidence of encasement to the celiac axis or superior mesenteric artery and no extra pancreatic disease suggests a resectable pancreatic tumor. The role of staging laparoscopy is controversial. Twenty to 40% of patients with stage I or II disease have unrecognized small metastases to peritoneal surfaces and can be detected laparoscopically, thus precluding a laparotomy.[24] In contrast it is argued that these patients can still benefit by performing prophylactic bilioenteric, and possibly gastroenteric, bypass. However, with the advent of laparoscopic ultrasound, biopsy, and peritoneal cytology it is now possible to detect the locally advanced disease.

Surgery

For resectable tumors of the head, neck, and uncinate process of the pancreas, pancreaticoduodenectomy, with or without preservation of the pylorus and proximal duodenum, is the surgical treatment of choice. Mortality rate for pancreaticoduodenectomy is 2 to 4%. Anastomotic leaks, intra-abdominal abscesses, gastrointestinal bleeding and delayed gastric emptying account for most of the perioperative complications after pancreaticoduodenectomy. Five-year survival rates of 15 to 20% have been reported.

For resectable tumors located in the body or tail of pancreas distal pancreatectomy with splenectomy is preferred. Complications include subphrenic abscess (5-10%) and pancreatic duct leak (up to 20%). Management of pancreatic carcinoma has been summarized in Figure 13.

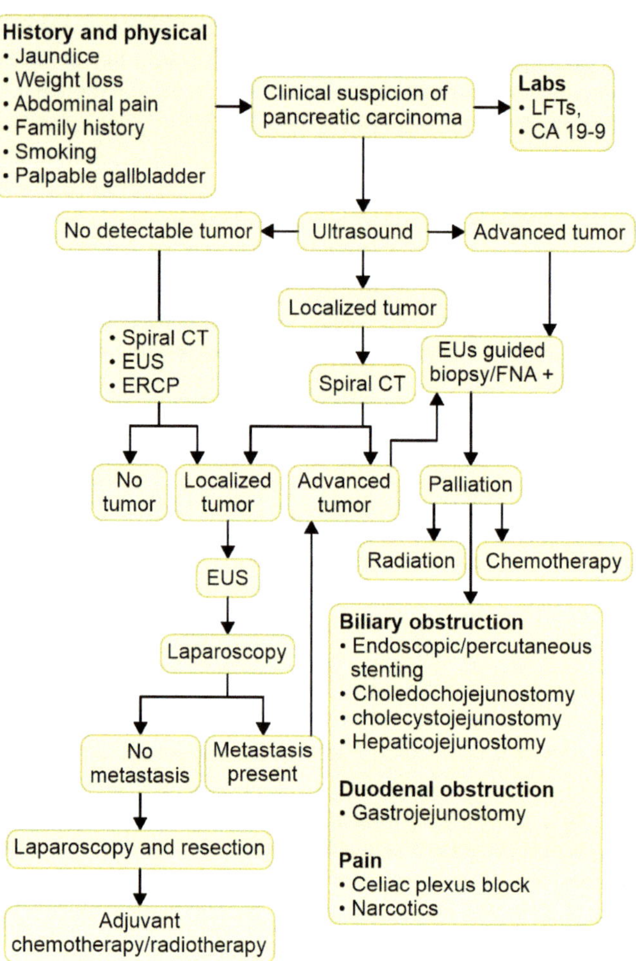

Figure 13: Algorithm summarizing the management of pancreatic carcinoma

Palliative Treatment of Pancreatic Cancers

Eighty percent of all pancreatic cancer patients present with unresectable disease at the time of diagnosis. Thus, most patients receive palliative care with the aim of establishing the diagnosis and to relieve symptoms of pain, jaundice, gastric outlet obstruction, depression, and weight loss. Tissue diagnosis is usually achieved by CT or ultrasound-guided percutaneous fine-needle aspiration of the tumor/ metastatic lesion. Transduodenal fine-needle aspiration of the tumor with endoscopic ultrasound guidance and duct cytology obtained by brushings is an alternative method of establishing the diagnosis.

For most patients with unresectable pancreatic cancer presenting with biliary tract obstruction, decompression can be achieved endoscopically or percutaneously. Endoscopic biliary decompression with plastic or expandable metal stents (Figure 14) are the preferred method. Endoscopic approach has a higher success rate and a low complication rate as compared to percutaneous transhepatic stenting. Alternative to endoscopic stenting include cholecystojejunostomy or a choledochojejunostomy. Cholecystojejunostomy is performed in patients who do not have dilated ducts and when the cystic duct-common bile duct confluence is far from the tumor. Choledochojejunostomy, is considered when bile duct is >1 cm in diameter[25] and the tumor is close to or at the cystic duct-common bile duct confluence. These drainage procedures often decrease the serum bilirubin levels in the majority of patients.

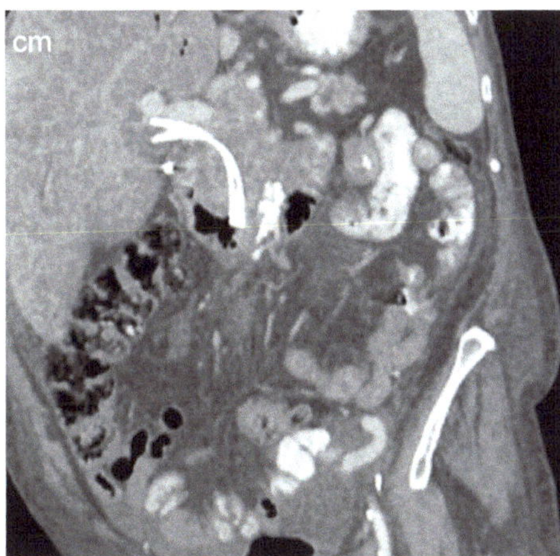

Figure 14: CT scan of the abdomen with 3D reconstruction showing a stent in the common bile duct

To relieve duodenal obstruction, expandable endoluminal metal stents are placed into the duodenum. Surgical gastrojejunostomy may be necessary when lesions cannot be fixed with stents. Role of prophylactic gastric bypass is debatable as only 20% of patients with pancreatic head tumors will ultimately develop gastric outlet obstruction (Figure 11).

Pain control is the most important aspect of palliative management and is oftentimes most difficult to control. NSAIDs, COX-2 inhibitors or opiates may be used. Percutaneous CT or EUS guided celiac plexus block eliminates/reduces pain in the majority of patients. This can also be done intraoperatively or via laparoscopically. Use of chemotherapy (especially gemcitabine) and radiation have also decreased pain in pancreatic cancer patients.

Radiation and Chemotherapy

For locally advanced pancertic cancer which is non-resectable may turn into a resectable tumor with neo adjucent chdemoradiation patients with locally advanced pancreatic cancer receive chemotherapy and/or radiation therapy, however the response rate is only 10-15% with a marginal improvement in survival. Chemo radiation therapy comprises radiation therapy combined with either 5-fluorouracil or gemcitabine. Intraoperative radiation therapy, as adjuvant treatment, has been evaluated, but has not shown to improve the survival rates.

PANCREATIC NEUROENDOCRINE TUMORS

Introduction

Pancreatic neuroendocrine tumors (PET) are rare neoplasms of the pancreas accounting for less than 5% of all primary pancreatic malignancies. They include insulinomas, gastrinomas, glucagonoma and somatostatinomas, all of which are classified as functional PETs. When a PET is not associated with hormone oversecretion resulting in a clinical syndrome, it is called a non-functioning PET.[26]

Nonfunctional Endocrine Tumors

They represent one third of all PETs but almost 90% of them are malignant. Unlike patients with functional PETs who clinically present due to hormone overproduction, non-functional PETs usually present with features of mass effect or metastatic lesions. Non-functioning PETs are pancreatic tumors with endocrine differentiation but do not have hormone hypersecretion and thus no clinical syndrome. Although hormonally “silent,” these tumors will sometimes produce a functionally inert precursor hormone or a level of hormone that is too small to cause symptoms. Nonfunctioning tumors are generally slow growing tumors in the pancreatic head.

Functional Endocrine Tumors

Insulinoma

Insulinomas are PETs that arise from islet beta cells, the insulin producing cell in the pancreas, and are the most common type of PET. Ninety percent of them are benign but can present with hypoglycemia due to the uncontrolled production of insulin. Hypoglycemia can manifest as confusion, behavioral changes, blurred vision, fatigue, seizures, and coma or even death. The classic Whipples’ triad of: (a) fasting hypoglycemia; (b) low serum glucose (<50 when symptomatic); and (c) relief of symptoms with IV administration of glucose. Diagnosis of an insulinoma consists of high serum insulin and low blood sugar. A ratio of plasma insulin to glucose >0.3 is diagnostic. Proinsulin levels more than 40% suggest malignant islet cell tumor. High resolution CT scan, MRI and EUS often help in localizing the insulinomas. Intraoperative ultrasound, surgeon palpation, and full pancreatic mobilization, results in localization of >95% of insulinomas. Enucleation is recommended for lesions <2 cm in size while a formal resection is advocated if lesion is >2 cm in size. For metastatic disease, the recommended treatments include streptozotocin, octreotide and 5-FU.

Gastrinoma (Zollinger-Ellison Syndrome)

Gastrinomas are the second commonest PET and arise from non-beta islet cells of the pancreas. They are most frequently diagnosed in the 5th and 6th decades of life. Fifty percent of gastrinomas are malignant and 50% are multiple. Seventy-five percent of these tumors occur spontaneously while 25% are associated with MEN I syndrome. Ninety percent of gastrinomas are located in the gastrinoma triangle consisting of the CBD, neck of the pancreas and third portion of the duodenum. Ten percent of the tumors may be found in ectopic sites including duodenum. Patients present with abdominal pain (refractory peptic ulcer disease) and diarrhea. The diagnosis is established by the demonstration of marked fasting hyper-gastrinemia and marked gastric acid hypersecretion. Serum gastrin levels are usually >200. Value >1,000 is almost diagnostic of gastrinoma. Secretin stimulation test increases the gastrin levels >200 in patients with suspected Zollinger-Ellison syndrome (ZES). High resolution CT scan, MRI and EUS often help in localizing the gastrinomas. Somatostatin receptor scintigraphy is the single best study for localizing the tumors. The symptoms of acid hypersecretion can be effectively controlled by proton pump inhibitors in the majority of patients with ZES. Enucleation is recommended for lesions <2 cm in size while a formal resection is advocated if lesion is >2 cm in size. High levels of gastrin may be present in G-cell hyperplasia. This can be distinguished from gastrinoma by the sharp rise of gastrin levels (>200%) in response to meals as compared to minimal or no increase in patients with gastrinoma.

Glucagonoma

Glucagonoma is one of the most malignant functional PET with the majority of tumors located in distal pancreas. They arise from pancreatic alpha cells. The patients usually present with diabetes, dermatitis, deep vein thrombosis and depression. The pathognomonic rash (necrolytic migratory erythema) is present in 70% of patients. Following treatment and normalization of glucagon levels, supplemented with zinc, amino acids, and fatty acids this rash generally resolves. Diagnosis is made with elevated plasma glucagon levels which increase paradoxically when challenged with intravenous tolbutamide. Symptomatic treatment consists of somatostatin analogues.

VIPoma (Verner Morrison Syndrome)

VIPoma is also one of the most malignant functional PET with the majority of tumors located in distal pancreas. Ten percent of the VIPomas may be extra pancreatic. VIPomas produce pancreatic cholera syndrome. Patients usually present with watery diarrhea, hypokalemia and hypochlorhydria or achlorhydria. The treatment is aimed at the correction of dehydration and electrolyte abnormalities. Similar to other PETs, the only cure is complete resection. Even when the VIPoma has metastasized, debulking aids with the postoperative management of VIP hypersecretion.

Somatostatinoma

Somatostatinoma is also one of the rare but most malignant functional PET with the majority of tumors located in the head of the pancreas. Fasting somatostatin level >14 mol/L is diagnostic. Patients present with diabetes, gallstones with a dilated gallbladder, steatorrhea, anemia and hypochlorhydria. Most of the patients have metastasis at the time of presentation. The diagnosis is established by demonstration of high serum levels of somatostatin. Surgery offers the only curative treatment by excising the primary tumor and all lymph node metastases. Cholecystectomy may be performed at the time of resection.

REFERENCES

1. Pannala Kidd RM, Modlin IM. Acute pancreatitis: a historical perspective. Pancreas 2009;38(4): 355-66.
2. Petrov MS. Early management of severe acute biliary pancreatitis: wind of change. Gut 2008;57(9):1337-8; author reply 1338.
3. Hasibeder WR, et al. Critical care of the patient with acute pancreatitis. Anaesth Intensive Care 2009;37(2):190-206.
4. Petrov MS, Pylypchuk RD, Uchugina AF. A systematic review on the timing of artificial nutrition in acute pancreatitis. Br J Nutr2009;101(6):787-93.
5. Bakker OJ, et al. Prevention, detection, and management of infected necrosis in severe acute pancreatitis. Curr Gastroenterol Rep 2009;11(2):104-10.
6. Werner J, et al. Management of acute pancreatitis: from surgery to interventional intensive care. Gut 2005;54(3):426-36.
7. Church NI, et al. Chronic pancreatitis: diagnosis and management of complications. Gut 2007;56(9):1189-90.
8. Tandon RK, Garg PK. Tropical pancreatitis. Dig Dis 2004;22(3):258-66.
9. Waljee AK, et al. Systematic review: pancreatic enzyme treatment of malabsorption associated with chronic pancreatitis. Aliment Pharmacol Ther 2009;29(3):235-46.
10. Forsmark CE. Antioxidants for chronic pancreatitis. Curr Gastroenterol Rep 2009;11(2):91-2.

11. Gachago C, Draganov PV. Pain management in chronic pancreatitis. World J Gastroenterol 2008;14(20):3137-48.
12. Buchler MW, Klar E. Introduction. Complications of pancreatic surgery and pancreatitis. Dig Surg 2002;19(2):123-4.
13. Johnson CD, Fitzsimmons D. Quality of life after surgery for chronic pancreatitis. Pancreatology 2006;6(5):497-8; author reply498.
14. Gourgiotis S, Germanos S, Ridolfini MP. Surgical management of chronic pancreatitis. Hepatobiliary Pancreat Dis Int 2007;6(2):121-33.
15. Singh S. Surgical management of complications associated with percutaneous and/or endoscopic management of pseudocyst of the pancreas. Ann Surg 2006;244(4):630.
16. Mahvi D. Defining, Controlling, and Treating a Pancreatic Fistula. J Gastrointest Surg 2009.
17. Greenhalf W, et al. Screening of High-Risk Families for Pancreatic Cancer. Pancreatology 2009;9(3):215-22.
18. Sipos B, et al. Pancreatic intraepithelial neoplasia revisited and updated. Pancreatology 2009;9(1-2):45-54.
19. Gonzalez Obeso E, et al. Pseudocyst of the pancreas: the role of cytology and special stains for mucin. Cancer Cytopathol2009;117(2):101-07.
20. Ng DZ, et al. Cystic neoplasms of the pancreas: current diagnostic modalities and management. Ann Acad Med Singapore 2009;38(3):251-9.
21. Freeman HJ. Intraductal papillary mucinous neoplasms and other pancreatic cystic lesions. World J Gastroenterol 2008;14(19):2977.
22. Pannala R, et al. New-onset diabetes: a potential clue to the early diagnosis of pancreatic cancer. Lancet Oncol 2009;10(1):88-95.
23. Saftoiu A, Vilmann P. Role of endoscopic ultrasound in the diagnosis and staging of pancreatic cancer. J Clin Ultrasound2009;37(1):1-17.
24. Pisters PW, et al. Laparoscopy in the staging of pancreatic cancer. Br J Surg 2001;88(3):325-37.
25. Hwang SI, et al. Surgical palliation of unresectable pancreatic head cancer in elderly patients. World J Gastroentero l2009;15(8):978-82.
26. O'Grady HL, Conlon KC. Pancreatic neuroendocrine tumors. Eur J Surg Oncol 2008;34(3):324-32.

❑❑❑

32
CHAPTER

Spleen

Austin Lee, BS
Lawrence Chen, BS
Kayla Umemoto, BA
Anthony Ma, BS
Shahini Ananth, BA
Dinesh Vyas, MD

INTRODUCTION

The spleen is an organ found in the left upper quadrant behind the 9th, 10th, and 11th rib of humans and plays an important role in the immune, lymphatic, and hematologic systems. It houses many antibody producing lymphocytes to help the immune response to pathogen attack, filters lymph and recycles heme and iron for hemoglobin, and synthesizes and stores red blood cells.[1]

The ancient Greeks once believed that the spleen was the source of melancholia and "black bile," one of the body's four humours that had to be kept in balance to maintain one's health. They believed that too much black bile caused someone to feel sad and depressed; too little would cause happiness and laughter (akin to what we today know as major depressive disorder and manic episodes). In Chinese Eastern medicine, the spleen is regarded as the source of yin, which balances the yang from the stomach. The spleen was misunderstood all the way up to the 19th century, when women who were down and depressed were often diagnosed "with spleen." In fact, it was so commonly used as a diagnosis that it was considered one of the two most prevalent diseases in the 1700s (the other was consumption, or tuberculosis).[2]

Our modern medical understanding of the spleen came about in the 1950s when the spleen's role in the immune system was better studied. The functional units of the spleen can be divided into the red and white pulp.[3] The red pulp, made up of complicated sinusoids and splenic cords, stores and filters red blood cells, and releases monocytes.[4] The white pulp regulates the active immune response and maturation of B and T lymphocytes. Similar to the liver, the spleen contains a central opening called the hilum, where the splenic vein, artery, and lymphatic vessels all traverse (Figure 1).[5]

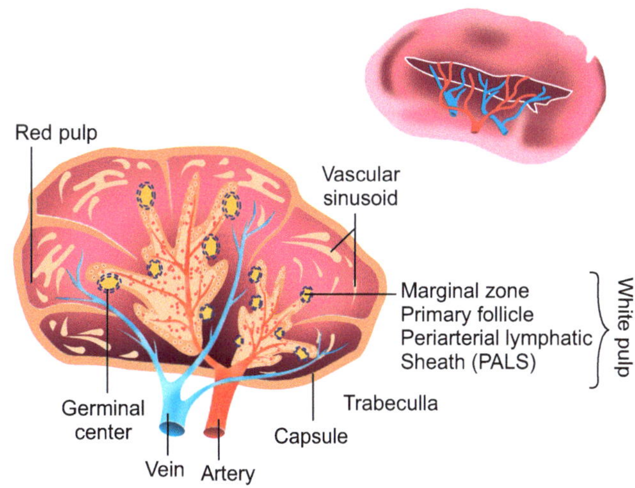

Figure 1: Spleen Anatomy

The spleen also plays an important role in the development of the fetus. Unlike other gastrointestinal organs, the spleen is derived from the mesoderm. Early in development, the spleen generates most of the blood cells and serves as a site of hematopoiesis until the bone marrow fully matures.[6]

Due to its large intertwinement with the circulatory and immune systems, diseases of the spleen can cause major hemorrhage and system-wide effects. Splenic infarction and abscesses can both lead to septic shock if left untreated. Acute trauma, such as motor vehicle accidents, can cause splenic rupture and hemorrhage.[8] Asplenia, which may be congenital or a result of splenectomy to treat hematological diseases, can create other complications. Patients without their spleen are majorly immunocompromised and cannot mount a response to infection. Vaccine recommendations for this group of patients must also be changed, especially with encapsulated pathogens.[9] Overwhelming post-splenectomy infection (OPSI), is a rare but life-threatening sepsis or meningitis most commonly due to Streptococcus.[10] Thus, proper care and attention intraoperatively and generous post-operative patient care and education are necessary to ensure that patients undergoing splenectomy avoid further complications.

Splenomegaly

The spleen enlarges in response to physiological stress or chronic processes, and abnormal enlargement of the spleen is called splenomegaly. The spleen hypertrophies due to an increase in function, congestion, or infiltration, causing splenomegaly.[11] Therefore, patients present with symptoms ranging from cytopenia, fever, lymphadenopathy, abnormal hepatic function, and additional organ dysfunction. The most common symptom is abdominal pain in the left upper quadrant, possibly with a referred left shoulder pain. Patients presenting with splenomegaly require a physical examination with thorough history to identify and diagnose the underlying cause.[12,13]

The spleen weighs between 50g-250g, and during splenomegaly, its weight increases to 400g-500g. Craniocaudal measurement increases as well from measuring less than 13cm to growing to a size of 12cm-20cm. Massive splenomegaly is an increase of splenic weight to over 1000g with the spleen measuring longer than 20cm craniocaudally. It is important to note that accepted values for normal and abnormal splenic dimensions and weight may vary slightly. Splenomegaly is best measured as an increase of splenic weight. However, splenic weight can only be determined post-splenectomy or post-mortem, posing a problem to accurately diagnose it.[12,13] Currently, the best way to diagnose splenomegaly in the clinic is palpating the spleen and using radiologic imaging to estimate its volume.[13]

Hematologic Conditions Causing Splenomegaly

Idiopathic Purpura and Autoimmune Processes

Patients with idiopathic purpuras present with signs of thrombocytopenia ranging from bruising, bleeding from skin/mucosal sites, and hemorrhage. In cases of idiopathic thrombocytopenic purpura (ITP) and thrombotic thrombocytopenic purpura, splenectomy is reserved for severe cases or after traditional first line therapies have been unsuccessful (Table 1).[18]

Particularly for ITP, first-line therapy for symptomatic patients or patients with platelet counts less than $3 \times 10^{10}/L$ consists of medical management with prednisone, intravenous immunoglobulin (IVIg), and/or anti-Rhd globulin. Prednisone should be dosed at 1 mg/kg every day for 2 to 4 weeks which should be tapered off over several weeks. If there is no response after 4 weeks, the patient should be rapidly tapered off the prednisone and discontinue the steroid. IVIg and anti-Rhd could be used to boost corticosteroid effect and could also be used for patients with corticosteroid contraindications. Dosing for IVIg is usually 1g/kg per day for 1 to 2 days. If these treatments fail, splenectomy is indicated. Pre-splenectomy platelet levels should be around $2 \times 10^{10}/L$ to $3 \times 10^{10}/L$ to help achieve hemostasis and help prevent postoperative bleeding. Therapies like corticosteroids, IVIg, and anti-Rhd could also be used to increase the patient's platelet levels pre-operatively.[19]

Thrombotic thrombocytopenic purpura (TTP) typically presents with weakness, dyspnea, and skin and mucosal hemorrhage. Other symptoms can include brain, heart, mesenteric, and renal ischemia, and infarction which can present with headache/confusion, myocardial infarction, abdominal pain, and proteinuria/hematuria, respectively. TTP is traditionally managed with plasma exchange therapy, glucocorticoids, and rituximab. Relapses in TTP can be life threatening in patients, and splenectomy significantly decreases these relapse occurrences (Table 1).[20]

Autoimmune hemolytic anemias (AIHA) present with mild to fatal anemia but differ slightly depending on whether hemolysis is IgG-mediated warm AIHA or IgM-mediated cold AIHA (cold agglutinin disease or CAD).[21] Specifically in CAD, patients can present with Raynaud's disease or acrocyanosis in addition to signs of anemia and hemolysis.[22] For patients with primary warm AIHA, a splenectomy is indicated as a third-line treatment, and in emergencies, partial splenic embolization or a splenectomy can be considered. In contrast, there are no indications for a splenectomy in patients with CAD (Table 1).[22,23]

Felty Syndrome is an extra-articular manifestation of rheumatoid arthritis that presents with neutropenia and splenomegaly.[24] Historically, splenectomy was the primary treatment for Felty Syndrome, but with the advent of DMARDs, biologic agents, and G-CSF, splenectomy is now reserved for patients with recurrent infection or patients who do not respond to these therapies. A splenectomy could also be considered in cases of severe anemia or thrombocytopenia with hemorrhage (Table 1).[25]

Table 1: Indications for splenectomy

Condition	Indication for Splenectomy
Idiopathic Thrombocytopenic Purpura	
Adults:	Second-line therapy after failing oral corticosteroids (prednisone), IVIG, and anti-RhD
Children:	Patients with life-threatening bleeds or severe ITP affecting quality of life[18]
Thrombotic Thrombocytopenic Purpura	Severe or refractory TTP after failing plasma exchange therapy, glucocorticoids, and rituximab[20]
Autoimmune Hemolytic Anemia	
Primary Warm:	Third-line therapy after steroids then rituximab In emergencies and severe hemolysis, partial splenic embolization or splenectomy used for patients not responding to IVIg or recombinant erythropoietin
Primary Cold:	No indications for splenectomy
Felty Syndrome	Patients with recurrent infections or not responsive to DMARDs, biologic agents, and G-CSF Severe anemia or thrombocytopenia with hemorrhage not responsive to standard treatment options

Red Blood Cell Disorders

Patients with hereditary spherocytosis, hereditary elliptocytosis, and pyruvate kinase deficiency present clinically with signs of anemia, jaundice, and venous ulcers. Red blood cells in these disorders are destroyed by macrophages in the spleen, thus a splenectomy will ameliorate the patient's clinical picture. Removing the spleen will not correct the underlying mechanism of these disorders but will help address the patient's hemolytic anemia and associated symptoms.[18,20,26]

In cases of thalassemia, patients present with splenomegaly and hypersplenism associated with ineffective erythropoiesis and hemolysis. Treatment of thalassemia consists of chronic blood transfusions which increases risk of hemochromatosis. With a splenectomy, the need for blood transfusions is reduced, and this procedure should be considered and performed before the patient is 6 to 8 years old. One risk is thrombotic complications after an average of 8 years post-splenectomy and should be considered before proceeding with the procedure.[18,27]

Patients with homozygous sickle cell anemia present with hemolytic anemia, dactylitis, and vaso-occlusive events leading to tissue infarcts, pain, and organ damage. Vaso-occlusive crises are particularly painful for patients with sickle cell disease and require prompt management with varying combinations of hydration, non-opioid analgesics, opioids, and adjunct therapies like hydroxyurea depending on the site of acute crises to prevent red blood cells from sickling. One potentially fatal complication of sickle cell disease is splenic sequestration, where the spleen enlarges and is filled with red blood cells.[28] A full splenectomy will prevent future splenic sequestration events, and a partial splenectomy could reduce the recurrence of these events.[29]

White Blood Cell Disorders

In cases of Hodgkin's Lymphoma, Non-Hodgkin's Lymphoma, Chronic Lymphoblastic leukemia, and Chronic Myeloblastic leukemia, and Primary Myelofibrosis, splenectomy is indicated as a palliative treatment for symptoms of massive splenomegaly. Along the same lines, if the case presents with thrombocytopenia, anemia, or neutropenia also due to splenomegaly, a splenectomy can be considered.[30]

For Hodgkin's lymphoma, while laparotomy used to be standard for staging, splenectomy is now usually not indicated. For Non-Hodgkin's Lymphoma, if the Splenic Marginal Zone lymphoma originates at the spleen, splenectomy is indicated as first-line treatment.[31] Splenectomy is rarely indicated now for Hairy Cell Leukemia as medical treatments with 2-CDA and pentostatin have been shown to be effective.

Myeloproliferative Disorders

In patients with Primary Myelofibrosis, splenectomy is indicated if the patient presents with signs of thrombocytopenia, hemolysis requiring numerous blood transfusions, painful massive splenomegaly, or multiple splenic infarcts. associated with a 15-30% risk of morbidity as well as a 10% risk of mortality, meaning the procedure is only indicated for a select group of patients.

For other bone marrow disorders, such as CML, polycythemia vera, PMF, and essential thrombocytopenia, splenectomy is indicated when the case presents with painful splenomegaly or cytopenia secondary to splenic sequestration. In polycythemia vera cases, splenectomy does not provide much benefit until myelofibrosis develops later in the disease process. Splenectomy is rarely indicated in essential thrombocytopenia.[32]

Tumors

In cases of primary Splenic Tumors, vascular tumors of the spleen, and malignant tumors of the spleen, splenectomy is used to manage symptoms or provide a definite diagnosis. Splenectomy is reasonable for almost all splenic tumors, particularly to relieve symptoms of fatigue, LUQ pain, and weight loss.

Malignant tumors, including NHL, HL, and CML, are all covered in previous sections. Generally, splenectomy is reasonable as a palliative treatment. Compared to lymphomas, primary splenic tumors are much rarer. Tumors may also metastasize to the spleen. The most common primary source organs for splenic metastases are the breast, lung, pancreas, and colon (Figure 2).

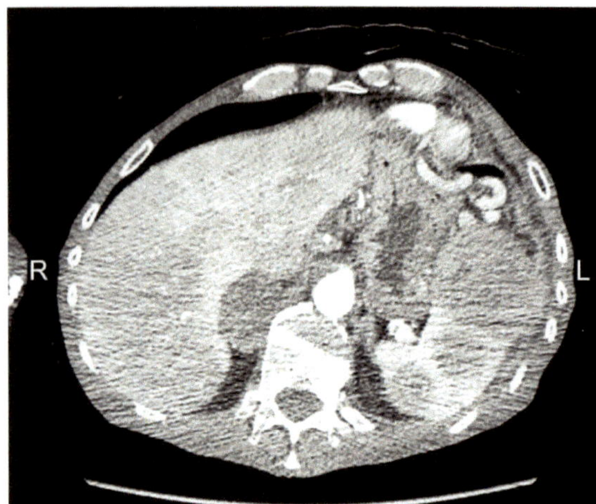

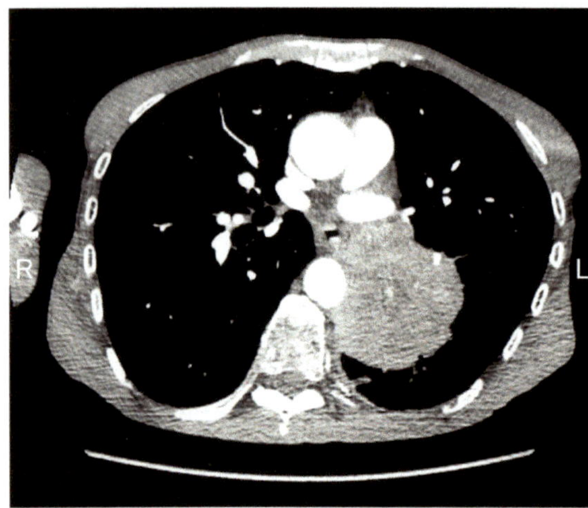

Figure 2: CT of primary small cell lung cancer metastasis to spleen

Regarding vascular tumors of the spleen, in addition to traditional lymphangiomas and hemangiomas, Sclerosing angiomatoid nodular transformation (SANT) is a rare hematological condition that is cause for splenectomy, although a diagnosis cannot be made until histologic exam post-resection (Figure 3).[33]

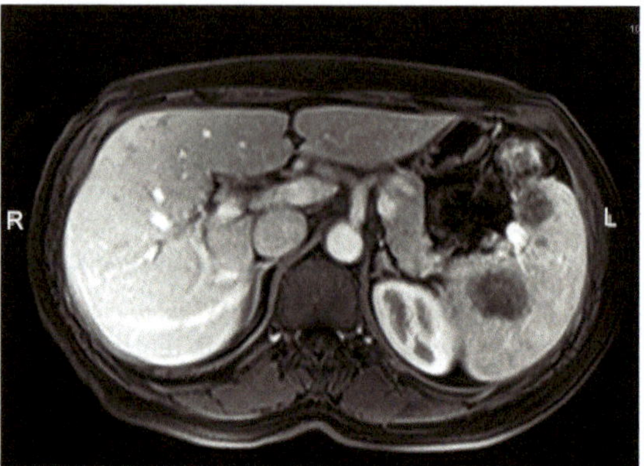

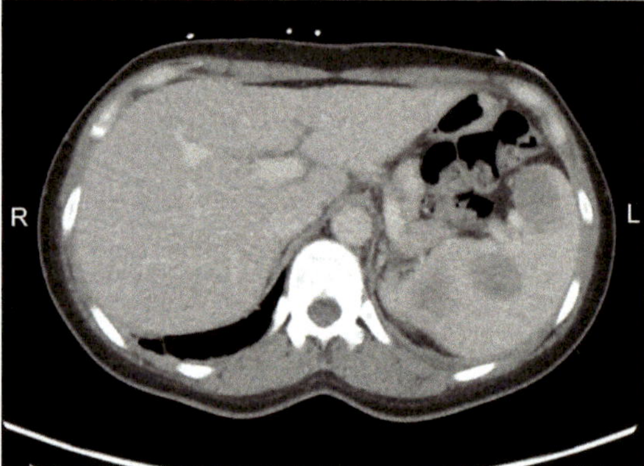

Figure 3: MRI without contrast of splenic lymphangioma (left) and CT of splenic lymphangioma (right)

Cysts and Abscesses of the Spleen

Overview

With the advancement and increased utilization of imaging modalities, more splenic lesions are being discovered incidentally. Most splenic cysts are secondary pseudocysts arising from trauma, infection, or infarction, while a smaller percentage are found to be either true primary cysts with epithelial lining or parasitic hydatid cysts. Regardless of etiology, preservation of functioning splenic tissue remains a goal of treatment.

Cysts

Splenic cysts, almost always discovered incidentally, are often asymptomatic, but can present with abdominal pain, LUQ discomfort, referred left shoulder pain, early satiety, or nausea and vomiting. If the cyst is greater than 5 centimeters, partial splenectomy, unroofing, or full splenectomy is indicated to prevent cystic rupture.[34]

These cysts can be categorized as parasitic versus nonparasitic. Parasitic cysts come in the form of echinococcal cysts, arising from infection from echinococcus granulosus, E. multilocaliaris, E. vogeli. Hydatid disease, often affecting the liver and the lungs may also cause splenic cysts due to infection from echinococcus species. Unless some preservation is feasible, total splenectomy is indicated.[35]

With regards to nonparasitic cysts, there is a further classification of primary versus secondary cysts. Primary cysts are mainly epidermoid. Secondary cysts, also known as pseudocysts, generally arise from trauma that causes hemorrhage.

If the cysts remain less than 5 cm in diameter, there is a low risk of spontaneous rupture, and nonsurgical techniques are recommended for treatment.

Abscesses

While lethal if left untreated, splenic abscesses are generally quite rare (Figure 4). These abscesses are normally caused by staphylococcus, streptococcus, salmonella, candida, or aspergillus and should be treated upon discovery. Intravenous drug users and immunocompromised patients are at greater risk for such infections. First-line treatment remains antibiotics, but procedural intervention may be required if refractory. Recently, imaging-assisted percutaneous techniques have been used with increasing success to address splenic abscesses, but a full splenectomy will provide definitive treatment for the abscess.[36]

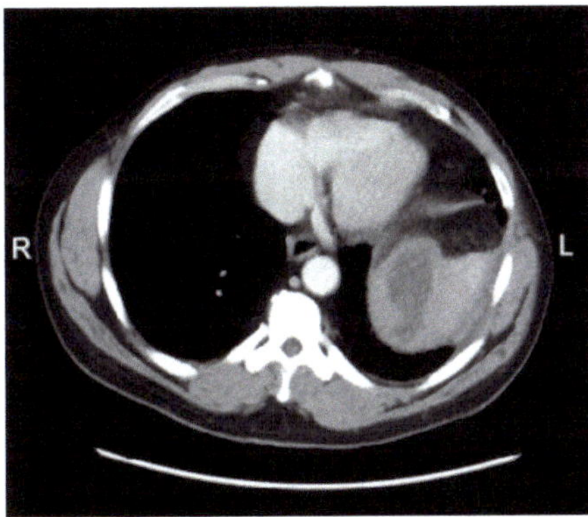

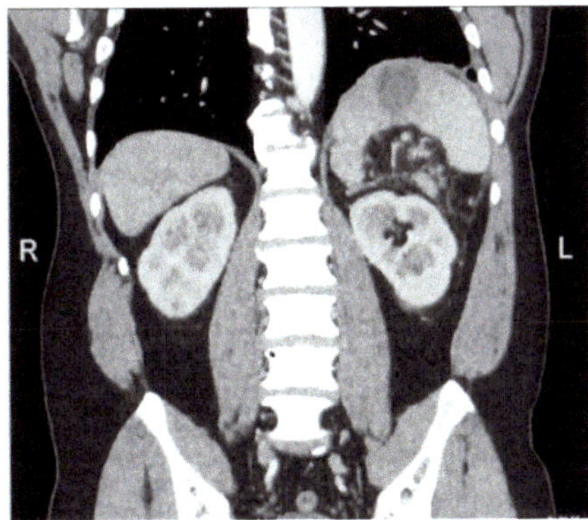

Figure 4: CT of Splenic Abscess

Splenic Trauma

Given the prevalence of splenic injuries and the highly vascular nature of the spleen, complete evaluation and management of splenic trauma are of prime importance. In terms of management, trauma resuscitation protocols must be followed. In particular, ABC's or airway, breathing, and circulation must be checked as assessment of circulation can provide information on hemodynamic stability; it can help identify potential hemorrhage and shock amongst patients, dictating treatment strategies such as resuscitation.[37]

After assessing hemodynamic stability, a thorough history and physical examination can be performed. Additionally, FAST (Focused Assessment with Sonography for Trauma) and CT (Computed Tomography) can be used to localize splenic injury and identify complications. FAST is a technique that employs sonography to examine the pericardiac, perihepatic, perisplenic, and pelvic acoustic windows. FAST can determine the presence of free intraperitoneal fluid or hemoperitoneum; a positive FAST finding in the backdrop of hemodynamic instability dictates immediate surgical intervention. However, CT can help image splenic damage including damage to the parenchyma and vasculature. Based on CT findings, an AAST grade can be determined. Within the AAST system, injuries are categorized from grades 1-5, with grade 1 being a less severe capsular tear, and grade 5 being a severely damaged spleen with avascularization. While the AAST is a useful system, studies have found that AAST alone does not determine surgical need.[37,38]

However, with the combination of imaging and examination findings, the need for nonoperative versus operative management can be determined. Importantly, if possible, nonoperative management is the preferred strategy due to the spleen's vital role in immune system functioning and the risk of a postoperative splenectomy infection.

Nonoperative Management

In terms of patient selection, patients are selected based on hemodynamic status; nonoperative management is currently considered the gold standard of care for hemodynamically stable patients. In fact, nonoperative management can be performed in patients with higher AAST grades if patients are hemodynamically stable.

Nonoperative management includes observation and monitoring, deep vein thrombosis prophylaxis, and or angioembolization.

Angioembolization

Splenic angioembolization was developed in the 1970's as a method to ensure splenic function and reduce the frequency of postoperative splenectomy infections. It was initially intended to serve pediatric populations; however, it is now used in a broader range of age groups.[39]

In terms of the technique, angioembolization involves gel foam, coiling, and catheters. The main splenic artery is catheterized to overcome vascular compromise via femoral access. A micro-puncture kit is used to access the femoral artery, and subsequently pass the celiac artery and enter the splenic artery.[40] Further, a distal or proximal embolization approach can be employed; in the distal approach catheterization is performed distally from the affected area to decrease bleeding risk. In contrast, the proximal approach decreases flow through the main splenic artery and maintains flow through collateral vessels; this technique also reduces the risk of bleeding and subsequent infarction.[40]

Risks of angioembolization include complications such as abscesses, pleural effusion, and infarcts. Interestingly, however, some studies suggest that angioembolization can improve the spleen's immune functioning.

Deep Vein Thrombosis

Deep Vein Thrombosis and pulmonary embolism are complications that can be encountered in trauma patients and increase the mortality rate of trauma injuries to 20%.[3] Given these statistics, non-operative management of splenic injuries may include deep vein thrombosis or venous thromboembolism prophylaxis. Thrombosis prophylaxis can be both mechanical and pharmacologic in nature. Examples of mechanical treatment include inferior vena cava filtration and compression stockings.[4] In contrast, pharmacologic treatments include typical anticoagulants and anti-platelet drugs. Unfractionated or low weight molecular heparin can also be administered.[4]

However, prophylaxis creates a treatment paradox through increasing the risk of bleeding and potentially decreasing the efficacy of nonoperative management. This creates a treatment challenge whereby timing of prophylaxis becomes a key parameter; timing of therapy has not been clearly defined as it is still an active area of research. Thus, timing of therapy is often left to clinical judgement.[3]

However, with regards to venous thromboembolism (VTE), studies have compared administration of prophylactic treatment at the 48-hour mark, comparing outcomes prior to and after 48 hours. Some studies have found that there is no difference between administration prior to and after the 48-hour mark, while other studies have found it beneficial to begin VTE therapy prior to the 48-hour mark. Interestingly, one study even found that VTE therapy could be administered within 24 hours of injury.[3]

Importantly, eliciting a thorough history and physical remains crucial in identifying patients at increased risk of developing VTE or DVT. New biomarkers are also currently being studied and are can potentially help determine a patients' ability to coagulate. A recent study found that increased severity of injury (determined by injury severity score), lower extremity fractures, and D-dimer levels after day 10 can help predict VTE risk. Such findings can augment traditional clinical reasoning and help identify a patient's coagulation status.[4]

Operative Management

While non-operative management is currently the preferred approach, non-operative management can have failure rates up to 40%. This is especially the case for elderly patients, patients who have a higher degree of injury, and patients who have a hemoperitoneum.[41]

When non-operative management cannot be employed, surgery becomes the main treatment modality: splenorraphy, partial splenectomy, and total splenectomy. Splenorraphy and partial splenectomy are spleen salvaging procedures that are intended to maintain some functioning of the spleen; this is of particular importance given the spleen's role in immune system functioning. However, there are cases where total splenectomy is still performed.

Splenectomy

In terms of surgical technique, open splenectomy is considered the mainstay technique; very few studies have compared open versus laparoscopic splenectomy. However, the studies that have been conducted demonstrate promising results.[41-43] The laparoscopic approach has advantages in that it allows for one to more easily discern the presence of diaphragmatic and visceral injuries. Studies have found that post-surgical outcomes are better; there is decreased blood loss during surgery, and there are fewer conversions to open surgery. Of note, in many of these studies patients were hemodynamically stable, but did not respond well to non-operative management. Thus, it has been proposed that those who are at risk of failing non-operative management, may be suitable candidates for laparoscopic surgery. Yet if patients present with hemodynamic instability, open surgery is preferred over laparoscopic surgery.[43-45]

Splenectomy can be considered for hematologic and neoplastic conditions as well as cysts and abscesses causing symptomatic splenomegaly.[14] For all cases except in trauma, laparoscopic splenectomy is preferred over open splenectomy, but longer operation times and more blood loss should be taken into consideration.[15] Another consideration before proceeding with a splenectomy is overwhelming post-splenectomy infection by encapsulated bacteria in the long-term for asplenic patients.[16] Vaccinations against haemophilus influenzae type b and meningococcus are recommended to be administered two weeks before splenectomy for patients older than two years old.[17] In cases of an emergency splenectomy, vaccinations should be administered after the procedure. Patients who are immunosuppressed should be given life-long antibiotics as a prophylactic measure against infections in addition to vaccinations.[14]

New Techniques and Technology for Splenectomies

In the late 1980s, the use of robotic and laparoscopic procedures for general surgeries began replacing open surgeries, this includes splenectomies.[46] Much of the success of these new technologies, in place of traditional open surgeries, is that they are minimally invasive. This results in the reduction of both intraoperative and postoperative complications such as decreased intraoperative bleeding, operating time, postoperative pain, hospital stay, and scarring.[47] Since their advent, both robotic and laparoscopic technology have continued to advance, finding ways to improve the technique. This section will discuss the newer laparoscopic techniques of hand-assisted laparoscopic splenectomy (HALS), single-incision laparoscopic splenectomy (SILS), and the electromechanical morcellator.

Hals

HALS is a surgical technique that combines both open and laparoscopic surgery. Due to the minimally invasive nature of laparoscopic surgery, there is a loss of tactile sensation that is often a valuable tool for the surgeon, especially for difficult procedures such as a massive splenomegaly.[47,48] In the HALS technique, the surgeon inserts their nondominant hand through an incision, the hand-assist device, and into the abdomen to maintain the pneumoperitoneum, while performing much of the procedure with the laparoscope.[47,48] Then they can more easily and quickly remove the spleen through this same incision made for the hand without the need for morcellation.[47] This enables the surgeon to still use their tactile sensation while also keeping many of the advantages provided by a laparoscopic procedure.[48] This technique has shown to improve intraoperative complications (i.e., hemorrhages), operating times, hospital stay, and postoperative pain.[47] Without the HALS technique, many massive laparoscopic splenectomies (> 22 cm in diameter) require conversion to an open procedure.[47]

The Electromechanical Morcellator

The electromechanical morcellator is a device that cuts tissue into small pieces so that they can be removed through the small incision initially created for the laparoscope.[49] This device is used for massive laparoscopic splenectomies to avoid the need for a larger incision to remove the spleen.[50] In a study by Jiang et al, 10 cirrhotic patients with bleeding portal hypertension and secondary hypersplenism underwent laparoscopic splenectomies assisted with the electromechanical morcellator.[50] The results demonstrated a successful procedure with no conversions to open surgery, and decreased operating time, blood loss, and perioperative complications.[50] These operating parameters resulted in better recovery for the patients and less pain and scarring.[50] Finally, this procedure avoids the need for an intracorporeal bag, an enlarged incision, and a hand-assisted incision.[50]

REFERENCES

1. Mebius R, Kraal G. Structure and function of the spleen. *Nat Rev Immunol* 5, 606–616 (2005). https://doi.org/10.1038/nri1669.
2. Bynum B. The spleen. The Lancet. 2002;359(9317):1624. doi:10.1016/s0140-6736(02)08479-9.
3. Sahin NE, Oner Z, Oner S, Turan MK. A study on the correlation between spleen volume estimated via cavalieri principle on computed tomography images with basic hemogram and biochemical blood parameters. *Anat Cell Biol.* 2022;55(1):40-47. doi:10.5115/acb.21.177.
4. Brender E, Burke A, Glass RM. The Spleen. *JAMA.* 2005;294(20):2660. doi:10.1001/jama.294.20.2660.
5. Swirski FK, Nahrendorf M, Etzrodt M, et al. Identification of Splenic Reservoir Monocytes and Their Deployment to Inflammatory Sites. Science. 2009;325(5940):612-616. doi:10.1126/science.1175202 https://www.science.org/doi/10.1126/science.1175202.
6. Jia T, Pamer EG. Dispensable But Not Irrelevant. Science. 2009;325(5940):549-550. doi:10.1126/science.1178329 https://www.science.org/doi/10.1126/science.1178329.
7. Vellguth S, von Gaudecker B, Müller-Hermelink HK. The development of the human spleen. *Cell Tissue Res.* 242, 579–592 (1985). https://doi.org/10.1007/BF00225424.
8. Brant WE. *Spleen.* Elsevier; 2012: p. 265-272.
9. Lee GM. Preventing infections in children and adults with asplenia. *Hematology Am Soc Hematol*

Educ Program. 2020;2020(1):328-335. doi:10.1182/hematology.2020000117.

10. Riva MA, Ferraina F, Paleari A, *et al.* From sadness to stiffness: the spleen's progress. *Intern Emerg Med* 14, 739–743 (2019). https://doi.org/10.1007/s11739-019-02115-2.
11. McKenzie CV, Colonne CK, Yeo JH, Fraser ST. Splenomegaly: Pathophysiological bases and therapeutic options, The International Journal of Biochemistry & Cell Biology, Volume 94, 2018, Pages 40-43, ISSN 1357-2725, https://doi.org/10.1016/j.biocel.2017.11.011.
12. Chapman J, Bansal P, Goyal A, Azevedo AM. Splenomegaly. In: StatPearls. StatPearls Publishing, Treasure Island (FL); 2020. PMID: 28613657.
13. Pozo AL, Godfrey EM, Bowles KM. Splenomegaly: Investigation, diagnosis and management, Blood Reviews, Volume 23, Issue 3, 2009, Pages 105-111, ISSN 0268-960X, https://doi.org/10.1016/j.blre.2008.10.001.
14. Weledji EP. Benefits and risks of splenectomy. Int J Surg. 2014;12(2): 113-9. doi: 10.1016/j.ijsu.2013.11.017. Epub 2013 Dec 3. PMID: 24316283.
15. Misiakos EP, Bagias G, Liakakos T, Machairas A. Laparoscopic splenectomy: Current concepts. World J Gastrointest Endosc. 2017 Sep 16;9(9):428-437. doi: 10.4253/wjge.v9.i9.428. PMID: 28979707; PMCID: PMC5605342.
16. Tahir F, Ahmed J, Malik F. Post-splenectomy Sepsis: A Review of the Literature. Cureus. 2020;12(2):e6898. Published 2020 Feb 6. doi:10.7759/cureus.6898.
17. Luu S, Spelman D, Woolley IJ. Post-splenectomy sepsis: preventative strategies, challenges, and solutions. Infect Drug Resist. 2019;12:2839-2851. Published 2019 Sep 12. doi:10.2147/IDR.S179902.
18. Weledji EP. Benefits and risks of splenectomy. Int J Surg. 2014;12(2):113-9. doi: 10.1016/j.ijsu.2013.11.017. Epub 2013 Dec 3. PMID: 24316283.
19. British Committee for Standards in Haematology General Haematology Task Force. Guidelines for the investigation and management of idiopathic thrombocytopenic purpura in adults, children and in pregnancy. Br J Haematol. 2003;120(4):574-596. doi:10.1046/j.1365-2141.2003.04131.x.
20. Manciu S, Matei E, Trandafir B. Hereditary Spherocytosis - Diagnosis, Surgical Treatment and Outcomes. A Literature Review. Chirurgia (Bucur). 2017 Mar-Apr;112(2):110-116. doi: 10.21614/chirurgia.112.2.110. PMID: 28463670.
21. Barcellini W, Fattizzo B. The Changing Landscape of Autoimmune Hemolytic Anemia. Front Immunol. 2020 Jun 3;11:946. doi: 10.3389/fimmu.2020.00946. PMID: 32655543; PMCID: PMC7325906.
22. Michalak SS, Olewicz-Gawlik A, Rupa-Matysek J, Wolny-Rokicka E, Nowakowska E, Gil L. Autoimmune hemolytic anemia: current knowledge and perspectives. Immun Ageing. 2020 Nov 20;17(1):38. doi: 10.1186/s12979-020-00208-7. PMID: 33292368; PMCID: PMC7677104.
23. Hill A, Hill QA. Autoimmune hemolytic anemia. Hematology Am Soc Hematol Educ Program. 2018 Nov 30;2018(1):382-389. doi: 10.1182/asheducation-2018.1.382. PMID: 30504336; PMCID: PMC6246027.
24. Rashba EJ, Rowe JM, Packman CH. Treatment of the neutropenia of Felty syndrome. Blood Rev. 1996;10(3):177-184. doi:10.1016/s0268-960x(96)90024-7.
25. Balint GP, Balint PV. Felty's syndrome. Best Pract Res Clin Rheumatol. 2004;18(5):631-645. doi:10.1016/j.berh.2004.05.002.
26. Grace RF, Barcellini W. Management of pyruvate kinase deficiency in children and adults. Blood. 2020 Sep 10;136(11):1241-1249. doi: 10.1182/blood.2019000945. PMID: 32702739.
27. Galanello R, Origa R. Beta-thalassemia. Orphanet J Rare Dis. 2010 May 21;5:11. doi: 10.1186/1750-1172-5-11. PMID: 20492708; PMCID: PMC2893117.
28. Bender MA. Sickle Cell Disease. 2003 Sep 15 [updated 2021 Jan 28]. In: Adam MP, Ardinger HH, Pagon RA, Wallace SE, Bean LJH, Gripp KW, Mirzaa GM, Amemiya A, editors. GeneReviews® [Internet]. Seattle (WA): University of Washington, Seattle; 1993–2021. PMID: 20301551.
29. Owusu-Ofori S, Remmington T. Splenectomy versus conservative management for acute sequestration crises in people with sickle cell disease. Cochrane Database Syst Rev. 2017 Nov 7;11(11):CD003425. doi: 10.1002/14651858.CD003425.pub4. PMID: 29112240; PMCID: PMC6486322.
30. Kehoe JE, Daly JM, Straus DJ, DeCosse JJ. Value of splenectomy in non-Hodgkin's lymphoma. Cancer. 1985 Mar 15;55(6):1256-64. doi: 10.1002/1097-0142(19850315)55:6<1256::aid-cncr2820550618>3.0.co;2-s. PMID: 2578865.
31. Sindel A, Al-Juhaishi T, Yazbeck V. Marginal Zone Lymphoma: State-of-the-Art Treatment. Curr Treat Options Oncol. 2019 Dec 5;20(12):90. doi: 10.1007/s11864-019-0687-5. PMID: 31807935.

32. Bonnet S, Guédon A, Ribeil JA, Suarez F, Tamburini J, Gaujoux S. Indications and outcome of splenectomy in hematologic disease. J Visc Surg. 2017 Dec;154(6):421-429. doi: 10.1016/j.jviscsurg.2017.06.011. Epub 2017 Jul 27. PMID: 28757383.
33. Jin Y, Hu H, Regmi P, Li F, Cheng N. Treatment options for sclerosing angiomatoid nodular transformation of spleen. HPB (Oxford). 2020 Nov;22(11):1577-1582. doi: 10.1016/j.hpb.2020.01.014. Epub 2020 Feb 13. PMID: 32063479.
34. Chin EH, Shapiro R, Hazzan D, Katz LB, Salky B. A ten-year experience with laparoscopic treatment of splenic cysts. JSLS. 2007 Jan-Mar;11(1):20-3. PMID: 17651551; PMCID: PMC3015798.
35. Golmohammadzadeh H, Maddah G, Shams Hojjati Y, Abdollahi A, Shabahang H. Splenic cysts: Analysis of 16 cases. Caspian J Intern Med. 2016 Summer;7(3):217-221. PMID: 27757209; PMCID: PMC5062182.
36. Kang M, Kalra N, Gulati M, Lal A, Kochhar R, Rajwanshi A. Image guided percutaneous splenic interventions. Eur J Radiol. 2007 Oct;64(1):140-6. doi: 10.1016/j.ejrad.2007.02.011. Epub 2007 Mar 19. PMID: 17374470.
37. Waseem M, Bjerke S. Splenic Injury. [Updated 2022 Jan 29]. In: StatPearls [Internet]. Treasure Island (FL): StatPearls Publishing; 2022 Jan-. Available from: https://www.ncbi.nlm.nih.gov/books/NBK441993/.
38. Coccolini F, Montori G, Catena F, et al. Splenic trauma: WSES classification and guidelines for adult and pediatric patients. World J Emerg Surg. 2017;12:40. Published 2017 Aug 18. doi:10.1186/s13017-017-0151-4.
39. Bankhead-Kendall B, Teixeira P, Musonza T, et al. Risk Factors for Failure of Splenic Angioembolization: A Multicenter Study of Level I Trauma Centers. Journal of Surgical Research. 2021;257:227-231. doi:10.1016/j.jss.2020.07.058.
40. Imbrogno BF, Ray CE. Splenic artery embolization in blunt trauma. Semin Intervent Radiol. 2012;29(2):147-149. doi:10.1055/s-0032-1312577.
41. Rodríguez-Luna MR, Balagué C, Fernández-Ananín S, Vilallonga R, Targarona Soler EM. Outcomes of Laparoscopic Splenectomy for Treatment of Splenomegaly: A Systematic Review and Meta-analysis. World J Surg. 2021;45(2):465-479. doi:10.1007/s00268-020-05839-x.
42. Tada K, Ohta M, Saga K, et al. Long-term outcomes of laparoscopic versus open splenectomy for immune thrombocytopenia. Surg Today. 2018;48(2):180-185. doi:10.1007/s00595-017-1570-2.
43. Feng S, Qiu Y, Li X, et al. Laparoscopic versus open splenectomy in children: a systematic review and meta-analysis. Pediatr Surg Int. 2016;32(3):253-259. doi:10.1007/s00383-015-3845-2.
44. Chen J, Ma R, Yang S, Lin S, He S, Cai X. Perioperative outcomes of laparoscopic versus open splenectomy for nontraumatic diseases: a meta-analysis. Chin Med J (Engl). 2014;127(13):2504-2510.
45. Romeo L, Bagolini F, Ferro S, et al. Laparoscopic surgery for splenic injuries in the era of non-operative management: current status and future perspectives. Surg Today. 2021;51(7):1075-1084. doi:10.1007/s00595-020-02177-2.
46. Vecchio R, MacFayden BV, Palazzo F. History of laparoscopic surgery. Panminerva Med. 2000 Mar;42(1):87-90. PMID: 11019611.
47. Misiakos EP, Bagias G, Liakakos T, Machairas A. Laparoscopic splenectomy: Current concepts. World J Gastrointest Endosc. 2017;9(9):428-437. doi:10.4253/wjge.v9.i9.428.
48. Targarona EM, Balague C, Cerdán G, Espert JJ, Lacy AM, Visa J, Trias M. Hand-assisted laparoscopic splenectomy (HALS) in cases of splenomegaly: a comparison analysis with conventional laparoscopic splenectomy. Surg Endosc. 2002 Mar;16(3):426-30. doi: 10.1007/s00464-001-8104-z. Epub 2001 Dec 10. PMID: 11928021.
49. Laparoscopic Power Morcellators. FDA. 2020 Dec.
50. Jiang G, Qian J, Yao J, Wang X, Jin S, Bai D. A new technique for laparoscopic splenectomy and azygoportal disconnection. Surg Innov. 2014 Jun;21(3):256-62. doi: 10.1177/1553350613492587. Epub 2013 Jun 26. PMID: 23804998.

❑❑❑

33
CHAPTER

Appendix

Armin Kamyab, MD
Binit Katuwal, MD
Vijay K. Mittal, MD

APPENDICITIS

Overview

The first successful appendectomy is credited to Claudius Amyand, a British surgeon, who performed an appendectomy during the repair of an inguinal hernia in 1735, in which the patient survived both the appendicitis and the surgery.[1] This gave rise to the term "Amyand's hernia", which defines an appendix-containing hernia.

The first appendectomy for appendicitis is credited to Reginald Fitz, who in 1886 identified an inflamed appendix as being the cause of a patient's right lower quadrant pain.[2] In 1889, Charles Heber McBurney described the characteristic migrating pain, initiating at the periumbilical region, and subsequently resting at a position two-thirds of the way from the umbilicus to the anterior superior iliac spine, hence terming the phrase "McBurney's point".[3] Of interest, the first laparoscopic appendectomy is credited to the gynecologist Kurt Semm in 1983.[4]

Acute appendicitis is one of the most common abdominal surgical emergencies. The diagnosis is sometimes clear-cut, but can also be challenging, especially in women of childbearing age. Early and accurate recognition is essential, as delayed diagnosis can be associated with perforation resulting in increased morbidity.

Although largely believed to be a clinical diagnosis, there are various imaging modalities widely used to assist in accurate diagnosis, including ultrasound and computed tomography (CT) scans. In certain cases of diagnostic uncertainty, a diagnostic laparoscopy may also be required.

Presentation and Pathophysiology

Both the clinical history and physical examination are of utmost importance in working up and evaluating patients with suspected appendicitis. The site of the pain, the timing, and any associated symptoms are crucial factors when assessing patients.

Appendicitis is believed to be most commonly due to obstruction of the appendiceal lumen.[5] Common attributed causes include fecaliths, lymphoid hyperplasia, dietary causes (e.g., seeds), parasites, or neoplasms. Subsequent luminal distention produces visceral pain experienced as periumbilical pain. Untreated, luminal distention causes obstruction of venous drainage, leading to mucosal ischemia and inflammation, with irritation of the adjacent peritoneum which causes localized right lower quadrant pain.

With prolonged appendiceal ischemia, transmural necrosis ensues, resulting in a gangrenous appendix which may lead to perforation. Appendiceal perforation can result in phlegmon formation or abscess formation. Depending on the location of the appendix, the abscess can be peritoneal or retroperitoneal.[5]

This classical presentation of acute onset periumbilical pain which subsequently migrates to the right lower quadrant is not always present, especially with a retrocecal appendix or in pregnant patients where the location of the appendix may have shifted. Therefore, the astute clinician will consider the wide array of differential diagnoses that may present with right lower quadrant pain, such as urinary tract infections, gastroenteritis, mesenteric adenitis, or gynecological conditions such as pelvic inflammatory disease. In the pediatric population, the differential diagnosis also included intussusception, Meckel's diverticulitis, and gastroenteritis.

Diagnosis

The hallmark of diagnosing acute appendicitis is based on a thorough history and physical examination findings. If the diagnosis is highly suspected, additional testing is not required. In equivocal cases however, additional objective findings can help narrow the differential diagnoses, and reduce the rate of negative appendectomies.

Laboratory Studies

There are no laboratory tests specific to acute appendicitis. Leukocytosis however is the hallmark of any acute inflammatory process and is present in most cases of appendicitis. A so-called left shift (neutrophilia) is neither sensitive nor specific in the absence of leukocytosis for the work up of acute inflammatory processes. Levels greater than 20,000/mL are believed to suggest complicated appendicitis. A beta-hCG level should be checked to rule out pregnancy, and therefore rule out ectopic pregnancy as the cause of acute onset lower quadrant abdominal pain. A urinalysis should be checked since urinary tract infections can also present as lower quadrant abdominal pain.

Studies have looked into identifying specific serum markers for diagnosing appendicitis. These include CRP, Granulocyte colony-stimulating factor, Leucine-rich α-2-glycoprotein, and riboleukograms.[6-9] However, these serum markers may not be any more sensitive than a WBC, are not widely available, are costly, and often take days to process making them impractical in the acute setting. A serum CRP is the only readily available serum marker. A CRP level greater than 3 mg/dL is associated with an increased likelihood of appendicitis, with an adjusted odds ratio of 3.44 for definite appendicitis.[6] However, a CRP alone cannot accurately diagnose appendicitis in light of negative physical and imaging findings. Studies assessing serum markers do however shed a glimpse into the future and show potential for aiding to diagnose appendicitis.

Radiography Studies

Radiographic findings have contributed a great deal in accurately diagnosing appendicitis. Most patients who have undergone an appendectomy have had some form of radiographic test performed. A CT scan and ultrasound remain the most common tests performed. MRI and barium enemas, although described, have limited value in evaluating suspected appendicitis in patients. Table 1 compares the aforementioned imaging techniques.

Computed Tomography

CT remains as the most sensitive imaging modality for diagnosing appendicitis, thus lowering the negative appendectomy rate.[10] A CT scan of the appendix appears as a tubular, pericecal structure that is filled with fluid, contrast, or air or collapsed (Figure 1).[5] Additionally, it has an outer diameter that does not exceed 6 mm, wall thickness less than 3 mm, and homogenous periappendiceal fat.[5] CT scan findings suggestive of appendicitis include a distended, thick-walled appendix, as well as periappendiceal fat-stranding, periappendiceal air, phlegmon or abscess, and adjacent bowel wall thickening.[5,11] The maximal cross-sectional diameter of the appendix is reported to be the most powerful CT sign in diagnosing acute appendicitis.[11]

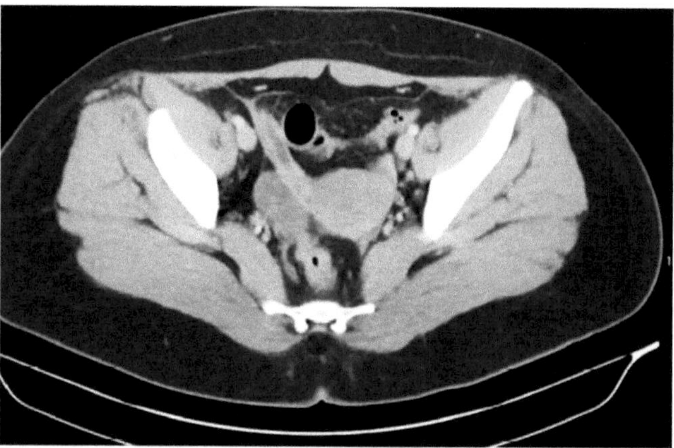

Figure 1: Acute appendicitis 11mm wide appendix, with fat stranding

Intravenous contrast is typically used, often supplemented with oral contrast and rectal contrast. Reported sensitivity and specificity ranges from 91% to 100%, and 91% to 99% respectively.[11] Studies have assessed the need for intravenous contrast. One study evaluated non-contrast CT scan performance[12] and yielded a sensitivity of 93% and a specificity of 96% in the diagnosis of appendicitis using CT scan. Other studies have concluded that CT without oral contrast appeared to be comparable with CT scans performed with oral contrast, and that IV contrast did not significantly improve the visualization of a normal appendix or the confidence in CT interpretation.[13,14]

In cases where the CT scan fails to visualize the appendix and secondary findings, the literature suggests that these cases should be interpreted as a true negative study.[10] This should be used with caution in patients with scant intra-abdominal fat, such as children, because of the decreased ability to see secondary signs of appendicitis such as periappendiceal fat-stranding.[10] Clinical judgment should be used with these patients based on other subjective and objective findings. If clinical suspicion remains high, an appendectomy is still warranted since non-visualization of the appendix on CT does not entirely exclude appendicitis.

The advent of CT scans has been associated with a decline in the number of negative appendectomies. Perhaps the greatest advantage of CT scanning is the ability to assess other organs and identify other disease processes. It should strongly be advised however that a CT scan should not be used routinely in the evaluation of patients with suspected appendicitis in the setting of characteristic symptoms and physical examination findings.

Ultrasound

Ultrasound has become the initial diagnostic imaging modality of choice[10] in the pediatric population. Advantages include noninvasiveness, no exposure to radiation, and no requirement for sedation of young children.[10] Recent studies report a sensitivity of 88% and a specificity of 94%.[10] However, ultrasound is not as sensitive as CT scan and can depend on who is operating it. In patients with peritonitis, compression sonography can be difficult. Furthermore, in obese patients, sonography can be very limited.

Sonography findings consistent with a normal appendix include a compressible, tubular, blind ending structure, with wall thickness of 3 mm or less, normal hyperechoic periappendiceal fat without inflammatory involvement of the cecum, and peristalsis absence.[5]

Sonography findings consistent with acute appendicitis include a dilated appendix 6 mm or greater, a thick-walled, non-compressible luminal structure, or the presence of an appendicolith.[5] Because appendicitis may be limited to the appendix tip, it is imperative to identify the blind end of the appendix to avoid missing early luminal or mural changes.[5] Sonographic findings suggestive of perforated appendicitis include loculated pericecal fluid, prominent pericecal fat, and circumferential loss of the submucosal layer.

A pelvic ultrasound also has the advantage of being able to exclude pelvic pathology like a tubal-ovarian abscess or an ovarian torsion. In cases when the appendix may extend into the pelvis, transvaginal sonography may be a useful adjunct.[5]

Magnetic Resonance Imaging

Concerns over CT related radiation exposure has led to research using magnetic resonance imaging (MRI) to evaluate suspected appendicitis. MRI has a high reported sensitivity and specificity of 97% and 92% respectively.[15] The motion artifacts and time required for imaging are limitations of MRI.[10] Furthermore, MRI is not widely available, and is more costly than other imaging modalities.

Barium Enema

Barium enemas were once used routinely in the evaluation of appendicitis. Since the advent of CT scans however, they are rarely used. Most of the literature regarding barium enemas are therefore from the 1970-80's, and barium enemas are now seldom employed in the workup of suspected appendicitis. In fact, there are even several reported cases of appendicitis caused by barium enema. Nonetheless, there are characteristic findings suggestive of appendicitis on barium enema that are worth mentioning. These include a mass impression on the cecum caused by an inflamed appendix, non-filling of the appendix secondary to appendiceal luminal obstruction, as well as cecal spasm due to local inflammation.[16,17]

It is important to note that a mass impression on the cecum can also be caused by other conditions such as pelvic inflammatory disorder, Crohn's disease, and endometriosis. Furthermore, normal appendices may fail to fill with barium, thereby rendering barium enema findings highly non-specific.[16]

Table 1: Comparison of imaging techniques in the evaluation of appendicitis

	Advantages	Disadvantages	Reported sensitivity	Reported specificity
CT	-Sensitive -Provides information on other organs	-Radiation exposure -Period of immobility required	91-100%	91-99%
Ultrasound	-Noninvasive -No radiation -Provides information on pelvic organs	-Low sensitivity -Operator dependent -Can be affected by body habitus	88-90%	90-94%
MRI	-Sensitive -No radiation	-Length of time needed -Motion artifact -Availability -Cost	97%	92%
Barium enema		-Non-sensitive -Nonspecific -Patient comfort -Provides no information on other organs		

Diagnostic Laparoscopy

In a small subset of patients, the history, physical exam, laboratory findings, and imaging findings may all be inconclusive or unconvincing. A diagnostic laparoscopy can provide direct examination of the appendix in these patients, as well as inspection of the peritoneal cavity for other possible causes of pain.

Management

The management of suspected appendicitis can be summarized in Figure 2. Patients with a high clinical suspicion should not undergo additional imaging and should undergo surgical appendectomy. Patients with low or intermediate clinical suspicion should undergo radiographic evaluation. Patients with positive CT scan or ultrasound findings should undergo surgery. Patients with negative imaging findings may be observed or discharged depending on the clinical correlation. Patients with inconclusive findings and intermediate clinical suspicion are candidates for diagnostic laparoscopy.

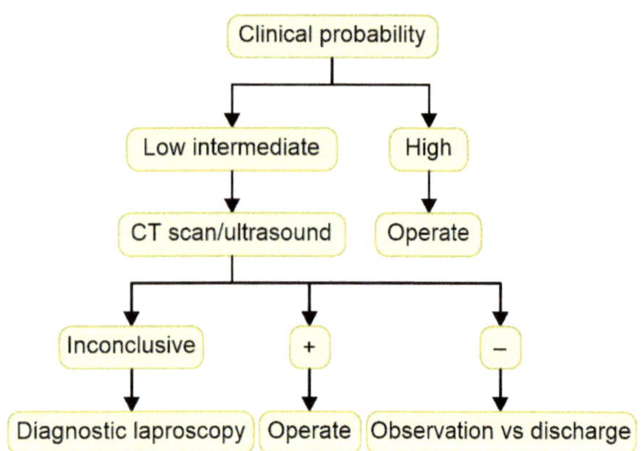

Figure 2: Algorithm for the evaluation and management of patients with suspected appendicitis

Nonperforated Appendicitis

Nonperforated appendicitis should be treated with appendectomy, either via an open or laparoscopic approach. To date, no evidence has shown a difference in outcome between the two approaches. The advantages of the laparoscopic approach however are shorter hospital stays, improved pain control, and a decrease in wound infection. These advantages are at the expense of increased operative cost, which may be counterbalanced by the decreased length of stay. Postoperatively, there is no data to support the use of therapeutic antibiotics for nonperforated appendicitis.

Immediate appendectomy is advocated by most to prevent perforation, but the timing of the appendectomy has been the subject of debate by some. Recent studies have supported a more semi-elective approach to acute appendicitis. Although a delayed appendectomy does not increase the risk of perforation, it does seem to be associated with an increased risk of surgical site infections, even in patients with nonperforated appendicitis.[18]

Nonoperative management has been suggested for nonperforated appendicitis. In one Turkish study, 107 out of 290 patients with presumed appendicitis were treated with antibiotics alone, and the remaining 183 underwent appendectomy. Of the 107 patients, 19 underwent appendectomy for failure to respond to treatment, and 9 had recurrence of appendicitis. This study demonstrated that 79 patients (73.8%) were successfully managed medically, thus the authors suggest medical management as an alternative.[19] In a similar Swedish study, the recurrence rate in patients treated non-operatively was 13.9%.[20] These studies shed light into the concept of managing appendicitis non-operatively. Limitations of these studies include the fact that the follow-up is not lifelong, as patients may develop recurrence later in life. The cost-effectiveness therefore has to be assessed, as performing an appendectomy at initial presentation eliminates the possibility of 'recurrence'. It should be emphasized that the findings in these studies are not validated. The standard of care for patients with uncomplicated appendicitis is still appendectomy.

Although it has generally been believed since the first descriptions of appendectomy that untreated appendicitis will eventually perforate, more recent studies suggest that the pathophysiology of perforated and nonperforated appendicitis is different.[21] Researchers have assessed epidemiological trends for perforated and nonperforated appendicitis and have noticed unassociated trends. They have both historical and immunological evidence to support their hypothesis that appendicitis is a more complex and heterogeneous disease than previously believed.[21] It is therefore possible that, in the near future, nonperforated appendicitis may not necessarily require surgery and can possibly resolve without perforation with nonoperative management. However, further research is needed to better understand this common disease, including the relationship between biomarkers and cases of appendicitis will not perforate.[21]

Perforated Appendicitis

The clinical status of patients with perforated appendicitis can vary from stable to sepsis requiring an initial period of resuscitation. As a result of the localized inflammation in perforated appendicitis, laparoscopic techniques may prove difficult, and switching to an open approach may be necessary depending on the ease of completing the appendectomy. Upon completion, the peritoneal cavity should be irrigated and the fluid aspirated. A closed-suction drain may be left in place, and antibiotics should be continued postoperatively, although the exact duration of antibiotic therapy is unclear. Many authors suggest antibiotics should be continued until the patient is afebrile postoperatively.

If the localized inflammation is deemed severe as noted on preoperative CT scan, or if the patient is septic, non-operative management with intravenous antibiotics should be initiated, with plans for an interval appendectomy. Although this may result in the interval development of an abscess, it avoids the unsafe attempt at an appendectomy in a severely inflamed operative field, and/or in a septic patient. Clinical judgment in this setting is paramount, as aggressive attempts at dissection in the context of severe inflammation increases the risk of injury to the surrounding viscera.

Appendiceal Abscess

Appendiceal abscesses develop from untreated perforated appendicitis. These patients should be initially managed conservatively with antibiotics and percutaneous abscess drainage, with ultimate plans for an interval appendectomy. Such patients should undergo colonoscopy prior to the scheduled interval appendectomy, to rule out colon cancer, which would alter the operative approach. The management of appendicitis with appendiceal abscess can be summarized in Figure 3.

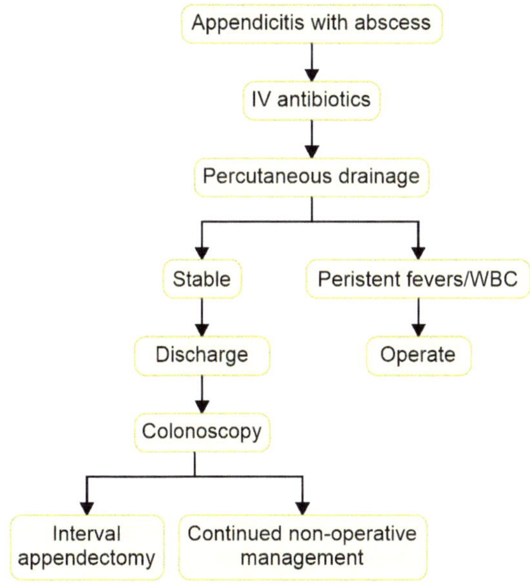

Figure 3: Algorithm for the management of patients with appendicitis with abscess

Interval appendectomy is associated with lower morbidity and shorter hospital stays than surgery in the setting of a perforated appendicitis with appendiceal abscess. If however fever and leukocytosis persists despite antibiotics and abscess drainage, surgical intervention may be required during the initial hospital stay.

Special Considerations

Appendicitis in Pediatrics

In the pediatric emergency department, one of the most common complaints is abdominal pain, and the most prevalent childhood surgical emergency is appendicitis.[10] Imaging studies such as ultrasound and CT scan have been shown to decrease the negative appendectomy rate. In certain centers, the initial diagnostic imaging modality of choice is now ultrasound.[10] Advantages include noninvasiveness, no exposure to radiation, and no requirement for sedation of young children.[10]

Even though CT scan is the most accurate modality for diagnosing appendicitis, radiation exposure in pediatric patients needs to be considered.[10] In a 5-year-old child undergoing abdominal CT, it is theorized that the lifetime risk for radiation-induced cancer is 26.1:100 000 in females and 20.4:100 000 in males.[22]

Appendicitis management in children is no different than in adults. Laparoscopy has proven feasible and safe in the pediatric population. The choice of operation is ultimately surgeon dependent.

Appendicitis During Pregnancy

During pregnancy, the most frequent abdominal surgical emergency is acute appendicitis.[23] It is more common in the first two trimesters of pregnancy, with incidence ranging from 0.05% to 0.2%.[23,24] Clinical, laboratory and physical examination findings may be atypical during pregnancy, but the treatment of choice remains to be an appendectomy.[23] Serious maternal and fetal complications can arise with delaying the diagnosis of appendicitis.[23]

During the first trimester, when the uterus is not larger, appendicitis usually presents with the same signs and symptoms as non-pregnant patients.[23] During the last two trimesters, diagnosing appendicitis becomes increasingly more challenging as the uterus rises out of the pelvis, displacing the appendix.[23] Therefore, tenderness might present in the right flank or right subcostal area instead of the classic right lower quadrant.[25]

Laboratory values are difficult to interpret during pregnancy because many signs and symptoms of appendicitis during pregnancy overlap with obstetric-related signs and symptoms, such as nausea, vomiting, and physiologic leukocytosis. A high degree of clinical suspicion is therefore needed, and obstetrical emergencies such as a ruptured ectopic pregnancy or abruptio placentae must first be eliminated.[23] A gynecological examination and ultrasound are useful adjunctive tests in this setting.

The surgical approach for appendicitis during pregnancy depends mainly on surgeon preference. With an open approach, the choice of incision can be challenging. A McBurney incision can be used during the first trimester, but an incision higher in the right abdomen should be used during the second and third trimester. The location of the pain can be used to guide the incision location. A laparoscopic approach is reported to be safe and possible at any gestational age.[26] Laparoscopic approach advantages include decreased postoperative pain, decreased ileus, and early mobilization.[26] Critics of the laparoscopic technique have pointed out the potential risk of damage to the gravid uterus by the passage of trocars, and fetal intolerance to carbon dioxide pneumoperitoneum.[23]

A delay in management and severity of the appendicitis results in a decline of the fetus and mother's prognosis.[23] The most important predictive factor for maternal morbidity has been shown to be perforation of the appendix.[27] For patients with appendicular peritonitis, mortality in fetuses reaches 35%[28] in contrast to 1% to 8% for uncomplicated appendicitis.[28] Spontaneous abortion and premature delivery are the main risks of the fetus, particularly during the first postoperative week.

Appendicitis in the Elderly

Acute appendicitis can occur at any age but is most common in the second and third decades of life.[29] Diagnosing appendicitis in older patients can be difficult. One-third of cases are assessed after significant delay in seeking medical attention, and upon admission, only half of these cases are correctly diagnosed.[30]

Older patients with acute appendicitis have significantly increased rates of morbidity and mortality post-operatively when compared to younger patients.[31] The risk of fatality in older patients is up to 14-fold more than the general adult population.[30] A late atypical presentation, more medical comorbidities, reduced physiological reserve, and impaired inflammatory response in older age are common reasons for this increase in mortaility.[30]

Early studies had suggested that a laparoscopic appendectomy carried increased risk due to carbon dioxide insufflation in a patient with reduced cardiopulmonary reserve, causing reduced venous return and cardiac output, and predisposing the patient to myocardial infarction and basal atelectasis.[29] New studies now suggest that there are less postoperative complications, inpatient stay length, and mortality associated with a laparoscopic appendectomy when compared with an open appendectomy in older patients.[29] No differences are noted in operative time or postoperative wound infections.[29]

NEOPLASMS

Primary tumors of the appendix are rare. The majority present as appendicitis and most cases undergo appendectomy for presumed appendicitis. The diagnosis is rarely made preoperatively since history and physical examination findings are usually non-specific, and imaging studies lack the sensitivity to diagnose appendiceal tumors. Many tumors are found incidentally on pathological evaluation of appendectomy specimens.[32]

Carcinoid

Carcinoid tumors are neuroendocrine tumors originating from enterochromaffin cells and are the most common appendiceal neoplasms.[32] Once believed to be the most common location of gastrointestinal carcinoids, more recent data suggests that the small intestine, followed by the rectum, are the most common sites of gastrointestinal carcinoids, followed by the appendix.[33]

Most carcinoid tumors of the appendix are located at the tip of the appendix, and therefore are often asymptomatic until they become metastatic.[34] Tumors positioned at the base of the appendix can occlude the lumen and result in similar signs and symptoms of appendicitis.[34]

Carcinoid tumors produce a number of hormones including serotonin, histamine, and bradykinin.[34] Patients can therefore present with signs and symptoms related to carcinoid syndrome which includes flushing, tachycardia, diarrhea, and hypotension.[34] The lungs and the liver are usually able to remove these agents, but in cases of carcinoid metastasis, the rate of production supersedes clearance of these substances. Therefore, carcinoid syndrome can ensue.[34] In patients with suspected carcinoid syndrome, appropriate workup begins with a 24-hour urine 5-HIAA and a serum Chromogranin A to confirm the diagnosis.

As with other carcinoid tumors of the gastrointestinal tract, appendiceal carcinoids often present with synchronous tumors of the gastrointestinal tract. Patients should therefore undergo screening colonoscopy and endoscopy when an appendiceal carcinoid is suspected.

The treatment of appendiceal carcinoids is based on the size and location of the tumor and the probability of nodal disease.[35] Nodal disease is apparent in fewer than 0.1% of cases where the original lesion measures less than 1 cm and in 30% of cases where it exceeds 2 cm.[35] Accordingly, tumors less than 1 cm or those at the tip of the appendix are therefore adequately treated with an appendectomy. Tumors greater than 1 cm, or those involving the base of the appendix are treated with a right hemicolectomy (Figure 4).

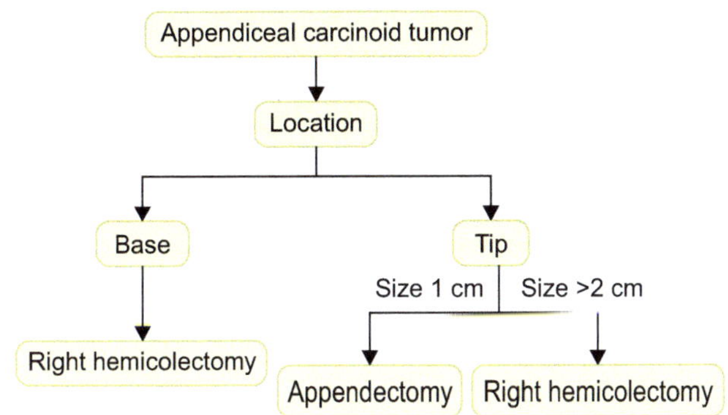

Figure 4: Algorithm for the management of appendiceal carcinoid tumors

The prognosis of carcinoid tumors of the appendix is good, as most are confined to the appendix. In such cases, the 5-year-survival is reported at 94%.[34] For distant metastasis, the 5-year-survival rate drops to 34%.[34]

Mucoceles/Mucinous Neoplasms

Appendiceal mucoceles are uncommon entities which arise with many different underlying pathologic processes. A subset of these mucoceles is associated with subsequent pseudomyxoma peritonei development.[36] The term mucocele denotes a dilatation of the appendiceal lumen as a result of abnormal accumulation of mucus.[36] This may be related to a neoplastic or non-neoplastic process.[36] It is a gross or macroscopic description, rather than a histopathologic diagnosis.[36] The pathologist must determine the underlying cause or process associated with the mucocele development for the pathologic diagnosis.[36]

Nonepithelial

Mucoceles of the appendix are divided into non-epithelial and epithelial processes. Nonepithelial processes associated with mucoceles include inflammatory, post-inflammatory or obstructive etiologies, such as appendicitis and fecaliths.[36] Hyperplastic or neoplastic changes in the residual epithelium are absent in these cases. The obstruction of the appendiceal lumen results in the intraluminal accumulation of mucoid material, resulting in the formation of a mucocele.

Epithelial

Mucinous hyperplasia, mucinous adenoma, mucinous neoplasms of low malignant potential, and mucinous adenocarcinoma are epithelial processes associated with mucoceles.[36]

Mucinous Hyperplasia

Mucosal hyperplasia is an uncommon cause of appendiceal mucoceles.[36] It is usually diagnosed incidentally after pathologic review of an appendectomy specimen.[36] Microscopically, mucosal hyperplasia of the appendix appears similar to hyperplastic polyps found in the intestine.[36] The diagnosis of mucosal hyperplasia of the appendix should be solely limited to benign, hyperplastic processes.[36] A diagnosis of mucinous adenoma or neoplasm should be considered if diffuse changes or minimal cytologic atypia are present.[36] Likewise, all appendices with hyperplastic mucosa should be attentively evaluated to factor out the presence of an adenomatous component.[36]

Mucinous Adenomas

Mucinous adenomas of the appendix were historically believed to be equivalent to adenomas occurring elsewhere in the gastrointestinal tract.[36] With increasing knowledge, it has become evident that mucinous adenomas of the appendix are unique as a result of their origin site in addition to their immunophenotypic and molecular genetic features.[36,37] Patients with mucinous adenomas may be asymptomatic, or might present with acute appendicitis, a palpable mass, chronic right lower quadrant pain, or intussusception.[36]

Microscopically, mucinous adenomas are composed of mucin-rich epithelium.[36] The extensive luminal mucin accumulation can cause luminal dilation and perforation.[36] Extravasated mucin triggers an inflammatory reaction with fibrosis, granulation tissue, chronic inflammation, and dystrophic calcification.[36] By definition, the epithelium does not infiltrate into the muscular wall and is not found in the extra-appendiceal mucin.[36] It is imperative to evaluate the whole appendix to confirm there are no undetected areas of malignancy determined by cytologic features that imply invasion or epithelium in the extra-appendiceal mucin.[36]

Appendectomy can cure mucinous adenoma of the appendix, as long as the resection margin at the base of the appendix is not involved.[36] Patients should be evaluated for synchronous lesions in the colon, as there is a strong association with synchronous colorectal adenoma or carcinoma.[38] Sometimes, differentiating a mucinous adenoma and a mucinous neoplasm is not straightforward.[36] Therefore, the diagnosis of mucinous adenoma should be abstained in cases where there is involvement of the proximal margin, where there is mucin with epithelium in the appendiceal wall, or when it is not certain if epithelium is present in the extravasated mucin.[36] In cases of diagnostic uncertainty, the term 'mucinous neoplasm of uncertain malignant potential' should be used.[36]

Mucinous Neoplasms of Low Malignant Potential

Mucinous neoplasms of low malignant potential are accountable for the majority of cases of pseudomyxoma peritonei.[36] They are macroscopically identical to mucinous adenomas, but microscopically, these cells penetrate the appendiceal wall and spread beyond the appendix as peritoneal implants and ovarian involvement.[36] Therefore, epithelium being present outside of the appendix in correlation with peritoneal implants is the critical discovery for these neoplasms.[36]

Fully developed peritoneal implants secrete voluminous, thick mucinous material, which distends the abdomen and creates the clinical condition called pseudomyxoma peritonei.[36] Surface implants can occur on the spleen, liver, and ovaries in female patients. In any women who present with a mucinous ovarian tumor or the clinical picture of pseudomyxoma peritonei, an appendiceal lesion should always be ruled out.[36] Likewise, in women with an appendiceal neoplasm, a cystic ovarian tumor should be ruled out.[36]

The clinical presentation of mucinous neoplasms of low malignant potential is frequently identified as an appendicitis or a vague abdominal mass.[36] Mortality is secondary to extensive peritoneal disease, with fibrosis and progressive loss of intestinal function and obstruction, rather than as a product of liver or lung metastases.[36] Despite peritoneal dissemination of tumor cells, nodal and liver metastases are uncommon, whereas locoregional recurrence is common and ultimately impairs small bowel function. Aggressive debulking and peritonectomy may improve survival.[36]

Mucinous Adenocarcinoma

Adenocarcinoma of the appendix is rare.[36] Mucinous adenocarcinoma represents a histologically distinct type of adenocarcinoma, alongside intestinal and signet-ring types. Mucinous adenocarcinoma of the appendix associated with the development of pseudomyxoma peritonei is[36] in contrast with mucinous neoplasm of low malignant potential.

Histologically, mucinous adenocarcinoma of the appendix exhibits destructive invasion of the appendiceal wall with architectural complexity and high-grade cytologic atypia with marked nuclear pleomorphism and brisk mitotic activity.[36] It is indistinguishable from mucinous adenocarcinoma elsewhere in the gastrointestinal tract.[36] It is therefore staged and treated similarly to cecal adenocarcinomas and appears to possess a similar prognosis.[36]

Table 2: Appendiceal mucinous neoplasms

	Cytology	Peritoneal implants	Metastasis to lymph nodes or distant sites	Treatment	Clinical behavior
Mucinous adenoma	Low grade	No	No	Resection curative	Cured by resection
Mucinous neoplasm of unknown malignant potential	Low grade	No	No	Complete resection with negative margins	Low potential for recurrence
Mucinous neoplasm of low malignant potential	Low grade	Yes	No	Complete resection and surgical debulking	Recurs often
Mucinous adenocarcinoma	High grade	Yes	Often present	Right hemicolectomy; debulking has little impact on survival	Poor prognosis

Pseudomyxoma Peritonei

Pseudomyxoma peritonei is a very uncommon clinical entity typified by grossly disseminated intraperitoneal mucinous tumors, with gelatinous ascites.[39] Most cases of pseudomyxoma peritonei originate from the appendix but occasionally mucinous tumors of other organs are implicated, like the colon,[40] ovaries[41] and pancreas.[42]

Since the chemical nature of the gelatinous substance in pseudomyxoma peritonei differs from that of mucous protein, this substance has been referred to as 'pseudo-mucous protein,' hence the term pseudomyxoma.[43] Pseudomyxoma peritonei reflects the clinical process and characteristics of the disease, and not a pathological diagnosis.[43]

Abdominal pain, abdominal swelling, and mucoid ascites are clinical characteristics of pseudomyxoma peritonei.[43] The tumor ultimately inhabits a majority of the abdominal cavity space, manifesting with "jelly belly syndrome."[43] Confirming a definitive diagnosis before surgery is challenging, and a majority of cases are diagnosed post-laparotomy.[43]

Pseudomyxoma peritonei associated with mucinous neoplasms of low malignant potential of the appendix has a low risk of nodal or liver metastases, but locoregional recurrence is common and multiple surgical resections are frequently needed. Even though it may progress slowly, it is often fatal.[43] Aggressive debulking such as peritonectomy and cytoreductive surgery are the two main operative treatment options. Hyperthermic intraperitoneal chemotherapy is used as an adjunctive treatment.

Many authors believe cytoreductive surgery with hyperthermic intraperitoneal chemotherapy to be the gold standard treatment.[43] In one of the first studies comparing debulking surgery with cytoreductive surgery, cytoreductive combined with hyperthermic intraperitoneal chemotherapy had a higher likelihood of achieving R1 surgery than debulking surgery combined with hyperthermic intraperitoneal chemotherapy.[44] Systemic chemotherapy has not been shown to prolong survival.[44]

Pseudomyxoma peritonei is the focus of active ongoing research. Much debate persists regarding the optimum therapeutic approach, and the possible role of adjunctive systemic therapy. As our understanding of this clinical entity improves, the prognosis will likely improve.

Lymphoma

Extranodal lymphoma is most often found in the gastrointestinal tract.[34] The most common site is the stomach, with the small intestine being the second most common site.[34] These extranodal lymphomas can be found anywhere in the gastrointestinal tract and are mostly non-Hodgkin's lymphoma (NHL).[45] Primary NHL of the appendix is rare and only represents 1.3% to 2.6% of all gastrointestinal tract lymphomas.[46]

The differential diagnosis of appendiceal lymphoma is difficult since there is often a large infiltrate of reactive inflammatory cells. Immunohistochemistry alone may be insufficient in differentiating between reactive lymphocytes and lymphoma cells. Molecular analysis may therefore be more useful in evaluating lymphoma cell monoclonality.[47]

As with other tumors of the appendix, patients usually present with similar symptoms to appendicitis or vague long-standing right lower quadrant discomfort.[34] Appendectomy with adjuvant chemotherapy remains the mainstay of treatment.[34]

OTHER CONDITIONS OF THE APPENDIX

Diverticula

Diverticular disease of the appendix is rare.[48] It was first described by Kelynack in 1893.[49] It is more common in males, and there is an increased incidence in cystic fibrosis.[50] It is most commonly identified on pathologic examination after appendectomy for suspected appendicitis and may therefore be underreported because identifying these small lesions is difficult in the setting of associated inflammation.

As with other gastrointestinal diverticula, appendiceal diverticula are classified as being either congenital or acquired.[48] Congenital appendiceal diverticula are extremely rare and involve all layers of the appendix.[48] Acquired appendiceal diverticula consist of mucosa and submucosal herniations through muscular defects covered with serosa.[48] The pathogenesis is believed to be focal weakness of the appendiceal wall at sites of blood vessel penetration, focal weakness after previous inflammation and necrosis, and obstruction of the lumen with resultant luminal distention and hypertension.[48]

Appendiceal diverticulitis is most often encountered in patients undergoing appendectomy for appendicitis. However, appendiceal diverticulitis clinically presents differently than acute appendicitis.[48] In contrast with acute appendicitis, appendiceal diverticula symptoms are usually weeks or months long, the pain is episodic and insidious, pain shifting is often absent, and it usually does not affect those less than 30 years of age.[48] Such atypical signs and symptoms suggestive of appendiceal diverticular disease should be treated with appendectomy, since acute appendicitis in the setting of appendiceal diverticulitis is associated with a higher incidence of perforation when compared to acute appendicitis without diverticular disease.[48] This is likely related to a thin diverticular wall being present.[48] Furthermore, several reports have proposed an association between appendiceal diverticula and appendiceal neoplasms, suggesting a role for appendiceal diverticula in the pathogenesis of pseudomyxoma peritonei.[51]

Preoperative imaging studies for appendiceal diverticulitis carries a low sensitivity. In a retrospective study, only 50% of appendiceal diverticulitis could be differentiated from acute appendicitis by using CT.[52] Ultrasound may be more sensitive in visualizing appendiceal diverticular disease.[53] Due to diverticula not filling in cases of luminal obstruction, barium enemas can miss appendiceal diverticular disease.[48]

The management of appendiceal diverticulitis is appendectomy because it is indistinguishable from acute appendicitis. Surgeons should be aware of this, especially in older patients with atypical clinical presentations.[48] Early diagnosis and treatment may prevent perforation and possibly pseudomyxoma peritonei.[48]

REFERENCES

1. Mlianchi S, Allins AD. Amyand's hernia: history, imaging, and management. Hernia. 2007;12:321-211.
2. Meljnikov I, Radojcic B, Grebeldinger S, Radojcic N. History of surgical treatment of appendicitis. Med Pregl. 2009;62(9-10):489-92.
3. McBurney C. Experience with early operative interference in cases of disease of the vermiform appendix. NY Med J. 1889:50;676-684.

4. Semm K. Endoscopic appendectomy. Endoscopy. 1983;15(2):59-64.
5. Chan L, Shin L, Pai R, Brooke J. Pathologic Continuum of acute appendicitis: sonographic findings and clinical management implications. Ultrasound quarterly. 27(2):71-79, June 2011.
6. Kwan KY, Nager AL. Diagnosing pediatric appendicitis: usefulness of laboratory markers. Am J Emerg Med 2010; 28:1009-1015.
7. Allister L, Bachur R, Glickman J, Horwitz B. Serum markers in acute appendicitis. J Surg Res 2009.
8. Kentsis A, Lin YY, Kurek K, et al. Discovery and validation of urine markers of acute pediatric appendicitis using high-accuracy mass spectrometry. Ann emerg Med 2010;55:62-70e4.
9. Muenzer JT, Jaffe DM, Schwulst SJ, et al. Evidence for a novel blood RNA diagnostic for pediatric appendicitis: the riboleukogram. Pediatr Emerg Care 2010;26:333-338.
10. Hennelly K, Bachur R. Appendicitis update; Current Opinion in Pediatrics. 23(3):281-285, June 2011.
11. Lai V, Chan W, Lau H, et al. Diagnostic power of various computed tomography signs in diagnosing acute appendicitis. Clin Imag 2012. 36:29-34.
12. Hlibczuk V, Dattaro JA, Jin Z, et al. Diagnostic accuracy of non-contrast computed tomography for appendicitis in adults: a systematic review. Ann Emerg Med 2010; 55:51-59e1;Epub2009 Sep 5.
13. Anderson Ba, Salem L, Flum DR. A systematic review of whether oral contrast is necessary for the computed tomography diagnosis of appendicitis in adults. Am J Surg. 2005;190(3):474.
14. Keyzer C, Pargov S, Tack D, et al. Normal appendix in adults: reproducibility of detection with unenhanced and contrast-enhanced MDCT. Am J Roentgenol 2008;191(2):507.
15. Chabanova E, Balslev I, Achiam M, et al. Unenhanced MR imaging in adults with clinically suspected acute appendicitis. Eur J Radiol 2010.
16. Fedyshin P, Kelvin F, Rice R. Nonspecificity of barium enema findings in acute appendicitis. AJR. 1984. 143:99-102.
17. Smith DE, Kirchmer NA, Stewart DR. Use of the barium enema in the diagnosis of acute appendicitis and its complications. Am J Surg. 1979 Dec;138(6)829-34.
18. Teixera PG, Sivrikoz E, Inaba K, et al. Appendectomy timing: waiting until the next morning increases the risk of surgical site infections. Ann Surg. 2012 Jul 26 Epub ahead of print.
19. Turhan AN, Kapan S, Kutukcu E, et al. Comparison of operative and non operative management of acute appenedicitis. Ulus Travma Acil Cerrahi Derg 2009;15:459-462.
20. Hansson J, Korner U, Khorram-Manesh A, et al. Randomized clinical trial of antibiotic therapy versus appendectomy as primary treatment of acute appendicitis in unselected patients. Br J Surg 2009;96:473-481.
21. Livingston E, Woodward W, Sarosi G, Haley R. Disconnect between incidence of nonperforated and perforated appendicitis. Ann Sureg. 2007:245(6);886-892.
22. Wan MJ, Krahn M, Ungar WJ, et al. Acute appendicitis in young children: cost-effectiveness of US versus CT in diagnosis – a Markov decision analytic model. Radiology 2009;250:378-386.
23. Miloudi N, Brahem M, Ben Abid S, et al. Acute appendicitis in pregnancy: specific features of diagnosis and treatment. J Visc surg. 2012. Epub ahead of print.
24. Cilo NB, Amini D, Landy HJ. Appendicitis and cholecystitis in pregnancy. Clin Obstet Gynecol 2009;52(4):586-96.
25. Hodjati H, Kazerooni T. Location of the appendix in the gravid patient: a re-evaluation of the established concept. Int J Gynecol Obstet. 2003;8:245-7.
26. Sadot E, Telem DA, Arora AM, et al. Laparoscopy: a safe approach to appendicitis during pregnancy. Surg Endosc 2012;24:383-9.
27. Yilmaz HG, Akgun Y, Bac B, Celik Y. Acute appendicitis in pregnancy: risk factors associated with principal outcomes: a case control study. Int J Surg 2007;5:192-7.
28. Lebeau R, Diane B, Koffi E, et al. Appendicite aigue et grossesse: a propos de 21 cas. J Gynecol Obstet Biol Reprod (Paris) 2005;34:600-5.
29. Southgate E, Vousden N, Karthikesalingam A, et al. Laparoscopic vs open appendectomy in older patients. Arch Surg. 2012;147(6):557-562.
30. Storm-Dickerson T, Horattas MC. What have we learned over the past 20 years about appendicitis in the elderly? Am J Surg. 2003;185(3):198-201.
31. Kraemer M, Franke C, Ohmann C, Yang Q. Acute appendicitis in late adulthood: incidence, presentation, and outcome: results of a prospective multicenter acute abdominal pain study and a review of the literature. Langenbecks Arch Surg. 2000;385(7)470-481.
32. McCusker ME, Cote TR, Clegg LX, et al. Primary malignant neoplasms of the appendix: a population based study from the surveillance, epidemiology and end results program. Cancer. 2002;94(12):3307-3312.

33. Maggard MA, O'Connell JB, Ko C. Updated population-based review of carcinoid tumors. Ann Surg. 2004;240(1):117-122.
34. Ruoff C, Hanna L, Zhi W, et al. Cancers of the appendix: review of the literature. ISRN Oncol. 2011. Epub ahead of print.
35. Whitfield C, Amin S, Garner J. Surgical management of primary appendiceal malignancy. Colorectal Dis 2012. Epub ahead of print.
36. Pai R, Longacre T. Appencieal mucinous tumors and pseudomyxoma peritonei. Adv Anat Pathol. 2005;12(6):291-311.
37. Kabbani W, Houlihan PS, Luthra R, et al. Mucinous and nonmucinous appendiceal adenocarcinomas: different clinicopathological features but similar genetic alterations. Mod Pathol. 2002;15:599-605.
38. Deans GT, Spence RA. Neoplastic lesions of the appendix. Br J Surg. 1995;82:299-306.
39. Smeenek RM, Verwaal VJ, Zoetmulder FA. Pseudomyxoma peritonei. Cancer Treat Rev .2007;33:138-145.
40. Bruin SC, Verwaal VJ, Vincent A, et al. A clinicopathologic analysis of peritoneal metastases of colorectal and appendiceal origin. Ann Surg Oncol. 20120;17:2330-2340.
41. Lee JK, Song SH, Kim I, et al. Retrospective multicenter study of a clinicopathologic analysis of pseudomyxoma peritonei associated with ovarian tumors. Int J Gynecol Cancer. 2008;18:916-920.
42. Imaoka H, Yamao K, Salem AA, et al. Pseudomyxoma peritonei caused by acute pancreatitis in intraductal papillary mucinous carcinoma of the pancreas. Pancreas. 2006;32:223-224.
43. Guo A, Li Y, Wei L. Pseudomyxoma peritonei of 92 chinese patients: clinical characteristics, pathological classification and prognostic factors. World J Gastroenterol. 2012;18(24):3081-3088.
44. Andreasson H, Nygren P, Glimelius B, Mahteme H. Outcome differences between debulking surgery and cytoreductive surgery in patients with pseudomyxoma peritonei. Eur J Surg Oncol. 2012.
45. Lewin KJ, Ranchod M, Dorfman RF. Lymphomas of the gastrointestinal tract. Cancer 1987,42:693-707.
46. Pascuale MD, Shabahang M, Bitterman P, et al. Primary lymphoma of the appendix. Case report and review of literature. Surg Oncol. 1994;3:243-248.
47. Kitamura Y, Ohta T, Terada T. Primary T-cell non-hodgkin's malignant lymphoma of the appendix. Pathol Internat. 2000;50;313-317.
48. Willems S, Vanhulle A, Deruyter L. Appendiceal diverticulitis: a rare cause of right iliac fossa pain syndrome. Acta Chir Belg. 2011;111:332-334.
49. Kelynack TN. A contribution to the pathology of the vermiform appendix. London: HK Lewis;1983;60-1.
50. George D. Diverticulosis of the vermiform appendix in patients with cystic fibrosis. Hum Pathol. 1987;18:75-79.
51. Lamps L, Gray G, Dilday B, Washington M. The existence of low-grade mucinous neoplasms of the appendix and appendiceal diverticula: a possible role in the pathogenesis of pseudomyxoma peritonei. Mod Pathol. 2000;13:495-501.
52. Lee K, Lee H, Park S, et al. Appendiceal diverticulitis: diagnosis and differentiation from usual acute appendicitis using computer tomography. J comput assist tomogr. 2007;31:763-769.
53. Barc RM, Rousset J, Maignien, et al. Diverticular of the appendix and their complications: value of sonography. J Radiol. 2005. Mar;86(3). 299-309.

34

CHAPTER

Bariatric and Metabolic Surgery

Elango Edhayan, MD
Vijay Mittal, MD
Michael Martin, MD
Abdelkader Hawasli, MD, FACS, FASMBS

INTRODUCTION

The basic definition of obesity is the accumulation of abnormal amounts or excess of body fat. The World Health Organization (WHO) defines obesity based on Body Mass Index (BMI). BMI closely correlates with adiposity and is calculated by dividing the weight in kilograms by the square of the height in meters (Kg/m^2). According to the WHO, patients are classified as follows:

Table 1: Weight categories based on BMI

BMI (Kg/m^2)	Classification
>18.5	Underweight
18.5-24.9	Normal
25-29.9	Overweight
30.0-34.9	Class I Obesity
35.0-39.9	Class II Obesity
>40	Class III Obesity

By the above definition 35% of the adult US population and 17% of the adolescent and teen population is obese. There is no difference in the prevalence between men and women. Obesity is associated with increased risk for type 2 diabetes mellitus, heart disease, dyslipidemia, osteoarthritis, sleep apnea, and some cancers (i.e., colon, rectum, prostate, and breast). In 2008, the increased cost to care for obese patients was estimated at 147 billion USD.[1]

The mainstay of obesity treatment has been diet and exercise. Even with recent advancements in pharmacological therapy, the weight loss and benefits are usually transient at best. To promote a consistent weight loss there must be a negative caloric balance between intake and energy expenditure. At a certain point in an obese patient's life, this balance has been lost and homeostasis has to be re-established.

PHYSIOLOGY OF OBESITY

Since the time of Pavlov, it has been shown that the thought of food produces anticipatory physiological changes. The act of eating and satiety produces a state of psychological well-being. These changes are mediated by complex entero-limbic networks that are activated by both the hormonal and neural systems. These systems constitute the entero-encephalic endocrine axis.[2] Hormones that promote appetite are known as orexins (Ghrelin, Neuropeptide Y) and hormones that decrease appetite are known as anorexins (Leptin, Polypeptide YY).

Ghrelin

Ghrelin is a polypeptide hormone produced by the P/D1 cells of the gastric fundus and the epsilon cells of the pancreas. Ghrelin levels are increased before meals and decrease in the fed state. Ghrelin acts on receptors in the arcuate nucleus and the lateral hypothalamus promoting a state of heightened hunger. The actions of ghrelin are believed to be mediated by the paracrine release of Neuropeptide Y (NPY) in the hypothalamus. Low ghrelin levels are associated with a state of satiety. Obese patients exhibit a loss of this negative feedback mechanism and instead ghrelin levels remain persistently elevated. Patients therefore continue to overeat as they do not experience a fed state.

In persons that are on a diet, ghrelin levels increase once the caloric intake is decreased leading to an increased appetite. The effect of ghrelin makes the control of obesity by diet alone physiologically difficult.

Leptin

Leptin is produced by the white adipose cells of the body and the levels are proportional to the amount of fat in the body. The action of Leptin is to counteract the effects of ghrelin by blocking the secretion of NPY in the arcuate nucleus. Leptin also stimulates the production of alpha melanocyte stimulating hormone and other peptides that counteract the effect of peptides produced by ghrelin. The presence of leptin allows the body to attain a state of satiety thereby giving the person the ability to reduce the craving for high calorie food.[3]

Leptin levels are high in obese individuals. Obese individuals seem to have lost the auto-regulatory function of leptin levels.[4] There seems to be no fluctuation in leptin levels and the brain does not reach a fed state resulting in overeating.

Neuropeptide Y

NPY is a ubiquitous peptide found in the central nervous system. It affects numerous functions such as circadian rhythm, increasing food intake, stress hormone release, and lowering blood pressure.[5] It is believed that NPY acts on food intake through the increased secretion of steroids and the concomitant effects of steroids on fat metabolism. There are numerous factors that interplay in the secretion of NPY and its role in the etiology and treatment of obesity is just beginning to be understood.

Peptide YY (PYY)

PYY is released by the L-cells of the terminal ileum and colon in response to food in the lumen. PYY counteracts the effects of NPY centrally and also forms an important part of the "Ileal Brake". PYY slows down the transit of food in the intestine and delays gastric emptying.[6] PYY levels are increased in patients that have had Roux-en-Y gastric bypass (RYGB) leading to improved satiety. It is believed that the early arrival of nutrients to the terminal ileum in patients that have had a RYGB leads to increased levels of PYY and a state of satiety.[7]

From studying the hormonal derangements of obese patients, it becomes obvious that obesity is due to a malfunctioning of the entero-encephalic axis. Bariatric surgery promotes the production of anorexins and inhibits the production of orexins leading to alterations in the entero-encephalic axis and thereby promoting more permanent weight loss.

Glucose-dependent Insulinotropic Peptide (GIP)

GIP is also known as Gastric Inhibitory Peptide (GIP). The hormone is secreted by the K cells of the duodenal mucosa in response to glucose in the lumen. The hormone promotes increased release of insulin from the pancreas as well as inhibiting gastric emptying. Some studies have suggested that alterations in GIP levels lead to resolution of Diabetes Mellitus (DM) although the mechanism is unclear.

Glucagon-like Peptide-1 (GLP-1)

GLP-1 is produced by the L cells of the terminal ileum in response to food in the lumen. The hormone leads to increased sensitivity of the beta cells to glucose levels, increased secretion of glucose, inhibition of glucagon, and early satiety by action on neural centers. It is postulated that the early arrival of food in the ileum in patients that have had RYGB leads to early resolution of DM by release of GLP-1.

Like the orexins and anorexins the role of incretins in symptom resolution following weight loss surgery is being studied. Although the final mechanisms of these hormones are being elucidated it is certain that they will play a greater role in our understanding of obesity going forward.

Surgery for Morbid Obesity

Diet and exercise have not proven to be effective in long term weight loss. There are no available drugs that can produce long lasting weight loss.[8,9] Further, they do not improve obesity related complications to the extent that surgery does.[10] In 1991, the National Institute for Health (NIH) established guidelines for surgical treatment of morbid obesity that led to the field of Bariatric Surgery. The NIH endorsed Bariatric Surgery for patients with a BMI >40 and patients with a BMI >35 with significant comorbid conditions.[11] These procedures can be divided into three different categories: malabsorptive, restrictive or a combination of both.

Early surgeries for weight loss were primarily procedures that created malabsorption. Dr. Viktor Henrikson[12] resected 105 cm of small bowel in the hope of creating permanent malabsorption. In the United States, Kerman and colleagues from the University of Minnesota performed a jejunoileal bypass. These procedures were followed by biliopancreatic diversion (BPD) and BPD with duodenal switch. Each of these procedures was associated with either failure due to adaptation by the body to the surgically altered state (small bowel resection) or with significant complications such as severe diarrhea, nutritional cirrhosis, and malnutrition. These failures prevented the field of bariatric surgery from advancing.

In the 1970's gastric restrictive procedures were in vogue. These procedures involved gastroplasty and gastric bands and the most common of these procedures was the Vertical Banded Gastroplasty. These procedures were associated with complications such as expansion of the pouch and erosion of the band into the stomach.

The Roux-en-Y gastro-jejunostomy was developed by Griffen and colleagues in 1977. They modified the previous gastro-jejunostomy technique to include a Roux loop to prevent bile reflux. The procedure created malabsorption by rapidly transporting food into the ileum and the small gastric pouch produced an element of restriction.

The development of laparoscopic surgery, endoscopic stapling devices and the adjustable gastric band led to an explosion in demand for obesity surgery in the 1990's. The laparoscopic approach was found to have significantly lower mortality, pulmonary, and wound complication rates with similar outcomes to those of the open surgical techniques.[13,14]

The most recent advances were the recognition of the sleeve gastrectomy, which was used as a step operation in the super morbidly obese patients who were going for BPD in the early 2000's, as a stand-alone operation in treating morbid obesity. This procedure has proven itself as a good restrictive operation without mal-absorptive complications.

Currently, in the United States, most bariatric surgery is done via the laparoscope. Laparoscopic Roux-en-Y gastric bypass remains the most commonly performed procedure, with laparoscopic sleeve gastrectomy and laparoscopic adjustable gastric bands still remaining common procedures as well. The biliopancreatic diversion is an option primarily reserved for the super obese (BMI >50 Kg/m^2).

Laparoscopic Roux-en-Y Gastric Bypass (LRYGB)

In 1966, Mason performed the first loop gastro-jejunostomy to the proximal stomach leaving the distal end of the stomach excluded in the abdomen. He based this on observations that women who had partial gastrectomy for ulcer disease had difficulty gaining weight. The loop jejunostomy was modified into a retro colic Roux loop by Griffen in 1977. This modification obviated the high incidence of Bile reflux in the loop gastro-jejunostomy. In 1980, Torres and colleagues created a vertical un-transected pouch of the stomach. The arrival of laparoscopic staplers accelerated the development of a fully laparoscopic Roux-en-Y Gastric Bypass (LRYGB). This procedure was first reported by Wittgrove and colleagues in 1994.[15]

Over the past decade multiple studies have shown the safety, efficacy, cost effectiveness and decreased complication rate of the LRYGB over the open Roux-en-Y gastric bypass.[16,17,18] The incidence of wound and pulmonary complications is significantly lower in the LRYGB group of patients.[19]

Patients are screened preoperatively to evaluate the indications for the procedure and undergo a medical weight loss program. They are brought into the operating room and 5 laparoscopic ports are used to access the stomach. The proximal stomach is transected along the lesser curve and the staple line is extended to the Angle of His. Care is taken to avoid stapling close to the esophagus as the leak rate increases from stapling onto the esophageal musculature. A 5 cm pouch of the proximal stomach is created.

The Roux limb of the intestine is prepared from the segment of jejunum 60 cm from the ligament of Treitz. The jejunal limb has been brought up to the stomach in either a retrocolic or antecolic fashion. An anastomosis is made between the transected stomach and the jejunum either with a trans-oral EEA stapler (EEA OrVil 21 mm Device; Covidien), or by linear reticulating endo stapler. A hand suture anastomosis is still being done as an option especially in the recently introduced Robotic approach to RYGB. The integrity of the anastomosis is checked for leaks by occluding the distal jejunum, immersing the anastomosis under water and insufflating air into the stomach. The other cut end of the jejunum is anastomosed to the roux limb distally. The distance of this anastomosis can vary from 75 cm to 150 cm from the gastro-jejunostomy. Greater distances produce greater degrees of malabsorption.

Efficacy of Laparoscopic Roux-en-Y Gastric Bypass

LRYGB combines elements of restriction with malabsorption. The reduced gastric pouch produces early satiety and filling preventing overeating. The small pouch reduces the production of ghrelin. In obese individuals, ghrelin levels may be persistently elevated without the typical waxing and waning with satiety and hunger. It is believed that sporadic elevations in ghrelin stimulate appetite, but constantly elevated levels do not stimulate appetite. The performance of a Roux limb rapidly transits food into the ileum. This causes the hormones of the ileal brake such as Polypeptide YY to be secreted.

LRYGP has been shown to be safe with a mortality rate below 1%. The complication rates reported are around 9.5%. The major immediate complications reported include wound complications, anastomotic leaks, gastrointestinal bleeding, and pulmonary embolism. Late complications include bowel obstruction, stomal (gastrojejunal or jejunojejunal) stenosis and perforation (Figure 1), and incisional hernias.[20,21]

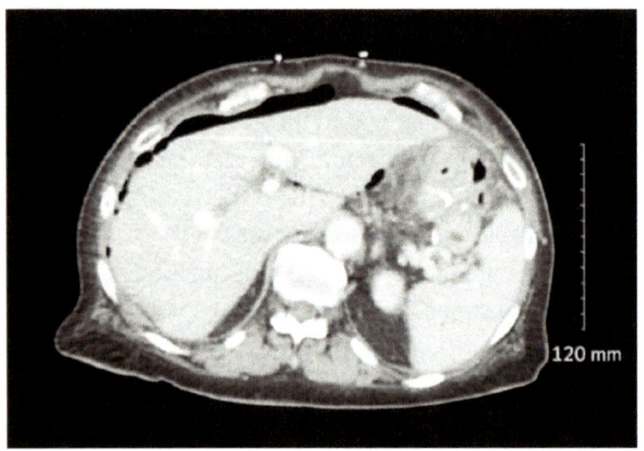

Figure 1: Gastrojejunal perforation

Patients that undergo LRYGP lose on an average 60% of their excess weight and keep it off at 3-year follow up. There is a marked decrease in co-morbid conditions. Over 80% are cured of Type 2 diabetes, 90 % show decrease in hypercholesterolemia, 75% show a reduction in high blood pressure and 85% improve their sleep apnea symptoms.[22,23] The reduction in co-morbid conditions leads to an overall reduction in 5-year mortality when compared to medically treated patients, despite the operative mortality risk.[24,25]

Complications of Laparoscopic Roux-en-Y Gastric Bypass

There is a significant learning curve associated with performing a LRYGB. These procedures are currently performed in Centers of Excellence for Bariatric Surgery with a strict tracking of surgeon performance by Bariatric Surgery Registries. There is a trend in the United States for specialized fellowships in bariatric surgery although this field is yet to be recognized by the Board of Medical Specialties.

Early Complications

Anastomotic Leaks

Anastomotic leaks remain the most dreaded complication from LRYGB. There is a learning curve to performing this procedure and authors have noted their leak rates going down as they perform more procedures.[26] Leaks can be from any one of the many staple lines, with the gastro-jejunostomy the most common site because of its technical difficulty. Other sites of leak are the 2 gastric staple lines and the site of the jejunojejunostomy. The reported incidence of anastomotic leaks is from 0-5.6% with a mortality rate as high as 37%.[27]

Symptoms can be subtle, and a high index of suspicion is needed to diagnose this potentially lethal complication. Any unexplained fever, tachycardia or general malaise with a patient not progressing as expected warrants investigation. Anastomotic leaks may present as myocardial infarctions from septicemia or respiratory distress. Diagnosis is made frequently by CAT scan and upper gastrointestinal (UGI) radiography showing a leak. A UGI may miss small leaks that a CAT scan will pick up as a fluid collection.

Small, contained leaks in hemodynamically normal patients can be managed conservatively by nothing per mouth, CAT scan guided drainage and antibiotics. Non-contained leaks are more ominous and require operative control of the leakage. In hemodynamically normal patients a laparoscopic approach is feasible, but an open approach should be used in hemodynamically unstable patients.

The operative principles are source control with stopping the leak with suture or an omental buttress, drainage of the area with external drains and antibiotics. It is important to drain the excluded stomach by a gastrostomy in case of leaks from the excluded stomach segment staple line.

Venous Thrombo-embolism (VTE)

Deep venous thrombosis (DVT) and subsequent pulmonary embolism (PE) are one of the most frequent complications of Bariatric surgery. VTE along with anastomotic leaks remain the 2 most common causes of post bariatric surgery mortality approaching 2% in some series.[28] This is despite the awareness of surgeons in instituting DVT chemoprophylaxis. Bariatric patients are predisposed to DVT due to many factors. Obese patients more often lead a sedentary lifestyle and have venous stasis. The operation is done under general anesthesia and the increased intra-abdominal pressure from pneumo-peritoneum also leads to increased femoral venous stasis.

Most surgeons initiate chemoprophylaxis before the operation and continue till discharge. Compression stockings and compression devices are routinely used intra-operatively. Some surgeons use chemoprophylaxis for extended periods after discharge, but that trend is not universal. The use of pre-operative Greenfield filters is being discouraged due to the risks associated with the filter.

Post-operative bleeding

Post-operative bleeding can be intra-abdominal or more frequently intra-luminal. The incidence of Gastro-intestinal bleeding (GIB) is around 1%. The increased incidence of bleeding is due to the lack of suturing to buttress staple lines, the thickness of the stomach that may be too thick for the available staple lines and due to the aggressive use of DVT chemoprophylaxis.[29]

Active bleeding in the unstable patient in the immediate postoperative period is usually managed by returning to the operating room to control the bleeder. Subtle signs of bleeding, without obvious hematemesis or hematochezia, in otherwise a stable patient, are possible from the excluded stomach or from staple line bleeds into the abdomen. A high index of suspicion is needed to diagnose and manage this complication. Patients that are hypotensive are managed by laparotomy while patients that are not hypotensive can be managed by initial re-laparoscopy.

Gradual ooze from staple lines may be diagnosed in 48 hours post operatively. This may be manifested by melena and a gradual drop in hematocrit. Slow ooze can be managed conservatively by replacement of blood and correction of coagulopathy if present.

Late Complications

Small Bowel Obstruction and Internal Hernias

Small bowel obstruction is usually a late complication of LRYGB. There is a higher incidence of small bowel obstruction from LRYGB (3-4%) than open gastric bypass. It is postulated that the increased incidence of small bowel obstructions could be because of the lack of adhesions that anchor the bowel internally. Internal hernias are the most common cause of bowel obstruction. The most common sites of obstruction are at the jejuno-jejunostomy, in the space between the roux limb and the mesocolon (Peterson's space) and through defects in the mesocolon in patients that have had a retrocolic LRYGB. The bowel obstruction is usually a late feature as these spaces enlarge with the loss of fat from weight loss.[30] Some patients may present with intermittent signs of bowel obstruction from sporadic filling of these spaces with small bowel. These patients may benefit from laparoscopic evaluation and closure of these spaces.[31] As with all laparoscopic procedures there is also potential for bowel obstruction from port site incisional hernias.

Small bowel obstruction should be treated aggressively. Early surgery is indicated in patients with complete obstruction to prevent strangulation.

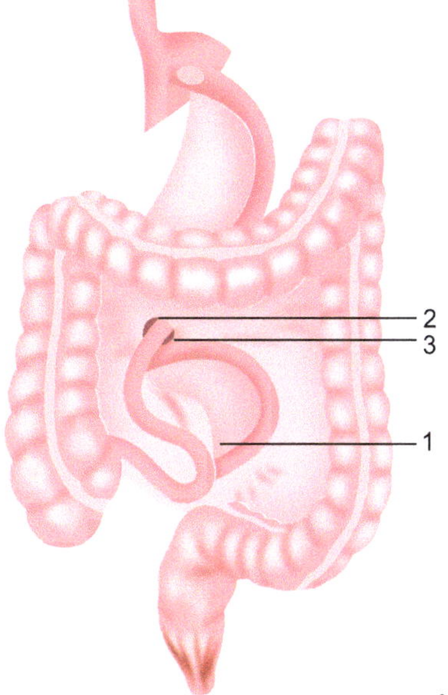

Figure 2: Location of potential hernia sites following RYGB

Marginal Ulceration (MU)

MU occurs in 1% of the patients at the gastro-jejunal anastomoses following LRYGB. MU has been associated with large pouch size, helicobacter pylori, tobacco use, NSAID usage and foreign body reaction from staple line.[32] Patients present with pain and if left untreated present with signs of gastric outlet obstruction from stricture formation. Diagnosis is by endoscopy and in the acute stage MU heals well with medical therapy. Unhealed MU may cause bleeding or perforation. Recurrent MU can lead to stenosis.

Stomal stenosis (SS)

SS occurs in 3% of patients at the gastro-jejunal anastomosis and this may occur as early as 3 weeks from surgery. Patients usually present with early satiety with vomiting and pain in the abdomen. The cause of stomal stenosis is multifactorial and includes marginal ulceration, ischemia, surgical technique, and proliferative scar tissue.[34] Diagnosis is by endoscopy to differentiate from MU. Treatment is endoscopic pneumatic balloon dilatation. Most patients respond to dilation, but refractory cases may need surgical revision of the anastomoses.

Cholelithiasis

Rapid weight loss associated with the alteration of the entero-hepatic circulation leads to elevation of cholesterol in the bile. This lithogenic bile leads to precipitation of cholesterol crystals. The incidence of gallstone formation is greater than 30% and can be reduced to less than 2% incidence with addition of ursodiol for the first 6 months.[35]

Dilatation of the Bypassed Stomach Remnant

Obstruction of the Y limb of the jejunum can lead to dilation of the gastric remnant. The remnant may dilate from loss of vagal innervations or for other, unknown reasons. Symptoms are hiccoughs, bloating and abdominal pain. Diagnosis may be made with a plain radiograph or by CT scan in case the stomach is filled with fluid. Treatment is percutaneous aspiration of the stomach under fluoroscopy. If the problem recurs a percutaneous gastrostomy tube for drainage will be needed.

Dilation of the proximal gastric pouch:

The most common cause of dilation of the proximal gastric pouch (Figure 3) is gastro-jejunal anastomotic stricture. However, this dilatation can occur without stricture due to patients' overeating which results in weight gain. This is treated by revising the gastric pouch.

In the remnant bypassed stomach, a bleeding, ulceration, or tumor formation may occur. The issue is the inability to diagnose these problems due to the isolation of this part from the endoscopic reach. A high index of suspicion, nuclear scanning for bleed, CT scan or MRI may lead to the proper diagnoses. A rare but life-threatening condition is the acute gastric distension of the ruminant stomach may occur.

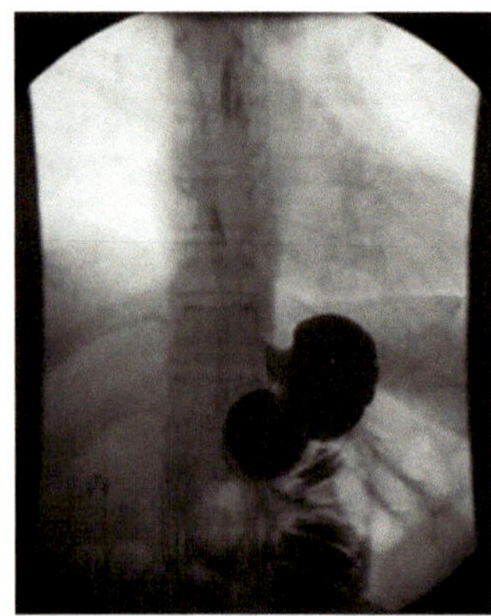

Figure 3: Dilated Gastric Pouch

Dumping Syndrome

70% of patients have symptoms related to dumping immediately following LRYGB. The rapid transit of high osmolar food into the ileum leads to symptoms of diarrhea, bloating, dizziness, abdominal cramping, and tachycardia. Most symptoms can be controlled by dietary modifications of small hypo-osmolar meals rich in complex polysaccharides.[36] Recent evidence places the etiology of dumping on the secretion of gastro-intestinal hormones like Polypeptide YY from the terminal ileum. Octreotide given 30 minutes before a meal controls the symptoms.[37]

Hyperinsulinemia Hypoglycemia

Hyperinsulinemia hypoglycemia is a rare complication following LRYGB. Pancreatic beta cells do not adjust to the decrease in absorbed nutrition and there is hyperplasia of the beta cells with autonomous production of insulin.[38] The loss of control of these cells has been attributed to Glucagon Like Peptide -1 (GLP-1) secretion by early bolus of food into the ileum.[39] Regardless of the etiology the condition is called Nesidioblastosis.

Treatment is initially conservative with dietary modifications. In cases of severe refractory hyperinsulinemia, surgical resection of the pancreas is considered. This will cause severe diabetes. Another option is the reversal of the LRYGB to a restrictive surgical procedure of gastric banding.[40]

Nutritional Complications of Gastric Bypass Surgery

LRYGB is both restrictive and malabsorptive to the regular digestive process. Nutrient supplementation is essential for these patients as they are unable to consume or absorb many essential nutrients. The unintended consequences are the loss of absorption of iron, calcium, protein, vitamins, and many micronutrients.

Iron deficiency anemia is the most common nutritional deficiency, found in 20-50% of LRYGB patients. The restrictive gastric pouch prevents the intake of large slices of meat that are rich in iron. The lack of gastric acid and the rapid transit into the ileum prevents exposure of iron to the duodenal and jejunal mucosa where iron absorption takes place.[41]

B12 absorption requires gastric acid and intrinsic factor from the stomach for absorption in the terminal ileum. Body stores of B12 are usually high enough that frank deficiency does not happen. Still, the serum levels of B12 are low and B12 should be given as a nutritional supplement.

Folate and thiamine deficiency occurs in patients with LRYGB. Fat soluble vitamin deficiency primarily happens in patients with Biliary Pancreatic diversion.

Patients with gastric bypass procedures can form macronutrient and macronutrient deficiency. Patients should be given daily multi-vitamins and iron pills.

Laparoscopic Sleeve Gastrectomy (LSG)

Vertical resection of the stomach is one of the two components of the biliopancreatic procedure with the duodenal switch. The vertical resection component was the restrictive component for the more efficacious malabsorptive portion of the operation. However, in some high-risk patients with BMI above 55 kg/m^2, the operation was offered as a staged procedure. Initially the patient was given the vertical gastric resection and followed by completion of the procedure one year later. However, it was noticed that there was significant improvement in co-morbidities associated with weight loss and an improvement in BMI during the interval between the two stages of the operation. This led to the development of LSG as an independent procedure for weight loss. LSG is gradually increasing in popularity as it is an easier operation to perform. It works by restricting the amount of food intake with decrease in appetite due to the great decrease of the Ghrelin hormone.

Surgical Procedure

The patient is placed in the reverse Trendelenburg position with or without the legs in a gentle lithotomy position (surgeon preference). The operating surgeon stands between the legs or on the side of the patient and 5 laparoscopic ports are used (Figure 4). The omentum is displayed and dissected off the greater curvature of the stomach. The gastro-phrenic ligament is divided to the left of the esophagus and freed from the diaphragm.

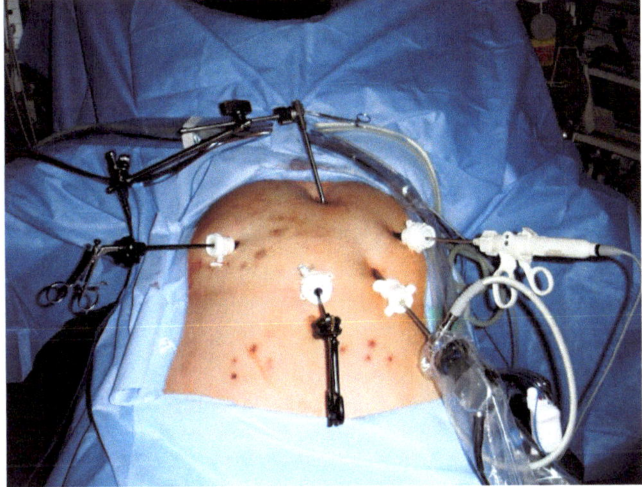

Figure 4: Five port sites used for LSG.

A 32 to 60 French (Fr) bougie is placed through the mouth and into the stomach. A stapling device is used to cut the stomach along the edge of the bougie taking care not to narrow the stomach at the incisura angularis. Using the bougie as a guide and taking care to not allow the staple line to rotate the stomach is vertically transected. At the superior edge, near the esophagus, care is taken to ensure that the final staple line is on the stomach and not on the esophagus or gastro-esophageal junction. Care is taken to ensure that the gastric pouch is not too large (Figure 5 to 7). The last step (Figure 6) may vary among surgeons where some surgeons prefer not to create any pouch.

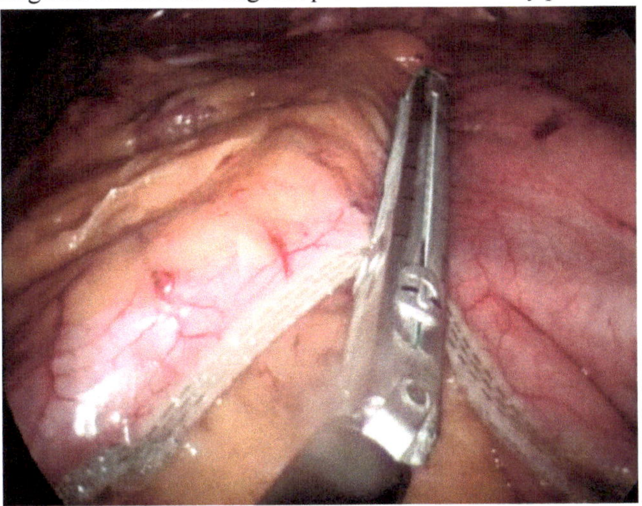

Figure 5: Transection of greater curvature along bougie (inside stomach lumen) during LSG.

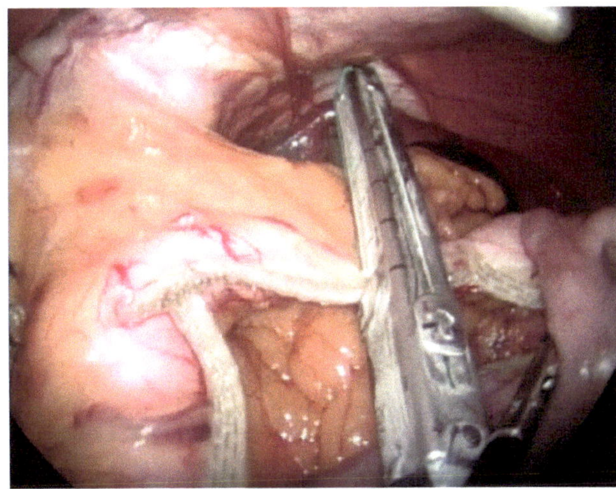

Figure 6: Creation of fundal gastric pouch during sleeve LSG.

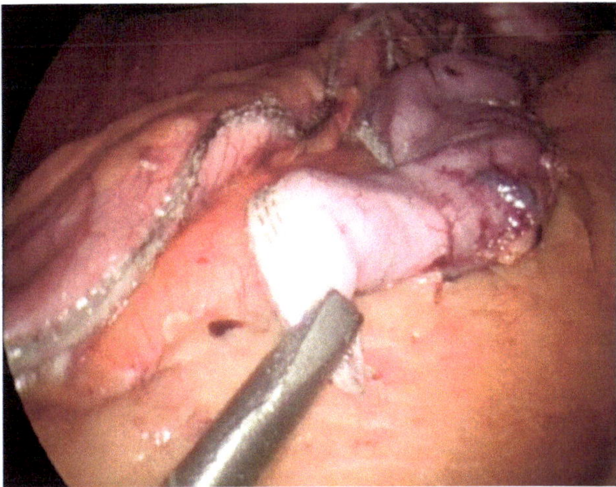

Figure 7: Grasper removing transected greater curve of stomach during LSG.

The integrity of the suture line is checked by either insufflating the stomach with air while the staple line is under water or using blue dye through an NG tube. An upper gastrointestinal series is done on postoperative day one prior to discharge to confirm the integrity of the suture line.

Efficacy of Laparoscopic Sleeve Gastrectomy

LSG has shown to be efficacious at 3- and 5-year follow up with a mean weight loss of 55%.[42] LSG has comparable rates to LRYGB in reduction of comorbidities such as Type 2 Diabetes Mellitus and metabolic syndrome.[43]

LSG works predominantly as a restrictive procedure. Reduction in Ghrelin levels and the rapid transit of nutrients into the small bowel led to earlier secretion of pancreatic polypeptide YY and its associated effects.

Complications of Laparoscopic Sleeve Gastrectomy

As with other laparoscopic procedures on the stomach the main complications are leakage and bleeding from the staple line and late formation of strictures. Leaking and bleeding complications are managed as for RNYGB.

A contained gastric leak after sleeve gastrectomy can be managed with placing the patient on nothing by mouth, total parenteral nutrition, and CT guided drainage of the collection. In addition, multiple methods were tried to close the leak side from inside the stomach by injecting fibrin glue or obliterating the leak site by using a gastric stent (Figures 8 and 9).

A non-contained leak requires laparoscopic or open drainage with attempt at either closing the leak site at the time of the operation or isolating the leak site using fibrin glue or stenting (Figure 8)

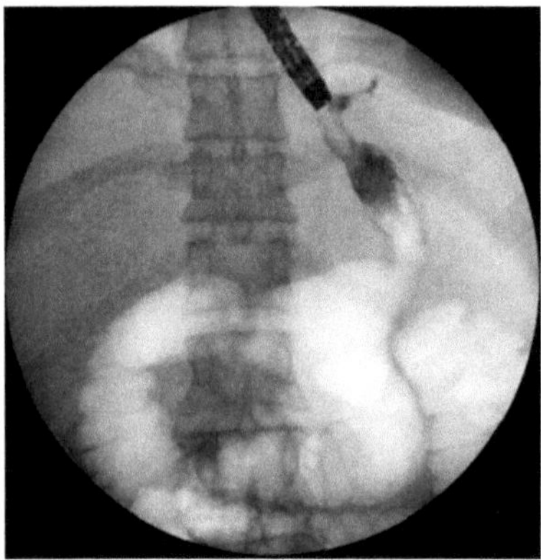

Figure 8: EGD showing gastric leak following LSG.

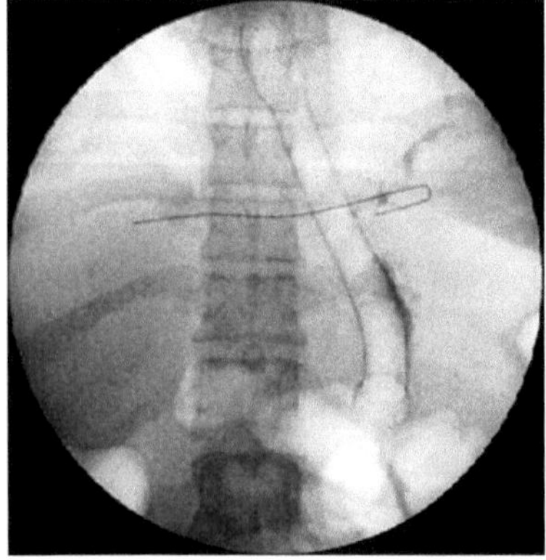

Figure 9: Placement of gastric stent to correct leak following LSG.

Late complications such as stricture may require stricturoplasty, or conversion to RNYGB. Dilatation of the proximal gastric pouch may lead to weight gain. Rare complications such as gastro-cutaneous or gastro-pulmonary fistulas (Figure 10) are difficult to manage and may require multiple procedures.

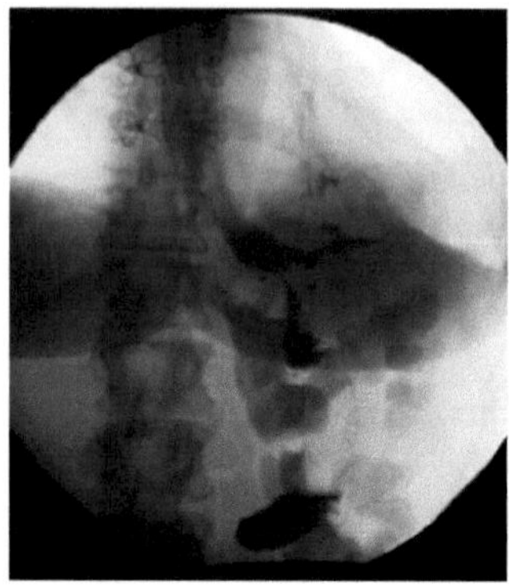

Figure 10: A Gastro-pulmonary fistula after Sleeve Gastrectomy

Gastro esophageal reflux disease is a unique complication of LSG. Reflux is diagnosed by endoscopy and managed by medical, dietary and lifestyle modification initially. This complication can occur in 28% of patients in the first year and usually drops to 3% after one year. This drop is thought to be due to the weight loss and the dilatation of the gastric body over time. Refractory reflux esophagitis may need reversal of LSG to LRYGB.

The gastric pouch may dilate over time leading to weight gain. Dilation may be due to gradual over-eating or idiopathic. In patients that develop recurrent obesity, repeat sleeve resection is an option (Figure 11 and 12).

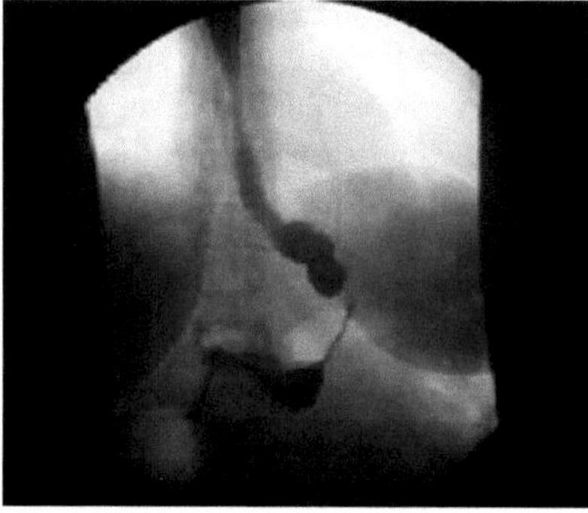

Figure 11: Normal postoperative upper GI contrast study of LSG.

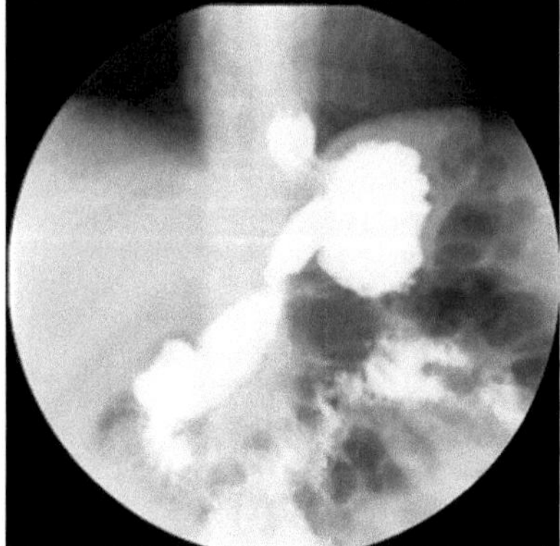

Figure 12: Upper GI contrast study showing dilated proximal gastric pouch after sleeve gastrectomy.

Laparoscopic Adjustable Gastric Band (LAGB)

LAGB is no longer a common weight loss surgery. Part of this was because LAGB does not transect or divert any of the GI tract. This meant no staple lines to leak or bleed. However, the long-term effect on permanent weight loss is less than that of patients who have had a LRYGB or LSG. The failure to produce long term success has led to the decreasing popularity of this procedure in the United States.

There are multiple types of gastric bands. In the United States there are two approved types; the Allergan band (by Allergan) and the Realize band (by Ethicon). Each type of band comes in two sizes to accommodate for the variability in the amount of tissue around the upper stomach. There are 2 components to the band. The sling, which contains multiple connected balloons, wraps around the stomach. The port is placed in the subcutaneous tissue that connects to the band by a catheter. The port is injected with saline which leads to filling of the balloons in the band and a reduction in the volume of the food passing rate from the proximal stomach.

In the United States the *pars flaccida* technique has become the standard method for placement of the band. First, the gastro-hepatic ligament is entered at the lesser curvature, followed by dissecting the greater curve at the Angle of Hiss. A retro-gastric tunnel is then made above the lesser sac leaving the stomach anchored to its retro-gastric attachments to the right and left crura of the diaphragm. The band is passed behind the proximal stomach and buckled, creating a small gastric pouch. A gastro-gastric plication suture is placed from the fundus of the stomach to the newly created gastric pouch above the band (Figure 13).

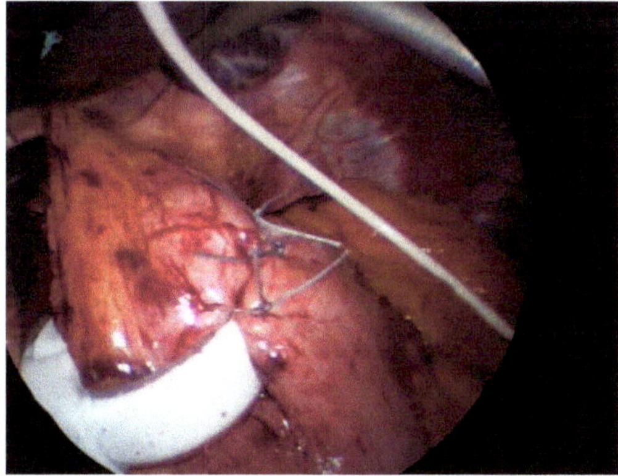

Figure 13: Successfully placed LAGB showing gastro-gastric plication.

The port for accessing the band is placed in the subcutaneous portion of the anterior abdominal wall for easy access. A barium swallow is done on postoperative day one prior to the patients discharge to ensure that there are neither leaks nor obstruction (Figure 14).

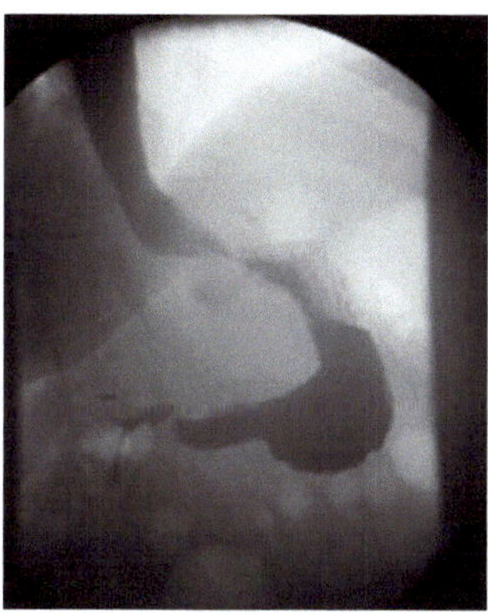

Figure 14: Upper GI contrast study postoperative day one after LAGB. Notice the band position pointing toward the left shoulder.

The patient is discharged home on a liquid diet and followed up in the office in a week. About 4-6 weeks after placement of the band, the port is accessed. The band is filled with saline under fluoroscopy to avoid complete obstruction of the band. The band can also be filled in small increments in the office to ensure reduction in the size of the passage of food from the gastric pouch. The final goal of the rate of food passage from the gastric pouch is achieving satiety for 3-4 hours after each meal. Patients gradually adjust their diet to accommodate the newly restricted stomach.

Efficacy and Complications following Laparoscopic Adjustable Band

Initial complication and patient satisfaction rates are good with LAGB. The adjustable nature of the surgery allows for patients to be eased into the lifestyle modifications that are needed to continue weight loss. However, the long-term incidence of weight gain, complications from the procedure and patient satisfaction rates are poor when compared to LRYGB.[44] In one study 72% of patients that had the band released or removed would never have consent to LAGB procedure again.[45]

Efficacy of Laparoscopic Adjustable Gastric Band

LAGB is primarily a restrictive procedure and patient cooperation, and motivation is needed to ensure long term success. While the average initial weight loss has been estimated to be around 35%, a large proportion of patients (up to 30%) fail to lose weight.[44,46]

When patients fail to lose weight, it is important to ensure that the device is working as intended. First, the port is aspirated to ensure integrity of the tubing. Once mechanical failure of the device is ruled out it is important to have a conversation with the patient regarding eating habits. Surreptitious eating of high calorie foods is a common cause of failure in the author's patient population.

Early Complications of Laparoscopic Adjustable Gastric Band

Perforation and Bleeding

Perforation and bleeding are intraoperative complications. Some steps in the procedure such as the retro-gastric passage of the band are blind. This step can lead to inadvertent injury to the stomach or the spleen. Symptoms of perforation may be missed as the leakage can be retroperitoneal in an obese patient that has post-operative pain. Fever, tachycardia, port site pain and fluid collections should be investigated aggressively. Re-operation with removal of the gastric band is needed in these conditions.

Esophageal Obstruction

Early esophageal obstruction is usually due to a combination of too tight a band, use of wrong size of band, post-operative edema at the band site and inclusion of perigastric fat pad.[47] Various modifications in technique and in the band have not eliminated this complication. In the presence of complete obstruction, the band should be re-adjusted or removed.

Late Complications of Laparoscopic Adjustable Gastric Band

Port and Tubing Related Complications

LAGB is dependent on the continued function of the mechanical catheter/band system, and like any mechanical device it will break down over time. Some studies have suggested the rate of mechanical failure is related to the degree of weight loss. This is expected as increased weight loss happens over extended periods of time, giving the device more time to fail.

The incidence of port and tubing related complications is between 4-24%.[48,49] The tubing may detach from the port which manifests by filling of the port does not cause a corresponding decrease in the opening size. This can be diagnosed by fluoroscopy or contrast study through the port. The patient will need to be explored to reattach the port and tubing.

The port may malfunction, flip, leak or get infected. Malfunctioning ports can be replaced. If a port infection is discovered early, it is likely from contamination. The port can be divided and removed. Late infection is usually from erosion of the band into the stomach. For this reason, late infections necessitate a gastroscopy to ensure that the band has not eroded into the stomach. If no erosion has taken place the port is removed and replaced once the infection is under control. A partially rotated port can still be accessed (Figure 15). However, a completely rotated port cannot be accessed and will require repositioning (Figure 16).

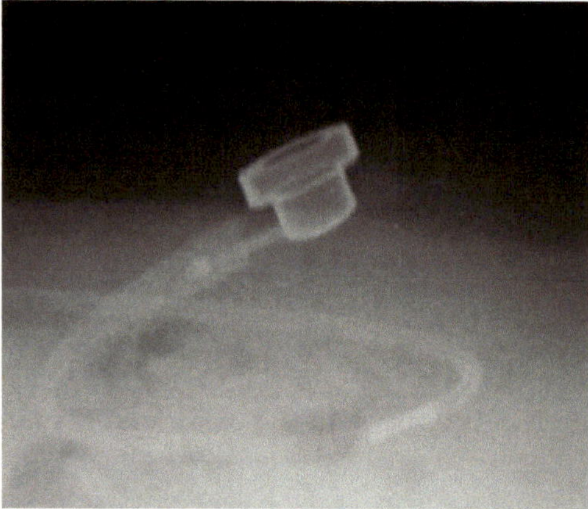

Figure 15: Lap-Band port slightly rotated.

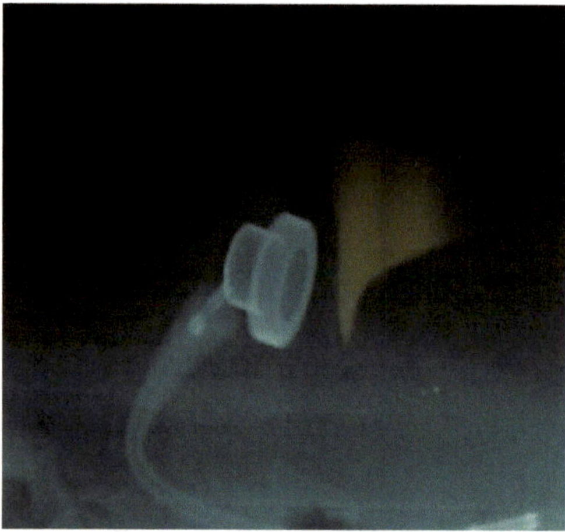

Figure 16: Lap-Band port completely flipped and cannot be accessed.

Esophageal Complications

Functional or anatomic complications of the esophagus are seen in over 50% of patients.[50] The abnormality may be a dilatation of the esophagus, gastro esophageal reflux, motility disorder of the esophagus, Barrett's esophagus, esophagitis or rarely adenocarcinoma of the esophagus.

Gastro-esophageal reflux is a common complication of LAGB. Pre-operative endoscopy is necessary to exclude patients with reflux disease of the esophagus. These patients should be offered LRYGB. In patients that develop reflux after LAGB, medical treatment is the mainstay. If medical treatment fails, LRYGB is the salvage procedure.

Esophageal motility disorders can develop in patients with normal preoperative esophageal manometry. Patients with abnormal esophageal manometry should be offered LRYGB. Patients that develop abnormal esophageal motility disorders after LAGB should be offered LRYGB.

Gastric Band Slip

The incidence of Gastric Band Slip has been variously reported as there is no consistent definition of pouch prolapse. Gastric Band Slip occurs when parts of the stomach prolapse above the band. Modification in surgical technique such as the *pars flaccida* operation and imbrication of the greater curvature on the band have decreased the incidence over time. Gastric band Slip can happen from overeating or too lose a band from weight loss. Symptoms are signs of obstruction with nausea, reflux, vomiting and pain in the abdomen. The prolapsed stomach can be superior to the band and strangulate.

Plain X-ray imaging will show the band to be tilted horizontally in cases of anterior prolapse. A gastrograffin UGI will confirm the diagnosis (Figure 17). A vertical position of the band will indicate a posterior prolapse (Figure 18 and 19).

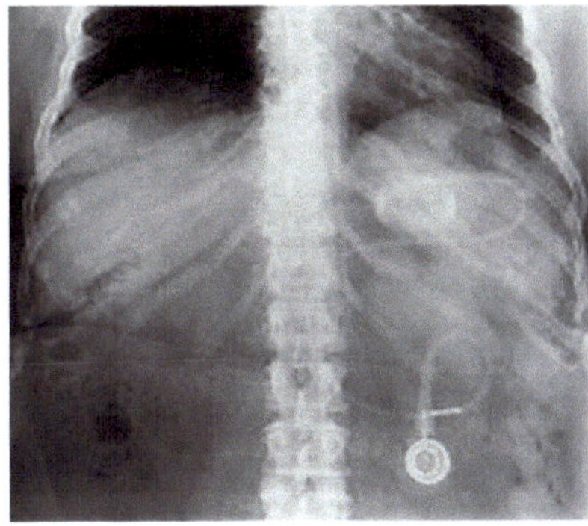

Figure 17: Slipped LAGB with horizontal orientation indicating anterior prolapse of stomach.

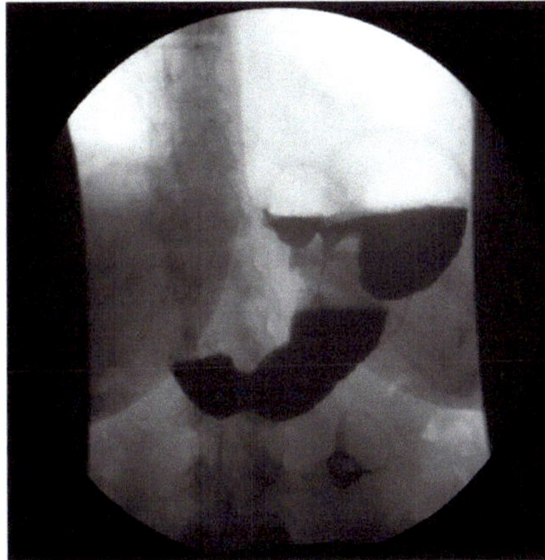

Figure 18: A gastrographic UGI study showing an anterior prolapse of stomach due to a lap-band slip.

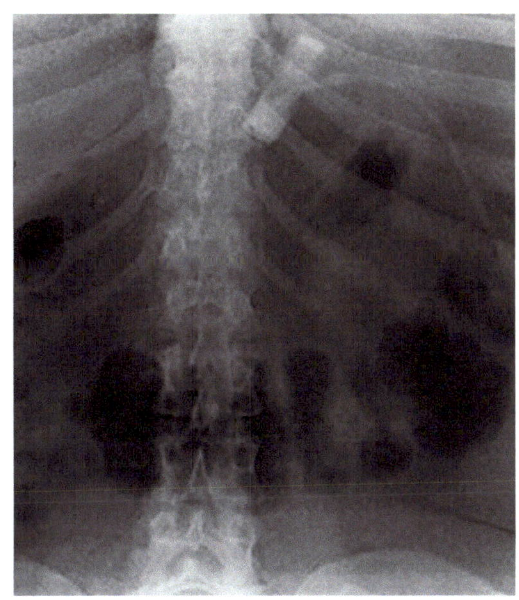

Figure 19: A more vertical position of the band indicating a posterior prolapse.

Treatment is to deflate the band initially. Once edema subsides and the obstruction is relieved the band can be inflated again. In cases of persistent or recurrent symptoms operative exploration is warranted. The band will have to be replaced through a different gap in the lesser and greater curvatures. Conversion to LRYGB or LSG is an option.

Pouch Dilatation

Pouch dilatation is an independent complication from band prolapse. The proximal stomach dilates in the face of chronic obstruction. Gastroscopy or imaging studies will show a smooth and concentric enlargement of the gastric pouch.

Symptoms are reflux esophagitis, vomiting, abdominal pain, and distension. A band holiday usually cures this condition. Fluid is removed from the band for a few weeks till the distension of the stomach has gone down. If pouch dilatation remains after slow fluid replacement, alternate surgical procedures such as LRYGB or LSG should be offered.

Erosion

Erosion of the band into the stomach remains a dreaded complication. Although the serosa of the stomach presents a stronger tissue against erosion when compared to the esophagus, erosion of the gastric band happens in 3-5% of patients. The etiology is postulated to be due to subclinical injury to the serosa of the stomach, over tightening of the band and the presence of a foreign body in contact with the stomach for extended period (Figure 20).

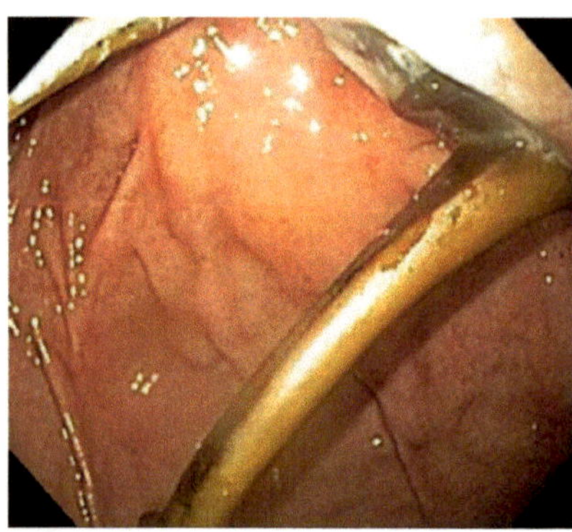

Figure 20: Band erosion with tube inside stomach lumen.

Symptoms are generally non-specific and can vary. Usually, the first sign of erosion is the loss of restriction of the band and beginning of weight regain. Other symptoms may range from general malaise, fever, or vague abdominal pain. Peritonitis is rare. The presence of port site infection despite a long period without accessing the port requires gastroscopy to evaluate for band erosion.

Treatment is removal of the band and laparoscopic approaches have been successful. It is not advisable to replace the band. If the patient desires further weight loss surgery, LRYGB or LSG should be offered, generally 6 months after removal of the band.

Biliopancreatic Diversion with Duodenal Switch (BPD-DS)

Essential elements of the BPD-DS consist of

- Sleeve gastrectomy with transaction of the duodenum in the first part
- Transection of the ileum at 250cm from the Ligament of Treitz
- Gastro-ileostomy of the stomach with the distal end of the ileum
- Illeo-illeostomy of the proximal ileum to a segment of ileum close to the ileocecal valve

The operation has not achieved widespread popularity in the USA probably because of the fear of metabolic consequences and the technical difficulty in performing the procedure. The operation was first performed as an open procedure and as a staged laparoscopic procedure with the sleeve gastrectomy as the first stage.

In studies from major centers the operative mortality has been comparable to the LRYGB. The weight loss has been greater with BPD-DS. In patients that had a BMI >50 kg/m^2, the incidence of resolution of comorbidities such as Type 2 Diabetes, hypertension and dyslipidemia were greater with the BPD-DS when compared to LRYGB. In the future, BPD-DS may have a role in patients that have a BMI > 50 Kg/m^2.[51,52]

Trends in Bariatric Surgery

Bariatric surgery is a nascent and evolving field. Innovation is rife with the aim of finding safer and more effective methods to handle the societal epidemic of obesity.

Laparoscopic Gastric Plication

Laparoscopic Gastric Plication is the reduction of the surface area of the lumen of the stomach without transecting. The stomach is first mobilized in the same fashion for a sleeve gastrectomy. This is followed by plication where the fundus is sutured over to the antrum. This leaves a lumen around the lesser curve open.[53] The operation is technically feasible but long-term results are still being studied. Plication has been combined with adjustable gastric bands to add a further restrictive procedure. Initial results have shown the procedure to be safe with weight loss similar to sleeve gastrectomy. Leak complications are not reported due to lack of gastric resection. However postoperative nausea and vomiting from obstruction due to edema has been seen.

Endoscopic Techniques

Intra-gastric Balloon

The intra-gastric balloon is a silastic balloon placed in the stomach and inflated with saline to 400-600 cc. The balloon mechanically fills the stomach and promotes satiety. The balloon has had limited exposure in Europe and has been found to be safe and efficacious. The main complications of the balloon are gastritis, gastric perforation, small bowel obstruction from balloon rupture, and gastric ulcers. The advantage of the balloon is its ease of insertion by endoscopy and the reversible nature of the intervention. Long term effects are needed as there is no physiologic change in the patient.

Endo-luminal Sleeves

These devices have a metallic frame with hooks to attach to the antrum of the stomach. A plastic sheet in the form of a lumen is attached to the frame and this sheath expands into the duodenum and small bowel. This sheath prevents the food in the lumen from coming into contact with digestive enzymes. Various anchor points for these sleeves have been manufactured. The safety and the efficacy of this procedure is under investigation.

Newer delivery platforms are continuously being pioneered with the goal of decreasing the invasiveness of the procedure while increasing the efficacy of the surgery. Newer methods include single incision laparoscopic surgery and robotic surgery for the current bariatric procedures. Newer techniques include a gastric pacer that can speed up gastric emptying.

Endoscopic techniques are being pioneered to suture a portion of the stomach shut using endoscopic sutures.

Bariatric surgery is currently just at the beginning of its transformative phase. With the obesity epidemic spreading to developing countries there is a pressing need to study the disease and fully understand the neuro-hormonal axis of obesity. The most effective procedures will be the ones that address the hormonal derangements that are associated with obesity.

REFERENCES

1. http://www.cdc.gov/obesity/data/adult.html
2. Park CW, Torquati A. Physiology of weight loss surgery. Surg Clin North Am. 2011 Dec;91(6):1149-61, vii. doi: 10.1016/j.suc.2011.08.009. PMID: 22054145; PMCID: PMC3382055.
3. Baicy K, London ED, Monterosso J, Wong ML, Delibasi T, Sharma A, Licinio J. "Leptin replacement alters brain response to food cues in genetically leptin-deficient adults". *Proc. Natl. Acad. Sci. U.S.A.* 2007 Nov. 104 (46): 18276–9.
4. Considine RV, Sinha MK, Heiman ML. "Serum immunoreactive-leptin concentrations in normal-weight and obese humans". *N. Engl. J. Med.* 1996 Feb. 334 (5): 292–295.
5. Tatemoto K. "Neuropeptide Y: History and Overview". 2004. In Michel MC. *Handbook of Experimental Pharmacology*. 162. Springer. pp. 2–15.
6. Hagan MM. "Peptide YY: a key mediator of orexigenic behavior". *Peptides.* 2002. 23 (2): 377–82.
7. le Roux CW, Welbourn R, et al. Gut hormones as mediators of appetite and weight loss after Roux-en-Y gastric bypass. Ann of Surg 2007; 246 (5): 780-5.
8. North American Association for the Study of Obesity and the National Heart, Lung, and Blood Institute. *The Practical Guide: Identification, Evaluation, and Treatment of Overweight and Obesity in Adults.* Bethesda, Md: National Institutes of Health; 2000. NIH publication 00-4084.
9. North American Association for the Study of Obesity (NAASO) and the National Heart. *Clinical Guidelines on the Identification, Evaluation, and Treatment of Overweight and Obesity in Adults: The Evidence Report.* Bethesda, Md: National Institutes of Health; 1998. NIH publication 98-4083.
10. Buchwald H, Avidor Y, et al. Bariatric Surgery: A systematic review and meta-analysis: *JAMA.* 2004;292(14):1724-1737. doi:10.1001/jama.292.14.1724.
11. National Institutes of Health Consensus Development Panel. Gastrointestinal surgery for severe obesity. *Ann Intern Med*1991;115:956-961.
12. Henrikson V. Can small bowel resection be defended as therapy for obesity? Obes Surg 1994;4: 54-5.
13. Jones KB Jr, Afram JD, Benotti PN, et al. Open versus laparoscopic Roux-en-Y gastric bypass: a comparative study of over 25,000 open cases and the major laparoscopic bariatric reported series. Obes Surg 2006;16:721-7.
14. Weller WE, Rosati C. Comparing outcomes of open versus laparoscopic bariatric surgery. Ann Surg 2008;248:10-5.
15. Surgical Treatment for Morbid Obesity: The Laparoscopic Roux-en-Y Gastric Bypass Surgical Clinics of North America - Volume 91, Issue 6. 2011 Dec.
16. Schauer PR, Ikramuddin S, Gourash W, et al. Outcomes after laparoscopic Roux-en-Y gastric bypass for morbid obesity. *Ann Surg* 232. 515-529.2000.
17. Higa KD, Boone KB, Ho T, et al. Laparoscopic Roux-en-Y gastric bypass for morbid obesity; technique and preliminary results of our first 400 patients. *Arch Surg* 135. 1029-1034.2000.
18. Nguyen NT, Goldman C, Rosenquist CJ, et al. Laparoscopic versus open gastric bypass: a randomized study of outcomes, quality of life, and costs. *Ann Surg* 234. 279-291.2001.
19. Westling A, Gustavsson S. Laparoscopic vs open Roux-en-Y gastric bypass: a prospective, randomized trial. *Obes Surg* 11. 284-292.2001.
20. Nguyen NT, Wilson SE. Complications of antiobesity surgery. *Nat Clin Pract Gastroenterol Hepatol* 4. (3): 138-147.2007.
21. Podnos YD, Jimenez JC, Wilson SE, et al. Complications after laparoscopic gastric bypass: a review of 3464 cases. *Arch Surg* 138. (9): 957-961.2003.
22. Buchwald H, Avidor Y, Braunwald E, et al. Bariatric surgery: a systematic review and meta-analysis. *JAMA* 292. (14): 1724-1737.2004,
23. Farrell TM, Haggerty SP, Overby DW, et al. Clinical application of laparoscopic bariatric surgery: an evidence-based review. *Surg Endosc* 23. (5): 930-949.2009.
24. Christou NV, Sampalis JS, Liberman M, et al. Surgery decreases long-term mortality, morbidity, and health care use in morbidly obese patients. *Ann Surg* 240. (3): 416-423.2004.
25. Sowemimo OA, Yood SM, Courtney J, et al. Natural history of morbid obesity without surgical intervention. *Surg Obes Relat Dis* 3. (1): 73-77.2007.
26. Wittgrove AC, Clark GW. Laparoscopic gastric bypass, Roux-en-Y—500 patients: technique and results, with 3-60 month follow-up. *Obes Surg* 10. 233-239.2000.

27. Fernandez AZ Jr, DeMaria EJ, Tichansky DS, et al. Experience with over 3,000 open and laparoscopic bariatric procedures: multivariate analysis of factors related to leak and resultant mortality. *Surg Endosc* 18. (2): 193-197.2004.
28. Sapala JA, Wood MH, Schuhknecht MP, et al. Fatal pulmonary embolism after bariatric operations for morbid obesity: a 24-year retrospective analysis. *Obes Surg* 13. (6): 819-825.2003.
29. Nguyen NT, Longoria M, Chalifoux S, et al. Gastrointestinal hemorrhage after laparoscopic gastric bypass. *Obes Surg* 14. (10): 1308-1312.2004.
30. Garza E Jr, Kuhn J, Arnold D, et al. Internal hernias after laparoscopic Roux-en-Y gastric bypass. *Am J Surg* 188. (6): 796-800.2004.
31. Gandhi AD, Patel RA, Brolin RE. Elective laparoscopy for herald symptoms of mesenteric/internal hernia after laparoscopic Roux-en-Y gastric bypass. *Surg Obes Relat Dis* 5. (2): 144-149.2009.
32. Rasmussen JJ, Fuller W, Ali MR. Marginal ulceration after laparoscopic gastric bypass: an analysis of predisposing factors in 260 patients. *Surg Endosc* 21. (7): 1090-1094.2007.
33. Swartz DE, Gonzalez V, Felix EL. Anastomotic stenosis after Roux-en-Y gastric bypass: a rational approach to treatment. *Surg Obes Relat Dis* 2. (6): 632-636.2006.
34. Nguyen NT, Stevens CM, Wolfe BM. Incidence and outcome of anastomotic stricture after laparoscopic gastric bypass. *J Gastrointest Surg* 7. (8): 997-1003.2003.
35. Sugerman HJ, Brewer WH, Shiffman ML, et al. A multicenter, placebo-controlled, randomized, double-blind, prospective trial of prophylactic ursodiol for the prevention of gallstone formation following gastric-bypass-induced rapid weight loss. *Am J Surg* 169. 91-97.1995.
36. Balsiger BM, Kennedy FP, Abu-Lebdeh HS, et al. Prospective evaluation of Roux-en Y gastric bypass as primary operation for medically complicated obesity. *Mayo Clin Proc* 75. 673-680.2000.
37. Ukleja A. Dumping syndrome: pathophysiology and treatment. *Nutr Clin Pract* 20. 517-525.2005.
38. Service GJ, Thompson GB, Service FJ, et al. Hyperinsulinemic hypoglycemia with nesidioblastosis after gastric-bypass surgery. *N Engl J Med* 353. 249-254.2005.
39. McLaughlin T, Peck M, Holst J, et al. Reversible hyperinsulinemic hypoglycemia after gastric bypass: a consequence of altered nutrient delivery. *J Clin Endocrinol Metab* 95. (4): 1851-1855.
40. Z'graggen K, Guweidhi A, Steffen R, et al. Severe recurrent hypoglycemia after gastric bypass surgery. *Obes Surg* 18. (8): 981-988.2008.
41. Halverson JD. Micronutrient deficiencies after gastric bypass for morbid obesity. *Am Surg* 52. 594-598.1986.
42. Brethauer SA, Hammel JP, Schauer PR. Systematic review of sleeve gastrectomy as staging and primary bariatric procedure. *Surg Obes Relat Dis* 5. 469-475.2009.
43. Vidal J, Ibarzabal A, Romero F, et al. Type 2 diabetes mellitus and the metabolic syndrome following sleeve gastrectomy in severely obese subjects. *Obes Surg* 18. 1077-1082.2008.
44. Angrisani L, Lorenzo M, Borrelli V. Laparoscopic adjustable gastric banding versus Roux-en-Y gastric bypass: 5-year results of a prospective randomized trial. *Surg Obes Relat Dis* 3. (2): 127-132.2007.
45. Lanthaler M, Strasser S, Aigner F, et al. Weight loss and quality of life after gastric band removal or deflation. *Obes Surg* 19. (10): 1401-1408.2009.
46. Suter M, Calmes JM, Paroz A, et al. A 10-year experience with laparoscopic gastric banding for morbid obesity: high long-term complication and failure rates. *Obes Surg* 16. (7): 829-835.2006.
47. Shen R, Ren CJ. Removal of peri-gastric fat prevents acute obstruction after Lap-Band surgery. *Obes Surg* 14. (2): 224-229.2004.
48. Keidar A, Carmon E, Szold A, et al. Port complications following laparoscopic adjustable gastric banding for morbid obesity. *Obes Surg* 15. (3): 361-365.2005.
49. Szold A, Abu-Abeid S. Laparoscopic adjustable silicone gastric banding for morbid obesity: results and complications in 715 patients. *Surg Endosc* 16. (2): 230-233.2002.
50. de Jong JR, Tiethof C, van Ramshorst B, et al. Esophageal dilation after laparoscopic adjustable gastric banding: a more systematic approach is needed. *Surg Endosc* 23. (12): 2802-2808.2009.
51. Prachand VN, Davee RT, Alverdy JC. Duodenal switch provides superior weight loss in the super-obese (BMI > or = 50 kg/m2) compared with gastric bypass. *Ann Surg* 244. (4): 611-619.2006.
52. Prachand VN, Ward M, Alverdy JC. Duodenal switch provides superior resolution of metabolic comorbidities independent of weight loss in the super-obese (BMI > or = 50 kg/m2) compared with gastric bypass. *J Gastrointest Surg* 14. (2): 211-220.2010.
53. Talebpour M, Amoli BS. Laparoscopic total gastric vertical plication in morbid obesity. *J Laparoendosc Adv Surg Tech A* 17. (6): 793-798.2007.

❑❑❑

35

CHAPTER

Small Bowel Neoplasms

Deepa Taggarshe MD
Vijay K. Mittal MD

INTRODUCTION

Although the small bowel itself accounts for approximately 80% of the total gastrointestinal tract and 90% of its mucosal surface area, neoplasms in the small bowel are quite rare. Small bowel neoplasms comprise less than 5% of all gastrointestinal cancers with an estimated incidence of 6,110 cases in the United States in 2008.[1] The possible reasons for this disparity include rapid transit of the luminal contents, limiting the contact time between carcinogens and mucosa, an alkaline environment due to the presence of pancreatic enzymes, high levels of IgA in the small bowel wall and the low bacterial counts in the small bowel luminal contents. The incidence of these neoplasms, however, is increasing especially with a four-fold rise in carcinoids.[2]

Small bowel cancers are more common in men and patients are usually diagnosed in their fifth or sixth decade. Most tumors of the small bowel are benign, which are usually asymptomatic and identified at autopsy. Malignant neoplasms on the other hand, comprise a majority of symptomatic lesions leading to surgery (Table 1).[3]

Risk factors for adenocarcinoma of small bowel include Crohn's disease, familial adenomatosis polyposis, hereditary nonpolyposis colorectal cancer (also known as Lynch Syndrome), Peutz-Jeghers syndrome, celiac sprue, and biliary diversion. Red meat, smoked, and cured food consumption has also been implicated. Recent studies have shown that carcinoid tumors are being increasingly seen and now constitute the most common primary malignant tumor in the small bowel.[2,4]

Table 1: Incidence of small bowel malignant neoplasms

Tumor Type	Frequency	Predominant Site
Adenocarcinoma	30% to 50%	Duodenum
Carcinoid	20% to 30%	Ileum
Lymphoma	15%	Ileum
GIST	15%	

Clinical Presentation

The clinical presentation of small bowel tumors is non-specific and ill defined. Most benign tumors are asymptomatic. Small bowel obstruction due to luminal narrowing or intussusception; associated with intermittent abdominal pain, distension, nausea, and vomiting can be seen. The second most common mode of presentation is intermittent gastrointestinal bleeding and anemia.

Patients with malignant tumors present with weight loss[3] and may already be malnourished at the time of surgery. Obstruction and bleeding can also be seen. Obstruction in case of malignant tumors is more likely to be reflective of extensive tumor infiltration and adhesions. A palpable mass may be felt in up to 25% of patients. Perforations from small bowel tumors are seen in 10%, usually due to lymphomas and sarcomas. Lesions in the periampullary duodenum can cause obstructive jaundice or pancreatitis.

Diagnosis

Laboratory tests are limited for diagnosis of small bowel tumors. Complete blood counts may show anemia. Elevated 5-hydroxyindoleacetic acid (5-HIAA) is seen in carcinoids. Elevated carcinoembryonic antigen (CEA) levels are seen in small bowel adenocarcinomas with liver metastasis.

Due to the rarity of small bowel neoplasms, a high index of suspicion must be kept for these tumors to be diagnosed. Keeping the radiologist informed of a suspected diagnosis improves the chances of diagnosis by imaging studies.

Upper GI series with small bowel follow through (SBFT) studies have been used for diagnosing small bowel neoplasms and have been reported to have a sensitivity of 30 to 44%.[5] Enterolysis has been reported to have a higher sensitivity at 90% and is the test of choice for distal small bowel tumors. Advanced stage small bowel adenocarcinomas can present as "apple-core lesions." These lesions are short, circumferentially narrowed segments with mucosal ulceration and overhanging proximal and distal borders. Malignant strictures are usually rigid, with a fixed, unchanging appearance during compression. The initial studies of carcinoid tumors may show some mucosal thickening, but with growth of the tumor into the mesentery, kinking of the bowel wall, narrowing of the lumen, and angulation of the involved small bowel may be seen. On barium studies, submucosal GISTs appear as smooth, round filling defects with or without ulceration.

Plain films may show small bowel obstruction but are ineffective at picking up tumors (Figure 1). Computed tomography (CT) is gaining more prominence in diagnosing small bowel neoplasms. It is particularly useful in picking up large tumors, extramural invasions of tumors and staging the cancer. The reported sensitivities vary from 57 to 63%. Adenocarcinomas may show as discrete small bowel mass causing intraluminal narrowing. With the improved quality of multidetector CT, even smaller carcinoids can now be diagnosed as submucosal lesions. Mesenteric extension of the carcinoid can be seen as an ill-defined calcified mesenteric mass in 70%.[6] The mass can also have a spiculated appearance due to desmoplastic reaction in the mesentery in response to serotonin. GIST may show up as a large smooth mass with central necrosis. Tumors of vascular origin can be diagnosed by angiography or Technetium-99mradioisotope-tagged red blood cells (RBC) scan.

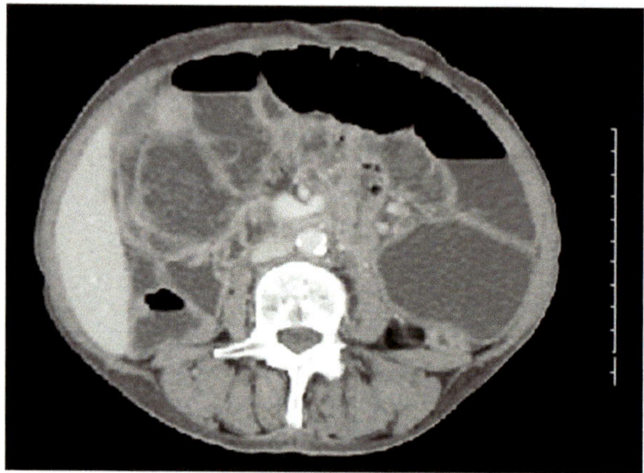

Figure 1: Small bowel obstruction

Flexible gastroduodenal endoscopy and small bowel enteroscopy are useful in diagnosing tumors of the duodenum and proximal jejunum. Terminal ileum can be visualized by advancing the colonoscope into the terminal ileum. The advantages of these techniques lay in the opportunity to biopsy the lesion and obtain a tissue diagnosis. Capsule endoscopy allows for visualization of the distal jejunum and ileum; however, it has its limitations mainly in the inability to reexamine the suspected area. It has a higher diagnostic yield than other tests at identifying small bowel tumors which present with GI bleeding.[7]

Staging

The staging of malignant small bowel neoplasms is according to the American Joint Committee on Cancer staging system.

Stage		Description
0	Tis	Cancer only in epithelium, no growth into deeper tissue layers
	N0	No spread to nearby lymph nodes
	M0	No spread to other parts of the body
I	T1 or T2	T1: Cancer has grown into lamina propria or submucosa OR T2: Cancer has grown through submucosa into muscularis propria The cancer has not spread to nearby lymph nodes (N0) or to distant parts of the body (M0).
	N0	No spread to nearby lymph nodes
	M0	No spread to other parts of the body
IIA	T3	Cancer has grown into the subserosa, no growth into any nearby organs or structures
	N0	No spread to nearby lymph nodes
	M0	No spread to other parts of the body

Stage		Description
IIB	T4	Cancer has grown through the outer layer of intestine tissue (serosa or visceral peritoneum), into nearby organs, or nearby structures
	N0	No spread to nearby lymph nodes
	M0	No spread to other parts of the body
IIIA	Any T	Cancer may have grown into any small intestinal wall layer
	N1	Spread to 1-2 nearby lymph nodes
	M0	No spread to other parts of the body
IIIB	Any T	Cancer may have grown into any small intestinal wall layer
	N2	Spread to at least 3 nearby lymph nodes
	M0	No spread to other parts of the body
IV	Any T	Cancer may have grown into any small intestinal wall layer
	Any N	Cancer may have spread to nearby lymph nodes
	M1	Cancer has spread to distant lymph nodes or organs (i.e., peritoneum, liver

* The following additional categories are not listed on the table above:

- TX: Main tumor cannot be assessed due to lack of information.
- T0: No evidence of a main tumor.
- NX: Nearby lymph nodes cannot be assessed due to lack of information.

BENIGN NEOPLASMS

Benign small bowel neoplasms include lipomas, adenomas, hamartomas, and GISTs, lipomas, hamartomas, benign GISTs, and mesenteric cysts (Figure 2). Although adenomas are the most common benign small bowel tumor, GISTs are the most common symptomatic benign tumor.

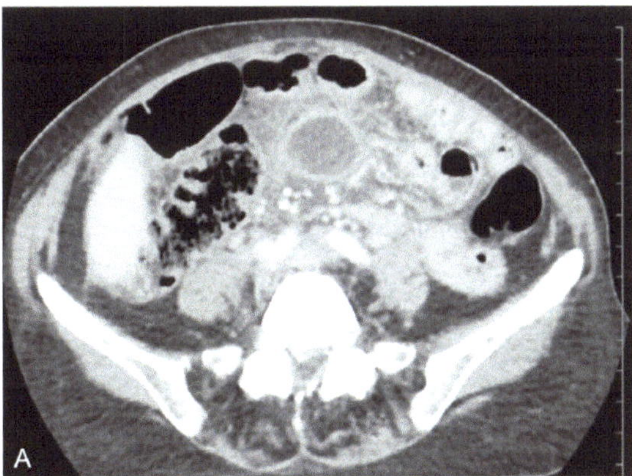

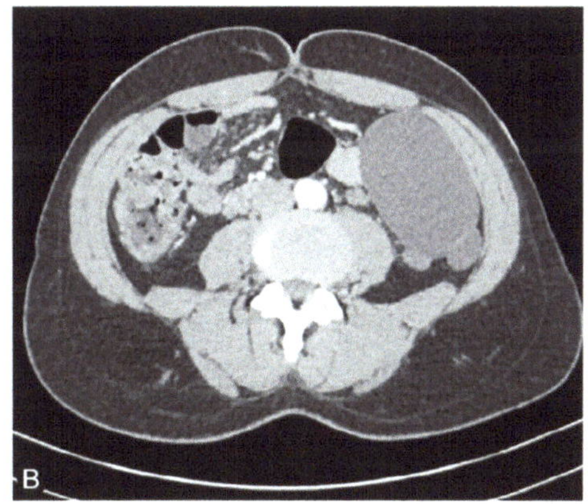

Figure 2: (A) Mesenteric cyst. (B) Large mesenteric duplication cyst with internal septation

Adenomas

Adenomas comprise about 15% of all benign small bowel tumors. They may be associated with familial adenomatous polyposis and Gardner's syndrome. There are three types: tubular adenomas, villous adenomas, and Brunner's gland adenomas. Nearly half of the small bowel adenomas are found in the ileum, with 20% in the duodenum and 30% in the jejunum. Majority of the lesions are asymptomatic. Most common presenting symptoms are bleeding and obstruction. The villous adenomas have high malignant potential, between 35% and 55%. The malignant potential increases with a size larger than 2 cm. Brunner's gland adenomas are hyperplastic lesions arising from the Brunner's glands in the duodenum. They do not have a malignant potential.

Adenomas can be diagnosed and treated with endoscopic measures. Diagnosis can be confirmed by biopsy. Tubular adenomas and Brunner's gland adenomas can be resected by simple endoscopic excision. However, with villous adenomas, especially if larger than 2 cm, endoscopic excision may be inadequate. Surgical options include segmental resection, transduodenal polypectomy and for tumors located near the ampulla of Vater, pancreaticoduodenectomy.

Lipomas

Lipomas are rarely found in the small intestine. Lipomas present as intramural lesions, located in the submucosa. They are mainly seen in the sixth and seventh decade and are seen more in men. Main symptoms include obstruction and bleeding due to ulceration. Lipomas can be identified in CT scans because of their high fat content. Treatment of symptomatic lipomas is excision.

Hamartomas

Hamartomas are seen as part of the Peutz-Jeghers syndrome, which is an autosomal dominant syndrome characterized by mucocutaneous melanotic pigmentation and gastrointestinal polyps. The pigmented lesions appear as 1 to 2 mm, black or brown lesions located in the circumoral region of the face, forearms, palms, soles, and the perianal region. These polyps are mainly located in the jejunum and ileum and have the potential to cause obstruction or intermittent intussusception. Patients present with colicky intermittent abdominal pain. Bleeding is less common, and patients may present with anemia.

Patients with Peutz-Jeghers syndrome have an increased risk of adenocarcinoma and should be followed closely. Extra-colonic cancers are also seen in 50 to 90% of these patients, mainly cancers of the small intestine, stomach, pancreas, lung, breast, ovary, and uterus. If patients are symptomatic, resection may be necessary, but should be limited to the segment of bowel involved in active disease. Due to the widespread nature of the disease, extensive resection is not curative and unnecessary.

Benign GISTs

Gastrointestinal stromal tumors are defined by their expression of the transmembrane tyrosine kinase receptor KIT (CD117). These tumors arise from the interstitial cells of Cajal, intestinal pacemaker cells, and are identified by staining with the monoclonal antibody for KIT.

Benign GISTs are three to four times more common than malignant GISTs. They are usually seen in the fifth decade with an equal incidence in men and women. The tumors can cause obstruction due to intramural growth, or bleeding. Patients may present with abdominal pain or symptoms of obstruction or GI bleeding. Due to the slow growth of these tumors, patients may remain asymptomatic for a long time. These tumors are submucosal and have a smooth appearance on barium studies. On CT scan, the tumor may appear smooth and if large, may show areas of central necrosis. Treatment is by surgical resection. Increased risk of local recurrence has been reported with tumors with mitotic counts higher than 2 per 50 high-powered fields.[8,9]

MALIGNANT NEOPLASMS

Carcinoid Tumors

Carcinoid tumors arise from the enterochromaffin cells (Kulchitsky cells) found in the crypts of Lieberkühn. These cells can be stained by silver compounds and hence are called Argentaffin cells. Carcinoid tumors may be derived from the foregut (respiratory tract, thymus), midgut (stomach, proximal duodenum, jejunum, ileum, and right colon), and hindgut (distal colon and rectum). The most common sites for gastrointestinal carcinoids are appendix, followed by the ileum. In the small bowel, nearly 80% of the carcinoids occur within the last two feet of the ileum. Carcinoids secrete various products, including 5-hydroxytryptamine (serotonin), 5-hydroxytryptophan, dopamine and somatostatin.

Carcinoids are small, submucosal tumors that are yellow in color. They can be multicentric in 20 to 30% of patients. As the tumors are slow-growing, most are found incidentally during surgery. Desmoplastic reaction is seen with the invasion of the tumor into the mesentery, secondary to the local effects of serotonin and other growth factors, leading to mesenteric fibrosis and obstruction.

Patients present with vague abdominal pain. Obstructive symptoms are more common than bleeding or perforation. Obstruction can be either due to intussusception of the tumor or the desmoplastic reaction mentioned earlier. Carcinoid syndrome is seen in 10% of patients with carcinoid tumors, and is caused by high levels of serotonin, 5-hydroxytryptophan, histamine, dopamine and other amines. Carcinoid syndrome is more commonly associated with small bowel carcinoids; these patients usually have widespread hepatic metastases at the time of presentation. Symptoms include diarrhea, flushing, sweating, wheezing and abdominal pain. The cutaneous flushing in patients may vary from short lived flushing of the face, neck, and chest to prolonged flashes lasting 2-3 days, involving the entire body and associated with hypotension and edema. Cardiac lesions include tricuspid and pulmonary stenosis. Carcinoid tumors utilize the majority of the body's tryptophan for serotonin production and patients may manifest symptoms of pellagra—dermatitis, dementia, and diarrhea.

Carcinoids can be diagnosed by elevated urinary levels of 5-hydroxyindoleacetic acid. 5-HIAA can be measured in a 24-hour urine collection, and it provides a summation of tumor secretory activity that may be missed by one-time urine samples. However, this test is time consuming and can be altered by various medications. Plasma levels of substance P and serotonin may be elevated. If these tests are equivocal, provocative tests, using calcium, epinephrine or pentagastrin may be employed, but with the advancement of current diagnostic tests, these are rarely used nowadays. On barium studies, carcinoid tumors present as smooth, solitary, intraluminal defects but may also exhibit narrowing, and obstruction. CT scan can show the extent of bowel and mesenteric involvement, hepatic metastases, and retroperitoneal extension. A spiculated mesenteric mass with radiating strands of fibrosis is pathognomonic for carcinoids.[11]

An Octreotide scan, using In-111 Octreotide (6 mCi administered intravenously) can identify carcinoids, which express serotonin receptors. This has a sensitivity of >90% and can also be used to detect metastases. Elevated Chromogranin A levels correlates well with metastatic disease and has also been shown to be indicative of a poor prognostic outcome in patients with liver metastases.[12]

Treatment of carcinoids (Figure 3) is based on tumor size and the presence of any metastases. Primary tumors less than 1 cm in diameter can be resected if there is no evidence of spread to lymph nodes. Wide excision of bowel and mesentery is employed for multiple tumors or lymph node involvement. Small duodenal tumors can be removed by enucleation; however larger tumors may require a pancreaticoduodenectomy. In ileal and jejunal carcinoids, en-bloc resection is required, with lymph node metastases. Debulking surgery has been shown to provide symptomatic relief.[13] Hepatic metastases are treated by surgical resection or ablation. In case of widespread hepatic metastases, embolization has shown good results. Carcinoid crisis may be precipitated by anesthesia, and hence Octreotide should be readily available in the operating room.

Medical therapy for carcinoids is directed towards symptomatic relief, by using somatostatin analogues like Octreotide. Adjuvant chemotherapy with streptozocin and 5-fluorouracil is used in patients with metastatic disease who are unresponsive to other treatments. The response rate to chemotherapy varies from 20-30%.

The overall 5 years survival rate is 60%. Patients with small, nonmetastatic disease, have 5 years survival rates of 100% after resection. Even with distant metastases, survival rates approach 25-35% and with resection of liver metastases, survival rates improve to 50%.

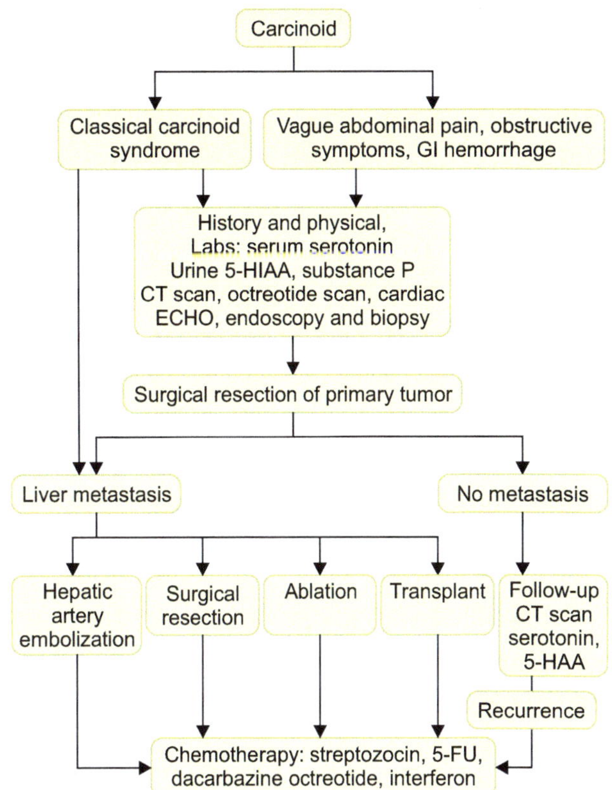

Figure 3: An overview of diagnosis and management of small bowel carcinoids

Lymphomas

Lymphomas are the third most common malignant type of small bowel neoplasm, accounting for about 15% of small bowel tumors. However, in children younger than 10 years, they are the most common intestinal neoplasms. They may be primarily from the GI tract or involve the small bowel as part of systemic involvement.

Most patients present in the fifth or sixth decade and it is slightly more common in men. Lymphomas are usually associated with immunosuppressive states like transplant recipients, AIDS, Crohn's disease, and systemic lupus erythematosus. These neoplasms are usually Non-Hodgkin's B-cell lymphomas with intermediate or high-grade,[14] and are more commonly found in the ileum.

Patients can present with abdominal pain, fatigue, malaise, and weight loss. With systemic involvement, patients may have fever. Patients may also present with features of obstruction or GI bleeding. About a quarter may have perforation. Generalized lymphadenopathy is suggestive of systemic involvement. Patients may have a palpable abdominal mass.

Diagnosis can be made using CT, where the lymphoma can sometimes be seen as a homogenous mass with mural thickening and enlarged nodes. Submucosal lymphomatous proliferation may show filling defects in barium studies.

Staging of Lymphoma (Ann Arbor Classification)

IE: Limited to the intestine with focal/multifocal spread.

IIE: Involvement of organ and regional nodes on the same side of the diaphragm

IIE1: Involvement of local nodes

IIE2: Involvement of non-continuous nodes.

IIIE: Involvement of organ and regional nodes on both sides of the diaphragm.

IVE: Involvement of distant organs and extra lymphatic organs.

Initial management of small bowel lymphomas involves surgical resection of the affected small bowel with its mesentery.[15,16] This can immediately palliate the symptoms, and prevent a potential perforation. A good exploratory laparotomy is essential at the time of surgery for staging the disease (Figure 4). Debulking is of benefit. Chemotherapy with CHOP (Cyclophosphamide, Doxorubicin, Vincristine, and Prednisolone) is used in patients with advanced staged tumors and has been shown to be of benefit in Stage IE and IIE.[17] Patients with stage IIE (regional nodal or extranodal involvement confined to one side of the diaphragm) chemotherapy with combined radiation is recommended. Combination chemotherapy is primarily used in patients with stage IIIE or IVE (involvement of nodes on both sides of the diaphragm or extra nodal involvement, i.e., of bone marrow or liver). Radiation therapy is used for bulky tumors and treatment of residual disease after chemotherapy.[18]

The overall prognosis is poor and dependent on the stage. Twenty to forty percent of patients with localized disease survive five years, whereas the survival for disseminated disease is less than a year.

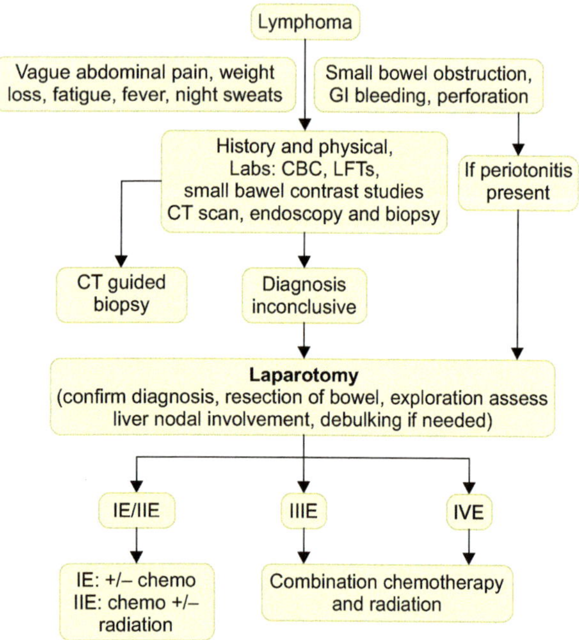

Figure 4: An overview of the diagnosis and management of small bowel lymphomas. Chemotherapy usually involves CHOP (Cyclophosphamide, Doxorubicin, Vincristine and Prednisolone)

Adenocarcinoma

Adenocarcinomas constitute about 30 to 50% of small bowel malignant neoplasms, although recent reports suggest that carcinoid may now outnumber adenocarcinoma in frequency. Epidemiologically, adenocarcinomas of the small bowel are similar to colorectal adenocarcinomas, with predominance in Western countries, and in patients with certain conditions like familial adenomatosis polyposis, Crohn's disease, hereditary nonpolyposis colorectal cancer, Peutz-Jeghers syndrome and celiac sprue.

KRAS mutation and p53 overexpression is common in small-bowel adenocarcinoma as in colorectal carcinoma. Mutation of the APC tumor suppressor gene, which is characteristic of colorectal carcinoma, however, does not commonly occur in small bowel adenocarcinoma.[19,20] Small bowel adenocarcinomas also show mutation of the SMAD/DPC4 gene.

Patients usually present in the seventh decade and there is a slight male preponderance. The most common location is the proximal small bowel, with a majority in the duodenum and jejunum. In contrast, patients with Crohn's disease have ileal adenocarcinomas. Patients with duodenal tumors may present with obstructive jaundice. Symptoms are otherwise non-specific, with vague abdominal pain, weight loss and feeling of fullness. Features of intestinal obstruction and GI bleeding may be present; however, perforation is uncommon. On physical examination, patients may have abdominal distension due to obstruction. Peritonitis if present is suggestive of perforation.

Laboratory investigations may show anemia due to blood loss, and in periampullary tumors, liver function tests may be deranged. Elevated carcinoembryonic antigen may be seen with small bowel adenocarcinomas. Duodenal tumors can be diagnosed by endoscopy and biopsy. In case of distal tumors, small bowel contrast studies show an "apple-core" or annular lesion with adenocarcinomas. Plain abdominal radiographs may show small bowel obstruction, but otherwise is unhelpful. On computed tomography (CT), small bowel adenocarcinomas may appear as a discrete tumor mass, with possible overhanging edges or as an ulcerative lesion. Sometimes annular narrowing of the lumen is present. The proximal tumors tend to be more polypoid, whereas distal tumors are more annular in nature. This narrowing of the lumen can cause partial or even complete small bowel obstruction over time Injection of intravenous contrast material will show moderate enhancement in the mass itself.

Treatment of small bowel adenocarcinomas primarily involves wide resection of the small bowel including the involved lymph nodes (Figure 5). Due to the higher local nodal involvement, a wide resection of the mesentery is essential. Removal of involved nodes has been shown to decrease the rate of local recurrence. Periampullary tumors need a pancreaticoduodenectomy (Whipple's procedure).

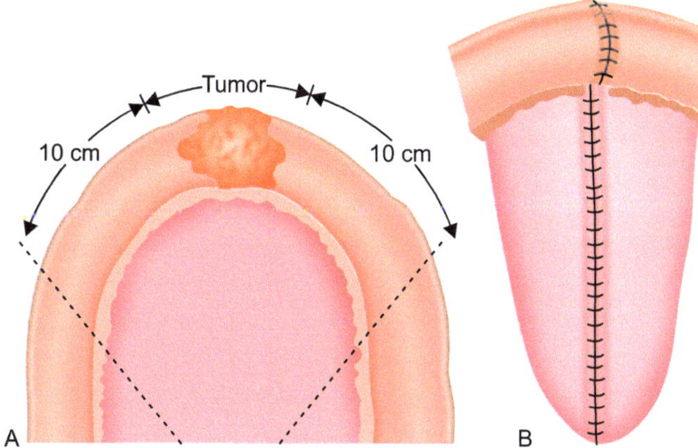

Figure 5: Small bowel resection for adenocarcinoma of the bowel with wide resection (A) and primary anastomosis (B)

Presence of liver or widespread peritoneal metastases is a contraindication to curative resection. However, patients can also present late, due to the indolent nature of the symptoms and surgical curative resection is not possible. In such cases, a palliative resection should be performed to prevent future episodes of obstruction and hemorrhage. If resection is not possible, a bypass procedure can provide symptomatic relief. Some studies involving small number of patients have shown minor response of small bowel adenocarcinomas to chemotherapy agents commonly used in colorectal cancers (i.e., 5-Fluorouracil, oxaliplatin, etc.). The role of adjuvant chemotherapy and radiation remains yet undefined.

Only 50% of patients have lesions amenable to a curative resection. About a quarter of the patients present with metastatic disease. In a National Cancer Database based review, by Howe et al the prognosis was dependent on age, site of tumor (worse in duodenal), stage and nature of surgical resection. In their review, patients who did not have a curative resection had a more than twofold increased risk of death related to the cancer, compared with patients who underwent curative surgery. A negative margin after curative surgery has been shown to be associated with longer survival. The overall 5-year survival remains poor at 25 to 30%.

Malignant GIST

Gastrointestinal stromal tumors are theorized to arise from the interstitial cells of Cajal and constitute a majority of GI sarcomas. These tumors occur because of mutation of the c-KIT oncogene, found on chromosome 4q, leading to increased expression of the tyrosine kinase receptor c-KIT (CD117). Expression of c-KIT is considered the most specific criterion for diagnosis. Activation of c-KIT leads to activation of other enzyme cascades which leads to cellular proliferation. This is a common feature to both benign and malignant GISTs. Malignant GISTs can be identified by the presence of metastases or local invasion. However, the aggressiveness of GISTs can be difficult to predict by pathology. The GIST workshop, convened by the NIH in 2000 proposed a criterion to grade the malignant risk of GISTs based on their size and mitotic rate as follows:

Most patients present with non-specific abdominal symptoms such as abdominal discomfort, GI bleeding, and with or without a palpable mass. GISTs are typically fast-growing neoplasms and hence develop a necrotic center due to outgrowing their blood supply. When this encroaches onto the lumen, profuse bleeding can occur. Small bowel GISTs may also cause obstruction, or jaundice if present in the duodenum.

On barium studies, GISTs are seen as smooth masses causing extrinsic compression. CT scan offers the best imaging modality for GISTs which appear as smooth masses with the presence of central ulceration. It provides information on the exact location, size and extent of the tumor, and presence of any metastases.

Surgery is the primary treatment modality for localized and advanced GISTs. Complete resection of the tumor with 2-3 cm margins, even in case of locally advanced tumors is associated with better survival. For small bowel GISTs, this entails a segmental resection of the small bowel with primary anastomosis. As these tumors do not spread by lymphatic dissemination, lymphadenectomy is not essential. Periampullary lesions may require a pancreaticoduodenectomy.

Table 2: Classification for GIST tumors

Risk	Size	Mitotic Count
Very low	Less than 2 cm	<5 per 50 hpf
Low	Between 2 and 5 cm	<5 per 50 hpf
Intermediate	Less than 5 cm	6-10 per 50 hpf
	Between 5 and 10 cm	<5 per 50 hpf
High	Greater than 5 cm	>5 per 50 hpf
	Greater than 10 cm	Any mitotic rate
	Any size	>10 per 50 hpf

Imatinib (Gleevec) is the first effective systemic therapy for patients with metastatic or locally advanced GIST. Imatinib which is a selective c-Kit inhibitor has been shown to decrease GIST cell proliferation and increase induction of apoptosis. It holds the progression of the tumor, and occasionally causes shrinkage, but complete response is rare. Dose is usually 400 mg per day, given orally and in the current setting lifetime therapy is indicated. Side effects include diarrhea, nausea, rash, abdominal cramps, and periorbital edema.

Recurrence rate of GIST is 20 to 50%, usually within the first two years after surgery. NCCN guidelines recommend abdominal and pelvic CT every 3 to 6 months for the first 5 years post-surgery. PET scan is also useful in identifying recurrences. Prior to the use of Imatinib, the overall 5 years survival rate was estimated to be 44%, and up to 64% with completely excised localized tumors.

Metastatic Neoplasms in Small Bowel

Metastatic neoplasms of the small bowel are more common than primary neoplasms of the small bowel. The primary sites for these metastases are usually other intra-abdominal organs, including the ovaries, colon, stomach, kidney, cervix, and pancreas. The small bowel involvement is due to direct extension of the tumor or implantation of tumor cells. Extra- abdominal tumors involving the breast, lung, and skin (melanoma) also metastasize to small bowel. The most common extra-abdominal source for small bowel metastases is melanoma of the skin, with small bowel involvement seen in more than half of the patients dying of metastatic melanoma. Patients may present with symptoms of small bowel obstruction, weight loss and bleeding. Diagnosis is usually made at surgery for obstruction or bleeding. Treatment involves small bowel resection. If the tumor is extensive or there are widespread metastases, either a palliative resection or bypass can relieve symptoms. Adjuvant therapy is dependent on the type of primary tumor.

REFERENCES

1. Jemal A, Siegel R, Ward E, Hao Y, Xu J, Murray T, et al. Cancer Statistics 2008. CA Cancer J Clin 2008; 58:71-96.
2. Bilimoria KY, Bentrem DJ, Wayne JD, Ko CY, Bennett CL, Talamonti MS. Small Bowel Cancer in the United States: changes in epidemiology; treatment, and survival over the last 20 years. Ann Surg 2009;249(1):63-71.
3. Mittal VK, Bodzin JH. Primary malignant tumors of the small bowel. Am J Surg 1980;140(3):396-9.
4. Maggard MA, O'Connell JB, Ko CY. Updated population-based review of carcinoid tumors. Ann Surg 2004;240(1):117-22.
5. Coit DG. Cancer of the small intestine: In: DeVita VT, Hellman S, Rosenberg SA (Eds): Cancer: Principles and Practice of Oncology, 6th edn. Philadelphia: Lippincott Williams and Wilkins, 2001, p1204.
6. Gore RM, Mehta UK, Berlin JW, Rao V, Newmark GM. Diagnosis and staging of small bowel tumors. Cancer Imaging 2006; 6:209-12.
7. Cobrin GM, Pittman RH, Lewis BS. Increased diagnostic yield of small bowel tumors with capsule endoscopy. Cancer 2006;107(1):22-7.
8. Kim CJ, Day S, Yeh KA. Gastrointestinal stromal tumors: analysis of clinical and pathological factors. Am Surg 2001;67(2):135-7.
9. Yao KA, Talamonti MS, Langella RL, Schindler NM, Rao S, Small W Jr, et al. Primary gastrointestinal sarcomas: analysis of prognostic factors and results of surgical management. Surgery 2000.128(4):604-12.
10. Modlin IM, Tang LH. Approaches to the diagnosis of gut neuroendocrine tumors: the last word (today). Gastroenterology 1997;112(2):583-90.
11. Pantongrag-Brown L, Buetow PC, Carr NJ, Lichtenstein JE, Buck JL. Calcification and fibrosis in mesenteric carcinoid tumor: CT findings and pathologic correlation. AJR Am J Roentgenol 1995;164(2):387–91.
12. Ahmed A, Turner G, King B, Jones L, Culliford D, McCance D, et al. Midgut neuroendocrine tumors with liver metastases. Results of the UKI NETS study. Endocr Relat Cancer 2009: May 20 epub ahead of print.
13. Kulke MH, Mayer RJ. Carcinoid tumors. N Engl J Med. 1999;340(11):858-68.
14. Ha CS, Cho MJ, Allen PK, Fuller LM, Cabanillas F, Cox JD. Primary non-Hodgkin lymphoma of the small bowel. Radiology 1999;211(1):183-87.
15. Romaguera JE, Velasquez WS, Silvermintz KB, Fuller LB, Hagemeister FB, McLaughlin P, et al. Surgical debulking is associated with improved survival in stage I-II diffuse large cell lymphoma. Cancer 1990;66(2):267-72.
16. Turowski GA, Basson MD. Primary malignant lymphoma of the intestine. Am J Surg 1995;169(4):433-41.
17. Daum S, Ullrich R, Heise W, Dederke B, Foss HD, Stein H, et al. Intestinal non-Hodgkin's lymphoma: a multicenter prospective clinical study from the German study group on Intestinal Non- Hodgkin's Lymphoma. J Clin Oncol 2003;21(14):2740-6.
18. Rawls RA, Vega KJ, Trotman BW. Small bowel lymphoma. Current Treat Options Gastroenterol 2003;6(1):27-34.
19. Arai M, Shimizu, Imai Y, Nakatsuru Y, Oda H, Oohara T, Ishikawa T. Mutations of the Ki-ras, p53 and APC genes in adenocarcinomas of the human small intestine. Int J Cancer 1997;70(4):390-5.
20. Wheeler JM, Warren BF, Mortensen NJ, Kim HC, Biddolph SC, Elia G, et al. An insight into the genetic pathway of adenocarcinoma of the small intestine. Gut 2002;50(2):218-23.

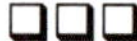

36
CHAPTER

Large Bowel Tumors

Deepa Taggarshe, MD
Vijay K. Mittal, MD

GENERAL CONSIDERATIONS

Cancer of the colon and rectum is the third most common cancer in the United States in both men (after prostate and lung cancer) and women (after breast and lung cancer). The estimated new cases of colon cancer in 2008 in the United States were 108,070 (53,760 men and 54,310 women). The predicted deaths in 2008 due to colon cancer were 49,960 with 24,260 men and 25,700 women predicted to die due to this condition in the United States.[1] According to the World Health Organization, 639,000 deaths occur every year across the world due to colorectal cancer. The incidence of colorectal cancer has decreased at an annual rate of 2.3% from 1998 to 2004 and similarly the mortality due to colorectal cancer decreased at an annual rate of 4.7% from 2002 to 2004.[2]

Tumors of the left side include those of the descending colon, sigmoid colon, rectosigmoid junction, and the rectum, and these account for more than half of all colorectal cancers.

EPIDEMIOLOGY

Some of the risk factors involved with colorectal cancer are as follows:

1. Hereditary risk factors: Colorectal cancer occurs in hereditary or familial forms. Hereditary syndromes of susceptibility to colorectal cancer are characterized by a strong family history, early onset, and the presence of specific genetic defects. Hereditary non-polyposis colorectal cancer (HNPCC) syndrome and familial adenomatous polyposis (FAP) are the two most common and widely researched forms of hereditary colorectal cancer.

   The familial form of colorectal cancer increases the risk for a person if one or more first-degree relatives have colorectal cancer, especially if diagnosed at an early age. The risk increases as the number of family members with colorectal cancer increases. An individual who is a first-degree relative of a patient diagnosed with colorectal cancer at an age younger than 50 is twice as likely as the general population to develop the cancer.[3]
2. Age: The incidence of colorectal cancer increases with age, with more than 90% of the patients diagnosed with colorectal cancer being over 50 years at the age of diagnosis. Colorectal screening programs in the United States are therefore geared towards asymptomatic people over 50 years.
3. Diet: Dietary fiber has been considered to be protective against colorectal cancer, by decreasing intestinal transit time, and acting as a diluent thus decreasing the exposure of the intestinal mucosa to potential carcinogens.[4] Studies have shown strong associations between dietary fiber intake and decreased incidence of colorectal adenomas and carcinomas.[5] A diet high in animal fat and saturated fat increases the risk of colorectal cancer whereas vegetable fiber is protective.
4. Inflammatory bowel disease: Patients with long standing colitis are at an increased risk of colorectal cancer, due to the chronic inflammation of the mucosa predisposing a malignant change. In ulcerative colitis, the risk of cancer is 2% after 10 years, 8% after 20 years, and 18% after 30 years. Patients with colitis due to Crohn's also have an increased risk of cancer. Patients with inflammatory bowel disease are therefore screened with an annual colonoscopy after 8-10 years of the disease.
5. Other factors: Lack of physical exercise, smoking and alcohol, have all been associated with a higher risk of

colorectal cancer. Altered bile metabolism after previous gastrectomy or vagotomy has also been implicated to increase the risk.[6] Patients with ureterosigmoidostomy also have an increased risk of colorectal cancer.[7]

COLORECTAL CARCINOGENESIS

Colorectal carcinogenesis constitutes the transition from normal epithelium to adenoma to invasive carcinoma and is associated with several characteristic genetic changes.

The human colon and rectum consist of millions of crypts and stem cells, which reside at the bottom of the crypts, divide slowly and asymmetrically, so regenerating themselves at the same time as producing the epithelial cells that will populate the rest of the crypts and the mucosal surface. The risk of mutational events increases with each cell division of the stem cells due to errors during DNA replication and chromosomal segregation and this can in turn increase the risk of colorectal carcinogenesis.

The genetic changes involved in the multistep process of colorectal carcinogenesis (adenoma-carcinoma sequence) were first described by Fearon and Vogelstein (Figure 1).[8] The accumulated genetic and epigenetic changes drive the progression to carcinoma and most of these tumors display some form of genomic instability.

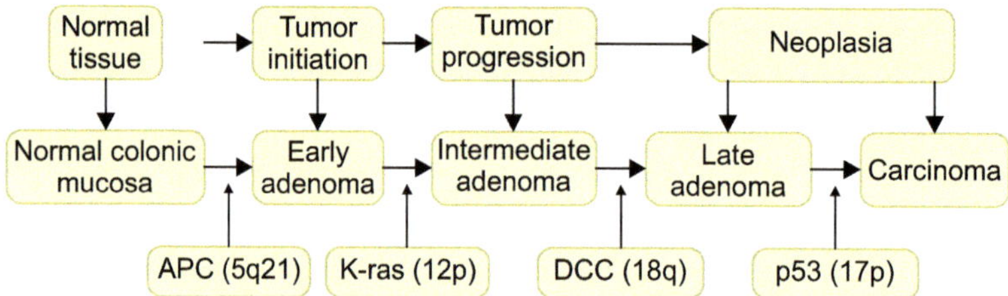

Figure 1: Genetic changes associated with the adenoma-carcinoma sequence in sporadic and hereditary colorectal cancers

The earliest event is the mutation of the adenomatous polyposis coli (APC) gene, which is a tumor suppressor gene located on 5q21. Mutations of the APC gene in colonic epithelial cells, very often resulting in truncated APC proteins very similar to those observed in Familial adenomatous polyposis patients, or deletions are also seen in about 80-85% of sporadic colorectal cancers.[9] APC acts as a "gatekeeper" of epithelial cell proliferation. Abnormal cells with mutations or deletions of both copies of APC accumulate in the crypt leading to the formation of a dysplastic polyp.

Accumulation of further mutations as in K-Ras, p53, and genes on 18q leads to the progression towards cancer. K-Ras is a proto-oncogene involved in intracellular signal transduction via the G-protein pathway. Ras proteins exist in two states: the active guanosine triphosphate (GTP)-bound state and the inactive state bound to guanosine diphosphate (GDP). GTPase-activating protein enhances the intrinsic capacity of Ras proteins to hydrolyze GTP into GDP, thereby returning Ras into the inactive form. Mutant Ras proteins have impaired GTPase activity, which makes them resistant to inactivation, thus leading to increased cellular division. Other genes involved in colorectal cancer include SMAD4, SMAD2, and possibly DCC located on chromosome 18q. The most frequently deleted gene is SMAD4, located on 18q21, encoding a protein, which is involved as a downstream regulator in the transforming growth factor α (TGF-α) signaling pathway that regulates epithelial cell growth and apoptosis and is a critical factor in sustaining the peripheral immunological tolerance that characterizes the microenvironment of many tumors.

Mutations in p53 are present in approximately 60% of colorectal cancers. This occurs late in the adenoma-carcinoma sequence. p53 is a tumor suppressor gene, which under normal conditions acts in response to cellular stress or damage such as DNA damage or hypoxia by either inducing apoptosis or cell cycle arrest.

This remains one of the best-known models for the multistep process of colorectal carcinogenesis. The supporting evidence for the adenoma-carcinoma sequence is as follows:

1. The prevalence of adenomas correlates well with that of carcinomas. The average age of patients diagnosed with adenomas is five to ten years younger than patients diagnosed with carcinoma.[10] A polyp larger than 1 cm has an estimated cancer risk of 8% in 10 years.
2. Benign adenomatous tissue is often found accompanying cancers, suggesting progression of the cancer from the adenomatous cells.
3. Patients with familial adenomatous polyposis (FAP) have a 100% risk of developing colorectal cancers. The adenomas found in sporadic colorectal cancers are histologically identical to those in FAP patients.
4. Larger adenomas are more likely to have cellular atypia than smaller ones and hence have a higher risk for cancer.[8] The risk also increases with the type of polyp; villous adenomas having a higher risk than tubular adenomas. The risk for cancer in a tubular adenoma smaller than 1 cm in diameter is less than 5%, whereas the risk for cancer in a tubular adenoma larger than 2

cm is 35%. A villous adenoma larger than 2 cm in size carries a 50% chance of containing cancer.

5. The incidenceate per 100000 of colorectal cancer has been decreasing with increased colorectal screening and polypectomy.[11]

There is a second pathway, the "mutator phenotype" pathway, which is due to early mutations in DNA repair genes responsible for maintenance of genomic stability (i.e., the DNA mismatch repair genes hMLH1 and hMSH2). This leads to accelerated accumulations of mutations in critical target genes and progression to neoplasia. The phenotype is recognizable by the presence of high frequency variation in microsatellites (regions of short repetitive DNA sequences) or microsatellite instability.[12] This is seen in patients with Hereditary Non-Polyposis Colorectal Cancer (HNPCC) syndrome and in 15% of sporadic colorectal cancers.

Genomic instability is a common feature of human cancer and is an important contributor to carcinogenesis. Two types of genomic instability have been described in colorectal cancer: chromosomal instability (CIN) and microsatellite instability (MSI). CIN is characterized by significant losses and gains of chromosomes or parts thereof and is detected as aneuploidy.

CIN is seen in 60-80% of all colorectal cancers, and has been claimed to be associated with a poor outcome.[13] Microsatellite instability (MSI) is the second major type of genomic instability, which can be detected as alterations in the length of short tandem repeat DNA sequences secondary to defects in the mismatch repair (MMR) system.[12] This is characteristic of tumors from patients with HNPCC syndrome, who have germline mutations in one of the mismatch repair genes, mainly in hMLH1 and hMSH2.[14] It is also seen in approximately 15% of sporadic colorectal cancers, where hMLH1 inactivation by promoter hypermethylation is often found. Sporadic MSI tumors are more often found in the right colon and have been suggested to have a better prognosis in some studies.[15]

COLORECTAL POLYPS

A polyp is any mass projecting into the lumen from the surface of the mucosa of the colon. Polyps can be classified into:

1. Hamartomatous polyps: These are polyps usually seen in childhood and associated with Peutz-Jeghers syndrome, Cronkhite-Canada syndrome, or Cowden's syndrome. These polyps are not usually premalignant and can sometimes present only in adulthood. Symptoms associated with these include bleeding and obstruction due to intussusception (Figure 1) and the treatment is polypectomy. Peutz-Jeghers syndrome is characterized by polyps of the small intestine and to a smaller extent of the colon and rectum. Patients also have pigmented lesions in the mucosa of the cheeks and lips. They have an increased risk of cancer and are therefore screened with a baseline colonoscopy and upper endoscopy at age 20 years, followed by annual flexible sigmoidoscopy thereafter. Cronkhite-Canada syndrome is characterized by gastrointestinal polyposis, alopecia, cutaneous pigmentation, and atrophy of nails. Patients present with diarrhea, vomiting and may develop malabsorption. Surgery is usually reserved for obstruction (Figure 2). Cowden's syndrome is characterized by gastrointestinal polyposis, facial trichilemmomas, breast cancer and thyroid disease.
2. Hyperplastic polyps: Hyperplastic polyps are the most common polyps in the colon. They are generally small and not premalignant and characterized by hyperplasia on histology. Treatment is polypectomy.
3. Inflammatory polyps: These are usually pseudopolyps seen in colitis due to inflammatory bowel disease, amebic or schistosomal colitis. These are removed as they sometimes cannot be distinguished from neoplastic polyps.
4. Neoplastic polyps: Neoplastic polyps or adenomas are premalignant as these polyps have dysplasia. They can be either sessile (flat or without stalk) or pedunculated (with a stalk). They are classified into three types: tubular (with branched tubular glands), villous (with long finger- like projections) and tubule-villous adenomas (with both patterns). Tubular adenomas are the most common and seen in 65 to 80% of patients with polyps, whereas villous adenomas are seen in only 5 to 10%. Tubular adenomas are more likely to be pedunculated and have fewer dysplastic changes, whereas villous adenomas are more likely to be sessile and have severe dysplastic changes. The risk of malignancy depends on the size and type of adenoma. Cancer is likely to be present in about 5% of tubular adenomas, whereas up to 40% of villous adenomas that may harbor cancer. This risk increases to 50% when the villous adenoma is larger than 2 cm.

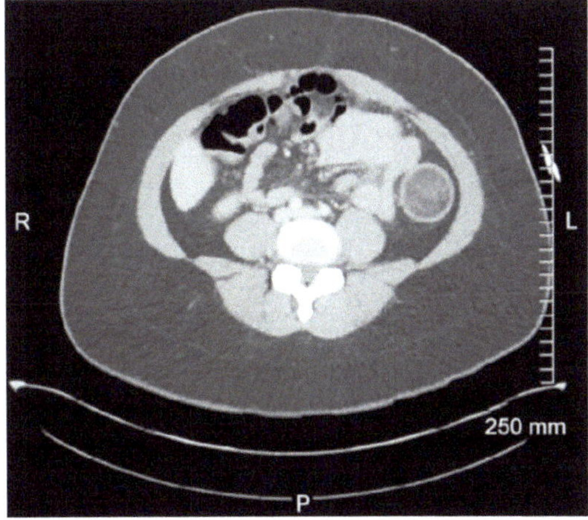

Figure 2: CT of a lipoma in the descending colon with intussusception

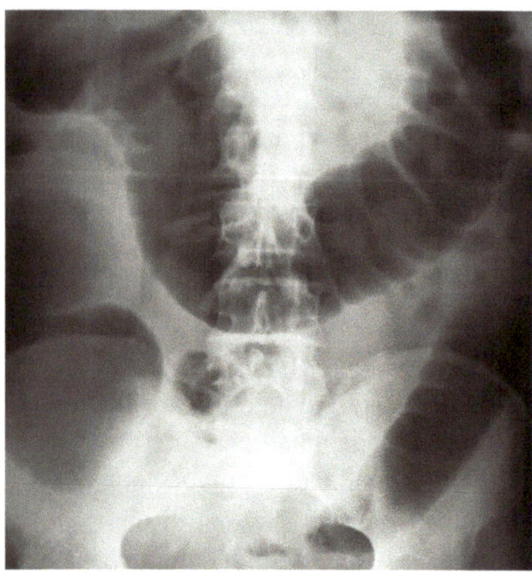

Figure 3: Large bowel obstruction

Treatment of polyps is with polypectomy. In case of pedunculated polyps, this can be performed by snaring with colonoscopy. Sessile polyps can be challenging and are elevated from the deeper layers using saline injection to enable polypectomy by endoscopic measure. If this is not feasible or there is a concern for perforation, a segmental colectomy is usually performed.

As mentioned before, adenomas are premalignant and may sometimes contain cancer. Carcinoma in situ is the condition when the malignant cells are confined to the mucosa. This cancer does not metastasize, and complete polypectomy is adequate.

Invasive cancer on the other hand is the condition in which the malignant cells have extended beyond the mucosa and through the muscularis mucosae of the polyp. These have a higher risk of lymph node involvement and local recurrence and may need more extensive surgery.

Haggitt's criterion classifies polyps with invasive cancer, depends on the level of invasion and is as follows:

- Level 0: Carcinoma in situ cancer limited to the mucosa.
- Level 1: Carcinoma invasion is through the muscularis mucosae and into the submucosa. Remains in the head of the polyp.
- Level 2: Carcinoma invasion is at the level of the polyp neck (the junction between the stalk and head).
- Level 3: Carcinoma invasion of any part of the stalk.
- Level 4: Carcinoma invasion into the bowel wall submucosa below the polyp stalk but above the muscularis.

Sessile polyps with invasive cancer are Level 4 by Haggitt's criteria, as by definition, they do not have a stalk. A polyp with poorly differentiated adenocarcinoma or with lymphovascular invasion has a risk of metastases of greater than 10%. Sessile polyps with invasive cancer have a 10% risk of involvement of lymph nodes. Complete polypectomy with clear margins of 2 mm, is adequate in case of well-differentiated adenomas without lymphovascular invasion, especially in case of pedunculated adenomas with invasion up to level 3 (Figure 2). For well or moderately differentiated sessile polyps in the colon with invasive cancer, with no lymphovascular invasion, prognosis after complete polypectomy depends on the level of invasion. All adenomas with the poor prognostic features and all sessile adenomas with invasive cancer in the rectum must be treated aggressively.

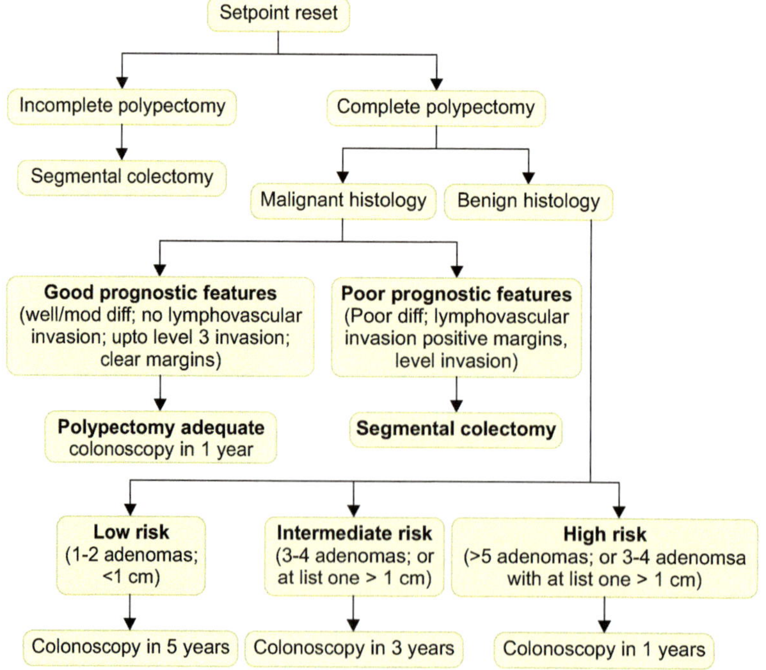

Figure 4: An algorithm showing the management of patients after polypectomy

INHERITED COLORECTAL CANCERS

Although most of the colorectal cancers are sporadic in nature, some are inherited. Two well-known familial syndromes are familial adenomatous polyposis (FAP) and hereditary non-polyposis colorectal cancer (HNPCC).

Familial Adenomatous Polyposis (FAP)

FAP is a rare autosomal dominant syndrome which has been well studied. The genetic abnormality in FAP is a mutation of the APC gene located on 5q21. The gene is expressed in 100% of the patients with the mutation. About 20% of the patients may have a negative family history, and in these cases the abnormality is due to a spontaneously acquired mutation.

Patients have multiple colonic polyps, gastric and duodenal polyps and may also have extra intestinal features such as osteomas (Gardner's syndrome), desmoid tumors, epidermoid cysts, and brain tumors (Turcot's syndrome). Patients will have hundreds to thousands of colonic polyps by puberty. The lifetime risk of colorectal cancer in these patients is 100%. APC gene testing is used to identify family members with the inherited mutation.

Family members with the mutation are then screened for colorectal and other cancers as follows:

- Colorectal cancer: Colonoscopy every year, starting at age 10-12 years.
- Duodenal cancer: Upper GI endoscopy every 1-3 years, starting at age 20-25 years.
- Pancreatic cancer: Abdominal ultrasound periodically.
- Thyroid cancer: Annual physical examination.
- CNS tumors: Annual physical examination.

Treatment once polyps are identified involves surgical excision of the affected colorectal mucosa. The most common recommended surgery is restorative proctocolectomy with ileal pouch-anal anastomosis (IPAA), with the anastomosis fashioned between the ileal pouch and the dentate line of the anal canal. A distal rectal mucosectomy is usually performed to decrease the risk of cancer by removing all the premalignant colonic mucosa. This procedure is usually satisfactory for patients and has a smaller incidence of pouchitis but is technically difficult due to the necessary pelvic dissection, with the accompanying risk of injury to the autonomic nerves. Alternative procedure is a total abdominal colectomy with ileorectal anastomosis. This procedure removes the risk of impotence due to autonomic nerve injury, but patients must be advised about the risk of developing new cancerous polyps in the rectum.

This risk has been shown to be 4%, 5.6%, 7.9%, and 25% at 5, 10, 15, and 20 years after the operation, respectively.[16] These patients should therefore have proper surveillance with proctoscopic examination every six months. COX-2 inhibitors (Sulindac, celecoxib) have been suggested to cause slowing or prevent the development of polyps.[17]

Attenuated FAP is a variant of FAP characterized by fewer colonic adenomas (typically less than 100), a high variability of polyp number, later age of onset of colorectal polyposis (15 years later than patients with classic FAP), later age of onset of colorectal cancer and a more limited expression of the extra-colonic features.[18] APC mutation may be positive in 60%, and then family members must be screened. Treatment involves total abdominal colectomy and ileorectal anastomosis.

Hereditary Non-polyposis Colorectal Cancer (HN-PCC)

HNPCC or Lynch syndrome is the most frequent occurring hereditary colorectal cancer and is seen in 3% of all colorectal cancers. It is characterized by replication errors or unstable microsatellites, due to defects in the mismatch repair systems. Mutations in hMLH1 and hMSH2 account for more than 90% of the mutations seen in patients with HNPCC. Defective mismatch repair facilitates malignant transformation by the accumulation of mutations in genes with key functions in the cell. Patients usually present at a younger age, with right sided tumors, mucinous or poorly differentiated adenocarcinomas, and have increased numbers of synchronous or metachronous lesions. Nevertheless, the prognosis is good after surgery. Extra colonic cancers are also common including gastric, endometrial, ovarian, and renal cancers. Lynch I syndrome has patients with proximal colonic cancers at an early age, whereas Lynch II syndrome is the presence of colorectal cancer and extra colonic cancers, including cancers of endometrial, ovarian, gastric, small intestinal, pancreatic, and ureteral and renal pelvic origin.

Modified Amsterdam Criteria

This is used as clinical criteria to identify patients with HNPCC syndrome. At least three relatives with colon cancer or any HNPCC associated cancer (endometrial, ovarian, gastric, small intestinal, ureteric, renal pelvis) and all the following:

- One affected person is a first-degree relative of the other two affected persons
- Two successive generations affected
- At least one case of cancer diagnosed before age 50 years
- Familial adenomatous polyposis excluded

Screening for HNPCC is as follows:

- Colon cancer: Colonoscopy every year, starting at either age 20 to 25 years or 10 years younger than the youngest age at diagnosis in the family, whichever comes first.

- Endometrial carcinoma: Transvaginal ultrasound or endometrial aspiration biopsy every year, starting at age 25 to 35 years.

Total colectomy with ileorectal anastomosis is recommended once adenomas or a colon carcinoma is diagnosed as there is a 40% risk of developing a second colon cancer. Annual proctoscopy is necessary because the risk of developing rectal cancer remains high. Similarly, prophylactic hysterectomy and bilateral salpingo-oophorectomy should be considered in women who have completed childbearing.

SCREENING FOR COLON CANCER

Colon cancer screening programs rely on early diagnosis and treatment of premalignant adenomas, as it is known that most cancers of the colon arise from adenoma. In addition, screening may diagnose asymptomatic cancers at an early stage, when they can be curable. Screening measures are for the asymptomatic population at-risk for cancer.

Fecal Occult Blood Test (FOBT)— Guaiac Test

This test detects the presence of blood in the stool by the pseudo-peroxidase activity of heme or hemoglobin. Individuals are advised to avoid non-steroidal anti-inflammatory agents, aspirin, Vitamin C, red meat, poultry, fish, and some vegetables prior to testing as these can interact and cause high false-positive and false-negative results. Studies have shown that FOBT has reduced cancer related mortality by up to 33%.[19] Sensitivity of the test varies from 37 to 79%; based on the brand and variant of test used.[20] Only up to 50% of the cancers are diagnosed in most series. Specificity is also variable. However, annual screening with FOBT, especially with the highly sensitive variants, have been shown to detect a majority of colon cancers and is recommended by national guidelines for screening in average-risk adults aged 50 years or above. Individuals who test positive should undergo a follow-up colonoscopy.

Flexible Sigmoidoscopy

This is an endoscopic examination of the distal colon (standard sigmoidoscope length is 60 cm). It has been associated with a 60 to 80% reduction in colorectal cancer mortality.[21,22] Flexible sigmoidoscopy is 60-70% as sensitive as colonoscopy,[23] but is less sensitive in African Americans compared to Whites. Current recommendations stated that flexible sigmoidoscopy performed for screening should be performed every five years by an endoscopist skilled at performing polyp biopsies; and the scope be inserted to 40 cm or beyond.[24] The main limitation of sigmoidoscopy is the inability to examine the proximal colon; hence all patients with polyps or cancers detected by sigmoidoscopy should undergo a colonoscopy.

Colonoscopy

Colonoscopy is the most complete examination of the mucosa of the colon from the appendiceal orifice to the dentate line. It allows biopsy and even treatment by polypectomy. Nevertheless, bowel preparation is critical for accuracy of colonoscopy and patients need sedation as the procedure can be very uncomfortable. Colonoscopy miss rate for large adenomas (≥ 1 cm) has been reported to be 6 to 12%[25,26] and the miss rate for cancer is about 5%.[25] Current recommendations for screening state that a colonoscopy should be performed every 10 years, starting at age 50.

Virtual Colonoscopy

Virtual colonoscopy is minimally invasive and uses computed tomography with image acquisitions of 1-2 mm thin slices and 3D reconstructions. Patients need a bowel preparation and air is then insufflated into the colon via a rectal catheter and both 2D and 3D images generated. Pickhardt et al. reported 94% sensitivity for large adenomas.[27]

Double Contrast Barium Enema (DCBE)

This test evaluates the entire colon by coating the mucosal surface with high-density barium and distending the colon with air introduced through a rectal catheter. It has high sensitivity (90%) for detecting large polyps (>1 cm). No randomized trials have been performed evaluating this test for screening for colon cancers. It requires bowel preparation, is uncomfortable for patients and does not provide for biopsy. DCBE every 5 years is acceptable for patients older than 50 years with an average risk for colon cancer.

In summary, the current national guidelines[24] recommend the following screening options for asymptomatic average risk individuals above 50 years.

1. Tests to detect adenomatous polyps and cancer:
   a. Every 5 years: flexible sigmoidoscopy or
   b. Every 10 years: colonoscopy or
   c. Every 5 years: double-contrast barium enema or
   d. Every 5 years: computed tomographic colonography
2. Tests to detect cancer primarily:
   a. Every year: guaiac-based fecal occult blood test with high test sensitivity for cancer or
   b. Every year: fecal immunochemical test with high cancer sensitivity or
   c. Uncertain interval: stool DNA test with high cancer sensitivity

SPORADIC COLON CANCER

Sporadic colorectal cancer generally occurs in the absence of a significant family history, mostly affects older people (60-80 years), and is usually seen as isolated colonic or rectal tumors.

Presentation

The symptoms of colon cancer can be non-specific and varied. Symptoms depend on the location of the tumor, and the degree of obstruction caused by it. Right sided tumors typically present with anemia, as the liquid stools and the wider diameter preclude obstructive symptoms. With left sided tumors, the most common symptoms are change in bowel habit and rectal bleeding. Although left sided tumors are more likely to cause obstruction, any advanced tumor will cause the same. Tumors of the sigmoid colon can cause colovesical or colovaginal fistulas. With advanced tumors, patients may have an abdominal mass.

Routes of Spread

Direct Spread

This can occur longitudinally, transversely, and radially spreading to organs close by. If located in the retroperitoneal colon, the spread may involve the ureter, duodenum, and posterior abdominal wall. It may also spread to the small intestine and the pelvic organs.

Lymphatic Spread

The cancer spreads initially to the paracolic nodes along the main blood vessels supplying the colon and then onto the para-aortic nodes. The risk of nodal metastases increases with poor differentiation, lymphovascular invasion and depth of invasion. Cancers limited to the bowel wall may have 5 to 20% associated lymph node metastases, whereas tumors that have invaded through the bowel wall or extended to adjacent organs, have >50% risk of associated nodal metastases.

Hematologic Spread

The most common site for distant metastases is the liver, due to spread via the portal system. Up to 37% of patients may have liver metastases at the time of surgery, and 50% are at risk of developing overt disease at some time.[28] Lung metastases are the next most common and seen in 10%.

Staging (TNM)

TNM staging is now widely used for staging colon cancers and is based on the tumor depth, presence, or absence of nodal or distant metastases.

Tumor Stage (T)

- Tx Primary tumor cannot be assessed.
- T0 No evidence of primary tumor.
- Tis Carcinoma in situ; tumor limited to mucosa.
- T1 Tumor invades the submucosa.
- T2 Tumor invades the muscularis propria.
- T3 Tumor invades through the muscularis propria into the subserosa or into non-peritonealized pericolic or perirectal tissues.
- T4 Tumor invades other organs or structures and/or perforates the visceral peritoneum.

Nodal Stage (N)

- Nx Regional lymph nodes cannot be assessed.
- N0 No regional lymph node metastasis.
- N1 Metastasis in 1 to 3 regional lymph nodes.
- N2 Metastasis in 4 or more regional lymph nodes.

Distant Metastasis (M)

- Mx Distant metastasis cannot be assessed. M0 No distant metastasis.
- M1 Distant metastasis.

Stage Grouping

0	Tis, N0, M0
I	T1-2, N0, M0
IIA	T3, N0, M0
IIB	T4, N0, M0
IIIA	T1-2, N1, M0
IIIB	T3-4, N1, M0
IIIC	Any T, N2, M0
IV	Any T, Any N, M1

PREOPERATIVE EVALUATION

Colonoscopy is the gold-standard test since it allows one to obtain a biopsy of the lesion. Even if a cancer is detected by other measures, a colonoscopy should be performed to evaluate the colon for synchronous tumors which may be present in

A CT scan of the abdomen and pelvis and a chest radiograph should be performed to detect any metastases. If a chest radiograph is positive, this can be further evaluated with a chest CT. Preoperative CEA is obtained and is more useful for postoperative follow-up. When patients present with obstruction, a water-soluble contrast enema is useful to understand the anatomic location of obstruction.

TREATMENT

Colon Resection

A curative resection entails complete removal of the primary cancer with anatomically complete lymphadenectomy of the regional nodes and en-bloc resection of any involved adjacent organs. About 80 to 90% of the patients are fit for a curative resection. The length of bowel resected depends on the vascular supply, as the lymphatics accompany the arterial supply. To achieve resection of the pericolic and paracolic nodes, the main vascular pedicles need to be ligated and divided. If this cannot be achieved, a palliative procedure may be considered, including colonic stenting for obstructive left sided tumors.

Tumors of the cecum and ascending colon are managed by a right hemicolectomy, which entails division of the ileocolic, right colic and right branch of the middle colic arteries. An extended right hemicolectomy may be used for hepatic flexure or proximal transverse colon tumors and involves extension of the standard right hemicolectomy to include division of the main middle colic vessel at its base. Transverse colectomy involves division of the middle colic vessel and resection of transverse colon with a colo-colonic anastomosis, but an extended right hemicolectomy with an ileo-colonic anastomosis is safer and preferred. For splenic flexure and descending colon tumors, a left hemicolectomy is performed, dividing the left branches of the middle colic, the left colic and the first branches of the sigmoid arteries. Sigmoid colectomy is used for sigmoid colon tumors and requires division of the sigmoid branches of the inferior mesenteric artery. Total abdominal colectomy which entails removal of the entire colon from the ileum to the rectum, with an ileorectal anastomosis is performed in patients with multiple tumors, HNPCC or rarely with obstructive sigmoid colon cancer.

In case of obstruction, the patients must be resuscitated and taken for an emergent laparotomy. If the tumor is in the right side, a right hemicolectomy with primary anastomosis can be performed in most cases, even with an unprepared bowel. Management of left sided tumors can be challenging. Traditionally, due to the higher risk of anastomotic leak with a primary anastomosis, these patients were managed by resection of the colon with the cancer, suture closure of the distal colon (sigmoid or rectum) and the creation of an end colostomy from the proximal colon (Hartmann's procedure). Recently, however the trend is towards a subtotal colectomy (removal of tumor and the entire colon proximal to it, with an ileosigmoid anastomosis) or a left hemicolectomy (performed after resection of the colon with cancer, and irrigation of the proximal colon with warm saline inserted through a catheter in the appendix or ileum).

Surgical Management of Metastases

About 20% of the patients with liver metastases can have a potentially curative resection. Survival in these patients is improved (20-40% at 5 years). Segmental resection of pulmonary metastases is also associated with 5-year survival rates of 20-40%.

Laparoscopic Colectomy

The results from three large randomized multicenter trials (COST, CLASICC and COLOR) show that the overall and disease-free survival rates of laparoscopic colectomy are similar to those achieved by open colectomy.[29-31]

Furthermore, laparoscopic colectomy resulted in shorter hospital stays, earlier return of bowel function and better pain management. The national guidelines do suggest that laparoscopic colectomy for cancer is acceptable in the hands of experienced surgeons who adhere to the surgical principles of colon resection for cancer.

LYMPH NODE ASSESSMENT

Lymph node assessment is not only important for accurate staging but plays an important role in further management as patients with nodal metastases from colon cancer need further adjuvant chemotherapy. The National Comprehensive Cancer Network (NCCN) recommends that a minimum of 12 nodes must be examined microscopically to determine the nodal status accurately. If fewer nodes are examined, this may lead to understaging of the patients.

ADJUVANT TREATMENT

Stage I and II: Majority of these patients are cured with a surgical resection. Few patients with stage I disease develop local or distant recurrence and hence adjuvant chemotherapy does not improve survival. More than 40% of Stage II patients, who have had a curative resection die from the disease. Adjuvant chemotherapy has therefore been recommended for few Stage II patients with poor prognostic features such as poorly differentiated tumors, lymphovascular invasion, bowel obstruction, <12 lymph nodes examined or T4 lesions.

Stage III: Current recommendations are that all medically fit Stage III patients should receive 5 FU based adjuvant chemotherapy. Treatment options include 5FU + leucovorin alone or FOLFOX 5FU+Leucovorin+Oxaliplatin. FOLFOX regime was shown to have improved disease-free survival over 5FU and Leucovorin by the MOSAIC trial.[32]

Stage IV: Chemotherapy regimens include FOLFOX with Bevacizumab, or FOLFIRI (5FU, leucovorin, irinotecan) with Bevacizumab (Figure 3).

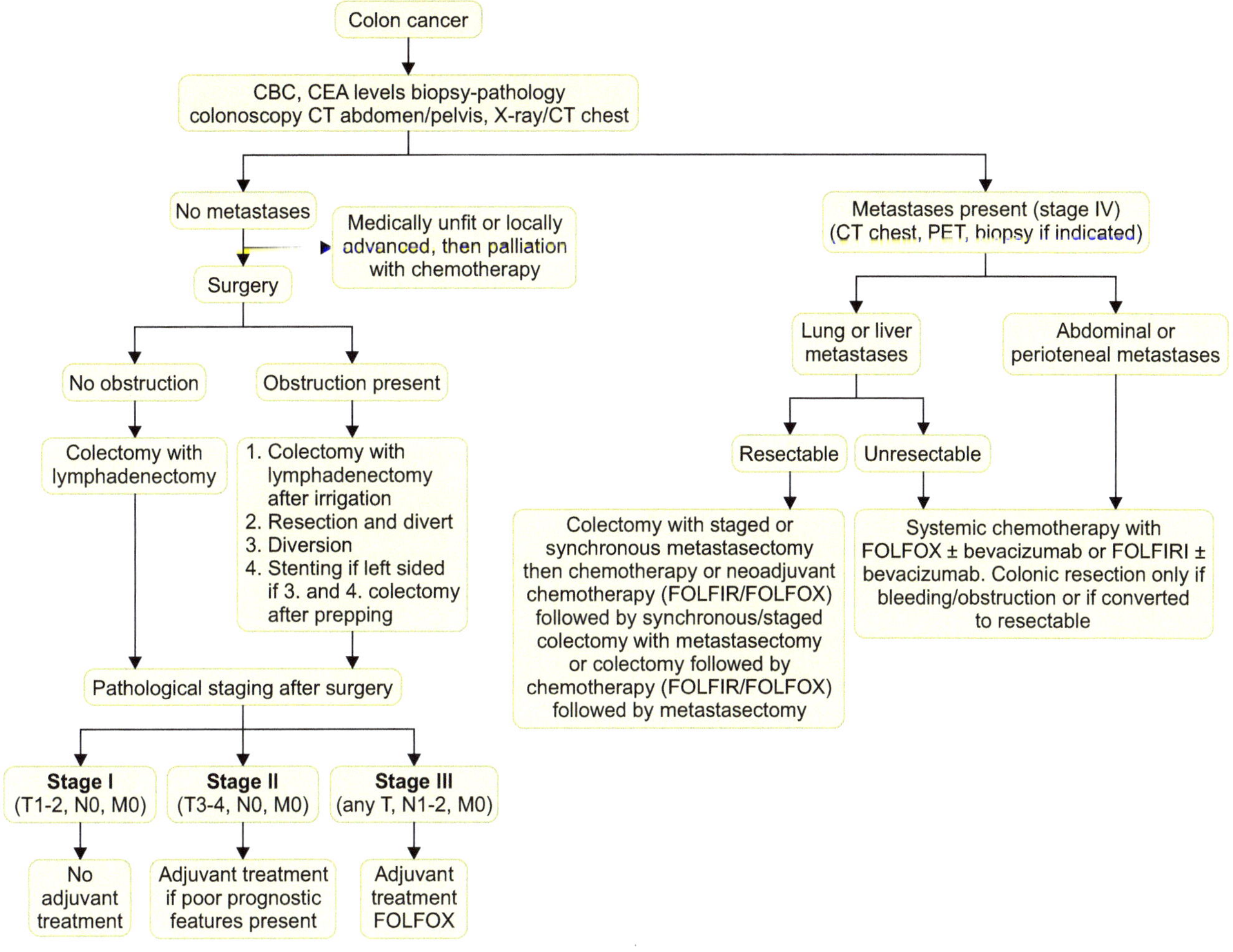

Figure 5: An algorithm showing the management of patients with colon cancer

SPECIAL CONSIDERATION FOR TREATMENT OF PATIENTS WITH MICROSATELLITE INSTABILITY/ DEFICIENT MISMATCH REPAIR TUMORS

Deficient mismatch repair tumors are characterized by many errors in DNA replication and of being highly immunogenic. However, about half of these tumors are susceptible to immune checkpoint inhibitors. Therefore, the treatment for patients with microsatellite instability tumors of deficient mismatch repair tumors includes an immune checkpoint inhibitor if they have not received it already. The immune checkpoint inhibitor can be given as either a monotherapy or a combination therapy. Monotherapy includes nivolumab or pembrolizumab which target the programmed cell death 1 (PD-1) receptor. If one of the drugs does not improve the cancer progression, then the other drugs should be tried. Combination therapy includes nivolumab and ipilimumab which is a monoclonal antibody against cytotoxic T lymphocyte antigen 4 (CTLA-4), another immune checkpoint. Currently, no randomized trials exist directly comparing these two treatment options.

PROGNOSIS

TNM staging and 5-year survival rates:[33]

Stage I	70-95%
Stage II	54-65%
Stage III	39-60%
Stage IV	0-16%

SURVEILLANCE

- History and physical: Every 3-6 months for 2 years; then every 6 months for a total of 5 years.
- CEA: Every 3-6 months for 2 years, then every 6 months for a total of 5 years.

- CT Chest/Abd/Pelvis: Every year for 3 years in patients with high risk of recurrence.
- Colonoscopy: In 1 year.
- PET scan: Not routinely recommended.

REFERENCES

1. Jemal A, Siegel R, Ward E, Hao Y, Xu J, Murray T, et al. CancerStatistics, 2008. CA Cancer J Clin 2008;58(2):71-96.
2. Toms JR. Cancer Stats Monograph 2004. Cancer ResearchUK: London 2004.
3. St John DJ, McDermott FT, Hopper JL, Debney EA, Johnson WR, Hughes ES. Cancer risk in relatives of patients with common colorectal cancer. Ann Intern Med 1993;118(10):785-90.
4. Burkitt DP. Epidemiology of cancer of the colon and rectum. Cancer 1971;28(1):3-13.
5. Bingham SA, Day NE, Luben R, Ferrari P, Slimani N, Norat T, et al. European Prospective Investigation into Cancer and Nutrition. Dietary fibre in food and protection against colorectal cancer. The European Prospective Investigation into Cancer and Nutrition (EPIC): an observational study. Lancet 2003;361(9368):1496-501.
6. Bundred NJ, Whitfield BC, Stanton E, Prescott RJ, Davies GC, Kingsnorth AN. Gastric surgery and the risk of subsequent colorectal cancer. Br J Surg 1985;72(8):618-9.
7. Woodhouse C. British Society for Gastroenterology; Association of Coloproctology for Great Britain and Ireland. Guidelines for monitoring of patients with ureterosigmoidostomy. Gut2002;51(Suppl V):v15-6.
8. Vogelstein B, Fearon ER, Hamilton SR, Kern SE, Preisinger AC, Leppert M, et al. Genetic alterations during colorectal -tumor development. N Eng J Med 1988;319:525-32.
9. Smith KJ, Johnson KA, Bryan TM, Hill DE, Markowitz S, Willson JK, et al. The APC gene product in normal and tumor cells. Proc Natl Acad Sci USA 1993;90(7):2846-50.
10. Muto T, Bussey HJ, Morson BC. The evolution of the cancer of the colon and rectum. Cancer 1975;36(6):2251-70.
11. Mandel JS, Church TR, Bond HJ, Ederer F, Geisser MS, Mongin SJ, et al. The effect of fecal occult-blood screening on the incidence of colorectal cancer. N Eng J Med 2000;343(22):1603-7.
12. Toft NJ, Arends MJ. DNA mismatch repair and colorectal cancer. J Pathol 1998;185(2):123-9.
13. Garrity MM, Burgart LJ, Mahoney MR, Windschitl HE, Salim M, Wiesenfeld M, et al. North Central Cancer Treatment Group. Prognostic value of proliferation, apoptosis, defective DNA mismatch repair, and p53 overexpression in patients with resected Dukes' B2 or C cancer: A North Central Cancer Treatment Group Study. J Clin Oncol 2004;22(9):1572-82.
14. Lynch HT, Smyrk T. Hereditary nonpolyposis colorectal cancer (Lynch Syndrome). An updated review. Cancer 1996;78(6):1149-67.
15. Parc Y, Gueroult S, Mourra N, Serfaty L, Flejou JF, Tiret E, et al. Prognostic significance of microsatellite instability determined by immunohistochemical staining of MSH2 and MLH1 in sporadic T3N0M0 colon cancer. Gut 2004;53(3):371-5.
16. Heiskanen I, Jarvinen HJ. Fate of the rectal stump after colectomy and ileorectal anastomosis for familial adenomatous polyposis. Int J Colorectal Dis 1997;12(1):9-13.
17. Steinbach G, Lynch PM, Phillips RK, Wallace MH, Hawk E, Gordon GB, et al. The effect of celecoxib, a cyclooxygenase-2 inhibitor, in familial adenomatous polyposis. N Engl J Med2000;342(26): 1946-52.
18. Knudsen AL, Bisgaard ML, Bulow S. Attenuated familial adenomatous polyposis (AFAP). A review of the literature. Fam Cancer 2003;2(1):43-55.
19. Mandel JS, Bond JH, Church TR, Snover DC, Bradley GM, Schuman LM, et al. Reducing mortality from colorectal cancer by screening for fecal occult blood. Minnesota Colon Cancer Control Study. N Engl J Med 1993;328(19):1365-71.
20. Allison JE, Tekawa IS, Ransom LJ, Adrain AL. A comparison of fecal occult-blood tests for colorectal-cancer screening. N Engl J Med 1996;334(3):155-9.
21. Selby JV, Friedman GD, Quesenberry CP Jr, Weiss NS. A case- control study of screening sigmoidoscopy and mortality from colorectal cancer. N Engl J Med 1992;326(10):653-7.
22. Newcomb PA, Norfleet RG, Storer BE, Surawicz TS, Marcus PM. Screening sigmoidoscopy and colorectal cancer mortality. J NatlCancer Inst 1992;84(20):1572-5.23. Imperiale TF, Wagner DR, Lin CY, Larkin GN, Rogge JD, Ransohoff DF. Risk of advanced proximal neoplasms in asymptomatic adults according to the distal colorectal findings. N Engl J Med 2000;343(3):169-74.
23. Lieberman DA, Weiss DG, Bond JH, Ahnen DJ, Garewal H, Chejfec G. Use of colonoscopy to screen asymptomatic adults for colorectal cancer. Veteran Affairs Cooperative Study Group 380. N Engl J Med 2000;343(3):162-8.

24. Levin B, Lieberman DA, McFarland B, Smith RA, Brooks D, Andrews KS, et al. American Cancer Society Colorectal Cancer Advisory Group; US Multi-Society Task Force; American College of Radiology Colon Cancer Committee. Screening and Surveillance for the Early Detection of colorectal cancer and adenomatous polyps, 2008: a joint guideline from the American Cancer Society, The US Multi-Society Task Force on Colorectal cancer and the American college of Radiology. CA Cancer J Cli2008;58(3):130-60.
25. Rex DK, Cutler CS, Lemmel GT, Rahmani EY, Clark DW, Helper DJ, et al. Colonoscopic miss rates of adenomas determined by back-to-back colonoscopies. Gastroenterology 1997;112(1):24-8.
26. Pickhardt PJ, Nugent PA, Mysliwiec PA, Choir JR, Schindler WR. Location of adenomas missed by optical colonoscopy. Ann InternMed 2004;141(5):352-9.
27. Pickhardt PJ, Choi JR, Hwang I, Butler JA, Puckett ML, Hildebrandt HA, et al. Computed tomographic virtual colonoscopy to screen for colorectal neoplasia in asymptomatic adults. N Engl J Med 2003;349(23):2191-200.
28. Cedermark BJ, Shultz SS, Bakshi S, Parthasarathy KL, Mittelman A, Evans JT. The value of liver scan in the follow-up study of patients with adenocarcinoma of the colon and rectum. Surg Gynecol Obstet 1977;144(5):745-8.
29. Jayne DG, Guillou PJ, Thorpe H, Quirke P, Copeland J, Smith AM, et al. UK MRC CLASICC Trial Group. Randomized trial of laparoscopic- assisted resection of colorectal carcinoma: 3-year results of the UK MRC CLASICC Trial Group. J Clin Oncol2007;25(21):3061-8.
30. The Clinical Outcomes of Surgical Therapy Study Group. A Comparison of laparoscopically assisted and open colectomy for colon cancer. N Engl J Med 2004;350(20):2050-9.
31. The Colon Cancer Laparoscopic or Open Resection Study Group.Survival after laparoscopic surgery versus open surgery for colon cancer: long term outcome of a randomised clinical trial. Lancet Oncol 2009;10(1):44-52.
32. Andre T, Boni C, Mounedji-Boudiaf L, Navarro M, Tabernero J, Hickish T, et al. Multicenter International Study of Oxaliplatin/5-Fluorouracil/Leucovorin in the Adjuvant treatment of Colon Cancer (MOSAIC) Investigators. Oxaliplatin, Fluorouracil, and Leucovorin as Adjuvant Treatment for Colon Cancer. N Engl J Med 2004;350(23):2343-51.
33. Greene FL, Page DL, Fleming, et al. AJCC Cancer Staging Manual (6th ed). New York: Springer-Verlag, 2002.

❑❑❑

37

CHAPTER

Anorectal Diseases

Vijay K. Mittal, MD
Alasdair MacKendrick, MD
Jasneet Singh Bhullar, MD

RECTAL DISEASES

Rectal Cancer

Cancers that occur within 12 cm of the anal verge, on a rigid proctoscopy are considered rectal cancer. They resemble colon cancer in their presentation, pathogenesis, and risk factors. Treatment of rectal cancer differs from colon cancer because of its location in the pelvis, proximity to the genitourinary organs, and its innervation which has a multitude of functions. Additionally, it is important to consider the location of the tumor within the rectum and the functional status of the sphincter during the treatment of rectal cancer.[1]

Anatomy

The rectum is 15 cm in length and extends from the recto sigmoid junction to the anal canal. The recto sigmoid junction is marked by the line fusing the three taenia coli into a complete circumferential muscular tube, and the anal canal is marked by the muscles of the pelvic floor. The rectum is intraperitoneal in the proximal two thirds and extraperitoneal in the lower one third. It is fixed posteriorly by Waldeyer's fascia and laterally by the lateral stacks.[2] In men, the rectum lies posterior to the Denonvillers fascia and in women it is clothed by the recto uterine pouch of Douglas. On the inside it has three valves of Houston, the inner valve corresponds to the anterior peritoneal reflection.

The rectum receives its blood supply from the superior hemorrhoidal artery and partly by the middle rectal artery when present. The venous drainage follows the arterial supply and empties in the inferior mesenteric vein.[3] The lymphatic drainage from the upper, middle, and lower rectum goes to the inferior mesenteric lymph nodes. The lymphatic drainage from the lower rectum can also travel along the middle-inferior hemorrhoidal vessels, which runs along the middle sacral vessels or via the recto uterine pouch to the inguinal lymph nodes and then to the para-aortic lymph nodes.[4-6]

The nerves around the rectum include the sympathetic and parasympathetic nerves which form a plexus around the rectum.

Diagnosis and Evaluation

A thorough history and physical exam must be done in all patients with suspected colon cancer. Rectal cancer resembles colon cancer in its presentation. History of changing bowel habits, narrow caliber stool, bloody bowel movement, weight loss, incontinence, painful defecation, and tenesmus all point to the possibility of an underlying colorectal cancer. The later three symptoms are more specific for rectal cancer and signify advanced disease. Additionally, these patients may present with palpable lumps at other body sites. Patients with metastatic disease to the lungs may present with cough, shortness of breath, effusions etc. Liver metastasis presents as jaundice, hepatomegaly, or liver failure. Family history of colon cancer may be present and point to a genetic cause of the cancer in as many as 20% of patients.[7] Inflammatory bowel disease also predisposes patients to colon cancer, this is true with both ulcerative colitis and Crohn's disease.[8] History of smoking also increases the risk of colon cancer. A complete physical must be done, and attention must be given in particular to the abdominal examination, or digital rectal exam (DRE).

On DRE attention must be given to any palpable lumps noting their size, location, mobility/fixity to the surrounding structures, and any palpable lymph nodes. Sphincter tone and distance from the anal verge or the dentate line are very important in determining the treatment. Distance from anal verge or dentate line is best done by rigid proctoscopy.[9] Inguinal nodes must also be assessed.

A complete colonoscopy must be completed in any patient suspected of having a colorectal mass. This will help find other synchronous colon cancer and provide tissue for diagnosis. For small lesions, the excision of the mass during colonoscopy may be therapeutic.

A CT scan of the chest, abdomen, and pelvis must be done in all patients to exclude metastatic disease. It is also important to evaluate for advanced disease by determining the extent of local invasion into the surrounding structures. If adenopathy is seen on CT scan, it is presumed to be malignant as benign adenopathy is rarely seen around the rectum.[10]

Endoluminal ultrasound or MRI (endo-coil or surface coil) helps evaluate the disease penetration into the bowel wall and perirectal lymph nodes. Ultrasound and MRI are equally sensitive, but ultrasound is more specific than MRI in evaluating the depth of invasion into the rectal wall. MRI may be of value in patients with anal stenosis and when endoluminal ultrasound may not be possible. A surface coil MRI may yield the same information in such patients. Endoluminal ultrasound usually under-stages the T lesion and over-stages the N lesion.[10]

Staging on the basis of endoluminal ultrasound

T1	Invasion confined to the mucosa and submucosa
T2	Penetration of the muscularis mucosa but not the perirectal fat
T3	Invasion of perirectal fat
T4	Invasion of adjacent organs
N0	No perirectal lymph node enlargement
N1	Enlarged perirectal lymph nodes

Labs including CBC, BMP, LFT, and CEA must be ordered on all patients. CEA helps in follow-up of these patients. Persistence of elevated CEA after surgery means residual disease. If CEA was normalized after surgery, future rising CEA is a predictor of cancer recurrence after surgery.

TNM classification of rectal cancer		
T stage Tis: In situ carcinoma T1: Invading the submucosa T2: Invading the muscularis propria T3: Invading the muscularis propria into the preperitoneal fat T4: • T4a: Invading the surface of visceral peritoneum • T4b: Invading adjacent organs	N Stage N1: • N1a: 1 lymph node involved • N1b: 2-3 lymph nodes involved N2: • N2a: 2-6 lymph nodes involved • N2b: 7 or more lymph nodes involved	M Stage M1: • M1a: Metastasis to 1 organ or other site (liver, lung, ovary, non-regional site • M1b: Metastasis to more than 1 other site or organ

Based on the above evaluation the patients are classified into clinical stages and treatment determined according to the AJCC/TNM classification.

Stage 1	T1N0M0 T2N0M0
Stage 2 a	T3N0M0
Stage 2 b	T4aN0M0
Stage 2 c	T4bN0M0
Stage 3 a	T1-2N1M0 T1N2aM0
Stage 3 b	T3-T4aN1 M0 T2-3N2aM0 T1N2bM0
Stage 3 c	T4aN2aM0 T3-4aN2bM0 T4bN1M0
Stage 4a	Any T Any N M1a
Stage 4 b	Any T Any N M1b

Treatment

The goal of rectal cancer treatment is to eradicate the primary tumor along with the adjacent meso-rectal tissue and the lymph nodes.[11-13] The patient will ideally have continuity of the gastrointestinal tract established with adequate oncological clearance and intact sphincter mechanism, otherwise the patient will receive a permanent colostomy.

Removal of the primary tumor is considered adequate with at least a 5 cm proximal and a 2 cm distal resection margin. A critical step in reducing local recurrence is by creating a negative circumferential or radial margin, which is a 4 cm edge of meso-rectal excision beyond the tumor. A positive circumferential margin is associated with higher local failure rates. Additionally, at least 12 lymph nodes must be removed for the specimen to be adequately staged. Less than 12 lymph nodes removed means that the cancer will be undersaged.[14]

Tumors Amenable to Local Excision

Local treatment involves excision of the tumor with adequate margins, trans-anally or via TEM/ TAMIS. It is not a preferred treatment but may be used in patients with contraindication for major laparotomy or in patients with extensive disease for local disease control. For a patient to be eligible for local excision of the tumor, the following criteria must be met.[15]

1. Lesion must be within 8 cm of the anal verge.
2. Lesion must be less than 3 cm in greatest dimension.
3. Lesion must involve less than 30% of the circumference of the bowel wall.
4. Lesion must be T1.
5. Lesion should not have any enlarged nodes on ultrasound (N0).
6. It must be a well differentiated tumor without any lymph or vascular invasion.
7. Margins must be clear (>3 mm).

Lesions seen on colonoscopy may be removed by snaring. Polyps can be adequately removed by colonoscopy, and if it does not have any high-risk features (i.e., poorly differentiated, positive margins, lymph or vascular invasion, not Sm3 type) removal can be therapeutic.[16]

Surgical options available for local disease control involve full thickness surgical excision of the rectal wall, with or without approximation of the edges. These options include the following:

1. Kraske Approach: Posterior midline approach involves the division of the sphincter in the midline and the division of the coccyx. It provides exposure to the posterior rectum. Lesions on the anterior wall can be approached by dividing the posterior wall and then arriving at the anterior wall from within the lumen. Lesions up to 3 to 5 cm above the dentate line (middle and distal rectum) can be approached by this approach.[17]

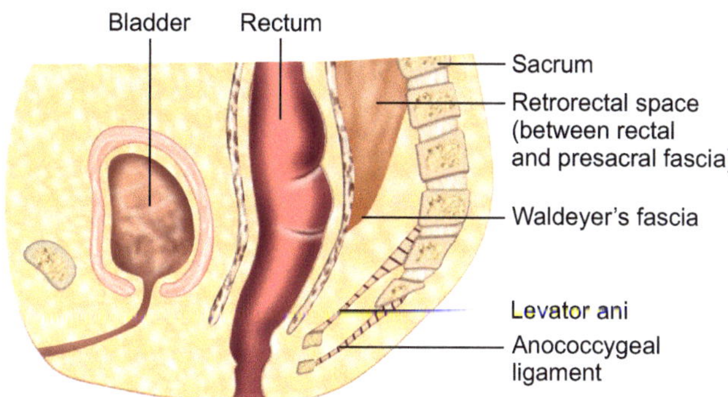

Figure 1: Kraske's approach for rectal lesions.

1. **York Mason Approach:** An oblique incision which includes the gluteus maximus muscle and the sphincter muscles. This approach requires a thorough approximation at the end of the surgery. It may provide access comparable to Kraske's approach.
2. **TEM/TAMIS:** Trans-anal endoscopic microsurgery (TEM) and Trans-anal minimally invasive surgery (TAMIS) are two techniques that have largely replaced other local surgical techniques.
   a. TEM uses a Wolf operating proctoscope, a binocular microscope, and CO2 insufflations with long operating instruments. For posterior lesions, the patient is placed in a prone jack-knife position. For anterior lesions, the patient is placed in a lithotomy position. For lesions on one side, the patient is placed with the involved side facing up.
   b. TAMIS uses a single incision surgery port and standard operating laparoscopic surgery instruments for the same procedure.

Low Anterior Resection with Meso-rectal Excision

Total meso-rectal excision is indicated for all mid or low rectal cancers with preservation of sphincter function. Appropriate bowel preparation such as GoLYTELY should be administered the day before surgery. Preoperatively, a single dose of broad-spectrum antibiotic is administered. After induction of general anesthesia, the patient is placed in a lithotomy position with their legs in padded stirrups at a 30-degree abduction. A bean bag is used to secure the patient, and shoulder gel pads are applied to prevent any pressure sores. An orogastric tube is placed to prevent gastric distention and is removed at the end of surgery. The urinary and ureteric catheter are placed to decompress the bladder and help in intraoperative localization of the ureter. Intraoperative rigid proctoscopy may be performed to determine the distal extent of the cancer. The surgery may be done laparoscopically or via laparotomy. The common arrangement of trocars in the surgical procedure is shown in Figure 2.

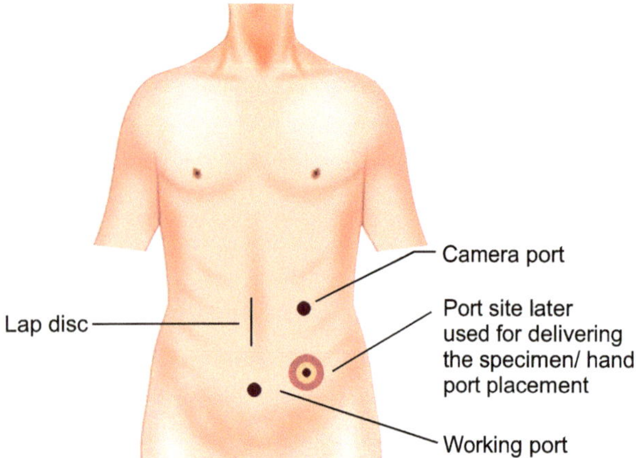

Figure 2: Port placement for laparoscopic colectomy.

After introduction of trocars, diagnostic laparoscopy is done to check for the feasibility of laparoscopic surgery. Presence of extensive adhesions from previous surgeries, invasion of surrounding structures, or aberrant anatomy (i.e., horseshoe kidney or pelvic kidney) may preclude laparoscopic surgery and early conversion is recommended. If laparoscopic surgery is feasible, the left colon is mobilized first to create the necessary length for a tension free anastomosis. The rectum and the sigmoid colon are then mobilized until an adequate margin free of tumor can be achieved. A 2 cm distal margin is considered adequate[5]. It may be necessary to divide the colon using an endo GIA stapler to mobilize the colon posteriorly from the pre sacral fascia (Waldeyer's). Next, a small vertical incision is placed on the trocar in the left iliac fossa, and the pneumoperitoneum is released. The colon is delivered through the incision and a wound protection device (Alexis) is used to isolate the wound from the bowel. Then using a TA stapler, the rectum is divided, and the specimen is delivered. The anastomosis is then performed to an EEA stapler in an end-to-end fashion. The quality of anastomosis is suggested by the following:

1. Complete doughnuts in the EEA stapler.
2. **Leak test:** The pelvis is filled with fluid, a rigid proctoscope is introduced from below, and air is insufflated to check for any leaks.
3. **Flexible colonoscopy:** Direct visualization of anastomosis.

At this point the colon is reposited in the abdomen and Alexis is removed. The wound is closed in layers. A drain is not used in the procedure. In the case of a patient with very low anastomosis or a previously irradiated pelvis, a diverting loop ileostomy is used to protect the anastomosis.

J pouch (transverse coloplasty) may be used to provide a reservoir to decrease the number of bowel movements and prevent incontinence.[18]

At the end of the procedure, preoperative ureteral catheters are removed and inspected for intactness, especially the catheter tip. The foley catheter is left in place for at least 24 hours after surgery.

In case of a laparotomy (open technique), the surgical steps are the same, but the incision tends to be larger, extending from the pubic symphysis to above the umbilicus.

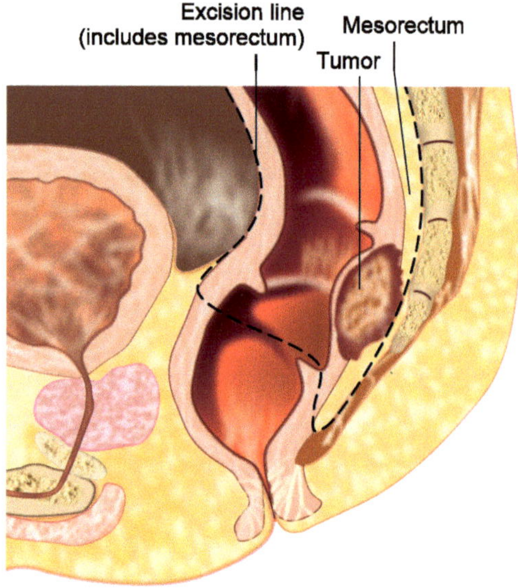

Figure 3: Total meso-rectal excision (TME).

A number of trials (CLASSIC[19], COLOR[20]) have failed to demonstrate any inferiority of laparoscopic surgery compared to laparotomy in terms of oncological outcome, survival, or tumor clearance. Laparoscopic surgery has proven beneficial to patients due to shorter hospital stay, less pain, and quicker return of bowel function. Prospective trials like the Barcelona trial demonstrated that laparoscopic surgery has a modest survival advantage, significantly faster recovery, and shorter hospital stay.[21]

Abdominoperineal Resection (Miles' Operation)[22]

Abdominoperineal resection (APR) was first described by Czerny in 1864 and later modified by Miles which is its current state. Miles' operation is meant for low rectal cancers which involve the pelvic floor, in patients with involvement of the anal sphincter, with recurrent rectal cancer after a previous LAR, or with persistent cancer after chemo-radiation.

Appropriate bowel preparation such as GOLYTELY should be administered the day before surgery. Preoperatively, a single dose of broad-spectrum antibiotic is administered. The permanent colostomy site is marked by an entero-stomal nurse preoperatively to ensure the best placement of the colostomy. After induction of general anesthesia, the patient is placed in a lithotomy position with the legs in padded stirrups at a 30-degree abduction. The coccyx is placed near the end of the table and elevated with a stack of towels. A nasogastric tube is placed to prevent gastric distention, and a urinary catheter is placed to decompress the bladder. The rectum is irrigated with povidone-iodine (Betadine) solution until clear. The anus is closed with a 0-silk purse-string suture.

After evaluating the extent of disease and ruling out metastasis to the peritoneum, the sigmoid colon is mobilized along the lateral visceral fascia covering the meso-sigmoid along the white line of Toldt. Then the medial visceral fascia is divided to mobilize the colon. Next, the presacral plane is developed at the level of sacral promontory and then extended to the other side. Finally, the lateral meso-rectal connections to the pelvic wall are divided, and the mobilization of the rectum is continued in the presacral plane. The inferior mesenteric artery is ligated at its origin after the left colic branch. The colon is transacted using an endo GI A stapler. A 2 cm skin opening is made at the site previously marked by the entero-stomal nurse to bring out the end colostomy.

Dissection is continued on the perineum starting in the ischiorectal fossa and then deepened to the level of the pelvic diaphragm. Branches of the inferior hemorrhoidal artery are ligated during the dissection. The distal sigmoid rectum and the anal canal are delivered through the perineal incision.

Neoadjuvant Therapy for Resectable Non-metastatic Rectal Cancer[23]

All patients with rectal cancer stage 11a and above need neoadjuvant therapy for better loco- regional control. Getting a good margin may be technically challenging in rectal cancer due the location of the rectum within the pelvis, absence of serosa, and proximity of the rectum to other important pelvic structures. Currently, preoperative chemotherapy, radiation therapy, and postoperative chemotherapy is recommended. 50-60% percent of patients undergo down staging and about 20% have complete response to chemotherapy.[24]

Recommendations on Follow-Up

All patients with colorectal cancer must be evaluated every 3 to 6 months for the first 2 years with history exams, physical exams, and repeat CEA levels. After 2 years, these patients can be evaluated every 6 months for a total of 5 years. Additionally, all patients need an annual CT scan of their chest, abdomen, and pelvis for 5 years (Figure 4). Postoperatively, repeat colonoscopy is done at 1 year. If normal, follow-up colonoscopy is done in 3 years, followed by every 5 years afterwards.[25] A proctoscopy is recommended for all patients with low anterior resection at every office visit to look for local recurrences.

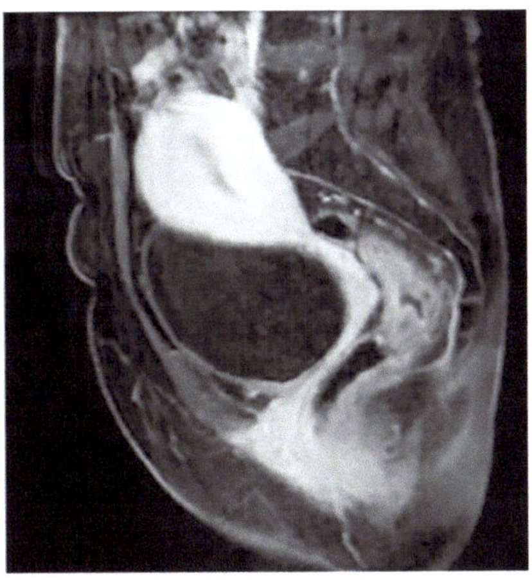

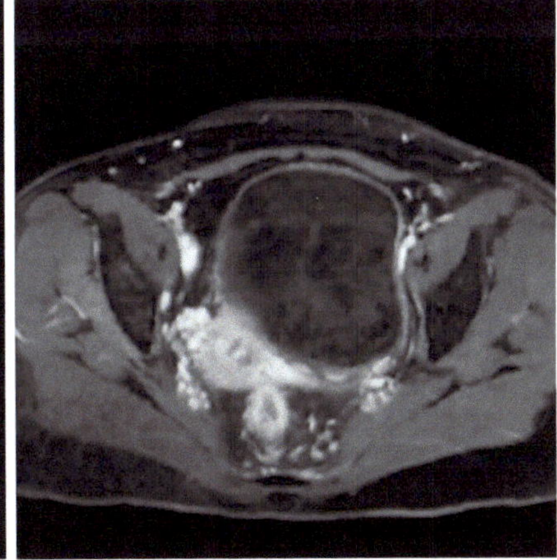

Figure 4: MRI showing residual rectal cancer after neoadjuvant chemoradiation therapy. The patient also has a large uterus fibroid.

ANAL DISEASES

Anal Cancer

Anal cancer is relatively uncommon and accounts for 3% to 5% of all large bowel malignancies. It has a slight male preponderance and is more common in the African American population. Its incidence is increasing in HIV positive people engaging in receptive anal intercourse. Squamous cell cancer is by far the most common variant, followed by the cloacogenic variant. Adenocarcinoma is the least common histological type.[26]

Anatomy

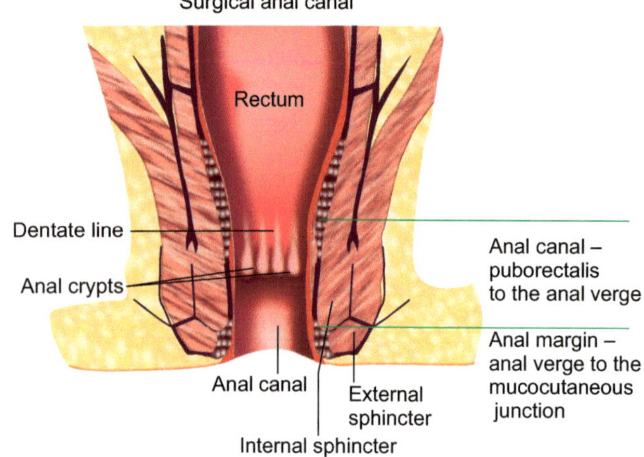

Figure 5: Anatomy of anal canal.

The anus is composed of the anal canal and the anal margin. Two definitions of the anal canal exist: the anatomic anal canal and the surgical anal canal. The anatomic canal extends from the dentate line distally to the anal verge. The surgical anal canal extends the length of the internal sphincter, from the pelvic floor (i.e., the anorectic ring) to the anal verge.

The anal margin is the perianal skin that extends radially from the anal verge. The anal verge is the junction of the specialized anoderm of the distal anal canal with the normal squamous epithelium of the anal margin. It contains the normal structures of the epidermis and is generally 2 cm distal to the dentate line. The anal verge defines the physiologic base of the anal canal and is therefore important in defining whether tumors can be excised without injury to the sphincter complex.

Histology

There are three types of epithelia within the anal complex. The anal margin consists of squamous keratinized epithelium containing all the structures of normal skin. The anoderm is a modified squamous epithelium without epidermal appendages and extends from the anal verge to the dentate line. Close to the dentate line, the anoderm merges with the transition zone, which is composed of distal rectal transitional and squamous epithelium.[27] The transition zone extends up approximately 2 to 3 cm from the dentate line, where it merges into rectal columnar epithelium. Multiple different types of cancers can arise in this area. The epithelium of the anal canal may give rise to epidermoid cancers, including squamous, cloacogenic, transitional, basaloid, mucoepidermoid, and round cell carcinoma. Epidermoid cancers tend to have similar responses to therapy and therefore have a similar prognosis. The anal canal also gives rise to adenocarcinomas and melanomas, although they are much rarer.

The anal margin, consisting of normal skin, gives rise to cancers seen elsewhere in the skin, with squamous cell carcinoma being the most common. Basal cell carcinoma and melanoma are common in other areas of skin but are very rare in the anal margin. Anal intraepithelial neoplasia (AIN) is believed to be a preinvasive form of squamous cell carcinoma, also called Bowen's disease[26].

The lymphatic drainage of the anal canal is threefold. Above the dentate line are the lymphatics which follow the superior hemorrhoidal artery to the pre-aortic and para-aortic nodes. The area directly around the dentate line drains through the internal pudendal, hypogastric, and obturator nodes. Distal to the dentate line, drainage is via the inferior hemorrhoidal vessels terminating at the inguinal nodes.[28] This trimodal drainage of the anal canal requires close monitoring of both the visceral and somatic lymph drainage sites in patients with anal canal carcinoma. Thus, physical examination includes palpation of the inguinal lymph nodes. Surveillance computed tomography (CT) scanning after treatment may indicate nodal areas of relapse within the pelvis.

Risk factors for anal cancer [29-31]

1. HPV infection (anal-genital warts)
2. Receptive anal intercourse or sexually transmitted diseases
3. Cervical, vaginal, or vulvar cancer
4. Immunosuppression after solid organ transplantation or HIV
5. Hematological malignancies
6. Smoking
7. Certain autoimmune disorders

Anal Intraepithelial Neoplasia (AIN)

AIN is a premalignant condition predisposing to anal cancer. It is historically known as Bowen disease. It is associated with infection with Human Papilloma virus. For the same reason it is more common in patients with anal condylomas and HIV.[32] AIN is graded into three categories depending on the extent of dysplastic changes in the epithelial. Grade 1 AIN is low grade dysplasia and refers to nuclear changes seen only in the lower third of the epithelium, grade 2 is defined as changes in the lower two thirds of the epithelium, and grade 3 describes changes throughout the epithelium. Grades 2 and 3 are together reported as high-grade dysplasia.

Most patients with AIN are asymptomatic or have nonspecific symptoms. The most common symptom is pruritus ani. These patients may also have discoloration of perianal skin. Evidence of skin breakdown or ulceration in a patient with a known history of AIN requires biopsy because it may represent progression to squamous cell carcinoma.

Diagnosis and Evaluation of Anal Cancer

Patients with anal cancer may be asymptomatic or they may present with nonspecific symptoms like perianal itching, discharge, bleeding, or pain. These symptoms may be attributed to incontinence, fistulas with the urinary tract or vagina, or constant severe pelvic pain. Patients may also present with metastatic disease to the inguinal nodes. Sexual history must also be taken, in particular a history of HIV.[33]

A complete physical examination is next. Attention is particularly paid to the inguinal nodes. This is followed by a detailed anorectal examination to assess the mobility of the mass, sphincter involvement and pararectal nodes. If the patient has excessive spasms during examination in the office, examination under anesthesia must be performed and a biopsy of the lesion must be obtained.[34]

Workup:

- Digital rectal examination (DRE)
- Inguinal lymph node evaluation
- Biopsy of FNA if suspicious nodes
- Chest x-ray or Chest CT
- Anoscopy
- Abdominal/pelvic CT or MRI
- Consider HIV testing + CD4 level if indicated
- Gynecological exam for women, including screening for cervical cancer
- Consider PET-CT scan

Routine labs including CBC, CMP, and UA, along with evaluation for HIV must be ordered. Additionally, CT scan of the abdomen, pelvis, and chest must be done. Endoanal ultrasound is recommended by some authorities for perirectal nodes. Women must also be evaluated for concurrent cervical cancer or dysplasia. Routine PET scan or PET-CT abdomen is not recommended.[34] Once the evaluation is done, the patient is staged according to the TNM classification by the AJCC.

American Joint Committee on Cancer/Union Internationale Contre le Cancer Staging System for Carcinoma of the Anal Canal and Anal Margin

Primary Tumor (T)	
Tx	Cannot assess primary tumor
T0	Cannot find evidence of primary tumor
Tis	Carcinoma in situ
T1	Greatest dimension is ≤2 cm
T2	Greatest dimension is >2 cm but ≤5 cm
T3	Greatest dimension is >5 cm
Anal Canal	
T4	Invading adjacent structures: urethra, bladder, or vagina (sphincter muscle involvement only is not classified as T4)
Anal Margin	
T4	Invading deep extra-dermal structure: bone or skeletal muscle
Involvement of Regional Lymph Node (N)	
Nx	Cannot assess regional lymph nodes
N0	Regional lymph nodes are not involvement
Anal Canal	
N1	Perirectal lymph nodes metastasis
N2	Unilateral unilateral inguinal +/- internal iliac lymph node metastasis
N3	Perirectal + inguinal +/- bilateral inguinal +/- bilateral internal iliac lymph nodes metastasis
Anal Margin	
N1 Ipsilateral inguinal lymph nodes metastasis	
Distant Metastases (M)	
Mx	Cannot assess distant metastasis
M0	Absence of distant metastases
M1	Presence of distant metastases

Clinical Staging			
Stage 0	Tis	N0	M0
Stage I	TI	N0	M0
Stage II	T2	N0	M0
	T3	N0	M0
Anal Canal			
Stage IIIA	T4	N0	M0
	T1-3	N1	M0
Stage IIIB	T4	N1	M0
	Any T	N2,3	M0
Anal Margin			
Stage III	T4	N0	M0
	Any T	N1	M0
Both			
Stage IV	Any T	Any N	M1

Treatment

Management of anal squamous cell carcinoma depends on its location with respect to the anal sphincter complex. Small lesions that are separate from the anal sphincters and without evidence of spread are typically excised. These lesions are generally found in the anal margin. In contrast, anal canal tumors tend to be larger, involve the anal musculature, and are therefore typically initially treated with chemoradiation therapy. The actual approach of surgical versus chemoradiation is determined more by the size of the lesion, its histology, the relationship of the lesion to the sphincter, and evidence of nodal spread rather than by its location in the canal or the anal margin.[35-36]

Small and well differentiated lesions on the anal margin are treated with local resection. All other lesions of the anal canal and the anal margin are treated with combined chemoradiation of 5-fluorouracil, mitomycin therapy, and radiation therapy. Patients with metastatic disease are best treated with fluoropyrimidine based chemotherapy combined with cisplatin.[37] Only scant data is available on the management of patients with metastatic disease, and, for this reason, it is recommended that these patients be treated in clinical trials.

All patients are reevaluated after 6 to 8 weeks of therapy and classified as having complete response, persistent disease, or progressive disease. Progressive disease requires histological confirmation and restaging with a CT scan of the chest, abdomen, and pelvis. Locoregional failure occurs in about 10% to 30% of patients.[38] Patients who have biopsy proven, locally progressive disease are candidates for salvage surgery with APR. Recurrence isolated to the groin can be treated with inguinal lymph node dissection followed with chemotherapy and/or radiation therapy depending on if they had prior radiation therapy.

All patients with persistent disease are evaluated based on their response to prior treatment. Patients who have responded at least partially are observed for an additional 4 weeks, unless they have progressive disease. In the case of regression on follow up, they are followed up every 3 months.

Follow up of patients in complete remission of the disease involves serial exam every 3 to 6 months. On each visit a DRE and anoscopy must be completed along with inguinal lymph node evaluation. Annual CT chest, abdomen, and pelvis must be done for 3 years after remission to detect recurrences.

Patients with HIV/AIDS who develop anal cancer early in the course of their disease are treated like any other patient with anal cancer. Patients with advanced HIV/AIDS and who develop anal cancer require dose modification of radiation and chemotherapy.[39-40]

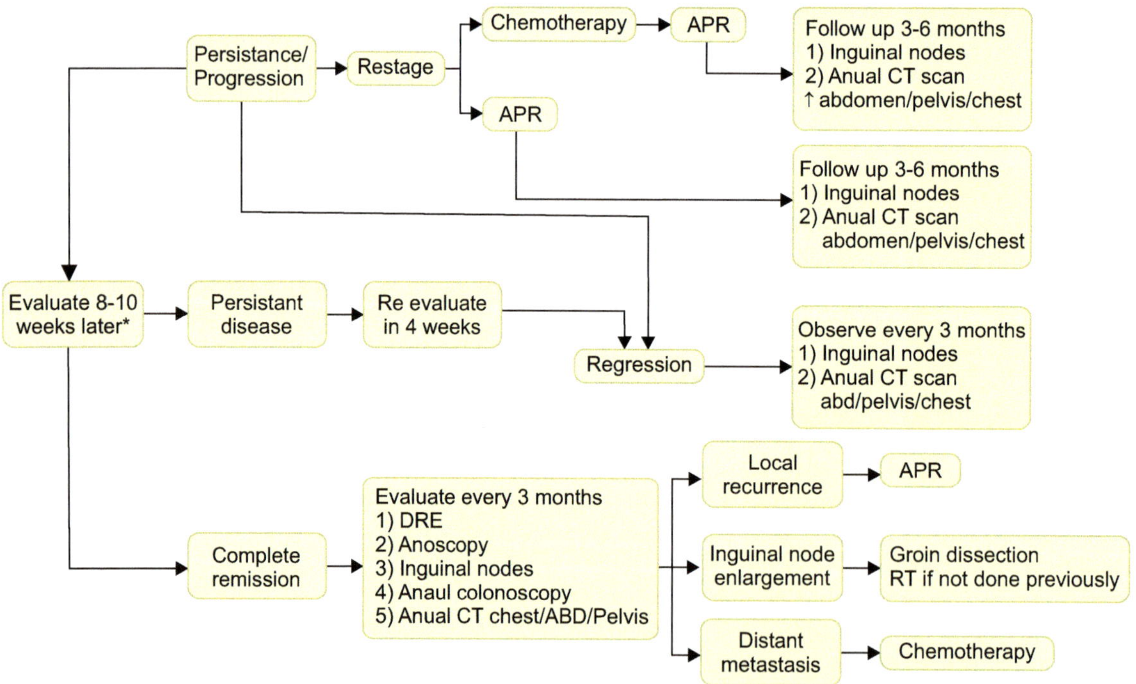

Figure 6: Follow-up of anal squamous cell cancer after chemoradiation therapy

* The diagnosis is confirmed by biopsy.

Factors depicting poor prognosis[41]

1. The patient is male by sex.
2. Positive inguinal nodes at the time of presentation.
3. Tumor size more than 5 cm at the time of presentation.

Risk reduction of anal cancer[38]

1. Early detection of AIN by anal cytology, high resolution anoscopy, HPV DNA analysis.
2. HPV Quadrivalent vaccine because it both reduces the incidence of CIN and decreases AIN.

Role of HAART: HAART has not been shown to reduce the progression of AIN to anal cancer.[40]

Less Common Anal Premalignant and Malignant Lesions

Paget's disease[42]

Paget's disease is an uncommon disease of elderly men, generally seen after 60 years of age. It presents with perianal pruritis, mass, bleeding, or incontinence. It may be associated with other cancers in the gastrointestinal tract or other body parts.

It consists of sharply demarcated lesions with silver scales like psoriasis. Histology will demonstrate large cells with clear cytoplasm and a large peripherally placed nucleus, resembling the signet cells but with a different staining pattern.

Management begins with biopsy of the perianal skin lesion to establish the diagnosis. Work-up for associated colorectal malignancy should include colonoscopy. If the Paget's lesion is isolated, wide local excision with skin graft or advancement flap reconstruction is performed. The deep margins of excision are the sphincter muscle and, proximally, the dentate line within the anal canal. An associated rectal cancer mandates abdominoperineal resection regardless of the level of the lesion in the rectum. Recent success has been obtained with imiquimod cream.

Melanoma

Anal melanoma is a rare tumor that accounts for 1% of malignant anal lesions. It is found more commonly in females and is usually seen in the 50- to 60-year-old age group. Bleeding is the most common symptom, and the lesions are often mistaken for thrombosed external hemorrhoids.

Local excision is recommended for small lesions and abdominoperineal resection for advanced lesions for local control or palliation. However, in a young patient, radical excision of a small lesion may be considered worthwhile for potential chance of cure. Immunotherapy may be considered in these patients since it is used for cutaneous melanoma.[43]

Basal Cell Carcinoma

Basal Cell Carcinoma (BCC) is an extremely uncommon lesion in the perianal skin. Generally seen in sun exposed areas. BCC in perianal areas is more common in men with a mean age of 65 years, and 60% of patients have BCC at other body sites.[43] Most can be treated with local therapy-resection, Mohs microsurgery, or electrodessication.

Adenocarcinoma of the Anal Canal

Adenocarcinoma of anal canal is a rare tumor.[43] It is more common in patients with Chron's disease and may also be seen in patients with chronic fistula-in-ano. It arises from the anal mucus glands and presents as a submucosal nodule.

There is no consensus on therapy and treatment options range from combined modality treatment (CMT), radiation therapy, neoadjuvant therapy followed by surgery, surgery alone including abdominoperineal resection.[43] The Rare Cancer Network performed a meta-analysis and concluded that CMT was associated with better survival than surgery alone. Similar findings were seen by papagikos et al who recommended neoadjuvant therapy followed by salvage abdominoperineal resection for patients. Further studies are required to make firm conclusions regarding the feasibility of CMT as the sole management of anal adenocarcinoma.

REFERENCES

1. Wei EK, Giovannucci E et al. Comparison of risk factors of rectal and colon cancer. Int J Cancer 2004;108:433-442.
2. Sato K , Sato T. Vascular and Neural composition of the lateral ligaments of rectum and the rectosacral fascia. Surg Radiol Anat. 1991;13:17-22.
3. Jones OM, et al. Lateral ligaments of the rectum: an anatomical study. Br J Surg.1999;86:487-489.
4. Scott N, et al. Total mesorectal excision and local recurrence and local recurrence: A study of tumor spread in the mesorectum distal to rectal cancer. Br J Surg. 1995;82:1031-1033.
5. Hida J, et al. Lymph node metastasis detected in the mesorectum distal to the carcinoma of the rectum by clearance method. Justification of the mesorectal excision. J Am Coll Surg.1997;184:584.
6. Ueno H, et al. Clinicopathological study of intra pelvic cancer spread to the iliac area in lower rectal adenocarcinoma by serial sectioning. Br J Surg. 199;86:1532-1537.
7. Hemminki K, Chen B. Familial risk for colorectal cancers are mainly due to heritable causes. Cancer Epidemiol Biomarkers Prev. 2004 Jul;13(7):1253-6.

8. Triantafillidis JK, Nasioulas G, Kosmidis PA.Colorectal cancer and inflammatory bowel disease: epidemiology, risk factors, mechanisms of carcinogenesis and prevention strategies. Anticancer Res. 2009 Jul;29(7):2727-37.
9. Schoellhammer HF, Gregorian AC, Sarkisyan GG, Petrie BA. How important is rigid proctosigmoidoscopy in localizing rectal cancer? Am J Surg. 2008 Dec;196(6):904-8.
10. Lahaye MJ, et al. Imaging for predicting the risk factors--the circumferential resection margin and nodal disease--of local recurrence in rectal cancer: a meta-analysis. Semin Ultrasound CT MR. 2005 Aug;26(4):259-68.
11. Steup WH, Moriya Y, van de Velde CJ. Patterns of lymphatic spread in rectal cancer. A topographical analysis on lymph node metastases. Eur J Cancer. 2002 May;38(7):911-8.
12. Schlag PM. Surgical Sphincter Preservation in Rectal Cancer. Oncologist. 1996;1(5):288-292.
13. Marr R, et al. The modern abdominoperineal excision: the next challenge after total mesorectal excision. Ann Surg. 2005 Jul;242(1):74-82.
14. Compton CC, et al. Prognostic factors in colorectal cancer. College of American Pathologists Consensus Statement 1999. Arch Pathol Lab Med. 2000 Jul;124(7):979-94.
15. Nash GM, et al. Long term surveillance after trans anal excision of T1 rectal cancer. Dis Colon Rectum.2009; 52:577-82.
16. Cooper HS, et al. Endoscopically removed malignant colorectal polyps: clinicopathologic correlations. Gastroenterology. 1995 Jun;108(6):1657-65.
17. Bleday R et al. Prospective evaluation of local excision of small rectal cancers. Dis Colon Rectum.1997;40:388-392.
18. Guillem JG. Ultra low anterior resection and coloanal pouch reconstruction for carcinoma of the distal rectum. World J Surg. 1997;21:721-727.
19. Jayne DG, et al . Randomized trial of laparoscopic-assisted resection of colorectal carcinoma: 3-year results of the UK MRC CLASICC Trial Group. J Clin Oncol. 2007 Jul 20;25(21):3061-8.
20. Colon Cancer Laparoscopic or Open Resection Study Group, Buunen M et al. Survival after laparoscopic surgery versus open surgery for colon cancer: long-term outcome of a randomised clinical trial. Lancet Oncol. 2009 Jan;10(1):44-52.
21. Lacy AM, et al. Laparoscopy-assisted colectomy versus open colectomy for treatment of non-metastatic colon cancer: a randomised trial. Lancet. 2002 Jun 29;359(9325):2224-9.
22. Miles WE. A method of performing abdominoperineal excision for carcinoma of the rectum and the terminal portion of the pelvic colon. Cancer, 1908;2:1812.
23. Sauer R, et al. Preoperative versus postoperative chemoradiotherapy for rectal cancer. N Engl J Med. 2004 Oct 21;351(17):1731-40.
24. Das P, Skibber JM, et al. Predictors of tumor response and downstaging in patients who receive preoperative chemoradiation for rectal cancer. Cancer. 2007 May 1;109(9):1750-5.
25. Pietra N, et al. Role of follow-up in management of local recurrences of colorectal cancer: a prospective, randomized study. Dis Colon Rectum. 1998 Sep;41(9):1127-33.
26. Johnson LG, Madeleine MM, Newcomer LM, et al. Anal cancer incidence and survival: the Surveillance, Epidemiology, and End Results experience, 1973–2000. Cancer 2004;101:281–288.
27. Fenger C. The anal transition zone. Acta Pathol Microbiol Immunol Scand. 1979;87:379-386.
28. Maruyama T, et al. Clinico-pathological study of intra pelvic cancer spread to the iliac area in lower rectal adenocarcinoma by serial sectioning. Br J Surg 1995;82:1031-1033.
29. Daling JR, et al. Human papillomavirus, smoking, and sexual practices in the etiology of anal cancer. Cancer. 2004 Jul 15;101(2):270-80.
30. Jiménez W, Paszat L, Kupets R, Wilton A, Tinmouth J. Presumed previous human papillomavirus (HPV) related gynecological cancer in women diagnosed with anal cancer in the province of Ontario. Gynecol Oncol. 2009 Sep;114(3):395-8.
31. Sunesen KG, Nørgaard M, Thorlacius-Ussing O, Laurberg S. Immunosuppressive disorders and risk of anal squamous cell carcinoma: a nationwide cohort study in Denmark, 1978-2005. Int J Cancer. 2010 Aug 1;127(3):675-84.
32. Holly EA, et al. The prevalence and risk factors of AIN in women . J Natl Cancer Inst.2001;93:843-849.
33. Ryan DP, Compton CC, Mayer RJ. Carcinoma of the anal canal. N Engl J Med. 2000 Mar 16;342(11):792-800.
34. Cummings BJ, Ajani JA, Swallow CJ. Cancer of the anal region . In DeVita Jr VT, Lawrence TS, Rosenberg SA et al. Cancer : Principles and practice of oncology, Eighth edition. Philadelphia PA: Lippencott , William and Winklins;2008.

35. Czito BG, Willett CG. Current management of anal canal cancer. Curr Oncol Rep. 2009 May;11(3):186-92.
36. Cummings BJ, et al. Epidermoid anal cancer: treatment by radiation alone or by radiation and 5-fluorouracil with and without mitomycin C. Int J Radiat Oncol Biol Phys. 1991 Oct;21(5):1115-25.
37. Nigro ND, Vaitkevicius VK, Considine B Jr. Combined therapy for cancer of the anal canal: a preliminary report. Dis Colon Rectum. 1974 May-Jun;17(3):354-6.
38. Schiller DE, et al, Outcomes of salvage surgery for squamous cell carcinoma of the anal canal, Ann Surg Oncol. 2007; 14(10):2780-9.
39. Frisch M, Biggar RJ, Goedert JJ. Human papillomavirus-associated cancers in patients with human immunodeficiency virus infection and acquired immunodeficiency syndrome. J Natl Cancer Inst. 2000 Sep 20;92(18):1500-10.
40. Chiao EY, Giordano TP, Richardson P, El-Serag HB. Human immunodeficiency virus-associated squamous cell cancer of the anus: epidemiology and outcomes in the highly active antiretroviral therapy era. J Clin Oncol. 2008 Jan 20;26(3):474-9.
41. Ajani JA, et al. Fluorouracil, mitomycin, and radiotherapy vs fluorouracil, cisplatin, and radiotherapy for carcinoma of the anal canal: a randomized controlled trial. JAMA. 2008 Apr 23;299(16):1914-21.
42. Delaunoit TH, Neczyporenko F, Duttmann R, et al. Perianal paget's disease : case report and review of literature. Acta GAstroentrol Belg. 2004,67: 228-231.
43. Billingsley KG, Stern LE, Lowey AM. Uncommon anal neoplasm. Surg oncol clinic North Am .2004;13: 375-388.

❑❑❑

SECTION 4: VASCULAR

38. Varicose Veins
39. Lymphedema
40. Endovascular Surgery
41. Carotid Artery Atheromatous Disease
42. Peripheral Vascular Diseases
43. Abdominal Aortic Diseases
44. Splanchnic Artery Aneurysms
45. Vascular Surgery Post-Operative Complications

38

CHAPTER

Varicose Veins

Saurabh Rai, FRCS

Morgan McMonagle, MD, FRCSI

Rajiv Vohra, Ph.D., FRCSEd, FRCSEng

INTRODUCTION

Venous diseases are amongst the most prevalent medical conditions and have been recognized for centuries. They have been mentioned in the Old Testament (Isaiah I:6), the Ebers papyrus in 1550 BC, and by Hippocrates five centuries before Christ.[1]

Varicose veins are dilated, incompetent subcutaneous veins measuring >3 mm in diameter while the patient is standing. Varicose veins are usually but not necessarily tortuous. Even a tubular vein, which meets the rest of the criteria, is called varicose. The size of the vein may vary in different circumstances. The vein may be dilated if the ambient temperature is high. Similarly, the presence of female hormones may make them appear larger in women. Therefore, the presence of incompetence rather than the size should be the essential criteria to classify a vein as varicose. Definitions and synonymous terms used for various venous conditions are described in Table 1. A case of varicose veins of the lower limbs is shown in Figure 1.

Table 1: Definitions and terms used for various venous conditions

Terms	Synonyms	Definitions
Telangiectasia	Spider veins, hyphen webs, thread vein, star bursts, matted veins	Confluence of dilated intradermal venule <1 mm in calibre
Reticular vein	Blue veins, subdermal varices, venulectasias	Dilated, tortuous bluish subdermal veins, 1-3 mm diameter
Varicose vein	Varix, varices	Dilated, incompetent, subcutaneous vein, >3 mm diameter (while standing), tortuous (usually but not necessarily)
Corona phlebectatica	Malleolar or ankle flare	A fan-shaped pattern made of small intradermal veins

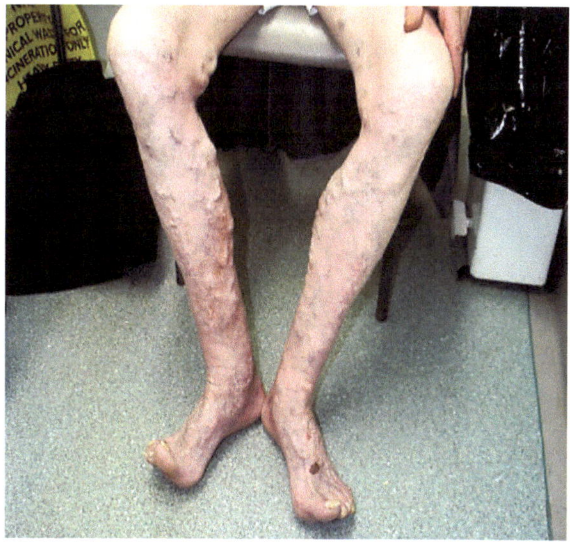

Figure 1: Varicose veins in the lower limbs

The spectrum of clinical presentations that are associated with varicose veins are defined in Table 2 and depicted in Figure 2.

Table 2: Spectrum of varicose veins

Terms	Definitions
Edema	Increase in the volume of fluid in the skin and subcutaneous tissue, characteristically palpable indentation following digital pressure
Pigmentation	Brownish darkening of the skin due to extravasated blood
Eczema	An erythematous dermatitis
Lipodermatoscle-rosis	Localized chronic inflammation and fibrosis of the skin and subcutaneous tissue
Atrophy blanche	Localized, circular whitish & atrophic skin area surrounded by dilated capillaries
Venous ulcer	Full thickness skin defect caused by venous disease

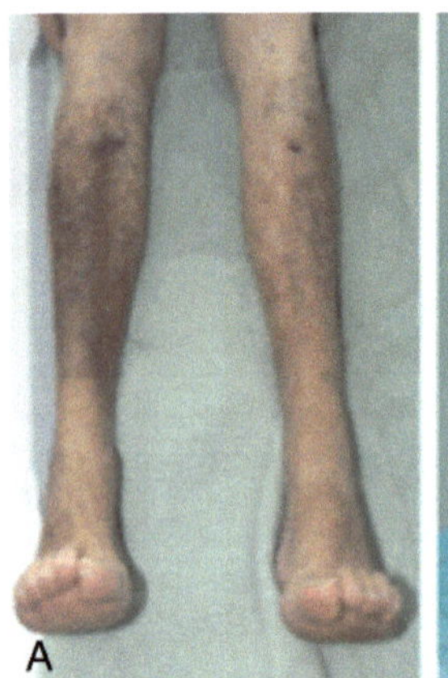

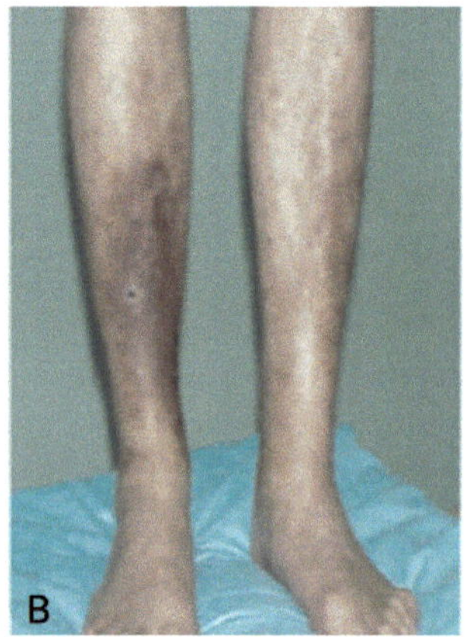

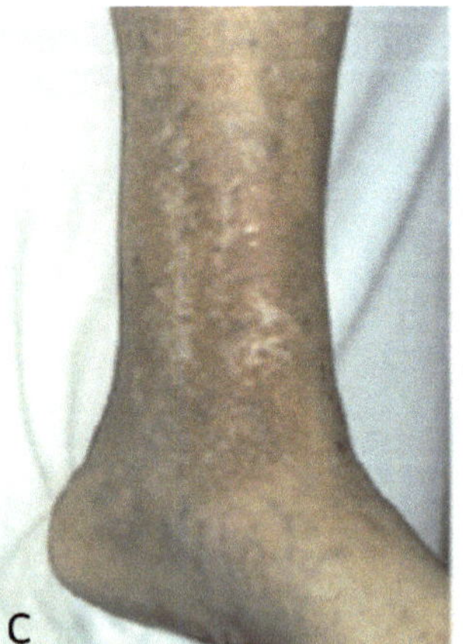

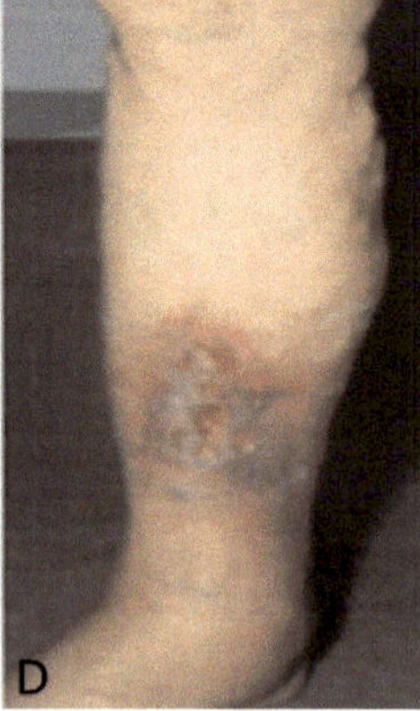

Figure 2: Clinical spectrum of varicose veins

A: pigmentation, **B**: lipodermatosclerosis, **C**: atrophy blanche, **D**: venous ulcer

The term 'chronic venous disease (CVD)' refers to any condition related to varicose veins. This may vary in presentation from visible small, dilated veins to venous ulcers. Whereas the term "chronic venous insufficiency" (CVI) refers to more advanced venous diseases that indicate the presence of venous edema, pigmentation, eczema, and ulceration.

Venous anatomy of lower limb

The deep fascia of the lower limb divides the veins into 2 main compartments; those superficial to this fascia are superficial veins, whereas those deep to this fascia are deep veins. "Perforators" are the veins that connect the two. Communicating veins are veins that connect the veins within the same compartment. Saphenous fascia surrounding the great saphenous vein (GSV) subdivides the superficial compartment as it separates the GSV from other veins of the superficial compartment.

In general, the superficial veins of the lower limbs are the most variable venous system of the human body. At the level of the metatarsal head, on the dorsum of foot there is a dorsal venous arch which drains the venous blood from superficial vein tributaries. Medial and lateral marginal veins continue from the medial and lateral end of this arch into the GSV and short saphenous vein (SSV) respectively.

Great Saphenous Vein

Beginning just anterior to the medial malleolus the GSV ascends in the leg and lies approximately a hand's breadth behind the medial border of patella at the knee level. In the lower two-thirds of the leg, the saphenous nerve runs in close proximity to the GSV. A cadaveric study has shown that the GSV is close to the saphenous nerve in 59.5% of legs in the middle-third, and in 83.1% of legs in the lower third of the leg.[2]

The GSV runs on the antero-medial aspect of the thigh above the knee and enters the fossa ovalis. Fossa ovalis, located 2.5 cm inferior and 2.5 cm lateral to the pubic tubercle, is an oval defect in the deep fascia of the thigh (fascia lata) covered by loose connective tissue strands, named as cribriform fascia. The GSV joins the confluence of superficial inguinal veins (i.e., superficial circumflex iliac, superficial epigastric and external pudendal veins) to form the saphenofemoral junction (SFJ). There is a valve in the GSV, present in 80% of population and located within 2.5 cm distance from SFJ which allows unidirectional flow from GSV to the femoral vein. The GSV rarely terminates on the lower abdomen or joins the femoral vein very low. The superficial inguinal veins empty individually into the femoral vein. Accessory GSVs, both in thigh and leg, are not uncommon. They can lie anterior, posterior, or superficial to the main trunk of GSV. The posterior accessory GSV of the leg (posterior arch vein or Leonardo's vein) begins posterior to the medial malleolus, runs on the postero-medial aspect of the leg, and joins the GSV below the knee. The anterior accessory GSV of the leg drains the anterior aspect of the leg below the knee. Similarly in the thigh, the anterior and posterior accessory GSVs of the thigh collect the blood from the antero-lateral and postero-medial aspect of the leg. Both veins join the GSV before the GSV joins the confluence of superficial inguinal veins.

Short Saphenous Vein

The SSV starts posterior to the lateral malleolus at ankle level, runs in the subcutaneous fat plane, and then pierces the fascia to run between the two heads of gastrocnemius muscle. In the popliteal fossa, the main trunk of the SSV drains into the popliteal vein (PV). The location of the sapheno-popliteal junction (SPJ) often varies. It may correspond to the knee skin crease, or it could be within a 1–2-inch distance above and below the knee. Instead of draining into the PV, the main trunk of SSV may continue upwards and empty into the GSV or femoral vein. There may also be a communicating vein connecting the SSV to the GSV in the postero-medial thigh, known as the inter-saphenous vein or Giacomini's vein. Ultrasound images in 39 of 40 limbs (97%) showed the sural nerve within the saphenous compartment. This nerve lies near the SSV, only in the distal third of the limb where the two components of the nerve join together, the medial calcaneal, a branch of the tibial nerve; and lateral calcaneal, a branch of the common peroneal nerve.[3]

Lateral Venous System

The superficial veins on the lateral aspect of the thigh and leg form the lateral venous system. This system drains either into the SSV or GSV, through multiple small tributaries, or into the deep system through the perforating veins.

Venous Valves

Veins have valves to prevent the backflow of blood. These valves are made of cusps which are bicuspid infoldings of the intima. The valves are covered by endothelium on either side with an intervening skeleton of connective tissue. The new terminology of lower limb veins is shown in Table 3.

Table 3: New terminology of lower limb veins

Historic Names, Old Names, Eponyms	New Terms
Superficial femoral vein	Femoral Vein
Long/greater saphenous vein	Great saphenous vein (GSV)
Short/lesser saphenous vein	Small saphenous vein (SSV)
Saphenofemoral junction (SFJ)	Confluence of the superficial inguinal veins
Leonardo's vein or Posterior arch	Posterior accessory great saphenous vein of the leg
Giacomini's vein	Intersaphenous vein
Cockett perforator (I, II, or III)	Posterior tibial perforators (lower, middle, and upper)
Sherman's perforator and "24 cm" perforator	Paratibial perforator
Boyd's perforator	Paratibial perforator (proximal)
Dodd's perforator and Hunter's perforators	Perforators of the femoral canal
May's perforator or Kuster's perforator	Ankle perforators

Classification of Venous Disease

In order to understand the clinical disease process and outline management of various stages of the disease process, the CEAP classification system was developed. In 1994 a sub-committee of world experts convened by the American Venous Forum created the "CEAP" (C, clinical: E, etiological; A, anatomy; P, pathophysiology) classification to provide a framework for precise scientific description, documentation, and comparing the outcomes of various treatment modalities for VV.[4] This classification was subsequently critiqued and slightly revised in 2004[5] by a new international committee who also added a simplified "basic CEAP" to create a more precise "full"/advanced CEAP classification. In simplified "basic CEAP", the single highest descriptor used for clinical classification and anatomic segments, is not included. The "full"/advanced CEAP that is essential for researchers and for reporting in scientific journals is depicted in Table 4. Further anatomic segment classification is shown in Table 5.

Table 4: CEAP classification

Classification			
C: Clinical	E: Etiologic	A: Anatomic	P: Pathophysiologic
C0 = Venous disease is not visible or palpable	Ec = It is congenital	A_s = In the superficial veins	Pr = There is reflux
C1 = Evidence of telangiectasia or reticular veins	Ep = It is primary	A_p = In the perforating veins	Po = There is obstruction
C2 = Evidence of a varicose vein	Es = It is post-thrombotic or secondary	A_d = In the deep veins	Pr,o = There is both reflux & obstruction
C3 = Evidence of edema	En = Venous etiology is not identified	A_n = Venous location is not identified	Pn = Venous pathophysiology is not identifiable
C4a = Evidence of eczema and/or pigmentation			
C4b = Evidence of atrophy blanche and/or lipodermatosclerosis			
C5 = Evidence of a healed venous ulcer			
C6 = Evidence of an active venous ulcer			
S Symptoms: tightness, heaviness, ache, pain, skin irritation, muscle cramps			
A Asymptomatic			

Table 5: Venous anatomic segments classification

Superficial veins (A_s)	Deep veins (A_d)	Perforating veins (Ap)
1. Telangiectasis/ reticular veins	6. Inferior vena cava	17. Thigh perforator veins
2. GSV above knee	7. Common Iliac vein	18. Calf perforator veins
3. GSV below knee	8. Internal iliac vein	
4. Small saphenous vein	9. External iliac vein	
5. Non saphenous vein	10. Pelvic: broad ligament veins, gonadal, other	
	11. Common femoral vein	
	12. Deep femoral vein	
	13. Femoral vein	
	14. Popliteal vein	
	15. Crural veins: peroneal vein, anterior tibial, posterior tibial (all veins are paired)	
	16. Muscular veins: soleal, gastrocnemius, other	

Incidence and prevalence

Studies examining the incidence of varicose veins (VV) are limited. The Framingham study found that the 2-year incidence of VV was 39.4 and 51.9 per 1000 men and women respectively.[6] The prevalence of VV in London in a 35-70 year age group was reported as 17% and 31% in men and women respectively.[7] A study conducted in Edinburgh of a 18-64 year age group found the prevalence of truncal varicosity to be 40% and 32% in men and women respectively.[8] This challenged the traditional belief that varicose veins are more common in women. The same study found the prevalence of reticular varicosity or telangiectasia to be greater than 80%. Another study reports that at any given time more than 20 million westerners have VV, 6 million some degree of edema, approximately 1 million have skin changes, and 500,000 people are estimated to have active venous ulceration.[9]

Etiology

The exact etiology of varicose veins is debatable. Some consider valvular incompetence to be the primary cause, whereas others consider valvular incompetence to be secondary to stretching of the vein as a result of other underlying factors. These factors may render vein valves incompetent due to the dilatation of the vein wall secondary to a structural abnormality, or due to recanalization of the vein after thrombosis. These primary and secondary venous insufficiencies are compared in Table 6. Varicose veins may be primary, secondary, or congenital. Most varicose veins are primary, while secondary varicose veins may be secondary to deep vein thrombosis or trauma causing arteriovenous fistulae.

Table 6: A comparison of primary and secondary venous insufficiency

	Primary	Secondary
Etiology	Degenerative (genetic?)	Acquired (inflammatory)
Feature	Reflux only	Obstruction-reflux
Intima	Retained	Destroyed
Valves	Atrophied, stretched	Destroyed, scarred
Site of occurrence	Primarily superficial vein	Primarily deep vein
Occurrence	Widespread	Localized
Treatment	Support &/ or surgery	Anticoagulant, support

The commonest source of reflux in the GSV is SFJ incompetence. Occasionally isolated mid-thigh perforator incompetence may cause GSV reflux. Similarly, the SSV may become varicose due to SPJ incompetence or less commonly due to gastrocnemius and Giacomini vein incompetence.

Congenital varicose veins may be associated with 'port-wine stains' on the skin, hypertrophy of soft tissue, presence of a congenital arteriovenous fistulae, and bone overgrowth. The affected limb may be longer on the contralateral side. A classic example of such a condition is 'Klippel-Trenaunay Syndrome'.

Risk factors

The risk factors for varicose veins include heredity, female gender, and ageing. Additional risk factors are summarised according to their location of abnormality in Table 7. One risk factor can cause varicose veins through multiple mechanisms. For example, pregnancy increases the chances of DVT, and causes an extrinsic obstruction to venous flow. Other proposed risk factors (smoking, hypercholesterolemia, leg crossing) have little or no evidence and are merely historical.

Table 7: Risk factors for varicose veins

Site of abnormality	Condition
Intraluminal	Deep vein thrombosis, malignancy, increased pressure due to prolonged standing or pregnancy, genetic
Vein wall pathology	Post-phlebitic scarring of valve cusps, genetic
Extrinsic obstruction to flow	Pregnancy, obesity, malignancy (pelvic/ intraabdominal)

Clinical features

Symptoms of varicose veins vary from cosmetic concerns about visible veins to complications such as skin changes and venous ulcers on the leg. Common symptoms include visible veins, heaviness, tension, ache, itching, and ankle swelling that worsen in the evening. Common symptoms and signs are summarised in Table 8.

Table 8: Symptoms and signs of varicose veins

Symptoms	Signs
Visible veins	Visible varicose veins
Heaviness, Tension, Ache,	Ankle flare
Itching in leg	Atrophy blanche
Ankle swelling	Champagne bottle shaped legs
Nocturnal cramps	Edema
	Hyperpigmentation
	Lipodermatosclerosis
	Stasis eczema
	Ulceration

Physical examination

The aim of the examination is to look for the presence of varicose veins, their likely source of origin, distribution, and any associated complications. It is important to examine and record the presence or absence of peripheral pulses in the extremity. One should look for visible varicose veins, scars of previous surgery for veins, characteristic 'champagne bottle legs', hyperpigmentation, lipodermatosclerosis, eczema, and ulceration. Palpation can demonstrate edema and the presence or absence of peripheral pulses in the lower limbs. Various clinical tests used for identifying the likely origin of venous reflux have been replaced by the hand-held Doppler examination. A few of the historical tests, their underlying aim, and a brief description are summarised in Table 9.

Varicose veins are generally examined with the patient standing in a comfortable, warm environment. One should expose the legs completely. The shape of the leg, area of distribution of varicose veins (whether in the great saphenous or short saphenous vein anatomical area), presence of ankle edema, pigmentation, ulceration, and scars of previous surgery in the legs are important points to be noted while examining these patients. For congenital varicose veins there could be limb length asymmetry associated with abnormal pigmentation. If an arterio-venous malformation is suspected, one should make a point to auscultate the prominent veins to check for any bruits.

Table 9: Special clinical tests used in varicose vein examination

Name of Test	Patient position	Method	Inference
Trendelenburg	Standing first then lies supine	Tourniquet below SFJ, elevate leg when patient lies, look for emptying of GSV if becomes less prominent	SFJ incompetent and perforators patent
Tourniquet Test (Mahorner-Ochsner Test, Pratt's Test)	Supine first then stands up	Empty the vein, tie many tourniquets, patient stands up, release tourniquet one by one starting from above	Incompetent perforator
Schwartz's Test (Tap sign, Wave Test)	Standing	Tap above and feel below, presence of thrill	Incompetent truncal vein valves
Perthes' Test	Standing	Tie tourniquet around proximal thigh, patient exercises, if VV becomes less prominent: Deep veins and perforators OK	Competence of deep veins and perforators
Linton Test	Stands first then lies down	Tie tourniquet, patient lies down then elevates leg	

Investigations

There are three main methods of investigating venous disease: duplex Doppler ultrasound, phlebography, and plethysmography. These methods are described here in some detail except plethysmography which is used for assessing the amount of reflux, calf muscle pump efficiency, obstruction, and is mainly used for research purposes.

Doppler examination

The hand-held Doppler (HHD) uses a continuous wave 8MHz Doppler. It has replaced all of the clinical tests. Duplex ultrasound is a combination of colour Doppler and B-mode imaging. For duplex ultrasound a 4-7 MHz linear array transducer is the most useful. Higher frequency probes give better resolution for superficial veins, whereas lower frequency probes are better for deeper veins (e.g., in the abdomen and pelvis.) Venous reflux can be physiological or pathological. The vein valve cusps take a fraction of a second to appose. The blood that refluxes prior to apposition of valve cusps generates physiological reflux. Larger veins have longer physiological reflux because they have fewer valves that take longer to appose. This is in comparison to smaller veins with more valves and a smaller lumen. As an international consensus, venous reflux >0.5 second is accepted as abnormal.

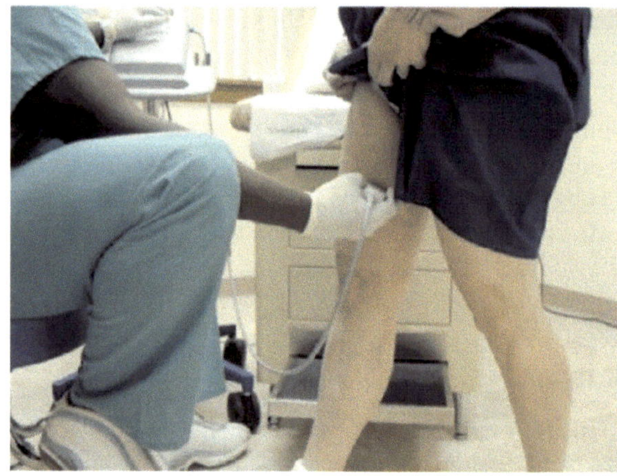

Figure 3: Venous duplex examination

For duplex examination, the patient should be standing as shown in Figure 3. To avoid spasm in the veins, the room temperature should not be too cold. The lower limb should be exposed and the body-weight should be transferred to the contralateral limb. The limb being examined should be slightly flexed at the knee and externally rotated. The examination starts at the common femoral vein and proceeds in an orderly manner to the saphenofemoral junction, great saphenous vein, popliteal vein, short saphenous vein, deep calf veins, and perforators. The great saphenous vein lies in the middle of two layers of fascia. During scanning, if the transducer looks at it transversely, this gives an appearance of a 'saphenous eye'.[10] In the transverse orientation, the short saphenous vein is surrounded by a triangle formed by the crural fascia and medial and lateral heads of the gastrocnemius muscle.[11]

There are two methods to demonstrate venous reflux: the Valsalva manoeuvre and augmentation. The Valsalva manoeuvre increases the intra-abdominal pressure. If valves are incompetent, this raised pressure can lead to reversal of flow. For groin valve reflux, this is a useful method. This method is not useful to demonstrate distal valve incompetence. The presence of any competent valve proximal to incompetent valve limits the reversal of venous blood-flow making this method unsuitable for demonstrating reflux at knee level. Augmentation, the other technique is where an ultrasound probe is placed and the limb muscle distal to the probe is compressed which increases the venous blood flow in the normal direction. On releasing the pressure on the muscle, the venous blood flows in the reverse direction. If the valves are competent this reverse-flow is minimal. An incompetent valve produces a larger reflux producing a 'whoosh' sound lasting >0.5 second in duration.

Coloured duplex Doppler sonography is particularly useful in cases of short saphenous vein reflux and recurrent veins in patients with a prior history suggestive of DVT. Due to its availability, coloured duplex is used nowadays, even in the case of primary varicose GSV. Duplex examination also helps in assessment regarding suitability of a vein for a minimal invasive endovenous ablation. Non-invasive imaging methods are accurate, relatively less expensive, and much safer than invasive methods.

Venography (Phlebography)

Contrast phlebography historically considered the 'gold standard' diagnostic test, currently plays no role in uncomplicated varicose veins.

Indications for venography include:

1. If planning an intervention (e.g., surgical thrombectomy or catheter-directed thrombolysis) during an acute setting when it is important to be sure of the upper extent of the thrombus. Such cases include an ilio-caval thrombus because iliac veins may be difficult to visualize with ultrasound due to interference from bowel gas and due to its deep location especially in patients who are obese.
2. If the results of duplex are not reliable. Duplex is not very reliable below the knee segment. The majority of DVTs start in this segment, but luckily does not progress higher up.
3. In chronic venous thrombosis cases where surgical intervention is planned. Phlebography provides reliable route-mapping prior to deep venous reconstruction.

Conventional venography is an invasive test with risks of inducing phlebitis. Non-invasive phlebography (i.e., CT or MR venography) are much safer and provide excellent resolution and anatomical details. CT venography is fast and provides information about calcification in the wall and tissue around vessels but carries the risk of iodinated contrast and radiation exposure. MR venography does not have these risks, but has problems in patients who have claustrophobia, metal implants, pacemakers, or aneurysm clips.

Depending upon where the contrast is injected and the direction in which it is followed, the invasive phlebography can be:

1. Ascending: puncture of the vein at foot level, and the contrast is followed towards the leg and/or the thigh.
2. Descending: contralateral femoral or upper limb veins are punctured, and the contrast is followed down the thigh and/or leg.

Treatment

Varicose veins are treated for cosmesis, primary symptoms, and complications as shown in Table 10.

Table 10: Indications for treating varicose veins

Primary symptoms	**Ankle swelling, itching, ache, heaviness**
Complications	Bleeding, ankle hyperpigmentation, eczema, atrophy, blanche, venous ulceration
Treatment for cosmesis	Visible veins

Though successful treatment of varicose veins allows ulcers to heal faster and decrease their likelihood of recurring, treating the varicose veins in the presence of active venous ulcer carries a slightly higher risk of wound infection. Often patients have unrealistic expectations especially when they do not have any complications due to varicose veins and are treated for primary symptoms or cosmesis. All patients should be warned that treatment may not be curative and there is a possibility of recurrence of varicose veins.

There are a variety of effective treatment modalities for various segments of the superficial venous system. In general, veins are treated in an orderly manner as shown in Table 11.

Table 11: Order and modalities of treating Varicose Vein

Order	Treated segment	Modality of treatment
I	Saphenous vein trunk	• Thermal ablation: laser or radiofrequency
		• Chemical ablation: (US guided sclerotherapy)
		• Ligation and stripping
II	Saphenous vein tributaries	• Ambulatory phlebectomy
		• Thermal ablation
		• Chemical ablation
		• Trivex
		• Sclerotherapy
III	Varicose vein not connected to saphenous vein trunk	• Ambulatory phlebectomy
		• Chemical ablation
		• Sclerotherapy
		• Trivex
IV	Reticular Veins	• Sclerotherapy
		• Ambulatory phlebectomy
V	Telangiectatic veins	• Sclerotherapy
		• Laser

Conservative management

The steps found potentially beneficial in all cases include exercise, ankle flexions, leg elevation, compression, and avoidance of high heeled footwear. Compression of the venous system is the underlying principle of conservative treatment. Compression can be applied in various forms.

From a historical perspective, Hippocrates said that it was better not to stand if an ulcer was on the leg. Romans knew the value of compression therapy for venous insufficiency. Even in the modern area, compression therapy is the most widely practised form of therapy to treat chronic venous insufficiency (CVI). The only contraindications are severe co-existing cardiac dysfunction and peripheral arterial occlusive disease (PAOD). Strong compression applied to both legs may squeeze the blood from the calves which a severely decompensated heart may not be able to handle. If ankle-brachial pressure index is < 0.7, indicating PAOD, compression therapy may further diminish limb-perfusion threatening gangrene and limb loss. A patient's understanding of their condition and compliance are the most important contributory factors for the success of compression therapy.

Elastic stockings

When elastic fibres became available in the 20th century, elastic stockings were made. In 1930, Conrad Jacobst, an engineer, developed venous ulcerations despite superficial venous ablation. His symptoms improved while standing in his swimming pool. Based on the conclusion that a natural graduated compression created by increasing depth of water improved his ulcers, he designed his own graduated compression stockings (GCS) which alleviated his symptoms. Today, GCS remains the most widely accepted therapeutic option for CVI. Graduated compression stockings are classified according to the pressure that they generate at the ankle. They are "graduated" as they exert 100% of the stated pressure at the ankle level, 70% at the upper calf, and 40% at the thigh level. The gradient created by the stockings facilitates venous outflow. The details of GCS including their indications are summarized in Table 12.

Table 12: Indications and Classes of Elastic Compression Stockings

Indications	Class	Pressure (mm Hg)
Ache, swelling, reticular, telangiectasia	I	20-30
CVI, Post-ulcer	II	30-40
CVI, Post-ulcer, lymphoedema	III	40-50
CVI, Post-ulcer, lymphoedema	IV	50-60

Though stockings are much easier to wear than other forms of compression therapies, compliance may still be poor. Elderly, frail, arthritic and obese patients may not be able to wear the stockings themselves. Younger patients, especially males, do not like wearing stockings. In hot climates compression stockings may not be comfortable to wear. However, patient education, application of a below-knee type stocking, and a gradual increase in the class of stockings may increase patient compliance.

Paste boots

Paul Gerson Unna, a German dermatologist, in 1896 developed this form of compression bandage. The first layer consists of a roller gauze bandage impregnated with calamine, zinc oxide, glycerine, sorbitol, gelatine, and magnesium-aluminium-silicate. The second layer consists of continuous gauze dressing. The third layer is made of elastic wrap. All these bandages are applied to exert a graded compression from the foot to the knee. After drying, it becomes rigid and exerts a pressure of 50-60 mmHg at the ankle. It needs to be changed on a weekly or biweekly basis by a trained professional. It has the usual problems of being bulky, heavy, labour-intensive, and operator dependent.

Compression bandages

Apart from the paste boots described above, inelastic compression can also be applied by other forms of multi-layered bandages. In theory, inelastic compression is more helpful in patients with venous ulceration, but it is more difficult to apply and maintain than elastic compression. One may use a short stretch of bandage which has a lesser degree of elastic in it. These "short-stretch" compression bandages are also effective in healing a majority of venous ulcers. In the four-layer technique, the ulcer is first covered by a non-adherent dressing, followed by a wool bandage that is applied from the base of the toes to just below the knee joint. Then, a crepe bandage is applied in a figure-eight fashion and is secured by a final cohesive layer. Expertise is required in applying short-stretch bandages. Until exudates and edema subside, bandages need to be changed more frequently at least twice a week. It can be maximally left on for 1 week. Usually, the compression bandaging obtains the result, and the compression stocking maintains it. If possible, one must try to correct the underlying cause of valvular incompetence to prevent recurrence. Compression leads to increased venous flow, decreased pathological venous reflux while walking, and an increased emptying of veins with activation of the calf pump. To maximize the benefit of compression, patients should incorporate at least 30 minutes of walking into their daily regimen.

Open Surgical treatment

Surgical treatment for saphenous incompetence includes surgery for the great saphenous vein, short saphenous vein, and recurrent varicose veins.

A well-informed consent is obtained. Veins in the leg are marked in standing position with an indelible marker pen. Some surgeons recommend tram-track marking for veins in the leg and making the incision in between two lines to minimise the chances of skin tabooing. Other surgeons may mark the vein with a single-line and make phlebectomy incisions on these marked sites. The surgery is mostly performed as a day-case under general, spinal, femoral nerve block, or under local anaesthesia.

Surgery for the Great Saphenous Vein

For surgery of the Great Saphenous Vein (GSV), the patient lies supine in a slight head-down position with the hip and knee partially flexed and externally rotated. An approximately 2.5 cm long incision is made in the groin crease. In obese and elderly patients, this incision is made just above the skin crease. Preoperative localisation with the help of ultrasound can aid in making a precise, smaller incision. Subcutaneous fat and fascia are incised. The great saphenous vein traversing through the cribriform fascia is traced up to the saphenofemoral junction (SFJ), the latter is characterised by a white line on the adventitial surface. All tributaries are then ligated and transected. The SFJ is divided and should either be ligated or transfixed. Trans-fixation minimizes the chances of ligature slippage. During trans-fixation one should not encroach beyond the SFJ or else it will result in constriction of the CFV causing an increased chances of femoral vein thrombosis. It is suggested by some surgeons that recurrence can be minimized by the closure of the SFJ with a non-absorbable suture and ligation of tributaries with absorbable suture material.[12] The superficial external pudendal artery passes deep to the GSV and in front of the CFV just proximal to the SFJ. This can be a useful guide to the SFJ as well as a source of bleeding if division is unrecognized during surgery. The GSV should be removed up to or just beyond the knee level. The close proximity of the saphenous nerve in the lower two-thirds of the leg increases the chances of nerve damage if the GSV is stripped up to ankle level.[13] For stripping, either a disposable plastic stripper or metallic PIN (perforation-invagination) stripper can be used. The stripped, evaginated GSV can be removed from a groin wound or a fresh, small, below-the-knee incision.

Varicosities in the leg are removed by multiple phlebectomies. Phlebectomies are avoided around ankle-level and near the head of the fibula to minimize the chances of nerve damage. Multiple 2-3 mm phlebectomy incisions are made in Langer's line using a size 15 blade, ophthalmic blades, or 19 G needle. Use of phlebectomy hooks allows phlebectomy to be performed with smaller incisions.

Avulsion wounds can be closed with steristrips. The groin wound is closed by approximating the cribriform fascia by interrupted absorbable stitches, subcutaneous fat with absorbable suture, and a subcuticular skin stitch with absorbable or non-absorbable suture. A long-acting local anaesthetic is infiltrated in the groin for better postoperative pain-control. The limb is then dressed with cotton wool and crepe bandage. This minimizes oozing and bruising. Some surgeons immediately put the leg in a thigh-length thrombo-embolic deterrent stockings (TEDS) which serves the dual purpose of minimizing bruising and DVTs.

Surgery for Short Saphenous Vein

The patient is placed in a prone position. A small transverse incision is made just over the sapheno-popliteal junction. The SPJ may not be at skin crease level. In almost equal proportion of cases, it is either above or below the skin crease. Preoperative localization of SPJ with duplex scan is helpful in making the incision precisely over the SPJ. Skin and subcutaneous fascia is incised to avoid injury to cutaneous nerves. The proximal SSV is then traced upward. Popliteal fascia is incised and the SPJ is exposed. The SSV is then transacted and the SPJ is transfixed or ligated. The sural nerve is very close to the SSV, and care should be taken to keep it out of harm's way. The SSV is not stripped but an 8-10-cm segment of the SSV is excised. Further, stripping is more likely to cause damage to the adjoining sural nerve. Hook phlebectomy should be performed carefully without damaging the sural nerve. The popliteal fascia is then closed with absorbable suture material, followed by closure of the skin incision with subcuticular stitches using absorbable or non-absorbable suture material.

Surgery for recurrent varicose veins

The most frequent causes of recurrent varicose vein are inadequate prior surgery (missed SFJ), neovascularization, and incompetent perforator veins. Neovascularization has been reported to be present in 39% of cases of recurrent varicose veins.[14] Surgery for recurrent varicose veins has less successful outcomes and may have a higher complication-rate. If the groin is re-explored the incision should be placed laterally and the femoral artery should be exposed with the femoral vein located just medial to it. All tributaries are ligated and the SFJ is transfixed with non-absorbable suture. If the GSV is found intact, it should be stripped. Re-do SSV surgery uses the same incision, if properly placed previously. A preoperative duplex localization of the SPJ is essential.

Complications

Complications of varicose vein surgery are either due to anaesthesia or surgery. They are summarized in Table 13. All of these complications are more likely to occur in recurrent varicose vein surgery. Incidence of groin wound infection is 1-2%. Nerve injury could vary from temporary to permanent neuropraxia. A temporary patch of numbness over the phlebectomy sites is very common. It results from pressure over the nerve from either a subcutaneous haematoma or damage to the cutaneous nerve branches during phlebectomy. Permanent numbness results from damage to the nerve during surgery. Saphenous nerve damage results in a patch of numbness over the medial side of the leg and foot. Sural nerve damage causes numbness over the posterior aspect of the leg and lateral aspect of the foot. Common peroneal nerve damage results in 'foot-drop'. Fibrosis resulting from healing of the wound could also result in late entrapment of the nerve. The incidence of true nerve injury can be up to 5%. Residual veins are visible veins usually present in the leg after phlebectomy. Sclerotherapy or re-do phlebectomy can be offered. Another complication is long-term recurrence following traditional surgery, which can occur in up to 30% of cases. Recurrence could be due to inadequate previous surgery, neovascularization, or progression of the underlying disease. Lastly, deep vein thrombosis can be recognised in 1-2% patients. Use of hormone-replacement treatment and oral contraceptive pills increases the incidence. Standard DVT prophylaxis steps include early mobilization, use of LMW Heparin, and TEDS.

Table 13: Complications of Open Varicose Vein Surgery

Early Complications	Late Complications
Bleeding	Residual veins
Bruising	Recurrent veins
Wound infection	Nerve injury
Deep Vein Thrombosis	
Nerve injury	
Seroma	
Lymphocele, lymph leak	

Endovenous Ablation of Varicose Veins

There are three established methods of achieving endovenous ablation of the saphenous vein: radiofrequency, endovenous laser ablation, and chemical ablation with ultrasound-guided foam sclerotherapy. The first two methods use electromagnetic energy. Chemical ablation uses a foamed chemical detergent which can be injected directly into the vein or delivered endoluminally via a catheter. There are other methods which utilize newer agents for endoluminal application (e.g., steam). This chapter will mainly discuss radiofrequency ablation (RFA) and endovenous laser ablation (EVLA) as these are well established methods that are currently used.

Radiofrequency Ablation

The radiofrequency (RF) energy delivered to the GSV via a probe abolishes the SFJ reflux without groin dissection. In a multi-centre study, the successful vein occlusion rates up to 5-years was between 83.5%-88.2%.[15] The percutaneous catheter-based radiofrequency closure procedure developed by VNUS Medical Technologies San Jose, CA, USA was started in Europe in 1998 and in the USA in 1999.

In RFA, the RF energy is used to heat the vein wall. A catheter is placed intraluminally in contact with the vein wall. The tip of the catheter has bipolar electrodes. Electric current flows between the tips of bipolar electrodes through the vein wall. By a phenomenon known as "resistive heating", this flow generates heat. A computerized generator monitors the electrodes' temperature. The heat results in the physical shortening of collagen fibrils, which are present in the sub-endothelial layer of the vein wall. This shortening of collagen fibril narrows down the vein diameter. The generated heat also denatures the blood proteins which congeal to obliterate the vein lumen. Over next 12-24 months the vein undergoes fibrosis.

The RFA procedure can be performed under general, spinal, or local anaesthesia. The disadvantage of general anaesthesia is the inability of the patient to describe nerve pain or temperature sensations in the skin, in the case that the RF catheter is too close to the nerve or skin, respectively.

After anaesthesia, the GSV is accessed with a 19–21-gauge needle. The sheath is introduced percutaneously using the Seldinger technique. If the access is difficult to obtain, a cut-down access to the vein may be obtained. The RFA catheter is passed into the GSV through the access sheath. Using the ultrasound guidance, the catheter tip is placed 2 cm proximal to the SFJ. This optimum positioning of the catheter potentially reduces the incidence of neovascularization thereby reducing the likelihood of recurrent varicose veins.[16] Tumescent anaesthesia is a solution made by mixing buffered lidocaine (1%) with adrenaline (100,000 diluted to strength of 0.1%). Tumescent anaesthesia is placed below the saphenous fascia and above the deep muscular fascia. This compresses the saphenous vein and its inflow branches. It also contains the heat within the treated vein and does not greatly affect adjacent cutaneous and sensory nerves.[17]

Prior to delivery of RFA the position of the RF catheter tip is reconfirmed. The patient is placed in a gentle Trendelenburg position. A gentle, manual pressure is exerted over the vein to help apposition between the vein wall and catheter. The RF energy is delivered for 20 seconds. The large diameter GSV or any large segment can be treated twice and then the RF catheter is withdrawn.

The method of treating the SSV is the same except that the catheter is placed in SSV and positioned at least 2.5 cm away from the SPJ. Tumescent anaesthesia is infiltrated around the SSV in the popliteal fascia. Inadvertent heating of the sural nerve is indicated by pain at the heel or in the foot at the beginning of the ablation procedure. After ablation, deep vein patency is confirmed with Doppler thus excluding any inadvertent damage.

After the RF treatment of the saphenous vein any adjuvant treatment (e.g., phlebectomy and sclerotherapy) for the small venous tributaries can be performed during the same sitting or in subsequent sittings if symptoms persist. The catheter entry-site is closed with steri-strips or stitches if a cut-down method is employed. The treated length of the limb is put in a class 2 graduated compression stockings for at least 2 weeks. Postoperatively, patients are encouraged to ambulate immediately but to avoid lifting heavy weights, hot-baths, and the sauna for 2 weeks.

Incompetent perforators can be treated using the ClosureRFS™ or the Closure RFSflex™ catheter. The incompetent perforator is directly accessed using ultrasound guidance, and RF energy is delivered through a small catheter placed at the sub-fascial level.

The advantage of RFA over other thermal ablation techniques is decreased postoperative pain and bruising. This is due to the fact that the RF catheter has a thermostat which controls the temperature and delivers the energy uniformly.

Endovenous Laser Ablation

Endoluminal application of laser energy was described by Bone in 1999.[18] The US Food and Drug Administration (FDA) approved endovenous laser treatment for varicose vein in 2002. In this technique the laser energy is delivered directly to the vein wall with the help of a laser-tip fibre. Lasers with wavelengths of 810, 940, 980, 1320 and 1470 have all been used successfully. There should be minimal blood between the laser fibre and the vein wall so that most of the laser energy is delivered to the vein wall resulting in thickness, eventual contraction, and fibrosis of the vein wall. Some amount of laser energy also gets absorbed by the haemoglobin (Hb) in the blood and water in the vein wall. Various wavelength lasers differ in the proportion of energy absorbed by water. The lesser the amount of energy absorbed by water, the better are the results. Higher wavelength lasers fare better in this aspect.

Most of the procedural details are the same as in the RFA. To avoid repetition the procedural differences are highlighted here. The access to the GSV is obtained by a smaller diameter 5F vascular sheath that has centimetre markings. With the help of the duplex scan, the tip of the catheter is placed 1-2 cm proximal to the SFJ (Figure 4) in the GSV. Tumescent anaesthesia infiltration and Trendelenburg position are the same as during RFA. The laser catheter and sheath are both pulled as one unit at approximately 1 cm every 8 seconds, delivering at least 70 J/cm of length of the GSV. Before taking the catheter out, the patency of the deep veins and successful occlusion of the GSV is confirmed with a duplex scan. Access-site is closed with steri-strips or stitches. Adjuvant procedures, if deemed necessary, can be performed after RFA.

Class 2 graduated compression stockings are applied immediately and worn for 2 weeks. The post operative advice, after-care, and follow-up should be the same as in RFA. EVLA can also be performed for SSV, perforators and accessory thigh veins. The successful occlusion rate of GSV was 98% up to 5-years follow up. Most Treatment failure seems to occur within the first year following treatment. [19]

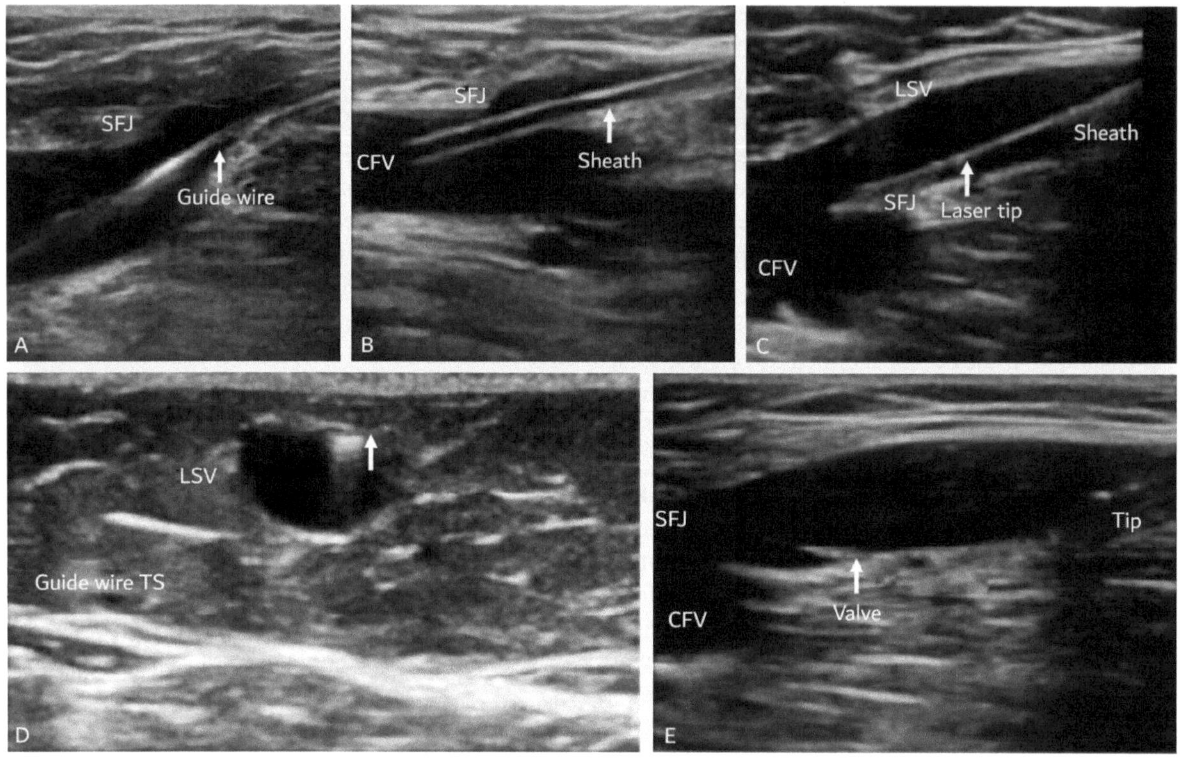

Figure 4: Endovenous Laser Ablation of the Great Saphenous Vein

A: guidewire placed across SFJ into common femoral vein; B: venous catheter sheath; C: exposed Laser tip beyond sheath but close to SFJ; D: guidewire in transverse section; E: final position, Laser tip placed in GSV proximal to SFJ, note the damaged SFJ valve cusp

Adverse events and complications can occur during or after endovenous ablation. During the procedure the cannulation of the vein can be challenging due to the small venous size or veno-spasm. With experience, smaller veins can be cannulated. RF and laser catheters can be passed over a much smaller diameter wire in difficult cases to negotiate the tortuous segment of the vein. Further, topical application of vasodilators can make access easier. Most of the venospasm is produced by the attempts to cannulate the vein. The difficulty could be in passing the wire, sheath, or treatment catheter due to tortuosity of the vein, aneurysmal segment in the vein or due to previous sclerotherapy. RF and laser catheters can be passed over a much smaller wire diameter in cases where it is difficult to negotiate the tortuous segment of the vein. Adverse events (e.g., vagal reaction and arrhythmia) can occur due to anxiety in patients, especially when the procedure is done under local anaesthesia.

Complications include phlebitis, clot extension, DVT, skin burn, haematoma, and wound infection. Some degree of phlebitis is inherent as the inflammation sets in the treated segment of the vein-wall. Usually, it settles down without any specific treatment. Some patients may describe a strange "pulling" sensation in the thigh or legs after 5-7 days. This could be due to inflammation in the treated vein which shrinks over a period of time. This also settles down in 2-3 weeks and only anti-inflammatory medication may be needed. The most serious complication of endovenous ablation is clot extension into the deep vein. If it is detected with duplex immediately after the procedure or in early follow-up days, treatment with LMW Heparin or thrombectomy should be offered. It is good practice to have an early duplex examination of the treated limb to exclude this possibility. Another complication is nerve injury which occurs when the heat is conducted to the nerve trunk which runs very close to the venous trunk especially in the lower third of the leg. The incidence of nerve injury even when GSVs are treated is low. The tumescent anaesthesia perhaps protects the nerve. Skin burns have diminished significantly since the introduction of tumescent anaesthesia.[20]

Table 14 and Table 15 summarise the percentage (not number) of complications following radiofrequency and endovenous laser ablation, respectively, for varicose veins published in the medical literature before and after 2008.

Table 14: Complications of Radio-frequency Ablation for Varicose Vein post 2008

Author (year)	Limbs treated	Follow-up (month)	Skin burn	Paraesthesia	Phlebitis	DVT/ PE	Recurrence/ Recanalization
Almedia (2009)	46	1	0	2.2	0	0 / 0	- / -
Gale (2010)	46	12	-	-	-	- / -	23.9 / -
Nordon (2011)	76	3	1.3	2.6	1.3	0 / 0	- / 3
Rasmussen (2011)	148	12	0	4	8	0 / 0	- / 4.8
Elkaffas (2011)	90	24+	0	10	6.6	0 / 0	13.3 / -

Table 15: Complications of Endovenous Laser Ablation for Varicose Vein post 2008

Author (year)	Limbs treated	Follow-up (month)	Skin burn	Paraesthesia	Phlebitis	DVT/ PE	Recurrence/ Recanalization
Darwood (2008)	62	12	0	1.4	12.6	0 / 0	5.6 / -
Fernandez (2008)	1985	24	-	2.43	2.9	0.13/0	21.7/ 1.8
Theivacumar (2009)	69	24	0	-	-	- / -	7 /4.3
Almedia (2009)	41	1	0	4.9	14.6	2.4 / 0	- / -
Rasmussen (2010)	69	24	0	-	-	-	26 / -
Gale (2010)	48	12	-	-	-	-	4 / -
Christenson (2010)	100	24	0	1	4	0 / 0	7 / -
Nordon (2011)	78	3	2.6	1.3	2.6	0 / 0	- / 4
Carradice (2011)	139	12	0	2.9	2.9	0 / 0	4 / 0.7
Rasmussen (2011)	144	12	0	2	2.8	0 / 0	- / 5.8
Wang (2011)	361	-	13	25	1.93	0.6 / 0	- / -

Ultrasound Guided Foam Sclerotherapy

Chemical sclerosing for treating varicose veins has been practised for quite some time. Its application for treating truncal venous reflux offers a simple, cheap, and affordable alternative. There is a renewed interest in foam sclerotherapy as an alternative to primary and recurrent truncal reflux in varicose veins.

All sclerosants produce a similar histological effect. Intravenous injection causes endothelial cell swelling and disruption, causing an acute inflammatory reaction and resulting in fibrous obliteration of the vessel lumen. The severity of the reaction depends upon the concentration and amount of agent. The selection of agent, concentration, and quantity depends upon the size and site of the vein to be injected. Smaller superficial veins should be injected with lower concentrations and smaller amounts of the sclerosant. The appropriately selected agent is injected intravenously in correct amounts, with a fine needle (after emptying the vein by leg elevation).

Sclerosing agents can be classified according to their mode of action into:

1. Osmotic: hypertonic saline 23.4%, glucose 65%, sodium salicylate.
2. Detergent: sodium tetradecyl-sulfate, polidocanol, sodium morrhuate, ethanolamine
3. Corrosive: sodium iodide, potassium iodide (both mixed with benzyl alcohol and chromated glycerine)
4. Chemical: ethanol

The detergent type of sclerosant can be injected as foam. Foam can be obtained by mixing a chemical detergent sclerosing agent with air or other gases (e.g., CO^2, O^2, or a combination of O^2 and CO^2). Foam is prepared by the Tessari's method[21] in which gas and sclerosing agent are mixed between two syringes connected with a 3-way connector, by at least 20 back and forth movements of the piston of the syringe. The ratio of sclerosing agent to gas can be 1:3 to 1:4. The sclerosing agent commonly used in the UK is sodium tetradecyl sulphate. In Europe polidocanol is also used. Higher amounts of foam are likely to result in an increased incidence of complications. The foam is superior to liquid sclerotherapy because once injected in the vein, it does not mix with the blood and pushes the blood away, maximizing contact with the vein wall. Therefore, smaller amounts of foam can induce more chemical irritation of venous endothelium, resulting in better obliteration of the venous lumen. The maximum total amount of sclerosant injected in one sitting should not exceed 4-6 ml of liquid sclerosants or 8-15 ml of foam.

Ultrasound guidance provides better access to veins which were not visible previously. A direct access to the vein is obtained by a needle mounted on a syringe. Freshly prepared foam is injected intravenously. The other method of foam delivery includes the "butterfly" needle, micro or long catheters with or without side-holes, and Seldinger sheaths.

Following the foam injection, thigh-length compression hosiery that exerts 20-30 mmHg of pressure at ankle level is recommended by most practitioners. The extremity could also be compressed in bandages with adequate padding and protection over the injected area and around the knee. Compression avoids trapping of blood and maintains the vein walls in apposition. This should be applied for at least 3-4 days without any interruption followed by compression hosiery. In most European countries a compression is applied for 3-4 weeks. Stockings have much better patient compliance, but full-thigh length stockings often roll-down unless worn with an appropriate waist support system. The evidence for compression is controversial.[22] A success-rate of 78-88% is quoted in the literature.[23]

Individualized sclerotherapy taking into account the risk-benefit analysis should be offered to pregnant women, elderly, sedentary, obese (body mass index >30), peripheral arterial occlusive disease (ankle brachial pressure index <0.7) patients, and patients who have underlying valvular or perforator incompetence. It can be offered to superficial veins of 1-3 mm diameter, postoperative residual veins, and congenital vascular (predominantly venous) malformations.

Absolute contraindications include allergy to sclerosing agent, severe impairment to general health, bed rest, deep vein thrombosis, and presence of a symptomatic patent foramen ovale. Relative contraindications include history of migraine with auras and active superficial thrombophlebitis.

Sclerotherapy can produce local or systemic adverse events which may be immediate or delayed in onset. Immediate systemic events include anaphylactic reaction and visual symptoms such as transient blindness and headache. These symptoms are more likely to occur with foam sclerotherapy and in the presence of a patent foramen ovale. Delayed local adverse events include ecchymosis, pigmentation, matting, thrombophlebitis, and skin necrosis. "Matting" or "Blushing" refers to the appearance of tiny red telangiectasias. They can appear spontaneously or following the treatment in the vicinity of an injected vein. Its cause is unknown. Microthrombectomy may be needed 2-3 weeks after injection to reduce the hyperpigmentation. Additionally, DVT can occur as a rare, delayed systemic adverse effect, especially if a large amount of sclerosants is injected in an immobile, obese patient.

Innovative Methods of Treatment of the Saphenous Vein

These methods include cryolysis, ambulatory bloodless catheter-delivered endovenous foam, obliteration of saphenous trunks with hyper-heated steam, and external ultrasound valvuloplasty. There is a clear shift towards less invasive treatment modalities.

Treatment of Telangiectasia

Patients with telangiectasia can be treated with sclerotherapy, laser, or intense pulsed light (IPL) therapy. IPL sources, unlike laser sources, do not use monochromatic or coherent light emission. Instead, a variety of lasers with wavelengths ranging between 532 and 1064 nm are used. Gradually the pulse-duration, fluence, and wavelengths of transcutaneous lasers are increasing. The laser and IPL do not involve needles, compression bandages, and are not dose limited.

Both legs can be treated at the same time. The success depends upon the physics of the light-tissue interaction. The correct selection of wavelength, amount of laser energy, and laser pulse duration is important for good outcomes.

Melanin found in the epidermis of human skin, also absorbs the light and in this aspect competes with haemoglobin in the dermis. If larger amounts of laser energy are absorbed by melanin, the skin will become hyperpigmented. Similarly, a tanned skin with higher melanin pigmentation is a relative contraindication for treating telangiectasia with a laser. Complications include idiopathic hypersensitivity, hyperpigmentation, matting, incomplete elimination of telangiectasia, treatment related pain, skin burn, and blister formation. Additionally, effective skin cooling prevents thermal skin damage.

REFERENCES

1. DeWeese JA: Treatment of venous disease: the innovators. J Vasc Surg 1994; 20:675-83.
2. Murakami G, Negishi N, Tanaka K, Hoshi H, Sezai Y. Anatomical relationship between saphenous vein and cutaneous nerves. Okajimas Folia Anat Jpn 1994;71(1):21-33.
3. Ricci S, Moro L, Antonelli Incalzi R. Ultrasound imaging of the sural nerve: ultrasound anatomy and rationale for investigation. Eur J Vasc & Endovasc Surg 2010;39(5):636-41.
4. Beebe HG, Bergan JJ, Bergqvist D et al. Classification and grading of chronic venous disease in the lower limbs: a consensus statement. Vasc Surg 1996; 30:5-11.
5. Eklof B, Rutherford RB, Bergan JJ et al. The American Venous Forum International Ad Hoc Committee for Revision of the CEAP Classification. Revision of the CEAP classification for chronic venous disorders: Consensus statement. J Vasc Surg 2004; 40: 1248-52.

6. Brand FN, Dannenberg AL, Abbott RD, Kannel WB. The epidemiology of varicose veins: the Framingham study. Am J Prev Med 1988; 4: 96-101.
7. Franks PJ, Wright DD, Moffatt CJ, Stirling J, Fletcher AE, Bulpitt CJ, McCollum CN. Prevalence of venous disease: a community study in West London. Eur J Surg 1992:158:143-47.
8. Bradbury A, Evans CJ, Allan P, Lee A, Ruckley CV, Fowkes FG. What are the symptoms of varicose veins? Edinburgh vein study cross sectional population survey. BMJ 1999; 318:353-6.
9. Coon WW, Willis PV, Keller JB. Venous thromboembolism and other venous diseases in the Tecumesh community health study. Circulation 1973;48: 838-46.
10. Caggiati A. Fascial relationships of the long saphenous vein. Circulation 1999; 100: 2547-9.
11. Caggiati A. Fascial relationships of the short saphenous vein. J Vasc Surg 2001; 34:241-6.
12. Frings N, Nelle A, Tran P, Fischer R, Krug W. Reduction of neoreflux after correctly performed ligation of saphenofemoral junction. A randomised trial. Eur J Vasc Endovasc Surg 2004; 28:246-52.
13. Negus D. Should the incompetent saphenous vein be stripped to ankle level? Phlebology 1986; 1:33-6.
14. Jones L, Braithwaite BD, Selwyn D et al. Neovascularisation is the principal cause of varicose vein recurrence: results of a randomized trial of stripping the long saphenous vein. Eur J Vasc Endovasc Surg 1996; 12: 442-5.
15. Lurie F, Creton D, Eklof B et al. Prospective randomised study of endovenous radiofrequency obliteration. J Vasc Surg 2003; 38:207-14.
16. Zikorus AW, Mirrizzi MS. Evaluation of set point temperature and pullback speed on vein adventitial temperature during endovenous radiofrequency energy delivery in an in-vitro model. Vasc Endovascular Surg 2004; 38:167-84.
17. Merchant RF, Pichot O. Long-term outcomes of endovenous radiofrequency obliteration of saphenous reflux as a treatment for superficial venous insufficiency. J Vasc Surg 2005:42:502-9.
18. Bone C. Tratmiento endoluminal de las varices con laser de diodo. Estudio preliminary. Rev Patol Vasc 1999; V:35-46.
19. Min R, Khilnani N. Endovenous laser treatment of saphenous vein reflux: long term result. J Vasc Interv Radiol 2003;14:991-6.
20. Merchant RF, DePalma RG, Kabnick LS. Endovascular obliteration of saphenous reflux: a multicentre study. J Vasc Surg 2002;35:1190-6.
21. Tessari L. Nouvelle technique d'obtention de la sclero-mousse. Phlebologie 2000; 53:129.
22. Breu FX, Guggenbichler S, Wollmann JC. 2nd Eouropean consensus meeting on foam sclerotherapy 2006, Tegernsee, Germany. Vasa 2008; 37 (Suppl 71):1-29.
23. Bergan J, Pascarella L, Mekenas L. Venous disorders: treatment with sclerosant foam. J Cardiovasc Surg 2006; 47:9-18.

❑❑❑

39

CHAPTER

Lymphedema

Gary Lambert, MD, MRCS, FRCS
Alok Tiwari, MS, FRCS
Rajiv Vohra, Ph.D., FRCSEd, FRCSEng

INTRODUCTION

Lymphedema is the term given to describe swelling due to the accumulation of protein rich fluid within the interstitium. The underlying cause of the accumulation is due to failure of the lymphovascular system to drain the affected area sufficiently. Lymphedema is characteristically associated with regional anatomical swelling, and subsequent trophic tissue changes in the affected area. It can affect any region of the body that undergoes lymphatic drainage. Although most commonly associated with limb swelling, it can affect organs and tissues throughout the body.

Pathophysiology

The lymphatic system consists of endothelial lined channels which drain into regional lymph nodes. It is from the nodes that the fluid is then returned to the circulating vascular system. Lymphedema results in the build-up of interstitial fluid with high protein content as a result of inadequate lymphatic drainage. The resultant elevation in the oncotic pressure further prevents fluid from being returned to the intravascular or intracellular state. Under normal conditions, the lymphovascular system is responsible for the drainage of this fluid and its return to the intravascular volume via the lymphatic channels and regional nodes. Any impairment of the lymphatic system therefore has the potential to cause lymphedema. Such failure can be due to occlusion, hypoplasia, aplasia, or fibrosis of any part of the lymphatic system.

The lymphatic system not only provides a mechanism for fluid homeostasis, but also plays an important role in immunity. Accumulation of lymphedema further impairs the immunological system, increasing susceptibility to infection within the affected region. The cumulative elevation of interstitial protein within the tissues also leads to inflammation, fibrosis, and scarring which further exacerbates the pre-existing lymphatic dysfunction.

Aetiology / Classification

Lymphedema is classified based upon the cause of the lymphatic failure. The most commonly used classification system describes the etiology as either primary or secondary lymphedema. Whilst this system categorises the cause of the condition, there is no bearing on the therapeutic modality, nor does it describe the severity of the condition.

Primary Lymphedema:

Primary lymphedema is considered to be developmental. It is further classified according to the age of onset (Table 1).

Classification	Onset
Congenital	• From Birth or before 1 year old • Familial (Milroy's syndrome)
Praecox	• Until the age of 35 • Most frequently during puberty • Familial (Meige's disease)
Tarda	• After the age of 35

Table 1: Classification of primary lymphedema

It is estimated that between 1/6000 and 1/10,000 live births are affected by congenital lymphedema, with 1.15/100,000 people under the age of 25 developing primary lymphedema. In addition, there are both familial and non-familial forms of primary lymphedema. Most forms are sporadic, but 10-15% are due to familial or syndromic causes.[1] Of these, the majority are autosomal dominant (Milroy's syndrome,

Meige's disease) and are linked to Vascular Endothelial Growth Factor (VEGF).

Primary lymphedema has been further classified by Browse into the functional abnormality leading to lymphedema.[2]

Table 2: Classification of Primary Lymphedema by Browse

A. Congenital primary lymphedema	1. Congenital hypoplasia or aplasia of peripheral lymphatics (the edema will be present at birth or will appear within 2 years)
	2. Congenital abnormalities of the thoracic or abdominal lymph trunks
	3. Congenital valvular incompetence (this will always be associated with megalymphatics and will often be associated with chylous reflux)
B. Acquired primary lymphedema	1. Intraluminal/intramural obstructive edema • *Distal:* this is an acquired obliteration of the distal lymphatics with an uncertain etiology • *Proximal:* this is an acquired obliteration of the lymphatics of the proximal limb, it is normally associated with distal dilation, the etiology is uncertain • *Combined:* this is an acquired obliteration of all the limb lymphatics
	2. Lymph node obstruction by hilar fibrosis; this may coexist with obstructive edema, and can be followed by acquired valvular incompetence

The classification into primary and secondary also creates the premise that the cause of lymphedema is one or the other. However, the development of secondary lymphedema in individuals with minimal causative risk has resulted in the understanding that there is an overlap between the two classifications. Patients may have a predisposing sub-clinical primary developmental abnormality that is exacerbated or exposed only through a secondary insult.

Secondary Lymphedema:

Secondary lymphedema is the more common form of lymphedema, potentially accounting for 99% of cases of lymphedema. There is considerable worldwide variation in the relative cause of secondary lymphedema. In the western world, the most common causes are malignancy related, either through direct infiltrative or mass effects of the malignancy, or through the damage caused to the lymphatic system as a result of surgery or radiotherapy. Infections of viral and, more commonly, bacterial origin can cause lymphatic obstruction due to recurrent or chronic inflammation and subsequent fibrosis. Within mosquito endemic areas, the risk of nematode related lymphedema (filariasis) is the leading cause of lymphedema, accounting for over 120 million cases of lymphedema worldwide, according to WHO figures. Filariasis is therefore the leading cause of lymphedema worldwide.[3]

Table 3: Causes of Secondary Lymphedema

Causes of Secondary Lymphedema	Mechanism
Filariasis	• Lymphatic invasion and obstruction by nematodes
Malignancy	• Direct Nodal Invasion • Mass effect and compression of lymphatics
Lymph Node excision / ablation	• Node excision for malignancy • Radiotherapy for malignancy
Infections Streptococcal Staphylococcus Aureus Tuberculosis	• Nodal and lymphatic scarring
Trauma	• Surgery • Curvilinear scars • Recurrent dissections
Obesity	• Elevated intra-abdominal / thoracic pressures • Lymphatic compression causing impeded lymphatic return

Filariasis

This is characterised by lymphedema secondary to lymphatic obstruction by adult nematodes. The disease is caused by roundworms of the family *Filarioidea* as listed below:

1. *Wuchereria bancrofti*, accounts for 90% of the cases
2. *Brugia malayi*, responsible for majority of the remaining cases
3. *Brugia timori*, which is also implicated

Mosquitoes act as the vector for transmission of the microfilaria, which then circulate within the host, migrating into the lymphatic channels as they mature. The lifecycle of the filarial nematode is approximately 6-8 years. The circulation of microfilaria within the bloodstream is adapted to coincide with the periods of peak activity in the relative mosquito vector. There is regional variability as to which mosquitoes act as vectors for the microfilaria (Table 4).

Table 4: Filariasis Vectors

Mosquito vector	Region
Culex	Urban and semi urban regions
Anopheles	Predominantly rural regions
Aedes	Pacific Islands

Studies have demonstrated that up to 85% of people with filariasis have clinical evidence of lymphedema, and that as many as 11% of endemic populations develop lymphedema secondary to filarial infection [3-6].

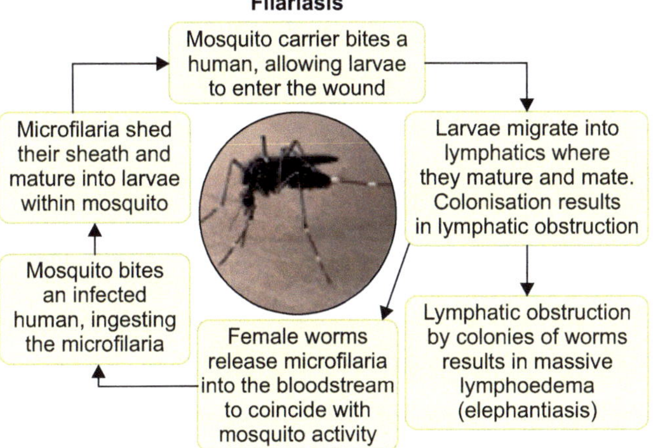

Figure 1: Filariasis Cycle

Clinical Assessment

History:

A detailed history will usually enable the diagnosis and classification of lymphedema to be made. It will permit the identification of potential causes for secondary lymphedema, confirm the likelihood of primary disease, and help determine whether there is a hereditary component. Features of the history will also help to exclude potential differential diagnoses. The pattern and nature of onset is of importance as lymphedema has a progressive onset and history of intermittent edema is rarely due to lymphedema.

A typical presenting history is of gradual onset, progressive swelling of a limb or region of the body such as the genitalia. Initially, it is rare for lymphedema to be painful. However, patients will often describe their limb as feeling heavy as the day progresses, with associated fatigue in the limb.

Recurrent infections both cause and result from lymphedema. It is important to ascertain the frequency and duration of any recurrent infections in the affected region, as this is prognostic. Infections that frequently recur can cause progression of the disease, exacerbating symptoms and limb volume. Frequent recurrence of infections should influence the management of the patient and consideration for more intensive therapy or the use of long-term prophylactic antibiotics.

Also, important and pertinent to the history of the condition is the patient's symptomatology. While the swelling is often initially pain free and therefore causes fewer symptoms, the psychosocial impact of the edema can be significant. With potential effects including fatigue, difficulty with clothing or footwear, and extending to social exclusion or stigma, it is important to assess the extent of the condition from a functional as well as clinical perspective.

Examination:

Crucial to the diagnosis of lymphedema is the physical presence of edema. Edema is due to the high oncotic pressure in the interstitial space. It does not result in pitting edema unless it is in the early stages. However, it is important to be aware that overlap exists with other conditions which may cause a degree of superimposed pitting. Most commonly the swelling is from distal to proximal, and there is unlikely to be any sparing of the distal region. By the end of the first year the edema usually becomes non-pitting due to the onset of fibrosis and hydrostatic pressure [1]. This progression can be staged using the International Society of Lymphology (ISL) staging criteria according to the clinical findings[7] (Table 5). In regions endemic with filariasis, the presence of genital and groin lymphedema is more common than in the western world.

Table 5: Clinical staging of lymphedema

Stage 0	• Latent or subclinical condition. Impaired lymph transport without evident swelling. This can exist for months or even years before overt edema is noticed.
Stage 1	• There is early accumulation of fluid that is fairly high in protein. The edema subsides when the limb is elevated. Pitting can occur.
Stage 2	• As tissue fibrosis develops, pitting can occur. • The tissue swelling is rarely reduced with limb elevated.
Stage 3	• Lymphostatic elephantiasis, pitting is absent. • Development of trophic skin changes (i.e., fat deposits, acanthosis, and warty overgrowths) occurs often.

Presence of non-pitting edema without distal sparing leads to a change in the architecture of the skin and subcutaneous planes. This can be demonstrated by Stemmer's sign (Figure 2), which is the inability to pinch the skin overlying the second metatarsal to form a tent. This sign is of potential use in differentiating lymphedema from lipoedema, as the foot is usually spared in lipoedema, allowing tenting to be demonstrated.

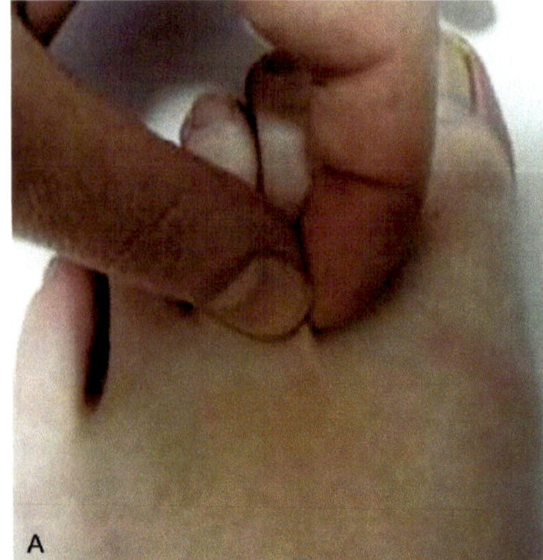

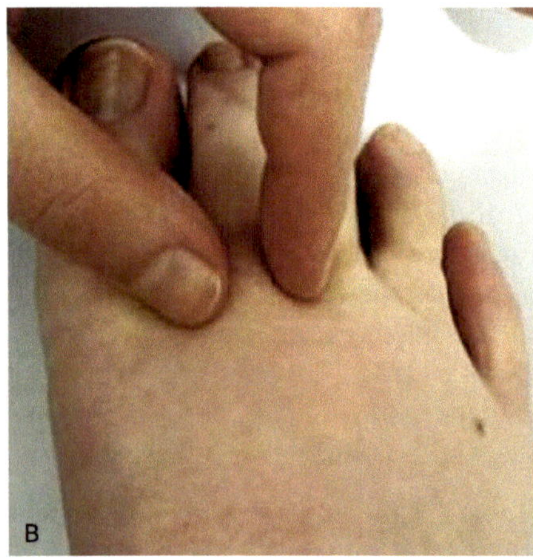

Figure 2: Stemmer's sign, negative in A, positive in B

It is also important to identify any evidence of complication such as infection or ulceration as a result of the presence of lymphedema. Many of the complications of lymphedema become evident only after a prolonged period of the condition (see 'Complications').

The extent of the swelling is important. Limb measurements using girth or displacement can be useful to distinguish subtle variations in deformity. In the case of filariasis, the extent of edema can be profound, with massive tissue deformity resulting in the classical appearances of elephantiasis.

Completion of the examination requires a directed systemic examination to exclude or confirm any relevant differential diagnoses or potential causes of secondary lymphedema. In particular, looking for regional lymphadenopathy in the groins, axillae, or cervical chains suggests lymphatic infiltration or inflammation. The limb or region in question, including interdigital web spaces, must be fully examined to exclude lesions which may otherwise be missed. Palpation of the abdomen may elicit pelvic masses as a cause of both venous and lymphatic obstruction, further guiding investigation.

Assessment of Limb Volume:

There are various methods used to assess the volume of affected limbs and to monitor the progress of the condition or its treatment. The most simple and widely used method is serial circumferential measurements of the limb at 4cm intervals from defined anatomical landmarks on the limb. Volume displacement utilises the Archimedes' principle of water displacement to estimate the volume of the limb when submerged in water; this remains the Gold Standard for volume assessment. More modern methods include bioimpedance analysis (BIA). A low-level electrical charge is passed and measured between electrodes, permitting analysis of the tissue fluid volume. Perometry involves the use of infra-red beam scanning of the limb to build a three-dimensional outline, allowing a computer to calculate the volume accordingly.

General Investigations

Basic laboratory investigations are aimed at assessing the possible systemic causes of peripheral edema (Table 6). They are only necessary to rule out remaining differentials following clinical assessment. The choice of investigations should be influenced by the clinical picture developed within the history and examination, aiming to exclude medical differential diagnoses.[8,9]

Table 6: General investigations

Standard blood tests	• Thyroid Functions • Liver Functions • Kidney Functions • Serum proteins • Inflammatory markers • Full blood count
Blood film	• Microfilariasis visualised • Optimal timing strategy needed to coincide with peak microfilaria circulation.
Polymerase Chain Reaction (PCR)	• Modern PCR testing for microfilariasis is available to some centres.

Radiological Investigations

Radiological investigations are both useful in finalising diagnosis as well as identifying potential causes of secondary lymphedema. There are several modalities available (Table 7). It is important to understand the limitations and indications for each modality in order to decide which is most appropriate for a case. The choice of modality, on its own or in combination, will yield far greater diagnostic information than a less systematic approach.

Lymphoscintigram

Lymphoscintigram is the investigation of choice in the diagnosis of lymphedema (Figure 3). It is considered to be the Gold Standard, with 100% specificity and 92% sensitivity.[8-12]

A subcutaneous injection of technetium Tc99m – labelled albumin, sulphur or antimony is injected into the interdigital webspace of both limbs. It is often also accompanied with an oral solution of Heptaminol Adenosine Phosphate, which has been shown to increase lymphatic uptake. The limbs are then imaged using a scintigraphic camera at intervals to allow comparison between the limbs. Images are taken at intervals up to 24 hours, if necessary, with early and late imaging being necessary in certain cases to provide adequate imaging for diagnosis.

Lymphedema is characterised by absent or delayed filling of the lymphatics and delay in proximal uptake via the regional lymph nodes. Dermal backflow within the skin is evidence of lymphatic reflux into the tissues as a result of lymphatic hypertension. The degree and intensity of dermal backflow potentially correlates with the response to manual and compressive lymphatic therapy.[8,9,13]

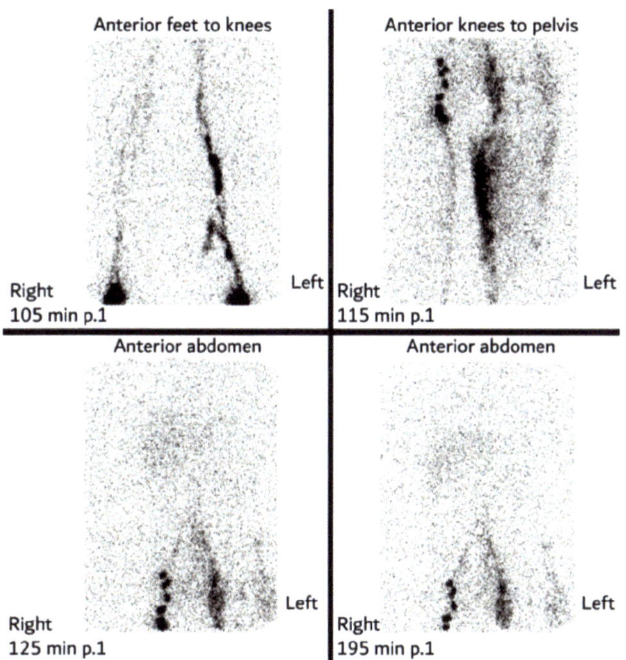

Figure 3: Lymphoscintigram showing delayed drainage and skin backflow in the lymphoedematous left leg in comparison with early uptake and inguinal node drainage on the right.

Ultrasound

Plain ultrasound scanning can be of use in non-invasive examination of the tissues within the affected region. In a skilled operator's hand, it is possible to identify some of the tissue and structural changes within the limb's tissues. This, however, is of less diagnostic value and is non-discriminatory. It is also possible to identify masses and nodal architecture on an ultrasound scan, which may help with both the diagnosis and identification of the cause of secondary disease.

Duplex Ultrasound is of little clinical use in the actual imaging of lymphatics and therefore non-diagnostic for lymphedema. Its main role is in the exclusion of superficial and deep venous insufficiency as a contributing factor. Evidence has demonstrated that lymphatic insufficiency is also associated with chronic venous insufficiency and can be present together.[8,9]

Magnetic Resonance Imaging

MRI imaging in lymphedema is very useful. It is able to identify and visualize the lymphatic system within the affected region. Although it is not effective in the differentiation between primary and secondary lymphedema, it is able to help clarify the cause of secondary disease such as nodal malignancy.[8,9]

The MRI is also able to provide information regarding the tissues affected and the extent of fibrosis and fascial involvement. This imaging of the tissues enables lymphedema to be distinguished from lipoedema and venous edema. The classical finding of lymphedema on MRI scanning is of circumferential edema within the epifascial plane, leading to the classic honeycombing pattern between the muscle and the dermis. In venous edema there is also edema within the subfascial plane and muscle, while lipoedema demonstrates swelling with an absence of edema fluid but the accumulation of fat, with normal lymphatic architecture.[9]

MRI is also useful in the monitoring of lymphedema. It is possible to calculate limb volumes using scans. MRI is also useful in the identification and staging of potential lymphangiosarcoma.

Computerised Tomography

CT scanning is of less clinical use than MRI. It can give similar information and diagnostic value with respect to tissue architecture. Unfortunately, it also involves the use of radiation. Similar to MRI, CT scanning demonstrates a honeycomb appearance of the tissue in lymphedema but not in venous or lipoedema [8,9].

Lymphangiography

Direct injection of lipid soluble contrast into the subcutaneous lymphatics following initial identification with patent blue dye, helps visualise and demonstrate the lymphatic anatomy. However, it has been replaced as a diagnostic imaging modality by lymphoscintigraphy which is technically easier to perform and carries less risk of lymphatic injury or pain. Its use is now limited to preoperative investigation of patients being considered for surgical intervention.

Radiological Test	Typical Findings	Useful differential findings
Ultrasound	• Skin and compartment thickening	• Pelvic mass • Lymphadenopathy not previously palpable • Lymphatic node structure • DVT • Venous reflux
CT scan	• Thickening of skin • Fibrosis in subcutaneous tissue • Honeycombing of tissue	• Presence of tumour • Vascular compromise • Lymphadenopathy
Lymphoscintigram	• Dermal backflow • Delayed or absent drainage	• Normal result has high negative predictive value
MRI scan	• Skin thickening • Increased interstitial fluid enhancement	• Identification of tumour or mass • Vascular information • Plane of edema • Lymphadenopathy

Table 7: Summary of investigations

Differential diagnosis

The potential list of differential diagnoses for lymphedema is extensive. In order to commence building a list of potential differentials, one can consider all causes of a swollen limb [8,9] (Table 8).

Condition	Features	Differentiation
Chronic Venous Insufficiency	• Failure of the ability to efficiently return blood from the region due to venous damage. • Can be bilateral or unilateral • Both deep venous insufficiency and varicose veins can result in peripheral edema	• Edema usually spares the foot • Skin changes consistent with venous disease • Negative Stemmer's sign • Duplex shows reflux >0.5 seconds
Deep Vein Thrombosis	• Occlusion of the deep vein preventing venous drainage. • Usually acute painful swelling of the limb. • Tender to palpate.	• Accompanying history with risk for DVT • Immobility, hypercoagulable state • Duplex identifying DVT • Visible on CT and MRI
Lipoedema	• Usually symmetrical swelling of the legs • Adipose deposition in the limbs. • Almost exclusively present in women	• Sparing of the feet. • Negative Stemmer's sign • Lymphoscintigraphy is normal • MRI demonstrates fat deposition as opposed to edema.
Obesity	• Morbid obesity results in symmetrical fat deposits in legs as well as the rest of the body. • It can progress to cause secondary superimposed lymphedema	• Normal lymphoscintigraphy. • Normal CT/MRI
Cardiac Failure	• Failure of the right ventricle • Pitting edema, bilateral • Associated symptoms, fatigue, reduced exercise tolerance, dyspnoea	• Edema is symmetrical and pitting • ECG may show evidence of LVH • CXR cardiomegaly potential evidence of LVF

Metabolic	• Myxoedema	• Deranged thyroid function tests
Hypoalbuminemia	• Protein loss; renal failure or enteropathy • Synthesis impairment; hepatic failure • Pitting edema due to reduced vascular oncotic pressure • Symmetrical	• Symmetrical pitting edema • Low serum protein levels on biochemistry • Impaired renal / hepatic function
Malignancy	• Lesions such as sarcoma, angiosarcoma • Swelling often associated with pain	• MRI demonstrates lesion and gives staging too • Pain is considerable feature of such malignancies, beyond that of lymphedema
Infection / Inflammation	• Arthritis, particularly in paediatrics • Osteomyelitis • Myositis • Associated systemic symptoms and pain	• Elevated inflammatory markers • MRI and USS can both demonstrate tissue inflammation, joint space increase
Arterio-venous Malformation	• Combined lymphatic venous and arterial malformations • Klippel-Trenaunay syndrome • Limb hypertrophy	• MRI demonstrates malformation • Involvement of muscular compartments as well
Hemihypertrophy	• Unilateral idiopathic enlargement of a limb	• Normal investigations • Diagnosis of exclusion

Table 8: Differential diagnosis of limb swelling

The potential differential diagnosis for regional or limb swelling is extensive. Much of the differentiation occurs at the clinical level during the history and examination of the patient.

Complications

Physical complications of lymphedema are related directly to the impairment of lymphatic drainage. Over time, the presence of the excess lymph results in fibrosis within the skin and subcutaneous tissues. This scarring results in excess keratinisation, and fissuring of the skin, progressing to a failure in the skin's ability to act as an immune barrier, thus permitting pathogens, commonly bacteria or fungi, to enter the skin through the fissures. Once bacteria, most commonly staphylococcus aureus and streptococcus,[14,15] enter via the fissure, the immune system is less able to mount an effective response due to the failure of the lymphatic system and inability to deliver lymphocytes to the region. Lymphatic failure further results in the accumulation of lymph, with its high protein content, which in turn acts as a perfect medium for bacterial culture. Therefore, bacteria can spread quickly within the cutaneous and subcutaneous planes. With an already impaired regional immune system due to the lymphatic failure, the body is less able to effectively clear the invading bacteria from the region in question.

Bacterial invasion within the subcutaneous tissues manifests as cellulitis/erysipelas or, if invasion of the lymphatic channel occurs, as lymphangitis. In both conditions, the onset of infection and resultant loco-regional acute phase response results in inflammation and edema. In turn, the acute phase response further impairs lymphatic drainage, resulting in persistent and progressive lymphedema, creating a vicious cyclical relationship between infection and lymphedema. Patients with lymphedema are at significantly increased risk of recurrent infections. The frequency and severity of recurrent infections may necessitate long term prophylactic antibiotic therapy to prevent recurrent infections and limit potential secondary damage to the lymphatics.[16]

Lymphangiosarcoma is a rare complication of chronic lymphedema. It was first described in 1948 in patients with secondary lymphedema of the arm following mastectomy. This description gave rise to the title of Stewart Treves Syndrome [1,17] which is a rare form of cancer, similar to Kaposi's sarcoma. It is usually an aggressive cancer with poor prognosis. Currently, approximately 400 cases have been described in the literature.

There are considerable psycho-social complications that are also associated with longstanding lymphedema. Cosmesis and functional impairment lead to feelings of isolation that often manifest themselves in actual social exclusion. Social Isolation is further exacerbated by the potential limitation of activity due to pain, recurrent infection, or reduced function of the limb or limbs affected. The reduced function limits activity and ability to mobilize in many instances.[18]

Treatment

Since there is no curative therapy for lymphedema, strategies must be directed wherever possible to prevent its development. In cases where prevention has failed, treatment centres on reduction or maintenance of limb volume for symptom relief and to reduce the risk of complications. Active treatment of lymphedema can be conservative, pharmacological, and surgical.

Prevention

Filaria: Filariasis is the leading cause of lymphedema worldwide and is caused by the proliferation of filarial nematodes transmitted via the mosquito vector. Interruption of this cycle is the single greatest opportunity to reduce the risk of lymphedema worldwide, especially within tropical endemic regions.

The WHO programme for prevention and management of filariasis was implemented in the year 2000 in the form of the Global Programme to Eliminate Lymphatic Filariasis (GPELF), with the aim of eliminating filariasis by 2020. The GPELF is based upon two key interventions. The first is Mass Drug Administration (MDA) which involves the interruption of vector transmission through large scale annual treatment programmes, implemented to cover the entire at-risk population within an area. The second intervention is through morbidity management and disability prevention in those with lymphedema due to filariasis.

Mass Drug Administration (MDA) is the method used to treat filaria prophylactically. In order to interrupt the transmission, the incidence within regions is mapped helping to determine where to administer MDA. With this information, single doses of albendazole plus either diethylcarbamazine or ivermectin is distributed in endemic regions, enabling the treatment of at-risk populations. In particular, the treatment regime for MDA is a single dose of albendazole (400 mg) plus either ivermectin (150-200 mcg/kg) in is given in areas where onchocerciasis (the filarial worm Onchocerca volvulus which causes river blindness) is also endemic, and diethylcarbamazine citrate (DEC) (6 mg/kg) in is given in areas where onchocerciasis is not endemic. The medication clears microfilaria from the bloodstream and kills a majority of the adult worms. To completely interrupt infection transmission, MDA should be continued for 4-6 years.

By 2010, mapping was completed in 59 endemic countries, and MDA started to be implemented in 53 countries. Between 2000 to 2010, over 3.4 billion treatments were delivered to 900 million people in 53 countries, greatly decreasing transmission in many regions. Since the year 2000, it is estimated that transmission of lymphatic filariasis in at-risk populations has decreased by 43%.[3,19]

Mosquito control is a complementary measure that is also required to assist transmission prevention. Measures such as insecticide-treated nets or indoor insecticide may help protect populations in endemic regions from primary infection and in conjunction with MDA provides greater protection.

Infection: Prompt appropriate management of acute infections such as cellulitis, reduces the degree of injury to the lymphatic system that results in the development of lymphedema. Management and prevention, reduction of occurrence, or frequency of infections in at-risk populations, such as those with diabetes, chronic venous, or arterial insufficiency—with or without ulceration—reduces the risk of developing secondary lymphedema. The presence of venous insufficiency in conjunction with lymphatic insufficiency creates a potential group who are at notable risk.

Iatrogenic: Advances in the management of malignancy have been accompanied by a reduction in the incidence of lymphedema in patients undergoing therapy, whether it is surgical or radiological. The move away from radical mastectomy to simple mastectomy and breast conserving surgery, and more recently to the node preserving surgery (i.e., sampling and sentinel node biopsy) in conjunction with improved imaging has reduced the necessity for radical nodal clearances, repeat surgical procedures,[20] and the associated morbidity from lymphedema.[21] The alteration of radiotherapeutic treatment regimes, both dose and field, have also resulted in a more localized targeted delivery of radiation, limiting the collateral damage to lymphatic regions.

Conservative Therapy

The majority of patients with lymphedema require only conservative therapy to maintain or reduce limb volume. Conservative therapies are most frequently used in combination to provide more beneficial results.

Skin Care

Skin care is vital to the management of lymphedema. The fibrosis associated with the condition and subsequent hyperkeratinization, when coupled with impaired immunity, greatly increases the risk of skin breakdown and subsequent infection. The lymphoedematous, hyperkeratinized skin becomes more prone to fissuring and injury, whilst the presence of hyperkeratinized squames permits a greater chance for bacterial and fungal colonization of the skin, wounds or fissures, and subsequent infection. Therefore, frequent and regular cleansing of the limb or affected region, with careful drying and moisturising of the skin is crucial to its maintenance. Protection of the skin through careful choice of clothing, particularly footwear, is essential. Foot care is important for those with lymphedema in a similar manner to that of diabetics, as their susceptibility to tissue injury and infection is increased due to the lymphedema. Correct footwear and protection from injury is very important.

Compression Hosiery

In combination with skin care, volume reduction is the second key to help prevent the development of fibrosis and progression. During early stages, this may be possible through simple elevation of the limb, exercises, or the use of static compression in the form of a medical grade compression garment, with a minimum compression rating of 40mmHg. Compression ratings up to 80 mmHg can be used. However, such compression is poorly tolerated, and compliance is reduced as a result. In most instances of grade 2 lymphedema, compression of 30-40 mmHg (or class 2 compression) is both adequate and better tolerated. Multi-layered compression bandaging is intensive and time consuming but is also effective in volume maintenance and reduction. Stockinette and foam padding is used to protect the joints and enable an even compressive force to be applied by the outer layer of short-stretch bandaging. Even compression throughout the limb is vital to prevent both pressure damage and exacerbation of the condition distal to any area of increased compression from a ring or band. There are also many further compression garments which work around the same principles of compression as the hosiery but utilizing different material and often strapping systems too. However, it is important to remember that elastic compressive hosiery has a finite life expectancy and will require routine replacement and measurement to ensure compression is maintained.

Manual Lymphatic Draingage (MLD)

This is a method of physical massage to assist lymphatic drainage. The aim is to utilise and recruit the remaining lymphatics within a region to help drain the tissue, usually through redirecting the lymphatic drainage to areas with preserved function. It is performed following a regime of good skin care with adequate moisturising. Massaging is started in the contralateral region of the main trunk of the affected limb. The aim is to start promoting lymphatic watershed activity. The massage is then continued through to the affected limb and then distally over the limb. MLD is usually applied on a daily basis across a one-to-six-week period. Each session is completed with application of a compression wrap or bandaging that is left in place until the following session of MLD. MLD has been shown to be effective in all stages of lymphedema, with up to 54% of patients demonstrating sustained benefit in terms of limb volume reduction.[8,9,22-23]

Intermittent Pneumatic Compression (IPC)

This is a method of applying a combination of compression and drainage techniques to a limb. Both single and multi-chamber IPC pumps exist and have been demonstrated to help reduce limb volume. As with MLD, compressive bandage or hosiery is required to help maintain the volume loss and prevent relapse. IPC pumps can develop pressures as high as 150 mmHg, although pressures of only 40 mmHg have also been demonstrated to have an effect as well. IPC has been demonstrated to reduce limb circumference measurements by almost 35-70% [25,26]. Due to the high pressures that can be utilised in IPC, it is of great importance to ensure the arterial supply to the limb under treatment is adequate to tolerate the pressure to be used, in order to prevent ischaemic risks. It has also been suggested that IPC can lead to fibrosis, particularly above the cuff, and that reduced pressures may have a lower risk of this fibrosis. Despite these potential hazards, IPC has been demonstrated to have relatively few side effects, though caution is advised in patients with pre-existing renal or congestive cardiac failure.

Complex Physical Therapy (CPT)

The term Complex Physical Therapy has been used to describe the combined therapeutic programme of skincare, volume reducing therapy such as IPC or MLD, and the subsequent use of compression bandaging or hosiery. CPT is often and most usually utilized in an intensive manner over relatively short periods of time to provide initial volume reduction, with maintenance via compression hosiery necessary to prevent relapse over time.[8,9]

Heat Therapy

The use of heat has been used as a method to aid volume reduction. Various methods of heat delivery have been used, including hot water immersion, microwaves, and electromagnetic irradiation, usually with the target of raising skin temperature to 39-49 C. Although the actual mechanism of action is not clearly understood, heat therapy has been shown to be effective in improving drainage of the limb and thus volume reduction.

Laser therapy

The use of Low-level Laser Therapy (LLLT) has been cited as a possible therapy, particularly for use in breast cancer related lymphedema.[27]

Pharmacological

Lymphedema is not responsive to diuretic therapy in the same way as peripheral edema due to renal, or cardiac failure. The presence of high oncotic pressure fluid in the interstitium due to the lymphatic failure renders the utilisation of osmotic pressures through manipulation of sodium and water ineffective.

A number of pharmacological interventions have been used, though none have gained widespread acceptance. Benzopyrones act through hydrolysing tissue proteins whilst stimulating their absorption. Their effect still remains to be proven and side effect profiles have been linked with hepatic failure, which has led to them remaining unlicensed in many countries [28]. The International Society of Lymphology does not endorse benzopyrones as substitutes for CPT [29].

Surgical

Surgical intervention is usually reserved for more severe cases where all other therapies have failed. It is important to carefully plan and assess the patient in order to provide the correct intervention for the individual concerned. Surgical intervention can be classified into two main forms: debulking procedures and bypass procedures. A third potential class of procedure is the prophylactic procedure, though this is rarely used with few potential indications, so is often not considered in the literature.

There is a wide array of potential surgical interventions, and there is no strong evidence to favour one over the other. This reflects the variability in outcomes with surgical treatment and all carry significant potential morbidity due to the underlying healing impairment caused by the condition. Conservative therapies are still considered the mainstay of therapy. Surgical intervention also poses the risk of exacerbating or creating its own secondary lymphedema due to scarring, excision, or injury to the lymphatics in the region operated upon and distally. Definitive evidence on the true risks and benefits is limited by the relatively small numbers of procedures that are performed and the many variations in technique [30].

Debulking Procedures: Debulking procedures are excisional procedures to remove excess lymphoedematous skin and subcutaneous tissue. Their main indications are for advanced fibrosis or elephantiasis due to filariasis. The most commonly used procedure is the Charles procedure.[9] Originally performed in 1912, this procedure has since been modified by a number of techniques. It involves the excision of skin, subcutaneous tissue, and the deep fascia. The defect is usually then skin grafted either primarily or as a delayed second stage procedure. The Homan/Miller procedure involves the raising of thin skin flaps and the excision of underlying lymphoedematous tissue, before trimming and closure of the flaps. The Servelle procedure is similar to that of the Homan/Miller procedure, but is staged in two parts, starting with the medial aspect first and then the lateral aspect. Liposuction has also been used, in conjunction with skin resection to reduce volume, though the long-term outcome is limited.

Debulking procedures are associated with limb deformity due to the excisional nature of the tissue and scarring. Complications such as sensory loss or impairment, exacerbation of distal lymphedema, graft and wound necrosis or infection can result from debulking.

Bypass Procedures: Bypass procedures are rarely performed, and this is reflected in the low numbers reported in literature. Bypass procedures are microsurgical procedures performed only in those patients who have failed conservative therapy and who are appropriate for bypass. They are performed to create either lympho-venous or lympho-lymphatic anastomosis to allow for drainage. As in vascular bypass procedures, it is necessary to demonstrate an adequate inflow in the form of patent, functioning distal lymphatics, and a patent run off site, with functioning, patent proximal lymphatics or venous system prior to considering any such procedure. In most instances the potential for bypass is therefore limited due to aplasia, hypoplasia, or injury to distal or proximal lymphatics occurring in secondary lymphedema, particularly through infection or inflammation.

Prophylactic procedures: Prophylactic lymphovenous anastomosis during inguinal node dissection for melanoma has been utilised, as has omentoplasty in the management of patients undergoing pelvic node dissection. In common with other surgical procedures, reported numbers are low despite suggestions of potential reduction in rates of secondary lymphedema, evidence remains inconclusive.

Liposuction: The use of liposuction has been trialled mainly in the management of secondary lymphedema in the arm following breast cancer surgery. Although not widely performed, there is evidence that it can potentially provide lasting improvement to patients' symptoms.[31,32]

Future Treatment Possibility

The endothelial structure of lymphatic channels lends itself to the possibility of molecular manipulation through the use of endothelial growth factors. VEGF is already implicated in the development of lymphatics and their subsequent aplasia or hypoplasia within primary disease [33]. Research is now centring on the possibility of its use in the treatment of lymphedema, though definitive therapies remain elusive.

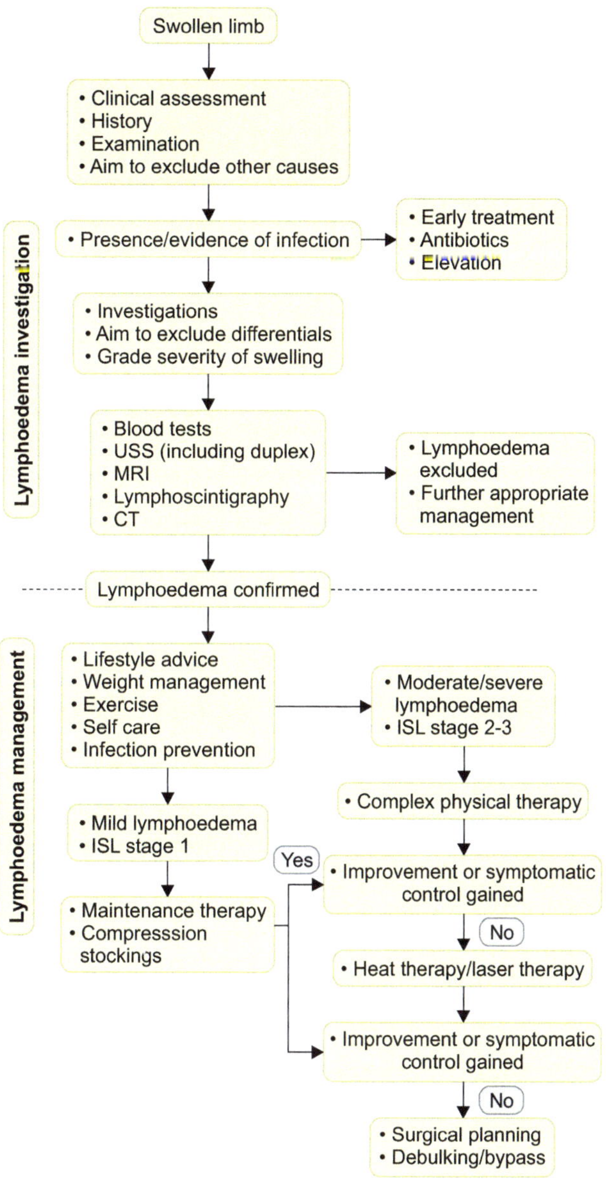

Figure 4: Investigation and management of the lymphoedematous limb.

SUMMARY

Lymphedema is a complex condition which can cause a number of physical and psychosocial complications. Whilst it is not curable, there exist treatment modalities which can be of benefit in preventing deterioration of both the condition and symptoms. Effective management requires timely and appropriate intervention with a multidisciplinary approach to optimise the long-term prognosis for those with the condition. Figure 4 describes a suggested flowchart for the investigation and management of the lymphoedematous limb.

REFERENCES

1. Lewis JM, Wald ER. Lymphedema praecox. J Pediatr 1984;104:641- 648.
2. Browse NL, Stewart G. Lymphoedema: pathophysiology and classification [review]. J Cardiovasc Surg 1985;26:91- 106.
3. World Health Organization (2010) WHO Global Programme to Eliminate Lymphatic Filariasis progress report for 2000–2009 and strategic plan 2010–2020.
4. Pani SP, Srividya A. Clinical manifestations of bancroftian filariasis with special reference to

lymphedema grading. Indian J Med Res 1995;102:114-18.

5. Pani SP, Krishnamoorthy K, Rao AS, Prathiba J. Clinical manifestations in Malayan filariasis infection with special reference to lymphoedema grading. Indian J Med Res 1990;91:200-07.
6. Srividya A, Pani SP, Rajagopalan PK, Bundy DA, Grenfell BT. The dynamics of infection and disease in bancroftian filariasis. Trans RSoc Trop Med Hyg 1991;85(2): 255-59.
7. The diagnosis and treatment of peripheral lymphedema: consensus document of the International Society of Lymphology. Lymphology 2003;36:84.
8. Szuba A, Rockson S, Lymphedema: classification, diagnosis and therapy. Vasc Med 1998;3:145.
9. Tiwari A, Cheng K, Button M, Myint F, Hamilton G. Differential Diagnosis, Investigation, and Current Treatment of Lower Limb Lymphedema. Arch Surg 2003;138(2):152-161.
10. Gloviczki P, Calcagno D, Schirger A. et al. Noninvasive evaluation of the swollen extremity: experiences with 190 lymphoscintigraphic examinations. J Vasc Surg 1989;9:683-689.
11. Stewart G, Gaunt JI, Croft DN, Browse NL. Isotope lymphography: a new method of investigating the role of the lymphatics in chronic limb oedema. Br J Surg 1985; 72:906-909.
12. Ter SE, Alavi A, Kim CK, Merli G. Lymphoscintigraphy: reliable test for the diagnosis of lymphedema. Clin Nucl Med 1993;18646- 654.
13. Szuba A, Strauss W, Sirsikar SP, Rockson SG. Quantitative radionuclide lymphoscintigraphy predicts outcome of manual lymphatic therapy in breast cancer-related lymphedema of the upper extremity. Nucl Med Commun 2002;23:1171–1175.
14. Chira S, Miller L.G. Staphylococcus aureus is the most common identified cause of cellulitis: a systemic review. Epidemiology and Infection 2010;138:313-317.
15. Cox N.H, Chapter 41, Streptococcal cellulitis / erysipelas of the lower leg in Williams H, Bigby M, Diepan T, Herxheimer A, Naldi L and Rzany B (Eds) Evidence-Based Dermatology, Second Edition 2009. Oxford, Blackwell Publishing.
16. Kilburn SA, Featherstone P, Higgins B, Brindle R. Interventions for cellulitis and erysipelas, Cochrane Database of Syst Rev 2010;6:CD004299.
17. Stewart FW, Treves N. Lymphangiosarcoma in postmastectomy lymphedema: a report of six cases in elephantiasis chirurgica. Cancer 1948;164-81.
18. Morgan PA, Franks PJ, Moffatt CJ. Health-related quality of life with lymphoedema: a review of the literature. Int Wound J 2005;2:47-62.
19. Lymphatic filariasis Fact sheet N°102 January 2012. WHO. Available at http://www.who.int/mediacentre/factsheets/fs102/en/.
20. Apostolopoulos A, Basit A, Kirby RM, Adjogatse JK, Lambert G, Chan KY, Hancock A, Hackney L, Wall M. Conservation of the Axilla: An Audit of Sentinel Lymph Node Biopsy After a New Start. Clinical Breast Cancer 2011;11(4):264-7.
21. Clarke D, Khonji NI, Mansel RE. Sentinel node biopsy in breast cancer: ALMANAC trial. World J Surg 2001;25(6):819-22.
22. Foldi M. Treatment of lymphedema [Editorial]. Lymphology 1994;27(1):1–5.
23. Foldi E, Foldi M, Weissleder H. Conservative treatment of lymphedema of the limbs. Angiology 1985;36(3):171–80.
24. Boris M, Weindorf S, Lasinski B, Boris G. Lymphedema reduction by noninvasive complex lymphedema therapy. Oncology 1994;8(9):95-106.
25. Richmond DM, O'Donnell TF, Zelikowski A. Sequential pneumatic compression for lymphedema: a controlled trial. Arch Surg 1985;120:1116-1119.
26. Boris M, Weindorf S, Leasinski BB. Persistence of lymphedema reduction after non invasive complex lymphedema therapy. Oncology 1997;11:99-109.
27. Omar MTA, Shaheen AAM, Zafar H. A systematic review of the effect of low level laser therapy in the management of breast cancer-related lymphoedema. Supportive care in cancer 2012; 20(11);2977-2984.
28. Badger CMA, Preston NJ, Seers K, Mortimer PS. Benzo-pyrones for reducing and controlling lymphoedema of the limbs. *Cochrane Database of Syst Rev* 2003; 4:CD003140.
29. Concensus Document of the International Society of Lymphology. The diagnosis and treatment of peripheral lymphedema. Lymphology 2009;42(2):51-60.
30. Cormier JN, Rourke L, Crosby M, Chang D, Armer J. The surgical treatment of lymphoedema: A systematic review of the literature (2004-2010). Annals of surgical oncology 2012;19(2):642-651.
31. Brorson H. Liposuction in arm lymphedema treatment. Scan J Surg 2003;92:287-295.
32. Brorson H. From Lymph to FatLiposuction as a Treatment for Complete Reduction of Lymphedema International Journal of Lower Extremity Wounds 2012;11(1):10-19.
33. Rockson S, Current concepts and future directions in the diagnosis and management of lymphatic vascular disease. Vasc Med 2010;15:223.

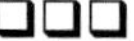

40

CHAPTER

Endovascular Surgery

***Mark Kay**, MS, FRCS*
***Martin Duddy**, FRCR*
***Rajiv Vohra**, Ph.D., FRCSEd, FRCSEng*

INTRODUCTION

Since the first superficial femoral angioplasty by the pioneering radiologist Charles Dotter in 1964[1], there has been significant evolution in endovascular techniques. There is an increasingly large array of wires, catheters, angioplasty balloons, and stents for the management of stenotic, occlusive, and aneurysmal disease. Endovascular treatment has revolutionised the management of cardiac, renal, and peripheral vascular disease, and has complimented even more traditional open surgical techniques.

As with all surgical interventions, preprocedural planning is a key concept for a successful outcome in endovascular treatment. The role of diagnostic angiography has now been surpassed in favour of non-invasive techniques such as duplex ultrasound, CT angiogram, and MR angiogram with catheter-based angiography being part of a treatment modality with angioplasty and stents.

All interventional procedures regardless of their complexity should be performed using simple guidelines. These guidelines include safe vascular access (the Seldinger technique), performing all procedures under vision, never forcing a guidewire (it should glide), and, once in place, never losing the wire which can easily occur when exchanging catheters over wires.

This chapter concentrates on endovascular treatment of arterial disease and covers core knowledge for the General Surgeon including recent evidence for procedures.

Seldinger Technique

This technique as described by the Swedish radiologist Seldinger in 1953, allows safe and easy access to a vessel and/or cavity. It involves a needle puncture either by manual palpation or under ultrasound guidance. The needle is hollow, allowing introduction of a guidewire. The needle can then be removed, and a catheter inserted over the guidewire, or a dilator passed over the wire to form a larger tract in the artery wall to accommodate a larger tube. This principle is a cornerstone of all endovascular procedures.

FUNDAMENTAL TOOLS FOR ENDOVASCULAR PROCEDURES

Needle Cannulation

Endovascular procedures commence with vessel cannulation. This may be performed under ultrasound guidance or by palpation and is traditionally performed with a 19-gauge needle as shown in Figure 1. The needle is passed at a 45° to 60° angulation to the skin and then levelled out once within the vessel lumen. A good back-bleed signifies a successful puncture, whilst a laboured back-bleed may suggest the needle is abutting the vessel wall which then requires repositioning or a diseased vessel proximally. The needle must then be held carefully in place to keep it within the vessel lumen whilst a guidewire is inserted before the needle can be removed. Ultrasound can be beneficial to detect calcified plaques which are best avoided during cannulation.

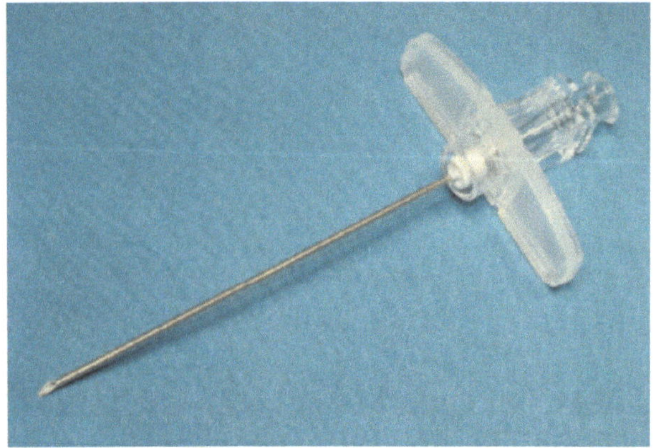

Figure 1: 9-gauge arterial puncture needle, this will accept an 0.035" guidewire

Guidewires

After vessel cannulation, a guidewire is passed. Guidewires have 2 main functions: (1) to act as a supportive rail, allowing passage of catheters to the site of disease and (2) to traverse stenoses and occlusions.

Guidewires may vary in stiffness, length, and wire tip, making each wire suited for particular tasks. Most wires have an atraumatic soft tip and a more rigid end as seen in Figure 2.

Guidewires may be classified as steerable and non-steerable. Non-steerable guidewires are used as a framework to allow passage of a catheter. Steerable wires are used to cross a stenosis. Commonly used non-steerable guidewires include the standard J wire (medium stiffness) and the Amplatz ® wire also known as the Cook Medical wire (stiff wires). These wires are used to pass stents and/or endografts. The most common steerable guidewire is the 0.035-inch Terumo® wire. It is hydrophilic so must be kept wet, highly mobile, and is used to either pass through stenoses or to select side branches with either an angled or straight tip. Such guidewires should not be used for the initial Seldinger access due to the risk of shredding the hydrophilic coating within the bevel of the needle.

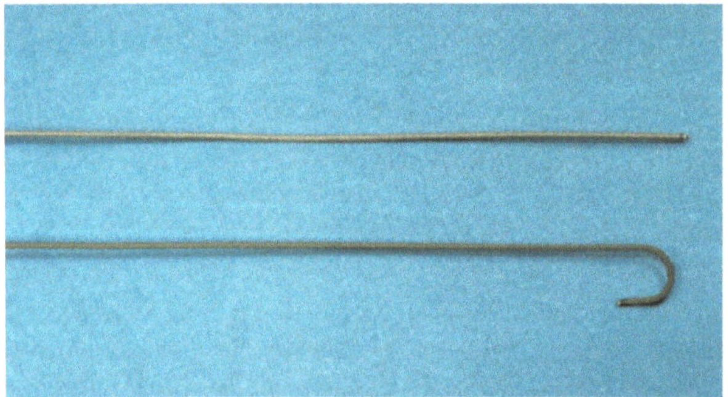

Figure 2: Braided 0.035" guidewires with PTFE coating. Above is an Amplatz Extra Stiff wire and below is a standard wire with an atraumatic J tip. Both have floppier distal segments to prevent vessel wall injury.

Sheaths

The sheath is a hollow plastic tube passed over a dilator with a valve for haemostasis and a side-arm to flush, shown in Figure 3. It allows the exchange of multiple wires and catheters during a procedure. It also facilitates contrast injection via the side-arm to perform angiography. The sheath size (French size) denotes the calibre size that the catheter will permit. Typically, a 5F or 6F sheath will be used for groin access procedures depending upon the size of the vessel, and hence balloon or stent required, to be treated.

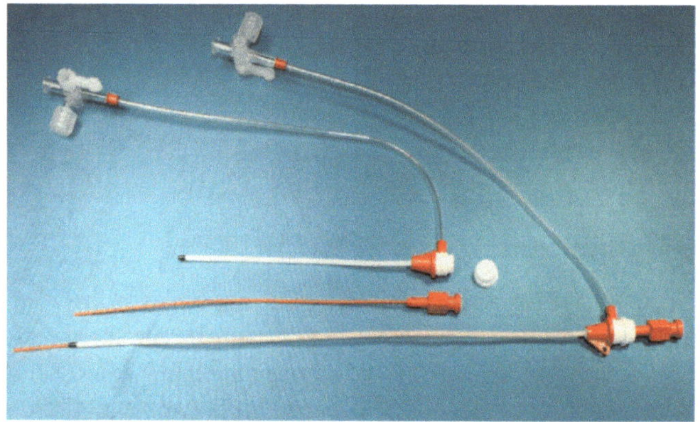

Figure 3: 4F vascular sheaths, 11 and 23 cm long. The shorter sheath has the 4F dilator (red) and the removable haemostatic valve removed. Each has a flushing side port with a 3-way tap.

Catheters

Catheters are used for contrast angiography or to allow cannulation of target vessels. A catheter also provides support for a guidewire during its advancement. They are available in a variety of sizes and shapes depending upon the need. Diagnostic angiography is traditionally performed using a pigtail catheter (non-selective catheter) which, as the name suggests, has a pigtail curled shape with multiple side holes. This shape allows widespread distribution of injected contrast and helps prevent inadvertent cannulation of branch vessels during passage. The multiple side holes also reduce the Venturi effect of a high-pressure injection that might cause vessel wall damage if a single end-hole catheter were used. Selective catheters have different shaped heads with an end hole as seen in Figure 4, which are used to approach angled branch vessels and permit their cannulation with steerable guidewires.

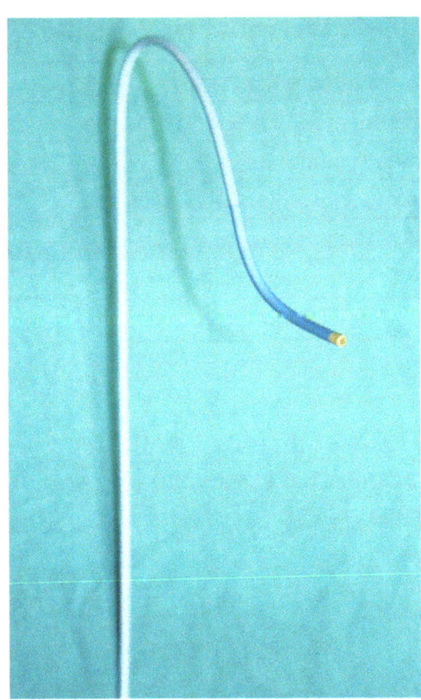

Figure 4: Sim-2 selective catheter with a single end-hole

Contrast

Contrast agents are commonly used in vascular radiology. Over the past few decades, there has been significant improvement in contrast agent composition, making them safer and better tolerated by patients. Modern intravenous contrast agents are typically based on iodine. These iodine-based contrast media are clear, colourless, water-soluble solutions whose concentrations are usually expressed as mg I/mL. All intravascular iodinated contrast agents are based on a tri-iodinated benzene ring. They can be classified as ionic and non-ionic.

1. Ionic: High-osmolar contrast media are monomers (single benzene ring) that ionize in solution. They are the oldest agents and have more side effects.
2. Non-ionic: Now more commonly used. These may be subdivided by their osmolarity.

a. Low-osmolar contrast media are monomers that dissolve in water but do not dissociate.

b. Iso-osmolar contrast media are dimers that consist of a two-benzene ring molecule, each with 3 iodine atoms. These larger molecules result in greater viscosity. This has clinical implications as the toxicity of contrast agents decreases and as the osmolality approaches that of the serum.

Complications of Contrast

Complications of contrast may be mild such as altered taste, urticaria, nausea, and vomiting. Severe complications are uncommon but significant including anaphylaxis, laryngeal oedema, hypotension, and contrast induced nephropathy.

Contrast-Induced Nephropathy

Contrast-induced nephropathy (CIN) is an acute renal function decline occurring 48 to 72 hours post intravascular injection of contrast medium. The most common definition is an increase in serum creatinine (SCr) of >25% of baseline value.[2] CIN is a complication of intravascular contrast medium use. It is linked with excess morbidity and mortality. Before administering contrast, patients should be fully assessed. Extra precautions must be taken in patients with renal impairment.

The risk of CIN increases with declining renal function. SCr and eGFR should be obtained prior to intervention. Other important risk factors include diabetes mellitus, sepsis or acute hypotension, dehydration or volume contraction, age >70 yrs, previous chemotherapy, organ transplant, myeloma, and vascular disease.

Patients with an eGFR of ≥60 mL/min have a relatively low risk of developing CIN. Therefore, they generally do not need preventive measures. For patients with eGFR <60, alternative imaging studies without iodinated contrast should be first considered. If contrast is necessary, then use of the lowest concentration of iodinated contrast needed for satisfactory images should be employed. Iodinated contrast can be diluted with normal saline without affecting image quality. Ionic and high-osmolar contrast media are associated with more adverse events overall and thus low-osmolar (Omnipaque®) and iso-osmolar (Visipaque®) media are more commonly used.[3]

Table 1: Common contrast agents

Generic Name	Trade name	Compound	Type	Iodine content mgl/mL	Osmolality mosm/kg H_2O
Diatrizoate	Hypaque 300	Ionic	Monomer	300	1570
Iohexol	Omnipaque 350	Non-ionic	Monomer	350	884
Iodixanol	Visipaque 320	Non-ionic	Dimer	320	290

Intraarterial injection of gadolinium carries a risk nephrogenic systemic fibrosis, a rare and potentially fatal disease.[4] Carbon dioxide (non-nephrotoxic) can be used instead of iodinated contrast in certain angiographic procedures, but it is technically more difficult to use, and also more challenging to interpret the image.

The most important measure to prevent CIN is adequate hydration. This should be administered intravenously with normal saline, which has been shown to be as efficacious as sodium bicarbonate.[5] Intravenous hydration should be given to patients with an eGFR <60 mL/min both pre- and post-procedure.

Nephrotoxic medications (i.e., NSAIDs) should be discontinued at least 48 hours prior to starting a procedure, and metformin should be withheld for the subsequent 48 hours. Using metformin does not include one's risk for developing CIN, but it may occasionally lead to lactic acidosis and subsequently acute kidney injury (AKI).

Table 2: Risk factors for contrast-induced nephropathy

Risk factors
Renal disease or solitary kidney
Diabetes Mellitus
Sepsis
Dehydration/ acute hypotension
Age >70 yrs
Vascular disease
Previous chemotherapy
Organ transplant
Myeloma

N-acetylcysteine (NAC) is an acetylated derivative of the amino acid cysteine. The role of NAC as a protective agent for CIN has been highly debated and with no consensus in the literature. Tepel *et al.* published the first clinical study on this subject in 2000, showing benefits for its use.[6] There have since been several published studies investigating the role of NAC for the prevention of CIN, but most studies are limited by small sample sizes and are underpowered. There are >11 meta-analyses published on this subject, seven of which have found a net benefit for NAC in the prevention of CIN. However, the results have been criticized for significant heterogeneity and thus questions the validity of the results.[7] Indeed the largest published randomized study was terminated early due to the lack of any trend showing benefit with NAC treatment.[8] There is no clear consensus on the use of NAC, but it is inexpensive, safe, and well tolerated by patients, thus its use in higher-risk patients requiring contrast is reasonable.

Table 3: Preventive measures for CIN

Preventive measures
Use alternative imaging where possible
IV fluids for patients with GFR <60 mL/min
Minimize contrast volume
Iso-osmolar and low-osmolar contrast media
Stop nephrotoxic medications (e.g., NSAIDS)
Administer N-Acetylcysteine (NAC)
Stop metformin for 48 hours

Angioplasty

This is the process of dilating a balloon across a stenosis or occlusion to recanalize a vessel and improve blood flow.

It involves 4 steps:

- Vascular access
- Traverse lesion
- Dilate lesion
- Completion angiography

The pre-procedure planning will dictate where vascular access should be obtained. It is sensible to avoid puncturing into a plaque or calcified area where possible as a flap may be created, and haemostasis may become an issue. Access can be from an anterograde approach (i.e., ipsilateral for infra-inguinal disease) into the common femoral artery or may be retrograde (contralateral) from the other groin. Where possible an anterograde approach should be used to minimise the number of angles to negotiate and to reduce the distance to the lesion being treated. A contralateral approach may be useful in an obese patient (can puncture below the inguinal ligament) or if there is a complication in the other groin (e.g., infection).

Traversing the lesion requires care and patience. An angiogram is used to define the anatomy from which there are a wide variety of catheters and wires to navigate through a stenosis. One should never use force on the wire and should avoid spiralling of the wire as this can induce a dissection flap. Once a lesion is crossed with a guidewire, an appropriately sized balloon (measured from the pre-angioplasty angiogram) is passed over the wire and inflated under pressure within the lesion.

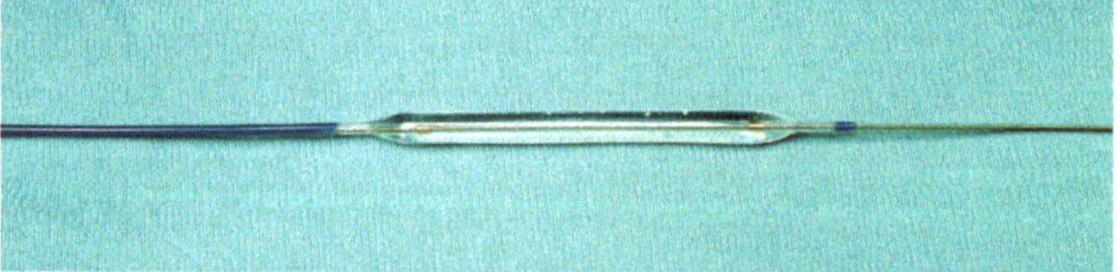

Figure 5: A conventional angioplasty balloon on a 5F catheter shaft. This would be mounted over a 0.035" guidewire.

Angioplasty balloons are introduced through a sheath to protect the arteriotomy site during removal and to allow multiple exchanges of wires and catheters. There are radio-opaque markers to denote the site of the balloon for successful placement. The balloon is then dilated using either manual pressure on a syringe or using an inflation device with a pressure gauge for more accurate reading. The balloon is filled with 50:50 contrast: saline to reduce resistance during inflation and deflation but is sufficient to demonstrate the angioplasty site on fluoroscopy.

A wire is kept in position during the completion angiography in case a repeat angioplasty is required or a bail out procedure necessary in the event of a complication. The completion angiography confirms successful treatment of a lesion and assesses the runoff vessels by checking for embolization.

Passage of the wires and balloon may be transluminal (i.e., within the vessel lumen) which is the preferred route seen in Figure 6 or subintimal seen in Figure 7. In subintimal angioplasty, the intimal vessel layer is deliberately punctured, and the guidewire is passed within the media to bypass the blockage and then re-enter the vessel lumen beyond the occlusion, like an aortic dissection with a false lumen. This method is usually performed for an occlusive disease or a very tight stenosis that is unsuccessfully crossed. The subintimal tract is dilated with balloon angioplasty and flow is re-established. Thus, an extraluminal neo-lumen is created which in theory is free of atheroma. This technique can be used to treat long occlusions and may avoid the need for bypass surgery. There is a risk of very distal re-entry, effectively excluding part of the native circulation, or non-re-entry from the tract and perforation. Collateral vessels can also be occluded which may be significant if the angioplasty fails. Newer developments have seen the production of specific catheters such as the Outback catheter® (Cordis) which are designed to guide the intimal dissection and re-entry beyond the lesion.

Figure 6a-d: Angioplasty of pedal arch occlusion

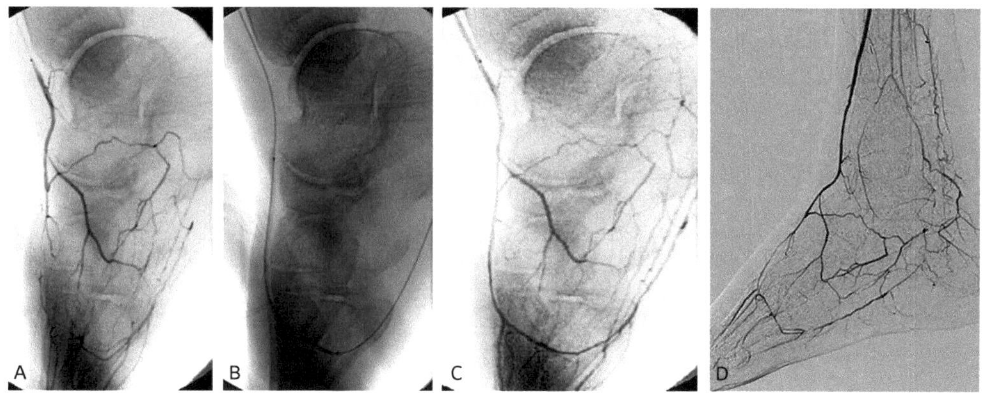

6a: DSA of a diabetic patient with ulceration of the fifth toe. The pedal arch is occluded. 6b: A guidewire passed around the pedal arch and a 2 mm balloon angioplasty of the pedal arch. The opaque markers demonstrate the borders of the balloon. 6c: DSA showing restoration of the pedal arch post angioplasty. 6d: DSA 2 years later. There is some recurrence of the pedal disease, but no foot ulcer.

Figure 7a-d: Subintimal angioplasty of an SFA occlusion

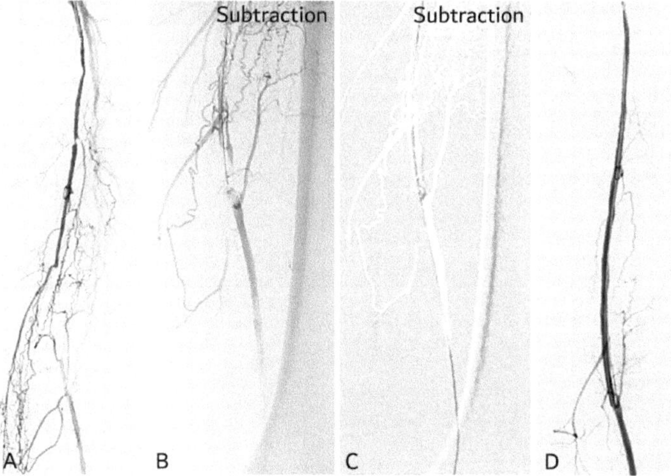

7a: Antegrade DSA showing SFA occlusion. 7b: DSA during placement of the re-entry device balloon. 7c: Road map image during re-entry with the stylette and guidewire. 7d: DSA following subintimal angioplasty.

Angioplasty causes the atherosclerotic plaque to split and the vessel wall to stretch which can cause patient discomfort particularly if subintimal. Balloon dilatation causes discomfort by stimulating nerve fibres in the adventitia. If severe it may indicate excess pressure or vessel rupture.

The benefits of angioplasty may be limited in cases of multi-segment disease, long occlusions, flush occlusions from the arterial bifurcation, elastic recoil, and restenosis. Restenosis following angioplasty can occur over time, as the damaged intima induced by angioplasty undergoes remodelling by neo-intimal hyperplasia, which when excessive, can result in restenosis. Further attempts at angioplasty can be made. If persistent, it may require placement of a stent or open surgical management. More recent advances have assessed the benefit of drug eluting balloons using Paclitaxel as a potential to combat restenosis. Early reports are promising compared to standard balloon angioplasty.[9] These drug eluting balloons may avoid the use of a stent and its inherent risks of stent thrombosis, stent fracture, and in-stent neo-intimal hyperplasia causing restenosis. The complications and their management is summarised in table 4.

Table 4: Complications of angioplasty and management

Bruising/bleeding	Choose smallest sheath possible
Recoil of stenosis	Repeat/prolonged angioplasty or stent
Vessel damage	Extravasation may need covered stent or open surgery
Emboli	Suction catheter to aspirate +/- thrombolysis
Vessel occlusion	Suction catheter/Stent/Open surgery
Balloon rupture	Remove with care

TASC classification

The Trans-Atlantic Inter-Society Consensus produced guidance in 2000 (TASC I) which was revised in 2007 (TASC II)[10] for stratifying aorto-iliac (Figure 8) and femoral-popliteal (Figure 9) lesions and their suggested management. This was produced to aid clinicians in treatment decisions. It essentially suggested that TASC A and B lesions were best managed by endovascular treatment whilst TASC C and D lesions were best managed (Table 5 and Table 6) surgically. In practice, many TASC C and D lesions are now treated by endovascular means as technical skills and equipment have developed, but it serves as a useful management guideline.

Table 5: TASC classification of aortoiliac lesions

	Lesion	Management recommendation
TASC A	CIA or EIA single stenosis (<3 cm) Uni or bilateral	Endovascular Treatment
TASC B	Single stenosis (3 to 10 cm), does not extend into CFA CIA or EIA with two stenoses (<5 cm), does not extend into CFA Unilateral CIA occlusion	Endovascular treatment
TASC C	Bilateral CIA or EIA stenosis (5 to 10 cm), CFA is involved Unilateral EIA occlusion, no CFA involvement Unilateral EIA stenosis, extension into CFA Bilateral CIA occlusion	Surgery
TASC D	CIA, EIA, and CFA diffuse stenosis (>10 cm) Unilateral CIA and EIA occlusion Bilateral EIA occlusion Iliac stenosis that is next to the aortic or iliac aneurysm	Surgery

The patient's comorbidities, fully informed patient preference and the local operator's long-term success rates must be considered when making treatment recommendations for Type B and Type C lesions.

Type A lesions • Unilateral or bilateral stenoses of CIA • Unilateral or bilateral single short (≤3 cm) stenosis of EIA	
Type B lesions • Short (≤3 cm) stenosis of intrarenal aorta • Unilateral CIA occlusion • Single or multiple stenosis totaling 3–10 cm involving the EIA not extending into the CFA • Unilateral EIA occlusion not involving the origins of internal iliac or CFA	
Type C lesions • Bilateral CIA occlusions • Bilateral FIA stenoses 3–10 cm long not extending into the CFA • Unilateral EIA stenosis extending into the CFA • Unilateral EIA occlusion that involves the origins of internal iliac and/or CFA	
Type D lesions • Infra-renal acrtoiliac occlusion • Diffuse disease involving the aorta and both iliac arteries requiring treatment • Diffuse multiple steroses involving the unilateral CIA, EIA, and CFA • Unilateral occlusions of both CIA and EIA • Bilateral occlusions of EIA • Iliac stenoses in patients with AAA requiring treatment and not amenable to endograft placement or other lesions requiring open aortic or iliac surgery	

Figure 8: TASC classification of aortoiliac lesions

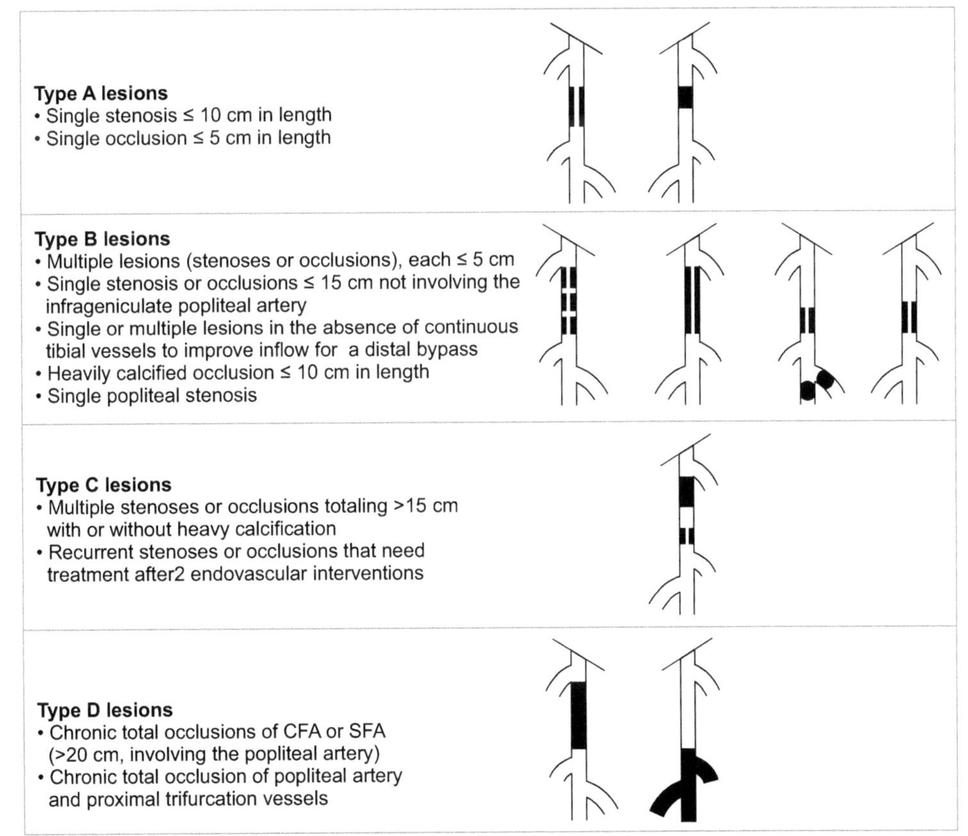

Type A lesions • Single stenosis ≤ 10 cm in length • Single occlusion ≤ 5 cm in length
Type B lesions • Multiple lesions (stenoses or occlusions), each ≤ 5 cm • Single stenosis or occlusions ≤ 15 cm not involving the infrageniculate popliteal artery • Single or multiple lesions in the absence of continuous tibial vessels to improve inflow for a distal bypass • Heavily calcified occlusion ≤ 10 cm in length • Single popliteal stenosis
Type C lesions • Multiple stenoses or occlusions totaling >15 cm with or without heavy calcification • Recurrent stenoses or occlusions that need treatment after2 endovascular interventions
Type D lesions • Chronic total occlusions of CFA or SFA (>20 cm, involving the popliteal artery) • Chronic total occlusion of popliteal artery and proximal trifurcation vessels

Figure 9: TASC classification of femora-popliteal lesions

Table 6: TASC classification of femoral popliteal lesions

TASC A	Single stenosis that is <10 cm Single occlusion that is <5 cm	Endovascular Management
TASC B	Multiple lesions (stenoses or occlusions) that are <5 cm each Single lesion (stenosis or occlusion) that is <15 cm. No involvement of the infra-geniculate popliteal artery Single or multiple lesions. No continuous tibial vessels that improve distal bypass inflow Heavily calcified occlusion <5 cm Single popliteal stenosis	Endovascular Management
TASC C	Multiple lesions (stenoses or occlusions) >15 cm. May have heavy calcification Recurrent lesions (stenoses or occlusions). Requires treatment after two endovascular interventions	Surgical Management
TASC D	Chronic total occlusions of CFA or SFA Occlusions >20 cm of the popliteal artery Chronic total occlusion of the popliteal artery and proximal trifurcation vessels	Surgical Management

Evidence for Angioplasty

Angioplasty is suitable for most anatomical sites except the common femoral artery which tends to have large, calcified plaques that respond poorly to angioplasty. These are best managed by surgical endarterectomy. The most common sites undergoing angioplasty include the iliac and superficial femoral arteries. Primary patency rates of 98% at 30 days and assisted primary patency rates of 80% to 90% at 5 years are achievable for iliac lesions.[11] Primary patency for shorter lesions of <5cm after SFA angioplasty is 77% at 1 year and 55% at 5 years.[12] Longer lesions, or occlusions have lower but acceptable patency rates in the iliac vessels. Endovascular management also avoids the morbidity of a bypass procedure in long SFA lesions.

Subintimal angioplasty has demonstrated 1 year patency rates of 70%[13] and limb salvage rates of 94% at 3 years follow up for below-knee lesions.[14]

There is minimal evidence to compare results of angioplasty and bypass surgery in the lower limb. The main multicenter randomized evidence is in the Bypass Versus Angioplasty in Severe Ischaemia of the Leg (BASIL) trial[15] which randomized 452 patients with severe lower limb ischaemia into two groups for the first revascularisation strategy: 228 patients undergoing bypass surgery and 224 patients undergoing balloon angioplasty. After 3 years follow up, only 45% of patients were alive and 38% of patients remained amputation-free. This highlights the high cardiovascular risk of such patients. Both strategies offered similar overall survival and amputation-free survival rates of 2 years, although both cost and morbidity were significantly higher with bypass surgery. For those patients who survived >2 years after intervention, bypass surgery offered a significant increase in overall survival of 7.3 months, and improved amputation-free survival of 5.9 months. The trial concluded that those patients expected to live <2 years are best managed with an angioplasty-first approach, and those patients expected to live >2years are best managed with bypass surgery. There is of course an inherent difficulty in making such a survival prediction.

The Angiography and Stenting for Renal Artery Lesions (ASTRAL) randomized trial[16] found no significant benefit in renal artery angioplasty or stent versus medical management in 806 patients for lowering creatinine levels and blood pressure.

Stents

A stent is a wire mesh tube used as a scaffold to support a vessel wall. They may be uncovered or covered (stent graft), balloon mounted or self-expanding. Stents may be deployed as a primary procedure or as a secondary procedure to treat recoil after angioplasty, restenosis, heavily calcification, or vessel wall dissection, detailed in Table 7 and Figure 10. The choice of stent depends upon the vessel and lesion to be treated. Most stents have radio-opaque markers to aid with positioning.

Table 7: Indications for stents

Primary Stent	Exclude aneurysm Treat bleeding Treat plaque dissection Prevent recoil post angioplasty
Selective Stenting	Recoil post angioplasty Persistent stenosis angioplasty >10mmHg 10mmHg should not be in a separate line but in the same sentence after angioplasty

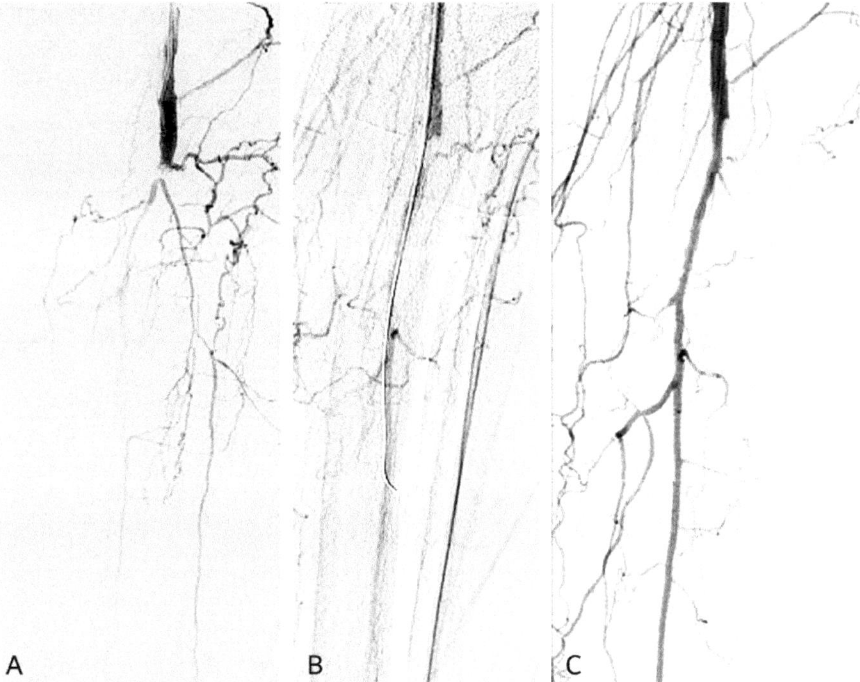

Figure 10. A: Embolic occlusion of trifurcation post angioplasty of a femoral occlusion in a Type I diabetic with ischaemic ulceration. B: Poor result after angioplasty with a 3 mm balloon. C: After placement of a 4 mm × 30 mm self-expanding stent into the Tibio-Peroneal artery

Balloon mounted (Figure 11) stents tend to be made of stainless steel or cobalt chromium alloy and are attached to a balloon which is then inflated once position is confirmed. It is common practice to oversize the stent by 1 mm although most have high radial force to prevent recoil and migration. These stents can be very accurately placed in relation to lesions and bifurcations. Stainless steel stents tend to be stiff and are best used for shorter lesions.

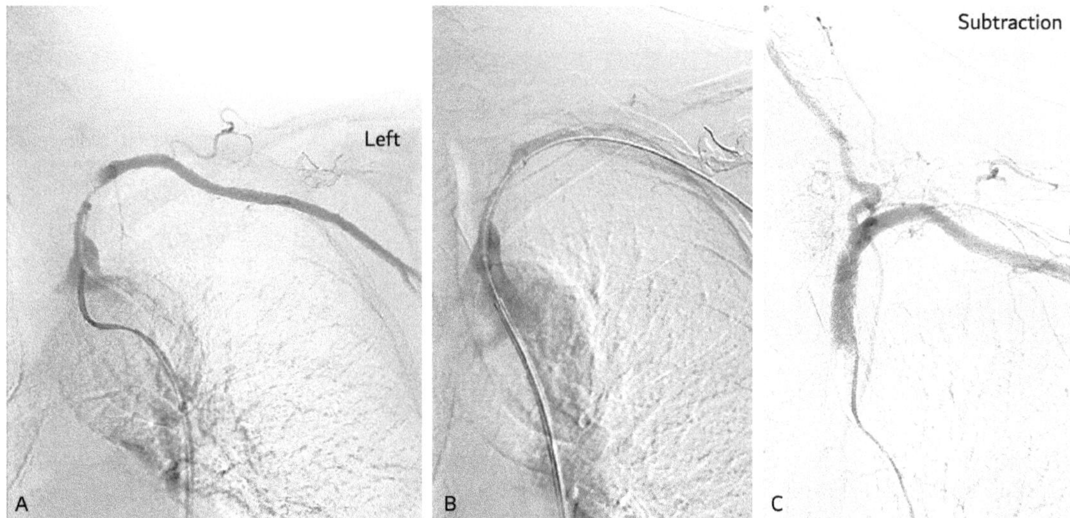

Figure 11. A: DSA of a tight subclavian artery stenosis. There is retrograde flow in the vertebral artery (subclavian steel). B: DSA during placement of a balloon mounted Palmaz® Stent on an 8 mm balloon. C: Completion DSA post stent deployment. Orthograde flow is redirected to the vertebral artery.

Self-expanding stents are mounted in a compressed state by a thin sheath which is withdrawn during deployment shown in Figure 12. These stents tend to shorten to a variable extent during deployment. They are commonly made of nitinol (a nickel-titanium alloy) and have inherent memory at body temperature, so once deployed, they adopt their normal size and exert radial force to the vessel wall. It is common practice to oversize by more than 1-2 mm. These stents tend to be more flexible than balloon mounted stents seen in Figure 13. They have a more complex helical framework structure that allows this greater flexibility and radial force. This is particularly useful in tortuous vessels and across joints. More recent advances have shown the use of drug eluting stents and biodegradable stents which aim to address the complications of stent-use including in-stent restenosis and stent fracture.

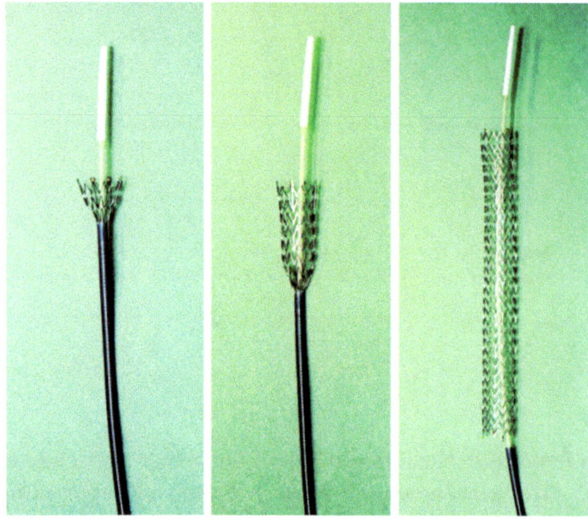

Figure 12: Deployment of a self expanding bare metal Nitinol Stent.

There are potential complications from placement of a stent detailed in Table 8. These include early complications such as vessel perforation, embolization as shown in Figure 14, stent thrombosis, and later complications including in-stent restenosis, stent migration, or kinking.

Table 8: Complications of stents

Complications
Access vessel injury/ dissection
Vessel perforation
Embolization
In-stent stenosis
Thrombus formation
Stent occlusion
Distal (run-off) vessel occlusion
Stent fracture
Stent kink

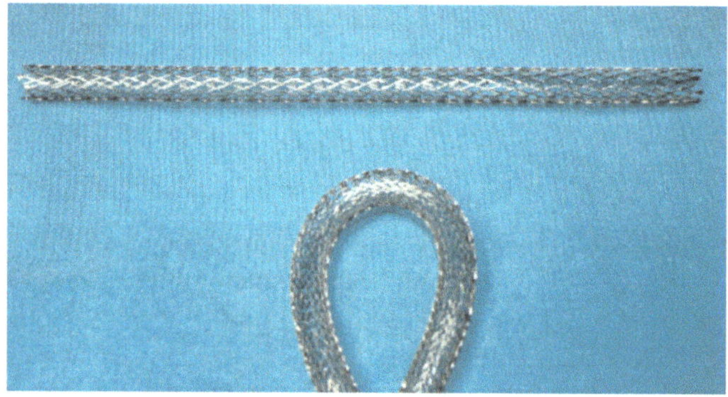

Figure 13: Two different self expanding flexible Nitinol Stents which might be used to treat an SFA occlusion.

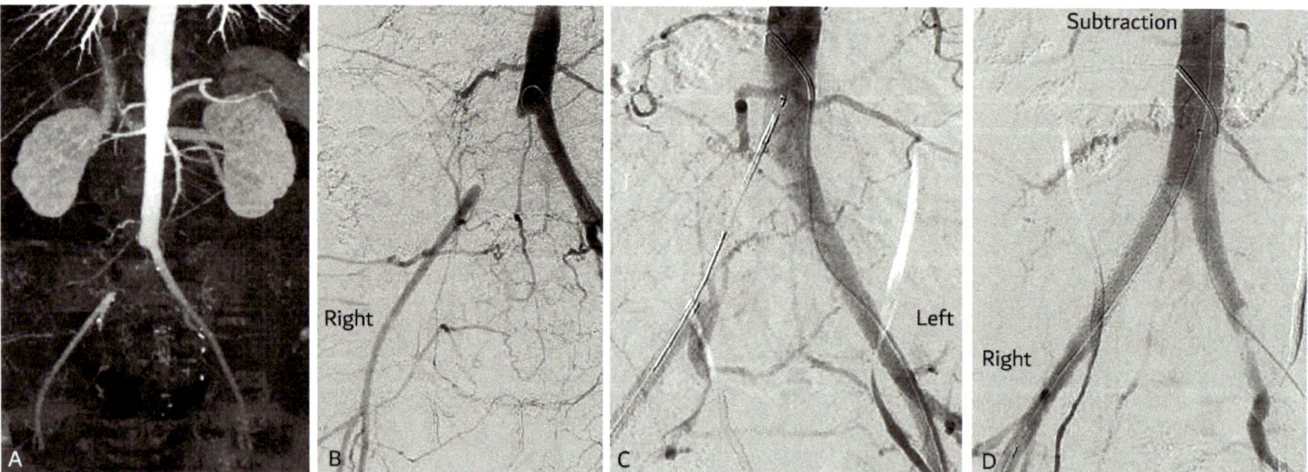

Figure 14 A: CT angiogram in a 50-yard claudicant, showing right common iliac occlusion. B: DSA confirming right common iliac artery occlusion. C: Subintimal passage through the lesion requiring a re-entry device at the aortic bifurcation. D: After balloon mounted stent grafting of the right common iliac artery. There is cross embolic occlusion of the left external iliac artery requiring aspiration and subsequent open femoral embolectomy.

Stent grafts

A stent graft comprises a stent framework with a fabric layer (i.e., covered stent) shown in Figure 15. They are used to treat false aneurysms shown in Figure 16, true aneurysms shown in Figure 17, and to manage vessel rupture during angioplasty or trauma. Covered stents also line the plaque and prevent plaque rupture. They are most commonly lined by Dacron or Polytetrafluoroethylene (ePTFE) but are uncovered at their proximal and distal ends to aid fixation. Stent-grafts are typically oversized by 10% to 20% of the vessel size. They may also be balloon mounted or self expanding.

One of the most commonly used stent grafts is the Viabahn® covered stent (WL Gore and Associates, AZ, USA). This is a flexible, self-expanding stent made of nitinol. It has an expanded PTFE lining with evidence of 91% 1-year patency and 95% secondary patency rates in iliac arteries.[17] It has also been demonstrated to have equivalent 1-year patency compared to synthetic femoro-popliteal bypass grafts.[18]

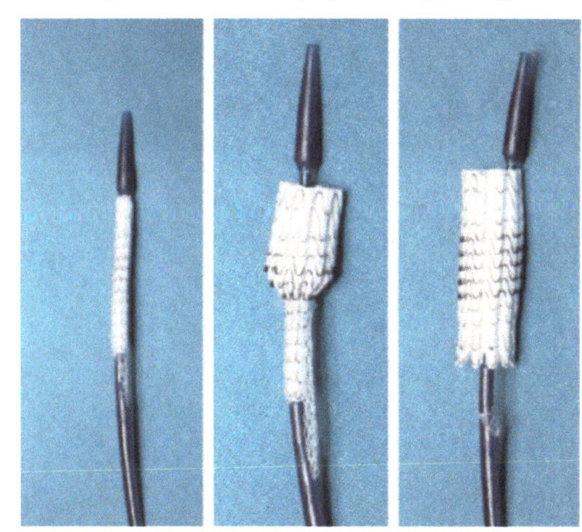

Figure 15: Deployment of a self expanding Covered Stent (Stent graft)

Figure 16: Covered stent to treat false SFA aneurysm.

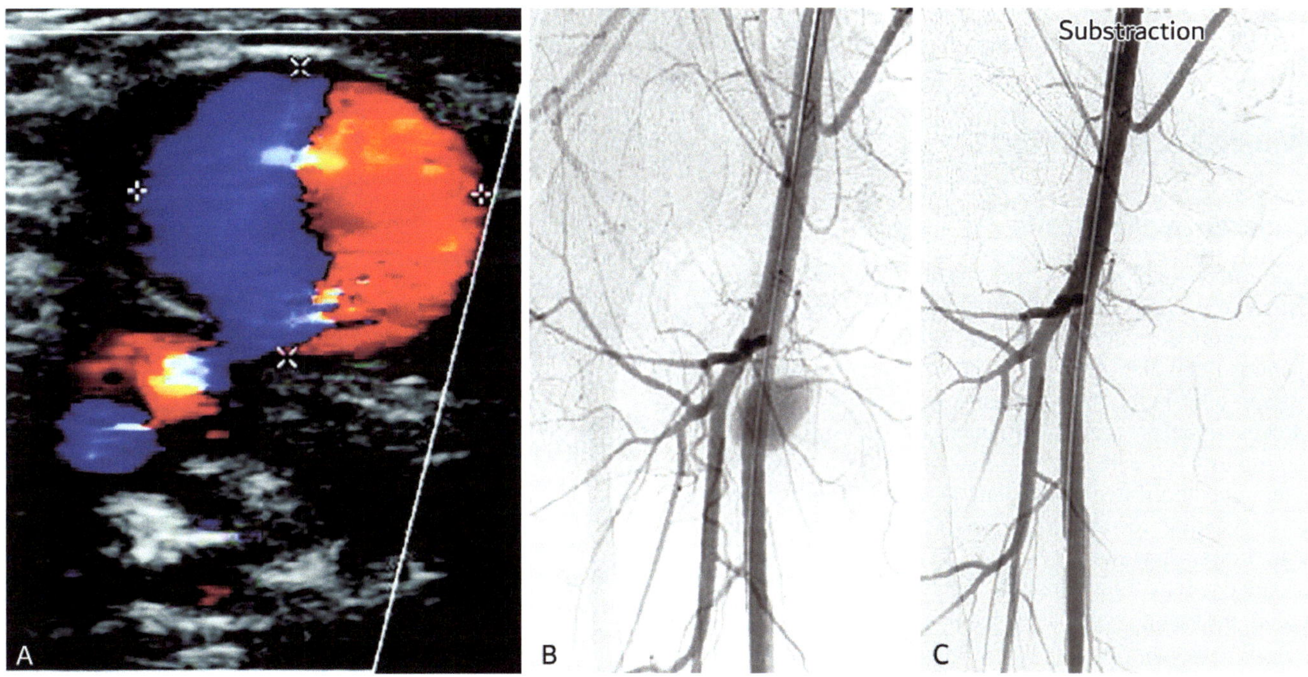

16 A: Colour Doppler ultrasound showing the typical 'yin-yang' appearance of flow within a 33 mm iatrogenic pseudoaneurysm sac. The neck was thought too wide for safe thrombin injection. B: DSA showing filling of the sac from an SFA defect. C: DSA after placement of a covered Viabahn® Stent.

Figure 17: Covered stent to treat true popliteal aneurysm.

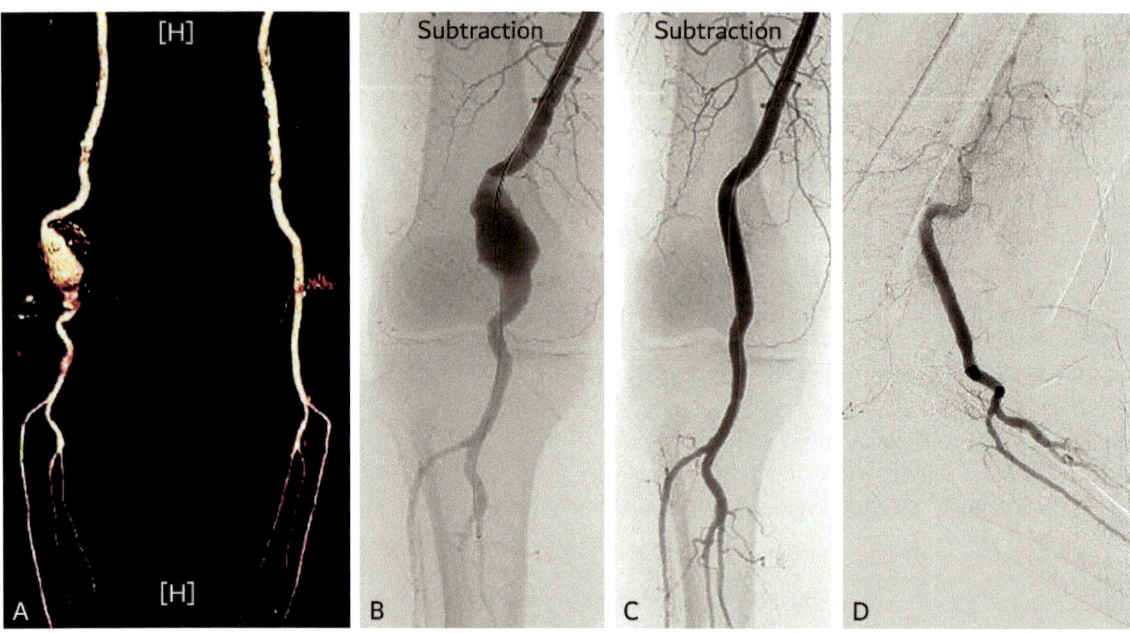

17 A: Planning CT angiogram of a 4cm right popliteal aneurysm. B: DSA at the time of intervention. C: DSA after placement of a 9 × 150 mm Stent graft. D: Lateral DSA in knee flexion with satisfactory flow.

EVIDENCE FOR STENTS

Evidence for Iliac stents

Iliac artery stenting is well established, showing good evidence to support its use with 93% to 95% clinical success rates reported.[19,20] A meta-analysis of iliac artery management demonstrated that the deployment of a stent reduced the risk of long-term failure by 39% compared to angioplasty alone.[21] However, debate persists whether to stent primarily after angioplasty or selectively. Advocates of primary stenting after uncomplicated angioplasty stress potential benefits of preventing recoil, fixing plaque, and hence preventing vessel dissection and preventing recurrent disease. Advocates of selective stenting stress the benefit of stents in cases of recoil post-angioplasty and persistent pressure gradient of >10 mmHg across the treated side post-angioplasty. There is evidence from randomized controlled trials and case series for selective use of stents demonstrating it to be equally as effective as primary stenting.[22,23] Selective stenting is also more cost effective but requires more re-interventions.

Evidence for SFA Stents

Endovascular treatment of superficial femoral artery (SFA) disease with stents is becoming increasingly common. Randomized studies using stainless steel stents have demonstrated no benefit for stenting[24,25] compared to plain balloon angioplasty. A comprehensive review of SFA stents demonstrated no significant benefit of a primary SFA stent over angioplasty[26], whilst a Cochrane database systematic review[27] showed a limited benefit to stenting lesions of the superficial femoral artery in addition to angioplasty but did not recommend routine placement. Early evidence with nitinol stents has been more encouraging, although the long-term results are pending.

The Vienna-ABSOLUTE trial[28] was the first randomized study that showed a benefit of SFA stenting compared to angioplasty for patients with severe, lifestyle-limiting claudication. The investigators used self-expanding nitinol stents. After 12 months, duplex ultrasonography assessment showed significantly lower rates of restenosis among the patients randomized to stenting (37% vs 63%; P=0.01) and this benefit persisted at 2 years.

There is evidence from the FAST trial[29] that shorter SFA lesions of <5 cm are effectively treated by angioplasty alone. Restenosis rates at 1 year were not significant, at 32% in the stenting group versus 39% in the angioplasty group.

Stenting was demonstrated to be superior to angioplasty for medium length lesions of <150 mm in the RESILIENT trial[30], with a primary patency rate of 81.3% for stenting versus 36.7% for angioplasty at 12 months.

Long SFA lesions are traditionally managed with bypass surgery, although such lesions are increasingly being managed with endovascular techniques. The main drawback with such lesions is the high incidence of restenosis. A retrospective study of 347 patients with long SFA lesions of >15 cm, demonstrated patency rates (freedom from restenosis) of 47% to 51% at 3 years with a variety of nitinol stents.[31]

Primary stenting of longer lesions may be considered a useful alternative to surgical bypass for patients with severe cardiovascular comorbidity whose life expectancy may be limited. However, failure of such stents may result in occlusion of the distal landing zone extending into the runoff vessels, making surgical bypass more challenging.

Drug-eluting stents may help address the issue of in-stent restenosis. The Zilver PTX® paclitaxel drug-eluting stent (Cook Medical, Bloomington, IN) is currently being investigated in a multicenter, prospective, randomized trial of 479 claudicants. 3-year data presented in 2012 showed significant improved primary patency over angioplasty and bare metal stents, 70.7% versus 49.1% respectively.[32]

Evidence for Carotid Stents

Carotid stenting is an alternative to open surgical endarterectomy for symptomatic carotid artery disease. It is particularly beneficial with distal internal carotid lesions which are difficult to access, and in those patients who have had radiotherapy to the neck. It comprises groin access in the CFA and, after crossing the stenosis with a fine steerable guidewire, the insertion of an uncovered stent (Figure 18). A cerebral protection device is commonly used to control cerebral embolization. The most notable trials include CREST and ICCS. Carotid Revascularization Endarterectomy versus Stenting Trial (CREST) is a randomized trial of 2502 patients which compared carotid stenting (CAS) with surgical endarterectomy (CEA).[33] It showed no significant difference for the composite primary endpoint of any stroke, myocardial infarct (MI), or death during the peri-procedural period, 7.2% CAS versus 6.8% CEA. However, there were individual endpoint differences, with incidence of stroke at 30 days significantly higher with stenting, 4.1% versus 2.3%. Conversely myocardial infarction (MI) was higher with CEA, 2.3 versus 1.1%. The report also demonstrated fewer events in younger patients with stenting. The International Carotid Stenting Study (ICSS) demonstrated a 3.3% higher risk of stroke, MI, or death with CAS compared to CEA.[34] The debate continues between these two modalities, where proponents of CAS maintain that their results at higher volume centers are better. There is certainly less morbidity with cranial nerve injury and wound complications. It is likely that the results of CAS will improve as clinicians become more skilled at performing it and that the treatment choice will reflect the type of lesion and the patient characteristics.

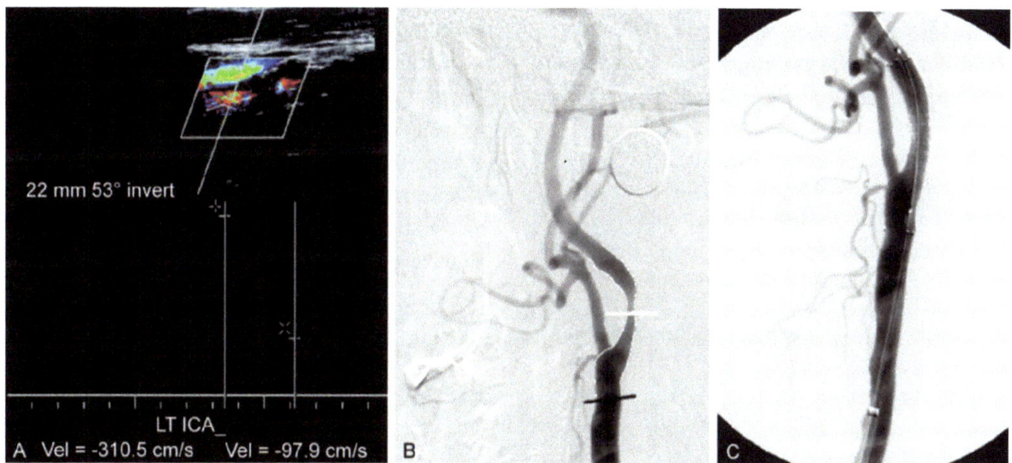

Figure 18 A: Duplex ultrasound scanning of a symptomatic left internal carotid stenosis. B: Left carotid angiogram demonstrating significant internal carotid stenosis. C: DSA after carotid Stent placement with a cerebral protection device in situ via a guide sheath in the common carotid artery.

EVAR

Parodi et al. introduced endovascular aortic aneurysm repair (EVAR) in 1991[35] and since then, it has been commonly used as an alternative to open repair for aneurysmal disease. The aim was to find a minimally invasive approach to aneurysm repair with faster recovery and reduced mortality and morbidity. The procedure involves access to the femoral arteries either by open 'cut down', percutaneous approach, introduction of sheaths, guidewires and catheters, angiogram to define the anatomy and placement of a covered stent-graft in the aorta to effectively exclude the aneurysm sac from the circulation. The aim is to prevent continued aneurysm growth and rupture. The stent-graft is anchored to the proximal and distal ends of the non-aneurysmal portion of the aorta and iliac vessels with the sac excluded. The proximal aortic neck is the section of non-aneurysmal aorta between the lowest renal artery and the aneurysm sac. The distal landing zone is typically the common iliac vessel at the iliac bifurcation to maintain perfusion of the internal iliac arteries.

There are numerous types of grafts available which have evolved and been modified over time. The stent framework is either made of stainless steel or nitinol depending upon the manufacturer, and both exert radial force on the aortic wall. Wire barbs at the proximal end of the graft or on an uncovered supra-renal stent, help fix the graft in position and resist movement shown in Figure 19.

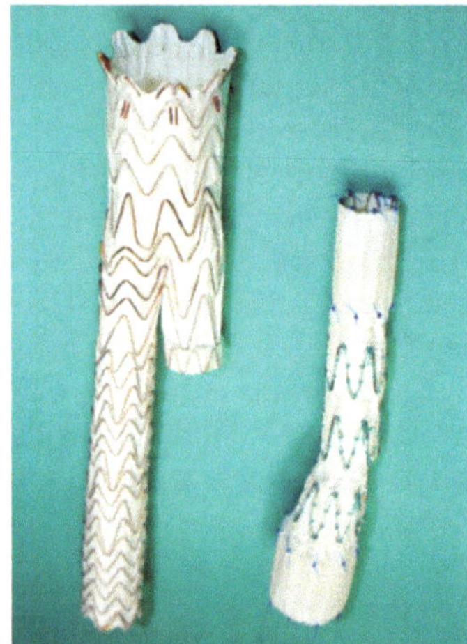

Figure 19: Conventional EVAR device (Gore) which has a long pant ipsilateral leg and a short pant contralateral leg. There are proximal hooks to prevent migration. A contralateral limb is shown by another manufacturer (Cook).

EVAR Planning

The most important step in successful endovascular treatment of aneurysms is careful planning. This is normally performed using multi-planer CT angiography with 1 mm slices (although MRA can be used) with software that allows centerline reconstruction. The morphology of the proximal and distal landing zones, access vessels, and the aneurysm are assessed. The length, diameter, and angulation of the aortic neck are of key significance during planning and assessment of suitability for endovascular repair. A centerline is drawn within the aorta along a "racing line" as this is normally the path the endograft will take. Adjustments need to be made for angulated vessels as these may often straighten once stiff guidewires are placed.

Once measurements are taken and anatomic suitability is confirmed, then graft selection takes place. Most centers prefer to use 1 or 2 types of graft to aid familiarity with sizes and handling, although there are a wide variety of endografts available.

General guidelines are to oversize the aortic neck diameter by using a graft 20% bigger and to oversize iliac diameters by 15% to 20%, but these differ slightly between the various device designs.

Table 9: Principal measurement requirements

Neck
• Diameter <32 mm (largest graft 36 mm)
• Length ≥15 mm (Endurant and Anaconda devices 10 mm)
• Flare <2 mm diameter over 15 mm of length
• Angulation <60° (Aorfix device licensed up to 90°)
• Minimal thrombus in aortic neck
• Minimal calcification
Bifurcation
• Diameter ≥20 mm (to allow graft to open)
Iliac
• Diameter 7 to 25 mm
• Minimal calcification
General Principle
• Oversize neck diameter by 20%
• Oversize iliac diameter by 15% to 20%

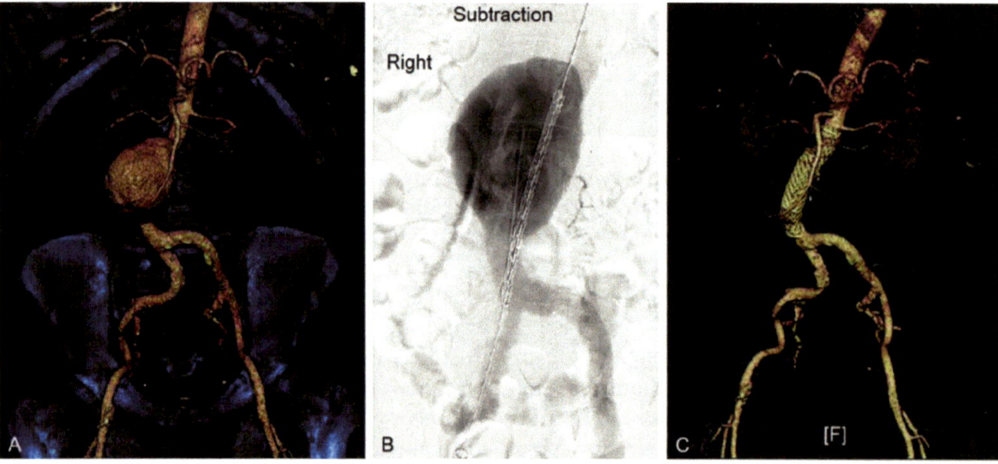

Figure 20 A: Planning CTA showing a 7.5 cm localized aortic aneurysm. This was treated with a straight stent graft. B: DSA during placement of two overlapping straight 'thoracic' Stent-grafts. C: 3-month follow-up CTA showing exclusion of the aortic sac.

Figure 21: Standard Bifurcated EVAR

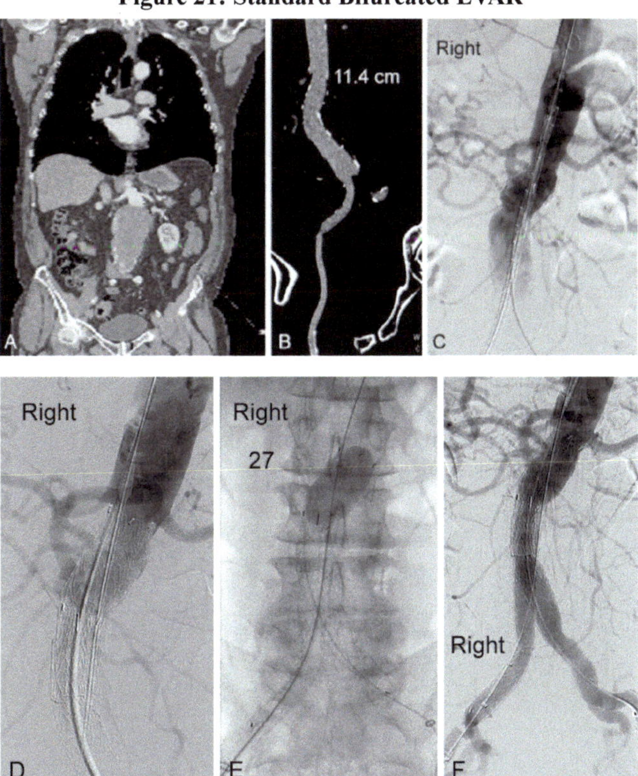

Figure 21 A: Coronal section showing aneurysm neck below lowest left renal artery (white line). B: Planning CT angiogram (curved center line reconstruction) of a 6 cm AAA. The distance from lowest renal artery to aortic bifurcation measures 11.4 cm. C: DSA during EVAR procedure. The un-deployed device is above the target left renal artery. D: DSA during deployment. The graft is aligned, flush with the target left renal arter E: Moulding of the proximal landing zone with a balloon for a small Type 1a endoleak. F: Completion DSA with no endoleak.

Endoleak

An endoleak is a recognized complication of endovascular repair and is defined as blood flow outside the stent graft but within the aortic sac. This may occur due to a leak at the proximal and distal ends of graft fixation (sealing zones, Type 1), retrograde flow from a branch vessel such as the inferior mesenteric artery (IMA) or lumbar vessels (Type 2), malfunction of the graft (e.g., Junctional separation of modular components), stent-graft fracture or fabric hole (Type 3), stent graft porosity (Type 4), or endotension (Type 5). Types 1 and 3 are considered sinister and, if persistent, require treatment by further stent graft placement. Type 2 leaks are common, and the management is controversial. Various techniques such as coiling, embolizing, or gluing the leaks can be performed, but many Type 2 leaks are benign and self limiting.

Endotension is defined as continued expansion of the aneurysm sac without evidence of an endoleak. It is a poorly understood phenomenon but likely reflects either an undiagnosed endoleak or may be due to excess transmitted aortic pressure. If the aortic sac continues to expand, then it is typically managed by relining with a further stent graft.

Table 10: Types of endoleak

Type 1	Sealing zone leak	1a - proximal end 1b - distal end
Type 2	Aortic sac filling via branch vessel	lumbar vessel or IMA
Type 3	Graft failure	Fracture/dislocation/Fabric hole
Type 4	Graft porosity	Fabric failure
Type 5	Endotension	Undiagnosed endoleak or transmitted aortic pressure

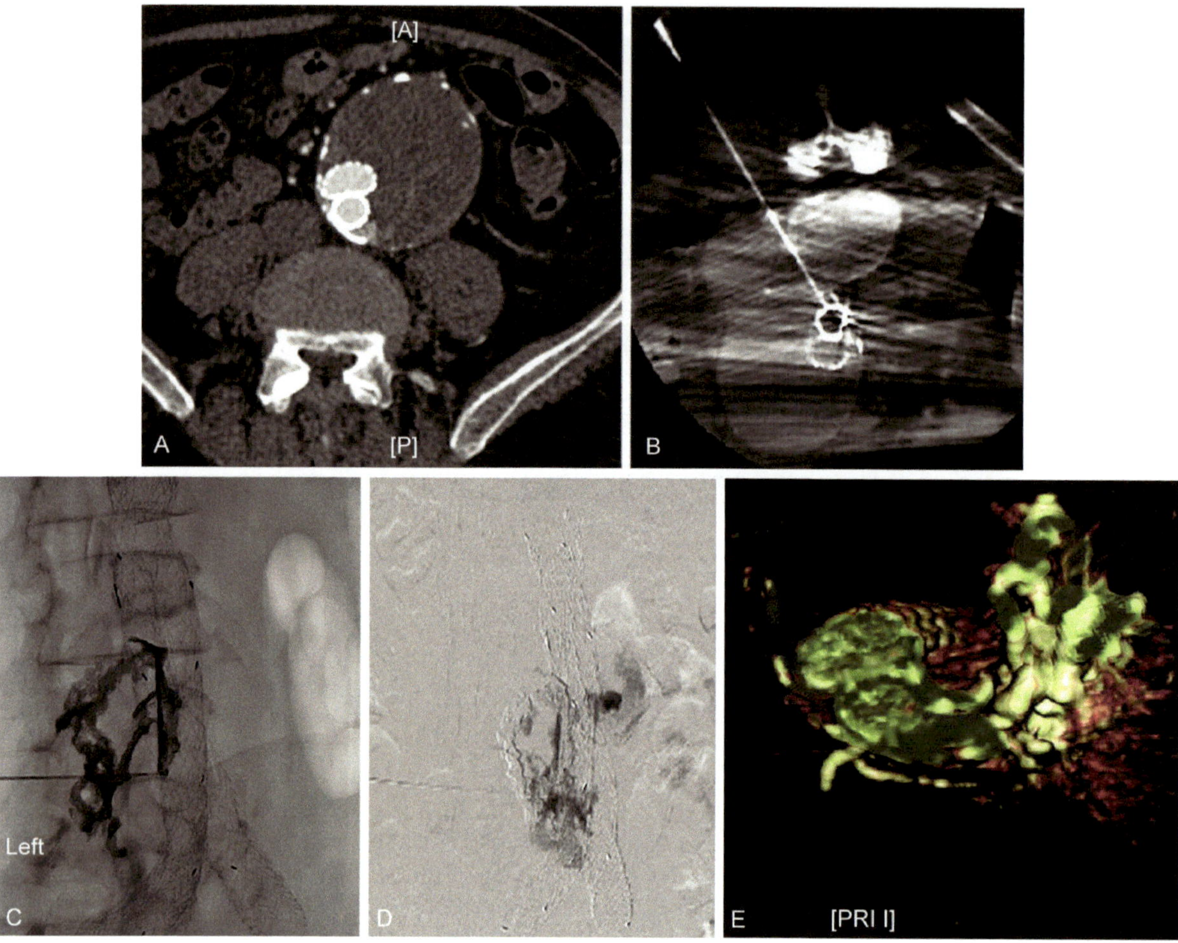

Figure 22 A: CTA showing posterior sac enhancement outside the EVAR device which was seen to communicate with the L4 Lumber arteries (Type 2 endoleak). The sac was continuing to increase in size. B: CT guided left trans-lumbar needle puncture of the sac at the point of enhancement. C: Fluoroscopic guided injection of a liquid embolic material (cyanoacrylate glue and/or lipiodol mixture). D: Injection during DSA acquisition shows glue exiting the sac via the L4 lumbar artery. E: Follow up CTA showing glue casts within both L4 lumbar artery branches.

Post EVAR Surveillance

Stent-graft surveillance is essential following endovascular repair to monitor for stent complications described in Table 11. Unlike open repair, the sac is only excluded from the circulation, but it still persists. A graft complication may allow sac reperfusion and hence risk of further rupture. In the longer-term data of EVAR 1, there were 25 aneurysm ruptures such that at 6 years the aneurysm-related mortality converged with open repair and with no added long-term benefit of endovascular repair.[36] The short-term benefit still persisted. This may be due to a variety of reasons such as older graft technology and inexperience, but the importance of surveillance is highlighted.

Surveillance may be performed with CT angiography, duplex ultrasound or MRA.

CT is the mainstay surveillance modality and is usually performed at 4 weeks and 3 months post-procedure. Increasingly subsequent imaging is performed by a combination of duplex ultrasound and plain x-ray if there are no signs of complication such as endoleak or sac size increase. Duplex ultrasound is sensitive to detect endoleaks and can accurately assess sac size changes. It is portable, safe, and inexpensive but user dependent. Plan x-ray is used to assess stent configuration for kinks or dislocations, strut fractures or device migration. This regime avoids the cumulative radiation exposure of repeat CT scans. The sensitivity of ultrasound for endoleak detection is improved with the addition of contrast (contrast-enhanced ultrasound) which may also be used to characterize an endoleak.

Table 11: Complications of EVAR

Endoleak
Stent migration / dislocation
Kinking of limb
Stent fracture
Iliac limb occlusion
Graft fabric holes

Evidence for EVAR

Several prospective randomized trials have compared EVAR and open repair of infra-renal aortic aneurysms. EVAR 1 was a randomized controlled trial for abdominal aortic aneurysms >5.5 cm undergoing either open or endovascular repair.[36] There were 626 patients in each group. The 30-day mortality rates were 4.3% for open repair compared to 1.8% for EVAR, clearly indicating a significant early advantage for endovascular repair. However, at 2 years, the all-cause mortality in the 2 groups converged and at 6 years aneurysm-related mortality converged. Increased late fatal graft rupture resulted in a decrease in early benefit of EVAR. Indeed 17 of 22 patients who experienced delayed rupture following EVAR had recognized graft complications that were not treated. Proponents of EVAR believe that these figures are outdated as newer improved grafts are now available, technical skills much improved, and the management of complications better understood.

The European DREAM trial of 351 patients observed statistically significant shorter procedure time, blood loss, hospital length stays, and intensive care stay for endovascular repair. 30-day mortality was 4.6% for open repair and 1.2% for EVAR.[37] However, reintervention rate was approximately 3 times higher in the first-year post procedure with EVAR.

The American OVER trial of 881 patients observed similar findings to the DREAM trial regarding procedure time, length of stay, blood loss, and 30-day mortality (3% open repair versus 0.5% EVAR).[38] After a 2-year follow-up, there was still an advantage evidenced by no late increase in mortality or morbidity in the EVAR group.

Complex Aneurysms

Complex aortic aneurysms at the level of the renal vessels (Juxta-renal) or suprarenal involving visceral branches, are not suitable for standard EVAR and are more challenging to treat. It is difficult to maintain perfusion of such vessels and maintain a seal. Fenestrated endografts are customized with scallops at the proximal end and fenestrations below. The fenestrations can be cannulated and stented to treat complex juxta-renal aneurysms seen in Figure 23. They require careful preoperative planning and precise placement to ensure the fenestrations align with the target vessels seen in Figure 24. Markers along the fenestrations and the graft, aid in positioning and graft deployment. Similarly, thoracoabdominal aneurysms can be treated through an endovascular approach using a longer device to treat the aneurysm and with branches for visceral vessels.

Iliac aneurysms may be treated with an iliac branch device, which has a side branch for the internal iliac artery and a main body that extends from the common iliac to external iliac artery.

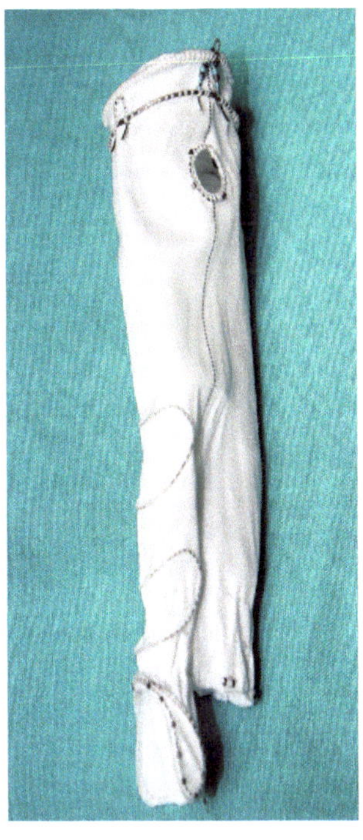

Figure 23: A fenestrated EVAR device. A round fenestration has been manufactured to accommodate a balloon mounted covered Stent which extends into one of the renal arteries. Proximal hooks engage the aortic wall to prevent device migration.

Aneurysms elsewhere can be similarly treated by exclusion with covered stents. These include isolated common or internal iliac aneurysms, popliteal aneurysms, and visceral artery aneurysms (e.g., splenic, hepatic, and renal). Pseudoaneurysms, either iatrogenic or acquired, occur by penetrating injury. They can happen in the community or on the battlefield and can be similarly treated by coil embolization and thrombin injection as appropriate.

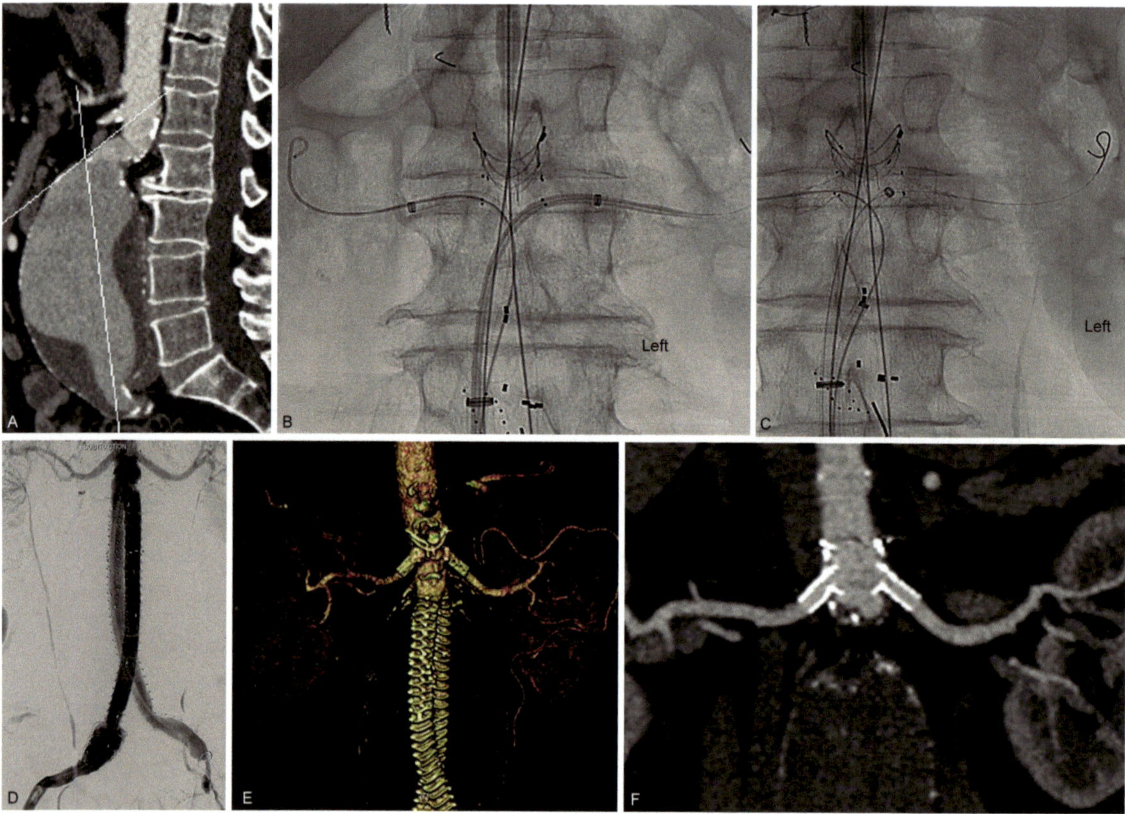

Figure 24 A: CT angiogram sagittal MPR of a 9 cm AAA with an angulated very short infrarenal neck unsuitable for conventional EVAR. B: Fluoroscopy image during fenestrated EVAR with vascular sheaths through the renal fenestrations into the renal arteries. C: Fluoroscopy image during fenestrated EVAR with balloon expandable covered Stent grafts in the renal arteries after flaring of the Stents within the EVAR fenestrations. D: Completed DSA showing patent renal arteries and no endoleak. E: Follow up volume rendered CTA at 1 month. F: Follow up curved MPR CTA image of the renal arteries at 1 month showing patent flared renal Stent grafts.

Aortic Dissection

Uncomplicated aortic dissections in patients who are asymptomatic are often treated medically by controlling blood pressure and pain. Symptomatic cases where the dissection includes branch vessels resulting in end-organ ischaemia or causing rupture requiring surgical treatment. Emergency open surgery is challenging and carries considerable risks of mortality and morbidity. Endovascular management offers an alternative in which the main goal is to cover and exclude the primary entry tear. Often the false lumen thromboses subsequently. In persistent cases, the stent graft can be extended distally to occlude the false lumen, but at the expense of increased risk of paraplegia due to coverage of spinal branches. The left subclavian artery may require coverage in order to achieve a proximal seal, in which case a carotid-subclavian bypass operation can be performed.

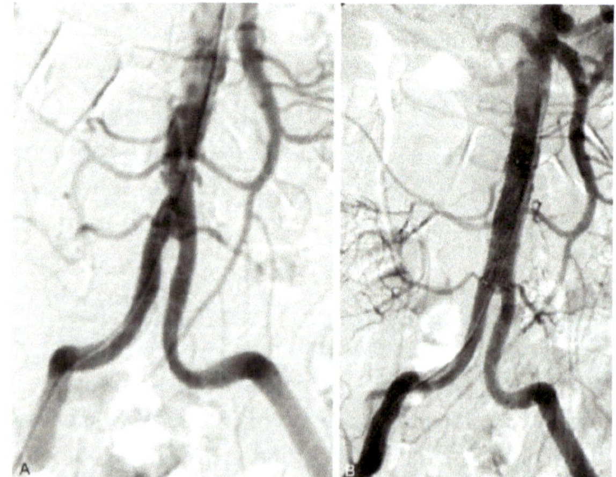

Figure 25 A: DSA of a focal dissection with narrowing of the aortic lumen. B: DSA after placement of an 18 x 54 mm self-expanding Stent

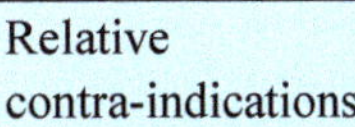

Thrombolysis and Thrombectomy

Thrombolysis is a useful technique to treat thrombosis and restore perfusion for an acute vessel, graft, or fistula occlusion. Most occlusions are secondary to an underlying stenosis which itself will require re-established perfusion and then treatment of angioplasty or bypass. However, other causes such as atrial fibrillation, mural thrombus and underlying thrombotic disorders (i.e., anti-phospholipid syndrome and thrombophilia) should also be excluded.

The technique involves an arterial and graft puncture, sheath insertion, delivery of a catheter into the thrombus, and local delivery of a thrombolytic agent (e.g., Alteplase®, Streptokinase®). This can be carried out through a Cragg McNamara catheter (ev3 Inc.) which has an active tip up to 20 cm long. It has multiple tiny side-holes and a terminal microvalve, either on table as a "pulse spray" technique, by slow pump infusion on the ward, or a combination of both. The aim of thrombolysis is to clear the thrombus and to treat distal run-off vessels. A continuous low-dose heparin infusion is given via the sheath to prevent peri-sheath thrombus formation. A repeat angiogram is usually performed at 12 to 24 hours to assess for effectiveness. Patients are usually managed on a vascular-skilled ward or high dependency unit due to the need for close observation of the limb and to patient observations. Complications include bleeding at a local puncture or distant site, stroke, distal embolization of thrombus, and reperfusion syndrome. Reperfusion syndrome is more likely in the event of a prolonged ischaemia and will manifest with renal failure, confusion, and respiratory distress. The timing and choice of patient for thrombolysis thus needs to be considered carefully.

Table 12: Indications and contra-indications of thrombolysis

Indications	• Dialysis fistula salvage • Bypass graft thrombosis • Thrombosed popliteal aneurysm • Acute myocardial infarction • Acute stroke • Post/peri-angioplasty thrombosis • Venous thrombosis (ileo-femoral/ axillary)
Absolute contra-indications	• Surgery or trauma within 2 weeks • Stroke (after 6 hours and within 2 months) • Pregnancy • Bleeding • Active gastric or duodenal ulcer
Relative contra-indications	• Age >80 years old • Early graft failure (usually technical) • Uncontrolled hypertension (systolic >180 mmHg or diastolic >110 mmHg) • The white limb- surgery best • Cardiac emboli

Mechanical thrombectomy

Mechanical thrombectomy comprises a rotating impeller driven by compressed air that creates a vortex and draws thrombus inside and breaks it down. It can also create a high-speed jet within a 'whistle tip' catheter side port producing a Venturi effect. It is passed into the most proximal thrombus and gradually advanced as the clot is broken down.

A commonly used example is the Angiojet device® (Medrad Interventional/Possis, Minneapolis, Minnesota). A multicenter, prospective, randomized trial comparing the technical success of Angiojet and surgical thrombectomy of thrombosed haemodialysis grafts demonstrated comparable results of 73.2% versus 78.8%, and similar complication rates of14.6% versus 14.1%.[39]

A further study investigated the AngioJet rheolytic mechanical thrombectomy system® (Possis Medical, Minneapolis, Minn) in terms of safety and effectiveness during treatment of acute infra-inguinal thromboembolism occurring during lower limb revascularization procedures. Technical success was 92.8% with adjunctive local thrombolysis and stenting used in 64.3% of cases.[40]

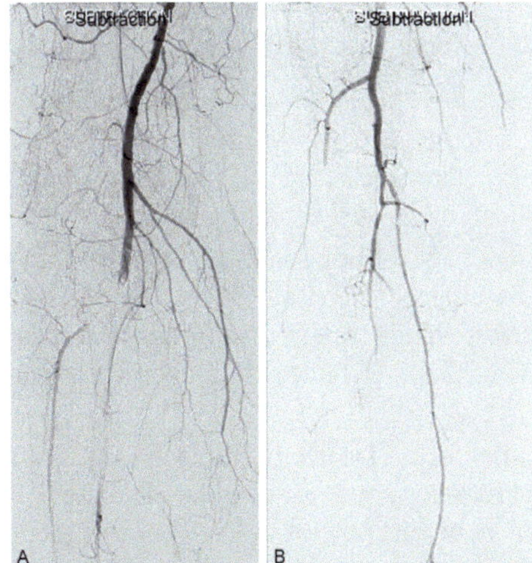

Figure 26 A: Embolization of the right popliteal trifurcation B: After AngioJet mechanical thrombectomy without thrombolysis

Thromboaspiration

Thromboaspiration is a technique using a straight wide lumen end-hole catheter to aspirate thrombus from occluded vessels and grafts, or distal emboli following angioplasty. It is an effective technique and adjunctive procedure to thrombolysis. It requires multiple passes of a catheter connected to a 50 mL syringe and aspiration of thrombus through a sheath. Clots may need to be cleared from the sheath via a removable hub. It requires a large bore catheter and hence large bore sheath of 6 to 8Fr depending upon the target vessel size, which can increase the risk of puncture site bleeding.

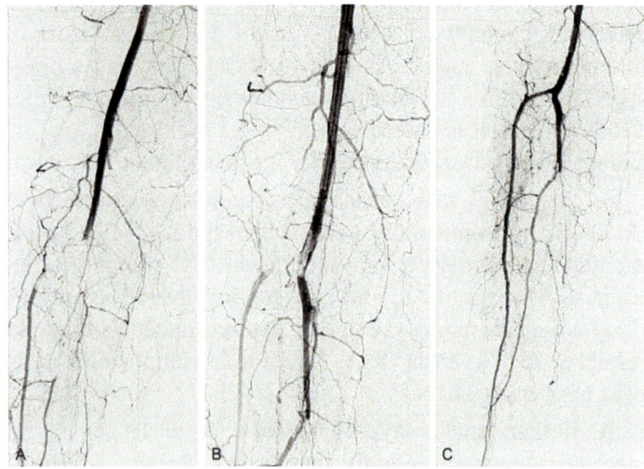

Figure 27 A: DSA of a popliteal embolus from the stump of an occluded right groin arteriovenous dialysis graft. B: Aspiration with a 6F big lumen aspiration catheter. C: DSA post aspiration showing restoration of the anterior tibial artery

REFERENCES

1. Dotter C, Judkins M. Transluminal treatment of arteriosclerotic obstruction. Description of a new technique and a preliminary report of its applications.1964 Circulation 1964, 30 (5): 654–70.
2. Morcos SK, Thomsen HS, Webb JA. Contrast-media-induced nephrotoxicity: a consensus report. Contrast Media Safety Committee, European Society of Urogenital Radiology (ESUR). Eur Radiol 1999; 9(8):1602-1613.
3. Heinrich MC, Haberle L, Muller V, Bautz W, Uder M. Nephrotoxicity of iso-osmolar iodixanol compared with nonionic low-osmolar contrast media: meta-analysis of randomized controlled trials. Radiology 2009; 250(1):68-86.
4. Cowper SE. Nephrogenic systemic fibrosis: an overview. J Am Coll Radiol 2008; 5(1):23-28.
5. Brar SS, Shen AY, Jorgensen MB, Kotlewski A, Aharonian VJ, Desai N et al. Sodium bicarbonate vs sodium chloride for the prevention of contrast medium-induced nephropathy in patients undergoing coronary angiography: a randomized trial. JAMA 2008; 300(9):1038-1046.
6. Tepel M, van Der GM, Schwarzfeld C, Laufer U, Liermann D, Zidek W. Prevention of radiographic-contrast-agent-induced reductions in renal function by acetylcysteine. N Engl J Med 2000; 343(3):180-184.
7. N-Acetylcysteine in the Prevention of Contrast-Induced Nephropathy Steven Fishbane Clin J Am Soc Nephrol 3: 281–287, 2008.
8. Webb JG, Pate GE, Humphries KH, Buller CE, Shalansky S, Al Shamari A, Sutander A, Williams T, Fox RS, Levin A: A randomized controlled trial of intravenous N-acetylcysteine for the prevention of contrast-induced nephropathy after cardiac catheterization: Lack of effect. Am Heart J 2004;148:422-429.
9. Fanelli F, Cannavale A, Boatta E, Corona M, Lucatelli P, Wlderk A, Cirelli C, Salvatori FM. Lower limb multi level treatment with drug-eluting balloons: 6-month results from the DEBELLUM randomized trial. Journal of Endovascular therapy 2012, Oct;19(5): 571-80.
10. Norgren L, Hiatt WR, Dormandy JA, Nehler MR et al. Inter-Society Consensus for the Management of Peripheral Arterial Disease (TASC II). European Journal of Vascular and Endovascular Surgery 2007;33 Suppl 1: S1-75.
11. Pulli R, Dorigo W, Fargion A, Innocenti, AA, Pratesi G, Marek J, Pratesi C. Early and long -term comparison of endovascular treatment of iliac artery occlusions and stenosis. Journal of Vascular Surgery 2011 Jan;53(1):92-98.
12. Karkos CD, Kaaramanos DG, Papadimitriou DN, Malkotsis DP, Demiropoulos KO, Papazoglou AG et al. Current Therapeutic Options in the Management of Superficial Femoral Artery Occlusive Disease. Acta Chir Belg 2007; 107:605-615.
13. Dorrucci V. Treatment of superficial femoral artery occlusive disease. Journal of Cardiovascular Surgery (Torino) 2004, 45: 193-201.
14. Ingle H, Nasim A, Bolia A, Fishwick G, Naylor R, Bell PRF, Thompsom MM. Subintimal Angioplasty of Isolated Infragenicular Vessels in Lower Limb Ischaemia: Long-term Results. Journal of Endovascular Therapy 2002;9(4): 411-416.
15. Adam DJ, Beard JD, Cleveland T, Bell J, Bradbury AW, Forbes JF, Fowkes FG, Gillepsie I, Ruckley CV, Raab G, Storkey H; BASIL trial participants Bypass versus

angioplasty in severe ischaemia of the leg (BASIL): multicentre, randomised controlled trial. Lancet. 2005 Dec 3;366(9501):1925-34.

16. The ASTRAL Investigators. Revascularization versus Medical Therapy for Renal-Artery Stenosis. N Engl J Med 2009; 361:1953-1962
17. Lammer J, Dake MD, Bleyn J *et al.*: Peripheral arterial obstruction: prospective study of treatment with a transluminally placed self-expanding stent graft. Radiology 2000;217:95-104.
18. Kedora J, Hohmann S, Garrett W, Munschaur C, Theune B, Gable D. Randomized comparison of percutaneous Viabahn stent grafts vs prosthetic femoral-popliteal bypass in the treatment of superficial femoral arterial occlusive disease. J Vasc Surg 2007; 45(1):6-10.
19. Rosanio S, Tocchi M, Uretsky BF, Stouffer GA: Use of intraluminal stents in the treatment of carotid, renal, and peripheral arterial disease. Am. J. Med. Sci 2000;319, 111–117.
20. Hassen-Khodja R, Sala F, Declemy S *et al.*: Value of stent placement during percutaneous transluminal angioplasty of the iliac arteries. J. Cardiovasc. Surg. 2001;42:369-374.
21. Bosch JL, Hunink MGM: Meta-analysis of the results of percutaneous transluminal angioplasty and stent placement for aortoiliac occlusive disease. Radiology 1997, 204; 87–96.
22. Tetteroo E, van der Graaf Y, Bosch JL *et al.*: Randomised comparison of primary stent placement versus primary angioplasty followed by selective stent placement in patients with iliac-artery occlusive disease. Dutch Iliac Stent Trial Study Group. Lancet 1998, 35; 1153–1159.
23. Uher P, Nyman U, Lindh M, Lindblad B, Ivancev K et *al*: Long-term results of stenting for chronic iliac artery occlusion. J. Endovasc. Ther. 2002, 9; 67–75.
24. Becquemin JP, Favre JP, Marzelle J, et al. Systematic vs. selective stent placement after superficial femoral artery balloon angioplasty: a multicenter prospective randomized study. J Vasc Surg. 2003;37:487–494.
25. Cejna M, Turnher S, Illiasch H, et al. PTA versus Palmaz stent in femoropopliteal artery obstructions: a multicenter prospective randomized study. J Vasc Interv Radiol. 2001;12:23–31.
26. Perrio S, Holt PJ, Patterson BO, Hinchliffe RJ, Loftus IM, Thompson MM. Role of superficial femoral artery stents in the management of arterial occlusive disease: review of current evidence. Vascular 2010 Mar-Apr;18(2):82-92.
27. Twine CP, Coulston J, Shandall A, McLain AD. Angioplasty versus stenting for superficial femoral artery lesions. Cochrane Database Syst Rev. 2009 Apr 15;(2).
28. Schillinger M, Sabeti S, Loewe C, et al. Balloon angioplasty versus implantation of nitinol stents in the superficial femoral artery. N Engl J Med. 2006;354:1879-1888.
29. Krankenberg H, Schluter M, Steinkamp HJ, et al. Nitinol stent implantation versus percutaneous transluminal angioplasty in superficial femoral artery lesions up to 10 cm in length: the femoral artery stenting trial (FAST). Circulation. 2007;116:285-292.
30. Laird JR, Katzen BT, Scheinert D, et al. Nitinol stent implantation versus balloon angioplasty for lesions in the superficial femoral artery and proximal popliteal artery: twelve-month results from the RESILIENT randomized trial. Circ Cardiovasc Interv. 2010;3:267-276.
31. Schlager O, Dick P, Sabeti S, Amighi J. Long-Segment SFA Stenting-The Dark Sides: In-StentRestenosis, Clinical Deterioration, and Stent Fractures J Endovasc Ther 2005;12:676–684.
32. Dake M. Zilver PTX Randomized Controlled Trial of Paclitaxel-Eluting Stents for Femoropopliteal Disease: Three Year Results, Presented at the Vascular Interventional Advances conference in Las Vegas, Nevada October 2012.
33. Stenting versus Endarterectomy for Treatment of Carotid-Artery Stenosis Brott TG, Hobson, II RW, Howard G, Roubin GS, Clark WM, for the CREST Investigators. N Engl J Med 2010; 363:11-23.
34. Carotid artery stenting compared with endarterectomy in patients with symptomatic carotid stenosis (International Carotid Stenting Study): an interim analysis of a randomised controlled trial. Ederle J, Dobson J, Featherstone RL, Bonati LH, van der Worp HB, et al International Carotid Stenting Study investigators. Lancet 2010 Mar 20;375(9719):985-97.
35. Parodi, JC, Palmaz, JC, Barone, HD. Transfemoral intraluminal graft implantation for abdominal aortic aneurysms. Ann Vasc Surg 1991; 5: 491–9.
36. Endovascular versus Open Repair of Abdominal Aortic Aneurysm The United Kingdom EVAR Trial Investigators N Engl J Med 2010; 362:1863-1871.
37. Long-Term Outcome of Open or Endovascular Repair of Abdominal Aortic Aneurysm**.** De Bruin JL, Baas AF, Buth J, Prinssen M., Verhoeven ELG et al for the DREAM Study Group. N Engl J Med 2010; 362:1881-1889.
38. Long-Term Comparison of Endovascular and Open

Repair of Abdominal Aortic Aneurysm. Lederle FA, Freischlag JA, Kyriakides TC, Matsumura JS, Padberg Jr FT et al for the OVER Veterans Affairs Cooperative Study Group. N Engl J Med 2012; 367:1988-1997.

39. Comparison of the angiojet rheolytic catheter to surgical thrombectomy for the treatment of thrombosed hemodialysis grafts. Peripheral AngioJet Clinical Trial. Vesely TM, Williams D, Weiss M, Hicks M, Stainken B, Matalon T, Dolmatch B. J Vasc Interv Radiol. 1999 Oct;10(9):1195-205.

40. Treatment of infrainguinal thromboembolic complications during peripheral endovascular procedures with AngioJet rheolytic thrombectomy, intraoperative thrombolysis, and selective stenting. Spiliopoulos S, Katsanos K, Fragkos G, Karnabatidis D, Siablis D. J Vasc Surg 2012 Nov;56(5):1308-16.

41

CHAPTER

Carotid Artery Atheromatous Disease

***Saurabh Rai**, FRCS*

***Morgan McMonagle**, MD, FRCSI*

***Rajiv Vohra**, Ph.D., FRCSEd, FRCSEng*

INTRODUCTION

The extracranial carotid arteries are vulnerable to several atheromatous and non-atheromatous disorders. In the western world, stroke is the third most common cause of death, only preceded by cardiac diseases and cancer. In the United Kingdom (UK), about 125,000 patients suffer their first stroke each year. It is the most common cause of disability in the United States (US) and Europe. The resulting disability has a crippling effect leading to socioeconomic burden to the patient, their family, and society. The American Heart Association estimated the financial impact of stroke in the US to be $57.9 billion in 2006.[1] Though the overall mortality due to stroke has decreased with improved survival-rate, the overall incidence of stroke may increase significantly in the next 20 years with an increasing elderly population.

Stroke is defined as an acute loss of focal cerebral function with symptoms exceeding 24 hours and no apparent cause other than that of a vascular origin. Stroke also includes acute loss of global cerebral function due to vascular origin (e.g., in cases of coma and subarachnoid hemorrhage). A transient ischemic attack (TIA) is defined as an acute loss of focal cerebral function or monocular visual loss (amaurosis fugax) due to vascular origin, with symptoms lasting less than 24 hrs. The risk of recurrent events after a TIA is highest in the first month showing rates of 8% to 10% risk at seven days and 11% to 15% at 30 days. Crescendo TIAs involve repeated TIAs within a short period of time in which the neurological deficit should have fully recovered before the onset of the next event. 'Stroke in evolution' means repeated episodes of stroke where the subsequent stroke occurs prior to the complete recovery of the previous stroke. Both of these clinical situations often imply that there is an acutely unstable intraarterial plaque with an overlying thrombus. Reversible ischemic neurologic deficit (RIND) describes a focal neurological deficit that lasts longer than 24 hours but resolves completely within 1 week.

About 36,000 patients suffer from a TIA in the UK each year. The incidence of stroke and TIA increases with age. In a typical western population of 200,000, approximately 168 TIAs or non-disabling strokes occur every year. Of these, 18 cases will have a carotid stenosis of greater than 70%. In the same community, 1,500 people will have an asymptomatic carotid stenosis.[2]

Anatomy of the Carotid Arteries

There is one common carotid artery (CCA) on each side of the neck. The right CCA originates from the brachiocephalic trunk while the left CCA originates directly from the arch of the aorta. After arising in the thorax, it runs through the neck towards the cranial cavity. At the upper border of the thyroid cartilage, which generally corresponds to the level of the fourth cervical vertebra, the CCA bifurcates into the external carotid artery (ECA) and internal carotid artery (ICA). The ECA usually arises medial and anterior to the ICA. There is a dilated segment at the level of the CCA bifurcation which is called the carotid sinus. The carotid sinus has extensive nerve endings which act as baroreceptors controlling blood pressure. The carotid body lies within the adventitia of the posterior aspect of the CCA bifurcation and works as a chemoreceptor. It is responsible for monitoring blood gases and pH. The ECA normally supplies extra-cranial muscles and the parotid gland through various branches. The ICA runs vertically upwards from its origin to the carotid foramen at the base of the skull. During its course through the neck, it is accompanied by the internal jugular vein (IJV) which lies posterolateral to the ICA and with the vagus nerve running in between. This segment of the ICA may have loops, kinks, or tortuosity. After entering the carotid foramen, the ICA runs vertically in the petrous part of the temporal bone for about 1 cm. Then it turns anteriorly and medially where it runs horizontal until it emerges at the apex of the petrous bone. The intracranial segment of the ICA has a pre-cavernous, cavernous, and supra-clinoid segment. The ICA bifurcates into the anterior and middle cerebral artery (ACA and MCA).

The vertebral artery (VA) arises from the proximal part of the subclavian artery in the neck. It ascends to enter the transverse process foramen of the fifth or sixth cervical vertebra. The pair of VAs unite to form the basilar artery, and later bifurcate into terminal the posterior cerebral arteries (PCA). Most of the brain is supplied by the central anastomotic network of the two internal carotids and vertebrobasilar arteries called the circle of Willis, shown in Figure 1.

In about 90% of cases, there exists some form of complete circular arterial channel between the ICA, PCA, and ACA. The greatest variation in length is found in the anterior communicating artery; and in diameter in the posterior communicating artery.

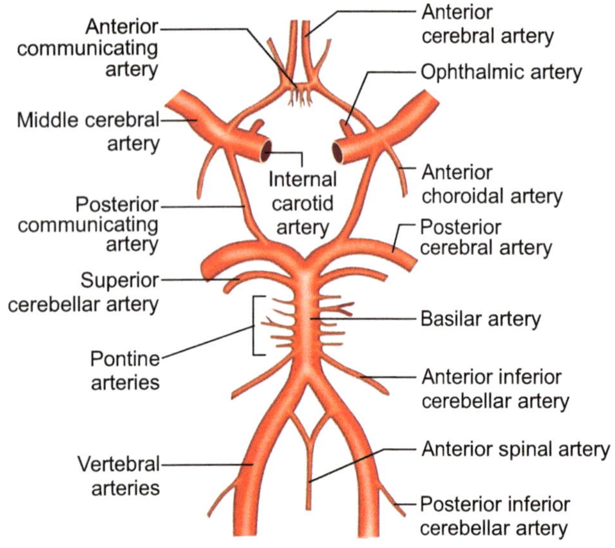

Figure 1: Circle of Willis

The nature and severity of the initial neurological deficit is unpredictable and depends upon the chronicity, degree of ICA stenosis, and the extent of collateral vessel development.

Etiology and Risk Factors

80% of all strokes are ischemic, 20% are hemorrhagic. Up to 80% of all ischemic strokes occur in the carotid territory. For every 100 patients who present with ischemic infarction in the carotid territory, 50 are due to thromboembolism of either the ICA or MCA, 25 are secondary to small vessel disease affecting lenticulostriate arteries, 15 are due to embolism from the heart, and the remaining 5-10 have a hematological or non-atheromatous condition accounting for the stroke. The risk factors for stroke are mentioned in Table 1.

Pathophysiology

Carotid atherosclerotic disease covers a wide spectrum of atherosclerosis from intima-medial thickness to complete occlusion. Various factors determine the evolution from one stage to the next. With increasing age, the incidence and degree of ICA stenosis due to atherosclerosis increases. Though the evolution of atherosclerosis is well-known, the triggers behind the transformation of carotid atherosclerotic plaque, shown in Figure 2A, from being asymptomatic to becoming symptomatic remain elusive. Similar to the concept of "vulnerable" coronary artery plaque leading to acute coronary event, a mechanism for cerebral manifestation due to carotid artery disease is evolving. An unstable (vulnerable) plaque carries a greater risk of stroke or recurrent TIAs due to embolization from the plaque. These plaques have a thin fibrous cap and a necrotic but biologically active lipid core seen in Figure 2B. There is a significant amount of inflammation with infiltration of T-lymphocytes and activated macrophages. Upon activation, these inflammatory cells secrete proteolytic enzymes including matrix metalloproteinases (MMPs) which degrade the collagenous extra-cellular matrix and weaken the plaque leading to an increase in the risk of plaque rupture. Direct interaction with the vascular smooth muscle cells (VSMC) also leads to the promotion of VSMC apoptosis which increases the vulnerability of the plaque by weakening the fibrinous cap. There have been attempts to utilize cellular and molecular biological events as markers of plaque instability. These markers are associated with various processes of atherosclerosis and plaque instability (e.g., inflammation, proteolysis, lipid accumulation, infection, and thrombosis). Important amongst these markers are MMP-2, MMP-9, soluble intercellular adhesion molecule -1 (sICAM 1), osteoprotegrin, fibrinogen, homocysteine, and anti-chlamydial pneumoniae antibodies.

It is debatable whether the elevated level of these biomarkers is an effect or a cause of the TIA or stroke. The fact is that most of these findings have not been tested on asymptomatic patients. Therefore, they cannot predict safely the occurrence of future TIAs or strokes. These biomarkers also lack the specificity for atherosclerosis affecting the ICA. There is a concern that the degree of stenosis alone may not be able to predict the risk of cerebral embolization, especially in asymptomatic patients, and thus cellular and molecular biomarkers may become particularly useful in the future for such patients.

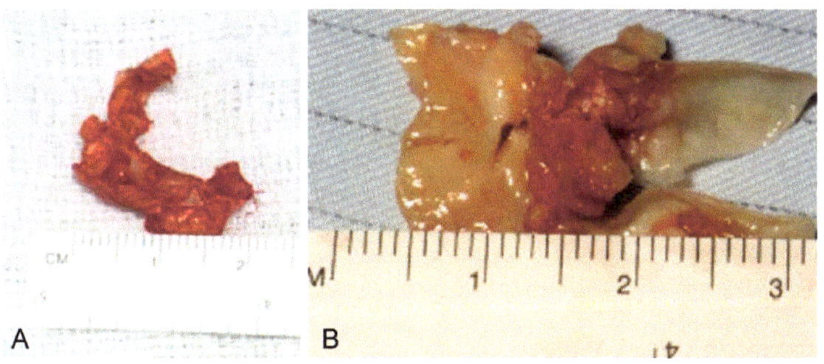

Figure 2: Left, ulcerated carotid plaque. Right, thin vulnerable carotid plaque

Table 1: Risk factors for stroke

Modifiable	Non-modifiable
• Hypertension • Cardiac diseases More common: AF, recent MI, mural thrombus, valvular heart disease Less common: Patent foramen ovale, aortic arch atheroma • Hyperlipidemia • Smoking • Diabetes mellitus • Physical inactivity • Carotid artery stenosis • Transient ischemic attack • Oral contraceptive pills • Substance abuse: crack cocaine, heroin	• Age >55 years (double every 10 years) • Race: African American, Hispanic > Caucasian • Family history

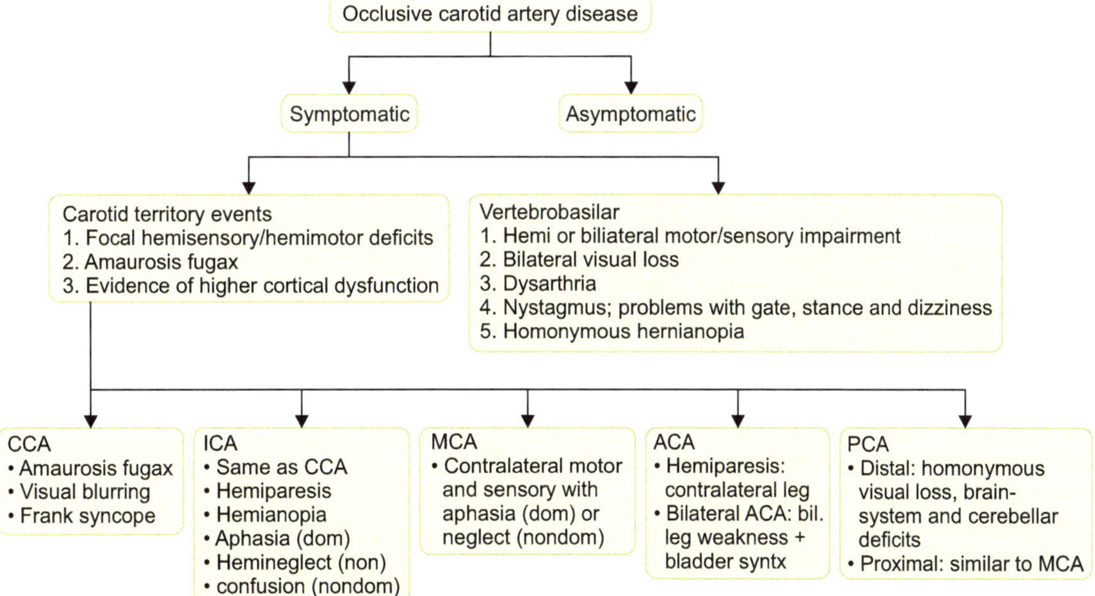

Figure 3: Clinical features of atheromatous carotid and large cerebral arteries disease

Presentation

Extracranial carotid artery disease can present in various ways as shown in Flow Chart 1 (Figure 3). The spectrum of presentation includes asymptomatic disease, TIA, RIND, and stroke.

Carotid territory TIAs involving only the eyes cause amaurosis fugax (transient monocular blindness) which refers to sudden loss of vision that is unilateral, transient in nature, and is due to ischemia or vascular insufficiency of the retina or optic nerve head. There is a loss of vision in the top or bottom half of the visual field, often described by patients as a curtain coming down over their eyes. This episodic loss may be partial or complete with a typical duration of several minutes but may vary from a few seconds to hours. The "curtain" may be perceived as black, gray, or white. The recovery of vision is as rapid as occurrence and is in reverse fashion. There are no positive visual phenomena such as flashes of light, bright shapes, or fortification spectra. These positive phenomena are more characteristic of visual loss due to a migraine and will also normally be bilateral and be followed by other features (e.g., headache, nausea, or photophobia). The risk of stroke after an episode of amaurosis fugax is 2% per year compared to 8% per year after a cerebral TIA. The causes of amaurosis fugax are listed in Table 2.

The diagnosis of TIA is based entirely on history, and it may not be straight forward in many situations. TIAs are sudden in onset with maximal symptoms at the onset. There is focal neurological deficit. Most TIAs last 5 to 15 minutes, thus, if symptoms last less than 30 seconds it is unlikely a TIA. TIA symptoms correspond to recognized neurological territory. Other information useful in differentiating a TIA is summarized in Table 3.

Table 2: Causes of amaurosis fugax

Ocular	• Giant cell arteritis • Congenital optic nerve abnormalities (e.g., nerve drusen) • Glaucoma • Anterior ischemic optic neuropathy • Retinal vein or artery obstruction • Tear-film abnormalities • Uhthoff's phenomenon (transient blindness due to increased body temperature, indicates demyelinating disease) • Dislocated lens • Optic disc edema • Vitreous or anterior chamber hemorrhage
Orbital	• Orbital mass (hemangioma, meningioma, osteoma) • Compressive optic neuropathy (thyroid/tumor related)
Intracranial	• Increased intracranial pressure • Aneurysm • Tumor
Carotid	• Embolism • Thrombosis • Dissection • Stenosis or occlusion
Cardiovascular	• Hypotension/bradycardia • Malignant hypertension • Arrhythmia
Hematological	• Anemia • Polycythemia • Thrombocytosis • Sickle cell disease • Plasma cell disorders (macroglobulinemia)
Miscellaneous	• Seizure • Migraine • Functional

Table 3: Exclusion and differential diagnosis of transient ischemic attacks[3]

Symptoms that don't suggest TIA	Conditions mimicking TIA
• Loss of consciousness • Acute confusion • Seizure • Loss of memory • Isolated dizziness, light-headedness, or vertigo • Gradual progression of symptoms • Multiple recurrent symptoms • Severe headache	• Migraine • Partial seizure • Syncope • Vestibular disorder • Neuropathy and radiculopathy • Ocular disorders • Hypoglycemia • Tumors of central nervous system

Management

The management algorithm for a TIA patient is outlined in Table 4. The carotid bruit is auscultated with the diaphragm of the stethoscope because it is a high-pitched bruit. It should be emphasized that the presence or absence of a carotid bruit is not of any diagnostic significance. The tightest stenosis may not have any audible bruit since the flow may be insufficient, whereas carotid bruit may be present in various other conditions apart from an ICA stenosis (e.g., ECA stenosis, CCA stenosis, subclavian artery stenosis, referred murmurs from the heart, and hyperdynamic circulation due to contralateral carotid artery stenosis/occlusion, anemia, hyperthyroidism, and pregnancy).

Table 4: Algorithm for the management of a TIA patient

A. General supportive measures (if applicable)
1. ABC (Airway, Breathing, Circulation)
2. Pulse oximetry and O_2 supplements
3. IV access
4. Obtain blood samples for: complete blood count, blood urea, serum creatinine, serum electrolytes, fasting blood sugar, lipid profile
5. Measure blood pressure
6. Cardiac monitoring
B. Examination
1. Check pulse rate and rhythm
2. Listen to heart sounds
3. Brief neurological examination including speech, cranial nerves, motor, sensory, coordination, gait
C. Investigations
1. Non-contrast head CT scan (to differentiate between ischemic and hemorrhagic infarct)
2. Carotid duplex Doppler (for ischemic infarct)
3. Echocardiogram (to detect embolic source)
4. MRI brain (to define infarct) and MRA of head and neck (to look at carotid artery and cerebral circulation)
D. Referral for further management
The $ABCD^2$ scoring system helps assess for stroke risk in patients who had a recent TIA. This ensures that high-risk patients are immediately identified, urgently assessed, and secondary prevention is quickly initiated.
$ABCD^2$ scoring systems:
• A – Age: ≥60 years old, 1 point.
• B – Blood pressure at presentation: ≥140/90 mmHg, 1 point.
• C – Clinical features: unilateral weakness, 2 points; speech disturbances with no weakness, 1 point.
• D – Duration of symptoms: ≥60 minutes, 2 points; 10 to 59 minutes, 1 point.
• E – patient has Diabetes: 1 point
The $ABCD_2$ score is the sum of the above points.
Patients with a score of ≥4 are considered at high risk of an early stroke.
This system excludes populations who are at a particularly high risk of early stroke, such as:
• ≥2 TIAs within 1 week – they are at higher risk for early stoke.
• Patients on anticoagulation treatment. In this case, patients require brain imaging to exclude intracranial bleeding.
• Patients who present days after a TIA.

After the initial management, it is important to stratify the patients according to their risk of future events. The $ABCD_2$ scoring system is a reasonable one. These recommendations are in line with guidelines issued by the National Institute for Health and Clinical Excellence (NICE), UK and the Royal College of Physicians Intercollegiate Stroke Working Party (RCP ICSWP), and are confirmed by various studies in different population-groups. On the basis of this evidence, the NICE Guideline Development Group defined a risk of >4% over 7 days as high risk requiring urgent referral to be seen within 24 hours.[4] This risk is equivalent to an $ABCD^2$ score of 4 or greater.

Investigations

The goal of the investigation for patients with suspected carotid atherosclerosis are: (1) to ascertain whether or not carotid stenosis is present, (2) to determine whether or not the patient's symptoms are due to a carotid lesion, and (3) to assess the severity of carotid stenosis, any unusual features, and its operability.

Duplex ultrasound is the current standard for non-invasive assessment of the carotid artery stenosis. "Duplex" is the combination of pulsed Doppler and B-mode ultrasound in the same device, where the "B" stands for "brightness". The transducer in the scan head of the ultrasound machine converts electrical energy into vibration energy and conversely converts vibration energy of returning echoes into electrical signals. A pulsed Doppler uses the same transducer to generate and receive echoes. For carotid examination, 5 to 7.5 MHz provides optimal tissue penetration. When sound waves encounter moving reflectors, such as red blood cells (RBCs), within the lumen of the carotid artery, the frequency of the reflected waves change from that originally made by the transducer. The frequency shift's magnitude depends upon the moving reflector's velocity and its angle with the sound wave. Traditionally, the examination is conducted at a Doppler angle of 60 degrees. This angle is used because few errors in velocity calculations secondary to misreading the Doppler angle occur. A color flow image is produced by assigning color to the Doppler shifts. The technician can adjust the color settings, usually making 'red' indicate flow towards the probe and 'blue' indicate flow away from the probe. The addition of color-flow scanning has made it easier to recognize an ICA occlusion and to differentiate between an ICA occlusion from very high-grade stenosis (string sign). Color-flow Duplex imaging also helps in seeing a tortuous ICA, carotid aneurysm, and carotid body tumor.

There are various spectral criteria for classifying stenosis in the ICA. The criteria developed at the University of Washington are, however, the most commonly used. These are mentioned in Table 5. The peak systolic velocity ratio between ICA to CCA of 4.0, detected a 70% to 99% stenosis by the NASCET criteria. A peak systolic velocity of >290 cm/s and end-diastolic velocity of >80 cm/s represents 60% stenosis of the ICA, which is the criterion used for offering CEA in the ACAS trial for asymptomatic patients.[5]

Table 5: University of Washington criteria for categorizing carotid artery stenosis

Stenosis (%)	PSV (cm/s)	EDV (cm/s)	Spectral analysis
0	<125	Here	Six lines in the 4th column should correspond against the six rows 0 Normal 1-15 No flow reversal in bulb 16-49 Spectral broadening during entire systole 50-79 Marked spectral broadening 80-99 Marked spectral broadening Occlusion No flow
1-15	<125		
16-49	<125		
50-79	>125	<140	
80-99	>125	>140	
Occlusion	–	–	

PSV = peak systolic velocity; EDV = end diastolic velocity

Duplex ultrasound also evaluates plaque density and surface morphology. There are two limitations of Duplex imaging: (1) it is operator dependent and (2) it does not show arch, great vessel origins, and intracranial vasculature. Intracranial vasculature can be seen noninvasively using trans-cranial Doppler (TCD).

Catheter angiography has been the gold standard for the evaluation of atherosclerotic disease. Figure 4 shows normal carotid digital substraction angiogram. The degree of stenosis in patients for possible CEA, seen in Figures 5 A to D. Intraarterial digital subtraction angiography (DSA) has allowed use of smaller contrast doses, catheter, and exposure time. DSA has largely replaced the cut-film angiography. Carotid angiography has evolved from direct percutaneous cervical arterial puncture to transfemoral catheterization. A variety of catheters and guide wires are available. It is worth noting that contrast angiography involves risks such as damage to artery secondary to puncture, dissection, plaque-embolization from the aortic arch or carotid bifurcation causing TIA/stroke (1%), and contrast-induced nephropathy and anaphylaxis.

MRA works on the principle of detecting the differences in emitted energy from moving compared to stationary protons after application of radiofrequency energy pulses within a magnetic field. The technique of differentiating energy released from stationary and moving protons is called 'time of flight' (TOF) technology. Two dimensional TOF MRA is better in detecting flow-related abnormalities whereas three dimensional TOF is better in detecting structural anatomy abnormalities including the degree of stenosis. MRI of the brain allows assessment of cerebral circulation along with structural assessment of the brain parenchyma. Although MRA is quite sensitive, it is not very specific. The assessment of the degree of stenosis can be erroneous because MRA often overestimates the degree of stenosis.

CT angiography (CTA) gives good anatomical detail including information about plaque morphology. However, it does need a significant contrast load and is not readily available. There is not enough data to support its routine use prior to CEA at present.

Newer non-invasive modalities (e.g., ultrasound, MRA, CTA) have replaced catheter angiography. With increasing expertise, patients can be offered CEA on the basis of duplex ultrasound alone. CT or MRI is not indicated routinely in patients requiring CEA. They are required in patients with acute, evolving stroke symptoms with atypical neurological features and patient with a prior history of a head injury or intracranial lesions.

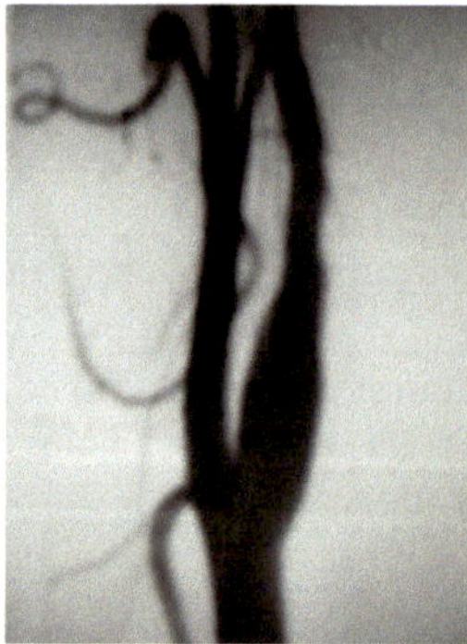

Figure 4. Normal carotid digital substraction angiogram

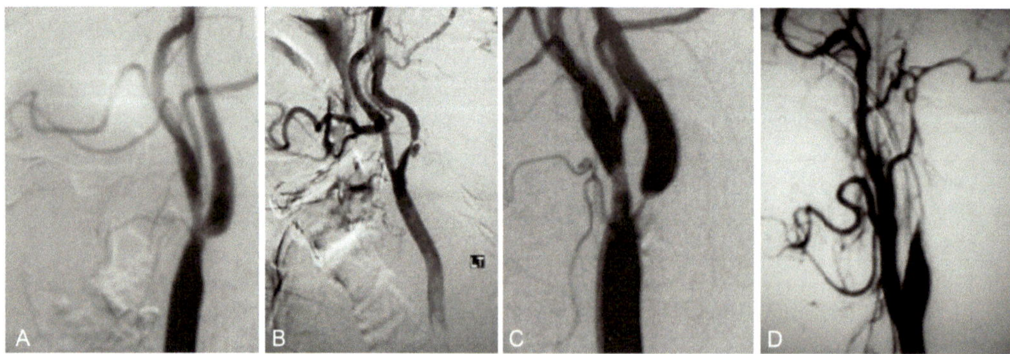

Figure 5 A: Stenosed internal carotid artery. B: Stenosed internal carotid artery with ulcerated plaque C: Severely stenosed internal carotid artery (string sign) D: Occluded internal carotid artery

Treatment

The optimal invasive treatment for the prevention of stroke has been a matter of much debate and controversy. Earlier debate was between using the best medical treatments alone versus using the best medical treatment with carotid endarterectomy (CEA). However, over the past 15 years carotid angioplasty and stenting (CAS) have emerged as alternative treatment modalities. It is important to understand: (1) the correct indications of carotid revascularization and (2) what constitutes the optimum carotid intervention.

Indications for treatment

Following a referral for an internal carotid artery (ICA) stenosis, the patient is assessed and listed for an intervention if they satisfy the well-defined criteria. The criteria for intervention are clearer in symptomatic patients compared to asymptomatic patients.

Symptomatic patients

Indications for intervention in symptomatic patients are relatively straightforward. All symptomatic ipsilateral ICA stenotic lesions pose a greater risk of subsequent disabling stroke and/or death in comparison to asymptomatic ICA stenotic lesions. Initially, there were two unsuccessful attempts to prove the benefit of CEA in symptomatic patients.[6,7] This was followed by two landmark randomized controlled trials (RCT) conducted in the 1980s which provided level I grade A evidence in favor of CEA. These studies were the European Carotid Surgery Trial (ECST) and the North American Symptomatic Carotid Endarterectomy Trial (NASCET). Although historical, 15 years down the line, these studies remain the "gold standard" in defining indications for CEA in symptomatic patients.

ECST was a randomized controlled trial conducted in 80 centers across Europe.[8] The degree of ICA stenosis was determined comparing the minimum residual lumen with the estimated normal lumen at greatest ICA stenosis (Figure 6). Symptomatic patients having 70% to 99% ICA stenosis treated with best medical treatment alone had a significantly higher risk of stroke and/or death compared to surgery. At three-years follow-up, risk of ipsilateral stroke and perioperative death was 10.3% in the CEA group compared to 16.8% in the best medical treatment group. Risk of stroke and/or death from any cause during follow-up was 12.3% for the surgical group and 21.9% in the medical group. Patients with 30% to 69% ICA stenosis who had CEA, did not benefit from medical treatment alone when followed for 4- to 5-years. Also, in patients with ICA stenosis of 0% to 29%, no benefit from CEA was seen.

NASCET analyzed the data from 50 centers in the US and Canada.[9] Only surgeons with a documented stroke/deathrate of <6% after CEAs for at least 50 consecutive cases over a 2-year period contributed to this trial. The degree of ICA stenosis was determined by comparing the diameter of the minimum residual lumen with the diameter at a point well beyond the region of greatest stenosis of the ipsilateral ICA (Figure 6). In severely stenosed ipsilateral ICAs, the diameter of the ipsilateral ECA or the contralateral ICA were used for comparison. In patients with 70% to 99% ICA stenosis, CEA was beneficial in comparison to best medical treatment alone. The 30-day stroke morbidity and mortality rate for the surgical group was 5.8% while in patients treated with best medical treatment was 11.2%. The cumulative risk of any ipsilateral stroke at 2 years was 9% for the surgical group and 26% for the medical group. The incidence of major or fatal ipsilateral stroke was 2.5% for the surgical group and 13.1% for the medical group. In patients with ICA stenosis of 50% to 69%, there was some benefit from CEA in men. The women with 50% to 69% ICA stenosis and who were symptomatic benefited only if they had one or more additional features such as age >70 years, severe hypertension, history of myocardial infarction, or a hemispheric event rather than a retinal event. Symptomatic patients with ICA stenosis of 30% to 49% and 0% to 29% had no significant difference between the surgical and best medical treatment groups.

Since the NASCET method of calculating the degree of stenosis was more accurate, the findings of the trials for symptomatic and asymptomatic ICA stenotic lesions were amalgamated by recalculating the degree of stenosis using the NASCET method in all patients. This data, now referred to as Carotid Endarterectomy Trialists Collaboration (CETC) data, is summarized in Table 6.

Table 6: Estimate of strokes prevented per 1000 cases[10]

	Trial	% Stenosis	Number of patients	30-day CEA risk	5-year risk: CEA	5-year risk: Medical	Strokes prevented per 1000 cases at 5 years
Symptomatic	CET	<30%	1749		2.6%	15.7%	0
	CETC	30-49%	1429	6.7%	22.8%	25.5%	26
	CETC	50-69%	1549	8.4%	20.0%	27.7%	78
	CETC	70-99%	1095	6.2%	17.1%	32.7%	156
	CETC	String	262	5.4%	22.4%	22.3%	0
Asympto-matic	ACST	60-99%	3120	2.8%	6.4%	11.8%	53
	ACAS	60-99%	1662	2.3%	5.1%	11.0%	59

Table 7: Approximate equivalent percentage of ICA stenosis in NASCET and ECST[14]

NASCET (%)	ECST (%)
30	65
40	70
50	75
60	80
70	85
80	91
90	97

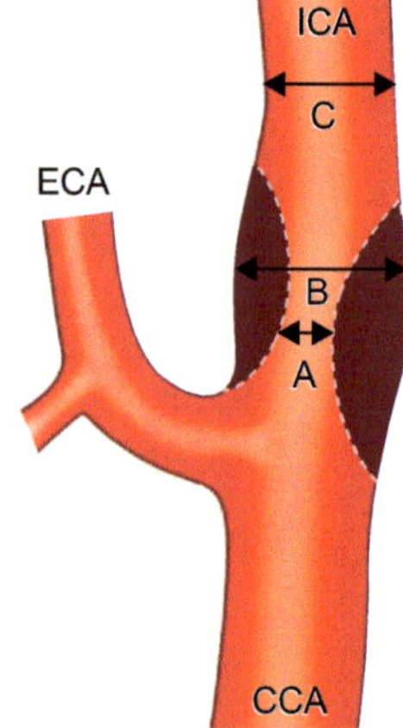

NACET % ICA Stenosis = C-A/C
ECST % ICA Stenosis = B-A/B

Figure 6: NASCET and ECST methods for calculating internal carotid artery stenosis

Interestingly it has been shown that the risk of stroke recurrence in the 'near occlusion' group was significantly lower than the 90% to 94% stenosis group, being 11% versus 35% respectively.[11] Subsets of patients with 94% to 99% stenosis in the NASCET and ECST pooled database had a stroke-risk of 14.1% on best medical therapy compared to 10.9% with surgery.[12] It is acceptable to offer CEA to patients with 95% to 99% stenosis if there is lack of collateral circulation from the contralateral carotid or ipsilateral/contralateral vertebrobasilar system.

In summary, despite differences in their design pattern, entry and exclusion criteria, methodology of estimating the degree of stenosis, and endpoints, the main findings of the trials for symptomatic patients have shown that:

1. For patients who are symptomatic and have a high degree of stenosis (70% to 99%), CEA is beneficial in both sexes.
2. For patients who are symptomatic and have stenosis of 50% to 69%, according to NASCET, CEA offered some benefit to men. For the same degree of stenosis, it did not offer any benefit to patients with diabetes and those with previous TIAs rather than strokes. Women benefited from surgery if they had one or more additional risk factor. According to ECST, there was no benefit from CEA in either sex. The major difference in this category between NASCET and ECST was explained by the different measuring criteria used for estimating the degree of stenosis shown in Figure 6. The ECST method overestimated the degree of stenosis as shown in Table 7. Therefore, what was calculated as an ICA stenosis of 50% to 69% in ECST was <50% ICA stenosis by NASCET measurement techniques. In <50% ICA stenosis there was no difference in either study.[13]
3. In patients with low-grade stenosis (<30%), whether symptomatic or asymptomatic, surgical treatment was actually harmful by increasing the risk of stroke and death.

Asymptomatic patients

In a general population aged 70 years and above, about 10% of people have an asymptomatic ICA stenosis of higher than 50%. If only patients with hypertension aged above 70 years are considered, this incidence will increase to 25%. In an aging population in the west, more asymptomatic lesions are likely to be identified. Usually, this lesion is found when the neck is auscultated, contralateral symptomatic side is scanned, or during other surgical procedures (i.e., coronary artery bypass graft (CABG)). This asymptomatic plaque can either remain stable or become problematic. The exact mechanism responsible for converting a stable plaque to a vulnerable one is not completely understood.

There have been two randomized controlled trials for asymptomatic patients: Asymptomatic Carotid Artery Stenosis study (ACAS) and Asymptomatic Carotid Surgery Trial (ACST). In ACAS there was an absolute risk-reduction of 5.9% in surgical patients with an ICA stenosis of > 60% demonstrated by duplex Doppler ultrasound.[15] The operative risk of stroke and/or death was only 2.3%. It showed that 20 CEAs were needed to prevent 1 stroke when followed for 5 years. Despite this, CEAs in asymptomatic patients were cost-effective. ACST included 3120 asymptomatic patients with ICA stenosis >60% as demonstrated by duplex Doppler ultrasound.[16] The 5-year stroke risk in surgical patients was 6.4% compared to 11.8% for patients in whom surgery was deferred. It showed a clear benefit for the patients aged <75 years. The efficacy of CEA in women compared to men was one-third due to their higher perioperative risk.

The ACAS trial recommended CEA for asymptomatic patients provided that the patient was anticipated to live in good health for 2 years or more, and the operating surgeon had an operative risk of stroke/death <3%. If the operative risk of an individual surgeon exceeds 4%, that surgeon should not recommend CEA for asymptomatic lesions. The summary points of ACAS are highlighted in Table 8.

Table 8: Summary of ACAS trial results

1. No apparent benefit in women (17% relative risk reduction versus 66% for men).
2. No evidence that CEA reduced the risk of disabling stroke.
3. No correlation between the degree of stenosis and late stroke.
4. Patients with bilateral disease do not have worse outcome.
5. To gain maximum benefit from CEA, patients should live at least for 5 years.
6. The cost per stoke prevented is extremely high.

The American Heart Association 2005 guidelines for CEA in asymptomatic ICA stenosis, based on the risk of operative intervention are summarized in Table 9 below:

Table 9: American Heart Association Guidelines (2005) for CEA in asymptomatic stenotic lesions

Patient characteristics	Proven indications	Acceptable indications	Uncertain indications
Surgical risk <3% and life expectance ≥5 years	Ipsilateral ICA stenosis >60% with/without ulceration and antiplatelet therapy irrespective of contralateral artery status	CEA simultaneous with CABG for >60% ICA stenosis	Unilateral stenosis >50%
Surgical risk of 3-5%	None	Ipsilateral ICA stenosis >75% with contralateral ICA occluded or stenosed >75%	ICA stenosis >75% contralateral artery status If CABG required: uni/ bilateral asymptomatic
Surgical risk of 5-10%	None	None	If CABG required: uni/ bilateral ICA stenosis >70%

If an interventionist's periprocedural stroke/deathrate is higher than 2% to 3%, it may be more harmful to intervene on an asymptomatic standard-risk patient. To date, no justifiable methods to identify the asymptomatic lesions with an increased risk of embolization have been identified. It has been suggested[17] that three group of patients will benefit from a revascularization procedure: (1) patients with plaque instability identified with MRA and/or duplex, with or without silent embolic signals, (2) patients with insufficient collateral circulation detected by transcranial Doppler, transcranial color-coded Doppler, and/or magnetic resonance arteriography, (3) or patients with severe metabolic compromise characterized by increased oxygen extraction fraction as measured with positron emission tomography.

The mainstay of the best medical treatment in these trials was Aspirin. Since then, there have been significant additions to the available treatment. Statins, beta-blockers, and clopidogrel are advocated more aggressively in these patients and have been shown to offer significant benefit. Due to more effective and aggressive medical management, the risk of ipsilateral TIA or stroke has dropped significantly in non-operated, asymptomatic cases with 50% to 75% stenosis.[18] Patients aged >79 years, who had a <5 years life-expectancy, or who suffered from conditions like unstable angina, atrial fibrillation, severe diabetes, uncontrolled hypertension, and renal insufficiency, were excluded from the NASCET and ACAS trials. Therefore, the findings of these trials cannot be extrapolated to this group. The true benefit of surgery for asymptomatic stenosis can be passed to the patients if the perioperative stroke-rate of the center and surgeon is low. Only high-volume surgeons performing >25 CEA per year with <6% combined perioperative stroke/deathrate participated in the NASCET trial. The complication-rate may be much higher in the hands of surgeons performing fewer cases.

Newer studies such as Transatlantic Asymptomatic Carotid Intervention Trial (TACIT) consist of three-way randomization of high and low-risk patients with a >70% asymptomatic stenosis. The groups include (1) best medical therapy with antiplatelets, statins, and anti-hypertensives and (2) CEA plus best medical therapy (3) CAS plus medical therapy. This will hopefully give better answers to the objections raised in these historical trials.

The Optimum Intervention

Best Medical Treatment

Optimal medical treatment includes control of blood pressure, hyperlipidemia, ischemic heart disease and diabetes, cessation of smoking, and commencing antiplatelets and statins. Hypertension is the most important treatable risk-factor for stroke. A gradual individualized control is necessary. Sudden lowering of blood pressure may be counterproductive because the carotid stenosis may require high blood pressure to maintain cerebral perfusion. Lowering of blood pressure reduces the chances of stroke and slows down the progression of atherosclerotic lesions. Similarly lowering the blood lipid by statins not only reduces the rate of progression of carotid stenosis but also exerts a plaque-stabilizing (pleotropic) effect which thereby minimizes the chances of cerebral embolization. Tobacco use increases the risk of stroke in proportion to duration and amount of smoking. If an average smoker quits smoking for five years, his risk of stroke drops to the level of a non-smoker. Use of recreational drugs including cocaine and amphetamines should be avoided. There are various antiplatelet pharmaceutical agents which helps patients with carotid stenosis, summarized in Table 10. Warfarin is only used if the TIA or stroke is due to embolization from the heart, usually due to atrial fibrillation.

Table 10: Antiplatelet agents used in patients of carotid stenosis

Name	Mode of action	Side effects	Comments
Aspirin	Cyclooxygenase inhibitor	Gastric irritation, peptic ulcer, GI bleeding, metabolic acidosis, renal insufficiency	Standard treatment, lower dose is as useful as larger dose but better tolerance
Dipyridamole	Phosphodiesterase inhibitor	Headache	Usually combined with aspirin
Ticlopidine	Inhibits the exposure of fibrinogen binding site GPIIa/IIIb receptor complex	GI irritation, diarrhea, allergic skin reaction neutropenia	More effective than aspirin, not used due to severe neutron/thrombocytopenia, especially in first 12 weeks
Clopidogrel	Adenosine diphosphate receptor antagonists	GI irritation and bleeding	An alternative to aspirin, but more expensive

Carotid Endarterectomy (CEA)

The first successful carotid revascularization was reported by Eastcott, Pickering, and Rob in 1954.[19] The durability of CEA is backed by level I grade A evidence, generated from randomized controlled trials and therefore remains to be the "gold standard".

Informed consent

It should be made clear to the patient and their family that CEA is a prophylactic surgery with the sole aim to minimize the chances of a disabling or fatal stroke. It does not improve the current state of health. The surgeon should be clear that, although the long-term stroke risk is lower with surgery, short-term postoperative risk is higher. Treating units should aim for a stroke/death rate of fewer than 5%. The possibility of complications should be discussed. Such complications include local injury such as wound hematoma requiring reoperation; nerve injury to the greater auricular, sensory branches of cervical plexus, glossopharyngeal, or recurrent laryngeal nerves; and systemic complications such as myocardial infarction (MI) and cerebral hyper-perfusion.

Timing of surgery

Patients with a TIA or minor stroke need to be referred, seen, and investigated for possible surgery as soon as possible, preferably within 2 weeks. But unfortunately, this is not possible even in the most developed countries. It was initially thought that if a patient has suffered a stroke, it is better to delay the surgery for an arbitrary time-limit of 6 weeks. The supportive reasons for this were two; (1) this period allows the ischemic penumbra to be reduced in size, thereby delaying the risk of perioperative stroke and (2) an early surgery may lead to hyper-perfusion and transform the ischemic penumbra into a hemorrhagic one. However, any delay may be risky as there is a higher risk of stroke in the first 8 weeks after the original presentation. This risk is higher in males. There is an increased frequency of TIAs if it occurs in the previous 3 months, coexists with peripheral vascular disease and hemispheric (rather than ocular) TIAs, is combined ocular and hemispheric symptoms, is in the presence of complicated carotid plaque morphology (ulceration or echolucency).

Preoperative medical treatment

All the patients who are scheduled to have CEA should be on antiplatelet treatment. This may increase the risk of hemorrhage during incision and at the endarterectomy site. On the other hand, if antiplatelet treatment is withheld, the chances of cerebral embolization and thrombosis at the endarterectomy site may increase. Aspirin, irrespective of dose, varying from 75 mg to 300 mg, should not be stopped preoperatively. There is uncertainty about clopidogrel. Either given alone or in combination with aspirin, it does increase hemostatic time, but there is no significant increase in postoperative haemorrhage.[20] If the patient is on dual antiplatelet therapy, most surgeons still stop clopidogrel 3 to 7 days prior to CEA. Patients receiving anticoagulants for atrial fibrillation or mechanical valve should stop warfarin 3 to 5 days preoperatively. To cover this period, they should be switched to IV heparin or low molecular weight heparin. Their International Normalized Ratio (INR) on the day of surgery should be <1.8. Irrespective of cholesterol level, all patients should be on statins which are continued uninterrupted throughout the perioperative period. Statins are beneficial by dual mechanisms, lowering the cholesterol level as well as exerting pleiotropic effect.

Once it is decided that a patient needs a CEA, it is worth going through a preoperative checklist to ensure that the correct operation is performed on the right patient for the correct indication. These points are listed in Table 11.

Table 11: Preoperative check list for CEA

1. What is the reason for surgery, especially for an asymptomatic lesion?
2. Does any atypical symptom warrant further investigation?
3. Is the degree of stenosis appropriate, considering the perioperative risk of surgery?
4. Is the patient on the best medical treatment?
5. If the patient is on antiplatelet therapy, does it need to be modified perioperatively?
6. Does the patient need rescanning of the carotid artery prior to surgery?
7. Is the operation side marked?
8. Is an informed consent obtained?
9. Does the patient need a bed in the ICU for postoperative care?

Technique of Carotid Endarterectomy

Choice of Anesthesia

CEA can be performed either under local anesthesia (LA) or general anesthesia (GA). For local anesthesia there are two techniques: cervical plexus block (deep and superficial) or infiltration. Local anesthesia allows conscious cerebral monitoring by talking to the patient and, in the event of inadequate cerebral perfusion, a shunt may be inserted. The disadvantage of local anesthesia is that the patient has to lie in a slightly uncomfortable position for a considerable period of time. Patient anxiety may lead to high catecholamine levels and a higher blood pressure. Initial non-randomized studies suggested that LA was associated with significant reduction in the odds of death, stroke, MI, and pulmonary complications within 30 days of the operation. However, these studies were too small to draw a definite conclusion. This led to the GALA (general anesthesia versus local anesthesia) trial, one of the largest randomized surgical/anesthetic trials ever performed. This trial recruited 3526 patients at 95 centers in 24 countries.[21] The results suggested that both GA and LA are equally safe, irrespective of age or comorbidities. Patients with contralateral carotid occlusion have a smaller chance of further neurological events if operated under LA. Therefore, the type of anesthesia used should be decided jointly between the surgeon, anesthetist, and patient.

Position

The operation site is marked preoperatively. The patient lies supine with their head extended and rotated away from the operation site. A head ring and sandbag beneath the shoulders stabilize this position. The head end of the table is raised to reduce venous congestion. It is good practice to mark the angle of the mandible, the lower border of the mandible, the tip of the mastoid process, the sternal notch, and the anterior border of sternocleidomastoid muscle. One dose of an antibiotic is given intravenously (co-amoxicillin-clavulanic acid, gentamycin). Usually there is no need to pass a urinary catheter unless the patient has symptoms of urinary frequency, takes diuretics, and cannot lie still comfortably (if having an awake CEA) on the operation table.

Incision

The skin incision is usually given along the anterior border of the sternocleidomastoid muscle. If the level of the carotid bifurcation is marked preoperatively with the help of the duplex Doppler, this point should be at the middle of the incision. Some surgeons give a transverse skin crease incision in the neck skin crease extending from the anterior border of the sternocleidomastoid towards the Adam's apple. It may be difficult to approach a high bifurcation of the carotid with the transverse incision. In terms of damage to sensory nerves by these incisions, there is no difference. After incising the platysma, the upper and lower flaps are raised. Below this level there is no difference between the two incisions. Both involve incising the deep cervical fascia between the anterior border of the sternocleidomastoid and the trachea. At this level, the common facial vein is a constant landmark. This is mobilized, ligated, and divided, bringing the carotid artery along with the internal jugular vein (IJV) into view. If the carotid artery is dissected with an approach posterior to the IJV (retro-jugular approach), the division and ligation of the common facial vein is not required. The retro-jugular approach also minimizes the chances of injury to the hypoglossal nerve. The CCA is mobilized circumferentially and encircled with a sloop or rubber sling. The carotid bifurcation is dissected carefully but not mobilized until the ICA is clamped. The carotid bulb is handled very gently, as a friable atherosclerotic plaque may dislodge and embolize, leading to stroke. The ECA and ICA are dissected and controlled with slings. The ICA should be dissected until a blue hue on the arterial wall is seen which indicates a healthy, plaque-free segment of the artery. Some surgeons block the carotid sinus nerve by injecting 1 to 2 mL of lidocaine, which blocks the reflex vagal response causing sinus bradycardia. Surgical exposure of the carotid arteries is shown in Figure 7.

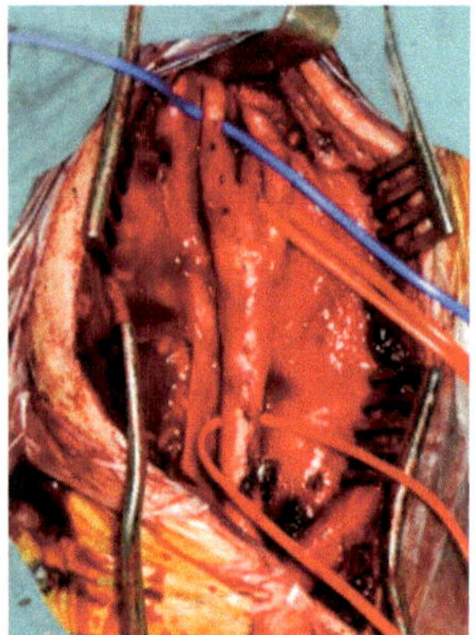

Figure 7: Surgical exposure of the carotid arteries

Optimal Intraoperative Antithrombotic Regimen

All the dissection is completed except for the mobilization of the carotid bulb. Before applying any clamp, systemic heparin (70 units/ kg body weight) is given. There is no evidence to support the use of systemic heparin, but most surgeons use it to minimize the chances of a MI and thrombosis of the ICA stump induced by clamping alone or by both clamping and shunting. Proponents of heparin highlight that the beneficial effects of heparin are not just confined to inhibition of coagulation. Heparin decreases platelet activation, thromboxane release, adhesion to collagen, and anti-inflammatory effects. Thus, heparin minimizes the ischemia-reperfusion injury to endothelial cells. A 2-minute time-gap is given to ensure that heparin has circulated in the system. Usually, a high dose heparin needs to be reversed by protamine 1 mg for 100 units of heparin. Because the half-life of heparin is 60 to 90 minutes, the dose of protamine is commonly calculated to reverse half the original heparin dose given. There is a slight increase in the chance of stroke by reversal of heparin. Patients may develop an allergic reaction to protamine which is higher in those who have used neutral protamine Hagedorn (NPH) insulin for diabetes or had prior vasectomy. Protamine should be avoided in these patients. Any allergic reaction should be treated by steroids and antihistamines.

Should the Patient be Shunted?

The best way to assess the safety of cross-clamping is by a temporary occlusion of the ECA, CCA, and ICA (in that order). In patients having CEA under local anesthesia, the speech and movement of the contralateral arm and leg are assessed after the clamping. If there is no evidence of weakness or disturbance of consciousness, intracranial circulation is judged to be adequate and the operation proceeds without any circulatory support (shunt). If the surgeon prefers GA, this technique cannot be employed. Surgeons fall into three categories of using shunts routinely in all cases, using shunts selectively, and never using shunts. There are different types of shunts as shown in Figure 8. There is no evidence that one type is better than another. Various pros and cons of deploying a shunt are listed in Table 12. If a shunt needs to be employed, a longitudinal arteriotomy is made on the anterior aspect of the CCA. This is extended to the ICA beyond the diseased intima. The distal end of the shunt is placed in the ICA, a back-bleed is allowed to fill the shunt. The proximal part of the shunt is now passed into the CCA. With the help of a handheld Doppler, the flow-signals in the shunt are detected to ensure proper functioning. It is important to remember that a shunt being in place does not equate to it working. Roughly 3% of shunts malfunction, often because of impaction on the distal ICA by kinks or coils.

Selective shunters use various techniques to identify patients who have inadequate collateral or contralateral cerebral circulation. These techniques are enumerated in Table 13.

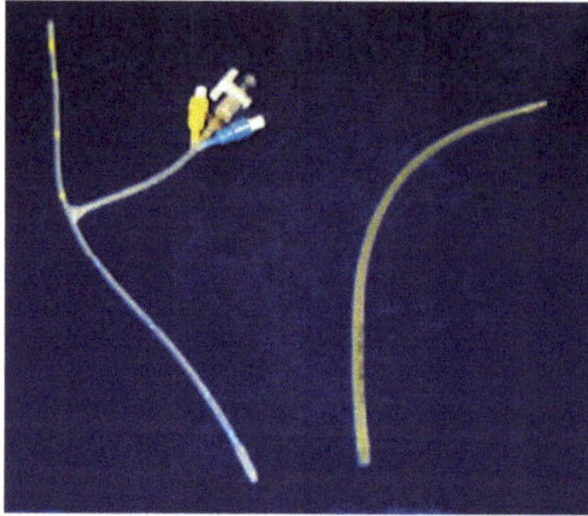

Figure 8: Carotid shunts. Left: Pruitt-Inahara shunt. Right: Javid shunt.

Table 12: Carotid shunting: pros and cons

Advantages	Disadvantages
1. Provides flow to all patients 2. Relieves surgeon of time-pressure 3. Optimizes the training opportunities for the trainee surgeons	1. Technically more cumbersome to perform endarterectomy 2. More difficult to visualize the distal endpoint of endarterectomy 3. Disruption of distal intima by shunt 4. Air/thrombotic embolization

Table 13: Methods of identifying inadequate collateral cerebral blood flow

Methods	Status	Reasons
1. Ipsilateral Jugular venous oxygen tension	Inaccurate	Venous drainage is a mixture of both cerebral hemispheres
2. Intraoperative Electro-Encephalogram	Inaccurate	Changes on EEG may be due to GA
3. Carotid stump pressure measurement	Useful	A stump-pressure >25 mmHg or >1/3rd of systemic pressure indicates acceptable collateral cerebral flow
4. Somatosensory-evoked potential		
5. Transcranial Doppler		
6. Near infrared spectrometry		

Only a stump-pressure monitoring technique is worth mentioning as it is validated by various researchers. There is a relationship between intracranial collateral blood flow and cerebral perfusion pressure. For measuring the stump pressure, a 19-gauge green needle is connected to a plastic tubing which is flushed with saline to ensure that there is no trapped air-bubble in it. This line is connected to the pressure transducer. After waiting for 3 minutes, the needle is inserted in the carotid bulb. It is ensured that a pulsatile reading is obtained, with the needle well-placed intra-luminally rather than abutting the arterial wall. The ECA and CCA are clamped. This leaves the needle in continuity with a static column of blood which is open to the ICA. Even though the needle is inserted proximal to the ICA stenosis, pressure will equalize on both sides of the carotid stenosis because there is no blood flow. As soon as the clamp is applied on the CCA, the pressure starts dropping down, and in a few minutes it stabilizes. This residual pressure in the carotid bulb (carotid stump pressure) is recorded. If this stabilizes at or above 25 mm Hg, or more than 1/3rd of systemic intraarterial pressure (checked in the radial artery), a shunt is not required.

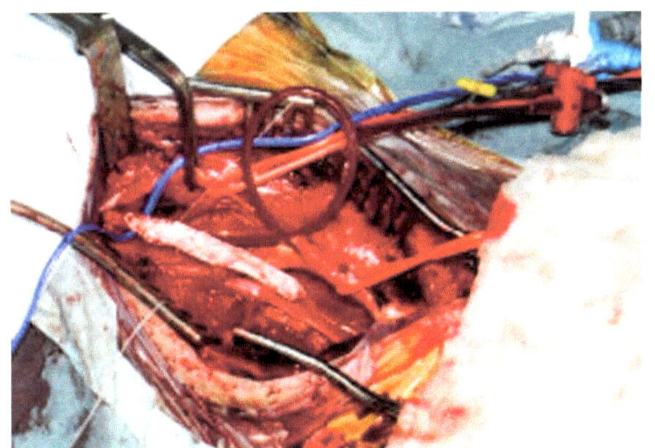

Figure 9: PTFE patch angioplasty

Bifurcation Endarterectomy

The optimal plane of dissection lies between the diseased intima and the circular fibers of the arterial media. The endarterectomy performed in this plane leaves a smooth distal tapering endpoint of plaque in the ICA.

Should it be Patched, if Yes What Patch to Use

On completion of endarterectomy, the closure is performed. Some surgeons close the arteriotomy without patch by using continuous, closely placed stitches. Other surgeons choose to patch either selectively or routinely. Primary closure avoids complications associated with patch angioplasty (e.g., patch blowout, pseudo aneurysm formation, prosthetic graft infection). The evidence supports the use of the patch to close the arteriotomy, especially in women who have smaller arteries and in the cases of restenosis. Patching increases the size of the artery and minimizes the chance of perioperative arterial occlusion and restenosis due to neo-intimal hyperplasia. The nature of the patch material is a matter of personal preference. The available options are knitted Dacron, polytetrafluoroethylene (Figure 9), bovine pericardium, and autologous (long saphenous, jugular, or cephalic) vein patch. Autologous vein patches minimize the chance of any patch infection. Bovine pericardium has a higher rate of developing a pseudoaneurysm. The results of PTFE and Dacron patches are comparable.

Eversion Carotid Endarterectomy

Another method called eversion carotid endarterectomy avoids the use of any patch. It involves an oblique transaction of the ICA at its origin of carotid bifurcation and endarterectomy by everting the ICA, endarterectomy of the carotid bifurcation and of the ECA, and reimplantation of the ICA on the CCA. Theoretical advantages of this technique include avoidance of longitudinal arteriotomy of the ICA, use of the patch, and a very effective correction of carotid kinks and tortuosity.

Once the arteriotomy is closed, one should wait to ensure that there is excellent hemostasis. Some surgeons leave a vacuum drain. The platysma and skin incision are closed using absorbable suture material or skin clips. Skin clips can be removed between the 3rd and 5th postoperative day.

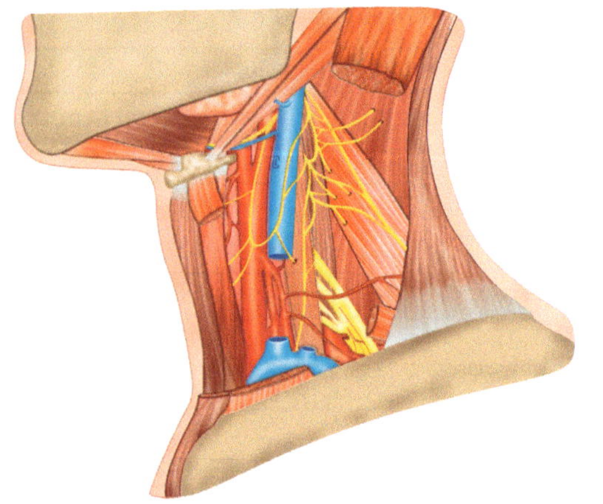

Figure 10: Distribution of relevant nerves (lateral profile)

Where Should Patients Recover

Usually, a patient's recovery is highly dependent on the area where invasive intraarterial blood pressure monitoring and close neurological observations are performed.

Special Scenarios

High Bifurcation

This is expected if the ultrasound examination fails to show the ICA above the stenosis clearly. High disease is when the plaque in the ICA extends above a line joining the tip of the mastoid process to the lower border of the ramus of the mandible. This corresponds to the lower border of the second cervical vertebra. To tackle high disease, patient should have nasopharyngeal rather than oropharyngeal intubation. This increases the available space between the mandible and the mastoid process. Division of the posterior belly of the digastric muscle makes access to higher segments of the ICA easier. By dividing the branch of the ECA which hooks the hypoglossal nerve, one brings at least 2 cm or more of the ICA into view. The subluxation of the temporomandibular joint has been described as another technique, but it increases the joint dysfunction later in life.

How to Avoid or Minimize Nerve Injuries

In order to avoid nerve injury, one must be aware of the anatomy. Figure 10 shows the distribution and course of the cutaneous and cranial nerves in relation to the carotid artery in a lateral profile.

The upper extent of incision should stop at least two fingers below the lower border of the mandible. In the case of high bifurcation, the incision needs to be extended, and should be curved posteriorly towards the mastoid process, running parallel to the lower border of the mandible. Diathermy should not be close to the nerves. Apart from the Ansa cervicalis, no other nerve-like structure that traverses the bifurcation should be divided. Dissection of the vagus should be performed carefully in the carotid sheath, and it should not be caught while applying the carotid clamps. Care should be taken to avoid over-stretching of the accessory nerve during the retro-jugular approach to the carotid artery.

When to Abandon a Planned CEA

If there is a significant delay between the duplex, revealing high-grade stenosis and planned CEA, one may find a totally occluded ICA on exploration. Such an occluded ICA should not be re-opened. If the ICA above the plaque is hypoplastic, and the patient is embolizing from this severely stenosed ICA, the ICA should be ligated, and no CEA should be performed. If there is no evidence of embolization, one should leave the stenosed ICA alone. There is no evidence to support either intervention. Either way, the patient should be anticoagulated for 6 months. If the plaque extends beyond the surgically accessible area, CEA should be abandoned.

How to Manage the Perioperative Neurological Deficits

Carotid thrombosis is the most common cause of early postoperative neurological deficit. If it occurs in less than 24 hours, the patient should return to the operating room immediately and the carotid should be reexplored. During re-exploration, one should be careful not to dislodge the friable thrombus into the brain. The patch should be reopened, and the thrombus removed. Once good back-bleed from the ICA is obtained, a shunt should then be inserted. Usually there is an underlying intimal defect which should be repaired and the arteriotomy site repatched. Neurological deficit which develops later could be due to cerebral hemorrhage or hyper-perfusion. Urgent CT scan of the head will be helpful in this situation. Cerebral hemorrhage is managed by carefully controlling the blood pressure with the input of a stroke physician specialist. Cerebral hyper-perfusion is also managed with accurate control of blood pressure and seizures.

When to Reoperate for Recurrent Stenosis

Restenosis of the ICA is attributed to neo-intimal hyperplasia within 24 months, or due to recurrent atherosclerosis >24 months later. The true incidence is ill-defined due to variable follow-up and diagnostic standards. The reported incidence in the literature is between 2% to 30%. A higher recurrence does raise the possibility of residual disease rather than a true recurrent stenosis. Patch angioplasty reduces the incidence of recurrent stenosis. There is a consensus that symptomatic recurrent stenosis needs to be reoperated. For asymptomatic patients, a careful surveillance alone is proposed. There could be restenosis beyond the original endarterectomy site making the dissection more difficult. Therefore, a repeated CEA has a higher incidence of cranial nerve injuries, wound hematoma, perioperative stroke, and death. Carotid angioplasty offers an alternative to a repeated CEA.

How to Manage an Infected Prosthetic Patch

Up to 1% of patients who had CEA with prosthetic patch angioplasty may develop patch infection. It may present early, within 6 months, or late. Clinically they present as a deep wound infection, discharging chronic sinus, or a false aneurysm. False aneurysms may occasionally rupture. Duplex or angiography or radioisotope-labelled white cell scan may be helpful in diagnosing and planning the reintervention. Presence of any abscess overlying the carotid incision should raise its suspicion. The mostly likely causative microorganisms are either staphylococci or streptococci. The optimal treatment involves patch removal and autologous venous reconstruction with either patch or bypass.

Perioperative Complications

Following CEA, the cerebral blood flow is increased. If this blood flow is well above the metabolic demand of the brain tissue, it may result in cerebral hyper-perfusion which is characterized by unilateral headache, face and eye pain, seizures, and focal neurological symptoms related to cerebral edema or intracerebral hemorrhage. Patients who have a high-grade stenosis, malignant hypertension, and poor collateral supply, or had a recent stroke and/or TIA are more likely to develop cerebral hyper-perfusion. It is important to maintain strict control of arterial blood pressure, keeping the systolic pressure below 160 mmHg.

The most common nerve injuries are sensory branches of the cervical plexus. Loss of sensation in men who shave may be more troublesome because they can easily cut their jaw and neck skin while shaving, resulting in profuse bleeding since they will also be on antiplatelets. Most of the time, the nerve injuries recover in 3 to 6 months. Damage to the unilateral right laryngeal nerve causes hoarseness of voice which also improves with time.

Pseudoaneurysms are rare and are most often due to breakdown of the suture line itself, rather than degenerative changes in the patch. Patch infection is another uncommon complication. Eversion endarterectomy avoids use of any patch. Autologous vein patch angioplasty carries a lower chance of infection. If the synthetic patch becomes infected, the patient needs to be treated with antibiotics and often requires replacing the synthetic patch with the autologous vein patch.

Carotid Angioplasty and Stenting (CAS)

The first balloon angioplasty for an ICA stenosis was performed in 1979, while the first balloon-expandable stent was deployed in the ICA in 1989.[22,23] Initially CAS was performed without a cerebral protection device and had a high risk of cerebral embolization. Carotid angioplasty with stenting using a cerebral protection device has evolved to be a viable alternative for treating ICA stenosis. Although it is still uncertain whether CAS is as effective and durable as CEA, the proponents argue various potential advantages with CAS (e.g., no incision, no nerve injury, improved cost-effectiveness, and possibly less cardiovascular comorbidity). CAS initially evolved to treat 'high-risk' patients who were excluded from the NASCET and ECST trials for various reasons, or for treating the carotid dissection. The term 'high-risk' is used in the medical literature without specifying the context and is hence confusing. 'High risk' patients for a surgeon could be defined by certain risk-factors which increase the probability of complications in the perioperative period. These may be classified as preoperative or intraoperative and are summarized in Table 14. Preoperative high risks include certain characteristics either in the carotid artery plaque or in the patient, whereas intraoperative risk factors are subdivided according to anatomical, surgical, or pathophysiological higher risks.

A number of nonrandomized and randomized controlled trials for CAS have been performed comparing CEA and CAS which are summarized in Table 15.

Table 14: High risk-factors

Preoperative risks	Intraoperative risks
1. Plaque-related	1. Anatomical
a. Degree of stenosis	a. Aortic arch and proximal carotid anatomy
b. Plaque morphology	b. High carotid bifurcation
2. Comorbidities	c. Contralateral recurrent laryngeal nerve dysfunction
a. Advanced age	2. Surgical
b. Cardiac disease	a. Hostile neck
c. Others: pulmonary disease, renal disease, diabetes, tracheostomy, neck immobility	b. Recurrent stenosis
	3. Pathophysiological
	a. Contralateral carotid occlusion

Table 15: Summary of CAS trials results[24]

Name of Trial	Number of patients	Patient characteristics	Primary end points (stroke and death)	CAS Results (%)	CEA Results (%)
Leicester	17	Low risk Symptomatic	30-day	7.0	0.0
Wall stent	219	Low risk Symptomatic	1-year	10.4	4.4
SAPPHIRE	334	High risk Symptomatic and Asymptomatic	30-day	12.2	20.1
Kentucky 1	104	Low risk Symptomatic	30-day	1.8	1.9
Kentucky 2	84	Low risk Asymptomatic	30-day	0.0	0.0
CAVATAS	504	Low risk Symptomatic and Asymptomatic	30-day	10.0	9.9
SPACE	1183	Low risk Symptomatic	30-day	6.8	6.3
EVA-3S	527	Low risk Symptomatic	30-day	9.6	3.9

Though there was a significant reduction in the risk of cranial neuropathy 30-days after CAS, CEA had a favorable outcome in terms of death or stroke at 30-days, 6-months, and 1-year time-points post-procedure.

Randomized controlled trials conducted thus far to evaluate CAS have had different designs, and the results have been heterogeneous. Whilst few trials favored CEA (e.g., EVA-3S), others have favored CAS (e.g., SAPPHIRE). A few other trials have been neutral, as they neither favored CAS nor CEA (e.g., CAVATAS and SPACE). There have not been uniform criteria about including or excluding the interventionist based on their experience and training. Most trials have included both symptomatic and asymptomatic patients, without any sub-analysis of each group. Therefore, the applicability of the results to the patient becomes unpredictable and remains open to the personal bias of the person either analyzing the results or offering the treatment. The results of CAS vary according to the patient's age. A subgroup analysis of the SPACE trial suggests that the risk of stenting may be higher in patients aged >75 years.[25] Four out of six symptomatic CAS trials were stopped prematurely either due to excess stroke rate after CAS or due to the lack of funding. Overall low recruitment has compromised the value of the calculations of all these trials, and therefore the inferences remain open to criticism.

Technique of CAS

Pre-requisites

A recent non-contrast head CT is mandatory to rule out intracranial hemorrhage. Unlike CEA, which is increasingly performed on the basis of duplex Doppler, CAS requires a diagnostic carotid cervical and cerebral angiogram. They should also have an ECG and chest x-ray done. Patients are given antiplatelet regimens such as clopidogrel, an adenosine diphosphate inhibitor, and aspirin for 2 to 4 days preoperatively. If possible, the level of platelet inhibition should be checked with an aggregometer with a target of 70% to 90% inhibition. CAS can be done under general or local anesthesia. General anesthesia gives the additional benefit of muscle paralysis and easier control of blood pressure. Peripheral venous access is gained for systemic heparinization and atropine, if bradycardia is necessary.

Procedure

The technique of high-magnification road-mapping allows superimposition of a stored image of the opacified blood vessel on a blank fluoroscopic image in real-time. Intraarterial access is obtained via femoral route. One should avoid excessive catheter manipulations into the aortic arch to minimize the chances of detaching an atheromatous plaque. Various types and shapes of catheters help in negotiating the origin of the great vessels. Intravenous heparin is given after an arterial puncture and a diagnostic angiogram is carried out. This allows size calibration for proper stent diameter and length in relation to the stenosis and native vessel diameters. If the stenosis is too tight, initial microwire manipulation and angioplasty may be needed. The stent diameter is oversized by 10% to 20% to avoid stent migration and/or embolization. The stent assembly is passed coaxially through the sheath and across the lesion as shown in Figure 11. If a Monorail stenting assembly is not used, an exchange length guide wire across the lesion is placed with its tip just proximal to the petrous ICA. This allows over-the-wire exchange of the stent assembly for an angioplasty balloon or other device without having to cross the stenotic the lesion twice. Avoidance of repeated crossing minimizes the chances of plaque-embolization. Self-expanding stents are more commonly used, but even these often require 'post-stenting in-stent angioplasty' also known as "touch-up angioplasty" which is done with standard angioplasty balloons. Angioplasty may stretch the nerves in the carotid sinus which may cause bradycardia. To counteract, this 0.5 to 1.0 mg of intravenous atropine may be required just prior to angioplasty. A completion angiogram is done. A closure device is used to minimize the chances of bleeding from the arterial puncture site as these patients are on dual antiplatelet therapy and heparinized. There is no need to reverse the heparin.

To minimize the risk of downstream, cerebral emboli, embolic protection devices (EPDs) are used. There are two broad families of these devices, balloon-based or filters. Two specific types of balloon-based protectors occlude flow or reverse flow. The detailed description of these devices is not within the remit of this chapter. However, pros and cons of various EPDs are summarized in Table 16.

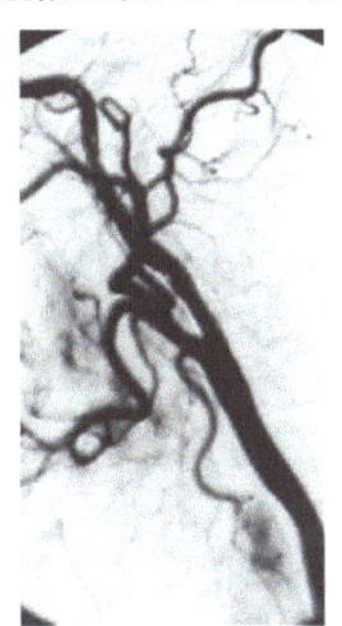

Figure 11: Carotid angioplasty with stenting

Post-procedure Care

A detailed neurological examination is carried out. Blood pressure is maintained at a mean arterial pressure of <85 mm Hg. Clopidogrel is continued for 6 weeks to minimize the risk of thromboembolic complications. Aspirin is continued for life. Follow-up carotid duplex is done at 6 months, 1 year, and 2 years to assess stent-patency. If the patient is in stent restenosis, or if it is suspected that they developed a tandem lesion, CT angiography is done.

Complications

The main complications are summarized in Table 17. It is worrying to note that CAS is increasingly being practised, especially for asymptomatic patients despite lacking strong evidence in the current era of evidence-based medicine. In the UK, the National Institute for Health and Clinical Excellence (NICE) recommendations (Sept 2006) about CAS with an embolic protection device state that:

1. Clinicians undertaking CAS should have adequate training.
2. Patients should understand that long-term safety is uncertain.
3. Selection should only be done by involving a multi-disciplinary team consisting of a surgeon, radiologist, and neurologist.
4. Preferably only symptomatic patients should be offered CAS.

Table 16: Advantages and disadvantages of various embolic protection devices concepts (ECA= external carotid artery, ICA= Internal carotid artery)

Features	Filters	Occluders	Flow reversers
Embolization during lesion crossing	+++	++	-
Cerebral flow decrease	+	++	+++
ICA protection from emboli	+	++	+++
Ability to perform angiography during protection	+++	-	+++
Embolization through ECA	-	+++	-
Potential spasm/damage to ICA	+++	+++	-
Tolerance	+++	+	+
Ease of use	+++	++	+

Table 17: Complications of CAS

Intraprocedural	Periprocedural	Delayed
• Thromboembolism • Stent mispositioning • Stent thrombosis • Intraarterial stent loss • Contrast-related: anaphylaxis, nephropathy • Puncture site: hematoma, pseudoaneurysm • Arterial dissection: carotid, femoral • Closure device related: stenosis, embolization	• Cerebral embolization • TIA/stroke • Myocardial infarction • Hemorrhagic event • Hypotension	• In-stent stenosis • Recurrent stenosis • Stent kind/fracture/migration

It is recommended that CAS with an embolic protection device should be offered only as part of a trial because thus far insufficient data is available about CAS. Outside the trial, CAS should only be considered if patients are unsuitable for CEA due to medical or surgical contraindications and if they have a high-risk of stroke with medical treatment alone. Irrespective of the modality of treatment offered to these patients, presence of various comorbidities increases the periprocedural complication rate. It should be emphasized that for many high-risk patients, one must question whether any form of revascularization is preferable to medical therapy alone. Extreme carotid artery elongation and tortuosity with coexisting stenotic disease, are more appropriately treated with open surgery than with CAS.

Summary Points

1. Stroke is the most common cause of disability in the western world.
2. Despite advances in management the incidence of stroke is likely to increase over the next 25 years.
3. The majority of strokes are ischemic.
4. The majority of ischemic strokes affect the carotid territory.
5. The commonest single cause of ischemic stroke is thromboembolism of the ICA or MCA.
6. Optimal medical care is very important for long term stroke prevention.
7. Carotid endarterectomy has an important role in the management of symptomatic patients with severe stenosis.
8. Carotid angioplasty and stenting with the use of a cerebral protection device is an alternative for patients with symptomatic stenosis and a hostile neck.

REFERENCES

1. Thom T, Hasse N, Rosamond W, et al. Heart disease and stroke statistics—2006 update: a report from the American Heart Association Statistics Committee and Stroke Statistics Subcommittee. Circulation 2006; 113(6): e85-151 Circulation 2006; 113:e85-151.
2. Dennis MS, Bamford JM, Sandercock PAG, et al. Incidence of transient ischaemic attacks in Oxfordshire, England, Stroke 1989; 20:333-9.
3. Adhiyaman V, Adhiyaman S. Trasient ischaemic attack: 10-minute consultation, BMJ 2009;338:a2343, 949.
4. NICE (June 2008). The diagnosis and acute management of stroke and transient ischemic attacks.
5. Moneta GL, Edwards JM, Chitwood RW, et al. Correlation of North American Symptomatic Carotid Endartetrectomy Trial (NASCET) angiographic definition of 70-99% internal carotid artery stenosis with duplex scanning. J Vasc Surg 1993; 17(1):152-9
6. Fields WS, Maslenikov V, Meyers JS, et al. Joint study of extracranial arterial occlusion: progress report of prognosis following surgery or nonsurgical treatment for transient cerebral ischaemic attacks and cervical carotid artery lesions. JAMA 1970;211:1993-2003.
7. Shaw DA, Venables GS, Cartlidge NE, et al. Carotid endarterectomy in patients with transient cerebral ischaemia. J Neurol Sci 1984;64:45-53.
8. European Carotid Surgery Trialists' Collaborative Group. Randomised trial of endarterectomy for recently symptomatic carotid stenosis: Final results of the MRC European Carotid Surgery Trial (ECST). Lancet 1998;351:1379-87.
9. Barnett HJM, Taylor DW, Eliasziw M, Fox AJ, et al. Beneficial effect of carotid endarterectomy in symptomatic patients with high-grade carotid stenosis. North American Symptomatic Carotid Endartectomy Trail Collaborators. N Eng J Med 1991;325:445-53.
10. Naylor AR. Is surgery still generally the first-choice intervention in patients with carotid artery disease? Surgeon 2008; 61:6-12.
11. Morgenstern LB, et al. The risks and benefits of carotid endarterectomy in patients with near occlusion of the carotid artery. North American symptomatic carotid endarterectomy (NASCET) group. Neurology 1997;48:911-5.

12. Fox AJ, Eliasziw M, Rothwell PM, et al. Management of patients with carotid artery near occlusion. Am J Neuroradiol 2005;26:2086- 94.
13. Shaw DA, Venables GS, Cartlidge NE, et al. Carotid endarterectomy in patients with transient cerebral ischaemia. J Neurol Sci 1984; 64:45-53.
14. Donnan GA, Davis SM, Chambers BR, et al. Surgery for prevention of stroke. Lancet 1998; 351:1372-3.
15. Executive Committee for the Asymptomatic Carotid Atherosclerosis Study. Endartrectomy for asymptomatic carotid artery stenosis. JAMA 1995:273:1421-8.
16. Asymptomatic Carotid Surgery Trial Collaborators. The MRC Asymptomatic carotid Surgery Trial (ACST): Carotid endarterectomy prevents disabling and fatal carotid territory strokes. Lancet 2004; 363:1491-1502.
17. Rijbroek A, Wisselink W, Vriens EM, et al. Asymptomatic carotid artery stenosis: past, present and future. Eur Neurol 2006;56:139- 54.
18. Abbot A, et al. What should we do with asymptomatic carotid stenosis? Int J Stroke 2007;2:27-39.
19. Eastcott HH, Pickering GW, Rob CG. Reconstruction of internal carotid artery in a patient with intermittent attacks of hemiplegia. Lancet 1954;67(6846):994-6.
20. Payne, et al. Beneficial effects of clopidogrel combined with aspirin in reducing cerebral emboli in patients undergoing carotid endarterectomy. Circulation 2004;109:1476-81.
21. GALA Trial Collaborative Group, Lewis SC, et al. General anaesthesia versus local anaesthesia for carotid surgery: a multicentre, randomised controlled trial. Lancet 2008;372:2132-42.
22. Bockenheimer SA, Mathias K. Percutaneous transluminal angioplasty in arteriosclerotic internal carotid artery stenosis. Am J Neuroradiol 1983;4:791-92.
23. Diethrich EB, Ndiaye M, Reid B. Stenting in the carotid artery: initial experience in 110 patients. J Endovasc Surg 1996;3:42-62.
24. Luebke T, Aleksic M, Brunkwall J. Meta-analysis of randomized trails comparing carotid endarterectomy and endovascular treatment. Eur J Vasc Endovasc Surg 2007;34:470-9.
25. Ringleb PA, Allenberg J, Bruckmann H, et al. 30-day results from SPACE trial of stent protected angioplasty versus carotid endartrectomy in symptomatic patients: a randomised non inferiority trail. Lancet 2006:368:1239-47.

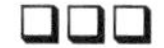

42

CHAPTER

Peripheral Vascular Diseases

Morgan McMonagle, MD, FRCSI
Saurabh Rai, FRCS
Rajiv Vohra, Ph.D., FRCSEd, FRCSEng

INTRODUCTION

The predominant lesion in peripheral arterial disease (PAD) is atherosclerosis. An atherosclerotic arterial plaque may progress, leading to chronic lower limb ischemia which may in turn progress to critical ischemia leaving a limb threatened. There are other rare causes of PAD giving rise to similar symptoms which the vascular surgeon needs to be aware of. These include persistent sciatic artery, cystic adventitial disease, popliteal artery entrapment, fibromuscular dysplasia and Buerger's disease. These conditions are summarized in Table 1. There are also other rheumatoid and vasculitic conditions that may present to a vascular service but are not covered in this chapter.

Table 1: Summary of the non-atherosclerotic causes of PAD

Non-atherosclerotic causes of PAD	Notes
Persistent sciatic artery	Congenital persistence of the embryonic sciatic artery. May be bilateral (22%). Proximal symptoms and iliofemoral hypoplasia. Prone to aneurysmal degeneration. Cowie's sign positive (absent proximal pulses with present distal pulses)
Cystic adventitial diseases (CAD)	Cystic degeneration of the tunica adventitia of the popliteal artery. May be in continuity with the synovium of the knee joint. Presents as claudication. Pulses present but disappearing on knee flexion. Results of angioplasty are poor with a high complication rate.
Popliteal artery entrapment	May be confused with CAD. Bilateral in 66%. Popliteal artery courses around the medial head of gastrocnemius (types I-III) or deep to popliteus muscle (type IV). Compression of artery on knee flexion. Prone to aneurysmal degeneration.
Fibromuscular dysplasia	Unknown etiology. More commonly affects the renal and carotid arteries. Classically beaded appearance on angiogram. May affect external iliac artery. Best treated with angioplasty (with or without stenting). Prone to aneurysmal degeneration.
Buerger's disease (thromboangiitis obliterans)	Classically affects younger males and heavy smokers. Also prevalent amongst people of Middle Eastern and Asian origin. Numerous thrombotic occlusions of small and medium sized arteries (i.e., below the knee). Vessels on angiogram are normal to a sudden point of occlusion with numerous, tortuous, cork-screw collaterals. Raynaud's phenomenon is also associated. Excellent prognosis with smoking cessation and exercise.

ATHEROSCLEROSIS

Atherosclerosis [from the Greek word 'athera', meaning 'lump of porridge' (International Classification of Diseases 10: I70)] is the commonest pathophysiological process leading to cardiovascular disease, including PAD. The resulting vascular lesion, almost ubiquitous in the western world, commonly affects the medium and larger sized arteries including the coronary arteries, aorta, carotid arteries, mesenteric arteries, and lower limb vessels. Histologically, the lesion primarily forms in the tunica intima of the arterial wall and consists of a nodular accumulation of soft, yellowish material at the centers of a harder plaque. It is composed of macrophages with cholesterol crystals and occasional calcified segments.[1]

The development of atherosclerosis is probably multifactorial. It may result from increased vascular permeability, perhaps due to injury that created 'Vascular leak'. This enables the entry of lipoproteins such as LDL and VLDL (low density lipoproteins and very low-density lipoproteins respectively) particles. They pass through the endothelium and enter the subendothelial space, at which point they are directly at the disease site. These lipoprotein molecules can then be further oxidized by endothelial cells and are then phagocytosed by macrophages via the 'scavenger' pathways leading to the formation of foam cells, which are pathognomonic of atherosclerosis.[1] Unless otherwise specified, this chapter will deal with the treatment and management of atherosclerosis as a cause of PAD.

PREVALENCE AND EPIDEMIOLOGY

PAD is caused by atherosclerotic occlusion or stenosis of the arteries in the lower limb. It is difficult to quantify the exact prevalence of PAD in the population, as in the majority it is silent and asymptomatic. However, studies, including the Edinburgh Artery Study, have suggested that the prevalence of asymptomatic PAD is 7 to 15 percent with the age-adjusted prevalence being about 12 percent and that the disorder equally affects men and women.[2-5] Using ultrasound criteria for the diagnosis of PAD, the British Regional Heart Study estimated a prevalence of 64 percent between the ages of 56 and 77 years, but only 10 percent of these were symptomatic.[6]

The Edinburgh Artery Study suggests that 7-15 percent of asymptomatic patients will go on to develop intermittent claudication over a 5-year period.[7] More importantly, patients suffering from PAD, even if asymptomatic have a higher risk of other cardiovascular events and death, including acute myocardial infarction (AMI) and stroke.[4] In fact, patients with PAD, even in the absence of a history of AMI and stroke, have approximately the same relative risk of cardiovascular all-cause death as those with a history of either documented coronary or cerebrovascular disease, regardless of whether the PAD is symptomatic or not.[7,8]

There is, however, a direct correlation between the severity of the PAD, as measured by the ankle-brachial index and the risk of cardiovascular events. Patients with critical limb ischemia and a very low ankle-brachial pressure index (ABPI) have an approximate annual mortality of 25 percent.[9-11] Hence, many of the treatments for patients with PAD are not only aimed at ameliorating the symptoms of the disease, but also aim to 'risk-modify' for other cardiovascular events that this population of patients are at higher risk for.

RISK FACTORS FOR PAD

Numerous epidemiological risk factors for the development of atherosclerosis (and thus PAD) have been identified. These include, advancing age, male gender, cigarette smoking, diabetes mellitus, hypertension, abdominal obesity (Table 2). It is also important to mention that PAD is also an independent risk factor for other vascular diseases such as coronary artery disease and stroke. The REACH (Reduction of Atherosclerosis for Continued Health) has shown that up to 40 percent of patients with symptomatic PAD also have evidence of coronary artery disease. In addition, this registry has identified numerous other risk factors for atherosclerosis, including diabetes (39%), hypertension (73%), hypercholesterolemia (59%) and history of smoking (46%).[12]

Table 2: Summary of the modifiable and non-modifiable risk factors for the development of PAD

Non-modifiable	Modifiable
Advancing age	Smoking male
Gender	Dyslipidemia
Diabetes Mellitus	Hypertension
	Obesity and sedentary lifestyle
	Glucose control
	Hyperhomocysteinemia

AGE AND GENDER

Advancing age and male gender are independent risk factors in the development of atherosclerosis. The traditional lifestyle choices of men over the last century (i.e., diet, lack of exercise, smoking habits), especially in the western world may be the contributing factors. The Framingham Heart Study showed that men have double the risk of PAD compared to women.[13] However, neither the Edinburgh Artery Study nor the Limburg study supported the findings of the Framingham

Heart Study.[14,15] Both the Framingham Heart Study and the Edinburgh Artery Study found advancing age to be an independent risk factor in the development of PAD.

SMOKING

Cigarette smoking is the leading contributor to the major mortalities in the Western World, including coronary artery disease, stroke, carcinoma (especially lung carcinoma) and respiratory disease. These disease categories form four out of the top five all-cause mortality for the Western World, thus making cigarette smoking perhaps the leading 'preventable' contributor to disease.

Smoking increases the risk of developing PAD by up to about three-fold.[16] Continued smoking in the face of established asymptomatic PAD is much more likely to progress to symptomatic disease compared to non-smokers, with worse clinical outcomes, including critical ischemic events and the risk of major limb amputation.[17] The Framingham Heart Study estimates that up to three quarters of cases of PAD are attributable to smoking.[13]

Although difficult to quantify, smoking cessation produces cardiovascular benefits even in those with established disease. The cardiovascular risk is halved within one year of cessation and is the same as non-smokers after about 5-15 years, or earlier in women.[18,19] Furthermore, cessation of smoking after intervention, especially coronary artery disease will significantly improve the medium and long-term outcomes for these patients.[20]

It would appear, therefore, that smoking cessation would be cost-effective with regard to health expenditure. Nicotine-replacement studies have demonstrated up to two-fold success rates in smoking cessation, with perhaps the nasal spray being most effective.[21]

DIABETES

Diabetes is an important independent risk factor in the development of atherosclerosis, which may be modifiable in the form of good glucose control. Lower limb arterial disease in diabetics tends to produce more diffuse and distal (below the knee) arterial disease. The UKPDS (UK Prospective Diabetes Study) showed that type 2 diabetic patients have a 3-5 fold increase risk of developing PAD compared to non-diabetics and that for every 1 percent rise in the HbA1C level, there was an associated 28 percent increase in PAD.[22,23] Diabetic patients also have a 10-16 fold increased lifetime risk of lower limb amputation and those who develop critical limb ischemia tend to have higher failure rates with revascularization attempts.[24,25] The high incidence of peripheral neuropathy contributing to ulceration and infection rates in the diabetic population also contributes to the poorer outcomes for these patients.

Work from the UKPDS has shown that glucose level is an independent risk factor for PAD in both type 1 and type 2 diabetes mellitus and that a reduction of 1 percent in the HbA1C is associated with a 21 percent reduction in complications.[22,26] However, the benefit of good glucose control on the modification of macrovascular disease does not appear to be as beneficial as the effect on microvascular disease.

HYPERLIPIDEMIA AND HYPERCHOLESTEROLEMIA

Hyperlipidemia and hypercholesterolemia are established risk factors for the development of atherosclerosis and coronary artery disease.[1] The Framingham Heart Study suggested that it is also a risk factor for PAD.[13] The post-hoc analysis showed that a fasting cholesterol >7 mmol/L doubled the risk of intermittent claudication. The ratio of LDL to HDL was also identified as an independent variable hence the term 'dyslipidemia'. These findings were supported by the Edinburgh Artery Study.[14]

HYPERTENSION

Hypertension is a common public health problem, affecting up to about 24 percent of the adult population suffering from this condition. The Framingham Heart Study identified hypertension as a risk factor for cardiovascular disease, especially coronary artery disease and stroke, but also as an independent predictor for PAD and intermittent claudication (by about three-fold).[13] Elevated blood pressure (>160/95) is associated with a 2.5-fold increased risk in men and a 4-fold increased risk in women of PAD. Other studies have also shown an increased risk in the incidence of PAD in untreated hypertensives by up to three-fold.[27]

The Framingham Heart Study also demonstrated that treatment of hypertension is associated with a reduction in the stroke rate by 38 percent, reduction in cardiovascular deaths by 14 percent and a reduction in peripheral vascular events by 26 percent. The Blood Pressure Lowering Treatment Trialists' Collaboration group have demonstrated that even modest reductions in blood pressure (10/5 mmHg) are associated with a reduction in stroke mortality (40%), coronary artery mortality (16%) and all cardiovascular causes (30%).[28] Further evidence was supplied by the UKPDS which showed that for every 10 percent decrease in systolic blood pressure, there is a 12 percent decrease in cardiovascular risk and a 16 percent decrease in lower limb amputation or PAD-related mortality amongst diabetics.[29] In fact, the blood pressure lowering beneficial effects on cardiovascular outcomes may be more important in the diabetic population, even more than glycemic control, which as mentioned earlier is less involved in the macrovascular changes associated with diabetes.[30,31]

OBESITY AND PHYSICAL EXERCISE

Obesity forms part of an arbitrary 'metabolic syndrome' including dyslipidemia and insulin resistance. Obesity is the dominant feature in this syndrome and is possibly best identified by the waist circumference (>102 cm in men and >88 cm in women).[32] Patients with this syndrome have a 20 percent increased risk of cardiovascular disease.

A sedentary lifestyle is a known risk factor for cardiovascular disease including PAD and the benefit of exercise has long been established in post-MI patients.[33] There are similar benefits seen in PAD (see section on Treatment).

HOMOCYSTEINEMIA

Elevated serum levels of homocysteine are associated with an increased risk of cardiovascular disease and PAD (four- fold increase compared to normal levels), especially the resting atheroma. Up to one-third of patients with PAD will have raised homocysteine levels.[34,35] One theory postulated, is that homocysteine-induced atheroma formation is secondary to impaired endothelial production of nitric oxide. Furthermore, vascular smooth muscle proliferation has been shown to be suppressed by dietary folic acid and vitamins B12 and B6.[36] Therefore, it would seem reasonable to treat elevated serum homocysteine (>5 mmol/L) with folic acid especially if associated with low levels of B12 and folate.

OTHERS

As described earlier in this chapter, the oxidation of lipoproteins plays a role in the development of atherosclerotic plaque formation. Thus, the use of antioxidants such as vitamin C and E may have a beneficial role. One systematic review failed to support their use as modifiers in vascular disease.[37] Similarly, chelation therapy using EDTA (ethylenediamine tetra-acetic acid) as an anti- oxidation agent has also failed to show benefit in the treatment of arterial disease.[38]

CLINICAL MANIFESTATIONS, SEVERITY AND PROGRESSION OF PAD

PAD may be asymptomatic or symptomatic. In symptomatic patients, the clinical manifestations and symptoms of PAD depend on the anatomical location and the extent of the disease. As with any ischemic symptoms, pain is the dominant presentation. In general, disease confined to the aorto-iliac system will give rise to buttock, hip, and thigh pain. Patients may also complain of impotence due to lack of blood flow in the internal iliac arteries. Concomitant femoropopliteal disease is quite common and therefore there may be associated calf pain. In general, patients will not get rest pain secondary to aorto-iliac disease, unless also accompanied by severe fem-pop disease. Leriche syndrome is a constellation of symptoms secondary to aortoiliac and femoropopliteal disease, including sexual impotence, buttock and leg claudication and muscle atrophy (usually the gluteal muscles).

In patients with femoral-popliteal and tibial disease, the classic presenting symptom is intermittent claudication (IC). IC is defined as a muscle cramp-like pain (usually in the calf muscles, but this depends on the site of occlusion) that is brought on by exercise and relieved with rest. This scenario is analogous to cardiac angina, where the arterial supply of blood and oxygen is insufficient to meet the demands of the working muscles (working muscle may require an increase in blood flow by an order of about 10-fold above the resting demands). This is non-critical ischemia, in that the tissues at rest have enough blood supply for viability and hence there is little immediate threat of gangrene and limb loss. In fact, the blood demand of resting muscles is so small that the resting blood flow in the common femoral artery is only in the order of 130-150 mL/min.

A crude measurement of the severity of disease in non-critical ischemia is the patient's 'claudication distance'. This is the distance on flat ground that the patient can walk before the symptoms of muscle cramp begin and the time taken on resting for the pain to subside enough so that walking may be recommenced. A change in the claudication distance also lets the physician know if the disease is improving with treatment (i.e., walking distance is increasing) or deteriorating (decreasing walking distance over time). Rather ironically, although it is the oxygen demand of muscle that leads to claudication, generally this will be well-tolerated when there is a bulky muscle bed, as the muscle groups can generate collaterals to bypass the occlusion that has led to the symptoms in the first place. Collaterals may develop adequately to supply the muscles of the calf with a more proximal occlusion (e.g., SFA occlusion with collaterals from the profunda and genicular branches). An occlusion within the iliac system may also generate collaterals around it. However, conservative management of an iliac stenosis is often less successful due to the larger muscle bulk in the lower limb distal to the iliac in-flow and hence higher oxygen demand from the exercising muscle.

Critical ischemia is present when the blood supply to the lower limb is severely reduced so that the demands of the resting limb cannot be met. This is characterized by rest pain, which typically starts at the most distal level, i.e., the forefoot with a risk of gangrene, infection, and tissue loss. A critically ischemic limb is under immediate threat, where the blood supply to the tissues is not capable of meeting the resting oxygen demand and may manifest as rest pain, tissue loss with wet (infected) or dry (not infected) gangrene. The limb is cool, mottled, dusky and usually pulseless in the affected field with variable amounts of gangrene (Figures. 1A and B).

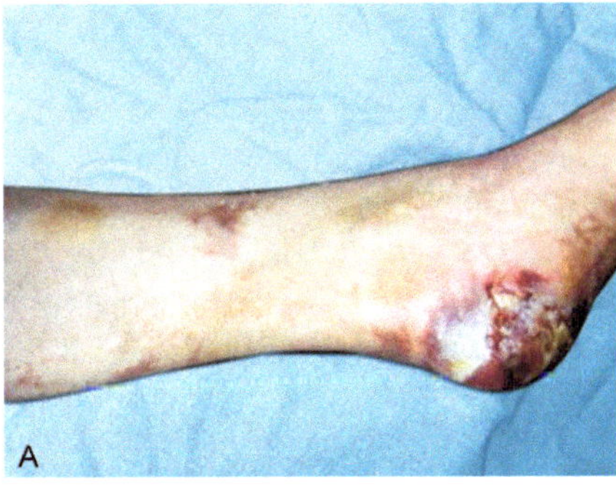

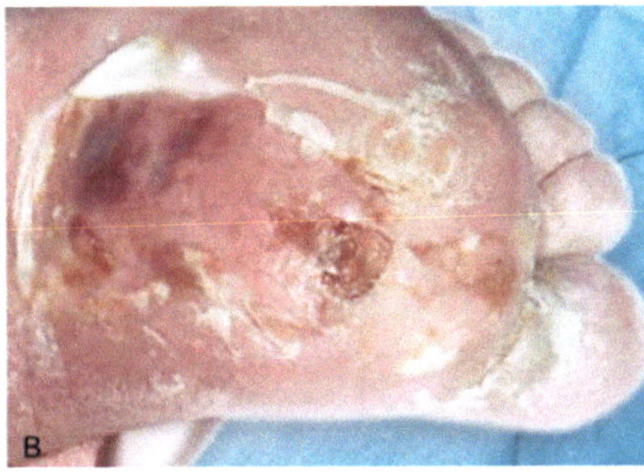

Figures 1A and B: Critically ischemic leg and foot with gangrene and tissue loss of the heel (A) and deep infection of the forefoot (B). Urgent revascularization is required if the limb is to be salvaged

Although somewhat arbitrary, the objective pressure at which a limb is considered critical is an ankle systolic pressure of < 50 mm Hg.[39] However, patients with symptoms and signs of critical ischemia may have pressures higher than this.[40] The rest pain and gangrene is usually in the distal arterial tree, hence foot pain and digital gangrene (Figure 2). The limb is under immediate threat and therefore revascularization is imperative. The prognosis is much worse in the patient with critical ischemia, as there is a high risk of amputation. As atherosclerosis is a systemic illness, these patients are also at a much higher risk of AMI and stroke.

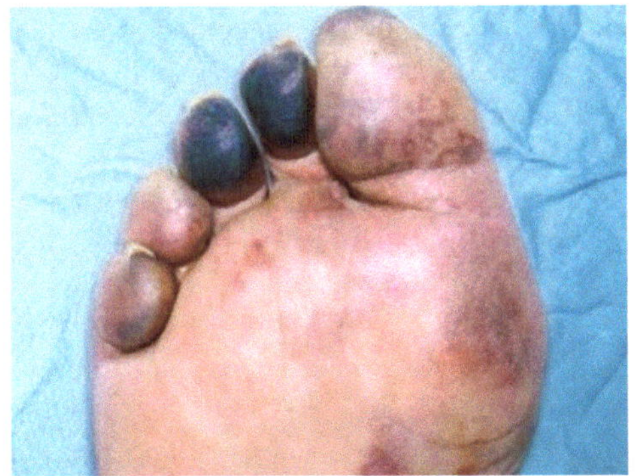

Figure 2: Forefoot ischemia with mottled skin, poor capillary refill, and digital gangrene (dry)

The goals of treatment will depend on the patient's level of symptoms. The treatment of patients with asymptomatic disease is controversial but given the increased risk of AMI and stroke that these patients have, it is certainly reasonable to treat them conservatively with 'risk factor modification' and best medical therapy. This has the potential to reduce progression of their PAD as well as reducing the risk of a serious cardiovascular outcome.

The severity of PAD can be classified according to the symptoms and signs of the disease, and the two most accepted classifications are by Fontaine or Rutherford, and these are outlined in detail in Table 3. Classifying the disease is less important as therapeutic decisions are made on the patient's symptoms and on whether the ischemia present is critical or non-critical, combined with the patient's general overall health (over 50% of the mortality after treatment of PAD is cardiac in origin). In patients suffering from claudication, the aims of treatment are to relieve the exertional symptoms, increase walking capacity and improve the quality of life. These goals are the same for patients with critical ischemia, but also to relieve rest pain, heal tissue loss and ulceration, treat infection and limb salvation.

Table 3: Classification of the severity of PAD using the Fontaine and Rutherford classification systems

Fontaine classification	Rutherford classification
I: Asymptomatic	0: Asymptomatic
II: Intermittent claudication	1: Mild claudication
IIA: Mild	2: Moderate claudication
IIB: Disabling	3: Severe claudication
III: Rest pain	4: Ischemic rest pain
IV: Non-healing ulceration; gangrene	5: Minor tissue loss; non-healing ulceration; focal gangrene
	6: Major tissue loss; extending above transmetatarsal level

CLINICAL EXAMINATION

Many of the findings on clinical examination will depend on the site and extent of the disease and also on whether the ischemia is critical or not. An outline of clinical examination and investigations is described in Table 4.

Table 4: Physical examination and relevant investigations for PAD

Clinical Examination	Investigations
Inspection	Shiny atrophic skin. Hair loss. Skin color (pallor cyanosis). Underfilled veins (guttering). Gangrene. Tissue loss. 'Sunset foot'
Palpation	Skin temperature (including gradient). Capillary refill (normal <2 seconds). Pulses (aorta, femoral, popliteal, AT, DP, PT)
Auscultation	Bruits (including aorta)
Adjuvant bedside tests	Blood pressure measurement. Hand-held Doppler examination. ABPI measurements. Buerger's angle*. Buerger's test and reactive hyperemia time. Examination pre- and post-exercise
Non-invasive (Bedside and vascular laboratory)	Hand-held Doppler and ABPI. Toe pressures. Continuous wave. Doppler. Segmental pressure studies. Duplex ultrasound
Non-invasive (specialized)	CT angiography. MR angiography
Invasive (specialized)	Angiography

*May be carried out during "Inspection"

INSPECTION

The affected limb will display variable degrees of hypoperfusion depending on the extent and severity of the PAD. In general, there may be a lack of hair growth (subjective and unreliable) with shiny, atrophic-looking skin over the shin and forefoot. The lower limb usually displays varying degrees of pallor, which is usually most severe distally in the foot and toes. The pallor is dependent on the position of the limb. If the severity of the disease is only mild, then the limb may only blanch on raising the leg. With more severe disease, the limb becomes white whilst lying on the flat. This finding is reflected in the Buerger's Angle. This is the angle to which the leg must be raised before it becomes white, which is directly related to the perfusion pressure of the limb. The height in centimeters between the sternum (with the patient lying flat) and the heel on elevation of the foot approximates to the perfusion pressure in the foot vessels in mmHg. An angle of 15 to 30 degrees corresponds with an ischemic leg. Below this would reflect a sub-critical perfusion pressure.

A pale limb may also display color changes associated with 'reactive hyperemia' and become suffused and red (see 'Adjunctive tests'). As the ischemia progresses, pallor may give way to cyanosis indicating a critical degree of deoxygenated blood in the limb, which may in turn progress to black, indicating gangrene. The veins on the dorsum of the foot may look underfilled, referred to as guttering of the veins. In fact, often after reperfusion of a limb, even if there is not a return of the pulse, the first sign of improved perfusion is 'filling of the veins. Figure 3 shows a typically sub-critically ischemic leg.

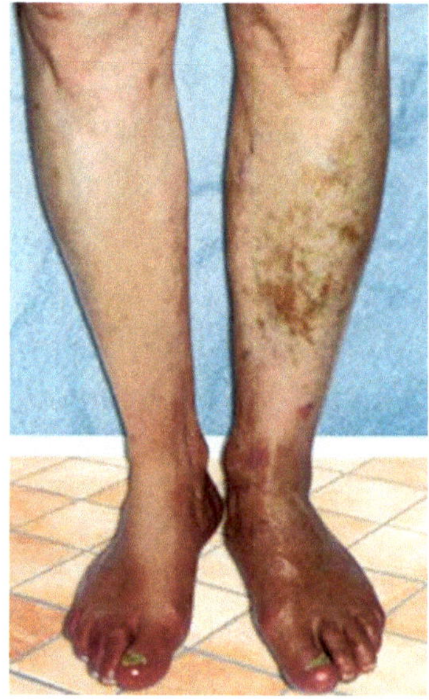

Figure 3: Typical appearance of sub-critical ischemia of the legs with shiny atrophic skin, hairlessness and suffused but poorly perfused feet

Finally on inspection there may be variable amounts of tissue loss with or without gangrene. Although gangrene is skin and tissue necrosis, ulceration may also develop in the limb with sub-critical ischemia as a result of infection or minor trauma. Here, although the blood supply is capable of meeting the resting demands of the limb, it cannot meet the demands necessary for normal tissue healing and repair after trauma and infection. Such tissue loss is an indication for a more aggressive approach to the management of the PAD. Classically, arterial ulceration occurs at the sites of repeated daily minor trauma, most notably 'pressure points', including the heel, between the toes and over the heads of the metatarsals, especially the 1st and 5th (Figures 4 and 5). Pressure changes in an ischemic foot may manifest early as hypertrophied skin, blistering, ulceration, and later frank gangrene. Gangrene may also manifest in an ischemic limb without preceding ulceration as a result of infection. This is especially problematic in diabetic patients.

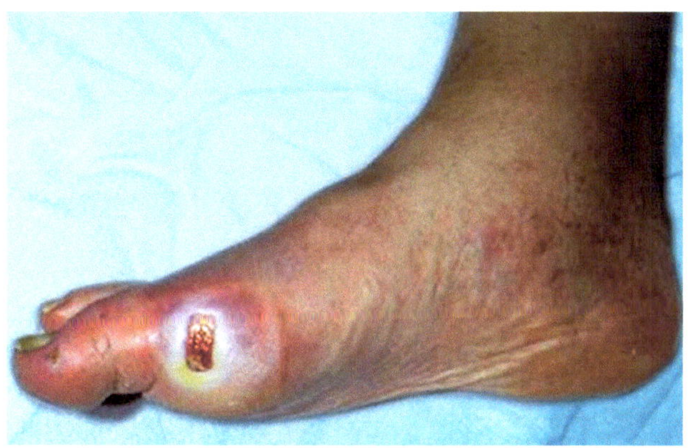

Figure 4: Pressure ulceration over the outer aspect of the head of the first metatarsal

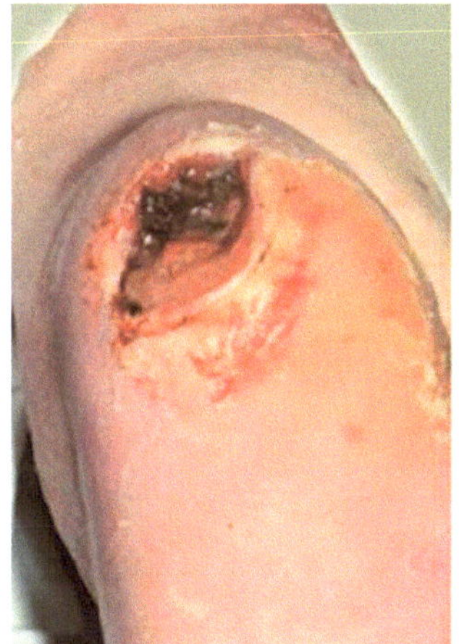
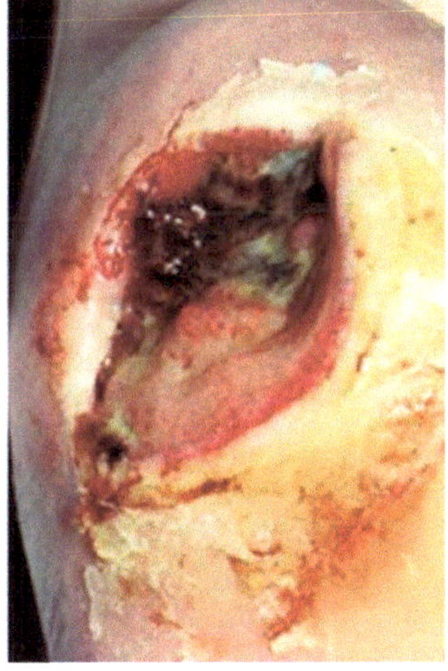

Figure 5: Severe ulceration secondary to critical ischemia affecting the heel area

One must not miss the 'sunset foot' on inspection. Here the foot, in particular the forefoot is cool and slightly cyanosed, but with a red, hyperemic look with demarcation between the critically ischemic forefoot and the better perfused proximal foot. This is a sign of critical ischemia, as the microcirculation is maximally dilated with little tolerance for further ischemia and must be investigated and treated aggressively.

PALPATION

The hypoperfused foot is cool and such skin temperature should be compared at the same points along the limb between both legs. A temperature gradient can often be appreciated as the palpating hand moves from the proximal portion of the limb towards the foot (using the dorsum of the fingers). The capillary refill time should also be palpated by pressing on the tip of the toe or the nail for 2-5 seconds, allowing it to blanch. Upon release of this pressure, count in seconds the time it takes for the skin to return to its pre-palpation color. Perfusion time longer than 2 seconds is considered abnormal.

All pulses should be palpated for, starting proximally with the aorta to exclude aneurysmal disease, and then progressing distally to the femoral artery, popliteal artery and the posterior tibial, anterior tibial and dorsalis pedis arteries. The corresponding arteries on both sides should be compared which may give an indication as to the level of disease in the affected limb. It is important to remember that a patient complaining of intermittent claudication may have palpable pulses at rest which disappear on exercise if the predominant occluding lesion is proximal iliac artery disease. In this situation, it may be necessary to palpate the pulses after exercise, for example after walking the patient or after tip-toe exercises (in a fairly immobile patient).

AUSCULTATION

After palpation, the aorta, femoral and popliteal arteries should be auscultated for bruits which may indicate a significant stenosis or aneurysmal disease with turbulent flow.

ADJUVANT TESTS

As described above, Buerger's angle should be sought and Buerger's test performed. Buerger's test is essentially pallor on elevation of the limb followed by abnormal rubor on dependency of the limb. A low angle corresponds to severe ischemia. Following this, the hyperemia test should be performed. Whilst lying flat, the patient's legs are elevated by the examiner to determine Buerger's angle. The patient is asked to plantar-dorsiflex the ankles repeatedly to simulate an increased exercise demand on the limb. This should be done for about 20 repetitions. Often the limb becomes even more pale, possibly cyanosed, and cold as the demand for blood outstrips supply. Immediately following this, the patient is asked to sit over the edge of the bed with the legs in a dependent position. The feet will become erythematous-looking like a result of reactive hyperemia. The time taken for this to occur reflects the severity of the occlusive disease. However, in severe cases, the limb may never become hyperemic looking like no blood can reach the foot. Also, in chronic, severe PAD, especially in diabetic patients, this hyperemic change may not occur, as the blood vessels have already lost their sympathetic tone and are already maximally dilated.

An exercise challenge may also be used to define the site and severity of an occlusion. This is often suited to the patient with a very proximal occlusion, e.g., aortoiliac disease where there is sufficient blood flow through the lesion, or via collaterals giving palpable pulses at rest and lying flat, but who still give a good history of intermittent claudication. The patient may be asked to take a walk, ideally as close to the distance that brings on symptoms, and the pulses are examined again. Alternatively, with the patient in the examining office, he/she may undergo repeated tip-toe exercises (about 20 repetitions) and then re-examined. With symptomatic proximal aortoiliac disease, there will be a loss or decrease of pulses distal to the occlusion after exercise. A femoral bruit may also become evident. The hand-held Doppler and ABPI measurement may also be performed at rest and subsequently post-exercise challenge (see below).

MEASUREMENT OF DISEASE SEVERITY AND IMAGING

The simplest bed-side test to obtain an estimation of the severity of PAD is the Buerger's test and measurement of Buerger's angle (see last section).

HAND-HELD DOPPLER AND THE ABPI

Pulses that cannot be palpated may be identified by insonation with a hand-held Doppler (4-8 MHz continuous- wave Doppler probe). Usually, some evidence of flow can be detected in the arterial tree, even in the presence of severe or critical ischemia. Therefore, insonation of pulses by hand-held Doppler alone is of limited use unless the pressures at which the pulses become audible are also measured. Normally about 90 mm Hg is needed to palpate the DP and PT pulses and about 70 mm Hg for the popliteal pulse. An ankle pressure less than 50 mm Hg is indicative of critical ischemia.

In an artery with normal compliance, the normal 'signal' using the hand-held Doppler probe is described as 'triphasic' in nature. This reflects the systolic pressure, kinetic changes, and finally Doppler pressures in the arterial system. Triphasic signals signify a healthy, elastic arterial wall with no significant resistance to flow. With more rigid vessel walls, the signal may become 'biphasic' in nature with the loss of arterial wall elasticity. A monophasic waveform indicates an increased flow resistance proximal to the point of insonation. Although not an absolute indication for intervention, when taken in the correct clinical context this will signify a potentially significant occlusion that may warrant further evaluation. A very dampened and monophasic signal may also be confused with a venous signal, which may be prominent in patients with venous insufficiency or congestive cardiac failure.

The ankle-brachial pressure index (ABPI) is the ratio of the pressure at which the highest foot pulse is measured compared to the brachial pulse (which is considered the perfusion pressure at the heart). The equipment needed to measure the ABPI is shown in Figure 6. Ideally the patient should be well-rested and lying supine for about ten minutes in a warm room. It is important that the patient is rested to mitigate any exercise effect on the measurements. Both brachial pressures are measured by placing a standard sphygmomanometer tourniquet on the arm as normal. The cuff must measure at least 2/3 the length of the humerus and be 50 percent wider than the limb diameter to minimize false positive artifacts. The cuff is inflated above systolic pressure to obstruct flow in the brachial artery and then slowly deflated whilst the hand-held Doppler probe is kept in position over the brachial pulse at the antecubital fossa. The pressure is recorded at the highest pressure when flow resumes in the brachial artery as detected by the probe. This is repeated for both arms and the highest value is taken for calculating the ABPI.

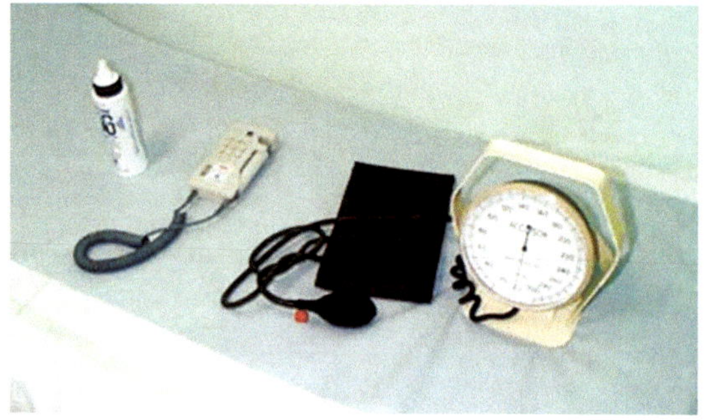

Figure 6: Equipment used to measure the ABPI, including the hand-held Doppler machine (with ultrasound gel) and a manual sphygmomanometer

The tourniquet is then placed around the calf of the affected limb. If there is ulceration in this area it should be covered with a simple non-adherent, non-porous material such as cling-wrap to protect the ulcerated area. Again, the same process is repeated by inflating the cuff to occlude the ankle arterial signals with the Doppler probe held in position. The pressures are measured with the Doppler probe over the DP pulse on the dorsum of the foot and PT pulse behind the medial malleolus respectively. As the cuff is deflated, the highest pressure at which a signal is insonated with the Doppler probe, is taken as the systolic pressure for the respective artery. The highest reading, DP or PT is taken to calculate the ABPI. To calculate the ABPI, the highest ankle pressure is divided by the highest brachial pressure. Although more cumbersome, occasionally the peroneal artery is also used. This can be located by placing the Doppler probe just above the lateral malleolus and slowly moving the probe in a cephalad direction along the line of the fibula until the pulse is detected.

The differential pressure gradient between the brachial pulse and the ankle pressures will reflect the severity of perfusion. The normal ABPI is 1.0 – 1.2. Less than 0.9 is considered abnormal and indicates arterial disease. Claudication will occur with an ABPI of less than 0.7 and less than 0.4 is associated with critical ischemia (Table 5). An exercise challenge (as described above) may also be performed on patients with normal or close to normal ABPI measurements, but with the clinical suspicion of proximal aortoiliac occlusion. The ABPI is then re-measured immediately on stopping exercise with no rest period and compared to those measured previously with the patient at rest.

Table 5: Summary of ABPI readings and their clinical significance

Normal	1.0-1.2
Claudication	<0.7
Rest pain	<0.4

Very calcified arteries may give rise to a falsely elevated ABPI as the occlusion pressure of the vessel is abnormally high due to increased arterial wall rigidity. This is typical of long-standing diabetes and chronic renal failure and therefore ABPI measurements are less helpful in this group of patients. In fact, it is not unusual to be unable to compress the arteries in the lower limbs due to extensive wall calcification, and hence, the ABPI cannot be measured. Another group of patients with whom the ABPI measured is not reliable is with subclavian artery occlusion (e.g., due to atherosclerosis or thoracic outlet syndrome). Therefore, both arms should be measured if there is a clinical suspicion.

Doppler signals may also be employed as part of Buerger's test. The pedal signal is measured with the patient supine and upon elevation of the limb. The angle of the limb at which the signal disappears is the ischemic angle. Obviously the smaller the ischemic angle, the more severe the ischemia.

Toe pressures may be useful in patients with incompressible, calcified arteries or when very distal disease is the likely source of ischemia. Again, a rested patient in a warm room is essential to avoid a false-positive reading. A specific digital occlusion cuff (2-3 cm wide) is placed around the proximal toe with a measuring device attached to the distal portion of the digit (e.g., photoelectric cell or mercury strain gauge plethysmograph). Photoplethysmography via the photoelectric cell is used to detect the disappearance and reappearance of the toe pulse as the cuff is inflated and deflated. The recorded toe pressure is expressed as a ratio to the brachial pressure similar to ABPI and is normally lower (0.8-0.9) but should be greater than 0.7. Critical ischemia may occur with a toe-brachial pressure < 0.3 or an absolute toe pressure of <30 mm Hg.

CONTINUOUS WAVE DOPPLER

Continuous wave Doppler uses the same principle as the hand-held Doppler except that it uses spectral analysis to study the waveforms created within the vessel. As described above, the resistance in a normal peripheral artery is high and triphasic in character. This triphasic component may be seen on the Doppler machine consisting of the high velocity of systolic forward flow, followed by the early flow reversal at the beginning of diastole (elastic recoil) followed by low velocity late forward flow of late diastole. With increasing stenosis of an artery, the waveform downstream will be 'dampened', becoming biphasic (distal to 50% stenosis) and later monophasic (distal to 70% stenosis) with a lower amplitude antegrade flow with loss of early reversal component. If the peak systolic velocity at the site of a lesion increases by more than 100 percent, then the lumen is likely to be narrowed by at least 50 percent.

The waveforms shape and characteristics displayed at a vessel lesion reflect both the degree of stenosis at the lesion as well as the level of resistance further downstream which is also affected by temperature, arterial dilatation, recent exercise, and the presence of multi-segmental disease.

SEGMENTAL PRESSURE STUDIES

Segmental pressures may also be used to map out and localize the site of significant stenosis. In this case, the blood pressure cuff (of an appropriate size) is placed around the leg at various points, including high calf, low thigh and high thigh and repeating the pressure measurements using the continuous wave Doppler as described above to see where the greatest drop in pressure is. A pressure drop of more than 20 mm Hg between two segments is considered significant. The same principle as measuring the ABPI can also be used, in that the three measurements taken during segmental pressure studies may be divided by the brachial pressure in an attempt to localize the greatest pressure drop, and hence, stenosis. If there is a fall in the ratio of greater than 0.2 between two cuff measurements, then this indicates a significant segment of disease.

ARTERIAL DUPLEX ULTRASOUND

Duplex ultrasonography uses a combination of gray-scale imaging, color flow Doppler mapping and pulse Doppler velocity measurements. Therefore, both visualization of the artery and hemodynamic assessment of the blood flow within the vessel is possible in a continuous fashion. Figure 7 shows a typical Duplex ultrasound machine that may be employed either in the out-patient setting or vascular laboratory.

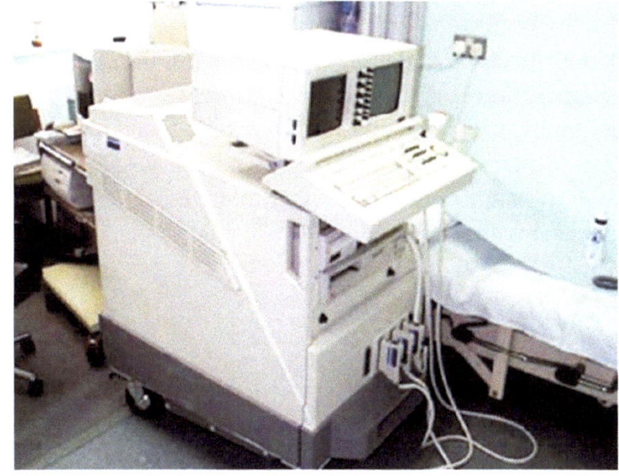

Figure 7: Typical Duplex Doppler machine used to visualize the arterial tree and flow-velocities.

Gray-scale imaging (B-mode) converts ultrasonic echoes from tissue into a two-dimensional image, the brightness of which is dependent on the intensity of the reflected signal. This allows the artery and its wall to be seen as well as the stenosis and character of the plaque. Both color-flow and pulsed Doppler are added to the images to gather information on blood flow within the tissues. Color-flow Doppler will enhance the image further by showing in color where there is blood flow versus non-moving areas such as thrombus. The color of the moving blood will also change with increasing blood flow velocities (e.g., across a stenosis). Hence, a picture of the vessel will be constructed on the computer screen in grayscale with the flowing blood as a mosaic of colors (changing velocities) in between. This gives a very accurate picture of the diseased segment of the artery. As blood flowing towards the probe moves faster than blood flowing away, these will register as differing colors. Traditionally if the image is red, then it is flowing towards the probe and blue if flowing away (Think: BART – Blue Away, Red Towards).

Pulsed (gated) Doppler allows the ultrasound signal to be directed to a specific depth. The change in frequency of the transmitted signal is determined by many factors, including the velocity of the blood flowing across a lesion. Hence, the peak systolic velocity may be measured in the normal proximal artery, across the lesion and distal to the lesion. The increase in velocity across a lesion is proportional to the severity of the stenosis. For example, an increase in velocity of two-fold corresponds to a stenosis of 50 percent. A 2.5-fold increase indicates a stenosis of greater than 50 percent. The distal velocity will in turn be reduced with a dampened waveform. In general, a ratio of 3 or greater is considered a clinically significant stenosis.

Duplex ultrasonography of the aortoiliac system can be difficult, even for experienced ultrasonographers, due to the depth of the vessels and the presence of overlying bowel gas and shadows cast by other pelvic organs. The sensitivity and specificity in this area has been reported as 89 percent and 90 percent respectively.[41] Duplex assessment of the leg vessels is considered more accurate and is comparable to conventional angiography, with a sensitivity and specificity of 84-87 percent and 92-98 percent respectively.[41-43] The calf vessels are more difficult to image compared to the thigh vessels, especially in the presence of proximal disease.[44,45]

ANGIOGRAPHY

Angiography is considered the 'gold standard' in the assessment of arterial disease. Since there are other less invasive techniques for assessment available now, angiography should really be confined to those patients who achieved it by angio-catheterization (Figure 8). Hence, there is now a greater tendency to perform both a diagnostic angiogram with a therapeutic procedure (e.g., angioplasty and/or stent insertion) at the same cath-lab visit. With conventional angiography, contrast media is injected directly into the vessel after needle catheterization (usually by the Seldinger technique) and usually via the transfemoral route (lower complication rate: 1.7%). The procedure is invasive with a risk of arterial wall damage and thromboembolism. Other risks include: subintimal dissection, inadvertent venous puncture, nerve trauma, arteriovenous fistula formation, infection, plaque and cholesterol embolization, limb loss and complications from the contrast medium used.

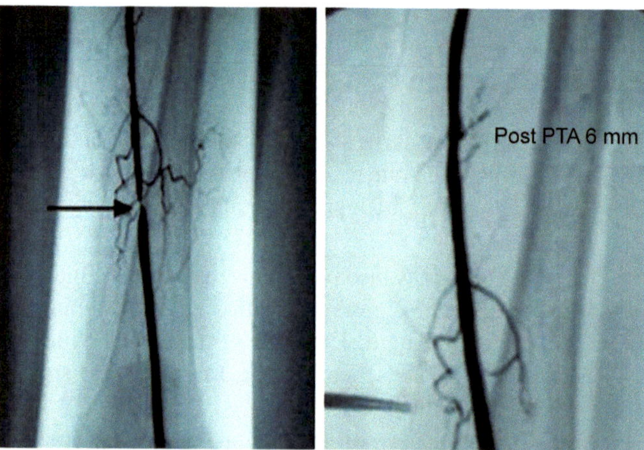

Figure 8: Angiogram pre- and post-angioplasty of distal SFA lesion (arrow)

Modern contrast media used are iodine-containing, non-ionic, hypo-osmolar agents (e.g., Omnipaque™). Although safer, these substances still carry a risk of both nephrotoxicity and allergic reaction of about 1/1000 (rash, urticaria and bronchospasm) and even anaphylaxis (1:40,000). The risk of an allergic reaction does not appear to be dose-related and is probably as a result of mast cell degradation (type 1 allergic reaction). The traditional ionic contrast media carried a risk of anaphylactic reaction of 0.01-0.02 percent, but the modern non-ionic, hypoosmolar agents are thought to be much safer. The risk of an allergic reaction is higher if the patient has a history of atopy (especially shellfish and iodine allergy) and therefore precautions should be taken (e.g., steroid prophylaxis). Treatment of an anaphylactic reaction, should it occur, includes oxygen therapy and airway management as appropriate, intravenous fluids to treat hypotension, intravenous steroid loading, nebulized B- agonists and epinephrine treatment. Further treatment may include the use of antihistamines, H1 blockers, H2 blockers and intravenous glucagon for refractory hypotension.

The nephrotoxicity seen after intravenous contrast injection is usually transient (peaks at about 48 hours post-procedure) and is of little significance in patients with previously normal renal function.[46] The degree of renal impairment seen after contrast administration is related to the extent of the pre-existing renal impairment, the dose of contrast material used and the state of hydration of the patient. Other risk factors include advanced age (>70 years), presence of congestive cardiac failure and concomitant use of other potentially nephrotoxic medications (e.g., nonsteroidal anti-inflammatories, ACE inhibitors). Thus, if possible, prior to angiography, any nephrotoxic agents should be temporarily stopped (but not aspirin) if safe to do so and the smallest dose of a low osmolar, non-ionic agent should be used. In general, good fluid management will mitigate the effects of the contrast material on renal function. If the patient has normal renal function, is generally well and hydrated, then normal oral fluid intake should suffice. If there is evidence of decreased renal function (raised creatinine), then intravenous fluid administration before (at least 6 hours) and after (for at least 12 hours) the injection of contrast should suffice. There is also some evidence that the administration (either orally or intravenously) of N- acetylcysteine has a nephroprotective effect in contrast- induced toxicity, especially with pre-morbid evidence of renal dysfunction.[47] With high creatinine levels > 300 mmol/L) an alternative imaging medium should be strongly considered (e.g., gadolinium, carbon dioxide) and the advice of a nephrologist sought. In all cases the risk/benefit ratio must be weighed up and full informed consent taken from the patient.

Patients taking metformin also need special consideration. A rare toxic side effect of metformin is metabolic acidosis secondary to lactic acid accumulation. As metformin is exclusively cleared by the kidneys, then the administration of contrast media may increase the risk of a lactic acidosis, especially if there is also a degree of renal impairment. As well as taking the precautions outlined above into consideration, the metformin should be stopped up to 48 hours prior to angiography or the patient switched to another diabetic treatment regimen. The advice of a diabetologist may be sought if in doubt.

Other potential side effects of contrast media administration include nausea and vomiting, flushing and feelings of a warm sensation, metallic taste in the mouth and rarely cardiac arrhythmias and pulmonary edema (rare and dose-related). As the contrast material is iodine-based, it should be avoided in patients suffering from hyperthyroidism. In patients with thyroid carcinoma, the use of iodinated contrast material will preclude the use of radio-iodine therapy for up to eight weeks post- administration.

The intra-arterial injection of contrast gives an outline of the arteries like a 'road-map' and any occlusion or stenosis may be visualized. Most angiographic suites are now computerized, where the contrast-enhanced image is displayed on a computer screen. 'Digital subtraction angiography' (DSA) may therefore be deployed, where a single 'mask image' is taken prior to injection of contrast. After the contrast-enhanced images are taken, the computer 'digitizes' these and they are 'subtracted' from the mask images in order to remove unwanted details, such as bony detail, giving a clearer, sharper image of the arterial system. DSA also has the advantages over older, conventional angiography, where smaller doses of contrast media are required.

The on-table angiogram should take images of the aorta (from the level of the renal arteries) down the affected limb including the foot and arch vessels. The images above a significant lesion are described as the 'in-flow', whereas the images below a lesion are described as the 'run-off'. Good in-flow and run-off are essential for successful revascularization.

CT ANGIOGRAPHY

CT angiography is non-catheter-based imaging modality and the newer spiral (helical) CT scanners and can process numerous images to give accurate detail as the computer 'reconstructs' them to give 3-dimensional detail. The computer can reconstruct 'maximum intensity projection' (MIP) images as well as subtracts unwanted detail to produce an angiographic-like image of the arterial tree. Detail such as vessel calcification, thrombus deposition and blood flow can also be appreciated on CT angiography. Disadvantages of this technique include the use of high dose ionizing radiation as well as the need for iodinated contrast agents (same potential risks as standard angiography described above). It is not necessarily available in every center and its accuracy over standard angiography has yet to be defined. Also, heavy calcification of a vessel is difficult to decipher from a stenosis, making a false-positive image more likely. However, it has the advantage of being non-invasive. This may be important in the older, infirm, and immobile patient where catheter-based intervention may be less.

MR ANGIOGRAPHY

Magnetic resonance imaging works by placing the patient in a very strong pulsed magnetic field and creates images from the radiofrequency pulse given off by hydrogen ions as they 'spin' from one axis (while the magnet is switched on) back to their normal axis and alignment (as the magnet is switched off), giving very accurate images.

Arteries and veins as well as flowing blood may be visualized on MRI. Phase-contrast angiography detects differences in the phase of spin of the protons in blood and shows flowing blood as white on the MR image. This can be determined from the stationary tissues (black images) and can help to provide flow quantitation in the vessels. Just like CT angiography, a 3D image can be created. However, turbulence created at the level of a lesion, may give rise to an overestimation of the severity of stenosis, as there will be a 'loss of signal' distal to the turbulence which may look like black and be misinterpreted as an occlusion in the vessel. Attempts to overcome this drawback of MR angiography include the use of gadolinium as a contrast agent. Gadolinium is a paramagnetic element and is used in a 'bolus-chase' technique. A 'time-of-flight' acquisition (or in-flow angiography) is obtained where images of the vessels are taken before and after administration of the gadolinium. There is a difference in the T1 relaxation time of blood versus gadolinium and therefore these images can be subtracted from each other to increase the signal ratio between the moving blood and stationary tissue.

Disadvantages of the use of MR angiography include the overestimation of a lesion as described earlier. Also, contrast material in the venous system, especially in the smaller vessels (i.e., calf vessels) may obscure the images. Many patients cannot undergo MR imaging (e.g., metal implants such as pacemakers) and may find the MRI tunnel too claustrophobic to withstand lying in a narrow space whilst the images are taken (about 10% of patients). MR angiography is less valuable at determining in-stent stenosis and although the stainless-steel stents are particularly prone to this problem, the nitinol ones also produce artifacts. Although small surgical clips in the tissues are generally safe (but may produce artifact mimicking an occlusion), the presence of intracranial aneurysm clips, cochlear implants or metallic intraocular foreign bodies are a contraindication to its use.

Nephrogenic systemic fibrosis (NSF) is a rare condition which has been linked to the use of gadolinium. Symptoms may start from the day of exposure up to 3 months post-exposure. Symptoms classically begin in the legs and include pain, pruritus, swelling and erythema. It may progress onto thickening of the skin and subcutaneous tissues with fibrosis of the internal organs including the heart, liver, lungs, and diaphragm. Patients can suffer contractures, cachexia, and death. High risk patients appear to be those with stage 4 and 5 chronic renal disease, acute renal failure, and those on dialysis as well as children under the age of 12 months, due to the immature excretion of the kidneys. No cases have been reported in patients with a GFR > 60 ml/min/1.73M2. Just like the use of other contrast agents, patients should be screened for the possibility of deteriorating renal function after which the risk/benefit ratio may be established. If the treating doctor continues with the examination, written informed consent should be sought and the lowest dose of agent to give optimum images should be used.

MANAGEMENT OF PAD

As stated previously, the goals in management will depend on whether the ischemia is critical or non-critical and on the general health of the patient and the ability to withstand invasive procedures especially surgery. Overall, all patients will undergo 'general management' and then the decision with regard to more invasive measures will depend on the degree of ischemia and the patient symptoms. The management of PAD is outlined in Figure 9 and described in more detail in the text below.

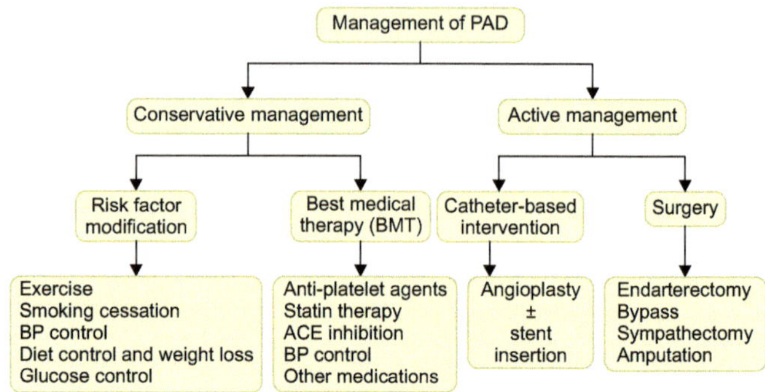

Figure 9: Overview of management of patients diagnosed with PAD. All patients should receive conservative management. Active management will depend on the severity of disease and patient symptoms.

GENERAL MANAGEMENT

Almost all patients will benefit from such disease modification approaches such as smoking cessation, exercise, good control of diabetes and hypertension as well as BMT. BMT aims to modify PAD by stabilizing plaque, reducing platelet aggregation, and preventing already-developed atherosclerotic lesions from progressing to complications. Even after more invasive treatment such as angioplasty, stent insertion and arterial bypass surgery, all patients should remain on the general conservative measures as well as disease-modifying medications. Such measures will not only potentially modify the course of the PAD and patient symptoms, but more importantly there will be an overall reduction in cardiovascular deaths including fatal MI and stroke.

RISK FACTOR/LIFE-STYLE MODIFICATION

Although many of the risk factors for PAD cannot be altered (e.g., gender, advancing age), there are other risk factors that may be improved on, including smoking cessation, strict diabetic control, blood pressure control and lifestyle improvements such as weight loss and exercise.

SMOKING CESSATION

Cessation of smoking is probably the single biggest modifiable risk factor that the patient can undertake. More importantly, stopping smoking will reduce the incidence of cardiovascular deaths including AMI and stroke, but may also help in reducing the patient's claudication symptoms. Smoking cessation will also improve the outcomes of any likely intervention.[20] As smoking is highly addictive, many patients find giving up very difficult. Nicotine replacement therapy has been shown to significantly affect smoking cessation habits in motivated patients, improving the odds of quitting by about 1.2-2-fold.[21]

BLOOD PRESSURE CONTROL

The Framingham Heart Study confirmed that hypertension is a predisposing factor for PAD, with BP measurements>160/95 mm Hg increasing the risk by ×2.5 in men and ×4in women over a 26-year period. Even modest reductions in blood pressure (i.e., 10/5 mm Hg) were associated with a decrease in stroke mortality by 40 percent, decrease in coronary artery disease mortality by 16 percent, decrease in all cause cardiovascular events by 30 percent and a decrease in PAD events by 26 percent. The conclusion from this study was to aim for a blood pressure of less than 140/85 mm Hg in treated individuals.

GLUCOSE CONTROL

This is a little more controversial, as the PAD disease seen in diabetics is already well established over many years of hyperglycemia and therefore, improving glucose control over a short period of time may not alter the disease course. The major benefits in glucose control in diabetic patients appear to be in the microvascular protection and prevention of neuropathy and secondary foot complications and not for the macrovascular disease.

EXERCISE

Exercise will improve overall cardiorespiratory health as well as a treatment for PAD. A meta-analysis of exercise regimens studies has demonstrated a benefit of walking in patients with PAD by up to 150 percent.[48] This improvement is certainly comparable to other treatments for PAD, including angioplasty and best medical therapy. The benefit of exercise is probably more important for general cardiac health and the recommended exercise routine is walking for up to 30 minutes at least three times per week for six months. This arbitrary routine has never been scrutinized properly. However, the Cochrane review did report that walking to near maximum pain produced best results, which is also supported by other studies.[49]

The conclusion from the Cochrane analysis that a prescribed exercise regimen had better outcomes than angioplasty was also supported by Perkins et al. This study concluded that exercise, especially when disease was confined to the superficial femoral artery, conferred a better outcome with regard to walking distance compared to angioplasty at 1 year. However, there was no difference on follow up at 70 months, perhaps due to reduced compliance in the exercise group.[50] Whyman et al showed that angioplasty was better at six months, but that there was no difference on follow up at 2 years.[51,52] Furthermore, iliac lesions are best treated with angioplasty than exercise alone.[50]

BEST MEDICAL THERAPY

Best medical therapy (BMT) refers to agents that have shown benefit in clinical studies in the treatment of PAD. These agents include angiotensin converting enzyme inhibitors, statins, and antiplatelet agents

ANGIOTENSIN CONVERTING ENZYME INHIBITORS

The renin-angiotensin system is an important regulator within the cardiovascular system, especially regarding blood pressure and homeostasis. However, it also exerts important autocrine effects within the vascular tree, where its effects are found in both the endothelium and smooth muscle cells.[53,54] Angiotensin-converting enzyme (ACE) is a membrane-bound dipeptidyl peptidase. The role of ACE is to convert inactive angiotensin I (ATI) to the active angiotensin II (AII) and inactivate bradykinin. AII binds to two receptors: AT1 and AT2. The AT1 receptor is primarily found on smooth muscle cells and the AT2 receptor on endothelial cells.[55,56] During periods of cardiovascular stress, injury and inflammation, levels of ACE increases within vascular tissue. In normal vascular tissue the ratio of AT1/AT2 is greater. However, there is a reversal of this ratio in vascular disease with an up-regulation of AT2.[57,58]

There is good evidence that patients with symptomatic PAD will benefit from ACE inhibitor therapy in addition to good blood pressure control. The HOPE study (Heart Outcomes Prevention Evaluation) conferred the protective effects of ACE inhibition (Ramipril) in reducing cardiovascular events in treated patients who had established vascular disease or were considered high risk (e.g., diabetic patients).[59,60] Interestingly, its benefits were irrespective of blood pressure control and normotensive patients with PAD also had significant reduction in cardiovascular outcomes when treated with ACE inhibition. Evidence from the PROGRESS trial also conferred the positive benefit in normotensive patients treated with an ACE inhibitor. ACE inhibition in diabetic patients also slows the onset of microproteinuria and renal disease, which in itself is an independent risk factor for vascular disease.[61]

Many patients are intolerant of ACE inhibition and instead, are more suited to angiotensin-receptor-2 blockade (A2RB). The ONTARGET study was a large randomized controlled trial comparing ACE inhibition with A2RB in patients with established cardiovascular disease of high-risk diabetic patients (evidence of end-organ damage).[62] The results were similar between both groups of patients with regards to efficacy, although hypotensive episodes were more common in the A2RB group. ACE inhibitors should be tried first and A2RB agents should be tried for those who cannot tolerate ACE inhibitors.

HMGCOA REDUCTASE INHIBITORS (STATINS)

HMG-CoA (3-hydroxy-3-methylglutaryl-coenzyme A) reductase inhibitors, also known as 'statins', have demonstrated enormous benefit in cardiovascular disease. Statins are specific, reversible competitive inhibitors of the enzyme HMG-CoA. This enzyme converts HMG-CoA to mevalonic acid, which is the rate-limiting step in the synthesis of cholesterol.[63] This inhibition leads to a decrease in liver cholesterol synthesis, which then results in an up-regulation of low-density lipoprotein (LDL) receptors. This then leads to an increased plasma clearance of LDL as well as decreased plasma cholesterol levels.[63] Although the main biochemical effect of statins is a reduction in plasma LDL, it also reduces plasma triglyceride concentrations and increases high density lipoproteins (HDL).[63]

More recently, the non-lipid lowering properties of statins have been described. These further contribute to their favorable cardiovascular profile. These auxiliary pleiotropic effects include anti-inflammatory properties (especially within the vascular endothelium), improved endothelial function, reduced platelet aggregation, atherosclerotic plaque stabilization, anti-thrombotic activity, and anti-proliferative properties.[64]

Hypercholesterolemia undoubtedly contributes to the development of atherosclerosis, including PAD. The Framingham Heart Study demonstrated that a fasting cholesterol level >7 mmol/L doubled the risk of intermittent claudication, and that the LDL/HDL ratio was as important as the actual serum cholesterol level in the prediction of PAD.[65]

Numerous trials have demonstrated the benefit of statins in the medical management of vascular disease. The British Heart Protection Study was a randomized controlled trial (n > 20,000) comparing simvastatin (40 mg) with placebo. Treatment with a statin significantly reduced late cardiovascular deaths and conferred a relative risk reduction for cardiovascular outcomes, including any major coronary event, stroke, and the need for revascularization at five years by almost 25 percent. These benefits were irrespective of age (up to about 80 years), gender or cholesterol levels, thus supporting the non-lipid-lowering benefits of statin therapy.[66]

The 4S Trial (Scandinavian Simvastatin Survival Study) and CARE Trial (Cholesterol and Recurrent Events study) studied simvastatin and pravastatin respectively in post-MI patients. These studies conferred a 30-40 percent decrease in fatal and non-fatal cardiovascular events and stroke. The incidence of new-onset or worsening claudication was also lower in the statin-treated groups compared to the placebo treated groups in the 4S Trial.[67,68] Although statins may help to stabilize PAD with improvement in symptoms,[69] the major benefit in using statins in this group of patients is in its cardiovascular and stroke outcomes.[70]

ANTIPLATELET AGENTS

Aspirin is a non-steroidal anti-inflammatory agent that acts by irreversibly inactivating both cyclooxygenase (COX) enzymes (COX-1 and COX-2). COX-1 is a principal enzyme involved in platelet aggregation. Once inactivated by aspirin, platelets will remain inactivated for up to 10 days.[71] The primary prostanoid produced by the action of COX-1is thromboxane A2 (TxA_2). TxA_2 is a potent vasoconstrictor and platelet aggregator. However, low dose aspirin (e.g.,75 mg once daily) will inhibit COX-1 more in platelets than endothelial cells, with higher doses inhibiting the endothelial cell derived PGI_2. As such, aspirin is both an antiplatelet agent and anti-inflammatory agent (albeit weak). PGI_2 inhibits platelet aggregation and disaggregates pre- formed platelet clumps (aspirin will potentially abolish this action). However, endothelial cells can quickly synthesize more PGI_2 after inhibition by aspirin, but platelets fail to synthesize more TxA_2, due to the lack of a cell nucleus (TxA_2 does not recover until the affected cohort of platelets is replaced in about 7-10 days), and thus the net effect of aspirin is platelet inhibition.[72]

The Antiplatelet Trialists Collaboration Study was one of the original studies to investigate the benefits of anti-platelet agents and cardiovascular disease. It demonstrated a significant reduction in non-fatal MI, non-fatal stroke and all vascular deaths when treated with low-dose aspirin.[73] In the subset of patients with PAD, there was a relative risk reduction in any serious vascular event by 23 percent. Just like with statin therapy, the major benefit with aspirin in patients with PAD is not in its ability to retard the progression of the PAD, but in the reduction of cardiovascular death, non-fatal MI, and stroke. However, there is some evidence, albeit weak that antiplatelet therapy may slow down the angiographic evidence of PAD.[74]

The recently published POPADAD Trial was a Scottish trial investigating the role of aspirin and/or antioxidants in high risk but asymptomatic vascular patients as a primary preventative agent.[75] The study included diabetics and asymptomatic patients with objective evidence of PAD (ABPI<1.0). Interestingly, aspirin did not significantly improve cardiovascular outcomes as compared to placebo in these patients. The findings of the POPADAD Trial were also substantiated by the JPAD Study and thus its role in cardiovascular disease is probably best restricted to symptomatic patients and/or patients with evidence of significant cardiovascular disease.[76]

Dipyridamole is a phosphodiesterase V and adenosine uptake inhibitor. This drug is a vasodilator and antiplatelet agent, but it has weak anti-thrombotic properties when used alone.[77] Dipyridamole can interfere with platelet function by increasing cellular cAMP concentrations. This is done by inhibiting cyclic nucleotide phosphodiesterase and/or blocking adenosine uptake. There is little benefit from using dipyridamole as a single antiplatelet agent, even in patients who are intolerant of aspirin. However, it has added benefits in addition to another antiplatelet agent, especially in the management of stroke. The European Stroke Prevention Study suggests that dipyridamole plus aspirin reduces the incidence of stroke in patients with prior stroke or transient ischemic attack.[78]

Ticlopidine and clopidogrel are thienopyridine compounds. They have anti-inflammatory and anti-platelet properties by inhibiting platelet activity through inhibiting the adenosine diphosphate receptor (ADP-selective, antiplatelet agent) on platelet cell membranes (the P_2Y1_2 receptor).[77] When this receptor is blocked, there is no activation of the glycoprotein IIb/IIIa pathway, thus inhibiting platelet aggregation and activation.[77] Clopidogrel is a ticlopidine analogue and a pro-drug and it has a potency that is seven times greater than ticlopidine, but with less documented side effects.[79]

In general, clopidogrel is used in the secondary prevention of vascular events, either in combination with other antiplatelet agents or alone, especially in patient who are intolerant of aspirin. The CHARISMA study suggested that clopidogrel used in combination with aspirin does not offer any advantage over aspirin alone, even in high-risk patients.[80]

The CAPRIE study enrolled >19,000 patients, including stroke, MI, and PAD. It demonstrated a small, but statistically significant net benefit of clopidogrel over aspirin for all composite vascular endpoints [absolute relative risk (ARR) 0.51%], which translates into a relative risk reduction of 8.7 percent and a number needed to treat (NNT) of 196. However, the largest benefit was in the subset of patients with PAD.[81] Currently, aspirin is the first line anti-platelet agent in the management of PAD, but for those intolerants or after endovascular intervention; clopidogrel is recommended, even in the short term. Recently, concerns regarding protein pump inhibitors (PPIs) and clopidogrel have come to light. Clopidogrel is a pro-drug, dependent on the cytochrome P450 enzyme CYP2C19 for activation, which is inhibited by PPIs. Two studies have now reported a higher risk of re-infarction and cardiac events in those on clopidogrel and a PPI (RR of almost 25% in one study!).[82,83] Therefore, patients taking clopidogrel who may also be taking a PPI should have their gastric protection agent changed to a H2 antagonist (although pantoprazole may be safe).

OTHERS

Cilostazol is a cAMP (cyclic adenosine monophosphate) phosphodiesterase (type III) inhibitor. It works by inhibiting platelet aggregation and is a direct arterial vasodilator. Currently, cilostazol is approved to treat intermittent claudication and has shown good improvements in both quality of life and walking distances.[84,85] Treatment with 50-100 mg twice daily may improve both the pain-free walking distance as well the maximum walking distance experienced by claudicants. Potential drawbacks of treatment include headache, flushing and diarrhea.

There is little data to support the use of other vasoactive agents in the treatment of symptomatic PAD such as pentoxifylline, inositol nicotinate and cinnarizine. However, the agent naftidrofuryl has shown some significant improvement in pain-free walking distance, although the absolute benefit is small.[86]

ADVANCED MANAGEMENT OF PAD: ENDOVASCULAR TREATMENT AND SURGERY

Advanced management of PAD includes interventional techniques (angioplasty and/or stent insertion) and surgery. Surgery may involve resection of an atherosclerotic lesion (i.e., endarterectomy) with or without patch grafting (to reduce stenosis) and bypass grafting. The results of both are comparable and will be discussed in more detail below.

ENDOVASCULAR TREATMENT

In general, this uses the same techniques as a diagnostic angiogram and should be done at the same time as the diagnostic study in order to minimize patient complications that would occur with two separate studies. The artery is accessed using the Seldinger technique, usually via the common femoral artery, which may be accessed on the ipsilateral or contralateral side of the lesion. Usually, the contralateral limb is preferred. Ultrasound may be used to gain access to the artery if it is poorly palpable and to minimize the risk of cannulating the common femoral vein, injury to the femoral nerve or extravasation of contrast into the subcutaneous tissues. Puncture may be described as 'antegrade' or 'retrograde' access. Antegrade puncture (used on the ipsilateral leg) aims the puncturing needle in the direction of arterial flow and is generally more difficult and also runs the risk of causing a retroperitoneal hematoma if cannulated above the level of the inguinal ligament. Retrograde puncture can cannulate the artery against the direction of flow. Occasionally retrograde puncture of the popliteal artery is necessary to gain access to the femoral artery. Transbrachial and occasionally transaxillary access may also be used.

After cannulation, a soft guidewire (PTFE coated), usually with a straight or J-tip (to minimize the risk of intimal damage) is inserted, and the catheter is passed over this and the guidewire removed. The standard size guidewire is 0.035 inches in diameter and 180 or 260 cm long. Generally, the tortuous nature of the vessels of the lower limb requires a stiff wire to negotiate the vessels (e.g., Amplatz wire). A sheath (11 cm long, 5-6 Fr) is placed over the guide wire and left in situ for further instrumentation with the angiocatheters as well as contrast medium injection via a side-arm. The one-way valve mechanism at the end of the sheath prevents back-flow of blood out through the sheath.

There are a wide variety of angioplasty balloons available (3-10 mm in diameter) and with varying balloon lengths. Treatment is then dependent on the site and type of lesion as well as the available equipment and experience of the personnel. Endovascular treatment is useful in treating aorto-iliac lesions, fem-pop lesions, and below-knee vessel occlusions and each of these will require a different size balloon and variable lengths. Ideally, the balloon should cover the entire length of the lesion for angioplasty, to reduce the number of attempts and potential complications, but clearly in long, complex lesions, this may not be possible. The guide wire is passed beyond the stenosis and the catheter-containing balloon passes along the guidewire and into position. After full heparinization, the balloon is then inflated (up to 3 – 20 atmospheres) for up to 1-3 minutes to widen the occlusion and allow blood flow.

The balloon should be seen to expand fully, thereby expanding the lesion. Occasionally the balloon is seen as only partially expanded at one section against the hard, calcified plaque and this is described as 'wasting' of the balloon. Generally, the success of the procedure is described by the radiographic findings at the time of treatment and may be 'fully successful' (<50% stenosis remaining after angioplasty) or 'partially successful' (>50% stenosis remaining after treatment). The angioplasty may be tried several times, but vessel wall recoil, arterial spasm as well as hard, calcified lesions may prevent a successful outcome. Specific complications (other than those already discussed in the section on 'angiogram') include distal embolization (of material from the atherosclerotic lesion, including thrombus or cholesterol) and de novo thrombus formation at the site of treatment. The clot formed may have to be removed with a 'suction' catheter. Similarly, for very hard non-compressible lesions, a 'cutting balloon' may be used to induce further trauma in the lesion to 'break it up'.

In general, angioplasty is more successful in larger vessels, such as the iliac vessels, as small, narrowed arteries (i.e., tibial vessels) have a higher rate of thrombosis and re- stenosis. The technical success rates are better for the treatment of a stenosis as opposed to a total occlusion, due to the difficulty traversing the lesion, but once traversed successfully the patency rates are similar. Following this therefore, long lesions have a higher failure rate from both a technical viewpoint as well as longer term outcomes. Calcified plaques are more difficult to angioplasty and cause more balloon wasting, and are more prone to complications, such as dissection and thrombosis.

As with all vascular lesion treatments, good inflow and run-offs are essential to maintain a vessel pressure gradient and hence flow. Females and diabetic patients seem to have worse outcomes also. The MIMIC Trial has compared angioplasty of lower limb arteries (either aortoiliac disease or fem-pop disease) with exercise regimen and BMT without intervention in patients with mild to moderate claudication. After two years, there were significant differences in favor of endovascular treatment regarding the initial claudication distance, absolute walking distance and ABPI measurements. These improvements were most marked for the group suffering from aortoiliac disease.[87]

SUBINTIMAL ANGIOPLASTY

Subintimal angioplasty is the technique first described by Bolia whereby the lesion undergoes angioplasty in the subintimal plane instead of directly within lumen, where the occluded vessel will not negotiate a guidewire.[88] The lesion is approached by a combined catheter-wire. The intima is deliberately dissected just at the beginning of the atherosclerotic lesion and the catheter-wire combination is manipulated into the subintimal space thereby developing a subintimal plane of dissection. Beyond the lesion, where the intima is healthy, the looped guide wire re-enters the lumen. The balloon may then be passed into this subintimal plane and angioplasty performed. Potential difficulties with this technique include perforation of the artery and difficulty re-entering the lumen distal to the lesion.

STENTING

Stents have allowed for the treatment of more complex lesions, especially where angioplasty alone has failed to maintain a good vessel caliber. Usually if a stent is required, it is deployed immediately following angioplasty of the lesion. A stent is a metallic structure designed to maintain patency of a vessel at the site of a stenosis by the radial force it generates on the arterial wall. In theory, elastic recoil of the vessel is minimized and hence re-stenosis, although in- stent restenosis can occur secondary to neointimal hyperplasia. Several types of stents are in use, including stainless steel (e.g., Palmaz stent), nitinol (e.g., SMART stent) and cobalt-chromium stent (e.g., Wallstent). Stents may be rigid and therefore 'balloon-expandable' (e.g., Palmaz stent) or flexible and self-expanding (e.g., Wallstent). The stainless steel Palmaz stent has high radial forces to keep a vessel open, but at the expense of flexibility. Nitinol on the other hand, is a nickel-titanium alloy which is also self-expanding, but with the properties of super-elasticity and thermal memory and is therefore best suited for very tortuous vessels (e.g., SMART stent; Shape Memory Alloy Recoverable Technology). The Wallstent is designed from numerous intercrossing wires, like a woven mesh and has good radial strength as well as flexibility. All stents are prone to thrombus formation. In order to minimize this, the surface of the stent is electrically charged or polished to minimize activation of the coagulation cascade.

All stents cause trauma to the arterial wall and hence can activate vascular smooth muscle cells and are prone to re-stenosis, in particular from neointimal hyperplasia.[89,90] Many attempts to combat this process have been tried, but to date there have been no great successes in suppressing its formation. Attempts to suppress or limit the neointimal hyperplasia seen after stent placement have been tried using anti-proliferative agents in the form of 'drug-eluting' stents. Drug-eluting stents (DES) are coated with a polymer matrix that can incorporate the anti-proliferative agent and control its release at the deployment site thus acting as a local reservoir for drug delivery. Commercially available DES incorporate such agents as rapamycin (sirolimus) and paclitaxel (Taxol) whose anti-proliferative properties are also exploited in anti-cancer therapy, but other non-commercially available DES have also been tried experimentally including heparin-coated and steroid-coated stents. These stents have mostly been tried in the coronary circulation, with good short-term and medium-term results, but with questionable long-term results. The SIROCCO trial was a double-blind, randomized trial (n=36) that studied the use of a Rapamycin- coated DES (SMART stent) with bare metal SMART stent for femoro-popliteal disease.[91] Follow up at six months failed to demonstrate any significant difference between the two groups with regards to the mean in-stent stenosis (P=0.29). However, the mean in-stent lumen diameter was larger for the DES treated groups, perhaps indicating more favorable longer-term results for DES (P=0.047). Late follow-up (2 years) in this study failed to show any advantage of DES over BMS in PAD, because the rate of in-stent restenosis was so low in both groups.[92]

In recent years, the long-term safety of the DES in the coronary circulation was called into question as there were reports of higher rates of death and myocardial infarction over BMS. However, a meta-analysis published in the Lancet has shown that the mortality rates for DES and BMS are similar, with slightly better clinical outcomes for sirolimus- eluting DES over both BMS and paclitaxel-eluting DES.[93,94]

Finally, some stents are described as 'covered stents' (e.g., Wallgraft), where they are covered with synthetic biomaterial material (e.g., PTFE), thus preventing cellular in-growth like in the conventional non-covered stents. These are useful in the treatment of vessel rupture during angioplasty, which is most likely to occur in the iliac vessels (e.g., 6-8 mm diameter, 8-10 cm long covered stent).

SURGERY

As a general rule, surgery is reserved for patients in whom other measures, including endovascular therapy have failed. This isn't entirely true as TASC have recommended that type C and D lesions should undergo surgery instead of endovascular intervention due to the high failure rate and complication rate of the latter. As a general rule, lesions longer than about 10 cm will not be successfully treated by angioplasty and/or stent insertion and therefore bypass surgery is the best option. However, the principal indications for surgery include limb salvage (often there is multilevel fem-pop-tibial disease), prevention of recurrent peripheral atheroembolization and incapacitating claudication. Good patient selection is important for good surgical outcomes.

Successful bypass surgery depends on many factors including inflow, and run-off (which should be treated or corrected either before or at the time of surgery) and the graft characteristics. In general, a vein graft is best, but its patency will also depend on the vein quality, diameter, and length. In general, for infrainguinal bypass, the long saphenous vein (LSV) should be used. Studies have shown that its patency rate is similar to using the larger superficial femoral vein for bypass at 3 years (60% vs. 64% respectively).[95] Similarly, there is no difference in patency rates for reversed and non-reversed vein grafts.[96,97] In general, the vein from the same leg should be used, but if this is unsuitable, then vein from the contralateral limb may also be used, remembering that up to 20 percent of patients will eventually go on to develop critical limb ischemia in the contralateral limb which may also need a bypass procedure.[98] In this situation, arm vein may be used, with patency rates of 70 percent and 49 percent at 1 and 3 years respectively, but with higher rates of aneurysm degeneration.[99] Synthetic grafts are either Dacron or PTFE and are best used for large diameter bypasses, as the patency rates are lower than for vein with smaller, diseased vessels.

DECIDING ON BEST INTERVENTIONAL TREATMENT AND THE ANATOMICAL CONSIDERATIONS

Numerous factors must be considered in deciding treatment for PAD, including patient fitness for a procedure especially surgery, how debilitating the symptoms are as well as the anatomical site of the lesion and whether it is amenable to endovascular treatment or surgery. As a general rule, endovascular treatment is often tried first and surgery reserved for failure of endovascular therapy, or after endovascular therapy where it as used as a 'bridge' to surgery (e.g., to improve in-flow and/or heal an ulcer before undertaking complex open reconstruction).

Anatomically, PAD and its treatment may be divided into lesions above the inguinal ligament (suprainguinal) and lesions below the inguinal ligament (infrainguinal). In practice of course, a treatment may involve both, but this arbitrary division helps in deciding if the problem is primarily an 'in-flow' or a 'run-off' problem or a combination of both.

SUPRA-INGUINAL TREATMENT

This is primarily concerned with the treatment of aorta, aorto-iliac and iliac disease. Treatment of aorto-iliac disease has the best long-term outcomes for both endovascular and open surgical treatment, especially if the lesion is short and confined to the iliac segment only with good run-off. An isolated aortic stenosis has excellent technical success rate and long-term patency rates for both angioplasty and stent insertion (90% for both). Surgery is generally not required because of the success of endovascular treatment and is probably confined to more complex situations, such as complete occlusion of the aorta and symptomatic distal thrombo-embolization. Complications of endovascular treatment include arterial wall dissection, vessel occlusion, distal embolization, and vessel rupture. Poor patency rates are generally associated with poor run-off.

The TransAtlantic Inter-Society Consensus (TASC) in 2000 generated recommendations to define iliac disease anatomically and morphologically into types A – D which is summarized in Table 6. In general, type A lesions are short (<3 cm) and generally amenable to endovascular treatment, whereas a type D lesion is longer and more complex, where endovascular treatment is more likely to fail and hence surgical treatment more appropriate. Simple iliac stenosis has excellent results with balloon angioplasty with excellent patency rates at 1 year (67-80%), 3 years (60-80%) and 5 years (55-80%) compared to 1 year (68%) and 3years (60%) for complete iliac occlusions. The technical success rate is lower for occlusive disease (83%) over stenosis (88-99%).[100]

Table 6: Transatlantic Inter-Society Consensus (TASC) lesions described for the aortoiliac and femoro-popliteal segments

	Iliac lesions	Femoro-popliteal lesions
TASC A	Single stenosis <3 cm of CIA or EIA	Single stenosis up to 3 cm not at SFA origin or distal popliteal
TASC B	CFA not involved Single stenosis 3-10 cm Two stenoses <5 cm in CIA or EIA Unilateral CIA occlusion	3-5 cm single stenosis or occlusion ≤3 cm Heavily calcified stenosis Multiple lesions ≤3 cm Single or multiple lesions with reduced run-off
TASC C	Bilateral 5-10 cm stenosis of CIA and/or EIA Unilateral EIA occlusion Unilateral EIA stenosis extending into CFA Bilateral CIA occlusion	Single stenosis or occlusion >5 cm Multiple stenosis or occlusion 3-5 cm with or without heavy calcification
TASC D	Diffuse, multilateral stenosis involving CIA EIA and CFA >10 cm Unilateral occlusion of CIA and EIA Bilateral EIA occlusions Diffuse disease of distal aorta and iliac vessels Iliac stenosis and abdominal aortic aneurysm	Complete CFA or SFA occlusions Complete popliteal and proximal trifurcation occlusions

The iliac vessels may also be stented, although the results from angioplasty alone are so good that this is usually not required, especially as stenting is associated with a higher complication rate compared to balloon dilatation alone (6.3% vs. 3.6%). Stenting may be reserved for longer, more complex lesions or when there is residual stenosis after balloon dilatation (i.e., residual luminal diameter reduction of >30 percent and/or residual pressure gradient >10 mm Hg) or a complication of angioplasty (e.g., intimal flap or vessel wall dissection). Stenting is associated with patency rates at 1, 3, and 5 years of 78 to 95 percent, 53 to 95 percent and 72 percent respectively. As with complete occlusion of the iliac vessel, stent placement gives lower success rates of 75 percent and 64 percent at 1 and 3 years respectively.

If a unilateral lesion is close to the aortic bifurcation, then there is a risk of distorting the contralateral iliac vessel after angioplasty or stent deployment (e.g., plaque fracture and dissection). Therefore, both sides should be stented, with so-called 'kissing stents' (or 'kissing balloons if balloon dilatation alone is carried out) to maintain patency on both sides, where there is partial projection into the distal aorta. Best published evidence has now suggested that the outcomes from balloon angioplasty alone versus angioplasty and stent placement is similar, but more costly in the stent group and therefore, stenting should be carried out on a selective basis.[101]

Occasionally after needle puncture with on-going retroperitoneal hemorrhage from rupture of the iliac artery on dilatation, a 'covered' stent may need to be deployed to maintain patency and stop the on-going bleeding. In this situation, the internal iliac artery is often sacrificed from circulation as its origin is covered by the stent.[100]

A selection of surgical procedures may be carried out for the treatment of aortoiliac disease, including aorto- bifemoral bypass, femoro-femoral crossover grafting and axillary-femoral bypass grafting (either Ax-unifem or Ax-bifem grafting). These can be done alone or in combination with endovascular treatment. Aortofemoral grafting (either aortobifem or aorto-unifem) is the preferred surgical option in low-risk patients. The procedure has high patency rates (95% at 5 years) and may be performed transperitoneal, through a lower midline incision (for aortobifemoral grafting) or retroperitoneal, via an oblique incision (for aorto-unifemoral bypass grafting). Aortoiliac surgery is associated with a higher mortality (1-4%) as cross-clamping or partial cross-clamping is required as well as retroperitoneal dissection and a higher morbidity (including impotence). The proximal anastomosis should be placed as high as possible on the aorta (usually infrarenal) as this is often associated with the least disease. If the patient is also suffering from an abdominal aortic aneurysm, then this may be repaired at the same time (either by in-lay technique or end-to-end anastomosis) with a trouser graft brought down to the femoral vessels. It is also important to remain vigilant for the heavily calcified aorta, which may make an anastomosis technically very difficult, if not impossible. Grafts used are typically Dacron grafts, although the superficial femoral vein may be used for unilateral disease, especially if a concomitant amputation is undertaken on the contralateral side.

Higher risk patients with unilateral disease may have a crossover graft performed with inflow from the asymptomatic contralateral artery (iliac or femoral arteries) to below the lesion on the symptomatic leg (iliac or femoral), constituting ilio-iliac (anatomical), ilio-femoral (anatomical) or femoro-femoral (extra-anatomical) cross-over grafting respectively (Figure 10). Although inferior to aorto-bifemoral grafting, these procedures still carry good 1-year and 5-year patency rates of 90 and 80 percent respectively. In general, an extra-anatomical bypass will have a lower patency rate, but also less morbidity as retroperitoneal dissection is not required. Cross-over grafts are typically Dacron or PTFE (8-10 mm), although vein may also be used. The tunnel may be created either subcutaneously or behind the rectus muscle.

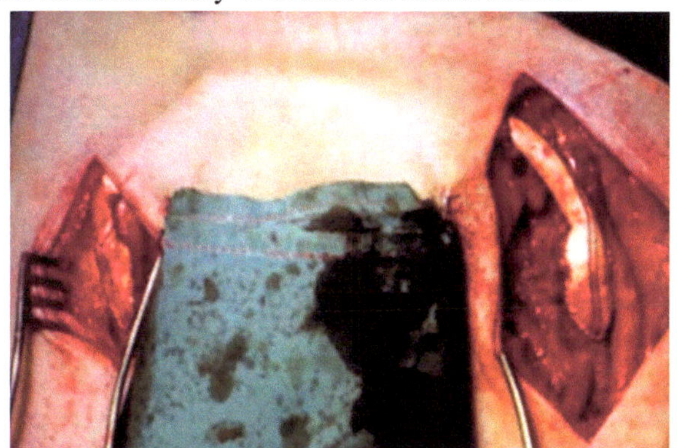

Figure 10: Both groins dissected to perform a femoro-femoral crossover graft using PTFE

Inflow may also be brought from the subclavian or axillary arteries (axillofemoral bypass) which may be uni-femoral or bifemoral for outflow. These extra-anatomical bypass grafts are best reserved for high-risk candidates (i.e.: there is no intra-abdominal or retroperitoneal exposure required) and are associated with lower patency rates (5-year patency rates of 33-85%) and are therefore not really recommended for patients whose symptoms may be managed by other means or for patients expected to live longer than 5 years. Blood pressure measurement in both arms should be undertaken and ideally the arm with the higher pressure used for inflow. The artery is approached via a mid- infraclavicular incision with separation of the fibers of the pectoralis major muscle. The pectoralis minor may be divided, or the vessel dissected out medial to it. The subclavian vein is retracted downwards to gain access to the artery. The artery must be handled with care as it is quite delicate in this region. A tunneller is used to create a subcutaneous tunnel from the axillary artery to the groin. Typical grafts used are 8-10 mm Dacron or PTFE, which should be reinforced externally to prevent compression. A general overview of the patency rates for the various treatment options are outlined in Table 7.

Table 7: 5-year patency rates after bypass surgery and iliac angioplasty

Aorto-bifemoral bypass	85-90% (15-20% if concurrent distal occlusive disease)
Axillo-bifemoral bypass	70-75%
Femoro-femoral bypass	80-85%
Percutaneous iliac artery angioplasty	80-90%

Aortoiliac endarterectomy is generally not recommended, despite the advantage of avoiding prosthetic material. It is a procedure fraught with danger and equally good results can probably be achieved with endovascular techniques. Iliac endarterectomy, however, may be performed as part of the treatment of infrainguinal disease to improve inflow to the leg.

INFRAINGUINAL TREATMENT

Treatment of infrainguinal disease may be divided into above knee (AK) arteries (common femoral artery, superficial femoral artery, profunda femoris and the AK portion of the popliteal artery) and below knee (BK) arteries (BK popliteal artery, tibio-peroneal stem, anterior tibial artery, posterior tibial artery, peroneal artery, dorsalis pedis artery and the lateral plantar artery).

AK Arterial Disease

Disease in the common femoral artery (CFA) that is causing a critical stenosis is usually treated by femoral endarterectomy. This may be done in isolation or as part of a more extensive procedure to improve inflow for a more distal bypass. Typically, it is carried out through a vertical incision, gaining access and control of the CFA, SFA and profunda arteries. The artery is opened vertically, and the occlusive lesion is dissected in its medial plane using a Watson-Cheyne instrument. Care must be taken to ensure an intimal flap is not left behind, especially at the distal intima, where the pressure gradient is likely to lift this up and occlude or thrombose the vessel. The procedure may be carried further into the profunda femoris as a profundoplasty. Usually, the vessel is then patched to keep it widely patent. Synthetic patch (PTFE or Dacron) may be used, but the close proximity of the superficial veins as they traverse the cribriform fascia to gain access to the CFV make a venous patch more attractive.

An iliac endarterectomy may also be undertaken if this is obstructing inflow. This may be performed via the same incision in the CFA, where the atherosclerotic lesion may be removed with the use of a heavy surgical clip (e.g., Roberts) through a separate, extraperitoneal approach to the iliac artery.

Stenting of the CFA is less successful, as is stenting of the profunda artery, although they may be angioplastied, usually as 'temporizing' measures before further treatment. The SFA is amenable to endovascular treatment, although the results are comparable to exercise and conservative measures and therefore may not be indicated for claudication unless very debilitating. The SFA is a smaller artery and more prone to extensive disease compared to the aorto-iliac system, and therefore the success rates for endovascular treatment are less favorable. Patency rates for SFA-AK popliteal artery balloon dilatation at 1, 3, and 5 years are 61, 51, and 48 percent respectively, but about 10 percent higher respectively if the primary failures (about 10% also) are excluded.100 Stenting the SFA-AK popliteal system has patency rates of 67 percent and 58 percent at 1 and 3 years respectively.[100] Thus it would appear that primary stenting for fem-pop disease yields disappointing results, especially as type D lesions are more likely in this system and therefore poor run-off due to extensive multilevel disease make endovascular treatment more unsuccessful. Stenting should only be carried out as a selective procedure for complicated situations such as significant residual stenosis after balloon dilatation, intimal dissection, etc. Balloon angioplasty and stent insertion may have a more important role to play for CLI as a 'bridge' to further treatment, as the benefit over risk is different for limb salvage. More recent evidence, however, suggests that primary placement of a self-expanding stent will yield better results in the intermediate term in 6 and 12 months than balloon dilatation alone.[102] However, this added expense may not make this approach justifiable.

The typical surgical intervention for AK infrainguinal PAD is the femoral-popliteal (AK) bypass procedure. Grafts that may be used include autologous vein or synthetic grafts (Dacron or PTFE). The best results are with autologous veins, usually the long saphenous vein (LSV) which may be reversed or non-reversed. If it is non-reversed, then it may be left in its anatomical bed (in-situ) or fully mobilized and placed deeper. By leaving it in its normal anatomical position, its nutrient supply is left fully intact, but the risk of missing a side branch on dissection is higher, thereby resulting in fistula which will need to be repaired. The other advantage of a non-reversed vein is that there is less of a size discrepancy on anastomosis. However, the intact venous valves will obstruct flow in the bypass graft and therefore need to be excised using a valvulotomy. This has the disadvantage of causing intimal injury or missing a valve which may later cause obstructive flow and thrombosis of the graft. The use of a reversed vein graft will obviously avoid these risks. Both configurations require the vein to be dissected from its bed and all side branches ligated, taking care not to tie the ligature too close to the base of a side branch which may 'kink' the vein. Any inadvertent tears in the vein are repaired with a 6/0 PROLENE suture.

Typically, the proximal anastomosis is to the CFA (after endarterectomy if needed) and the distal anastomosis to the AK popliteal artery. The AK popliteal artery may be approached from the medial side, making an incision at the lower edge of the vastus medialis muscle, which is felt as a 'groove' by the palpating hand. One may also go a little posterior to this groove if the long saphenous vein is to be harvested. The fascia is divided below vastus medialis and above the anterior border of sartorius muscle to enter the popliteal fossa. Care must be taken to avoid the saphenous nerve. The space is deepened and widened to gain access to the popliteal artery with care not to damage the popliteal vein and sciatic nerve. After the vein is prepared, a tunneler is used to create a tunnel deep to the sartorius muscle and the distal anastomosis is completed using 5/0 or 6/0 prolene. Just like other procedures, the success of this operation is largely dependent on the inflow and run-off.

The patency results are comparable for both autologous vein and synthetic grafts at two years (75-80%), but the 4-year patency rates were 61 percent and 38 percent for vein and prosthetic grafts respectively.[103] Others have shown 5-year patency rates of 62 percent and 43 percent for vein and prosthetic grafts respectively.[104] Kumar et al compared vein grafts with both Dacron and PTFE synthetic grafts and showed 4-year patency rates of 73, 47 and 54 percent respectively.[105] The patency rates and outcomes are similar for both reversed and non-reversed vein grafts.[106,107] There appears to no advantage of PTFE over Dacron and vice versa, and therefore the choice often comes down to the surgeon's preference.[108,109]

Below Knee (BK) Arterial Disease

This includes disease in the BK popliteal artery, tibio-peroneal trunk (trifurcation disease) and any of the three run-off arteries, AT, PT and peroneal or a combination of these. In general, the patency rates and success rates are lower for BK disease and in general treatment is reserved for critical limb ischemia (rest pain, tissue loss and gangrenous ulceration) or limb salvage as opposed to claudication alone. The principle of balloon angioplasty in this region is to restore axial flow to the foot arch vessels. Smaller balloon diameters (e.g., 5 Fr) can be used for this purpose and vessels down to a diameter of 2-3 mm may be treated, by both transluminal and subintimal techniques. Limb salvage rates of 60 to 88 percent have been reported up to 2-year post-angioplasty, but the success is largely dependent on the 'run-off'.[100] Vessel spasm is more common here and is treated with vasodilators such as GTN and papaverine. Acute arterial damage and thrombosis, which if recognized at the same time, may be treated with suction thrombectomy and anticoagulation. Stenting in this region is generally unsuccessful as is stenting of the popliteal artery, due to the repeated flexion at the level of the knee joint.

Surgical bypass procedures are also less successful in the BK segment, and therefore are confined to selected patients who either have critical limb ischemia or debilitating claudication who will maintain good post-operative mobility (Figure 11). BK bypasses have a 5-year graft patency rates of 68 percent and 27 percent for venous and synthetic grafts respectively. Furthermore, up to 30 percent of successful BK vein bypass grafts will require further intervention in the future. Often when a BK graft occludes, this may be associated with a worsening of symptoms, due to a combination of factors including damage to collaterals at the time of surgery, neointimal hyperplasia at the distal anastomosis causing worsening run-off of the limb in general and a loss of pressure gradient after successful bypass resulting in a loss of collateral supply. If possible, the vein graft may be taken from the SFA instead of the CFA to minimize the length of the graft required. If a prosthetic graft is to be used, then an adjuvant venous cuff (e.g., Miller cuff, Taylor patch or St Mary's boot) should be constructed to maintain distal patency and reduce the incidence of neointimal hyperplasia and re-stenosis which are believed to result from the compliance mismatch where graft is anastomosed directly onto artery. The use of a vein cuff is associated with higher 2-year patency rates in BK-bypasses (but not AK-bypasses) compared to synthetic grafts without a vein patch (52% vs.29% respectively).

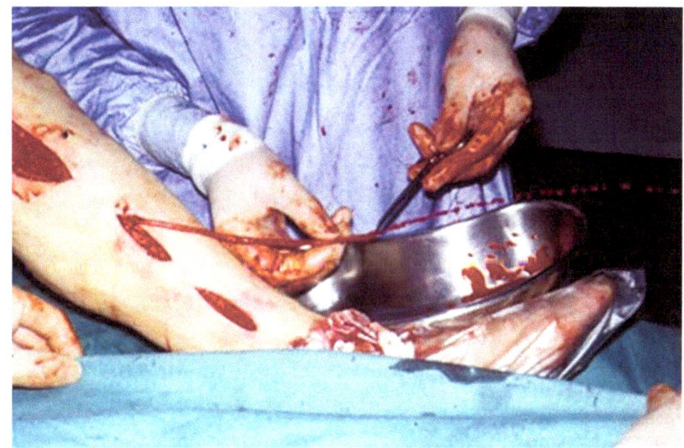

Figure 11: Lower end of vein graft demonstrating excellent forward flow for anastomosis onto the posterior tibial artery

Patency rates for BK bypasses are lower than for AK bypasses. Data from TASC has shown the 1, 3, and 5-year patency rates for tibial bypasses using vein as 85, 80 and 70 percent respectively and 70, 35, and 25 percent respectively for prosthetic grafts.[100] Other evidence has supported this and work by Hunink et al has demonstrated 5-year patency rates for vein graft (AK or BK) of 66 percent, but 47 percent for AK PTFE and 33 percent for BK PTFE.[111]

The approach to the BK vessels for bypass grafting is largely dependent on the target artery, but in general, the incision is made on the medial side. From here the BK popliteal artery, trifurcation, anterior tibial artery and peroneal artery can be approached. Usually, with the knee slightly flexed with a degree of external rotation of the hip joint, a longitudinal incision is made beginning at the level of the knee joint, just posterior to the medial femoral condyle and running straight downwards about a finger breadth posterior to the medial edge of the tibia. The BK saphenous vein can also be dissected through this incision for use in the bypass. The fascia just posterior to the tibia is then incised and the popliteal fossa entered. Usually, the popliteal artery can be accessed deep in the knee recess. However, lower down to the level of the trifurcation may require dissection and division of the upper fibers of soleus muscle. The vessels can then be looped and manipulated, remembering that the popliteal vein usually covers the lower portion of the popliteal artery down to the origin of the AT artery and thus needs to be retracted to gain access. By applying downward traction on the artery with vessel loops at different levels, the AT artery will become more apparent, as it passes anteriorly from the popliteal artery in an attempt to enter the anterior tibial compartment. The interosseous membrane may need to be opened for 2-3 cm to gain further access to the AT, taking care to ligate the small veins and venae comitantes that accompany it.

Inferior to the origin of the AT is the tibioperoneal trunk. The popliteal vein may need to be retracted upwards to adequately expose the peroneal and PT artery, taking care not to damage the posterior tibial nerve which lies close by. If the PT artery is to be exposed further down (i.e.PT2 or PT3 level), then a similar longitudinal incision just posterior to the medial edge of the tibia is necessary (Figure 12). On dividing the fascia and separating the gastrocnemius muscle from the tibia, the PT may be exposed as it runs between the muscle and posterior surface of the bone. If the peroneal artery is to be exposed, then dissection deeper behind the tibia will be necessary from the same medical approach. The peroneal artery is seen lying between the soleus muscle and the posterior tibialis muscle in the deep posterior compartment of the leg. The vein for bypass (whether reversed or non-reversed) may be tunneled sub-sartorially (if coming from the CFA) as described earlier, or lower down from the SFA (if this has good inflow). Occasionally the inflow is taken from the profunda artery, exposed by a medical incision, about halfway along the thigh, but above the sartorius muscle. The vein should then be tunneled through the popliteal fossa, by blunt finger dissection, so that the distal end may be anastomosed to the BK popliteal artery. If the distal anastomosis is the PT2/PT3, then it may be tunneled subcutaneously from the BK popliteal fossa to come to rest at the distal anastomosis site.

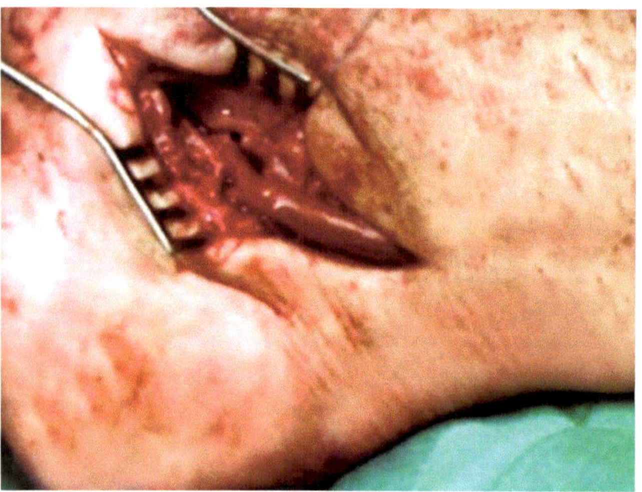

Figure 12: Vein graft anastomosis onto the distal posterior tibial artery

If the distal anastomosis is to be the AT, in particular AT2 or AT3, then this portion of artery should be approached via an anterolateral incision. Again, the knee joint is flexed, but internal rotation of the hip joint is less amenable. A similar medial exposure of the BK popliteal artery will still be necessary to tunnel the vein from above the knee and through the popliteal fossa. An incision is made on the lateral edge, about halfway between the fibula and tibia, in the natural groove that demarcates the tibialis anterior muscle from the extensor digitorum longus muscle. The AT is easily exposed on separation of these two muscles along the natural plane. A tunnel may be created for the graft passing from the medial popliteal exposure to the antero- lateral AT exposure in the anterior compartment. This may be achieved using a blunt clamp to pierce the interosseous membrane, staying close to the tibia bone. The division in the membrane should be extended for a few centimeters cephalad and caudally to avoid kinking or pinching of the vein graft as it passes through.

The peroneal artery may also be approached from the lateral side, and this is probably best reserved for re-operations, where re-exposure medially is too difficult. A segmental fibulectomy is usually necessary. On exposure of the bone, a periosteal elevator is used to remove the periosteum and then using a Gigli saw, the section of fibula is removed to allow greater exposure. The peroneal artery lies beneath the removed section of bone. The vein graft is tunneled to this position as for the AT exposure.

ADJUVANT THERAPY AFTER ENDOVASCULAR TREATMENT

Acute arterial thrombosis is a risk during endovascular treatment in a freshly angioplastied lesion or after stent deployment; therefore, the patient should be fully heparinized for the duration of the procedure, with a bolus and repeat if necessary. In more complex cases, or where acute thrombosis occurs, on-going post-procedure heparinization may be necessary.

It goes without saying that BMT should also be continued for these patients, especially aspirin. However, other antiplatelet agents are also used, most notably the platelet GPIIb/IIIa receptor inhibitors (e.g., tirofiban, abciximab), but use of these after treatment of PAD is not widespread. If a stent has been deployed, dual antiplatelet therapy with aspirin and clopidogrel should be undertaken for 4-6 weeks post-procedure to reduce the short-term thrombosis risk.

Numerous other therapies in the suppression of neointimal hyperplasia have been studied, but to date with little clinical success. One recent study investigated the efficacy of using locally delivered paclitaxel during angioplasty to inhibit restenosis during lower limb angioplasty.[94] Paclitaxel-coated balloons and paclitaxel dissolved in contrast medium were analyzed in patients who had femoropopliteal disease. Six-months follow-up demonstrated a significant difference in the mean late-lumen loss in favor of the paclitaxel-coated angioplasty balloons, but no significant difference in the paclitaxel-contrast media. Additionally, 6-month target revascularization rates showed great benefit for the paclitaxel-coated balloon catheters, but not for the paclitaxel-contrast media.

ADJUVANT THERAPY AFTER SURGERY

All vascular patients should be maintained on BMT after surgery, as this reduces the risk of cardiovascular death (AMI and stroke) and probably 'modifies' further atherosclerosis development which may slow down the disease process in the peripheral vessels. However, it remains an area of some controversy that following a technically successful bypass, whether anything else (i.e., pharmacotherapy) can be done to maintain graft patency. Certainly, preoperative platelet inhibition is important in improving patency as it reduces platelet deposition on prosthetic bypass grafts and areas of arterial wall injury.[112] Furthermore, statin therapy appears to improve graft patency and limb salvage rates.[113]

Antiplatelet therapy in combination with warfarin appears to improve graft patency in high risk patients (e.g. limb salvage, poor run-off) over aspirin alone or warfarin alone.[114,115] Anticoagulation with low molecular weight heparin, treated for three months has also been shown to improve the 1-year patency rates in patients undergoing lower limb bypass surgery for CLI, over dual antiplatelet therapy alone.[116] It would seem reasonable therefore that both anti-platelet therapy and anticoagulation be used in selected patients at high risk of graft failure or after limb salvage surgery.

COMPARING ENDOVASCULAR THERAPY WITH SURGERY

Endovascular intervention is often the preferred option over open surgery as it is less invasive. However, not all lesions are amenable to successful balloon dilatation and/or stent insertion. For those lesions that are, there does not appear to be any difference in the patency rates for either technique.[117,118]

The BASIL Trial (n=452) compared angioplasty with bypass surgery in patients with CLI, with the primary end-point of amputation-free survival. After 6 months, there was no difference between the two groups regarding the 30-day mortality or health-related quality of life. There was no difference with regard to the primary outcome variable at 30 days, 6 months, 1 year or 3 years. The two therapies appeared to be equivalent up to 2 years and post-hoc analysis of data seems to suggest that surgery is preferable if the patient is expected to survive for 3 years or more.[119] Although there is a tendency to favor surgery, it is reasonable to undergo endovascular therapy first as it is less invasive and to proceed to surgery thereafter if the patient is fit.

GRAFT SURVEILLANCE

The general patency rates of various bypass techniques are summarized in Table 7. The role of graft surveillance is controversial. However, up to 30 percent of vein bypass grafts will develop a stenosis requiring treatment. Clinical examination is poor at detecting a stenosis as often the graft has become completely occluded when clinically detectable. Therefore, graft surveillance is generally recommended using duplex ultrasound and many vascular centers have protocols in place to detect a re-stenosis early so that it can be treated, before a complete occlusion occurs, which is more difficult to treat. In general, a peak systolic ratio >3 (i.e., 70% stenosis) is considered significant to warrant further treatment. Significant improvements in patency rates have been reported with a surveillance programme.[120]

OTHER TREATMENTS

For many patients with critical limb ischemia, the disease is considered 'unreconstructable' and symptoms are treated with a variety of analgesics (e.g., NSAIDs, opiates) and other neuromodulator agents such as gabapentin and amitriptyline.

Other vasodilators may be tried to 'open up' small vessels and improve overall circulation in the resting limb. The prostacyclin (PGI_2) analogue iloprost has a short half-life (about 30 mins) and may be given by intravenous infusion. It has antiplatelet and vasodilatory properties and has been shown to have lower mortality rates and lower amputation rates at 6 months when used for CLI.[121]

Lumbar sympathectomy is another way to abolish sympathetic control over vasoconstriction thereby leaving vasodilatation as the dominant effect. This may be done by chemical means (chemical sympathectomy), whereby sclerosant is injected translumbar into the sympathetic chain on the affected side, or by open surgery (surgical sympathectomy), where the lumbar sympathetic chain is excised via a retroperitoneal approach, often with mixed results with regard to pain relief and ulcer healing.[87] A sympathectomy is less likely to work in the diabetic population, as many of these already have an 'auto- sympathectomy' secondary to diabetic autonomic neuropathy and therefore, the blood vessels may already be maximally dilated despite the critical level of ischemia.

Numerous other therapies exist including spinal cord stimulation, hyperbaric oxygen, topical wound oxygen therapy and intermittent compression therapy. Many of these have not gained wide acceptance in clinical practice or are not readily available commercially.

AMPUTATION

In many patients with non-reconstructable disease or failed treatment of critical limb ischemia, an amputation may be necessary. Other indications may include deep necrosis and/or infection of the foot, especially over a pressure area (e.g., non-healing ulcer of the heel), or a flexion contracture of the limb that is not correctable.

In general, the lowest level of amputation should be chosen, and amputation sites are generally either below knee amputation (BKA) or above knee amputation (AKA). A BKA will generally allow the patient to ambulate on an artificial limb as the knee joint is preserved. Also, general movement and transfer are better due to longer limb preservation. The independent ambulatory rates with prosthesis are summarized in Table 8. An AKA if necessary is much more difficult to ambulate and the energy demand is much higher for these patients to try to walk. Energy required for walking increases by about 50 percent after a unilateral BKA, but by up to 100 percent after an AKA.

Table 8: Independent (prosthetic) ambulation rates after various amputations

Unilateral	BKA	66-80%
	AKA	35-50%
Bilateral	BKA	45%
	AKA	10%

Occasionally an AKA is selected instead of a BKA, even if a BKA is feasible. This is usually in the patient who is already wheelchair bound, as to leave a BKA stump will only result in a painful contracture and /or a pressure ulceration on the stump secondary to sitting in the chair. Also, an AKA wound is more likely to heal than a BKA wound, and this must be considered before surgery to avoid infection and necrosis of the stump (Figures 13 and 14). In general, a popliteal pressure of 70 mm Hg is required to heal a BKA. Advice from a rehabilitation specialist should be sought regarding a patient's potential to rehabilitate and ambulate successfully. However, it must also be remembered, that due to underlying generalized atherosclerotic disease, survival after amputation is greatly reduced being approximately 75, 50 and 35 percent at 1, 3 and 5 years post-amputation respectively.

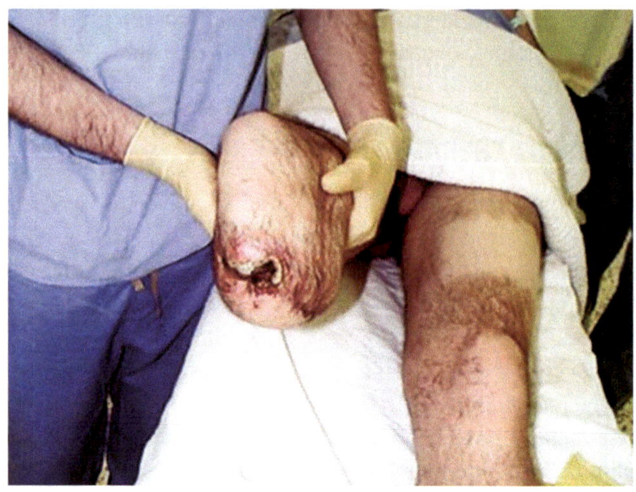

Figure 13: Infected BK stump

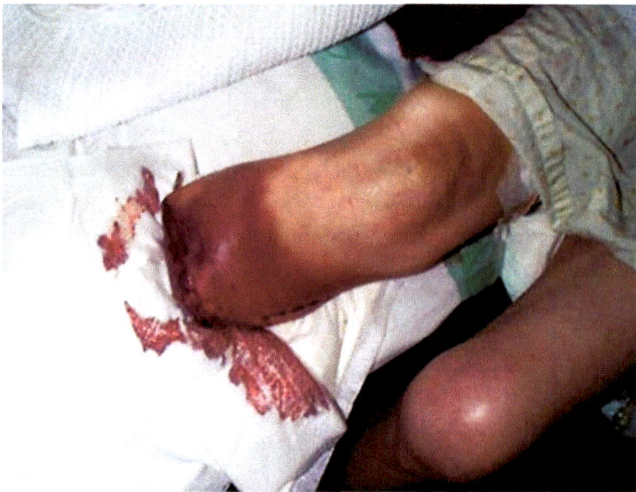

Figure 14: Necrosis of BKA flaps needing revision to an AKA

REFERENCES

1. Ross R. The pathogenesis of atherosclerosis: a perspective for the1990's. Nature 1993;362:801-9.
2. Criqui MH, Fronek A, Barrett-Connor E, Klauber MR, Gabriel S, Goodman D. The prevalence of peripheral arterial disease in a defined population. Circulation 1985;71:510-5.
3. Hiatt WR, Hoag S, Hamman RF. Effect of diagnostic criteria on the prevalence of peripheral arterial disease: the San Luis Diabetes Study. Circulation 1995;91:1472-9.
4. Fowkes F. Edinburgh Artery Study: prevalence of asymptomatic and symptomatic peripheral arterial disease in the general population. Int J Epidemiol 1991;20:384-92.

5. Newman AB. Ankle-arm index as a marker of atherosclerotic disease in the Cardiovascular Health Study. Cardiovascular Heart Study (CHS) Collaborative Research Group. Circulation 1993;88:837-45.
6. Leng GC. Femoral atherosclerosis in an older British Population:prevalence and risk factors. Atherosclerosis 2000;152:167-74.
7. Leng GC. Incidence, natural history and cardiovascular events in symptomatic and asymptomatic peripheral arterial disease in the general population. Int J Epidemiol 1996;25:1172-81.
8. Newman AB, Shemanski L, Manolio TA, et al. Ankle-arm index as a predictor of cardiovascular disease and mortality in the Cardiovascular Health Study. Arterioscler Thromb Vasc Biol1999;19:538-45.
9. McKenna M, Wolfson S, Kuller L. The ratio of ankle and arm arterial pressure as an independent predictor of mortality. Atherosclerosis 1991;87:119-28.
10. Vogt MT, McKenna M, Anderson SJ, Wolfson SK, Kuller LH. The relationship between ankle-arm index and mortality in older men and women. J Am Geriatr Soc 1999;12:142-7.
11. Dormandy JA, Heeck L, Vig S. The fate of patients with critical leg ischemia. Semin Vasc Surg 1999;12:142-7.
12. Cacoub CC, Abola MT, Baumgar tner I, Bhatt DL, et al.Cardiovascular risk factor control and outcomes in peripheral artery disease patients in the Reduction of Atherothrombosis for Continued Health (REACH) Registry. Atherosclerosis 2009;e86-92.
13. Maurabito JM, D'Agostino RB, Silbershatz H, et al. Intermittent claudication. A risk profile from the Framingham Heart Study. Circulation 1997;96:44-9.
14. Fowkes F. Edinburgh Artery Study: prevalence of asymptomatic and symptomatic peripheral arterial disease in the general population. Int J Epidemiol 1991;20:384-92.
15. Hooi JD. Incidence of and risk factors for asymptomatic peripheral arterial occlusive disease: a longitudinal study. Am J Epidemiol 2001;153:666-72.
16. Hiatt WR, Hoag S, Hamman RF. Effect of diagnostic criteria on the prevalence of peripheral arterial disease. The San Luis Valley Diabetes Study. Circulation 1995;91:1472-9.
17. Hirsch AT. The role of tobacco cessation, antiplatelet and lipid- lowering therapies in the treatment of peripheral arterial disease. Vasc Med 1997;2:243-51.
18. Doll R, Peto R, Wheatley K, Gray R, Sutherland I. Mortality in relation to smoking: 40 years' observations on male British doctors. Br Med J 1994;309:901-11.
19. Rosenberg L, Palmer JR, Shapiro S. Decline in the risk of myocardial infarction among women who stop smoking. N Engl J Med 1990;322:213-7.
20. Cavender JB, Rogers WJ, Fisher LD, et al. Effects of smoking on survival and morbidity in patients randomized to medical or surgical therapy in the coronary artery surgery study (CASS): 10-year follow-up. J Am Coll Cardiol. 1992;20:287 91.
21. Silagy C. Meta-analysis on efficacy of nicotine replacement therapies in smoking cessation. Lancet 1994;343:139-42.
22. UK Prospective Diabetes Study (UKPDS) Group. Intensive blood glucose control with sulphonylureas or insulin compared with conventional treatment and risk of complications in patients with type 2 diabetes (UKPDS 33). Lancet 1998;352:837-53.
23. Adler A. UKPDS 59: hyperglycemia and other potentially modifiable risk factors for peripheral arterial disease in type 2 diabetes. Diabetes Care 2002;25:894-9.
24. Fowkes FG. Epidemiological research on peripheral vascular disease.J Clin Epidemiol 2001;54:863-8.
25. da Silva A. The management and outcome of critical limb ischemia in diabetic patients: results of a national survey. Audit committee of the Vascular Surgical Society of Great Britain and Ireland. Diabetic Med 1996;13:726-8.
26. Stratton IM, Adler AI, Neil HAW, et al. Association of glycaemia with macrovascular and microvascular complications of type 2 diabetes (UKPDS 35): prospective observational study. Br Med J.2000;321:405-12.
27. Hiatt WR. Medical treatment of peripheral arterial disease and claudication. N Engl J Med 2001;344:1608-21.
28. Neal B, MacMahon S, Chapman N. Effects of ACE inhibitors,calcium antagonists, and other blood-pressure-lowering drugs: results of prospectively designed overviews of randomised trials. Blood Pressure Lowering Treatment Trialists' Collaboration. Lancet 2000;356:1955-64.
29. Adler A. Association of systolic blood pressure with macrovascular and microvascular complications of type 2 diabetes (UKPDS 36): prospective observational study. Br Med J 2000; 321:412-19.
30. Hansson L. Effects of intensive blood-pressure lowering and low- dose aspirin in patients with hypertension: principal results of the Hypertension Optimal Treatment (HOT) randomised trial. HOT Study Group. Lancet 1998; 351:1755-62.

31. Beckman J, Creager M, Libby P. Diabetes and atherosclerosis:epidemiology, pathophysiology and management. JAMA 2002;287:2570-81.
32. Khunti K, Davies M. Metabolic syndrome. BMJ 2005; 331:1153-4.
33. Housley E. Physical activity and risk of peripheral arterial disease in the general population: Edinburgh Artery Study. J Epidemiol Community Health 1993; 47:475-80.
34. Cheng SW, Ting AC, Wong J. Fasting total plasma homocysteine and atherosclerotic peripheral vascular disease. Ann Vasc Surg 1997;11:217-23.
35. Graham IM, Daly LE, Refsum HM, et al. Plasma homocysteine as a risk factor for vascular disease: the European Concerted Action Project. JAMA 1997; 277:1775-81.
36. Rauwerda JA, de Jong SC. Homocysteinemia and vascular disease.Critical Ischemia 1999; 9:53-7.
37. Kleijnen J, Mackerras D. Vitamin E for intermittent claudication.In: The Cochrane Library, issue 1. Chichester: John Wiley & Sons, 2005.
38. Ernst E. Chelation therapy for peripheral arterial occlusive disease:a systematic review. Circulation 1997; 96:1031-3.
39. Second European Consensus Document on Chronic Critical LegIschemia. Eur J Vasc Surg 1992; 6:1-4.
40. Thompson MM, Sayers RD, Varty K, et al. Chronic critical leg ischemia must be redefined. Eur J Vasc Surg 1993; 7:420-6.
41. Kohler TR, Nance DR, Cramer MM, Vandenburghe N, Strandness DE Jr. Duplex scanning for the diagnosis of aortoiliac and femoro- popliteal disease: a prospective study. Circulation 1987; 76:1074-80.
42. Cossman DV, Ellison JE, Wagner WH, et al. Comparison of contrast arteriography to arterial mapping with color-flow duplex imaging in the lower extremities. J Vasc Surg 1989; 10:522-9.
43. Moneta GL, Yeager RA, Antonovic R, et al. Accuracy of lower extremity arterial duplex mapping. J Vasc Surg 1992; 15:275-84.
44. Larch E, Minar E, Ahmadi R, et al. Value of color duplex sonography for evaluation of tibioperoneal arteries in patients with femoropopliteal obstruction: a prospective comparison with antegrade intra-arterial digital subtraction angiography. J Vasc Surg 1997; 25:629-36.
45. Grassbaugh JA, Nelson PR, Rzucidlo EM, et al. Blinded comparison of preoperative duplex ultrasound scanning and contrast angiography for planning revascularization at the level of the tibia. J Vasc Surg 2003; 37:1186-90.
46. Waybill MM, Waybill PN. Contrast media-induced Nephrotoxicity: identification of patients at risk and algorithms for prevention. J Vasc Intervent Radiol 2001;12:3-9.
47. N-acetylcysteine and contrast-induced nephropathy in primary angioplasty. N Engl J Med 2006; 354:2773-82.
48. Gardner AW, Poehlman ET. Exercise rehabilitation programs for the treatment of claudication pain. A meta-analysis. JAMA 1995;274:975-80.
49. Leng GC, Fowler B, Ernst E. Exercise for the treatment of intermittent claudication. Cochrane Database Syst Rev 2000(2); CD000990.
50. Perkins JM, Collin J, Creasy TS, Fletcher EW, Morris PJ. Exercise training versus angioplasty for stable claudication. Long and medium term results of a prospective, randomised trial. Eur J Vasc Endovasc Surg 1996; 11:409-13.
51. Whyman MR, Fowkes FG, Kerracher EM, et al. Randomised controlled trial of percutaneous transluminal angioplasty for intermittent claudication. Eur J Vasc Endovasc Surg 1996; 12:167-72.
52. Whyman MR, Fowkes FG, Kerracher EM, et al. Is intermittent claudication improved by percutaneous transluminal angioplasty? A randomized controlled trial. J Vasc Endovasc Surg 1997; 26:551-7.
53. Dzau VJ. Evolving concepts of the renin-angiotensin system. Focus on renal and vascular mechanisms. Am J Hypertens 1988;1:334-7s.
54. Dzau VJ. Implications of local angiotensin production in cardiovascular physiology and pharmacology. Am J Cardiol 1987;59:59-65A.
55. Griendling KK, Lassegue B, Murphy TJ, Alexander RW. AngiotensinII receptor pharmacology. Adv Pharmacol 1994;28:269-306.
56. Griendling KK, Murphy TJ, Alexander RW. Molecular biology of the renin angiotensin system. Circulation 1993;87:1816-28.
57. Rakugi H, Wang DS, Dzau VJ, Pratt RE. Potential importance of tissue angiotensin converting enzyme (ACE) inhibition in preventing neointimal formation. Circulation 1994;90(1):449-55.
58. Rakugi H, Kim DK, Krieger JE, Wang DS, Dzau VJ, Pratt RE.Induction of angiotensin converting enzyme (ACE) in the neointima after vascular injury. Possible role of restenosis. J Clin Invest 1994;93(1). 339-46.
59. Yusuf S, Sleight P, Pogue J, Bosch J, Davies R, Dagenais G. Effects of an angiotensin-converting-enzyme-inhibitor, ramipril, on cardiovascular events in high-risk patients. The Heart Outcomes Prevention

Evaluation (HOPE) Study Investigators. NEJM 2000;342:154-53.

60. Heart Outcomes Prevention Evaluation (HOPE) Study Investigators.Effects of ramipril on cardiovascular outcomes in people with diabetes mellitus: results of the HOPE Study and MICRO-HOPE Substudy. Lancet 2000;355:253-9.
61. PROGRESS Collaborative Group. Randomised trial ot perındopril- based blood pressure-lowering regimen among 6,105 individuals with previous stroke or transient ischemic attack. Lancet 2001;358:1033-41.
62. Telmisartan, ramipril, or both in patients at high risk for vascular events. ONTARGET Investigators, Yusuf S, Teo KK, Pogue J, Dyal L, et al. NEJM 2008;358:1547-59.
63. Mahley RW, Bersot TP. Drug therapy for hypercholesterolemia and dyslipidemia. In: Goodman & Gilman's The Pharmacological Basis ofTherapeutics: Brunton LL, Lazo JS, Parker KL, (Eds). (11th edn). McGraw-Hill. Philadelphia, PA, 2006.
64. Laws PE, Spark JI, Cowled PA, Fitridge RA. The role of statins in vascular disease. Eur J Vasc Endovasc Surg 2004;27:6-16.
65. Kannel WB. Intermittent claudication. Incidence in the Framingham Study. Circulation 1970;41:875-83.
66. Heart Protection Study Collaborative Group. MRC/ BHF Heart Protection Study of Cholesterol-lowering with simvastatin in 20,536 high-risk individuals. Lancet 2002;360:7-22.
67. Scandinavian Simvastatin Survival Study (4S). Randomised trial of cholesterol Lowering in 4444 patients with coronary heart disease. Lancet 1994;244:1383-9.
68. Sacks FM. The effect of pravastatin on coronary events after myocardial infarction in patients with average cholesterol levels. Cholesterol and Recurrent Events Trial Investigators. N Engl J Med 1996;335:1001-9.
69. Pederson TR, Kjekshus J, Pyorala K, et al. Effect of simvastatin on ischemic signs and symptoms in the 4S study. Am J Cardiol 1998;81:333-5.
70. Leng GC, Price JF, Jepson RG. Lipid-lowering for lower limb atherosclerosis. Cochrane Database Syst Rev 2000(2); CD000123.
71. Smyth EM, Burke A, Fitzgerald GA. Lipid-derived autacoids: eicosanoids and platelet-activating factor. In: Goodman & Gilman's The Pharmacological Basis of Therapeutics (11th edn). Brunton LL, Lazo JS, Parker KL, (Eds). McGraw-Hill. Philadelphia, PA.
72. Cheng Y, Austin SC, Rocca B, Koller BH, Coffman TM, Grosser T, et al. Role of prostacyclin in the cardiovascular response to thromboxane A2. Science 2002;296:539-41.
73. Antiplatelet Trialists' Collaboration. Collaborative overview of randomised trials of antiplatelet therapy. Prevention of death, myocardial infarction, and stroke by prolonged antiplatelet therapy in various categories of patients. Br Med J 1994;308:81-106.
74. Goldhaber SZ. Low-dose aspirin and subsequent peripheral arterial surgery in the physicians' Health Study. Lancet 1992;340:143-5.
75. Belch J, MacCuish A, Campbell I, Cobbe S, Taylor R, et al. The prevention of progression of arterial disease and diabetes (POPADAD) trial: factorial randomised placebo controlled trial of aspirin and antioxidants in patients with diabetes and asymptomatic peripheral arterial disease. BMJ 2008; 337:1840.
76. Ogawa H, Nakayama M, Morimoto T, et al. Low-dose aspirin for the primary prevention of atherosclerotic events in patients with type 2 diabetes: a randomized controlled trial. JAMA 2008;300:2134-41.
77. Majerus PW, Tollefsen DM. Blood coagulation and anticoagulant, thrombolytic and antiplatelet drugs. In: Goodman & Gilman's The Pharmacological Basis of Therapeutics. Brunton LL, Lazo JS, Parker KL, Eds. 11th Edition. McGraw-Hill. Philadelphia, PA.
78. Diener HC, Cunha L, Forbes C, Sivenius J, Smets P, Lowenthal A.European Stroke Prevention Study 2. Dipyridamole and acetylsalicylic acid in the secondary prevention of stroke. J Neurol Sci 1996;143:1-13.
79. Hollopeter G, Jantzen HM, Vincent D, Li G, England L, Ramakrishnan V, et al. Identification of the platelet ADP receptor targeted by antithrombotic drugs. Nature 2001;409:202-7.
80. Bhatt DL, Fox KA, Hacke W, Berger PB. Clopidogrel and aspirin versus aspirin alone For the prevention of atherothrombotic events. CHARISMA Investigators. N Engl J Med 2006; 354:1706-17.
81. CAPRIE Steering Committee. A randomised, blinded, trial of clopidogrel versus aspirin in patients at risk of ischemic events (CAPRIE). Lancet 1996;348:1329-39.
82. Juurlink DN, Gomes T, Ko DT, et al. A population-based study of the drug interaction between proton pump inhibitors and clopidogrel. CMAJ 2009;180:713-8.
83. Ho MP, Maddox TM, Wang Li, Fihn SD, et al. Risk of adverse outcomes associated with concomitant use of clopidogrel and proton pump inhibitors following acute coronary syndromes. JAMA2009;301:937-44.
84. Dawson DL, Cutler BS, Meissner MH, Strandness DE Jr. Cilostazol has beneficial effects in treatment of

intermittent claudication: results from a multicenter, randomized, prospective, double-blind trial. Circulation 1998;98:678-86.

85. Money SR, Herd JA, Isaacsohn JL, et al. Effect of cilostazol on walking distances in patients with intermittent claudication caused by peripheral vascular disease. J Vasc Surg 1998;27:267-74.
86. Lehert P, Comte S, Gamand S, Brown TM. Naftidrofuryl in intermittent claudication: a retrospective analysis. J Cardiovasc Pharmacol 1994;23(suppl 3):S48-S52.
87. Greenhalgh RM, Belch JJ, Brown LC, Gaines PA, et al. The adjuvant benefit of angioplasty in patients with mild to moderate intermittent claudication (MIMIC) managed by supervised exercise, smoking cessation advice and best medical therapy: results from two randomised trials for stenotic femoropopliteal and aortoiliac arterial disease. Eur J Vasc Endovasc Surg 2008;36:680-8.
88. Bolia A, Miles K, Brennan J, Bell P. Percutaneous transluminal angioplasty of occlusions of the femoral and popliteal arteries by subintimal dissection. Cardiovasc Intervent Radiol 1990;13:357-63.
89. Palmaz JC, Tio FO, Schatz RA, et al. Early endothelialization of balloon expandable stents: experimental observations. J Intervent Radiol 1988;3:119-24.
90. Fischman DL, Leon MB, Baim DS, et al. A randomised comparison of coronary stent placement and balloon angioplasty in the treatment of coronary artery disease. Stent Restenosis Study Investigators. N Engl J Med 1994;331:496-501.
91. Duda SH, Pusich B, Richter G, et al. Sirolimus eluting stents for the treatment of obstructive superficial femoral artery disease: 6- month results. Circulation 2002;106:1505-9.
92. Duda SH, Bosiers M, Lammer J, et al. Drug-eluting and bare nitinol stents for the treatment of atherosclerotic lesions in the superficial femoral artery: long-term results from the SIROCCO trial. J Endovasc Ther 2006;13:701-10.
93. Stettler C, Wandel S, Allemann S, et al. Outcomes associated with drug-eluting and bare-metal stents: a collaborative network analysis. Lancet 2007;370: 937-48.
94. Tepe G, Zeller T, Albrecht T, Heller S, et al. Local delivery of paclitaxel to inhibit restenosis during angioplasty of the leg. N Engl J Med 2008;358:689-99.
95. Schulman ML, Badhey MR, Yatco R. Superficial femoral-popliteal veins and reversed saphenous veins as primary femoropopliteal bypass grafts: a randomized comparative study. J Vasc Surg 1987;6:1-10.
96. Wengerter KR, Veith FJ, Gupta SK, et al. Prospective randomized multicenter comparison of in situ and reversed vein infrapopliteal bypasses. J Vasc Surg 1991;13:189-97.
97. Moody AP, Edwards PR, Harris PL. In situ versus reversed femoropopliteal vein grafts. Long-term follow-up of a prospective, randomized trial. Br J Surg 1992;79:750-2.
98. Tarry WC, Walsh DB, Birkmeyer NJ, et al. Fate of the contralateral leg after infrainguinal bypass. J Vasc Surg 1998;27:1039-47.
99. Holzenbein TJ, Pomposelli FB Jr, Miller A, et al. Results of a policy with arm veins used as the first alternative to an unavailable ipsilateral greater saphenous vein for infrainguinal bypass. J vasc Surg 1996;23:130-40.
100. Trans-Atlantic Inter-Society Consensus (TASC) Working Group.Management of peripheral arterial disease (PAD). J Vasc Surg 2000;31:S1-S296.
101. Tetteroo E, Van der Graaf T, Bosch JL, et al. Randomised comparison of primary stent placement versus primary angioplasty followed by selective stent placement in patients with iliac-artery occlusive disease. Dutch Iliac Stent Trial Study Group. Lancet 1998;1153-9.
102. Schillinger M, Sabeti S, Loewe C, et al. Balloon angioplasty versus implantation of nitinol stents in the superficial femoral artery. N Engl J Med 2006;354:1879-88.
103. Veith FJ, Gupta SK, Ascer E, et al. Six-year prospective multicenter randomized comparison of autologous saphenous vein and expanded polytetrafluoroethylene grafts in infrainguinal arterial reconstructions. J Vasc Surg 1986;3:104-14.
104. Michaels JA. Choice of material for above-knee femoropopliteal bypass graft. Br J Surg 2003;90:57-8.
105. Kumar KP, Crinnon JN, Ashley S, Gough MJ. Vein, PTFE orDacron for above knee femoropopliteal bypass. Int Angiol 1995;14:200-5.
106. Harris PL, Veith FJ, Shanik GD, et al. Prospective randomized comparison of in situ and reversed infrapopliteal vein grafts. Br J Surg 1993;80:173-6.
107. Watlet J, Soury P, Menard JF, et al. Femoro-popliteal bypass: in situ or reversed vein grafts? Ten-year results of a randomized prospective study. Ann Vasc Surg 1997;510-19.
108. Abbott WM, Green RM, Matsumoto T, et al. Prosthetic above- knee femoropopliteal bypass grafting: results of a multicenter randomized prospective trial. Above-Knee Femoropopliteal Study Group. J Vasc Surg 1997;25:19-28.

109. Robinson BI, Fletcher JP, Tomlinson P, et al. A prospective randomized multicenter comparison of expanded polytetra- f luoroethylene and gelatine-sealed knitted Dacron grafts for femoropopliteal bypass. Cardiovasc Surg 1999;7:214-18.

110. Stonebridge PA, Prescott RJ, Ruckley CV. Randomized trial comparing infrainguinal polytetrafluoroethylene bypass grafting with and without vein interposition cuff at the distal anastomosis. The Joint Vascular Research Group. J Vasc Surg 1997;26:543-50.

111. Hunink MG, Wong JB, Donaldson MC, Meyerovitz MF, Harrington DP. Patency results of percutaneous and surgical revascularization for femoropopliteal arterial disease. Med Decis Making 1994;14:71-81.

112. Antiplatelet Trialists' Collaboration. Collaborative overview of randomised trials of antiplatelet therapy. II. Maintenance of vascular graft or arterial patency by antiplatelet therapy. Br Med J 1994;308:159-68.

113. Henke PK, Blackburn S, Proctor MC, et al. Patients undergoing infrainguinal bypass to treat atherosclerotic vascular disease are under prescribed cardio protective medications: effect on graft patency, limb salvage and mortality. J Vasc Surg 2004;39:357-65.

114. Sarac TP, Huber TS, Back MR, et al. Warfarin improves the outcome of infrainguinal vein bypass grafting at high risk for failure. J Vasc Surg 1998;28:446-57.

115. Arfvidsson B, Lundgren F, Drott C, Schersten T, Lundholm K.Influence of coumarin treatment on patency and limb salvage after peripheral arterial reconstructive surgery. Am J Surg 1990;159-60.

116. Edmonson RA, Cohen AT, Das SK, Wagner MB, Kakkar VV.Low-molecular-weight heparin versus aspirin and dipyridamole after femoropopliteal bypass grafting. Lancet 1994;344:914-8.

117. Wolf GL, Wilson SE, Cross AP, Deupree RH, Stason WB. Surgery or balloon angioplasty for peripheral vascular disease: a randomized clinical trial. J Vasc Intervent Radiol 1993;4:639-48.

118. Holm J, Arfvidsson B, Jivegard L, et al. Chronic lower limb ischemia. A prospective randomised controlled study comparing the 1-year results of vascular surgery and percutaneous transluminal angioplasty (PTA). Eur J Vasc Surg 1991;5:517-22.

119. Adam DJ, Beard JD, Cleveland T, et al. Bypass versus angioplasty in severe ischemia of the leg (BASIL): Multicenter, randomised controlled trial. Lancet 2005;366:1925-34.

120. Lundell A, Lindblad B, Bergqvist D, Hansen F. Femoropopliteal- cural graft patency is improved by an intensive surveillance program: a prospective randomised study. J Vasc Surg 1995;21:26-33.

121. Loosemore TM, Chalmers TC, Dormady JA. A meta-analysis of randomized placebo control trials in Fontaine stages III and IV peripheral occlusive arterial disease. Int Angiol 1994;13:133-42.

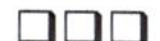

43

CHAPTER

Abdominal Aortic Diseases

Nav Yash Gupta, MD, FACS

INTRODUCTION

Although it is true that the art and science of vascular surgery has many basic universal tenants, from a practical standpoint (1) variance in specific disease patterns, (2) the set up for delivery of health care, and (3) the availability of resources and devices specific to vascular and endovascular procedures necessitates that the practice of vascular surgery be tailored to locations such as India and other developing countries.

Vascular surgery, as a separate specialty, has been slow to develop in India. This is related to several factors including the fact that the disease processes are not well recognized and remain under-diagnosed. In addition, most peripheral vascular procedures have traditionally been performed by cardiothoracic surgeons and endovascular procedures currently are often performed by interventional radiologists in India. Only a few centers provide dedicated training in the field of vascular surgery and endovascular techniques, which have become an integral part of the treatment options for vascular diseases in most western countries. These techniques have not been widely disseminated in India.

ANATOMY AND EXPOSURE

The aortic root originates at the ventricular outflow tract of the heart and includes the aortic valve, the sinuses of Valsalva, and the left and right coronary arteries. The aorta ends at the aortic bifurcation in the abdomen and divides into the right and left common iliac arteries, approximately at the level of the second lumbar vertebral body. The ascending aorta curves posterior and to the left as the aortic arch and the brachiocephalic vessels originate from the aortic arch. They include the brachiocephalic (innominate), left common carotid and left subclavian arteries. The descending thoracic aorta begins just beyond the left subclavian artery and ends at the 12th intercostal space. The descending thoracic aorta gives off intercostal, bronchial, and esophageal arteries. The artery of Adamkiewicz, which is the main source of blood supply to the lower part of the anterior spinal artery, has a variable origin but generally branches from an intercostal artery that originates between the 9th and 12th intercostal spaces. This artery supplies much of the blood flow to the spinal cord. The aorta exits the thorax and enters the abdomen through the aortic hiatus.

Exposure of the brachiocephalic vessels is usually accomplished through a median sternotomy approach. A limited or "mini" sternotomy can also provide exposure to all these vessels other than the first portion of the left subclavian artery. The mini sternotomy requires a partial median sternotomy and then a transverse transaction of the sternum at the third intercostal space. Exposure of the left subclavian artery for reconstruction of traumatic injuries requires a left anterolateral thoracotomy through the fourth intercostal space. If it is anticipated that distal control of the left subclavian artery will be required, a supraclavicular incision is often added.

Wide exposure of the thoracoabdominal aorta is best accomplished via a thoracoabdominal incision going through the fourth or fifth intercostal space. The patient is positioned in a right lateral decubitus position with the aid of a beanbag and support of the left upper extremity on a cushioned stand. The level of the rib interspace incision is determined by the extent to which the aorta needs to be exposed and if access is only required to the distal thoracic aorta this can be done through the seventh or eighth intercostal space.

In the abdomen, the visceral vessels originate (i.e., the Celiac and superior mesenteric arteries). The renal arteries originate below the superior mesenteric artery, and then the inferior mesenteric artery comes off below this level. The aorta ends at the aortic bifurcation in the abdomen and divides into the right and left common iliac arteries, approximately at the level of the second lumbar vertebral body. The common iliac arteries divide into the internal and external iliac arteries and the external iliac artery becomes the common femoral artery at the level of the inguinal ligament.

Small arteries arising from the supraceliac aorta include the inferior phrenic and left adrenal arteries. The main branches of the abdominal aorta include the celiac trunk which branches into the left gastric, the splenic artery, and the common hepatic artery. The superior mesenteric artery arises more inferiorly, and the renal arteries traverse in a posterolateral direction. The left renal vein crosses anteriorly over the aorta. Exposure of the proximal renal arteries at this level requires mobilization of the left renal vein including ligation and division of draining venous tributaries.

Exposure of the infrarenal aorta can be accomplished via a midline transperitoneal approach with retraction of the small bowel to the right side and mobilization of the third and fourth portions of the duodenum. This segment of the aorta can also be exposed through an oblique incision in the left subcostal region with division of the left rectus, oblique, and transversus muscles. Medial visceral rotation is then performed by mobilization of the spleen, pancreas, and left colon with or without mobilization of the left kidney.

CONGENITAL ANOMALIES

Aortic anomalies generally involve various branching patterns of the brachiocephalic vessels. The most common branching pattern is the brachiocephalic trunk, followed by the left common carotid artery, and then the left subclavian artery (75%). A bovine arch describes the pattern in which the brachiocephalic trunk and left common carotid arteries share a common origin off the aortic arch (20%), followed by branching of the left subclavian artery. Infrequently (3%), there are separate origins for the brachiocephalic, left common carotid, left vertebral, and left subclavian arteries.

Other more rare anomalies are associated with an anomalous aortic arch and can result in a partial or complete ring around the trachea or esophagus with symptoms related to compression. A right-sided aortic arch and a left ligamentum arteriosum associated with a left retroesophageal subclavian artery can result in an esophageal diverticulum known as Kommerell's diverticulum. Another anomaly involves an aberrant right subclavian artery which arises from the descending thoracic aorta (0.5%), distal to the left subclavian artery. The right subclavian artery then traverses posterior to the trachea and esophagus which can result in compression of the esophagus by the aberrant blood vessel and causes dysphagia (dysphagia lusoria).

Although a patent ductus arteriosus is the most common vascular anomaly (5-10% of all congenital heart diseases), coarctation, which refers to a narrowing of the aortic wall lumen, accounts for 5-8% of congenital heart diseases. Coarctation most commonly occurs distal to the ligamentum, but it can occur just proximal to a patent ductus arteriosus. Chronic coarctation results in extensive formation of collateral intercostals arteries, proximal hypertension, and rib notching. Traditionally these patients are treated with resection of the aortic isthmus and primary anastomosis. More recently balloon angioplasty has emerged as an alternative treatment, although the long-term results are unknown.

Abdominal aortic coarctation and hypoplasia is an uncommon entity and may be focal or diffuse in nature. The cause of abdominal aortic coarctation may be related to intrauterine developmental events. Often multiple renal arteries are seen in these patients and the majority of these patients have associated renal artery stenosis which can lead to renovascular hypertension from activation of the renin-angiotensin system. Splanchnic artery occlusive disease is less commonly associated with this disease process. Additionally, it may not be as clinically relevant as renal artery stenosis because of the extensive mesenteric collateral network. Treatment can be medical management of hypertension, as well as operative approaches tailored to the specific disease process of the patient. Again, more recently, percutaneous balloon angioplasty has been advocated by some, but is not widely accepted as an appropriate treatment for this disease process.

VENOUS ANOMALIES

The most common venous anomaly is a persistent left superior vena cava, which drains into the right atrium through an enlarged orifice of the coronary sinus. This anomaly can be important to recognize during surgical procedures requiring central venous access. The most common anomaly of the inferior vena cava is an interruption of its course in the abdomen, with drainage to the heart via the azygos or hemiazygos venous system. Anatomic variants of the left renal vein are estimated to be present in up to 10% of patients and the most common variants include a retro-aortic vein and a circumaortic venous collar encircling the aorta. If these variants are not recognized at the time of aortic dissection the result can be a significant venous injury and substantial hemorrhage.

AORTIC DISEASE

Atherosclerotic aortic disease is generally divided into occlusive disease and aneurysmal disease. Current treatment concepts and understanding of the treatment of aortic disease should be attributed to various pioneers including Rudolph Matas. In the 1880s, Matas described the technique of endoaneurysmorrhaphy in which the aneurysm sac is actually opened, and the contents evacuated. Alexis Carrel is credited with perfecting the technique of repairing a blood vessel and performing an end-to-end anastomosis using suture and the triangulation technique. He also described patch angioplasty to prevent luminal narrowing of a longitudinal arteriotomy. Rene Leriche, a student of Carrel's, described aortoiliac occlusive disease. In an article published in 1940, Leriche described the constellation of symptoms seen typically in men with severe aortoiliac occlusive disease: absent femoral pulses, lower extremity muscle atrophy, and impotence.

In France in 1951, Charles Dubost performed the first aneurysm resection and replacement with an aortic homograft. In the late 1950's Arthur Vorhees worked extensively on developing appropriate synthetic substitutes and in 1957 Charles DeBakey described a successful treatment of aortic aneurysms using a knitted Dacron graft as the replacement. The description of endovascular treatment of aortic aneurysms by Juan Parodi in 1991 revolutionized the treatment of abdominal aortic aneurysms.

AORTOILIAC OCCLUSIVE DISEASE

Overview

Risk factors for the development of atherosclerotic disease in general include tobacco abuse, diabetes mellitus, hypertension, and dyslipidemia. In addition, advanced age, male gender, and a family history seem to be non-modifiable risk factors for this. There is some evidence to suggest that race, hypercoagulable states, and chronic renal insufficiency also play a role. Atherosclerotic disease of the abdominal aorta and iliac arteries is a common cause of lower extremity ischemia in middle-aged and elderly patients in Western society, however its prevalence in India is not known. Claudication is pain or discomfort that occurs in large muscle groups in the lower limbs with exercise. This discomfort is typically reproducible and resolves with rest. Because of the level of occlusion, aortoiliac occlusive disease usually results in claudication of the more proximal muscle groups including the buttocks, hips, and thighs, although these patients can also complain of calf claudication. In male patients, limitation of blood flow to the internal iliac artery circulation can result in impotence. The constellation of symptoms in men including diminished femoral pulses, buttock claudication, muscle atrophy, and impotence is known as Leriche syndrome.

Although claudication is a common symptom in these patients, because of the extensive collateral circulation that can develop around chronic aortoiliac occlusive disease, they rarely present with rest pain or ischemic tissue loss and gangrene. Rest pain is a sign of advanced ischemia that typically occurs in the forefoot across the metatarsal heads. Often patients describe this pain as occurring at night when they are in a recumbent position, and it may be relieved by dangling the affected extremity in a dependent position. Typically, multilevel occlusive disease such as that affecting the aortoiliac segment as well as the femoro-popliteal segment can result in rest pain and tissue loss. In addition, embolization of an atherosclerotic plaque from the diseased aorta can result in painful patches of ischemic tissue in the digits, although the perfusion to the feet at baseline may appear to be adequate. In these patients, studies such as CT angiography may confirm a more proximal source of atheroemboli.

The disease process usually affects the distal abdominal aorta and the proximal common iliac arteries, but it can progress to complete occlusion of the aorta with preservation of flow into the renal arteries. The supra-renal aorta, renal vessels, and visceral vessels are less commonly involved.

Diagnosis

The importance of the history and physical exam cannot be understated. Symptoms suggestive of claudication combined with diminished or absent femoral pulses suggest an aortoiliac occlusive disease. As noted previously, tissue loss is uncommon and at rest the legs may appear quite well perfused. However, muscle atrophy may be seen and a history of impotence in a male patient can also aid in the diagnosis.

Segmental Doppler pressures are usually noted to be abnormal at all levels including the high thigh level. Measuring ankle pressures at rest and after a period of exercise may help unmask the more proximal inflow disease. The ankle pressures are noted to drop significantly after exercise. If available, Doppler waveform analysis or pulse volume recordings (PVR) can also help in the diagnosis, although these are not essential.

Surgical Treatment

Treatment varies depending on the severity of the symptoms and the co-morbidities of the patient. Consensus guidelines for management of patients with aorto-iliac occlusive disease include the Trans-Atlantic Inter-Society Consensus Document on the Management of Peripheral Arterial Disease (TASC) published in the year 2000[1,2] and the Inter-Society Consensus for the Management of Peripheral Arterial Disease (TASC II) published in the year 2007.[3] Patients with severe, diffuse aortoiliac occlusive disease or complete occlusion of the aorta (Figure 1) are best treated with aortobifemoral bypass. This is an involved operation using a bifurcated prosthetic graft (knitted Dacron or ePTFE), requiring either an end-to-end or end-to-side anastomosis between the infra-renal aorta and the graft, and an end-to-side anastomoses between the graft and the femoral arteries in the groin which may need to be endarterectomized if there is significant plaque at this level. This procedure requires appropriate patient selection, a skilled surgeon, and adequate anesthetic and post-operative support, initially in an intensive care setting. The mortality rate associated with this procedure in the literature ranges from

2-4%, with an excellent 5-year patency rate of over 90%.[4] Correction of the proximal (aortoiliac) occlusive disease is sufficient to result in resolution of symptoms, unless the patient has extensive tissue loss in which case an outflow procedure such as a femoropopliteal bypass may need to be added at the same time. This adds to the length of the procedure and potentially the morbidity and mortality associated with it. If the patient is considered to be too high-risk for a transabdominal aortic procedure, an alternative may be an axillary-femoral or bifemoral procedure for bilateral occlusive disease. If only a single iliac artery is involved, a cross-over femoro-femoral bypass may be an acceptable option. These bypasses can be performed with an 8mm externally supported ePTFE graft or a 7mm Dacron graft. Another reasonable option may be a unilateral ilio-femoral bypass performed via a retro-peritoneal incision, but it is critical to ensure that there is adequate inflow from the aorta into the native iliac artery.

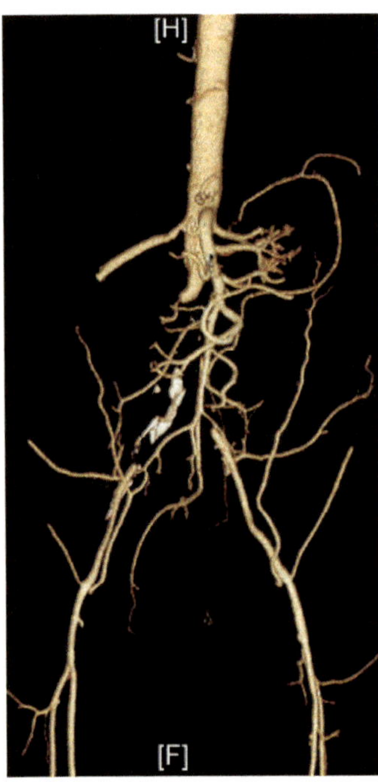

Figure 1: 3-Dimensional CTA image showing occlusion of the aorta below the renal arteries with reconstitution of the iliac arteries

Endovascular Treatment

Percutaneous endoluminal treatment of atherosclerotic disease of blood vessels was introduced by Dotter in 1963. However, this technique did not gain widespread acceptance until 1976 when Gruntzig introduced the angioplasty balloon made of polyvinyl chloride. With the rapid evolution of the technology, stents, and endovascular techniques, endoluminal treatment of atherosclerotic occlusive disease has become an important modality in the treatment of this disease process.

Stents

Often balloon angioplasty alone is not sufficient to treat these chronic atherosclerotic occlusive lesions. In this situation, stents may be used. A stent provides a mechanical scaffold within the diseased segment of the blood vessel to maintain patency. Stents should be relatively flexible and durable with a small profile prior to deployment so they can be introduced into the vascular system percutaneously with the aid of a sheath. A sheath is first introduced into the blood vessel to protect it, minimize blood loss, and help with introduction of wires, catheters, balloons, and stents into the vascular system. Fluoroscopic imaging, preferably digital subtraction imaging, is generally required for proper positioning of the balloons and deployment of stents. Stents are categorized as self-expanding and balloon expandable. Self-expanding stents are usually constrained within a delivery sheath, and after introduction into the vascular system over a guide wire, the constraining sheath is withdrawn allowing the stent to expand within the vessel. Although these stents are more flexible than balloon-expandable ones, they have lower radial force against the blood vessel. Some self-expanding stents are made of nitinol (a nickel-titanium alloy) which has a unique temperature associated memory and, while the stent can be constrained at cool temperatures, when it is exposed to warm body temperatures it assumes the original coil spring shape that it had when it was manufactured at elevated temperatures. Balloon-expandable stents are initially mounted onto a balloon and once positioned within the diseased segment of the blood vessel, the stent is deployed by inflating the balloon. These stents can generally be expanded to larger diameters with larger balloons. They have better radial force against the blood vessel but tend to be more rigid and less suited for tortuous blood vessel segments.

Stents can be used to treat occlusive diseases in the aorta, common iliac arteries, and external iliac arteries. Focal atherosclerotic lesions can be adequately treated with balloon angioplasty alone. However, if there is a residual stenosis, or an intimal tear with a flap or dissection, a stent may be indicated. A residual stenosis is considered hemodynamically significant if there is a greater than 10 mmHg pressure gradient across the area of stenosis. Short-segment complete-occlusions of the iliac arteries can also be treated endovascularly if the lesion can be traversed with a wire and the true lumen of the blood vessel can re-enter beyond the occlusion. In this scenario, a stent is generally necessary, however, pre-dilation of the occluded area may ease passage of the stent. If the level of disease is in the very proximal common iliac segment, it essentially represents aortic disease that extends into the iliac arteries. In this situation, treating just one of the iliac arteries may result in compromise of the lumen of the contralateral iliac artery by plaque being pushed over to that side. A reasonable option in this case would be to treat both proximal common iliac arteries with stents (Figure 2). Although the patency of endoluminal treatment of aortoiliac disease has improved in the past several years, the long-term patency is limited by the development of intimal hyperplasia leading to re-stenosis. The advantages of endovascular therapy include a high technical success rate with a low morbidity and mortality. Endovascular procedures in the more proximal arterial beds appear to be more durable than those in the distal arteries and, even if the initial endovascular therapy fails, the possibility of re-intervention (either endovascular or operative) remains an option in these patients. Review of the literature suggests that the 2-year primary and secondary patency rates for the treatment of complex aortoiliac occlusive disease range from 69-76% and 85-96% respectively.[5,6,7]

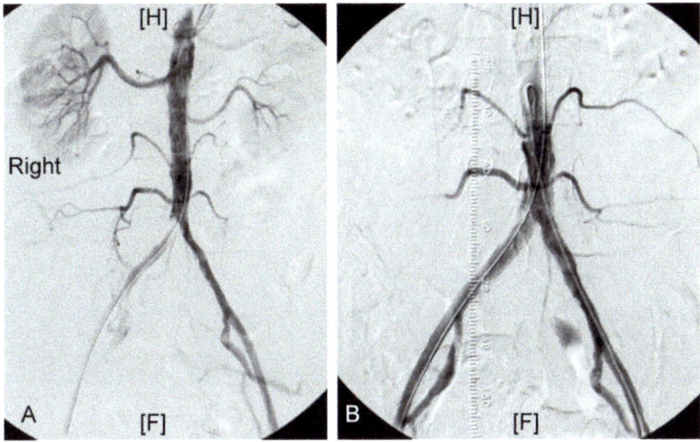

Figure 2: Digital subtraction angiograms showing bilateral iliac occlusive disease pre (A) and post (B) iliac stenting

AORTIC ANEURYSMAL DISEASE

Overview

Aneurysms of the abdominal aorta are relatively common in the Western world with an increasing incidence, it is less common in Asian and African populations, and the incidence of aortic aneurysmal disease in India is unknown. The disease entity does exist, and the true incidence is probably underestimated. An aneurysm is defined as a focal dilatation of an artery to at least 1.5 times its normal diameter. Most abdominal aortic aneurysms (AAAs) are true aneurysms that include all three layers of the arterial wall and are atherosclerotic in origin. False or pseudoaneurysms of the abdominal aorta can occur and are related to trauma, infection, or can occur at anastomotic sites from prior surgical procedures. The aneurysms can be fusiform in nature with diffuse dilation, or saccular in nature with an abrupt outpouching of the vessel. The majority of AAAs are infrarenal (over 90%) and patients with an AAA are more likely to have aneurysms of other blood vessels. It is estimated that up to 15% of patients with an AAA have popliteal artery aneurysms and 40-50% of patients with a popliteal artery aneurysm have an AAA. In addition, the majority (50-60%) of patients with a popliteal artery aneurysm will have a contralateral popliteal artery aneurysm.

Pathophysiology

Most (90%) AAAs are associated with atherosclerotic disease of the aorta. Risk factors associated with the development of aortic aneurysms include hypertension, tobacco abuse, advanced age, and being male (Table 1). Men significantly outnumber women by a factor of greater than 4 to 1.[8,9] Studies in the past decade have indicated that a decreased amount of elastin and collagen as well as increased levels of matrix-metalloproteinase (MMP)-2 and MMP-9, which may promote arterial wall degeneration, also play a role in the development of aneurysms. Rarer causes of AAA formation include various connective tissue disorders (i.e., Marfan's syndrome, Ehlers-Danlos syndrome), cystic medial necrosis, and syphilis.

Table 1: Risk factors associated with the development of aortic aneurysms

Risk Factors for Development of Aortic Aneurysms
Tobacco use
Hypertension
Dyslipidemia
Male gender
Family history

The natural history of an AAA is growth over time and, if left untreated, they rupture. The growth rate of an AAA in a particular patient cannot be predicted, however, on average most AAAs expand by about 3-4mm per year. The growth rate can be explained by the law of Laplace which essentially describes the relationship between the tangential stress (T) which causes disruption of the wall, and the radius (R) and the transmural pressure (P):

$$T = P \times R$$

As a general principle, the larger the aneurysm diameter, the higher the risk of rupture. AAAs less than 5cm in maximal diameter have a low risk of rupture (less than 2% per year). Once an AAA gets to 7cm or greater in diameter, the risk of rupture is estimated to be 20-30% per year. Women tend to rupture at slightly smaller sizes compared to men.

Diagnosis and Clinical Findings

Most aneurysms are asymptomatic until the aortic wall begins to become disrupted. Unfortunately, once an AAA causes symptoms with abdominal or back pain, the patient is usually quite critical. Most patients in this situation do not survive and may not even make it to the hospital because of the large volume of blood loss and subsequent cardiovascular collapse. A ruptured AAA should be suspected in a patient with severe abdominal or back pain, hypotension, and abdominal distention, or possibly a pulsatile abdominal mass. These patients should be rushed to the operating theater for an urgent laparotomy. In this situation, the rupture may be contained in the retroperitoneum but will eventually progress to free intraperitoneal rupture if not treated. In some instances, the AAA may cause symptoms such as distal embolization of the thrombus to the lower extremities, thrombosis of the aneurysm with acute arterial insufficiency of the lower extremities, or pain prior to rupture. In the elective setting, the diagnosis can be made by palpation of a pulsatile abdominal mass on physical exam if the aneurysm is of a significant size. These patients should be examined for possible iliac, femoral, or popliteal artery aneurysms as well. To properly determine the size of the aneurysm and the anatomical relationship to the renal arteries and visceral vessels, imaging techniques such as ultrasonography and computed tomography (CT) are useful. For screening purposes and follow-up of known aortic aneurysms, B-mode ultrasonography is sufficient, however a trained technician or physician should perform the test to get accurate information. This imaging modality is relatively inexpensive and does not involve any radiation. Limitations of ultrasound include poor visualization secondary to bowel gas and somewhat imprecise measurements of aneurysm size. CT can give more detailed information regarding the size and extent of the aneurysm, its relationship to the renal and visceral vessels and the iliac arteries, and assess for the presence of retroperitoneal hemorrhage. Contrast-enhanced CT scans can give very detailed information regarding the patency of branch vessels and can allow for detailed measurements that are needed for endovascular treatment of aneurysms (Figure 3). Aortography has limitations in the detection of aortic aneurysms and the evaluation of the true diameter of the aneurysm. This is because many aneurysms are filled with chronic laminated thrombus that lines the walls of the aneurysm sac to varying degrees. The iodinated contrast agent flows only in the lumen of the blood vessel and this can significantly underestimate the size of the aneurysm. Several studies including the UK Small Aneurysm Trial [10] and the US-based Aneurysm Detection and Management (ADAM) trial[11] have demonstrated that yearly surveillance is adequate for AAAs up to 4.5cm in diameter and surveillance at 6-month intervals should be performed for AAAs measuring between 4.5 and 5.5 cm in diameter. New recommendations in the United States suggest an AAA screening ultrasound for all men over the age of 65 who have smoked, or for men and women who have a family history of aneurysms. This may be impractical in countries such as India where health care resources are scarce and health insurance coverage for the majority of the population is non-existent. In patients that present with symptoms, the test of choice is a rapid CT scan with contrast if the patient is hemodynamically stable. If the patient is unstable then the diagnosis is made based on history and presentation and the patient should be rapidly transported to the operating room for repair of the AAA. Although CT scanning can confirm the diagnosis of a ruptured AAA with retroperitoneal hemorrhage, there are no other specific CT scan findings that have been shown to accurately predict "impending" rupture. [12]

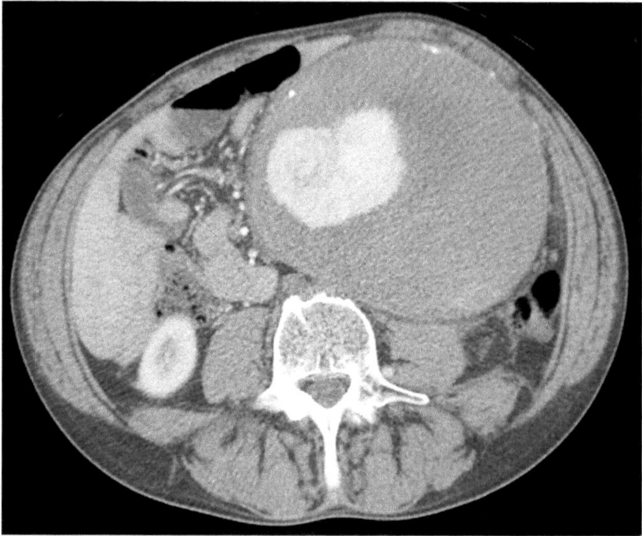

Figure 3: Cross-sectional CT image showing a large abdominal aortic aneurysm

Treatment

The decision for treatment of aortic aneurysmal disease can be complex due to factors such as the anatomy of the aneurysm, patient co-morbidities and life expectancy, and the risk of the operative procedure. In general, infra-renal AAAs should be considered for elective repair at a diameter of 5cm in women and 5.5cm in men. A rapid aneurysm growth rate of over 5 mm in a 6-month period has also been suggested as reason to proceed with aneurysm repair. Other factors that mandate repair (Table 2) in the appropriate clinical setting include symptomatic aneurysms, need for concomitant iliac or thoracic aneurysm repair, mycotic aneurysms, and significant saccular aneurysms (Figure 4). A thorough medical and surgical history allows for a more complete preoperative evaluation of the patient as well as appropriate surgical planning. Pre-operative evaluation should include a thorough cardiopulmonary evaluation. Underlying cardiac dysfunction is the leading cause of mortality after AAA repair[13] and patients with severe coronary artery disease (CAD), unstable angina, a diminished ejection fraction in the range of 25-30%, severe valvular heart disease (aortic valve area < 1 cm^2), and congestive heart failure are considered very high risk for operative repair. These patients may benefit from pre-operative cardiac stress testing and intraoperative use of a trans-esophageal echocardiography (TEE) may help guide management in the operating room. Perioperative heart rate control with beta blockade may be of benefit, and several randomized, controlled studies have demonstrated that beta-blockade in high risk patients reduces cardiac morbidity and death.[14,15] Other factors that adversely affect outcomes after AAA repair include chronic renal insufficiency with a serum creatinine of greater than 2.5 mg/dL and severe pulmonary dysfunction.[16,17,18] Smoking is probably the most important risk factor for the development of aortic aneurysms and also predisposes to aneurysm expansion and rupture. Patients that are smokers should be strongly encouraged to cease smoking for at least 2 weeks prior to elective aneurysm repair. Patients with significant comorbidities should only undergo repair after optimizing their medical status and in the setting of adequate anesthetic support and peri-operative intensive care monitoring. Patients with ruptured AAA (Figure 5) should be rapidly transported to the operating room for operative repair. Aggressive resuscitation should be avoided in these patients and their abdomen should be prepared prior to induction of anesthesia as they may become profoundly hypotensive upon induction of anesthesia. Rapid proximal control of the aorta in the supra-celiac position is recommended. Endovascular repair should only be attempted if there is an adequate setup including equipment, imaging, and endovascular devices readily available. Studies have demonstrated that surgeons who perform higher volumes of these procedures is associated with lower mortality in patients with ruptured AAA.[19] Hence transport of these critically ill patients to a higher volume center is probably warranted.

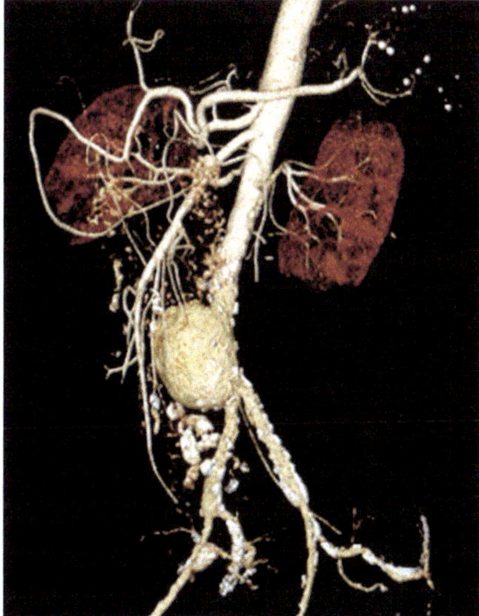

Figure 4: 3-D CTA showing a saccular aneurysm of the distal abdominal aorta

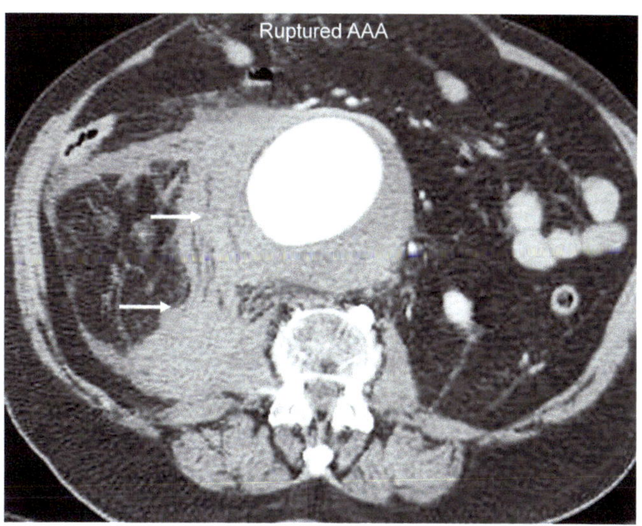

Figure 5: Cross-sectional CT image showing a ruptured abdominal aortic aneurysm. Note the large retroperitoneal hematoma (arrows)

Table 2: Indications for repair of abdominal aortic aneurysms

Indications for Repair of Aortic Aneurysms
Aortic aneurysm ≥ 5.5 cm in diameter in men
Aortic aneurysm ≥ 5 cm in diameter in women
Aneurysm expansion rate of ≥ 1cm per year
Symptomatic aneurysm
Need for concomitant iliac or thoracic aneurysm repair
Mycotic aneurysm
Saccular aneurysm

Open Repair

Traditional open surgical repair of AAAs involves either a midline trans-peritoneal incision or a left-sided retro-peritoneal incision with medial rotation of the visceral contents. A retro-peritoneal approach may be more suitable when the aneurysm extends to the juxta-renal segment or when the visceral vessels have to be addressed. The more normal infra-renal aortic neck and the common iliac arteries are exposed and prepared for clamping. The level of clamp application may vary depending on the extent of the aneurysm and the amount of calcification in the wall of the vessel, and the burden of atheromatous debris. After a systemic bolus of heparin, the vessels are clamped, the aneurysm is incised, the laminated thrombus contents is evacuated, there is back-bleeding from lumbar vessels and the inferior mesenteric artery is controlled, and either a straight tube or bifurcated Dacron or ePTFE graft is sewn in place using a permanent monofilament suture. The proximal anastomosis should be performed as close to the renal arteries as is practical to avoid leaving a long segment of native infra-renal aorta that may degenerate and become aneurysmal over time. If, for purposes of exposure, the left renal vein has to be divided, it should be divided as close to the inferior vena cava as possible to allow for collateral venous drainage of the kidney via the gonadal, adrenal, and lumbar veins. Significant aneurysmal disease of the iliac arteries generally requires placement of a bifurcated graft with the iliac limbs anastomosed to relatively healthy, non-aneurysmal iliac arteries. If the iliac arteries are healthy and non-aneurysmal, a tube graft can be sewn in place. It is important to maintain blood supply to the left colon and pelvis to avoid sexual dysfunction, buttock claudication, colonic ischemia, and rarely, spinal cord ischemia. In most patients the inferior mesenteric artery (IMA) can be ligated with impunity. However, in certain circumstances such as the presence of significant visceral occlusive disease or when hypogastric circulation cannot be directly maintained, consideration should be given for re-implantation of the IMA into the graft. This is aided by preserving a small island of native tissue around the orifice of the IMA (Carrel patch) to facilitate re-implantation. The residual aneurysm sac is then closed over the graft to protect the visceral contents and exclude the graft from the peritoneal contents. This can also aid in hemostasis. The operative mortality for elective repair of infra-renal AAAs is under 5% in low-risk patients.[20,21,22,23] If there is associated intra-abdominal pathology, it is generally left alone unless it has a life-threatening nature. Repair of gastrointestinal or genitourinary pathology is avoided to prevent bacterial contamination of the prosthetic graft. If there is a colonic malignancy causing obstruction, significant bleeding, or perforation, then it should be treated prior to aneurysm repair, generally with a diverting colostomy. In most other circumstances, aneurysm repair takes precedence.

Endovascular Repair

The development of endovascular techniques has led to the treatment of AAAs with endoluminally placed stent-grafts (Endovascular Aortic Aneurysm Repair – EVAR) and this modality is now gradually replacing open surgery for treatment of AAAs (Figure 6). In the United States, more than half of all AAAs are repaired endovascularly, however long-term durability is not well established. Although a significant number of AAAs are repaired with stent-grafts in Western countries, this technology has not gained widespread application in India and other developing countries. Several reasons can account for this including the need for sophisticated imaging equipment, the expense of procuring the stent-graft itself, and knowledge of the sophisticated wire and catheter techniques required to safely accomplish EVAR. Although in its infancy in India, EVAR could become much more widespread if surgeons are taught the endovascular skills and patients are not forced to bear the entire cost of these expensive devices. It is now well established that EVAR is associated with a lower perioperative mortality (<2%). The mortality rate for EVAR was noted to be significantly lower than for open repair in the DREAM and the EVAR -1 trails, which were both prospective, randomized trials. Specifically, the in-hospital mortality rates in the DREAM and EVAR-1 trials for EVAR were 1.2% and 1.7% compared to 4.6% and 6% for open repair, respectively.[24,25] Other benefits of EVAR include decreased blood loss, a shortened hospital stay, and a more rapid return to normal activities. Open aneurysm repair requires general anesthesia; however, it has been demonstrated that EVAR can be safely performed under regional and local anesthesia. EVAR requires an adequate segment of non-aneurysmal vessel at the proximal and distal fixation sites.[26] Various devices are commercially available on the market and there are advantages and disadvantages to each device. Some provide suprarenal fixation and others provide infrarenal fixation. Most of the devices are modular, but there are variances in radial force and fabric as well as the range of sizes available. In regards to sizes, the specific device are chosen by the physician based on the specific anatomy and measurements of the patient's aorta from CT imaging. The rapid advance of technology in this area holds the promise to significantly expand the future possibilities for endovascular repair in most patients with aneurysms. If the common iliac artery is aneurysmal, extension of the endograft to the external iliac artery is required. This involves exclusion of the hypogastric artery and several studies have shown that unilateral exclusion of a hypogastric artery is well tolerated.[27,28] Bilateral hypogastric artery occlusion can result in severe buttock claudication and erectile dysfunction, and in rare instances severe pelvic or colonic ischemia. The disadvantage of EVAR is that a small percentage of patients can have problems with sealing of the stent-graft against the normal blood vessel. This results in continued perfusion of the sac and pressure (endoleak) leading to growth of the sac over time, and potentially even rupture if left untreated. In addition, there can be issues with access to vessel injury, graft limb occlusion, and graft migration or disruption. Because of these issues, patients require regular follow-up and imaging studies (i.e., CT angiography) to detect any problems. The 30-day re-intervention rate is higher following EVAR (15-20%)[29] than with open surgical repair. Most of the problems can be treated via an endovascular means. Follow-up can be an issue in non-compliant patients or in patients that live a significant distance from the treatment center. There is also a monetary cost associated with the required follow-up imaging studies, and there is the potential for progressive renal dysfunction secondary to the contrast agents used in the CT or angiographic imaging studies.

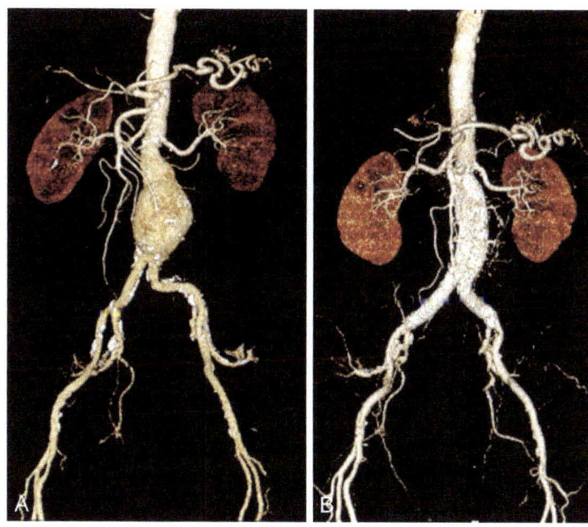

Figure 6: 3-D CTA of AAA pre (A) and post (B) placement of a modular bifurcated stent graft

Para-Visceral and Thoracoabdominal Aortic Aneurysms

When the aneurysmal aorta also involves the para-visceral or thoracic aorta, this presents a challenging situation both from a technical standpoint as well as perioperative care and management. Endovascular and hybrid (open and endovascular) techniques for repair of these types of aneurysms are evolving and these techniques have been employed to treat descending thoracic aortic aneurysms and traumatic aortic transaction.[30] More complex thoracoabdominal aortic aneurysms are best treated with open repair. These aneurysms are best approached with a left sided retroperitoneal incision and medial rotation of the visceral contents to expose an adequate amount of the normal supra-renal or supra-celiac aorta. The complications associated with paravisceral aortic aneurysm repair are similar to those seen with infra-renal AAA repair except that the incidence of complications is higher in patients with para-visceral aneurysms. This is related to the need for supra-renal or supra-celiac aortic clamping, which is associated with a period of renal and or visceral ischemia as well as increased cardiac stress. Complications include renal insufficiency, cardiac ischemia, respiratory failure, spinal cord ischemia, and mesenteric ischemia. These patients are also more likely to develop intraoperative coagulopathy and post-operative bleeding complications requiring re-exploration. As would be expected, the mortality rate associated with this repair is also higher (5-20%).[31]

Peri-Operative Care of Patients

Open aneurysm repair is performed under general anesthesia with muscle relaxants to allow for adequate retraction of the abdominal wall. Placement of an epidural catheter for infusion of analgesic medication after surgery may assist not only in pain control, but also in enabling a shorter time on the ventilator and early mobilization of the patient. EVAR can safely be performed under general, local, or regional anesthesia.

Blood loss during an open aneurysm repair can be significant. Pre-operative donations of autologous blood by the patient for elective operations may be of benefit, especially in countries where banked blood supply is limited. In addition, returning autologous blood to the patient intra-operatively using various blood cell salvage devices can preserve resources and minimize the need for banked blood transfusion. Use of transesophageal echocardiography can prove to be helpful in unstable patients or those who have a severely diminished cardiac reserve. It is critical to maintain body temperature during the aneurysm repair procedure to prevent acidosis, coagulopathy, and diminished cardiac function. In this regard, use of intravenous fluid warmers and forced air warming blankets are helpful. Nasogastric tube decompression is often performed after open aneurysm repair because of the laparotomy and presumed ileus; however, some studies have indicated that this is not necessary and may even be detrimental to the patient from a pulmonary standpoint.[32] Appropriate and adequate pain management after surgery can minimize cardiac and respiratory complications and allow for early extubation and mobilization. Deep venous thrombosis (DVT) prophylaxis is appropriate in this group of patients and can be performed with unfractionated heparin or low-molecular-weight heparin administered subcutaneously.

Long-Term Care of Patients

With open repair, concerns include incisional ventral hernia formation and bowel obstruction. Over time if the anastomosis is disrupted, para-anastomotic pseudoaneurysms can develop. These pseudoaneurysms can be difficult to treat, especially if they occur in the para-visceral segment of the abdominal aorta, and infection may predispose to the development of these false aneurysms. True aneurysms occur more frequently and can involve the supra-renal or paravisceral aorta, the iliac arteries, as well as the femoral and popliteal arteries. For this reason, patients should be seen at regular intervals for follow-up with imaging studies. Graft infection is an extremely rare but devastating complication of aneurysm repair.[33] If a bifurcated graft is used then limb occlusion can occur. This seems to be more common in women and in situations where the graft limb extends to the femoral artery. Limb occlusion can occur with both open and endovascular repair, however, there are certain complications that are unique to endovascular repair. The most frequent of these complications is endoleak where there is persistent blood flow into the aneurysm sac around the endograft. It is estimated to occur in as many as 25% of patients undergoing EVAR.[34] Endoleaks are classified based on the source of blood flow into the aneurysm sac (Figure 7). Type I endoleaks occur when there is an incomplete seal between the endograft material and the normal native vessel. Type IA describes a seal problem proximally and Type IB describes a lack of appropriate seal distally. In this situation, there is still significant pressurized blood entering the sac and the natural progression is that the sac will continue to enlarge and eventually rupture if left untreated. Once detected, these endoleaks should be fixed, either endovascularly or via an open procedure. Type II endoleaks occur because of retrograde flow into the sac either from lumbar arteries, the inferior mesenteric artery, or both. Although these types of endoleaks are much more common, they rarely need to be treated and usually resolve spontaneously. Type III endoleaks refer to blood flow into the sac from modular junctions, various components of the endograft that overlap with each other. These should be treated when detected. Type IV endoleaks are related to graft material porosity and these resolve without treatment. Another concern with EVAR is graft migration, either during deployment of the endograft, or detected in subsequent follow up imaging studies. If the migration results in an endoleak, it should be treated. For many of the above reasons, patients with the endograft implanted should be followed with routine imaging studies, typically a contrast enhanced CT scan, to detect problems. Some studies have shown the utility of color Duplex ultrasonography in the detection of endoleaks. However, at this time CT imaging remains the gold standard.

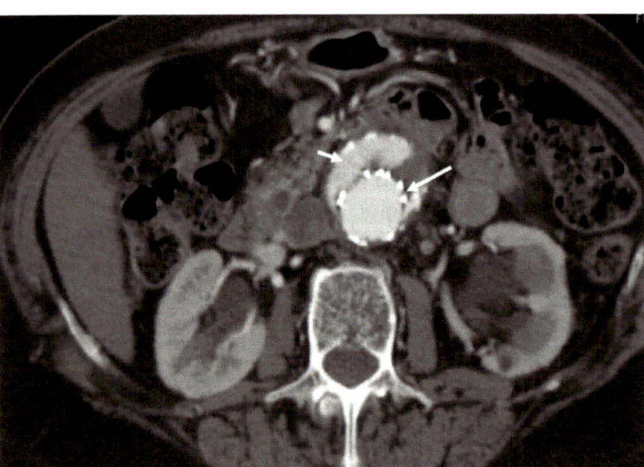

Figure 7: Cross-sectional CT image showing an endograft (arrow) in the aneurysm sac with persistent flow in the aneurysm sac demonstrating an endoleak (arrowhead)

Inflammatory Aneurysm

Inflammatory aneurysms are rare and typically have a thickened aortic wall and a dense fibrous rind around the aneurysm. The etiology of inflammatory aneurysms is poorly understood, and possibilities include infection, autoimmune response, or lymphatic obstruction. Patients may present with flank pain and weight loss and a majority of patients will have an elevated erythrocyte sedimentation rate. On CT imaging, the peri-aortic inflammatory tissue can be well visualized. Repair of these aneurysms can be technically challenging. Because of the fibrotic process, nearby structures such as the duodenum, left renal vein, vena cava, and ureters are often stuck to the aneurysm and can be easily injured in the process of mobilization. In fact, it is best to avoid extensive mobilization of the duodenum if possible. Preoperative placement of ureteral stents can help identify the ureters and prevent injury. EVAR may be a preferred approach if feasible. Following repair, the inflammatory process is noted to subside.

Aortocaval Fistula

Aortic aneurysms have been reported to perforate into the inferior vena cava or iliac vein in a small percentage of patients, estimated to occur in about 2-4% of all ruptured aneurysms. The mortality rate is estimated at about 30%. Patients can present with high-output cardiac failure as well as signs of venous hypertension including lower extremity edema, hematuria, and rectal bleeding. Hypoperfusion of the lower extremities with cyanosis can also be seen. On exam, these patients may have a palpable abdominal mass with a very loud murmur. Surgical treatment is required in these patients, and closure of the fistula is best accomplished from within the aneurysm sac. There is a high risk of bleeding and air embolism. Maneuvers that can assist with control of the venous bleeding during closure include manual compression with sponge sticks or use of a large balloon catheter. Following repair of the fistula, the aneurysm is repaired in the standard fashion.

Primary Aortoenteric Fistula

Primary aortoenteric fistulas are quite rare. Patients can present with gastrointestinal bleeding and abdominal pain. The majority of these patients have an AAA, and the patients can present with repeated episodes of sudden gastrointestinal bleeding or exsanguinating hemorrhage. CT scan may aid in the diagnosis, and upper endoscopy should include the 3rd and 4th portions of the duodenum as the fistula often involves this portion of the bowel. The recommended treatment is extra-anatomic bypass and repair of the intestinal defect. However, if the patient is unstable, an in-situ repair with an ePTFE graft can be performed. In this situation, a pedicle of omentum may be used to buttress the vascular anastomosis. Post-operative antibiotic treatment should be initiated.

Primary Mycotic Abdominal Aortic Aneurysm

Primary mycotic abdominal aortic aneurysms are another rare entity and can result from primary aortitis, septic emboli, or an adjacent infection that spreads to the aorta. Typical organisms include salmonella and staphylococcus. A CT scan can aid in the diagnosis with findings such as peri-aortic inflammation, rapid expansion or development of an aneurysm, and rupture. The treatment approach is similar to that for an aortoenteric fistula. As expected, EVAR is not a definitive treatment for this disease process as it does not treat the infected tissue. Additionally, reports in the literature describe a poor outcome for treatment of mycotic AAAs solely with EVAR.[35]

Horsesoe Kidney and AAA

This is an uncommon anomaly but when noted in the presence of an AAA appropriate planning is required to avoid renal ischemia. The kidney mass may be fused anterior to the aorta and often the ureters are displaced inferiorly. The isthmus of the kidney does not need to be divided and is generally avoided as it could result in injury to the renal collecting system. In this case, the isthmus can be mobilized, and the graft tunneled beneath it. In addition, multiple anomalous renal arteries may arise from the aorta and preservation of these arteries is essential for re-implantation into the graft. A retroperitoneal approach may facilitate management of the multiple renal arteries as the majority of the renal tissue can be displaced anteriorly. Endovascular repair is usually not feasible in this setting unless there are individual main renal arteries originating above the aneurysm.

Iliac Artery Aneurysms

Most iliac artery aneurysms are atherosclerotic in origin, occur in conjunction with aortic aneurysms, and are generally repaired at the same time. Isolated iliac aneurysms are rare and most iliac aneurysms occur in older males. Because of their pelvic location, iliac aneurysms may not be palpable on routine physical exam, but compression of adjacent structures including the bladder, rectum, lumbosacral nerves, and pelvic veins can often result in symptoms such as flank and groin pain. These aneurysms can remain undetected until imaging studies are performed, and the operative mortality rate of ruptured iliac aneurysms is quite high. Small isolated iliac aneurysms measuring less than 3.5cm in diameter can generally be observed while larger aneurysms should be repaired. When iliac aneurysmal disease is seen in association with an AAA, the disease is treated concomitant with repair of the AAA.

Femoral and Popliteal Artery Aneurysms

The most common peripheral artery aneurysms are popliteal and femoral artery aneurysms, and they are atherosclerotic in nature. These aneurysms are often bilateral in up to 50% of patients, and these patients often have an associated aortic aneurysm.

True femoral artery aneurysms can result in thromboembolic complications or rupture if they become large, and are generally repaired when they become larger than 2cm. Repair usually involves an interposition prosthetic graft, and all attempts are made to preserve the profunda femoral artery. False (pseudo) aneurysms of the femoral artery can occur secondary to percutaneous interventions (i.e., catheterization) and these may thrombose spontaneously. However, if they persist, they can be treated with open surgical repair or ultrasound guided thrombin injection of the active pseudoaneurysm cavity. Pseudoaneurysm of the femoral artery can also occur at the site of disruption of a graft to native artery anastomosis. Mycotic (infected) femoral artery aneurysms can occur in IV drug users or at the anastomotic site of a prosthetic graft to the native vessel. Repair in this situation may require resection, debridement, and replacement with autogenous tissue such as a vein graft, or possibly an extra-anatomic bypass.

Complications arising from popliteal artery aneurysms are thromboembolic in nature and can eventually result in limb loss. Rarely large aneurysms can cause symptoms related to compression of the adjacent structures such as the tibial nerve and the popliteal vein. Most of these patients are male, and over 50% have bilateral disease. Diagnosis can be made on careful physical exam and can be confirmed with Duplex imaging. Conventional contrast angiography helps with operative planning. Aneurysms larger than 2cm in diameter and those with a significant amount of laminated mural thrombus should be considered for repair. Traditionally, open surgical repair is performed with ligation of the aneurysm and bypass using the saphenous vein from either a posterior or medial approach. More recently, endovascular repair with covered stent-grafts has been performed in selected patients with decent proximal and distal landing zones and patent, relatively un-diseased tibial runoff vessels.

REFERENCES

1. TASC. Management of peripheral arterial disease (PAD). TransAtlantic Inter-Society Consensus (TASC). Eur J Vasc Endovasc Surg 2000;19(Suppl A):Si-xxviii. S1-250.
2. TASC. Management of Peripheral Arterial Disease (PAD) TransAtlantic Inter-Society Consensus (TASC). J Vasc Surg 2000;31(1 part 2):S1-287.

3. Norgren L, Hiatt WR, Dormandy JA, Nehler MR, Harris KA, Fowkes FG. Inter-Society Consensus for the Management of Peripheral Arterial Disease (TASC II). J Vasc Surg 2007;45(suppl S):S5-67.
4. de Vries SO, Hunink MG. Results of aortic bifurcation grafts for aortoiliac occlusive disease: a meta-analysis. J Vasc Surg 1997;26:558-69.
5. Dyet JF, Gaines PA, Nicholson AA, Cleveland T, Cook AM, Wilkinson AR, et al. Treatment of chronic iliac artery occlusions by means of percutaneous endovascular stent placement. J Vasc Interv Radiol 1997;8:349-53.
6. Henry M, Amor M, Ethevenot G, henry I, Mentre B, Tzvetanov K. Percutaneous endoluminal treatment of iliac occlusions: a long-term follow-up in 105 patients. J Endovasc Surg 1998;5:228-35.
7. Kashyap V, Pavkov M, Bena J, Sarac T, O'Hara P, Lyden S, Clair D. The management of severe aortoiliac occlusive disease: Endovascular therapy rivals open reconstruction. J Vasc Surg 2008;48:1451-57.
8. Vardulaki KA, Walker NM, Day NE, Duffy SW, Ashton HA, Scott RA. Quantifying the risks of hypertension, age, sex, and smoking in patients with abdominal aortic aneurysm. Br J Surg 2000;87:195-200.
9. Johnston KW. Influence of sex on the results of abdominal aortic aneurysm repair. J Vasc Surg 1994;20:914-23; discussion 923-6.
10. United Kingdom Small Aneurysm Trail Participants. Long-term outcomes of immediate repair compared with surveillance of small abdominal aortic aneurysms. N Engl J Med 2002;346:1445-52.
11. Lederle FA, Johnson GR, Wilson SE, Chute EP, Hyn RJ, Makaroun MS, et al. The aneurysm detection and management study screening program: validation cohort and final results. Aneurysm Detection and Management Veterans Affairs Cooperative Study Investigators. Arch Intern Med 2000;160:1425-30.
12. Boules TN, Compton CN, Stanziale SF, Sheehan MK, Dillavou ED, Gupta N, Tzeng E, Makaroun MS. Can computed tomography scan findings predict (impending" aneurysm rupture? Vasc and Endovasc Surg 2006; 40(1): 41-47.
13. Roger VL, Ballard DJ, Hallett JW Jr, Osmundson PJ, Gersh BJ. Influence of coronary artery disease on morbidity and mortality after aortic aneurysmectomy: a population-based study, 1971-1987. J Am Coll Cardiol 1989;14:1245-52.
14. Auerbach AD, Goldman L. Beta-Blockers and reduction of cardiac events in noncardiac surgery: clinical applications. JAMA 2002;287:1445-7.
15. Yang H, Raymer K, Butler R, Parlow J, Roberts R. The effects of perioperative beta-blockade: results of the Metoprolol after Vascular Surgery (MaVS) study, a randomized controlled trail. Am Heart J 2006;152:983-90.
16. Johnston KW. Multicenter prospective study of nonruptured abdominal aortic aneurysm. Part II. Variables predicting morbidity and mortality. J Vasc Surg 1989;9:437-47.
17. Axelrod DA, Henke PK, Wakefield TW, Stanley JC, Jacobs LA, Graham LM, et al. Impact of chronic obstructive pulmonary disease on elective and emergency abdominal aortic aneurysm repair. J Vasc Surg 2001;33:72-6.
18. Upchurch GR Jr, Proctor MC, Henke PK, Zajkowski P, Riles EM, Ascher MS, et al. Predictors of severe morbidity and death after elective abdominal aortic aneurysmectomy in patients with chronic obstructive pulmonary disease. J Vasc Surg 2003;37:594-9.
19. Cho JS, Kim JY, Rhee RY, Gupta N, Marone LK, Dillavou ED, Makaroun MS. Contemporary results of open repair of ruptured abdominal aortic aneurysms: Effect of surgeon volume on mortality. J Vasc Surg 2008; 48:10-18.
20. Brewster DC, Cronenwett JL, Hallett JW Jr, Johnston KW, Krupski WC, Matsumura JS. Guidelines for the treatment of abdominal aortic aneurysms. Report of a subcommittee of the Joint Council of the American Association for Vascular Surgery and Society for Vascular Surgery. J Vasc Surg 2003;37:1106-17.
21. Conrad MF, Crawford RS, Pedraza JD, Brewster DC, Lamuraglia GM, Corey M, et al. Long-term durability of open abdominal aortic aneurysm repair. J Vasc Surg 2007;46:669-75.
22. Ernst CB. Abdominal aortic aneurysm. N Engl J Med 1993;328:1167-72.
23. Hirsch AT, Haskal ZJ, Hertzer NR, Bakal CW, Creager MA, Halperin JL. ACC/AHA 2005 practice guidelines for the management of patients with peripheral arterial disease (lower extremity, renal, mesenteric and abdominal aortic). Circulation 2006;113:1474-1547.
24. Prissen M, Verhoeven EL, Buth J, Cuypers PW, van Sambeek MR, Balm R, et al; Dutch Randomized Endovascular Aneurysm Management (DREAM) trial group. A randomized trail comparing conventional and endovascular repair of abdominal aortic aneurysms. N Engl J Med 2004;351:1607-18.
25. Greenhalgh RM, Brown LC, Kwong GP, Powell JT, Thompson SG. Comparison of endovascular aneurysm repair with open reapir in patients with abdominal

aortic aneurysm (EVAR trail 1), 30-day operative mortality results: randomized controlled trail. Lancet 2004;364:843-8.

26. Dillavou ED, Muluk SC, Rhee RY, Tzeng E, Woody JD, Gupta N, Makaroun MS. Does hostile neck anatomy preclude successful endovascular aortic aneurysm repair? J Vasc Surg 2003; 38: 657-663.
27. Schoder M, Zaunbauer L, Holzenbein T, Fleischman D, Cejna M, Kretschmer G, et al. Internal iliac artery embolization before endovascular repair of abdominal aortic aneurysms: Frequency, efficacy, and clinical results. Am J Roentgenol 2001;177:599-605.
28. Cynamon J, Lerer D, Veith FJ, Taragin BH, Wahl SI, Lautin JL, et al. Hypogastric artery coil embolization prior to endoluminal repair of aneurysms and fistulas: buttock claudication, a recognized but possibly preventable complication. J Vasc Interv Radiol 2000;11:573-7.
29. Wilt TJ, Lederle FA, MacDonald R, Jonk YC, Rector TS, Kane RL. Comparison of endovascular and open surgical repairs for abdominal aortic aneurysm. Evidence report. Rockville, MD: AHRQ Publication No. 06-E017; 2006.
30. Go MR, Barbato JE, Dillavou ED, Gupta N, Rhee RY, Makaroun MS, Cho JS. Thoracic endovascular aortic repair for traumatic aortic transaction. J Vasc Surg 2007; 46: 928-933.
31. Sarac TP, Clair DG, Hertzer NR, Greenberg RK, Krajewski LP, O'Hara PJ, Ouriel K. Contemporary results of juxtarenal aneurysm repair. J Vasc Surg 2002;36:1104-11.
32. Goueffic Y, Rozec B, Sonnard A, Patra P, Blanloeil Y. Evidence for early nasogastric tube removal after infrarenal aortic surgery: a randomized trail. J Vasc Surg 2005;42:654-9.
33. Lehnert T, Gruber HE, Maeder N, Allenberg JR. Management of primary aortic graft infection by extra-anatomic bypass reconstruction. Eur J Vasc Endovasc Surg 1993:7:301-7.
34. Hobo R, Buth J. Secondary interventions following endovascular abdominal aortic aneurysm repair using current endografts. A EUROSTAR report. J Vasc Surg 2006;43:896-902.
35. Kan CD, Lee HL, Yang YJ. Outcome after endovascular stent graft treatment for mycotic aortic aneurysm: A systematic review. J Vasc Surg 2007;46:906-12.

❑❑❑

44

CHAPTER

Splanchnic Artery Aneurysms

Sarah D. Hans, MD
Jimmy Haouilou, MD, FACS
Sachinder Singh Hans, MD, FASC

1.1 INTRODUCTION

Splanchnic artery aneurysms (SAAs) are a rare, but important component of vascular surgery. An aneurysm is defined as a permanent and localized dilatation of a blood vessel that is more than 1.5 times the normal diameter. A true aneurysm involves all three layers, the intima, media, and adventitia of the vessel wall. A false, or pseudoaneurysm, is a disruption of the vessel wall and is lined by adventitia or perivascular soft tissue. Splanchnic aneurysms include both of these types. A splanchnic aneurysm is an intra-abdominal aneurysm that is not part of the aortoiliac system. These aneurysms include dilatations of the celiac, superior mesenteric, or inferior mesenteric arteries and their branches. SAAs may be fusiform, involving the entire vessel circumference, or saccular, affecting a portion of the circumference.

SAAs comprise 5% of all intraabdominal aneurysms. Literature demonstrates a 0.1% to 0.2% prevalence of these diseases in the general population.[1] Some studies have found splanchnic aneurysms to be more common than abdominal aortic aneurysms on autopsy.[2,3] Recent studies have shown an increase in these conditions, likely secondary to an increase in the use of cross-sectional imaging, such as computed tomography (CT) and magnetic resonance imaging (MRI) to evaluate vascular and non-vascular disease. Moreover, technical improvements in both CT and MRI have allowed these imaging modalities to detect aneurysms that were previously too small or positioned in a way that precluded diagnosis on imaging.

Table 1: Anatomic Distribution of Splanchnic Artery Aneurysms[4,5]

Anatomic Location of Aneurysm	Percentage of all Splanchnic Aneurysms
Splenic artery	60%
Hepatic artery	20%
Superior Mesenteric artery	6%
Celiac artery	4%
Gastric/Gastroepiploic artery	4%
Jejunal/Ileal/Colonic artery	3%
Pancreaticoduodenal/Pancreatic artery	2%
Gastroduodenal artery	1.5%
Inferior Mesenteric artery	<1.0%

With rare exceptions, the distribution detailed in Table 1 has remained consistent in the literature. Some studies found the incidence of hepatic artery aneurysms to be greater than that of splenic artery aneurysms, likely due to increased pseudoaneurysms associated with abdominal trauma and iatrogenic injuries to the liver and biliary tree.[4,6,7]

It is necessary to understand the diagnosis and treatment of splanchnic artery aneurysms because these aneurysms often present secondary to rupture, which carries significant morbidity and mortality. Studies have demonstrated that between 22% to 25% of splanchnic artery aneurysms present with intraperitoneal rupture or significant gastrointestinal hemorrhage at initial diagnosis.[5,8] Another study found that 25% of splanchnic artery aneurysms are complicated by rupture at some point in their clinical course.[9]

Risks of rupture vary with anatomic location of an aneurysm. For instance, hepatic artery aneurysms have a 20% to 44% risk of rupture, whereas celiac and gastric or gastroepiploic artery aneurysms have a 13% and 90% risk of rupture respectively.[4] Current and historic data does not demonstrate many consistent factors that influence the chances of aneurysmal rupture. Some studies demonstrate that larger size increases chances of rupture and that calcifications in an aneurysm protect against rupture.[4] However, these results are not consistent in the literature.

Splanchnic artery aneurysms can present in many different ways. Many are asymptomatic or present with vague abdominal pain. Furthermore, aneurysmal rupture includes a multitude of clinical presentations, because aneurysms can rupture into different locations within the abdomen. For instance, these aneurysms can rupture (1) into the peritoneal cavity and present as hemorrhagic shock, (2) into the gastrointestinal tract and present as massive or intermittent gastrointestinal bleeding, or (3) into the biliary tree and present as haemobilia. The mortality rate after rupture ranges from 25% to 100%.[9] Carr and Shanley found the mortality rates after intraperitoneal rupture of hepatic artery, splenic artery, and celiac artery aneurysms to be 21%, 36%, and nearly 100% respectively.[7,10] Other studies have corroborated the finding of extremely high mortality with celiac artery aneurysm rupture, especially in pregnant women.[4]

The increased incidence of rupture and its devastating consequences necessitate an understanding of the incidence, presentation, diagnosis, and management of SAAs. Furthermore, up to 1/3 of visceral aneurysms are associated with other non-splanchnic artery aneurysms, including those of the thoracic aorta, abdominal aorta, renal, iliac, lower extremity, and intracranial arteries.[10,11] Thus, healthcare professionals need to think about SAAs when evaluating patients for aneurysmal disease.

Each type of splanchnic artery aneurysm requires individual attention because of differences in presentation and management. The following sections in this chapter describe splenic, hepatic, superior mesenteric, celiac, gastric, gastroepiploic, jejunal, ileac, colonic, pancreaticoduodenal, pancreatic, and gastroduodenal aneurysms in more detail.

SPLENIC ARTERY ANEURYSMS

Epidemiology

Splenic artery aneurysms (SPAAs) are the most common splanchnic artery aneurysm. Studies report the overall incidence in the general population to be around 0.01%,[12] but can be up to 10% in patients over 60 years of age.[2] SPAAs comprise 0.78% of aneurysms incidentally noted on angiography.[5] These aneurysms are usually less than 2 cm and are saccular. Many SPAAs affect the mid or distal splenic artery, especially at bifurcation points. SPAAs affect women 4 times as often as men.[5,13] One study found a male predominance when SPAAs exceeded 10 cm in size.[14] The mean age at diagnosis is 52 years.[4]

Pathogenesis and Risk Factors

Many factors lead to development of an SPAA. Common causes of these aneurysms include local hemodynamics, hypertension, hormones, and medial degeneration. Most of these causes lead to blood vessel dilation by increasing splenic artery blood flow, which increases stress on the vessel wall and eventually leads to aneurysmal dilatation. Histological changes found at surgery and on autopsy include atherosclerosis, calcification, intimal hyperplasia, arterial dysplasia, fibromuscular dysplasia, and cystic medial degeneration. Less common causes of SPAAs include polyarteritis nodosa, lupus, and anomalous origin of the splenic artery. Blunt trauma and pancreatitis can cause pseudoaneurysms of the splenic artery.

The most common clinical risk factors for SPAAs are female gender, multiple pregnancies and portal hypertension.[13,15] Several physiologic changes during pregnancy contribute to splenic artery aneurysmal formation. These changes include increased blood volume, increased cardiac output, and portal hypertension. Each of these alterations in physiology increases splenic artery blood flow, which contributes to aneurysmal formation. Furthermore, the estrogen and progesterone released during pregnancy impair elastin formation and lead to degeneration of the internal elastic lamina. These occurrences weaken the vessel wall and predispose a woman to aneurysm formation. Lastly, relaxin impairs the elasticity of the vessel wall.

Clinical Presentation and Diagnosis

Most SPAAs are asymptomatic and found incidentally on imaging performed for unrelated symptoms. Patients can present with vague abdominal pain. The physical exam is usually normal in asymptomatic patients. It is rare to auscultate bruits over the aneurysm. Classic x-ray findings include calcifications in the left upper quadrant.

SPAAs may also present with rupture. Pregnancy is associated with 20% to 50% of all ruptures.[16,17] There is a further increase in incidence of rupture in the third trimester.[13] These patients often present with sudden onset of left sided abdominal pain. SPAAs can also present with a "double-rupture." In this instance, initially the rupture is contained within the lesser sac and the patient often remains hemodynamically stable. This contained rupture converts to a free intraperitoneal rupture within 48 hours.[18-20] In addition to the "double-rupture," SPAA may rupture into the gastrointestinal tract, the splenic vein, a pancreatic pseudocyst, or into one of the pancreatic ducts. Overall mortality rates with rupture approach 25%,[18,20] which is lower than mortality rates associated with rupture of other splanchnic artery aneurysms.[4] However, mortality rates for pregnant women and their fetuses range between 80% and 90%.[21,22]

Indications and Techniques for Treatment

Current evidence includes absolute and relative indications for treatment of SPAAs. Absolute indications for treatment include aneurysms that are symptomatic, have ruptured, or are found in pregnant women or women of childbearing age. Relative indications consist of aneurysms larger than 2 cm, and those that are enlarging. Some studies advocate treating SPAAs found in individuals with portal hypertension and in liver transplant candidates.[15,23] As further sections of this chapter demonstrate, surgeons possess more specific indications for treatment of SPAAs than they do for other splanchnic artery aneurysms. Indications for treatment of other splanchnic aneurysms include treating all aneurysms unless operative risks outweigh the benefits of intervention. It is likely that the lower rate of mortality and incidence of SPAA rupture is responsible for surgeons' more selective intervention for these patients.

One can repair SPAAs using open, laparoscopic, or endovascular approaches. Patient presentation, aneurysmal characteristics, and anatomic location determine the type of surgical intervention. Traditional open surgical management is classified based on the anatomic location of the aneurysm. For aneurysms of the proximal and middle splenic artery, one can perform proximal and distal ligation of the artery, aneurysmectomy, or both. Most of the time, it is not necessary to revascularize the distal splenic artery due to adequate collateral circulation to the spleen provided by the short gastric arteries. For distal and intrasplenic aneurysms one should perform a splenectomy. Depending on the specific location of the distal aneurysm and the patient's anatomy, it may also be necessary to perform a distal pancreatectomy.

Recent data has described laparoscopic approaches to SPAA repair. It is possible to perform a laparoscopic repair of an SPAA utilizing intraoperative ultrasound to assist with aneurysmal clipping or exclusion. Moreover, retro pancreatic SPAAs are difficult to access using an open surgical approach. One study found some success with laparoscopic occlusion of these aneurysms using coil embolization.[24]

Endovascular treatment options include coil embolization, cyanoacrylate glue embolization, occlusion with thrombin injection, and stent-grafting. Embolization and thrombin occlusion trap the aneurysm and prevent further expansion and rupture. Most studies illustrate success with endovascular techniques for saccular SPAAs.[4,25] Stent-grafting has been used for mid-artery saccular aneurysms. Complications of stent-grafting include splenic infarct and pancreatitis. These complications are more common when the SPAA is distal.

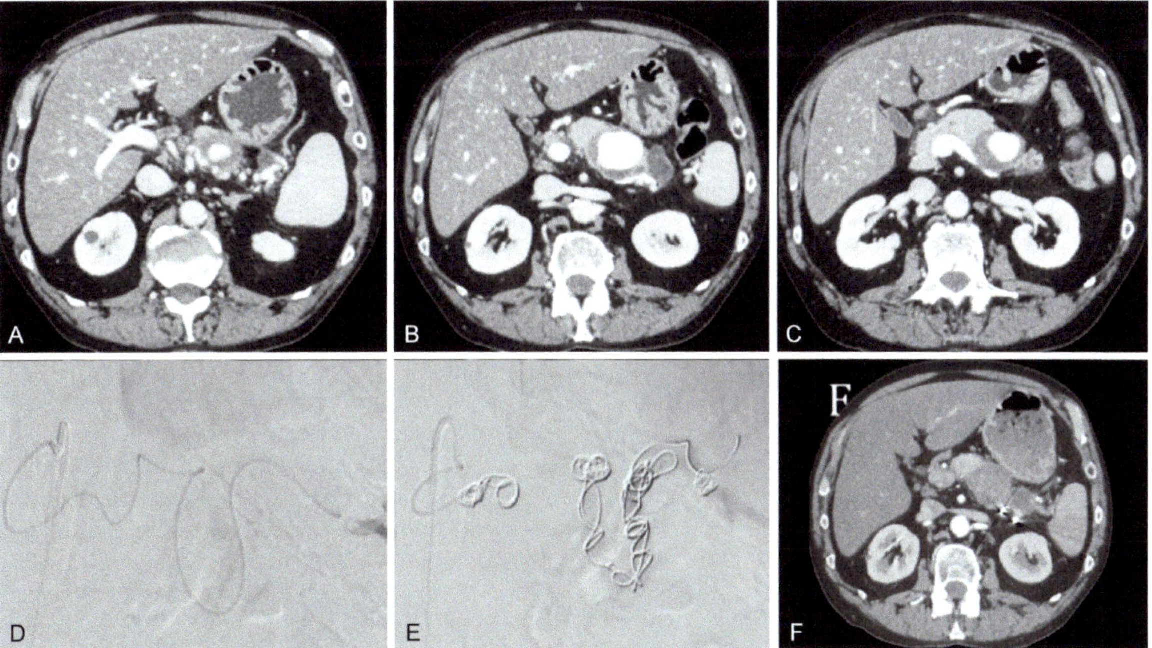

Figure 1 A-C: Large splenic pseudoaneurysm on a patient with history of recurrent alcoholic pancreatitis. D-E: Endovascular coil embolization of splenic artery. F: Post embolization with no flow of splenic pseudoaneurysm.

HEPATIC ARTERY ANEURYSMS

Epidemiology

Hepatic artery aneurysms (HAAs) are the second most common type of splanchnic artery aneurysm. The prevalence of these aneurysms on autopsy is 0.1%.[26,27] Recently, there has been an increase in the incidence of HAA. It is likely that this increase is due to improved cross-sectional imaging, as there is also an increase in incidence of other splanchnic artery aneurysms. However, several factors are unique to the increased incidence of HAAs. For instance, recent studies have documented an increased incidence of intrahepatic pseudoaneurysms secondary to blunt liver trauma and iatrogenic injuries from PTC and ERCP.[4,28] One review noted that 50% of HAAs diagnosed between 1985 and 1995 were intrahepatic false aneurysms secondary to trauma.[28] The mean age at diagnosis is 60 years.[4] Traumatic pseudoaneurysms are more likely to be found in younger individuals because blunt and penetrating liver injuries are more common in this population. There is a 2:1 male to female ratio.[4]

As is true with other splanchnic artery aneurysms, HAAs are commonly associated with other aneurysms. One study found that 20% patients with HAAs also had an abdominal aortic aneurysm.[29] Moreover, 31% and 42% of patients with HAAs also have aneurysmal disease in other splanchnic and non-splanchnic vessels, respectively.[4] 80% of HAA are extrahepatic and 20% are intrahepatic.[29,30] Of the extrahepatic lesions, 63% are found in the common hepatic artery, 28% in the right hepatic artery, 5% in the left hepatic artery, and 4% affect both the left and the right hepatic arteries.[29,30]

Pathogenesis and Risk Factors

HAAs are caused by many different factors. The following list describes causes of HAAs:

1. Atherosclerosis/degenerative changes
2. Medial degeneration
3. Fibro-dysplasia
4. Trauma
5. Infection
6. Biliary disease and associated ERCP/PTC
7. Polyarteritis Nodosa
8. Connective tissue disease
9. Periarterial inflammation caused by cholecystitis or pancreatitis

Other procedure-related causes of HAAs include hepatic tumor embolization and orthotopic liver transplantation. It is thought that the embolic agent is responsible for aneurysmal formation.

Clinical Presentation and Diagnosis

Up to 60% of HAAs are symptomatic at the time of initial diagnosis.[31] One study from the 1990s disputed this finding and found most HAAs to be asymptomatic.[28] Symptoms include epigastric pain, right upper quadrant pain, gastrointestinal bleeding, and jaundice. The literature describes a classic triad of Quincke, which includes abdominal pain, haemobilia, and obstructive jaundice. One study found that this triad is seen in less than 1/3 of patients.[32] If the aneurysm grows to a significant size, it may be possible to auscultate a bruit on physical exam.

In addition to the above mentioned symptoms, HAAs can also present with rupture into the peritoneal cavity, the gastrointestinal tract, or the biliary tree. Studies have found the rate of rupture to be around 21% to 65%.[4,31] The mortality rate associated with rupture ranges from 21% to 40%.[28,29,33] Hepatic artery aneurysm location determines symptoms associated with rupture. For instance, extrahepatic aneurysms often rupture into the abdominal cavity. Intrahepatic aneurysms are more likely to rupture into the biliary tree and cause Quincke's triad.[28] 10% of all patients with ruptured HAAs will present with hemorrhagic shock.[28]

It is possible to diagnose HAAs on a variety of imaging modalities. First, curvilinear calcifications in the right upper quadrant on x-ray can indicate a HAA. On ERCP, PTC, and UGI an HAA may be seen as a filling defect in or near the duodenum. HAAs are most commonly diagnosed using ultrasound and CT. Ultrasound will show a discrete fusiform or round lesion in the right upper quadrant that is hypoechoic. It is also used to follow aneurysms in asymptomatic patients. CT may demonstrate hepatic artery dilation, vessel wall calcification, or a clot in the vessel. Angiography is helpful in surgical planning. This imaging can diagnose the presence of other intraabdominal aneurysms and feeding vessels. Angiography can also provide anatomic detail necessary for endovascular treatment.

Indications and Techniques for Treatment

Indications for treatment of HAAs depend on clinical presentation, size, etiology, growth, and type of aneurysm. Current indications for intervention include HAAs that are symptomatic, larger than 2 cm, have rapid growth, false aneurysms, and those caused by fibromuscular dysplasia and polyarteritis nodosa. All pseudoaneurysms need to be repaired because these aneurysms have a higher incidence of rupture and a more unpredictable clinical course. As the section on splenic artery aneurysms showed, and future sections will demonstrate, aneurysms may not be repaired if the risks of the intervention outweigh the benefits of the surgery.

Both open and endovascular treatment options exist for HAAs. The method of intervention depends on the anatomic location, morphology, and underlying etiology of the aneurysm, as well as the health of the liver. It is possible to utilize both open and endovascular techniques to repair common hepatic artery aneurysms. If the gastroduodenal artery (GDA) provides adequate collateral circulation to the liver, one can ligate the common hepatic artery or occlude the vessel with coil embolization. If there is GDA disease the patient may need arterial revascularization or may be treated with a stent graft. Usually hepatic artery aneurysms require arterial reconstruction secondary to poor collateral circulation. It is difficult to utilize an open approach to access intrahepatic true and false aneurysms; therefore, many surgeons treat these aneurysms with coil or particle embolization. In addition to avoiding a difficult open exposure procedure, these endovascular approaches avoid liver parenchymal resection.

SUPERIOR MESENTERIC ARTERY ANEURYSMS

Epidemiology

Superior mesenteric artery aneurysms (SMAAs) represent 5.5% to 7% of all splanchnic artery aneurysms.[34] Most studies demonstrate that the incidence in males and females are equal. However, one center found a 2:1 male to female ratio.[34] The mean age at presentation is 59 years.[34] The majority of these aneurysms are found within 5 cm of the artery's origin from the aorta.

Pathogenesis and Risk Factors

Unlike other splanchnic artery aneurysms, infection causes the majority of SMAAs. Sixty percent of SMAAs are mycotic, often due to nonhemolytic streptococcal subacute bacterial endocarditis.[4] Two recent studies dispute the role of infection in SMAA.[18,34] It is postulated that the branching of the SMA from the aorta predisposes lodging of septic emboli. Other causes include connective tissue disease, atherosclerosis, and cystic medial dysplasia. In one study, researchers were unable to determine a cause of SMAA in 52% of patients.[34] Pancreatitis, SMA dissection, and trauma can cause false SMA aneurysms.

Clinical Presentation and Diagnosis

Many studies have shown that 70% to 90% of SMAAs are symptomatic at the time of diagnosis.[34-36] One study found 48% to be asymptomatic at the time of diagnosis.[34] Common presenting signs and symptoms include generalized abdominal pain, gastrointestinal bleeding, fever, and a tender, pulsatile abdominal mass. As with most other splanchnic artery aneurysms, a significant portion of SMAAs present with rupture. Studies have found rupture rates ranging from 38% to 50%.[34-36] The mortality associated with rupture ranges from 30% to 90%.[34-36] Rupture can lead to intestinal ischemia and intraperitoneal hemorrhage, thus resulting in associated high mortality.

One can diagnose SMAAs preoperatively or during laparotomy performed for hemodynamic instability and/or gastrointestinal bleeding. Common methods of preoperative diagnosis include angiography, CT, and MRI. Fewer SMAAs are diagnosed using ultrasound and plain abdominal radiographs.

Indications and Techniques for Treatment

Current evidence recommends treating all SMAAs, unless operative risk precludes intervention. This recommendation comes from the high mortality rates associated with rupture. Moreover, there is less than a 15% mortality rate with elective repair.[35] Options for open treatment consist of ligation of the artery and excision of the aneurysmal sac without arterial reconstruction. It is possible to utilize this method of treatment if there is adequate collateral circulation to the small and large intestines from the celiac and inferior mesenteric arteries. If collateral circulation is inadequate, one can perform aneurysmectomy with arterial reconstruction using a reverse saphenous vein or a prosthetic graft. In an emergent situation one can ligate the superior mesenteric artery and not remove the aneurysmal sac. For saccular aneurysms it is possible to perform anuerysmorrhaphy. If patients present with bowel ischemia, or if the bowel is not viable after aneurysm repair or ligation, then it is necessary to resect these sections of the intestine.

Endovascular treatment options consist of coil or glue embolization and stent grafts. It is difficult to utilize stent grafts to repair SMAAs because these aneurysms often affect the proximal SMAs and do not have an adequate landing zone for the stent graft.[37] Endovascular treatment is more common in elective repair, but studies have demonstrated that up to 12% of endovascular repairs occur during emergent situations.[34]

CELIAC ARTERY ANEURYSMS

Epidemiology

Celiac artery aneurysms (CAAs) are the fourth most common SAA, representing 5% of all visceral aneurysms.[38] One study found a 1 out of 8000 prevalence of CAAs on autopsy.[38] The mean age of diagnosis is 56 years.[39,40] There is a 2:1 male predominance.[5] 40% are associated with other SAAs and 20% are associated with abdominal aortic aneurysms.[41,42]

Pathogenesis and Risk Factors

Historical data reveals that many CAAs were caused by syphilis.[43] More recent data demonstrates that medial degeneration and atherosclerosis are the two most common causes of CAAs. Less common causes include trauma, collagen vascular disease, celiac artery dissection, and anomalous splanchnic circulation.

Clinical Presentation and Diagnosis

CAAs can present in many different ways. Most are symptomatic. Common complaints include epigastric pain, nausea, and vomiting. Other clinical presentations include hemorrhagic shock secondary to rupture, gastrointestinal bleeding, and jaundice. Literature describes a 10% to 20% risk of rupture with an associated 50% mortality rate.[18,33,40] Similar to splenic artery aneurysms, CSAs can present with a double rupture. In this situation, a patient initially complains of epigastric pain and is hemodynamically stable because the aneurysm ruptured into the lesser sac. Once the rupture extends through the foramen of Winslow, and free intraperitoneal hemorrhage occurs, a patient will often become hemodynamically unstable and require emergent intervention.

Indications and Techniques for Treatment

Indications for treatment are based on size and symptoms. Current evidence recommends intervention on all symptomatic aneurysms and on all asymptomatic aneurysms greater than 1.5 cm. These indications are not absolute. Each patient with a CAA requires an individual approach to treatment. Ultimately, the decision to intervene is based on size, etiology, and anatomy of the aneurysm, as well as patient comorbidities.

Both open and endovascular techniques are used in clinical practice. Current options for open repair include aneurysmectomy, aneurysmorrhaphy, and ligation. In most instances, it is possible to ligate the celiac artery because the superior mesenteric, gastroduodenal, and pancreaticoduodenal arteries provide adequate collateral circulation. It is not possible to ligate the celiac artery without performing distal revascularization in patients with underlying hepatic disease.[44] Ultimately, the strength of collateral circulation determines the need for distal arterial revascularization. The standard revascularization procedure is aneurysmectomy followed by aorto-celiac bypass with a synthetic graft.[4] It is possible to perform aneurysmorrhaphy for isolated saccular aneurysms.[18]

Improvement in cross-sectional imaging has increased the preoperative diagnosis of celiac artery aneurysms, which has increased the opportunities for endovascular treatments of these aneurysms. Current endovascular options include coil embolization, thrombin injection, and stent grafts.

GASTRIC AND GASTROEPIPLOIC ARTERY ANEURYSMS

Epidemiology

Gastric and gastroepiploic artery aneurysms (GAAS and GEAAs) are very rare and represent only 4% of all splanchnic artery aneurysms. Gastric artery aneurysms are 10 times more common than those of the gastroepiploic arteries. Both of these aneurysms are more common in men than in women and are usually diagnosed in the sixth or seventh decade of life. There is a 10% to 40% chance that an individual with a GAA or GEAA will have an additional intraabdominal aneurysm.[45]

Pathogenesis and Risk Factors

Table 2 describes the frequency of common causes of gastric and gastroepiploic artery aneurysms. Less common causes of these aneurysms include septic emboli and medial dysplasia.

Table 2: Causes of Gastric and Gastroepiploic Artery Aneurysms[46,47]

Etiology	Frequency
Degenerative	30%
Traumatic	25%
Inflammatory	15%

Clinical Presentation and Diagnosis

GAAs and GEAAs most commonly present with rupture. For instance, one study found that more than 90% of GEAAs presented with rupture at initial diagnosis.[45] When aneurysms present with rupture, they are often diagnosed as hemoperitoneum of unknown source at the time of surgery. The mortality rate associated with rupture of these aneurysms is 70%.[18]

Indications and Techniques for Treatment

Since the majority of GAAs and GEAAs present with rupture and need emergent repair, specific indications for treatment of these aneurysms do not exist. It is possible that the incidence of these aneurysms diagnosed preoperatively will increase with the improvement in cross-sectional imaging techniques. It is also possible that an increase in diagnosis may provide adequate sample sizes for future research and eventual indications for elective treatment of these aneurysms. The specific surgical approach that a physician should take when repairing these aneurysms depends on anatomic location. For aneurysms located outside of the stomach, one can ligate the artery and may or may not perform an aneurysmectomy. For lesions inside the stomach wall, in addition to vessel ligation, a surgeon must excise the portion of the stomach wall containing the aneurysm. The stomach has significant collateral circulation; therefore, in most cases it is unnecessary to perform arterial revascularization after ligation and aneurysmectomy. It is uncommon for surgeons to use endovascular approaches to repair of GAAs and GEAAs. However, one study showed promising results with thrombin injection.[48]

JEJUNAL, ILEAL, AND COLONIC ARTERY ANEURYSMS

Epidemiology

Small bowel and colonic splanchnic artery aneurysms are exceedingly rare. These aneurysms comprise of only 2% of splanchnic artery aneurysms.[4] The incidence is equal in males and females. The majority of these lesions are solitary.

Pathogenesis and Risk Factors

It is difficult to characterize the pathogenesis of jejunal, ileal, and colonic artery aneurysms. Current research reveals several potential causes of these lesions. In descending order of incidence, causes include: atherosclerosis, medial degeneration, inflammation, infection, trauma, congenital, and iatrogenic from recent abdominal surgery.[49,50] Polyarteritis nodosa can also cause these aneurysms.

Clinical Presentation and Diagnosis

The majority of small bowel and colonic artery aneurysms are asymptomatic. Colonic artery aneurysms are more likely to rupture than those affecting the jejunal vessels. As with other splanchnic artery aneurysms, many of these aneurysms are diagnosed on CTA or MRA which are performed due to vague abdominal complaints.

Indications and Techniques for Treatment

It is recommended to treat all jejunal, ileal, and colonic artery aneurysms unless the operative risk is great enough to preclude intervention. Treatment options include open and endovascular approaches. Open treatment involves ligation of the artery and resection of an affected small bowel or colon if non-viable. Endovascular treatment includes microcatheter embolization. When performing endovascular treatment, it is important to avoid occlusion of adjacent vessels because it can lead to resulting intestinal ischemia. If these aneurysms are larger than 1 cm and proximally located, it is advised to perform arterial revascularization to avoid significant bowel resection.

PANCREATIC, PANCREATICODUODENAL, GASTRODUODENAL ARTERY ANEURYSMS

Epidemiology

Each of the aneurysms discussed in this section are exceedingly rare entities yet are important because they are all surgical emergencies. Pancreatic and pancreaticoduodenal artery aneurysms (PAAs, PDAAs) comprise of 2% of all SAAs. Gastroduodenal artery aneurysms (GDAAs) represent 1.5% of all SAAs.[51-53] As with other splanchnic artery aneurysms, these three include both true and false aneurysms. Interestingly, pseudoaneurysms of the pancreatic and pancreaticoduodenal arteries are much more common than true aneurysms of these vessels. Typically, these pseudoaneurysms are seen in 50-year-old individuals and have a 4:1 male to female ratio.[54-58] There is no gender difference in the incidence of true aneurysms of the pancreatic circulation.

Pathogenesis and Risk Factors

The majority of PAAs, PDAAs, and GDAAs are associated with pancreatic and biliary disease. Specifically, 60% of GDAAs and 30% of PDAAs/PAAs are related to pancreatitis.[54] Pseudoaneurysms of the pancreatic and pancreaticoduodenal arteries are associated with pancreatic necrosis, pseudocyst expansion and erosion, septic emboli, trauma, and ERCP/PTC. True PDAAs, PAAs, and GDAAs are related to increased flow through the pancreatic circulation. Causes of this increased flow include celiac occlusive disease and median arcuate ligament syndrome.

Clinical Presentation and Diagnosis

In contrast to other SAAs, most aneurysms of the pancreatic circulation are symptomatic. Individuals present with epigastric pain, often with radiation to the back. This pain can be sudden in onset, especially if the aneurysm has ruptured. PAAs, PDAAs, GDAAs can also present as bleeding into the duodenum or pancreatic duct.[52,59,60] 62% to 75% of PDAAs present with rupture.[61] These aneurysms have a 21% mortality rate with rupture.[4] GDAAs have a higher mortality rate with rupture.[4]

PDAAs, PAAs, and GDAAs can be diagnosed using many different imaging techniques. CTA, MRA, and arteriography are the most common methods of diagnosis. Furthermore, these aneurysms can be diagnosed during an exploratory laparotomy for uncontrolled gastrointestinal bleeding.

Indications and Techniques for Treatment

All true and false PAAs, PDAAs, and GDAAs should be treated due to high rates of rupture. Surgeons can utilize open and endovascular repair techniques. If one of these aneurysms is diagnosed preoperatively it is essential to perform an angiography prior to surgical intervention. This test delineates the anatomic location and the number of branches and feeding vessels of the aneurysm. Standard open surgical technique consists of aneurysmal exclusion through ligation of all branches. It is difficult to perform this maneuver to repair a PDAA because these aneurysms often have many branches. It is best to approach the branches from within the aneurysmal sac. GDAAs have fewer branches and are generally easier to repair. However, both GDAAs and PDAAs have difficult surgical exposures.

The abovementioned difficult surgical exposure is one reason that the use of endovascular repair has increased in recent years. Current endovascular techniques include coil embolization and thrombin injection. Studies have demonstrated favorable outcomes with both techniques.[62-65] Complications with coil embolization include aneurysmal sac reperfusion and rupture. A surgeon can inject thrombin percutaneously or with ultrasound guidance. Thrombin injection is especially useful in patients with PAAs, PDAAs, and GDAAs associated with pancreatitis.

SUMMARY

In conclusion, splanchnic artery aneurysms are a rare but important clinical problem. The incidence of these lesions is increasing due to improvements in cross-sectional imaging and more frequent non-operative management of traumatic solid organ injury. Many of these aneurysms are asymptomatic until rupture. Common treatment techniques include open aneurysmectomy and ligation of the artery with or without arterial reconstruction. As more of these aneurysms are diagnosed preoperatively and with improvements in technique, there is increased use of endovascular therapy to treat these aneurysms, such as coil embolization and stent grafting. It is important to note that each aneurysm requires an individualized approach to treatment based on the etiology, size, and anatomy of the aneurysm, as well as patient comorbidities. Ultimately, the increase in incidence of these aneurysms necessitates an understanding of the epidemiology, etiology, clinical presentation, diagnosis, and management of splanchnic artery aneurysms.

REFERENCES

1. Saltzberg SS, Maldonado TS, Lamparello PJ, et al. Is endovascular therapy the preferred treatment for all visceral artery aneurysms? Annals of vascular surgery 2005;19:507-15.
2. Bedford PD, Lodge B. Aneurysm of the splenic artery. Gut 1960;1:312-20.
3. Darling RC, 3rd, Cordero JA, Jr., Chang BB, et al. Advances in the surgical repair of ruptured abdominal aortic aneurysms. Cardiovascular surgery 1996;4:720-3.
4. Cronenwett JL, Johnston, W. Rutherford's Vascular Surgery. 7th ed: Saunders; 2010.
5. Messina LM, Shanley CJ. Visceral artery aneurysms. The Surgical clinics of North America 1997;77:425-42.
6. Nosher JL, Chung J, Brevetti LS, Graham AM, Siegel RL. Visceral and renal artery aneurysms: a pictorial essay on endovascular therapy. Radiographics : a review publication of the Radiological Society of North America, Inc 2006;26:1687-704; quiz
7. Shanley CJ, Shah NL, Messina LM. Common splanchnic artery aneurysms: splenic, hepatic, and celiac. Annals of vascular surgery 1996;10:315-22.
8. Carr SC, Mahvi DM, Hoch JR, Archer CW, Turnipseed WD. Visceral artery aneurysm rupture. Journal of vascular surgery : official publication, the Society for Vascular Surgery [and] International Society for Cardiovascular Surgery, North American Chapter 2001;33:806-11.
9. Pasha SF, Gloviczki P, Stanson AW, Kamath PS. Splanchnic artery aneurysms. Mayo Clinic proceedings Mayo Clinic 2007;82:472-9.
10. Carr SC, Pearce WH, Vogelzang RL, McCarthy WJ, Nemcek AA, Jr., Yao JS. Current management of visceral artery aneurysms. Surgery 1996;120:627-33; discussion 33-4.
11. Busuttil RW, Brin BJ. The diagnosis and management of visceral artery aneurysms. Surgery 1980;88:619-24.
12. Moore SW, Guida PM, Schumacher HW. Splenic artery aneurysm. Bulletin de la Societe internationale de chirurgie 1970;29:210-8.
13. Dave SP, Reis ED, Hossain A, Taub PJ, Kerstein MD, Hollier LH. Splenic artery aneurysm in the 1990s. Annals of vascular surgery 2000;14:223-9.
14. Pescarus R, Montreuil B, Bendavid Y. Giant splenic artery aneurysms: case report and review of the literature. Journal of vascular surgery : official publication, the Society for Vascular Surgery [and] International Society for Cardiovascular Surgery, North American Chapter 2005;42:344-7.
15. Lee PC, Rhee RY, Gordon RY, Fung JJ, Webster MW. Management of splenic artery aneurysms: the significance of portal and essential hypertension. Journal of the American College of Surgeons 1999;189:483-90.
16. Stanley JC, Fry WJ. Pathogenesis and clinical significance of splenic artery aneurysms. Surgery 1974;76:898-909.
17. Trastek VF, Pairolero PC, Joyce JW, Hollier LH, Bernatz PE. Splenic artery aneurysms. Surgery 1982;91:694-9.

18. Stanley JC, Wakefield TW, Graham LM, Whitehouse WM, Jr., Zelenock GB, Lindenauer SM. Clinical importance and management of splanchnic artery aneurysms. Journal of vascular surgery : official publication, the Society for Vascular Surgery [and] International Society for Cardiovascular Surgery, North American Chapter 1986;3:836-40.
19. Mattar SG, Lumsden AB. The management of splenic artery aneurysms: experience with 23 cases. American journal of surgery 1995;169:580-4.
20. de Vries JE, Schattenkerk ME, Malt RA. Complications of splenic artery aneurysm other than intraperitoneal rupture. Surgery 1982;91:200-4.
21. Holdsworth RJ, Gunn A. Ruptured splenic artery aneurysm in pregnancy. A review. British journal of obstetrics and gynaecology 1992;99:595-7.
22. Barrett JM, Van Hooydonk JE, Boehm FH. Pregnancy-related rupture of arterial aneurysms. Obstetrical & gynecological survey 1982;37:557-66.
23. Sachdev-Ost U. Visceral artery aneurysms: review of current management options. The Mount Sinai journal of medicine, New York 2010;77:296-303.
24. Hassen-Khodja R, Declemy S, Batt M, et al. Visceral artery aneurysms in Von Recklinghausen's neurofibromatosis. Journal of vascular surgery : official publication, the Society for Vascular Surgery [and] International Society for Cardiovascular Surgery, North American Chapter 1997;25:572-5.
25. Huang IH, Zuckerman DA, Matthews JB. Occlusion of a giant splenic artery pseudoaneurysm with percutaneous thrombin-collagen injection. Journal of vascular surgery : official publication, the Society for Vascular Surgery [and] International Society for Cardiovascular Surgery, North American Chapter 2004;40:574-7.
26. Arneson MA, Smith RS. Ruptured hepatic artery aneurysm: case report and review of literature. Annals of vascular surgery 2005;19:540-5.
27. Kibbler CC, Cohen DL, Cruicshank JK, Kushwaha SS, Morgan MY, Dick RD. Use of CAT scanning in the diagnosis and management of hepatic artery aneurysm. Gut 1985;26:752-6.
28. O'Driscoll D, Olliff SP, Olliff JF. Hepatic artery aneurysm. The British journal of radiology 1999;72:1018-25.
29. Abbas MA, Fowl RJ, Stone WM, et al. Hepatic artery aneurysm: factors that predict complications. Journal of vascular surgery : official publication, the Society for Vascular Surgery [and] International Society for Cardiovascular Surgery, North American Chapter 2003;38:41-5.
30. Luebke T, Heckenkamp J, Gawenda M, Beckurts KT, Lackner K, Brunkwall J. Combined endovascular-open surgical procedure in a great hepatic artery aneurysm. Annals of vascular surgery 2007;21:807-12.
31. Zachary K, Geier S, Pellecchia C, Irwin G. Jaundice secondary to hepatic artery aneurysm: radiological appearance and clinical features. The American journal of gastroenterology 1986;81:295-8.
32. Harlaftis NN, Akin JT. Hemobilia from ruptured hepatic artery aneurysm. Report of a case and review of the literature. American journal of surgery 1977;133:229-32.
33. Funahashi S, Yukizane T, Yano K, et al. An aneurysm of the right gastroepiploic artery. The Journal of cardiovascular surgery 1997;38:385-8.
34. Stone WM, Abbas M, Cherry KJ, Fowl RJ, Gloviczki P. Superior mesenteric artery aneurysms: is presence an indication for intervention? Journal of vascular surgery : official publication, the Society for Vascular Surgery [and] International Society for Cardiovascular Surgery, North American Chapter 2002;36:234-7; discussion 7.
35. Lorelli DR, Cambria RA, Seabrook GR, Towne JB. Diagnosis and management of aneurysms involving the superior mesenteric artery and its branches--a report of four cases. Vascular and endovascular surgery 2003;37:59-66.
36. Lindberg CG, Stridbeck H. Aneurysms of the superior mesenteric artery and its branches. Gastrointestinal radiology 1992;17:132-4.
37. Ballard JL, Reiss J, Abou-Zamzam AM, Teruya TH, Bianchi C. Two-graft repair of very proximal superior mesenteric artery aneurysms: a technical note. Annals of vascular surgery 2005;19:465-9.
38. Haimovici H, Sprayregen S, Eckstein P, Veith FJ. Celiac artery aneurysmectomy: case report with review of the literature. Surgery 1976;79:592-6.
39. Deterling RA, Jr. Aneurysm of the visceral arteries. The Journal of cardiovascular surgery 1971;12:309-22.
40. Stone WM, Abbas MA, Gloviczki P, Fowl RJ, Cherry KJ. Celiac arterial aneurysms: a critical reappraisal of a rare entity. Archives of surgery 2002;137:670-4.
41. Hossain A, Reis ED, Dave SP, Kerstein MD, Hollier LH. Visceral artery aneurysms: experience in a tertiary-care center. The American surgeon 2001;67:432-7.
42. Carmeci C, McClenathan J. Visceral artery aneurysms as seen in a community hospital. American journal of surgery 2000;179:486-9.
43. Graham LM, Stanley JC, Whitehouse WM, Jr., et al. Celiac artery aneurysms: historic (1745-1949) versus contemporary (1950-1984) differences in etiology and clinical importance. Journal of vascular surgery : official publication, the Society for Vascular Surgery [and] International Society for Cardiovascular Surgery, North American Chapter 1985;2:757-64.

44. Wagner WH, Allins AD, Treiman RL, et al. Ruptured visceral artery aneurysms. Annals of vascular surgery 1997;11:342-7.
45. McDermott VG, Shlansky-Goldberg R, Cope C. Endovascular management of splenic artery aneurysms and pseudoaneurysms. Cardiovascular and interventional radiology 1994;17:179-84.
46. Montisci R, Cuccu G, Serra F, Lantini V, Cocco G, Brotzu G. Spontaneous rupture of an aneurysm of the left gastroepiploic artery. European journal of vascular surgery 1992;6:95-7.
47. Rohatgi A, Cherian T. Spontaneous rupture of a left gastroepiploic artery aneurysm. Journal of postgraduate medicine 2002;48:288-9.
48. Chandran S, Parvaiz A, Karim A, et al. Ruptured left gastric artery aneurysm successfully treated by thrombin injection: case report and literature review. TheScientificWorldJournal 2005;5:20-3.
49. Huang YK, Hsieh HC, Tsai FC, Chang SH, Lu MS, Ko PJ. Visceral artery aneurysm: risk factor analysis and therapeutic opinion. European journal of vascular and endovascular surgery : the official journal of the European Society for Vascular Surgery 2007;33:293-301.
50. Diettrich NA, Cacioppo JC, Ying DP. Massive gastrointestinal hemorrhage caused by rupture of a jejunal branch artery aneurysm. Journal of vascular surgery : official publication, the Society for Vascular Surgery [and] International Society for Cardiovascular Surgery, North American Chapter 1988;8:187-9.
51. Chiou AC, Josephs LG, Menzoian JO. Inferior pancreaticoduodenal artery aneurysm: report of a case and review of the literature. Journal of vascular surgery : official publication, the Society for Vascular Surgery [and] International Society for Cardiovascular Surgery, North American Chapter 1993;17:784-9.
52. Bageacu S, Cuilleron M, Kaczmarek D, Porcheron J. True aneurysms of the pancreaticoduodenal artery: successful non-operative management. Surgery 2006;139:608-16.
53. Iyomasa S, Matsuzaki Y, Hiei K, Sakaguchi H, Matsunaga H, Yamaguchi Y. Pancreaticoduodenal artery aneurysm: a case report and review of the literature. Journal of vascular surgery : official publication, the Society for Vascular Surgery [and] International Society for Cardiovascular Surgery, North American Chapter 1995;22:161-6.
54. Eckhauser FE, Stanley JC, Zelenock GB, Borlaza GS, Freier DT, Lindenauer SM. Gastroduodenal and pancreaticoduodenal artery aneurysms: a complication of pancreatitis causing spontaneous gastrointestinal hemorrhage. Surgery 1980;88:335-44.
55. Stanley JC, Frey CF, Miller TA, Lindenauer SM, Child CG, 3rd. Major arterial hemorrhage: a complication of pancreatic pseudocysts and chronic pancreatitis. Archives of surgery 1976;111:435-40.
56. White AF, Baum S, Buranasiri S. Aneurysms secondary to pancreatitis. AJR American journal of roentgenology 1976;127:393-6.
57. Hildebrand P, Esnaashari H, Franke C, Burk C, Bruch HP. Surgical management of pancreaticoduodenal artery aneurysms in association with celiac trunk occlusion or stenosis. Annals of vascular surgery 2007;21:10-5.
58. Mandel SR, Jaques PF, Sanofsky S, Mauro MA. Nonoperative management of peripancreatic arterial aneurysms. A 10-year experience. Annals of surgery 1987;205:126-8.
59. Gangahar DM, Carveth SW, Reese HE, Buchman RJ, Breiner MA. True aneurysm of the pancreaticoduodenal artery: a case report and review of the literature. Journal of vascular surgery : official publication, the Society for Vascular Surgery [and] International Society for Cardiovascular Surgery, North American Chapter 1985;2:741-2.
60. Krmpotich PT, Makdisi WF. Superior pancreaticoduodenal artery aneurysm rupture presenting with hemorrhage from the ampulla of Vater into the gastrointestinal tract. The American journal of gastroenterology 1995;90:2046-7.
61. Sessa C, Tinelli G, Porcu P, Aubert A, Thony F, Magne JL. Treatment of visceral artery aneurysms: description of a retrospective series of 42 aneurysms in 34 patients. Annals of vascular surgery 2004;18:695-703.
62. Carroccio A, Jacobs TS, Faries P, et al. Endovascular treatment of visceral artery aneurysms. Vascular and endovascular surgery 2007;41:373-82.
63. Tulsyan N, Kashyap VS, Greenberg RK, et al. The endovascular management of visceral artery aneurysms and pseudoaneurysms. Journal of vascular surgery : official publication, the Society for Vascular Surgery [and] International Society for Cardiovascular Surgery, North American Chapter 2007;45:276-83; discussion 83.
64. Neschis DG, Safford SD, Golden MA. Management of pancreaticoduodenal artery aneurysms presenting as catastrophic intraabdominal bleeding. Surgery 1998;123:8-12.
65. Boudghene F, L'Hermine C, Bigot JM. Arterial complications of pancreatitis: diagnostic and therapeutic aspects in 104 cases. Journal of vascular and interventional radiology : JVIR 1993;4:551-8.

45

CHAPTER

Vascular Surgery Post-Operative Complications

Sachinder Singh Hans, MD, FACS, FRCS(C)

INTRODUCTION

Complications following arterial reconstructions offer one of the greatest challenges to the vascular surgeon and if not managed promptly may lead to catastrophic results, in terms of limb or life-threatening event, as well as major morbidity. Intraoperative complications such as major venous injury during open AAA repair or cranial nerve injury during distal exposure for high plaque for carotid endarterectomy should be avoided by meticulous operative technique. On the other hand, some complications such as post carotid endarterectomy stroke, graft thrombosis and hemorrhage are often first diagnosed in the recovery room. These patients required rapid assessment by the surgeon and return to the operating room in most instances. With the adoption of endovascular therapy in managing vascular disease, a different set of complications occur despite lower morbidity and mortality and shorter length of stay for these procedures. During the performance of endovascular procedure, knowledge of "bail out" techniques are essential in the hands of an interventionalist, and close follow-up of these patients is necessary as patients may require secondary interventions.

COMPLICATIONS OF CAROTID ENDARTERECTOMY

Carotid endarterectomy (CEA) is an established surgical procedure in the treatment of asymptomatic (severe) extracranial carotid stenosis. In order to justify carotid endarterectomy (CEA), incidence of complications must be less than the risk of stroke for untreated carotid stenosis. Combined stroke/death rate should be less than 3% in asymptomatic patients and less than 6% in symptomatic patients.

POSTOPERATIVE STROKE

Commonest causes of postoperative stroke following carotid endarterectomy are:

1. Thromboembolism.
2. Cerebral ischemia during carotid artery clamping.
3. Thrombosis of carotid endarterectomy due to a technically imperfect endarterectomy.
4. Embolization of the plaque or thrombotic material can occur during manipulation of the carotid artery bifurcation.
5. Intracerebral hemorrhage.
6. Stroke from contralateral carotid artery or posterior circulation.

If stroke occurs following carotid endarterectomy, immediate assessment should be performed by carotid duplex study (portable) and emergency non-contrast CT scan of the head. If the patient was awake following carotid endarterectomy and subsequently developed neurological deficit, the patient should be presumed to have post carotid endarterectomy thrombosis. Satisfactory neurological outcome can be expected in more than half the patients if they come back to the operating room for re-exploration of CEA site.[1,2] Occasionally, the patient can be unresponsive following carotid endarterectomy. Immediate assessment of arterial blood gasses should be performed as acute respiratory acidosis superimposed on a patient with chronic obstructive pulmonary disease (COPD) can result in an unresponsive state.

Table 1: Post-op Stroke following Carotid Endarterectomy

1. Carotid duplex AND		
2. CT scan of the head (non-contrast)		
↓ Post CEA thrombosis	↓ Intracerebral hemorrhage/occlusion MCA	↓ Occlusion distal branches of MCA
↓ Suspected by clinical scenario and carotid duplex workup	↓ If carotid duplex shows normal flow in the CCA and ICA and if CT scan of the head shows MCA sign	↓ If CT scan is negative and carotid duplex study shows normal carotid endarterectomy site
↓ Re-exploration/removal of the intimal flap patch graft and completion arteriogram	↓ Interventional Neuroradiology consult for retrieval of the plaque	↓ Medical management for embolization to small branches of MCA
	↓ If CT scan of the head shows intracerebral hemorrhage	
	↓ Immediate Neurosurgery consult for possible craniotomy	

Cerebral ischemia during CEA (carotid clamping) and the indwelling shunt is necessary in about 10% of patients undergoing CEA under cervical block anesthesia (patient awake), and 12-18% under general anesthesia with EEG monitoring.[3,4] Ischemic infarct with contralateral neuro deficit may occur due to malfunction of the shunt or its non-usage in patients with incomplete Circle of Willis.

CEREBRAL HYPERPERFUSION SYNDROME

Cerebral hyperperfusion syndrome is defined as an increase in cerebral blood flow in excess of metabolic demand following carotid endarterectomy or stenting. Reported incidence is as high as 2.2% following carotid endarterectomy and as high as 5.5% following carotid artery stent placement. Cerebral hyperperfusion syndrome is a particularly feared complication of carotid revascularization as permanent disability or death may result from cerebral hemorrhage or ensuing seizures. Initial symptoms include unilateral headache, facial and ocular pain, seizure, or focal neurological deficit. Discrete quantitative criteria for the development of cerebral hyperperfusion syndrome presently do not exist. However, cold xenon or single photon emission CT scanning to compare preoperative versus postoperative, as well as operative side versus non-operative side cerebral blood flow has been described. Risk factors include postoperative hypertension, high-grade stenosis, poor collateral flow, and contralateral carotid occlusion. Clamping of the internal carotid artery during carotid endarterectomy can contribute to the development of this condition by inducing hyperperfusion post-operatively, although prolonged clamp time has not been found to place patients at increased risk of cerebral hyperperfusion. Specifically, the generation of reactive oxygen species as the clamp is released from the internal carotid artery causes a reperfusion injury to the cerebrovascular endothelium and leads to subsequent edema.[5,6] The use of a shunt at time of clamping may help to mitigate this phenomenon. Patients who go on to develop cerebrovascular hyperperfusion syndrome following carotid endarterectomy have been consistently shown to exhibit decreased pre-operative cerebrovascular reactivity to acetazolamide. General anesthesia with continued post-operative propofol sedation may confer significant protection against this complication in high-risk patients, as propofol has been shown to reduce cerebral perfusion. Strict blood pressure control can be maintained with this technique, although the possibility of missing a perioperative stroke exists. Two-stage carotid artery angioplasty is presently under investigation as a method to reduce the incidence of cerebral hyperperfusion syndrome following carotid stenting among patients with elevated operative risk for carotid endarterectomy. An initial angioplasty is performed with an undersized balloon, with subsequent stenting following approximately one month afterward. Initial results have shown promise, with one small series reporting manifestation of cerebral hyperperfusion syndrome in 56% of patients treated with traditional carotid artery stenting versus 0% among those treated with the two-stage approach.

CERVICAL HEMATOMA

Postoperative cervical hematoma has a reported incidence of 2-15%.[7] Cervical hematoma following carotid endarterectomy is associated with multiple other perioperative complications, including cranial nerve injury, myocardial infarction, infection, stroke, respiratory compromise, and death. Inpatient length stay is increased by a week, on average, for patients who develop hematoma after carotid endarterectomy. Combined aspirin and clopidogrel platelet inhibition therapy carries an increased risk for hematoma, with an odds ratio of 1.82.[7] Patients with symptomatic stenosis have been shown to be at increased risk. However, these are the patients most frequently placed on combined antiplatelet regimens. The use of dextran has been more strongly implicated as a risk factor, with an odds ratio of 2.72 for subsequent hematoma.[7]

Postoperative hypertension, with systolic blood pressure in excess of 160 mm Hg, has shown to be associated with hematoma formation in carotid endarterectomy patients. The use of closed suction drainage has not reduced the rate of re-exploration of the neck following carotid endarterectomy, but may help to recognize bleeding patients. Blood loss can be significant, with a decrease in postoperative hemoglobin on an average of 20%. When hematoma is recognized, prompt evaluation of the airway is critical. Endotracheal intubation should be performed if there is any evidence of impending airway compromise.[8] Approximately 0.7-5% of patients with evidence of hematoma will require re-exploration, and relatively few patients will have a readily addressable source of bleeding. The majority will have diffuse oozing from the operative site and anastomosis. Topical administration of thrombin to the anastomosis and wound bed may help mitigate this phenomenon. Reversal of heparin with protamine sulfate reduces the risk of cervical hematoma three-fold when compared with patients whose anticoagulation at time of carotid clamping is not reversed.

CRANIAL NERVE PALSY

Hypoglossal is the most common nerve injured during carotid endarterectomy, followed by vagus and ramus mandibularis. The most common cause of injury is clamp trauma or stretch injury, the transection of the nerve is uncommon.[9] Glossopharyngeal nerve injury may occur in patients undergoing CEA for high plaques. Incidence of nerve injury is higher in patients undergoing redo carotid surgery.

PATCH GRAFT RUPTURE

Saphenous vein patch rupture is a thankfully rare complication of patch angioplasty performed in conjunction with carotid endarterectomy because of the usage of saphenous vein as patch material of choice for CEA. Vein patch has been supplanted by synthetic material (Dacron or PTFE) or bovine pericardial patch. Aseptic necrosis of the vein patch typically occurs without warning two to seven days after surgery.[10] Patients may experience pain or swelling at the operative site exacerbated with respirations. Stroke or death may ensue if the condition is not recognized promptly. Pathologically, this process is characterized by central aseptic necrosis of the graft without anastomotic disruption. While perioperative hypertension is thought to contribute to the development of patch graft rupture, the primary risk factor is felt to be technical. Nearly all cases of saphenous vein patch rupture have occurred with graft specimens harvested at the level of the ankle, with a reported incidence of aseptic necrosis and rupture of 4%. The rate of aseptic necrosis among saphenous patch grafts harvested from the groin or thigh approaches 0%. This is most likely due to the increased diameter and thickness of the vein in its proximal portion. It has been suggested that width of saphenous vein patch grafts be kept below 4 mm to prevent aneurysmal dilatation. Careful surgical technique to minimize damage to the intima and media may also be key in preventing this lethal complication.

PATCH GRAFT INFECTION

Infection of carotid patch graft angioplasty is a phenomenon that is, for the most part, specific to synthetic graft material. Dacron graft material implanted for carotid endarterectomy has a reported infection rate of as high as 0.5%. *Staphylococcus epidermidis* and *Staphylococcus aureus* are the most common pathogens isolated from culture. The majority, approximately 80%, of infections will occur in the first sixty days following CEA. The remainder may present much later, up to several years postoperatively. Development of cervical hematoma is an independent risk factor for graft infection. Patients will present with a cervical pseudoaneurysm, swelling of the neck, or a draining sinus tract. Treatment options include incision and drainage with appropriate antibiotic coverage, Dacron patch excision with saphenous vein patch angioplasty, or patch excision with vein interposition graft. Sternocleidomastoid muscle flap reconstruction may be necessary to achieve adequate tissue coverage for patients with extensive soft tissue necrosis (Figures 1, 2, 3).

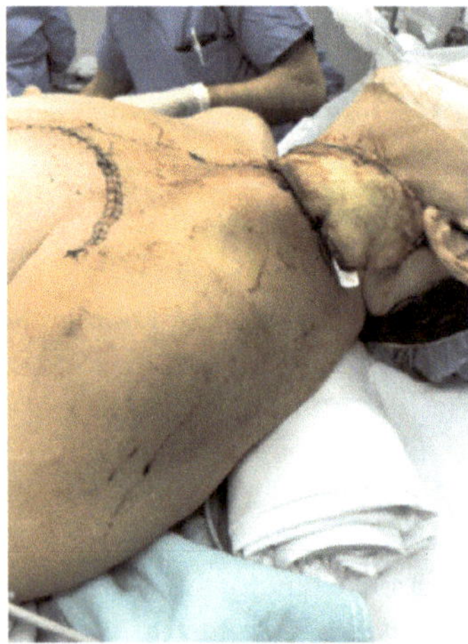

Figure 1: Pectoralis major myocutaneous flap for prosthetic patch graft infection following CEA in a patient with radiation induced carotid stenosis

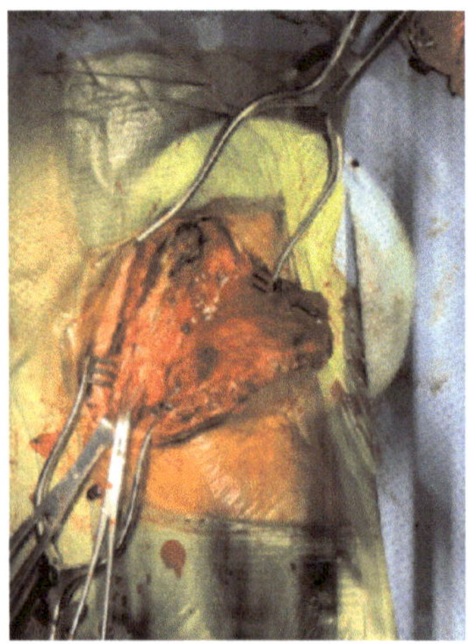

Figure 2: Exposed carotid endarterectomy site with Dacron patch and pectoralis major patch following secondary hemorrhage

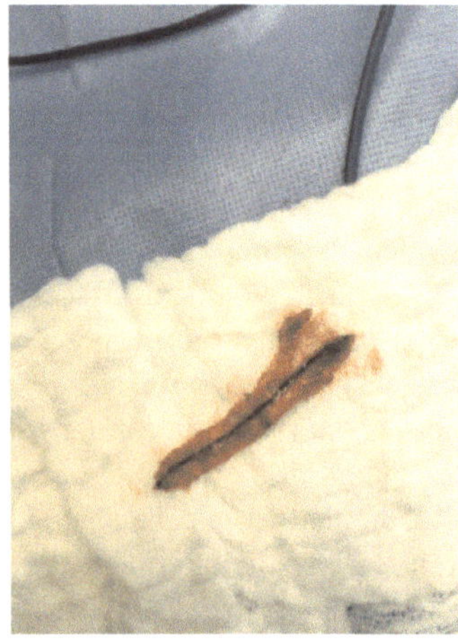

Figure 3: Removed infected Dacron patch used during CEA

POSTOPERATIVE MYOCARDIAL INFARCTION

Postoperative myocardial infarction remains a serious complication of surgical intervention in the medically debilitated population that is typically in need of carotid revascularization. The Carotid Revascularization Endarterectomy Versus Stenting Trial (CREST) has demonstrated a higher risk for postoperative MI following carotid endarterectomy as compared with carotid artery stenting, with a hazard ratio of 0.50 and 95% confidence interval, after review of 2502 patients.[11] The CREST investigators defined myocardial infarction as an elevation of biomarkers to greater than twice the upper limit of normal in conjunction with either chest pain lasting greater than fifteen minutes or evidence of ischemia on ECG obtained six to eight hours following endarterectomy.[11] Among patients suffering from postoperative MI, the majority occurred within twenty-four hours of surgery. At two-year follow-up, patients with evidence of postoperative MI demonstrated increased mortality versus those with no such event, with a hazard ratio of 3.40 and 95% confidence interval. Estimated four-year mortality was 7.1%, approximately three times higher than that of patients who had not suffered postoperative MI. Mortality rate was equivalent between genders as well as between symptomatic versus asymptomatic preoperative status. The Endarterectomy Versus Angioplasty in Patients with Symptomatic Severe Carotid Stenosis (EVA-3S) trial describes a postoperative MI rate of 0.4% for carotid artery stenting versus 0.8% for carotid endarterectomy. The Stenting and Angioplasty with Protection in Patients at High Risk for Endarterectomy (SAPPHIRE) trial reported a higher MI rate for both patients undergoing carotid artery stenting and carotid endarterectomy, 2.4% and 5.9% respectively. Patients with pre-existing coronary artery disease or renal impairment were at increased risk. It has been suggested that a similar approach to carotid artery stenting, with high dose statins or dual antiplatelet therapy, may be reasonable. While the rate of major perioperative bleeding is increased by 0.4-1% when clopidogrel antiplatelet therapy is used in conjunction with aspirin when compared to aspirin alone, this may be justified in patients with known coronary artery disease or renal impairment. The potential benefit of CEA versus stenting with respect to decreased postoperative stroke rate must be weighed against the cardiac risk, given the concordance of the findings of increased cardiac events associated with carotid endarterectomy as compared with carotid stenting among the current major prospective trials.

CAROTID RESTENOSIS

Carotid restenosis, as defined in the CREST trial, represents reduction in diameter of the carotid artery of at least 70% with peak systolic velocity of at least 3.0 m/s. Carotid duplex ultrasound performed on patients who have undergone carotid endarterectomy with patch angioplasty may show an increased peak systolic velocity just distal to the patch angioplasty at the origin of internal carotid artery due to a relative narrowing of the lumen as the reconstructed vessel tapers at the end of the graft. As such, peak systolic velocity criteria for stenosis in preoperative patients may not hold true for detecting restenosis in those who have undergone carotid endarterectomy with patch angioplasty. Secondary analysis of the CREST randomized controlled trial showed a nearly equivocal restenosis rate of 6.0% for carotid stenting versus 6.3% for carotid endarterectomy at two-year follow-up.[12,13] Female gender, diabetes mellitus, dyslipidemia, and tobacco abuse were independent risk factors. Although nearly half of such patients were asymptomatic, those with restenosis were at increased risk of ipsilateral stroke versus those without restenosis at two-year follow-up with a hazard ratio of 4.37 at 95% confidence interval. There are, at present, no universally accepted guidelines for revascularization in patients with restenosis. Treatment remains at the discretion of the patient and surgeon given the established risks of restenosis and individual comorbidities. Revascularization options include balloon angioplasty, carotid stenting, and repeat carotid endarterectomy. Carotid artery stenting for restenosis has been shown to have a decreased rate of embolic complications versus primary stenting and is felt to be as safe as repeat carotid endarterectomy for treatment of restenosis.

CAROTID ANEURYSM

Extracranial carotid aneurysm is a relatively uncommon entity. It represents, at most, 2% of all carotid surgical procedures. Presenting symptoms may mirror that of carotid stenosis or may be complicated by an acute stroke or a painful, pulsatile mass in the neck. The majority of patients are asymptomatic at time of diagnosis. Carotid aneurysm arises most frequently at the level of the common carotid artery, with approximately half of all carotid aneurysms being of the saccular type and the remainder fusiform.[14-16] Atherosclerosis is thought to be the most common etiology. Trauma, previous carotid endarterectomy, infection, cystic medial necrosis, Marfan syndrome, syphilis, and Takayasu arteritis may also contribute to the development of carotid aneurysm. Attempted internal jugular access with inadvertent puncture of the carotid artery is a known iatrogenic cause for carotid pseudoaneurysm. Preferred imaging modalities are similar to that of carotid stenosis, with most lesions being discovered initially on carotid ultrasound. CT angiography, magnetic resonance angiography or angiography, are useful adjuncts for pre-operative planning. Carotid aneurysm carries a risk or rupture, embolic stroke, thrombosis, and possible cranial nerve impairment due to mass effect on adjacent structures. Intervention is frequently warranted and typically consists of interposition graft placement consisting of autologous saphenous vein, internal iliac artery, or synthetic graft material. Surgical exposure is similar to that of carotid endarterectomy. Carotid ligation, innominate to carotid artery bypass, aneurysmectomy with primary repair, and endovascular exclusion with deployment of a stent-graft, has also been described. Interposition graft placement carried a reported 6% incidence of permanent cranial nerve injury, 2% perioperative stroke rate, and a stroke free rate of 87% at twenty-year follow-up in a series of 57 patients.[14-16] Carotid aneurysms that extend to the base of the skull represent a challenge for the surgeon attempting open repair and may be exposed with double mandibular osteotomy and subsequent mini plate osteosynthesis reconstruction. In particular, mycotic aneurysms can be amenable to ligation due to the increased risk of subsequent graft infection if stump pressures are 70 mm Hg or greater. Otherwise, the risk of perioperative stroke becomes prohibitive. An endovascular approach may be preferred in those patients with high cardiac risk or previous radiation treatment to the neck. A prospective case control trial on endovascular versus open surgical treatment of carotid aneurysm has yet to be conducted, owing to the relative rarity of this condition as well as the unexpected nature of its discovery.

THORACOABDOMINAL ANEURYSM REPAIR

Open repair of thoracoabdominal aortic aneurysm is probably the most challenging operation in all vascular surgery. Operative mortality (within 30 days) ranges from 5 to 12%.[16-20] The main factor determining the mortality following thoracoabdominal aneurysm repair is:

1. Increasing age.
2. Extent of thoracoabdominal aortic aneurysm (higher in type 1 and type 2).
3. Urgency of the repair.

High rates of complications are usually observed in patients who undergo emergency or urgent thoracoabdominal aneurysm repair.[16-20]

Complications include:

1. Renal failure, preoperative renal dysfunction and post-op renal failure adversely affect operative mortality.
2. Cardiac and pulmonary complications. Respiratory failure is the commonest complication following thoracoabdominal aneurysm repair. Therefore, diaphragm-sparing techniques and slow weaning following ventilatory support should be carried out.
3. Spinal cord ischemia. This is the most feared and dreaded complication of thoracoabdominal aneurysm repair and usually results from multiple factors. But one

common denominator is ischemic injury to the spinal cord due to temporary or permanent interruption of the spinal cord blood supply. If the deficit is partial, good recovery may occur. However, patients who undergo urgent repair of thoracoabdominal aneurysm and have proximal extent of the thoracoabdominal aneurysm repair (type 1 and type 2) have higher incidence of spinal cord ischemia.

Five-year survival following thoracoabdominal repair is 67.2% +/- 5%.[18]

COMPLICATIONS OF RUPTURED ABDOMINAL AORTIC ANEURYSM REPAIR

Repair of ruptured AAA has a mortality of 30-70% depending upon the type of rupture (contained or frank). Preoperative shock (duration) and age of the patient are important factors in determining the morbidity/mortality.[21] Patients presenting in the ER with normal blood pressure, age less than 80 years, and hemoglobin equal or more than 10g% have better outcomes. The most important factor determining the mortality of ruptured AAA is the time interval between rupture and the time of aortic cross clamping.[21]

1. Repair of a ruptured abdominal aortic aneurysm is technically challenging and injury to the surrounding veins (left renal vein, iliac veins, and inferior vena cava) can result in profound blood loss and increasing the morbidity and mortality of the operation.[22]
2. Lower extremity ischemia. This could be the result of inadequate anticoagulation or embolization with failure of properly flushing the graft as the anastomoses are being completed. In patients with suspected distal embolization, Fogarty catheter should be passed distally, and embolic material retrieved before the distal anastomosis is completed.[22,23]
3. Colon ischemia (40%) and is usually associated in patients with shock and massive transfusion.[22,23] If colon ischemia is suspected, (prolonged ileus, metabolic acidosis, and diarrhea with passage of mucus or blood) immediate flexible sigmoidoscopy should be performed. Colectomy should be performed for full-thickness necrosis of the bowel and supportive treatment with patient being kept nothing by mouth, total parenteral nutrition (TPN) and correction of fluid and electrolytes.
4. Abdominal compartment syndrome can occur in 30-40% of patients following repair of ruptured abdominal aortic aneurysm and can result in multiple organ failure. If abdominal compartment syndrome is suspected, (pressure measurements with the help of Foley catheter in the urinary bladder), one should leave the abdomen open and cover the abdominal wall with mesh and consider performing delayed closure. Contributing factors for abdominal compartment syndrome include:[24]
   1. Duration of aortic occlusion balloon or proximal clamp.
   2. Massive blood transfusion.
   3. Coagulopathy at the completion of the operation.

COMLICATIONS OF NON-RUPTURED ABDOMINAL AORTIC ANEURYSM REPAIR

The mortality of abdominal aortic aneurysm repair varies from 3-5% and morbidity of 20-25%. Pulmonary complications are the most common (8-15%), however, MI is the leading cause of early and delayed deaths following open repair of abdominal aortic aneurysm (MI 98%, renal failure 5-15%, or dialysis dependent 1-6%), colon ischemia 1-2%, DVT 5-8%, bleeding 2-5%, distal embolization 1-4%, ureteral injury and spinal cord ischemia less than 1%.[25]

READMISSION FOLLOWING OPEN REPAIR OF AAA

Wound complications are the commonest, followed by bowel obstruction. Graft-related complications after endovascular aneurysm repair develop in about 10-15% of patients and in 2% of patients undergoing open AAA repair.

COMLICATIONS OF ENDOVASCULAR REPAIR OF RUPTURED ABDOMINAL AORTIC ANEURYSM

Endovascular repair of ruptured abdominal aortic aneurysm is better tolerated and has better outcome than open repair of ruptured AAA. However, there is a high incidence of abdominal compartment syndrome and incidence of colon ischemia is similar to open repair.[24]

COMPLICATIONS OF AORTOBIFEMORAL BYPASS GRAFT

Mortality should be less than 5% (range 1-2%). Major complication rate should be less than 10%. Common complications following aorto-femoral bypass procedure are pulmonary (commonest), followed by cardiac, renal failure, and pancreatitis.[26,27] Complications can be reduced by preoperative assessment and meticulous surgical technique. Complications pertaining to the procedure itself include[26,27]:

1. Colon/pelvic ischemia.
2. Atheroembolization with lower extremity ischemia.
3. Male sexual dysfunction.

4. Wound complications in the groin.
5. Pelvic ischemia is rare, but a very serious complication and results in either:
   a. Colon ischemia.
   b. Infarction of the buttock musculature/skin.
6. Cauda equina/lumbar plexopathy with neurological deficit.

Therefore, flow to one of the hypogastric arteries should be maintained either by considering the end-to-side anastomosis to the hypogastric artery or a jump graft to the hypogastric artery. Atheroembolization occurs during dissection and clamping and if it is major, thromboembolectomy will become necessary and if flecks of microembolization, it presents as blue toenail syndrome which would be treated with antiplatelet medications and pain control and observation. Many lesions which appear to be severe at the time of presentation (microembolization), will improve at follow up and local amputation of the toes is rarely necessary. Rigorous flushing of the distal vessels into the pelvic and the femoral artery before establishing the flow distally is important. Thrombosis of a limb or entire graft is usually due to technical errors resulting from the kink in the graft or narrowing of anastomosis. Male sexual dysfunction can result from inadequate pelvic perfusion or interruption of autonomic nerves coursing over the distal aorta and proximal iliac arteries and the incidence is 5-15%, with the disruption of the internal urinary sphincter resulting in retrograde ejaculation.[26,27] Wound complications occur in 15% of the patients due to wound breakdown with healing problems. The wound infections are uncommon. Patency of aortobifemoral graft at 5 years is 80-90%.[26,27] Patency of the aortoiliac endarterectomy is comparable to that of aortobifemoral graft with its attendant complications and avoids the insertion of a prosthetic material, but the procedure is technically demanding. Late deaths following aorto-femoral grafts are due to cardiovascular causes, therefore, aggressive management of risk factors for atherosclerosis is important. Five percent of patients following aorto-femoral graft procedure develop femoral anastomotic aneurysm. Incidence may be higher depending upon the duration of follow-up. These are usually caused by suture breakage, graft infection, degeneration of the native artery, and rarely due to technical errors. Incidence of prosthetic graft infection is 1-2%. The prosthetic graft exposure in the groin will require appropriate antibiotics and muscle flap reconstruction. The most commonly used flap for exposed graft in the groin is sartorius myoplasty (Figures 4 and 5).

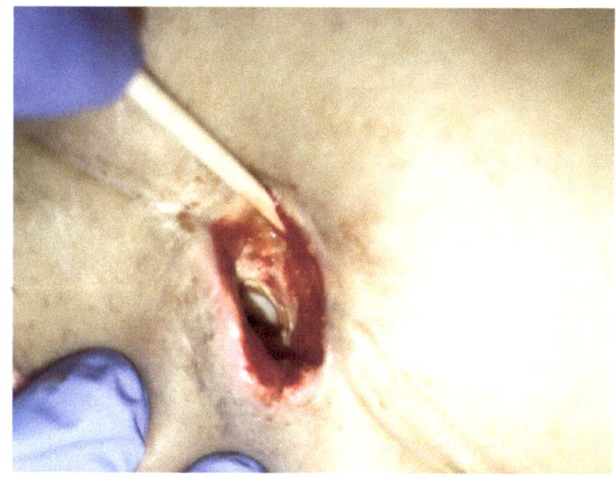

Figure 4: Exposed graft in the left groin following repair of left femoral anastomotic aneurysm

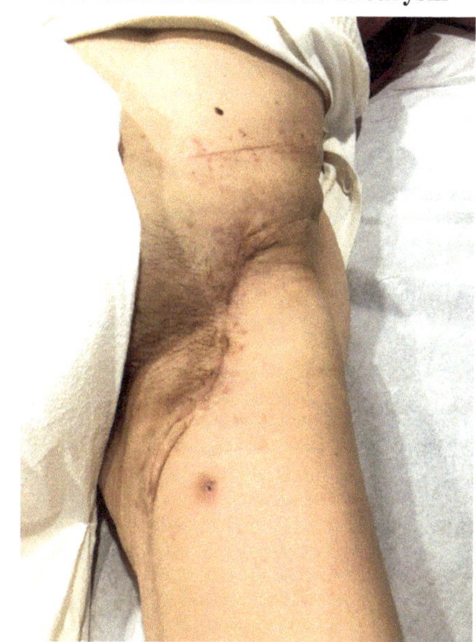

Figure 5: Satisfactory healing 3 months later following sartorius myoplasty

COMPLICATIONS OF EXTRA-ANATOMIC BYPASS GRAFTS (AXILLOFEMORAL AND FEMORAL-FEMORAL CROSSOVER GRAFT)

1. Graft occlusion. Five-year patency is slightly inferior to aorto-femoral graft (69-75%).
2. Five-year patency of femoro-femoral graft is 60-80%.

Incidence of proximal graft disruption is 5%. Repeated shoulder abduction associated with infraclavicular pain and swelling may result in proximal graft disruption. Another interposition graft may become necessary with a new anastomosis to the axillary artery. Thromboembolization to the donor upper extremity artery (25%) may occur during re-operation or due to embolization from the blind segment of the occluded axillofemoral graft.

COMPLICATIONS AFTER EXTRA-ANATOMIC BYPASS GRAFT

1. Infection. Infection in the groin needs CT scan evaluation to determine the extent of infection. If the entire graft is involved, removal of the graft with a new extra-anatomic bypass graft will be necessary. If there is a partial graft infection, removal of the involved portion of the graft may help in resolving the graft infection, although there is always a danger of infection involving the remaining portion of the graft.
2. Perigraft seroma. Sterile perigraft fluid collection surrounded by fibrous pseudocapsule. Worst cases resolved with conservative therapy. May need graft and perigraft cyst excision. Five-year survival following axillofemoral graft is 52%, five-year patency 71%.[27,28]

COMPLICATIONS OF ENDOVASCULAR PROCEDURES FOR AORTOILIAC OCCLUSIVE DISEASE

Due to increasing experience of the interventionalists, iliac stenting for iliac artery occlusion is being increasingly performed. These procedures have inferior primary patency, but equivalent secondary patency and shorter length of stay with lower morbidity than open reconstruction.

Arterial access complications include:

1. Bleeding = 2%.
2. Thrombosis at the access site.
3. Pseudoaneurysm.
4. Arteriovenous fistula.

Access complications are higher for brachial artery access, larger sheath, multiple exchanges, and small diameter arteries particularly in women.[29-32] In patients with chronic occlusions, there may be a fresh thrombus superimposed on a stenotic artery. Patients may need preliminary thrombolysis (with TPA) before considering iliac stenting; otherwise, distal embolization may occur. Rupture of an iliac artery (and heavily calcified arteries) may occur during iliac angioplasty and stenting and can be treated with:

1. Prolonged balloon inflation.
2. Covered stent placement.
3. Patients may need emergency aorto-femoral grafting.

Primary patency of endovascular procedures for aortoiliac occlusive disease is 69-76% at two years, secondary patency 85-95% at two years, and overall complication rate of 1.4-4.8%. Many series have shown that primary patency of endovascular therapy for aortoiliac occlusive disease is lower than aorto-femoral grafting. However, secondary patency is equivalent in both endovascular and open reconstruction groups.

COMPLICATIONS BYPASS GRAFT TO POPLITEAL AND INFRAPOPLITEAL ARTERIES

1. Thrombosis within less than 30 days is caused by technical error or poor choice of arterial conduit. If a graft thrombosis develops, immediate thrombectomy should be performed. Factors contributing to graft thrombosis include age less than 60 years, African American race, non-diabetics, and bypass to tibial artery have a higher incidence of graft thrombosis. Late graft thrombosis is usually not due to technical factors. Vein grafts develop intimal hyperplasia (20-23%) significant graft stenosis, solitary and focal within two years of implantation.[33] Routine duplex surveillance identifies and monitors such lesions. They are treated either by percutaneous intervention or open repair.
2. Bleeding during infrainguinal bypass is uncommon, as small branches of the vein conduit should be ligated and may need suture ligature with a fine monofilament suture. Hemostatic clips should usually be avoided. Bleeding in the graft tunnel may occur during passage of a tunneler. Anastomotic bleeding should be treated with re-do anastomosis. This bleeding usually results from technical factors or due to anticoagulation and antiplatelet therapy.
3. Infection and lymphatic leak are more common if the bypass is performed for critical limb ischemia (ulceration and gangrene) and patients should be treated with systemic antibiotics and may need local debridement. Surgical site infection often is superficial. Wound care and antibiotics are useful. Deep infection can lead to graft exposure and rupture. Aggressive treatment by debridement and muscle flap closure is often necessary. Prosthetic graft exposure, complete graft removal and replacement with either autogenous vein or cryopreserved vein may become necessary. Lymphatic leak increases the risk of late graft infection.

COMPLICATIONS PROSTHETIC GRAFTS FEMORAL, POPLITEAL AND INFRAPOPLITEAL

1. Occlusion and infection. If graft occlusion occurs within less than six months is due to technical reasons where the causes are compliance mismatch, thrombogenicity, poor hemodynamics and progression of the disease. Compliance mismatch often results in intimal hyperplasia, anastomotic stenosis and decreases the patency of the conduit. Since the prosthetic grafts lack the functional intima, there is an increased incidence of thrombosis. Endothelializing of the graft and heparin bonding have not yielded superior results. Patency rate

at three years for below-knee femoropopliteal grafts varies from 25-40% and some series have reported only patency of about 12%.[33]

2. Infection of the prosthetic graft. Entire graft removal is often necessary, although segmental resection of the infected prosthesis can be used in selected cases. Rifampicin-soaked Dacron graft has yielded some success following removal of the infected prosthetic graft.
5. Seroma following ePTFE graft. Seepage of serous fluid can result in infection. Patency of femoropopliteal vein bypass at five years is 60-75% and below-knee patency (vein graft) at three years 76-78%.

COMPLICATIONS OF INFRAPOPLITEAL BYPASS

Complications of dorsalis pedis bypass:

1. Higher mortality than femoropopliteal bypass (4.2%, post-op wound infection in 2%).
2. Re-operation for graft thrombosis, post-op bleeding or infection is required in 4-7% of patients. Primary patency of dorsalis pedis bypass is 56.6% and secondary patency of 62.8% with lymph salvage rate of 78.2% at five years. Secondary patency of peroneal bypass = 78%. Patency of dorsalis pedis and plantar bypasses at two years is 70%.[34-36]

REFERENCES

1. Hans SS. Extracranial Carotid and Vertebral Artery Aneurysms. In Extracranial Carotid and Vertebral Artery Disease: Contemporary Management. Hans SS (ed.) Springer 2018. 135-147.
2. Hans SS. Results of carotid re-exploration for post-carotid endarterectomy thrombosis. J Cardiovasc Surg (Torino). 2007 Oct;48(5):587-91.
3. Hans SS, Jareunpoon O. Prospective evaluation of electroencephalography, carotid artery stump pressure, and neurologic changes during 314 consecutive carotid endarterectomies performed in awake patients. J Vasc Surg. 2007 Mar;45(3):511-5.
4. Schneider JR, Droste JS, Schindler N, Golan JF, Bernstein LP, Rosenberg RS. Carotid endarterectomy with routine electroencephalography and selective shunting: Influence of contralateral internal carotid artery occlusion and utility in prevention of perioperative strokes. J Vasc Surg. 2002 Jun;35(6):1114-22.
5. Suga Y, Ogasawara K, Saito H, Komoribayashi N, Kobayashi M, Inoue T, Otawara Y, Ogawa A. Preoperative cerebral hemodynamic impairment and reactive oxygen species produced during carotid endarterectomy correlate with development of postoperative cerebral hyperperfusion. Stroke. 2007 Oct;38(10):2712-7.
6. Kawamata T, Okada Y, Kawashima A, Yoneyama T, Yamaguchi K, Ono Y, Hori T. Postcarotid endarterectomy cerebral hyperperfusion can be prevented by minimizing intraoperative cerebral ischemia and strict postoperative blood pressure control under continuous sedation. Neurosurgery. 2009 Mar;64(3):447-53; discussion 453-4.
7. Comerota AJ, Difiore R, Tzilinis A, Chahwan S. Cervical Hematoma Following Carotid Endarterectomy is Morbid and Preventable: A 12-Year Case-Controlled Review. Vasc Endovascular Surg. 2012 Nov;46(8):610-6.
8. Shakespeare WA, Lanier WL, Perkins WJ, Pasternak JJ. Airway management in patients who develop neck hematomas after carotid endarterectomy. Anesth Analg. 2010 Feb 1;110(2):588-93.
9. Schauber MD, Fontenelle LJ, Solomon JW, Hanson TL. Cranial/cervical nerve dysfunction after carotid endarterectomy. J Vasc Surg. 1997 Mar;25(3):481-7.
10. Scott EW, Dolson L, Day AL, Seeger JM. Carotid endarterectomy complicated by vein patch rupture. Neurosurgery. 1992 Aug;31(2):373-6; discussion 376-7.
11. Blackshear JL, Cutlip DE, Roubin GS, Hill MD, Leimgruber PP, Begg RJ, Cohen DJ, Eidt JF, Narins CR, Prineas RJ, Glasser SP, Voeks JH, Brott TG; CREST Investigators. Myocardial infarction after carotid stenting and endarterectomy: results from the carotid revascularization endarterectomy versus stenting trial. Circulation. 2011 Jun 7;123(22):2571-8.
12. Lal BK, Beach KW, Roubin GS, Lutsep HL, Moore WS, Malas MB, Chiu D, Gonzales NR, Burke JL, Rinaldi M, Elmore JR, Weaver FA, Narins CR, Foster M, Hodgson KJ, Shepard AD, Meschia JF, Bergelin RO, Voeks JH, Howard G, Brott TG; CREST Investigators. Restenosis after carotid artery stenting and endarterectomy: a secondary analysis of CREST, a randomised controlled trial. Lancet Neurol. 2012 Sep;11(9):755-63.
13. Vos JA, de Borst GJ, Overtoom TT, de Vries JP, van de Pavoordt ED, Zanen P, Ackerstaff RG; Antonius Carotid Endarterectomy, Angioplasty, and Stenting Study Group. Carotid angioplasty and stenting: treatment of postcarotid endarterectomy restenosis is at least as safe as primary stenosis treatment. J Vasc Surg. 2009 Oct;50(4):755-761. e1.
14. Garg K, Rockman CB, Lee V, Maldonado TS, Jacobowitz GR, Adelman MA, Mussa FF. Presentation and management of carotid artery aneurysms and

pseudoaneurysms. J Vasc Surg. 2012 Jun;55(6):1618-22.
15. Huyzer M, Reijnen MM, Sybrandy JE, Buth J, Zeebregts CJ. Interposition grafting of large extracranial carotid aneurysm._Tex Heart Inst J. 2011;38(1):52-5.
16. Hans SS. Extracranial Carotid and Vertebral Artery Aneurysms. In Extracranial Carotid and Vertebral Artery Disease: Contemporary Management. Hans SS (ed.) Springer 2018. 261-266.
17. Conrad MF, Ergul EA, Patel VI, Cambria MR, Lamuraglia GM, Simon M, Cambria RP. Evolution of operative strategies in open thoracoabdominal aneurysm repair. J Vasc Surg. 2011 May;53(5):1195-1201.
18. Conrad MF, Crawford RS, Davison JK, Cambria RP. Thoracoabdominal aneurysm repair: a 20-year perspective. Ann Thorac Surg. 2007 Feb;83(2):S856-61; discussion S890-2.
19. Patel VI, Ergul E, Conrad MF, Cambria M, LaMuraglia GM, Kwolek CJ, Brewster DC, Cambria RP. Continued favorable results with open surgical repair of type IV thoracoabdominal aortic aneurysms. J Vasc Surg. 2011 Jun;53(6):1492-8.
20. Svensson LG, Crawford ES, Hess KR, Coselli JS, Safi HJ. Experience with 1509 patients undergoing thoracoabdominal aortic operations. J Vasc Surg. 1993 Feb;17(2):357-68; discussion 368-70.
21. Hans SS, Huang RR. Results of 101 ruptured abdominal aortic aneurysm repairs from a single surgical practice. Arch Surg. 2003 Aug;138(8):898-901.
22. Dardik A, Burleyson GP, Bowman H, Gordon TA, Williams GM, Webb TH, Perler BA. Surgical repair of ruptured abdominal aortic aneurysms in the state of Maryland: factors influencing outcome among 527 recent cases. J Vasc Surg. 1998 Sep;28(3):413-20; discussion 420-1.
23. Dueck AD, Kucey DS, Johnston KW, Alter D, Laupacis A. Survival after ruptured abdominal aortic aneurysm: effect of patient, surgeon, and hospital factors. J Vasc Surg. 2004 Jun;39(6):1253-60.
24. Mehta M, Darling RC 3rd, Roddy SP, Fecteau S, Ozsvath KJ, Kreienberg PB, Paty PS, Chang BB, Shah DM. Factors associated with abdominal compartment syndrome complicating endovascular repair of ruptured abdominal aortic aneurysms. J Vasc Surg. 2005 Dec;42(6):1047-51.
25. Chaikof, E. L., Brewster, D. C., Dalman, R. L., et al. The care of patients with an abdominal aortic aneurysm: the Society for Vascular Surgery practice guidelines. J Vasc Surg. 2009 Oct;50(4), S2-S49.
26. De Vries SO, Hunink MG. Results of aortic bifurcation grafts for aortoiliac occlusive disease: a meta-analysis. J Vasc Surg. 1997 Oct;26(4):558-69.
27. Hertzer NR, Bena JF, Karafa MT. A personal experience with direct reconstruction and extra-anatomic bypass for aortoiliofemoral occlusive disease. J Vasc Surg. 2007 Mar;45(3):527-535; discussion 535.
28. Passman MA, Taylor LM, Moneta GL, Edwards JM, Yeager RA, McConnell DB, Porter JM. Comparison of axillofemoral and aortofemoral bypass for aortoiliac occlusive disease. J Vasc Surg. 1996 Feb;23(2):263-9; discussion 269-71.
29. Hans SS, DeSantis D, Siddiqui R, Khoury M. Results of endovascular therapy and aortobifemoral grafting for Transatlantic Inter-Society type C and D aortoiliac occlusive disease. Surgery. 2008 Oct;144(4):583-9; discussion 589-90.
30. Kashyap VS, Pavkov ML, Bena JF, Sarac TP, O'Hara PJ, Lyden SP, Clair DG. The management of severe aortoiliac occlusive disease: endovascular therapy rivals open reconstruction. J Vasc Surg. 2008 Dec;48(6):1451-7, 1457.e1-3.
31. Norgren L, Hiatt WR, Dormandy JA, Nehler MR, Harris KA, Fowkes FG; TASC II Working Group. Inter-Society Consensus for the Management of Peripheral Arterial Disease (TASC II). J Vasc Surg. 2007 Jan;45 Suppl S:S5-67.
32. Klinkert P, Schepers A, Burger DH, van Bockel JH, Breslau PJ. Vein versus polytetrafluoroethylene in above-knee femoropopliteal bypass grafting: five-year results of a randomized controlled trial. J Vasc Surg. 2003 Jan;37(1):149-55.
33. Sachwani GR, Hans SS, Khoury MD, King TF, Mitsuya M, Rizk YS, Zachwieja JA, Sayed L. Long-term results of iliac stenting and aortofemoral grafting for iliac artery occlusions. J Vasc Surg. 2012 Nov 21. [Epub ahead of print]
34. Andros G, Harris RW, Salles-Cunha SX, Dulawa LB, Oblath RW. Lateral plantar artery bypass grafting: defining the limits of foot revascularization. J Vasc Surg. 1989 Nov;10(5):511-9; discussion 520-1.
35. Ascer E, Veith FJ, Gupta SK. Bypasses to plantar arteries and other tibial branches: an extended approach to limb salvage. J Vasc Surg. 1988 Oct;8(4):434-41.
36. Berceli SA, Chan AK, Pomposelli FB Jr, Gibbons GW, Campbell DR, Akbari CM, Brophy DT, LoGerfo FW. Efficacy of dorsal pedal artery bypass in limb salvage for ischemic heel ulcers. J Vasc Surg. 1999 Sep;30(3):499-508.

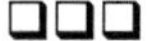

SECTION 5: TRAUMA

46

CHAPTER

Surgical Critical Care

Sanjeev V. Chhangani, MBA, MD, FCCM

INTRODUCTION

Critical care medicine, or Intensive care medicine, is a discipline of medicine concerned with the provision of specialized care to critically ill patients. Critical care originally began with the close monitoring of wounded soldiers in the Crimean war by Florence Nightingale and evolved through the polio epidemic in 1952 into its current multi-disciplinary and multi-professional model. The current multi-professional model of critical care utilizes a team approach (intensivist, nurse, respiratory therapy, pharmacy, physical therapy, nutrition, etc.) to deliver timely, safe, and efficient patient-centered care.

Critical care involves immediate stabilization of abnormal physiology and organ support, followed by definitive therapy and continued care. End-of-life care is part of critical care. Critical illness or injury acutely impairs one or more vital organ systems such that there is a high probability of imminent or life-threatening deterioration of the patient's condition. Although the critically ill are typically cared for in an intensive care unit (ICU) where a high degree of monitoring, attention, and therapy is provided, critical care can be initiated at any place where the patient is determined to be critically ill. Some of the common conditions and concepts in surgical critical care are presented in this chapter. The reader is referred to many treatises in this area for an extensive review.

ACUTE RESPIRATORY FAILURE AND MECHANICAL VENTILATION

Acute respiratory failure is one of the common reasons for admission to ICU and is associated with increased postoperative mortality. Acute respiratory failure, defined as the inability of the lungs to oxygenate the blood and/or eliminate carbon dioxide (CO_2) due to inefficiency of oxygenation and imbalance of respiratory load and capacity, is a non-specific condition and often associated with an underlying process (local: injury/trauma, pneumonia, worsening chronic lung disease; systemic: inflammation, injury/trauma, sepsis). The nature of the underlying process often determines prognosis.[1-2]

Clinical Signs and Symptoms

Tachypnea is an important sign of critical illness and should not be ignored. Dyspnea, as a result of compensatory increased work of breathing, and cyanosis are commonly present. Crackles and other adventitious breath sounds may be heard during auscultation of the chest. These signs and symptoms are a result of a decrease in functional residual capacity (FRC) and lung compliance, as well as an increase in intrapulmonary shunting due to interstitial and alveolar edema, gravity, and weight-based dependent atelectasis. Other signs and symptoms of associated systemic disease may be present. Risk factors for postoperative respiratory failure are listed in Table 1. Phosphorus level should be evaluated as hypophosphatemia can play a significant role in postoperative respiratory failure in a patient with poor respiratory reserve.

Table 1: Risk factors for postoperative respiratory failure

Patient-Related Risk factor for postop pulmonary	
• Age > 50 yrs	• Smoking (OR 1.40-1.73)
• 50-60 (OR 1.50)	
• 60-70 (OR 2.28)	• Emerging risk factors
• 70-80 (OR 3.90)	• OSA (OR 1.37-1.95)
• >80 (OR 5.63)	• Pulmonary HTN
• ASA class ≥ 2 (4.87)	• Asthma is not a risk factor
• Heart failure (OR 2.93)	
• Total functional dependence (OR 2.51)	• Obesity is not a risk factor
• COPD (OR 2.36)	

Diagnosis

Initial diagnosis is made clinically, based on good history and physical examination. This is complemented by laboratory and radiological testing. An important goal in the diagnosis of acute respiratory failure is to determine the degree of its severity and compensation. The pulse oximeter is a useful monitor to assess the adequacy of peripheral arterial hemoglobin saturation. Pulse oximetry, however, does not assess the adequacy of ventilation. An arterial blood gas (ABG) is useful in this regard.

Alveolar-arterial (A-a) oxygen gradient can be calculated using the equation:

(A-a) oxygen gradient = $FiO_2 (P_B - PH_2O) - \underline{PaCO_2} - PaO_2 R$

FiO_2 = fraction of inspired oxygen; P_B = barometric pressure; PH_2O= partial pressure of water; R= respiratory quotient; $PaCO_2$= partial pressure of carbon dioxide in arterial blood; PaO_2= partial pressure of oxygen in arterial blood.

A normal alveolar-arterial (A-a) oxygen gradient (less than 10 mm Hg on room air) suggests pure hypercapnic respiratory failure due to hypoventilation. An increased (A-a) oxygen gradient is present in the presence of hypoxemia due to ventilation/perfusion (V/Q) mismatch, diffusion defect, or intrapulmonary shunt. Criteria for diagnosis of acute lung injury (ALI) and acute respiratory distress syndrome (ARDS) are summarized in Table 2. ALI/ARDS is an acute inflammatory condition of the lungs caused by direct (pneumonia, aspiration, contusion, inhalation of toxic gasses, drowning) or indirect (sepsis, massive trauma, ischemia, cardiopulmonary bypass, systemic inflammation due to major surgery) injury. The ABG in ALI/ARDS will typically show hypoxemia with an acute respiratory alkalosis (low pCO_2) due to hyperventilation. The presence of acute respiratory acidosis in ALI/ARDS is a late sign and indicates respiratory decompensation and impending respiratory arrest. In contrast, respiratory acidosis is common in acute-on-chronic respiratory failure, and hypoxemia is a late sign.

Table 2: Criteria for diagnosis of acute lung injury (ALI) and acute respiratory distress syndrome (ARDS)

Clinical Variable	ALI	ARDS
Onset	Acute	Acute
Hypoxemia	$PaO_2/FiO_2 \leq 300$	$PaO_2/FiO_2 \leq 200$
Chest X-ray	B/L infiltrates Consistent with pul. Edema	B/L infiltrates Consistent with Pul. Edema
Non-cardiac cause	No clinical e/o left atrial HTN or pulm pressure ≤ 18 mm Hg	No clinical e/o left atrial HTN or pulmartery occulusion pressure ≤ 18 mm Hg

Chest radiograph and computed tomography (CT) are commonly performed in the diagnosis of acute respiratory failure. Chest radiograph, in ALI/ARDS, commonly shows bilateral interstitial infiltrates, often diffuse and fluffy, and basal atelectasis. CT scan can accurately define lung pathology (distribution of infiltrates, consolidation, effusions, atelectasis, and pneumothorax).[3] The radiological findings are subject to change due to the evolving nature of the disease process and the effects of PEEP and lung recruitment.

Management

The primary goal in the management of acute respiratory failure is to restore adequate oxygenation and ventilation. Supplemental oxygen should be immediately provided to improve oxygenation. Treatment of the underlying cause of respiratory failure is initiated simultaneously. The need for a low-flow/low FiO_2 (nasal cannula or face mask) Vs high-flow/high FiO_2 (non-rebreathing mask with reservoir) delivery system is dependent on the degree of hypoxemia and the patient's flow demand. A patient with severe hypoxemia and high minute ventilation, for example, should receive a high-flow/high FiO_2 non-rebreathing mask with a reservoir. Ventilatory assistance in acute respiratory failure can be provided noninvasively (noninvasive positive pressure ventilation, NIPPV) or invasively (mechanical ventilation).

Noninvasive Positive Pressure Ventilation (NIPPV)

NIPPV is administered using an interface to the upper airway and does not require endotracheal intubation. NIPPV has a significant role in the management of acute respiratory failure, especially in certain settings. There is strong evidence to support the use of NIPPV in acute respiratory failure due to COPD exacerbation,[4-6] acute cardiogenic respiratory failure,[7-9] in immunocompromised patients, and to facilitate ventilator weaning in intubated COPD patients. Several studies and meta-analyses have shown significant reductions in intubation and mortality rates and reduced hospital length of stay in patients treated with NIPPV through respiratory muscle unloading and improvement in gas exchange.[5,6] NIPPV may be considered in postoperative respiratory failure, patients with do-not-intubate (DNI) status, and as a bridge to extubation and prevent extubation failure. Although NIPPV has shown to be effective in the above settings, its use in acute hypoxic respiratory failure remains controversial.[12,13] Contraindications to NIPPV are listed in Table 3. The patient on NIPPV should be monitored for improvement or deterioration in respiratory status based on close clinical examination and blood gasses.

Table 3: Contraindications to NIPPV

Contraindications to NIPPV
• Cardiac or respiratory arrest
• Nonrespiratory organ failure
• Severe encephalopathy (e.g., GCS < 10)
• Severe upper gastrointestinal bleeding
• Hemodynamic instability or unstable cardiac arrhythmia
• Facial surgery, trauma, or deformity
• Upper airway obstruction
• Inability to cooperate/proted the airway
• Inability to clear respiratory secretions
• High risk for aspiration

Interface & Settings

Success of NIPPV depends on a multitude of factors; interface (or mask), ventilator setting, and skills of providers (physician, nursing, respiratory therapy). Nasal or full face (oronasal) masks are commercially available. Both masks perform equally well, although nasal masks may be associated with an excessive leak from the mouth. When using these interfaces, the bony facial prominences and ear cartilage should be well padded and closely monitored for erythema and pressure necrosis. Most critical care ventilators are designed to deliver invasive or noninvasive ventilation. Pressure-limited (pressure support) mode is most commonly used and is well accepted by patients. This can be delivered in a continuous (continuous positive airway pressure, CPAP) or bi-level (Bi-level airway pressure, BiPAP) mode. Whatever the chosen mode, initial settings should be low (8-10 cm H_2O) for better patient tolerance and can be titrated in 2 cm H_2O increments. Typical starting BiPAP setting consists of inspiratory pressure (inspiratory positive airway pressure, IPAP) of 8-10 cm H_2O and EPAP (expiratory positive airway pressure, EPAP) of 4-5 cm H_2O. IPAP may be increased to improve ventilation and EPAP may be increased to improve oxygenation or prevent upper airway collapse or apnea. Other advanced modes such as mandatory backup minute ventilation (set tidal volume and rate) and proportional assist ventilation (PAV) are available on some critical care ventilators. Although gastric decompression using a nasogastric tube is not routinely advised in a patient receiving NIPPV, it should be strongly considered to prevent the possibility of abdominal compartment syndrome when high settings (≥ 20 cm H_2O) are used during NIPPV.[14]

Mechanical Ventilation

The goals of mechanical ventilation include the provision of adequate gas exchange (arterial oxygenation and carbon dioxide clearance), the reduction of work of breathing, and the prevention of iatrogenic harm to the patient. Often, the goals are conflicting and depend upon the clinical setting. Specific therapy for the underlying cause of respiratory failure is instituted simultaneously. The decision to intubate and institute mechanical ventilation is most often clinically based. Indications for mechanical ventilation are listed in Table 4.

Table 4: Indications for mechanical ventilation

Indication	Definition	Examples/Etiologies
Inadequate oxygenation	• Acute hypoxemia • PaO_2 < 60 mm Hg	• Atelectasis • Small-airway or parenchymal disease/infection • PARDS
Inadequate ventialtion	• Acute hypercapnia • $PaCO_2$ > 50 mm Hg	• Obstructive lung disease (i.e., asthma)
Airway protection	• No underlying lung disease	• Trauma • Traumatic brain injury • Postictal state • Intoxication

Ventilation Strategy versus Modes

It is important to consider that mechanical ventilation strategy, and not the mode(s), determines the outcome in a mechanically ventilated patient. A protective mechanical ventilation strategy should include considerations for the following:

Tidal Volume: Tidal volume (V_T) used in mechanical ventilation is based on predicted body weight (PBW), and not actual body weight, especially in obese patients. In patients with ALI/ARDS, V_T of 6 ml/kg PBW when compared with V_T of 12 ml/kg PBW has been shown to reduce mortality, the release of inflammatory markers, and dependence on a mechanical ventilator.[15-17] In at-risk patients, one should not, however, wait for ALI/ARDS to occur before considering a low V_T strategy. In most circumstances low V_T allows to keep plateau pressure (P_{plat}) lower than 30 cm H_2O. Application of high V_T and P_{plat} has been associated with high mortality in critically ill patients requiring mechanical ventilation in a variety of non-ALI/ARDS settings, e.g. pulmonary edema, COPD, CHF, trauma, aspiration, and following surgery. A low V_T strategy may also result in many positive circulatory effects (improved venous return and cardiac output) by reducing intrathoracic pressure and right ventricular afterload, and the resultant hypercapnia. Consequences of low V_T and P_{plat} include hypercapnia, atelectasis, and hypoxia if respiratory rate and PEEP are not sufficiently increased.

Positive End Expiratory Pressure (PEEP): PEEP, when applied appropriately, should prevent atelectasis and improve oxygenation in a mechanically ventilated patient. Therefore, PEEP may have a protective effect by preventing lung derecruitment and promoting alveolar recruitment. Unfortunately, the effects of PEEP on arterial oxygenation and pulmonary mechanics are not as simple as they may seem. High PEEP/low FiO_2 compared with low PEEP/high FiO_2 in the ARDSnet trial failed to improve mortality in patients with ALI/ARDS.[18] Alternatively, in ALI/ARDS PEEP may be titrated using a static pressure-volume (P-V) compliance curve or by measuring lung compliance (or elastance). It is difficult to identify lower inflection points on the P-V compliance curve in every patient with ALI/ARDS. Similarly, the effect of PEEP on lung compliance (or elastance) depends upon the underlying etiology of ALI/ARDS (pulmonary or extrapulmonary). Therefore, the strategy to select an adequate level of PEEP is quite complex in an individual patient.

Patient-ventilator Synchrony: Ideally, the patient's inspiratory time (neural input) and ventilator inspiratory time should be matched to establish patient-ventilator synchrony. During spontaneous ventilation, patient-ventilator interaction is complex and dependent upon the respiratory drive, muscle strength, timing, and respiratory mechanics. In order to optimally reduce the work of breathing and provide sufficient alveolar ventilation, mechanical breaths must proportionally support the patient's spontaneous inspiratory effort and respiratory rate/minute ventilation. These features are available as assist controlled ventilation (ACV), automatic tube compensation (ATC), pressure support ventilation (PSV), and proportional assist ventilation (PAV) in most contemporary mechanical ventilators. Providing optimal sedation, sleep, and anxiolysis is also important in ensuring patient-ventilator synchrony.

Spontaneous breathing & Weaning: Using partial support and less sedation encourages spontaneous breathing in a patient on a mechanical ventilator. Spontaneous ventilation improves V/Q matching, reduces atelectasis, and results in better gas exchange and oxygenation. Cardiovascular effects of spontaneous ventilation include better venous return, cardiac output, and oxygen delivery. Therefore, encouraging spontaneous breathing during mechanical ventilation is associated with better perfusion and organ function, less need for sedation, and quicker weaning and discontinuation from mechanical ventilator support. Patients with left ventricular dysfunction should be watched closely during spontaneous breathing trials as depressed left ventricles may not tolerate an increase in ventricular filling and afterload associated with spontaneous breathing.

Modes: Positive-pressure mechanical ventilatory support, partial or total, provides pressure and flow to the airway. The basic ventilator modes are classified based on three features of a mechanical breath: *trigger* (ventilator or patient), *target* (volume or pressure), and *cycle* (transition from inspiration to exhalation).

Weaning and Extubation: All patients supported on mechanical ventilators should be evaluated on a daily basis for their ability to breathe spontaneously, weaning, and eventually for extubation. The weaning process involves decreasing support from the ventilator and allowing the patient to increase the work of breathing. Common criteria for weaning include reversal or resolution of acute respiratory failure, ability to make an inspiratory effort, cardiovascular stability, and adequate gas exchange indicated by pH (>7.25), PaO_2 (>60 mmHg, FiO_2 <0.6), PEEP <10 cm H_2O.[19] Patients considered weanable should undergo a short period (30-120 minutes) of spontaneous breathing trial (SBT). SBT may include breathing with a T-tube, CPAP, or PS. Close clinical observation is important during SBT. Rapid shallow breathing index (RR ÷ V_T (L)) between 60 and 105 has been shown to be highly predictive of weaning success. Weaning does not necessarily mean that the patient can be extubated. Adequate mental state and amount of secretions should be evaluated before extubation. Tight fluid balance or forced diuresis, bronchodilators, and physiotherapy may improve weaning success during SBT.

HEMODYNAMIC SUPPORT & RESUSCITATION

Shock is a state of inadequate supply or inappropriate utilization of oxygen and nutrients by the cells. Unless reversed by resuscitation, this can lead to multiple organ failures, irreversible tissue damage, and death. The goal of hemodynamic support and resuscitation is to restore the balance between oxygen supply and utilization and prevent tissue death. Multiple studies have shown that perioperative hemodynamic optimization and early goal-directed resuscitation improves outcome in high-risk surgery patients.

Clinical Presentation and Characterization

The classical clinical picture of shock such as hypotension and altered tissue perfusion (oliguria, altered mental state, decreased skin perfusion) may not be present in all patients, especially the young and during the compensatory phase. "Cryptic shock" is present with normotension despite decreased tissue perfusion. Elevated blood lactate level is one of the important biochemical markers of shock. The Weil and Shubin classification of shock is based on underlying pathophysiological mechanisms. *Hypovolemic shock* is the most common form of shock seen in surgical and trauma patients. Common causes of hypovolemic shock include hemorrhage and dehydration. Capillary leak with loss of intravascular volume can result in hypovolemic shock in the early postoperative period. *Cardiogenic shock* is the result of cardiac pump failure. This may be due to postoperative myocardial infarction, cardiomyopathy, cardiac valvular disease, or arrhythmia. *Obstructive shock* is the result of obstruction to the flow of blood into or out of the heart. The common causes include massive pulmonary embolism and cardiac tamponade. *Distributive shock* may be due to capillary leak due to mediator-induced systemic inflammation, vasodilation, and loss of sympathetic tone. Sepsis, anaphylaxis, neurogenic, and acute adrenal insufficiency are causes of distributive shock. Shock due to sepsis is complex in nature and includes features of all four types of shock.

Management

Management of shock includes treatment of the underlying cause, resuscitation, and hemodynamic monitoring to evaluate guide and response to therapy. Supplemental oxygen should be provided to treat hypoxemia. Intubation and mechanical ventilation, when considered, should be performed early. The importance of initial fluid loading is common to all types of shock irrespective of its underlying cause. In patients with hemorrhagic shock, bleeding must be stopped. Often the source of bleeding is obvious from drains in the postoperative period. Correction of coagulopathy and hypothermia must be actively pursued in a patient with postoperative bleeding. In patients with postoperative myocardial infarction, anticoagulation and thrombolytic therapy must weigh the risk of bleeding. Percutaneous coronary intervention and intraaortic balloon counterpulsation may be used as appropriate. In patients with obstructive shock, percutaneous pericardiocentesis for cardiac tamponade may be performed at bedside with echocardiography, and thrombolytic therapy or surgical thromboendarterectomy may be considered for massive pulmonary embolism. In patients with septic shock, timely administration of antibiotics and removal of sources are crucial.

Hemodynamic Monitoring and Resuscitation

Basic non-invasive monitoring with electrocardiogram (ECG), arterial blood pressure (BP), and pulse oximetry (SpO_2) is initiated in all patients with shock. Invasive hemodynamic monitoring, in addition to repeated clinical assessment, may be required for the assessment of global and regional tissue perfusion. Early goal-directed therapy using hemodynamic monitoring has been shown to improve outcomes in septic shock.[20] Direct beat-to-beat BP monitoring using an intraarterial catheter is indicated in presence of persistent severe hypotension despite fluid loading and when frequent sampling of arterial blood gasses and titration of vasoactive drugs is required. The exact target value for arterial pressure (systolic or mean arterial pressure) is not known and should be determined for an individual patient based on age, comorbidities, and adequacy of global oxygen delivery. Measurement of oxygen delivery and consumption, cardiac output (flow), or their surrogate or determinants may be considered in a patient with persistent signs of organ hypoperfusion with or without hypotension. Key determinants of oxygen delivery include hemoglobin (total (gm/dl) and percent saturation (SaO_2)) and cardiac output. The role of the pulmonary artery catheter, a gold standard cardiac output monitor, for hemodynamic management in critical care practice has been extensively scrutinized in the literature and even considered as harmful. Central venous pressure (CVP) alone may be used as a trend monitor for the assessment of right heart preload and volume responsiveness. Both CVP and pulmonary artery occlusion pressure (PAOP), however, are reliable only half the time as a guide for fluid therapy. Therefore, approximately 50% of the patients may receive excessive amounts of fluids based on CVP or PAOP as a preload monitor. Often, simple straight leg raising tests may demonstrate fluid responsiveness in a spontaneously breathing patient with hemodynamic instability. Dynamic physiological parameters (pulse pressure variation (PPV), systolic pressure variation (SPV), and stroke volume variation (SVV)), derived from arterial pressure waveform analysis have been shown to be more sensitive indicators of preload/fluid responsiveness in mechanically ventilated patients. There has been a recent resurgence of a plethora of minimally invasive cardiac output monitors. Although based on good physiological principles, their clinical application is fraught with a lack of accuracy, precision, and outcome data. Measurement of mixed venous oxygen saturation (S_VO_2) can provide information on the adequacy of resuscitation and systemic oxygenation, i.e. balance between oxygen consumption and oxygen delivery. More recently, based on a landmark study by Rivers et al.,[20] central venous oxygen saturation ($S_{CV}O_2$) monitoring, as compared with true S_VO_2 from the pulmonary artery, is used as an endpoint (S_VO_2 >65%) to guide goal-directed resuscitation in the critically ill patient.

Since no single hemodynamic parameter can provide all the information necessary to determine the adequacy of resuscitation in a critically ill patient with shock, integrated multiple hemodynamic parameters along with repeated clinical examination should be used to assess response to therapy. The Surviving Sepsis Campaign Guidelines recommend that the goals of initial resuscitation in septic shock should include a CVP of 8-12 mm Hg, a MAP >65 mmHg, and a urine output of >0.5 ml/kg/hr, and a $S_{CV}O_2$ >70%.[21] These endpoints of resuscitation can also be applied in high-risk patients undergoing major surgery.

More recently, attention is drawn to the state of microcirculation in patients with shock, independent of systemic hemodynamics. Microcirculatory alterations, such as decreased capillary density, stagnation, sludging, and shunting of blood, can result in tissue hypoperfusion and hypoxia. Impairment of microcirculation is more severe in non-survivors and its persistence is associated with the development of organ failure and death. Technology to visualize and assess microcirculation has improved over the years. Nevertheless, it is not readily available in most ICUs. Lactate measurement has been used to assess tissue hypoperfusion and is considered a biochemical marker of the state of microcirculation. Although hyperlactatemia could be due to aerobic and anaerobic pathology, mitochondrial dysfunction and oxygen supply dependency in severe sepsis and septic shock is commonly associated with hyperlactatemia. Increased blood lactate level and a lack of decrease during therapy carry poor prognosis in critically ill patients.[22-23] Therefore, blood lactate level should be used in goal-directed therapy and may be used as a resuscitation endpoint.

Fluids versus Pressors

Fluid administration is the first line of treatment in most types of shocks. The goal of fluid administration is to improve cardiac output by increasing preload (plasma volume). Fluids should be given as a "bolus." Crystalloid solutions are commonly used for fluid resuscitation. The common considerations in fluid administration include, crystalloid solution (250- 1000ml) infused rapidly over 30 minutes with physiological endpoints (BP, HR, urine output, CVP, etc.) and keeping safe limits in mind. The total amount of fluids required for adequate resuscitation is variable in each patient. One must carefully watch for potential complications of excessive fluid administration, such as pulmonary edema, hypoxemia, and abdominal compartment syndrome. The biological properties of crystalloids and colloids may be considered when choosing fluids for resuscitation. Normal saline and synthetic colloids have been shown to induce inflammation by neutrophil activation. Starch solutions may cause coagulopathy by inhibiting platelet function and impairing fibrin polymerization and should be avoided in the perioperative period in patients with coagulopathy, severe sepsis, or at risk for bleeding.[24]

Vasopressor therapy may be required in patients with shock to treat hypotension refractory to or in addition to fluid therapy and to maintain adequate perfusion pressure. Central venous access should be established as early as possible when vasopressor use is considered in the treatment of shock. The choice of vasopressor agent may vary with the underlying etiology of shock. Current Surviving Sepsis Guidelines recommend dopamine or norepinephrine in the initial management of septic shock.[21] Phenylephrine, epinephrine, or vasopressin is not considered the initial vasopressor in septic shock. Physiological doses of vasopressin (max. dose 0.04 units/min) may be used in addition to norepinephrine infusion to treat persistent hypotension due to septic shock. A prospective, randomized controlled trial performed by Levy et al. compared the effects of norepinephrine and dobutamine to those of epinephrine in dopamine-resistant septic shock.[25] Despite the equal hemodynamic response, deleterious effects on splanchnic perfusion and rise in lactate were more likely observed with epinephrine infusion. Epinephrine is, however, the drug of choice in anaphylactic shock. Inotropic agents are used to treat conditions associated with reduced myocardial contractility. Dobutamine is considered the inotrope of choice to improve cardiac output in patients with impaired ventricular function due to septic shock.

Adjuvant Therapy in Shock

Drotrecogin alfa (activated) and low-dose steroids have been used with improved outcomes in most severe forms of septic shock. Intraaortic balloon counter pulsation may be used to improve coronary perfusion in patients with cardiogenic shock. Renal replacement therapy (RRT) is considered to manage fluid overload and electrolyte abnormalities associated with acute kidney injury in patients with shock and multiple organ dysfunctions. However, the correct timing, mode, and dose of RRT remain controversial. Physiological doses of steroids may be considered in the patient with vasopressor-dependent septic shock.

ABDOMINAL COMPARTMENT SYNDROME

The abdomen is a closed space lined by compliant (abdominal wall and diaphragm) and non-compliant (ribs, spine, and pelvis) structures. Normally, intra-abdominal contents include solid organs, hollow viscera, and little fluid (ascites). The abdomen behaves as a hydraulic system whereby the pressure measured at one point may be assumed to represent the intra-abdominal pressure (IAP) throughout the abdomen. IAP, measured in mmHg, is the intrinsic pressure within the abdomen at steady-state. Normal IAP ranges from subatmospheric to 0 mm Hg. Morbid obesity and pregnancy may be associated with chronic elevations in IAP (10-15 mm Hg). IAP is slightly elevated (5-7 mm Hg) in critically ill adults on mechanical ventilators. Normally, IAP varies with respiration (increases during inspiration and decreases during exhalation) and body position (increases with the elevation of the head of the bed or reverse Trendelenburg). Clinical understanding and research into the effects of elevated IAP (intra-abdominal hypertension, IAH) on physiology and organ function, as well as morbidity and mortality in the critically ill, has increased significantly over the past decade. The development of intra-abdominal hypertension and abdominal compartment syndrome during the ICU period is an independent risk factor for death. Although initially considered a disease of traumatic injury, IAH/ACS is now recognized as a cause of significant organ failure (Figure 1), morbidity, and mortality in all critically ill populations. This section presents a brief review of the diagnosis and management of abdominal compartment syndrome (ACS). In 2007 The World Society of Abdominal Compartment Syndrome (WSACS, www. wsacs.org) published definitions and recommendations from the international conference of experts on ACS.[26-27]

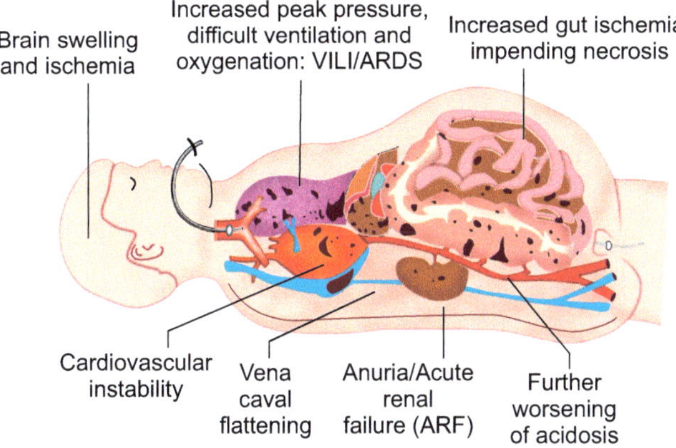

Figure 1: Onset of multiple organ dysfunction syndrome due to intra-abdominal pressure >20 mmHg

Definitions related to IAP and its critical care implications are summarized in Figure 1. Due to its simplicity and minimal cost, bladder pressure measured after installation of 25 ml volume of sterile saline via Foley catheter is considered the reference standard for intermittent IAP measurement. IAP is expressed in mmHg and measured at end-expiration in the supine position and with the transducer zeroed at the level of the mid-axillary line. Bladder pressure should be measured intermittently every 4 hours in patients at risk of developing IAH/ACS. The sensitivity of physical examination in detecting IAH has been demonstrated to be too low.

Diagnosis

Incidence and prevalence of IAH and ACS is reported to be high and can occur in a wide variety of critically ill populations. Numerous risk factors for the development of IAH/ACS have been identified in large-scale prospective trials. A high index of suspicion and low threshold for serial IAP measurement should be considered in high-risk post-surgical patients with acute onset organ dysfunction. Unrecognized and untreated ACS has been shown to be associated with progressive multi-organ failure and a high risk of death.

Management

The best treatment for ACS is prevention. Screening patients at risk for ACS, monitoring IAP, goal-directed fluid resuscitation guided by defined end-points and early recognition of ACS, and possibly keeping the abdomen open in some situations are useful preventative strategies. The reader should be referred to an algorithm for the management of IAH/ACS, proposed by the World Society of Abdominal Compartment Syndrome. Key principles in the management of IAH/ACS include resuscitation for optimization of systemic and splanchnic perfusion, serial monitoring of IAP (bladder pressure), medical management to reduce IAP, and early surgical decompression of IAH/ACS refractory to medical therapy.

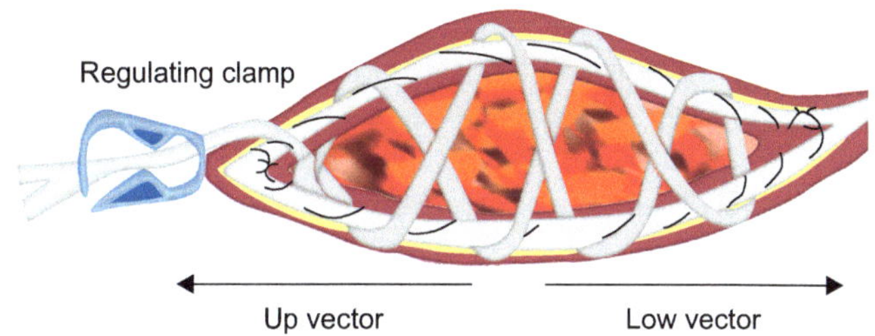

Figure 2: Open abdomen with a wound closure device

Resuscitation: Fluid resuscitation to maintain adequate intravascular volume and preload is important in IAH/ACS and should be initiated early. A combination of hypovolemia (relative or absolute) and elevated intrathoracic pressure due to positive pressure ventilation tends to aggravate hypotension in IAH/ACS. The total amount of crystalloid administered must be closely monitored. Interactions between heart and lung become more complex in IAH/ACS due to changes in lung mechanics. It is important to keep in mind that CVP and PAOP may be falsely elevated in IAH/ACS and are not reliable monitors to guide fluid therapy. Dynamic measures of volume responsiveness (SVV, PPV, or SPV) may be considered to guide fluid therapy in IAH/ACS. There is some evidence that the use of hypertonic saline may be associated with significantly decreased fluid requirement, lower inspiratory pressure, and higher abdominal perfusion pressure (APP). Inotropes may be considered to improve cardiac output and myocardial contractility in patients with LV dysfunction. The concept of APP, defined as MAP minus IAP, is an important consideration for resuscitation in IAH/ACS. The goal is to maintain adequate splanchnic perfusion. APP has been studied as a resuscitation end-point in several trials. APP value of $\geq$ 50-60 mmHg is suggested as an appropriate resuscitation goal. This can be achieved through a balance of judicious fluids and vasoactive drugs. Maintaining adequate APP appears to predict improved survival from IAH/ACS.

Mechanical Ventilation: IAH/ACS is associated with increased intrathoracic pressure, pleural pressure, and chest wall stiffness with resultant alveolar collapse, atelectasis, and hypoxemia. Peak inspiratory pressures rise with volume-control and tidal volume drops during the pressure-control mode of ventilation due to decreased compliance in IAH/ACS. Plateau pressure and ΔP (P_{Plat} – PEEP) should be closely monitored. High airway pressures are usually needed to maintain adequate ventilation due to a stiff chest wall. Titrating PEEP to overcome atelectasis and improve oxygenation can be challenging in IAH/ACS. Probably the best strategy includes incrementally increasing the PEEP to a level equal to IAP (which closely reflects pleural pressure). As opposed to ALI/ARDS, high airway pressure (P_{Plat}) is less concerning in ACS because the transpulmonary swing in pressure (ΔP-PEEP) is less when PEEP is equal to IAP. Frequent blood gas monitoring and close attention to intravascular volume status are required with this strategy. PEEP and P_{Pla} should be immediately reduced once the abdomen is decompressed and ACS has resolved.

Surgical Decompression: Surgical decompression of the peritoneal cavity (decompressive laparotomy) coupled with the open abdomen management technique remains the gold standard for the management of ACS. A variety of temporary abdominal closure techniques have been described. Whatever the technique used, commercial or customized, it is important to avoid tension on the fascia, provide sufficient sterile cover over abdominal contents, and prevent recurrent ACS by allowing visceral expansion during ongoing resuscitation. Timing and method of abdominal closure following resolution of the ACS and improvement in organ failure are variable for each case.

Medical Management: Several non-surgical (medical) treatments may be used in the treatment of IAH/ACS. These are usually temporizing measures, especially for lower grades of IAH, and to facilitate the transport of the patient. The stomach and rectum may be decompressed using a nasogastric and rectal tube. Prokinetic motility agents (erythromycin, neostigmine, or metoclopramide) may be considered to improve ileus and evacuate intraluminal contents. Pseudomembranous colitis or surgical etiology of ileus, however, should be excluded before using prokinetic agents. Fluid management using diuretics or venovenous hemofiltration or ultrafiltration may be considered once fluid and vasopressor requirement has ceased. Controlled paracentesis may be used in patients with chronic ascites. Sedation and neuromuscular blockade may be helpful by decreasing airway and IAP, especially during transport.

PREVENTING ERRORS AND IATROGENIC COMPLICATIONS

"Primum non nocere", first do no harm, is one of the fundamental aspects of medical practice. Reports, such as "To Err is Human" and "Crossing the Quality Chasm", have shown that medical errors are common and adversely affect patient outcomes.[28-29] *Napoleon Bonaparte (1820)* once said "I do not want two diseases-One nature made, one doctor made." Safety and performance have become the main focus of attention in recent years in healthcare, including in ICU. An ICU, where multiple, often complex, interventions by multiple providers occur, is a stressful and error-prone environment. It is not uncommon to have a situation in the ICU similar to the holes in a stack of "Swiss Cheese" line up resulting in an error.[30] The holes represent failures. Most errors result from a combination of active failures and latent conditions (system). Fortunately, not all errors result in a complication or patient harm. This is often called "near miss" or "sentinel event." Patient safety is the result of a series of checks and balances that ensures safe practices within the framework of an ICU. Establishing a culture of safety is among the major challenges faced by current ICUs.

Several approaches have been advocated by many Quality & Safety organizations and evidence-based research to improve safety and quality of care in ICU. First and foremost, the ICU must create a safety culture, as proposed by Pronovost, whereby the collective attitudes and beliefs of the caregivers take into account the effect of local culture on safety outcomes.[31] All caregivers must be empowered to speak up without hesitation, increase awareness and create protective barriers whenever they notice safety practices being breached by another provider. Secondly, structure (how care is organized) and process (how it is delivered) of care are important to the quality of care. Intensivist-led multidisciplinary and multi-professional ICU team recognizes each team member's contribution toward patient care. Recently there is increased emphasis on organizing the goals and process of care in the form of goal-sheet, checklists, and bundles. This ensures that the team has shared and common goals of care for the patient and important elements of the treatment plan and procedure are followed consistently. This has been shown to reduce errors and complications and improve patient outcomes. Examples include daily goal-sheet, procedure checklist, and various disease bundles (e.g. sepsis, central line care, and ventilator-associated pneumonia bundle). Although this may at first seem very labor-intensive, however, once incorporated into the daily practice, it becomes part of the ICU safety culture and daily routine. Finally, one must recognize that errors are bound to occur and each ICU should have a system of measuring, reporting, and analyzing errors in a non-threatening manner. Figure 3 lists common strategies to reduce errors and complications in the ICU.

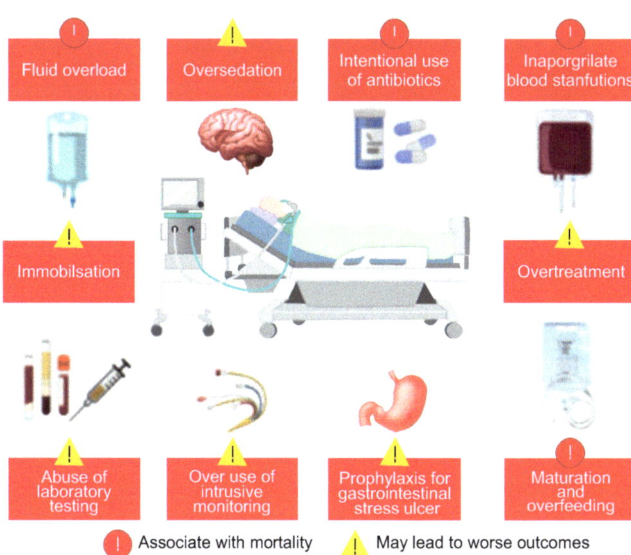

Figure 3: Common strategies to reduce errors and complications in the ICU

LESSONS FROM COVID-19

The COVID-19 pandemic surge has changed the way hospitals approach the critical care setting. One of the more serious presentations of a COVID-19 infection is a rapidly progressing acute respiratory failure, which is often treated initially with a mechanical ventilator. Mechanical ventilation is quite invasive, and the still high mortality rate of patients on ventilators leads some to hypothesize that other mechanisms of oxygenation may be preferred. Invasive mechanical ventilation is associated with ventilator-induced lung injury and ventilator-associated pneumonia. Furthermore, ventilation is often unpleasant for both the patient and the patient's family, and the pandemic has pushed healthcare decision-makers to take the "human factor" into account.[32]

FUTURE DIRECTION

Critical care has made significant advancements over the last 50 years and is still evolving. In addition to providing excellent clinical care, the current focus is on ICU organization and management, communication, accountability, and error prevention. In the future, the practice of critical care medicine will be collaborative, recognizing regional and cultural differences; see no geographic boundaries or barriers to communication. Future critical care will utilize technology in the diagnosis and delivery of critical care, e.g., telemedicine. In the future, accountability will be important in every aspect of care for the critically ill in the ICU. Finally, it is important to create a balance between the professional and spiritual aspects of critical care.

REFERENCES

1. Brun-Buisson C, Minneli C, Bertolini G, et al. ALIVE Study group. Epidemiology and outcome of acute lung injury in European intensive care units. Results from the ALIVE study. Intensive Care Med 2004; 31(1):51-61.
2. Rubenfeld GD, Caldwell E, Peabody E, Weaver J. Incidence and outcomes of acute lung injury. N Engl J Med 2005; 353(16); 1685-93.
3. Pesenti A, Tagliabue P, Patroniti N, Fumagalli R. Computerized tomography scan imaging in acute respiratory distress syndrome. Intensive Care Med 2001; 27: 631-37.
4. Brochard L, Isabey D, Piquet J, Amaro P, Mancebo J, Messadi AA, et al. Reversal of acute exacerbations of chronic obstructive lung disease by inspiratory assistance with a face mask. N Engl J Med. 1990;323(22): 1523–30.
5. Plant PK, Owen JL, Elliott MW. Early use of non-invasive ventilation for acute exacerbations of chronic obstructive pulmonary disease on general respiratory wards: a multicentre randomised controlled trial. Lancet. 2000;355(9219):1931–5.
6. Keenan SP, Sinuff T, Cook DJ, Hill NS. Which patients with acute exacerbation of chronic obstructive pulmonary disease benefit from noninvasive positive-pressure ventilation? A systematic review of the literature. Ann Intern Med. 2003;138(11):861–70.
7. Masip J, Betbese AJ, Paez J, Vecilla F, Canizares R, Padro J, et al. Non-invasive pressure support ventilation versus conventional oxygen therapy in acute cardiogenic pulmonary oedema: a randomised trial. Lancet. 2000; 356(9248):2126–32.
8. Nava S, Carbone G, DiBattista N, Bellone A, Baiardi P, Cosentini R, et al. Noninvasive ventilation in cardiogenic pulmonary edema: a multicenter randomized trial. Am J Respir Crit Care Med. 2003;168(12):1432–7.
9. L'Her E, Duquesne F, Girou E, de Rosiere XD, Le Conte P, Renault S, et al. Noninvasive continuous positive airway pressure in elderly cardiogenic pulmonary edema patients. Intensive Care Med. 2004;30(5):882–8.
10. Nava S, Ambrosino N, Clini E, Prato M, Orlando G, Vitacca M, et al. Noninvasive mechanical ventilation in the weaning of patients with respiratory failure due to

chronic obstructive pulmonary disease. A randomized, controlled trial. Ann Intern Med. 1998;128(9):721–8.

11. Girault C, Daudenthun I, Chevron V, Tamion F, Leroy J, Bonmarchand G. Noninvasive ventilation as a systematic extubation and weaning technique in acute-on-chronic respiratory failure: a prospective, randomized controlled study. Am J Respir Crit Care Med. 1999;160(1):86–92.
12. Evans TW. International Consensus Conferences in Intensive Care Medicine: non-invasive positive pressure ventilation in acute respiratory failure. Organised jointly by the American Thoracic Society, the European Respiratory Society, the European Society of Intensive Care Medicine, and the Societe de Reanimation de Langue Francaise, and approved by the ATS Board of Directors, December 2000. Intensive Care Med. 2001; 27(1):166–78.
13. Schettino G, Altobelli N, Kacmarek RM. Noninvasive positive-pressure ventilation in acute respiratory failure outside clinical trials: experience at the Massachusetts General Hospital. Crit Care Med. 2008; 36(2):441–7.
14. De Keulenaer BL, De Backer A, et al. Abdominal compartment syndrome related to noninvasive ventilation. Intensive Care Med (2003) 29:1177–1181.
15. Brower RG, Shanholtz CB, Fessler HE, et al. Prospective, randomized, controlled clinical trial comparing traditional versus reduced tidal volume ventilation in acute respiratory distress syndrome patients. Crit Care Med 1999; 17: 1492–98.
16. The Acute Respiratory Distress Syndrome Network. Ventilation with lower tidal volumes as compared with traditional Tidal volumes for acute lung injury and the acute respiratory distress syndrome. N Engl J Med 2000; 342: 1301–8.
17. Parsons PE, Eisner MD, Thompson BT, Matthay MA, Ancukiewicz M, Bernard GR, et al. Lower tidal volume ventilation and plasma cytokine markers of inflammation in patients with acute lung injury. Crit Care Med 2005; 33: 1–6.
18. Brower RG, Lanken PN, MacIntyre N, Matthay MA, Morris A, Ancukiewicz M, et al. Higher versus lower positive end expiratory pressures in patients with the acute respiratory distress syndrome. N Engl J Med 2004; 351: 327–36.
19. MacIntyre NR, Cook DJ, Ely EW Jr, Epstein SK, Fink JB, Heffner JE, et al. Evidence-based guidelines for weaning and discontinuing ventilatory support: a collective task force facilitated by the American College of Chest Physicians; the American Association for Respiratory Care; and the American College of Critical Care Medicine. Chest 2001; 120:375S-95S.
20. Rivers E, Nguyen B, et al. Early goal-directed therapy in the treatment of severe sepsis and septic shock. N Engl J Med 2001; 345(19): 1368–77.
21. Dellinger RP, Levy MM, et al. Surviving Sepsis Campaign: International guidelines for management of severe sepsis and septic shock: 2008. Intensive Care Med (2008) 34:17–60.
22. Trzeciak S, Dellinger RP, Chansky ME, Arnold RC, Schorr C, Milcarek B, et al. Serum lactate as a predictor of mortality in patients with infection. Intensive Care Med. 2007;33:970–977.
23. Howell MD, Donnino M, Clardy P, Talmor D, Shapiro NI. Occult hypoperfusion and mortality in patients with suspected infection. Intensive Care Med. 2007;33: 1892–1899.
24. Westphal M, et al. Anesthesiology 2009; 111(1):187-202.
25. Levy B, et al. Comparison of norepinephrine and dobutamine to epinephrine for hemodynamics, lactate metabolism, and gastric tonometric variables in septic shock: a prospective, randomized study. Intensive Care Med. 1997;23(3):282–7.
26. Malbrain ML, et al. Results of the international conference of experts on intra-abdominal hypertension and abdominal compartment syndrome. I. Definitions. Intensive Care Med 2006;32:1722-1732.
27. Cheatham ML, et al. Results of the international conference of experts on intra-abdominal hypertension and abdominal compartment syndrome. I. Definitions. Intensive Care Med 2007; 33:951-962.
28. Institute of Medicine. To err is human: Building a safer healthcare system. Washington DC. National Academy Press, 2000.
29. Institute of Medicine. Crossing the quality chasm: a new health system for the 21st century. Washington, DC. National Academy Press, 2001.
30. Reason J. Human Error: Models and management. BMJ 2000; 320 (7237): 678-70.
31. Pronovost PJ, Goeschel CA, et al. Framework for patient safety research and improvement. Circulation 2009; 119(2): 330-7.
32. Turan S, Sevim Yakin S, Yamanel L. The timing of intubation and principles of ICU care in COVID-19. Turk J Med Sci. 2021 Dec 17;51(SI-1):3340–9. doi: 10.3906/sag-2106-182. PMID: 34461685; PMCID: PMC8771050.

47

CHAPTER

Acute Care Surgery

Elango Edhayan MD FACS
Patrick Collier MD

INTRODUCTION

Acute Care Surgery is a surgical subspecialty that includes aspects of trauma surgery, emergency medicine, general surgery and surgical critical care. The emergence of Acute Care Surgery as a specialty is the direct result of a lack of surgeons available to care for patients in an emergency.[1]

History and Introduction

In the United States, there is an impending crisis with regards to the availability of trained general surgeons who are willing and able to care for surgical patients in an emergent setting. This has created the need for the identification and training of surgeons willing to care for these patients. The American Council of Graduate Medical Education (ACGME) work hour restrictions have reduced time available for training surgeons by over a year. This reduction in training may have led to recent graduates being underprepared and less willing to care for emergency surgical problems. The increased use of non-operative treatment modalities for traumatic injuries has decreased the number of operations performed by trauma specialists, further decreasing the interest amongst graduating surgical residents in this field. In addition, the emergence of technology such as laparoscopy has increased the allure of technical fields of surgery in the eyes of graduating surgeons. These and other factors have led to an overall decrease in the general surgeon population, which was 2.3% between 1996 and 2006 with only about 300 new general surgeons graduating each year.[2] Lifestyle choices are now limiting surgeons' interest in taking call or being available after hours and on weekends. The demand, however, has increased as hospitals have begun to embrace "Centers of Excellence" standards in surgical subspecialties. These centers have been created with the existing surgical staff, further diminishing the workforce available to care for patients with emergent surgical problems. Patients presenting with surgical emergencies are more likely to be uninsured or underinsured, reducing the allure of caring for these patients. These factors combined with high stress, declining reimbursement rates, and higher rates of patient non-compliance with care plans, as well as increased drug and alcohol abuse in this patient group has led to reluctance amongst surgeons to care for these patients.

The Institute of Medicine (IOM) in its report "Hospital Based Emergency Care: At the Breaking Point (2007)" underscores this emerging trend. Currently, emergency surgical care is provided by board certified general surgeons assisted by a group of surgical subspecialists. Vascular surgeons, orthopedic surgeons, and neurosurgeons provide the vast majority of surgical subspecialty coverage essential for providing high acuity surgical emergency care. Akin to the number of available general surgeons decreasing over the past six years, there has been a decrease in the numbers of surgical subspecialists willing and able to care of emergent surgical problems.[3]

Acute Care Surgery Training Programs

One of the proposed solutions to the above problems is the creation of a new surgical subspecialty: Acute Care Surgery (ACS). In March 2003, the leadership of the American Association for Surgery for Trauma (AAST), the Western Trauma Association (WTA), Eastern Association for Surgery in Trauma (EAST), and the American College of Surgeons Committee on Trauma (ACS-COT) met to develop a non-ACGME accredited fellowship in Trauma, Emergency General Surgery, and Surgical Critical Care. In 2005 the AAST established a standing committee on Acute Care Surgery designed to oversee development of ACS and promote research in the field. The AAST and other trauma leaders saw the creation of an ACS fellowship as necessary to enhance the brand of trauma and emergency surgery, thereby increasing the attractiveness of the field to new graduates. The primary goals of the AAST sub-committee are 3 fold: increase surgeon operative experience in times of declining operative trauma, improve work satisfaction amongst trauma surgeons, and create a solution to declining emergency room coverage by surgeons and surgical subspecialists. With the creation of this program, the AAST is attempting to create a niche for these specialists in the healthcare continuum.

The AAST has created a curriculum for ACS training, and has approved sites with accredited fellowships. Currently, there are 30 Acute Care Surgery training programs which are all at major university training centers. Critical care training is at the center of Acute Care Surgical Training. All ACS programs need an ACGME approved Surgical Critical Care fellowship as a prerequisite for program accreditation. These programs vary in their curriculum offered and the level of exposure in elective rotations can differ substantially. Currently, there is no matching program akin to the National Residency Matching Program (NRMP) to assign candidates to these programs. Each program accepts individual applications and enrolls desirable candidates.

Training in Acute Care Surgery takes place after completion of a five year ACGME approved General Surgery residency. The ACS fellowship is two years, with one of these years spent in surgical critical care. The second year is spent in emergency surgery along with desirable rotations in orthopedics, neurosurgery, and other surgical specialties that mimic a general surgical residency curriculum. It is expected that the ACS fellow will be exposed to advanced technical skills in burn care, great vessel exposure and control, imaging, and interventional radiology. The ACS fellow is expected to take Trauma and Emergency Surgery calls for 12 months of fellowship training.

Currently, there are no immediate plans to seek ACGME accreditation of this fellowship, and there is no Board Certification offered in Acute Care Surgery. However, a graduating ACS fellow can sit for the Critical Care boards and take a certification exam in ACS sponsored by the AAST. The graduate is also expected to be board certified in General Surgery as well as possess competency to assess and manage complex airway and vascular injuries, be proficient in damage control surgery, and adept at managing all modalities of operative trauma. In the present curriculum, it is not essential that the graduate operatively manage orthopedic or neurosurgical injuries, however, a few programs provide at least some training in these fields.[4]

Acute Care Surgery in Clinical Practice

In clinical practice, the Acute Care Surgery model has been implemented predominantly in the university setting. Declining revenues due to reduced operative procedures for trauma have accentuated this shift. By combining emergency general surgery calls and trauma surgery calls amongst surgical critical care specialists, acute care surgery services have been created. An acute care surgeon is expected to work shifts of emergency room calls combined with shifts in the Intensive Care Unit. Upon completion of the shift, the acute care surgeon signs off the service to their colleague on call. This differs from traditional emergency surgery wherein in the ACS model the ACS service cares for the patient from admission to discharge. The operating surgeon does not necessarily follow the patients they have operated upon. This method of reorganization of services has led to increased reimbursement for trauma services, while providing job satisfaction.

Acute Care Surgical services are set up with the premise that they will provide initial stabilization of the critically ill or injured surgical patient. The ACS service is expected to interact with the surgical subspecialties of orthopedic, vascular and neurosurgery by providing initial damage control surgery for these providers to deliver definitive care in a semi-elective situation. In practice, the paradigm is, at best, evolving. There has been reluctance by neurosurgeons and orthopedic surgeons to entrust initial surgical care of complex injuries in their specialties to surgeons with minimal formal training. These injuries are, by nature, complex, and their treatment is nuanced and requires experienced surgeons with formal training. Hospital credentialing boards have been reluctant to grant orthopedic and neurosurgical operating privileges without a formal residency training. This ACS paradigm for immediate neurosurgical and orthopedic care may yet be successful in the future, as the number of sub-specialists taking emergency calls has not kept up with population growth. For example, there are currently fewer neurosurgeons taking call than there are emergency rooms in the country.[3]

In community hospitals across the United States, the ACS model has not taken hold as of yet. Currently, board certified general surgeons provide most of the call coverage for trauma and emergency surgery needs. This trend is expected to continue as the number of ACS programs and interest in ACS fellowships has not kept up with population and hospital growth.[5]

The Future of Acute Care Surgery in the United States

The AAST has been promoting Acute Care Surgery by providing leadership, accreditation of programs, and supporting research in this nascent field. The AAST clearly sees ACS as how trauma services will evolve in the near future. Just as there is evidence that trauma centers improve outcomes in trauma patients, there is increasing evidence that

ACS services improve outcomes, are cost effective, and create interest in the field.[2] That said, almost all of this evidence is from university hospitals which operate on different models than community hospitals.

Development of Acute Care Surgical services has led to regionalization of emergency surgical care in some parts of the country. This paradigm is similar to regionalization of trauma care into American College of Surgeons verified trauma centers and the development of state-wide and regional trauma networks. Multiple studies have proven that better outcomes can be expected in a number of different aspects, mortality included, when trauma patients are cared for at verified trauma centers.[2] It is believed that this prototype could be expanded to include other aspects of acute care surgery where patients needing emergency surgical care are transferred to regional hospitals where ACS specialists are readily available.

Health care delivery in the United States is bound to change with the passage of the Affordable Care Act. As resources are reallocated there is a push to deliver affordable acute care in the form of Regional Acute Care Centers. The impact on patients in terms of accessibility and the cost of these centers is still unclear.

The development of Acute Care Surgery is not without detractors who have questioned the need for this specialty outside of large metropolitan centers. They have questioned if Acute Care Surgery is essentially emergency surgery currently performed by general surgeons in a different brand name. The argument is that trauma surgeons provide a specialized coordination of care, and do not have large clinical practices to gain the operative experience needed to maintain sustained competency. This model calls for reorganization of surgical residencies to ensure that graduating residents are adept at emergency surgery rather than create a new layer of specialization.

International Efforts in Acute Care Surgery

The Acute Care Surgery model has not been confined to the United States of America. The ACS trend is evident in Canada where 13 programs offer training in Urgent Surgical Care. In European countries such as Austria, Germany, and Switzerland, the trauma surgeon does both orthopedic and abdominal surgery. In some centers in these countries, the trauma surgeon also performs neurosurgical and thoracic procedures. The training of these traumatologists is primarily orthopedic with additional training in visceral or abdominal surgery.

SUMMARY

The field of Acute Care Surgery, as it exists today, is still seeking a final definition of its scope as well as a place where it fits into surgical health care delivery. At present, an acute care surgeon is a general surgeon who is also board certified in Surgical Critical Care, and is willing and able to take trauma and emergency general surgery calls. ACS's success or failure depends on the surgeon's ability to deliver improvements in process and outcomes in health care at an affordable cost.

REFERENCES

1. Britt LD. Acute Care Surgery: Whats in a name? J Trauma 2012; 72(2):319-20.
2. Jurkovich GJ. Regionalized Health Care and the Trauma System Model. J Am Coll Surg 2012; 215(1):1-11.
3. Hospital-Based Emergency Care: At the Breaking Point. National Academy of Sciences, 11 Oct. 2009.
4. Acute Care Surgery. The American Association for the Surgery of Trauma, 2012.
5. Napolitano L, et al. Challenging Issues in Surgical Critical Care, Trauma, and Acute Care Surgery: Report From the Critical Care Committee of the American Association for the Surgery of Trauma. J Trauma 2010; 69(3):1619-33.
6. Bosse MJ, et al. Acute Care Surgery. J Trauma 2005; 59:1035-6.
7. Austin MT, et al. Creating an emergency general surgery service enhances the productivity of trauma surgeons, general surgeons and the hospital. J Trauma 2005; 58:906-10.
8. Urenues S, Lamont E. Acute Care Surgery: The European Model. World J of Surgery 2008; 32:1605-1612.
9. Acute Care Surgery: Trauma, Critical Care, and Emergency Surgery. A report from the committee to develop the reorganized specialty of trauma, surgical critical care, and emergency surgery. J Trauma 2005; 58:614–616.
10. MacKenzie EJ, et al. A national evaluation of the effect of trauma center care on mortality. N Engl J Med 2006; 354:366–378.

❑❑❑

48

CHAPTER

Abdomen and Thoracic Trauma

Khanjan Nagarsheth, MD
Scott Marshall, MD
Mayur Narayan, MD, MPH, MBA, FACS, FICS

INTRODUCTION

The majority of trauma injuries around the globe are a result of blunt injury. These injuries include, but are not limited to, motor vehicular and motorcycle crashes, pedestrian struck, falls, and blast injuries. Blunt trauma is a complex entity in which the extent of a patients' injuries may not all be readily apparent during the initial evaluation. Pre-hospital reports from the scene identify the mechanism of injury. Logistics of a crash can help provide crucial information to the injury sustained. Physical exam and imaging studies also play a much larger role in the correct diagnosis and workup of patients after blunt trauma. These patients are more likely to have injury to multiple body cavities simultaneously. The physics behind blunt trauma is significantly more complicated than penetrating trauma and a good working knowledge of mechanics will greatly help understanding injury mechanisms. Another helpful skill is pattern recognition. Certain patterns of injury occur frequently after blunt trauma. In this chapter, we will review the mechanics that are relevant to blunt trauma, discuss the most common mechanisms of injury, outline an approach to patient management, and then address organ specific injuries.

Kinematics of Blunt Trauma

In order to fully understand the impact of blunt injury, it is helpful to recall Sir Isaac Newton's laws of motion, on which the study of mechanics is based.[1] These laws govern how we think about objects in motion and the forces that act upon them. *Newton's first law of motion* states that every object continues to either remain in a state of rest or motion in a straight line until an external force compels it to do otherwise. *Newton's second law* states a force (F) is defined as the product of its mass (m) and acceleration (a): $F = ma$. The second law combined with the *law of conservation of energy* explains how energy cannot be created or destroyed, it merely changes forms. This has clear implications for understanding blunt trauma and will become apparent as we discuss further. To further assess the impact of forces, we recall *Newton's third law of motion*, which states that when two bodies apply a force to each other, the action and reaction forces occur in equal but opposite directions.

Velocity is defined as the product of acceleration and time. This is represented as: $v = at$ and this relationship is important to understand in order to appreciate an object's kinetic energy. *Kinetic energy* is the energy of an object in motion. Kinetic energy is a function of an object's mass and velocity. The actual relationship is represented as: $KE = \frac{1}{2} mv^2$. Here KE is kinetic energy, m is mass and v is velocity. This relationship illustrates that the velocity of an object plays a much larger role in determining the object's kinetic energy, compared to its mass.

This understanding of kinetic energy is important for the understanding of an object's momentum. For this discussion we will be referring to linear momentum as momentum. *Momentum* is defined as $p = mv$, where p is momentum, m is again mass, and v is again velocity. In a closed system, linear momentum is conserved; the initial momentum of an object must equal the ending momentum of an object as it interacts with another object. When we look at this in terms of Newton's third law of reciprocal forces, this means that the forces between the two objects are exactly the same in magnitude but opposite in sign. This is due to the *law of conservation of momentum*. This law is visually represented as $p_1 = p_2$ or $m_1v_1 = m_2v_2$ and is important in understanding the damage due to either blunt or penetrating trauma.

In penetrating trauma, the initial momentum with respect to a gun and its projectile, will be zero, as both will be at rest. After the gunpowder is ignited, the bullet is propelled forward into tissue until it eventually comes to rest. As a result, the final momentum of the bullet and tissue will be zero. The kinetic energy from the bullet will be transferred to the tissue in multiple forms, thus energy will also be conserved.

In blunt trauma, motor vehicle collisions (MVC) can also help illustrate this energy transfer. The kinetic energy from one vehicle is transferred into another vehicle. Assuming that the vehicle being hit is at rest and is in a perfectly inelastic collision, the momentum of the first vehicle will be transferred to the second vehicle, and both cars will be in effect "fused." Following the *law of conservation of momentum*, the mass of the two vehicles together is larger than either one alone, whereas the velocity of both fused cars after the collision will be less than the velocity of the initial moving car, thus conserving momentum in the system.

With this understanding of force (F) and acceleration (a), we can begin to understand the physics of a falling object. When describing falling objects, it is helpful to ignore the concept of air resistance, or *drag force, for illustration purposes.* The falling object can be thought of as falling in a vacuum. This helps to simplify the discussion and allow us to focus on the energy transfers that occur on the object or in the area of blunt trauma, the victim. In a vacuum, where there is no air resistance, the rate of falling is not dependent on the object's mass. Therefore, the only factor that affects the object is the acceleration; on Earth this is a constant of 9.80665 m/s^2 denoted by the letter g. The constant g allows for determination of potential energy stored in an object before it falls. The potential energy (PE) is a product of the object's mass (m), g and the height from which it falls (h). This is represented by the equation $PE = mgh$. Knowing the object's PE can help determine its velocity at impact. This is again determined through the *law of conservation of energy*, since as the object falls, its PE is converted into KE. Therefore $PE = KE$ or $mgh = ½ mv^2$.

In any trauma, it is important to understand that damage is caused by energy transfer. Although energy is conserved, it changes forms and the amount that is imparted to the victim will determine the extent of their injuries. The amount of energy that is exchanged is dependent on the density of the objects involved and the size of the contact area between two objects. *Density* is defined as the number of a given particle in a given volume. The area of contact is defined as the measured area on the victim's body that comes into contact with a given force. A greater force over a smaller area of contact will cause a penetrating injury. If the same force is given over a much larger area of contact, this will likely result in a blunt injury. Now that density and area of contact have been defined, we can understand an example. If a person falls off a ladder at a given height and lands into either a large pile of feathers or onto a concrete slab, there would be a difference in the amount of injury sustained. In this situation, if the person was to fall in the exact same way and make contact in the same position with either substance, then the area of contact would be the same. The difference is in the density of the material upon which the person lands. The object with less density will absorb more of the energy being transferred. In this example, when the person falls onto the concrete slab, since their body is less dense, it will absorb more energy, thus causing more damage to the person than the concrete. When they fall onto the pile of feathers, their body is denser than the feathers they are landing on, resulting in more energy being transferred to the feathers, with less resultant damage to their body.

Taking our understanding of blunt mechanics further, the next important concept to understand is work. *Work* is defined as a force applied through a distance. This is represented by the equation $W = Fd$, where W is work, F is force and d is distance. The *work-energy principle* is a basic principle in mechanics which explains that the net work done on an object is equal to its change in kinetic energy. Therefore $W_{net} = KE_2 - KE_1$. This can be rewritten as $Fd_{net} = ½ mv^2_2 - ½ mv^2_1$. This relationship is now important for the discussion of impact force. Based on the work-energy principle the impact force or F is equal to the final KE divided by the distance traveled. The distance is the distance the body travels into the surface upon falling. All surfaces will deform upon impact, based on the densities of both the falling body and the surface being struck. If a body strikes a less dense surface, the surface deforms more and the distance (d) increases. This will therefore decrease the force of impact. If the density of the surface is higher than the density of the body falling, the distance of impact is much smaller and therefore the impact force will be greater.

Mechanisms of Blunt Trauma

Motor Vehicle Crash

It is critically important, and often overlooked, to understand on-scene observations from first responders. The extent of vehicular damage, the angle and direction of the impact, whether restraints or airbags were deployed, difficulties during extrication, and other environmental information can all provide insight to the injuries sustained by a patient. There are five distinct patterns of impact for motor vehicle collisions. These include frontal impact, rear impact, lateral impact, rotational impact, and rollover. Each pattern is associated with its own specific injuries and mortality. Data from the United States shows that the associated mortality for frontal impact can be up to 60%. For side impact collisions, the mortality is up to 35% and for rollovers up to 15%.[1] Although contrary to expectation, MVCs that involve vehicle rollover have a lower rate of mortality due to the dispersion of momentum, and thus the force directed at the passenger is often reduced.

In any MVC, three identifiable collisions occur due to rapid deceleration. The first collision is either the vehicle on vehicle, or the vehicle on victim collision. In this instance, a moving object transmits its force to either another moving or stationary object, eventually coming to rest. The next is when the unrestrained occupant keeps moving at the same velocity and then collides with the inside of the vehicle. The third and final collision is when the occupant's organs continue to move at the same velocity as the vehicle and then collide with the body wall, with other organs within the body, or are sheared from fixed points.

Frontal impact occurs when a motor vehicle's forward motion is slowed or stopped by another object or a person. This impact results in damage to the front of the vehicle as it continued to move forward while another force was trying to stop its forward motion. This same energy transfer is transferred to the passengers of the vehicle. They will continue in their forward motion and will have a sudden deceleration when the second collision occurs.

Rear impact occurs when a motor vehicle is hit from behind by a faster moving vehicle. For this situation, recall the laws of conservation of energy and momentum: the car that hits from behind will have a higher velocity. It will impart some of its energy and momentum to the other vehicle in this system. If there is a large difference in momentum of the two vehicles, there is potential for greater damage. The injury pattern in a rear impact accident is not only from the rear impact but also from the vehicle being hit, from hitting another object, or from pressing on the brakes abruptly. This results in both rear impact injuries as well as frontal impact injuries.

Lateral impact typically occurs at an intersection or when a vehicle loses control and strikes a stationary object sideways. The impact can occur on either side of the vehicle being hit, leading to significant intrusion into the vehicle. Momentum is transmitted to the vehicle being struck as well as the passengers within, leading to injuries secondary to lateral acceleration.

Rotational impact MVCs occur when the corner of a vehicle strikes or is struck by another object. This results in the corner that is struck decelerating while the rest of the vehicle continues to move forward. This forward motion is now around the fixed point of the corner and leads to rotation of the vehicle; much like a pinwheel moving around its fixed central point. The injury pattern is a combination of those seen in frontal impact and lateral impact, and the passengers closest to the point of impact will be most severely injured.

Rollover MVCs are a complex type of impact where there is no longer just impact along the *x*- and *y*-axes, but additional impact along the *z*-axis (Figure 1). This type of MVC results in a combination of injury patterns that are seen with all the collisions noted above. The rolling nature of the MVC leads to even more shearing injury in restrained passengers. This is where injuries to organs occur at fixed points because they also follow *Newton's first law of motion*. Ejection of unrestrained passengers also occurs most frequently in these types of MVC. Although rollover MVCs have a relatively reduced mortality, ejection can cause the victim to be hit by oncoming traffic resulting in increased mortality. Ejection carries a four-fold increase in intensive care unit admission and a five-fold increase in average Injury Severity Score (ISS) (Table 1). These patients also have a three-fold increase in brain injury and a five-fold increase in mortality secondary to injuries sustained in the crash.[1]

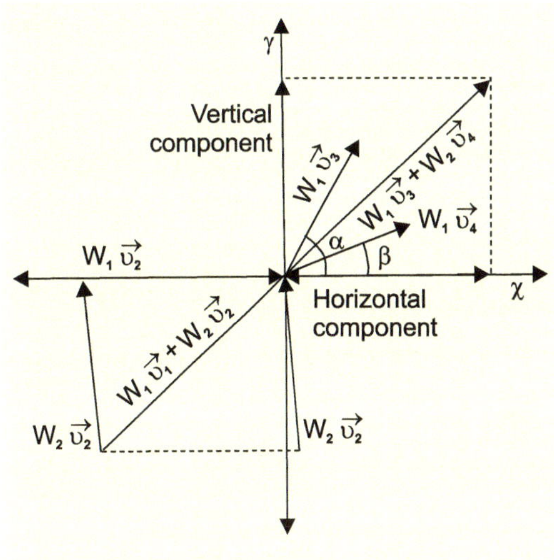

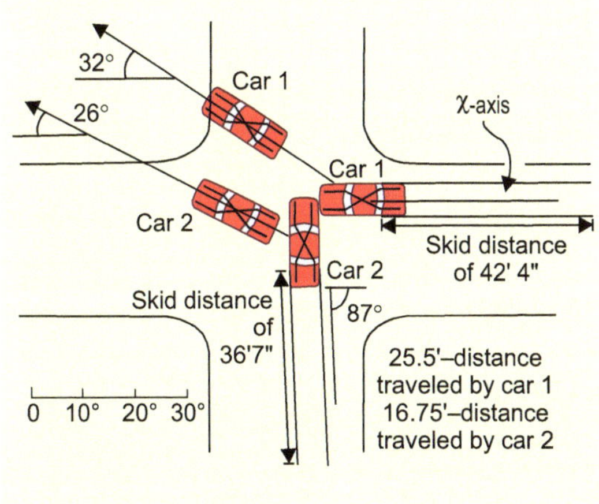

Figure 1: Motor vehicle crash kinetics

Table 1: Injury Severity Score; ISS

Region	Injury Description	AIS	Square Top Three
Head & Neck	Cerebral Contusion	3	9
Face	No Injury	0	
Chest	Flall Chest	4	16
Abdomen	Minor Contusion of Liver	2	
	Complex Rupture Spleen	5	25
Extremlty	Fractured femur	3	
External	No Injury	0	
	Injury Severity Score:		50

AIS Score	Injury	ISS	
1	Minor	1-8	Minor
2	Moderate	9-15	Moderate
3	Serious	16-24	Serious
4	Severe	25-49	Severe
5	Critical	50-74	Critical
6	Survivable	75	Maximum

Motorcycle/Two-Wheeler Crash

Motorcycle crash (MCC) is another commonly seen form of blunt trauma and can be associated with serious morbidity and mortality. Though the physics of the injuries remain the same, the way injuries occur can significantly differ from MVCs. The lack of an external frame and body to protect the victim also contribute to potentially worse injuries.

Head-on impact involves the motorcycle moving forward into another object. With MCC, the center of gravity for the motorcycle changes with the type of impact. In this particular type of collision, the center of gravity is behind the front axle and just as with the rotational impact MVC, this now becomes a fixed point around which the bike and passenger will rotate. This will send the rider headfirst over the handlebars or the mid thighs will get caught on the handlebars and they will then absorb the majority of forward force.

Angular impact MCC is another type of crash where the rider and motorcycle either strike or are struck at an angle. This results in the bike either falling on the rider or the rider being pinned between the bike and the object that is struck. In both cases, there is a high possibility of a crush injury occurring.

Ejection occurs with greater frequency after MCC than after MVC because of a lack of restraints on motorcycles. Once ejected, the rider will continue to travel until they come into contact with another object such as a motor vehicle, the street, or a lamp post. There is a significant likelihood of internal organ injury with this mechanism.

MCC remains a major cause of morbidity and mortality, especially in developing countries such as India. Helmet use can significantly reduce head injury. Unfortunately, many states lack laws mandating their use. In the United States, only 19 states have mandatory helmet laws, and the number is declining to the disappointment of public health experts. In many developing countries, states have no laws mandating helmets. Some states only mandate helmets for the driver, leaving passengers exposed to traumatic brain injury in the event of a crash. Enforcement of helmet laws has also been an issue. Much work remains in the area of injury prevention to avoid these types of injuries. Helmet laws for driver, passenger, or both are weak. In places where laws do exist, their limited enforcement also plays a role in the continued morbidity and mortality seen from these types of injuries.

Pedestrian Struck

Pedestrian injuries typically follow a predictable pattern depending on the height of the victim and the height of the vehicle's bumper (Figure 2). Three distinct phases of pedestrian versus automobile trauma have classically been described. The first phase is the initial contact. An automobile traveling at a given speed will hit the victim's lower extremities as this corresponds to the height of the vehicle's bumper. If the vehicle is a truck or has a higher front end, the initial contact will be relatively higher on the victim's body. This phase is characteristically associated with lower extremity fractures and injuries. The second phase is described as the torso and upper body due to rolling up onto the hood of the vehicle or hitting the windshield. This occurs also in accordance with Newton's first law. The body at rest has a tendency to stay at rest, but now the vehicle has imparted momentum to the victim's body. This results in the lower half of the body being pushed out, thus causing the upper half of the pedestrian's body to fall forward onto the vehicle itself. The vehicle with its initial kinetic energy and momentum will continue to move forward and so the victim's body will roll up onto the hood of the vehicle. Provided the lower extremities are not trapped, this also will sometimes result in the head, neck, and upper torso potentially hitting the windshield. The third phase of this type of blunt trauma results in the pedestrian being thrown from the hood of the vehicle onto the ground. This collision is an inelastic collision, where momentum is conserved but not kinetic energy. When the motor vehicle comes to an abrupt stop, the less massive pedestrian will be thrown forward as they will have the initial momentum of the vehicle that struck them. This phase can cause any number of traumatic injuries due to the variable nature of how the pedestrian will land and the possibility of being struck by another motor vehicle.

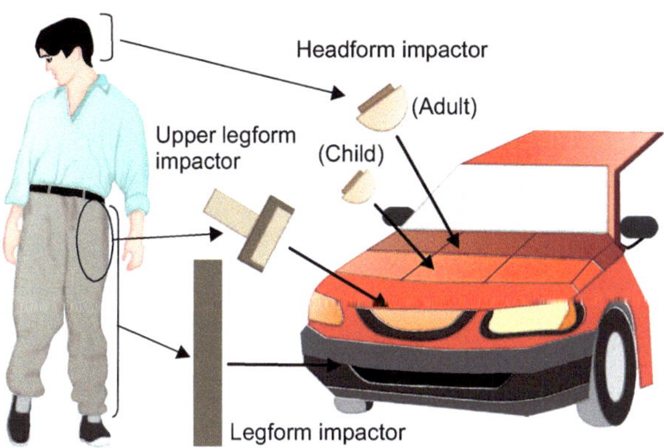

Figure 2: Pedestrian struck kinetics

Falls

Falls represent a common form of blunt trauma that can result in a complex set of injuries. These injuries are also a major source of disability and may be the initiating event for developing multi-system organ failure, especially in elderly patients. As mentioned earlier, a falling body converts its gravitational potential energy into kinetic energy. The impact force is the impact kinetic energy divided by the distance the body travels into the surface that it strikes at the time of impact. The injuries sustained in falls will be dependent upon how the victim lands and from what height they fell (Figure 3). A classically sustained injury pattern is when a patient falls from a height and lands on their feet. Energy is transmitted from the ankles up to the spine leading to bilateral calcaneal injuries, pelvic fracture, and thoracolumbar spinal injury.

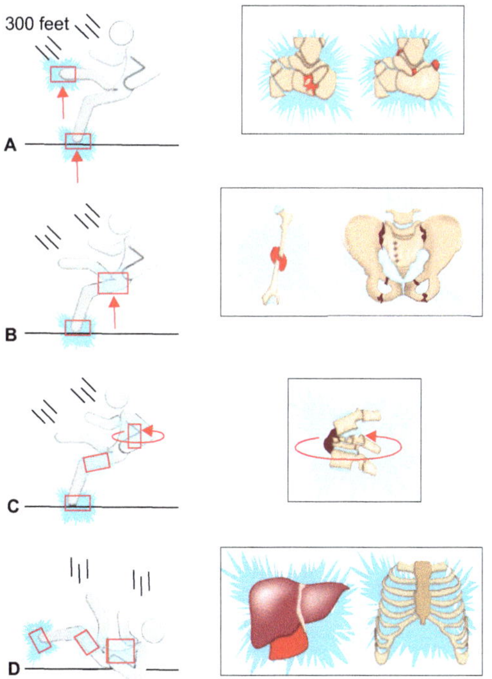

Figure 3: Injuries from different types of falls.

Approach to the Patient with Blunt Trauma

Any trauma patient that arrives at the ED or trauma resuscitation unit should undergo a rapid but thorough primary and secondary survey with appropriate adjunct studies. If there is a clear indication for immediate operative intervention, such as in the hypotensive patient with a positive abdominal ultrasound revealing free fluid, further adjunctive studies such as CT scan, should be avoided as this will unnecessarily delay the patient from definitive management and potentially expedite death. In hemodynamically stable patients, further adjunct studies can help clarify the extent of injury and can aid in determining treatment options, whether that be watchful waiting, interventional angiography, or operative intervention. These adjuncts can include radiographs, CT scans, and ultrasound examinations.

Pattern recognition is especially important in the blunt trauma victim. Certain mechanisms of trauma will present with predictable injuries and so a high index of suspicion is necessary to drive the decision making in patients with blunt trauma. In the hemodynamically stable patient, a complete medical and surgical history complementing a thorough physical exam can prove very valuable. A detailed report from the prehospital provider about the scene of the accident and type of vehicular damage are essential in determining the possible injuries to these patients as described above. For patients sustaining intra-abdominal injury requiring exploration, the initial operative plan will remain the same for any blunt trauma case. This includes adequate exposure, controlling of arterial hemorrhage, packing of venous hemorrhage followed by definitive repair versus ligation, control of gross contamination, thorough exploration and assessment of wounds, damage control, and resuscitation of the patient if necessary. Patient physiology will help determine the need for damage control resuscitation and damage control laparotomy.

Site Specific Injury

Thorax

Chest Wall

Common causes of chest wall injury in blunt trauma can be secondary to MVCs, MCCs, and falls. Blunt chest wall trauma is often associated with rib fractures and studies show that an increasing number of rib fractures are a predictor of morbidity and mortality (Figure 4). Three or more rib fractures on initial chest X-ray have been shown to be a marker of solid organ and visceral injury, and increased mortality.[1] In another study of 7,000 patients, 10% had rib fractures and of those, 94% had associated injuries. Half of these patients were admitted to the intensive care unit or needed an emergent operation.

In this study, there was a 12% mortality rate in patients with rib fractures.[1] Significant chest wall trauma, rib fractures, and flail segments have been associated with higher Injury Severity Scores, increased need for mechanical ventilation, increased need for blood transfusions, higher mortality, and longer intensive care unit and hospital stays.

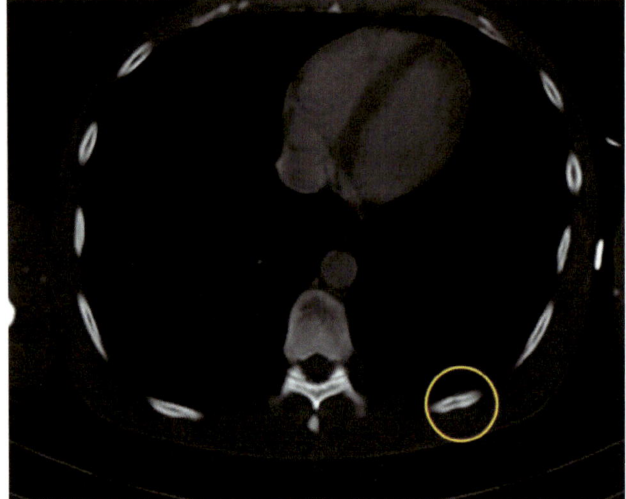

Figure 4: Un-displaced fracture of the posterior rib

Blunt trauma to the chest wall can lead to multiple complications which include extreme pain, bleeding complications, and chest wall instability. Pain in patients with chest wall trauma can be excruciating. It is a common belief that significant pain leads to 'splinting' or poor inspiratory effort. This poor effort is believed to be associated with poor pulmonary toilet, pooling of secretions, increased atelectasis, and possibly associated with higher incidences of pneumonia. Appropriate pain control is necessary in these patients to avoid these complications.

Hemothorax associated with rib fractures after blunt chest wall trauma can typically be managed with tube thoracostomy. Associated parenchymal injury can occur due to laceration by a fractured rib and can lead to further bleeding or an air leak. CT scan of the chest can show lacerations of the lungs and contrast can reveal signs of contrast extravasation. This indicates that there are lacerated vessels which are actively bleeding and may need either surgical or radiographic intervention. Retained hemothorax is a source of morbidity after trauma. The concern with retained hemothorax is that the patient undergoes a systemic inflammatory response which can prevent the body's ability to absorb the hemothorax. The blood and chest wall injury create a local inflammatory state in the pleural space that causes an influx of neutrophils but also results in decreased phagocytic activity.[1] This is a rich medium that can promote infection and bacterial growth.

Chest wall instability refers to multiple rib fractures or *flail segments* where ribs are fractured in multiple locations. The prevailing belief about flail segments and unstable chest walls is that there is a greater number of pulmonary contusions and injury that occur due to the paradoxical movement of the flail segment. This paradoxical movement is due to the negative intrapleural pressure during inspiration. On inspiration, as the thoracic rib cage moves outward, the flail segment is pulled inward, potentially worsening the underlying *pulmonary contusion*. On exhalation, as the thoracic rib cage moves inward and the abdominal contents push up on the diaphragm, the flail segment moves outward causing significant pain. Historically, these patients were intubated and mechanically ventilated, but it has been shown that respiratory failure after chest wall trauma is not due to mechanical dysfunction as seen with a flail segment. Instead, this is likely due to the underlying pulmonary contusion. The contusion will lead to worsened lung compliance and worsen a physiologic shunt. This can lead to hypoxemic respiratory failure and require intubation. Therefore, it is the underlying lung pathology and not the chest wall instability that leads to respiratory failure. The role of chest wall stabilization procedures such as rib plating is still controversial and cannot be recommended as a gold standard therapy at the time of this publication.

Lung

Blunt trauma can cause lung injury in the form of contusions and hematomas. Contusions are bruising of the lung parenchyma and are being appreciated more in the era of chest CT scan for trauma. On chest X-ray they may not manifest for several hours to days and are said to 'blossom' much as bronchopleural pneumonia does over time. Though they may not be readily apparent on radiograph initially, they can still result in impaired gas exchange which can manifest as decreased oxygen saturation or abnormal arterial blood gas values. Uncomplicated pulmonary contusions will usually resolve with supportive care. If there is major disruption of the chest wall or significant pulmonary laceration or hemorrhage, this may require prolonged mechanical ventilation or possibly extracorporeal membrane oxygenation (ECMO) to help with gas exchange.

Pulmonary hematomas are a result of parenchymal disruption and are a space occupying lesion within the lung. They may appear to be a pulmonary contusion on chest X-ray but are in fact blood within the lung. These can cause the same problems with gas exchange as a contusion and will typically resolve with the same supportive measures but will usually take longer to heal than a contusion.

Blunt Cardiac Injury

Although blunt cardiac injury (BCI) has been reported in the literature dating back to 1764, it was not until 1958 that a large review of this injury had been reported. Parmley et al.

reviewed 207,548 autopsies from the Armed Forces Institute of Pathology and found the incidence of 0.1%. This translated into 546 patients who had sustained a blunt cardiac injury. Out of 353 patients with cardiac chamber ruptures, 80 were associated with aortic ruptures. The distribution of injury per chamber was found to be 66 right ventricle ruptures, 59 left ventricle ruptures, 41 right atrium ruptures, and 26 left atrium ruptures. Additionally, he found that 106 patients had BCI in multiple chambers.[1]

BCI includes a spectrum of injuries that can range from simple cardiac contusions to chamber rupture, and even cardiac arrest and cardiogenic shock from sternal injury. The actual incidence of BCI is difficult to determine based on the literature but it is noted that any blunt trauma that transmits force through the chest wall to the heart can cause BCI. The most common cause of BCI is high speed MVCs that have associated steering wheel and column deformity. Part of the difficulty in determining the true incidence of BCI is due to the variability of presentation. Patients can present without any signs or symptoms of cardiac injury, they can have significant chest wall tenderness overlying the heart, they can present with cardiac tamponade, or they can present with heart failure and cardiac arrest. Patients with a suspected BCI typically will have an electrocardiogram (EKG) performed. In a hemodynamically stable patient with a normal EKG, no further workup is required. However, if electrical disturbances are observed, further investigation is warranted. Abnormalities on EKG can range from sinus tachycardia to complete heart block with signs of myocardial ischemia. It is uncommon to see conduction abnormalities on a screen EKG.

The next area of controversy in the diagnosis of BCI after an abnormal EKG is measuring blood levels of creatine phosphokinase (CPK) or creatine kinase (CK) with myocardial band (MB). Although these lab values have been said to be specific for BCI, multiple studies in the literature have shown this not to be the case. These studies show that the levels of these labs do not correlate with BCI.[1] Troponins are proteins found in the contractile units of the myocardium. Since the discovery of high troponin levels in patients with myocardial infarctions, this has carried over to the trauma world to help diagnose BCI. There has been work trying to show that EKGs and troponin levels in patients with blunt injury could effectively rule-in and rule-out BCIs, but the individual sensitivities and predictive values of troponin I and troponin T have been found to be low.[2]

Since the literature has shown such controversy in the definition of BCI and since there is not a gold standard diagnostic modality of choice to identify BCI, the Eastern Association for the Surgery of Trauma (EAST) has created a set of practice management guidelines to help identify patients with BCI. A Level I recommendation is to obtain an EKG on admission for anyone suspected of having BCI. A Level II recommendation states that, if there is an abnormality on the admission EKG, the patient should be admitted for continuous EKG monitoring for 24 to 48 hours and have a transthoracic echocardiography (TTE). If suboptimal, a transesophageal echocardiogram (TEE) should be obtained. The last level II recommendation was that nuclear medicine studies were not useful if an echocardiogram was performed. If the admission EKG was normal, no further workup to identity BCI was needed. A level III recommendation states that geriatric patients with heart disease, unstable patients, or patients with abnormal admission EKGs could be taken to the operating room if necessary and if monitoring equipment was present and placement of a pulmonary artery catheter was a reasonable means of monitoring them. Additionally, the presence of sternal fractures alone does not necessitate BCI workup. Decision making should be based on a combination of EKG and clinical suspicion. Cardiac isoenzymes were not helpful in determining the presence of BCI.[3]

As mentioned earlier, blunt cardiac injury can range from myocardial contusion or bruising to cardiac chamber rupture. Pericardial injury after blunt trauma is due to a high energy collision or transmitted from a sudden increase in intra-abdominal pressure. Pericardial rupture typically occurs on the left side parallel to the left phrenic nerve or along the diaphragm. Patients can present in any condition from being completely stable to having cardiovascular collapse. It is possible to have the heart herniated out of the pericardium into the thorax or abdomen depending on the site of injury. These kinds of herniations also put the great vessels on stretch and can cause torsion injuries. Chest X-ray, EKG, and echocardiogram should all be part of the workup for suspected pericardial injury. If there is no associated cardiac injury, and the patient is hemodynamically stable, this may not require surgical intervention.

Injury to cardiac valvular structures is uncommon after BCI. The typical signs of valvular injury may not be noticed due to other more apparent injuries. The most common valves injured are the aortic and mitral valves. The patient may present with a new onset of cardiac murmurs and cardiovascular collapse in the form of left heart failure and shock. The proposed mechanism of injury is from force applied to the thoracic cage, transmitted to the heart. This causes the blood in the ventricle to be rapidly displaced during diastole. This then leads to laceration or rupture of the papillary muscles, chordae tendineae, and/or cardiac valve leaflets. Blunt cardiac injury leading to injury of the coronary arteries is usually to the left anterior descending artery (LAD) or the right coronary artery (RCA). The LAD is directly beneath the sternum and blunt injury can lead to stretch or intimal disruption, leading to acute thrombosis of a coronary artery. Typically, this will present as a myocardial infarction. Long term complications of this include ventricular failure, aneurysmal dilation of the ventricle with thrombus formation, arrhythmias, embolism, and rupture.

Cardiac chamber rupture after blunt trauma is another form of BCI. One hypothesized mechanism of rupture is pressure transmission through a fluid column of blood, from the abdomen to the heart via the venous system. This would account for right atrial rupture. Another theory is acceleration and deceleration injury causing separation from the great vessels leading to ventricular rupture. Most patients who do not expire at the scene of the accident will present with hypotension and possibly pericardial tamponade. The tamponade is protective, and release of the tamponade can result in very rapid decompensation and cardiovascular collapse. Right sided ruptures appear to occur with greater frequency than left sided ruptures, presumably due to the lower pressure system and the thinner walls of the right heart compared to the left heart.

Great Vessel Injury

The majority of great vessel injuries are secondary to penetrating traumas. Vessels most commonly injured by blunt trauma include the innominate artery, the pulmonary veins, the vena cava, and the thoracic aorta. Blunt injury to the great vessels likely occur secondary to shearing forces at the junction of fixed and mobile portions of the vessels, compression injury by direct injury to overlying structures, or intimal injury due to intraluminal hypertension. Intraluminal hypertension could possibly be due to transmitted forces from other compartments being injured during blunt injury. A classic example of this last mechanism would be significantly increased intra-abdominal pressure being transmitted to the vena cava leading to intraluminal hypertension and possible caval injury.

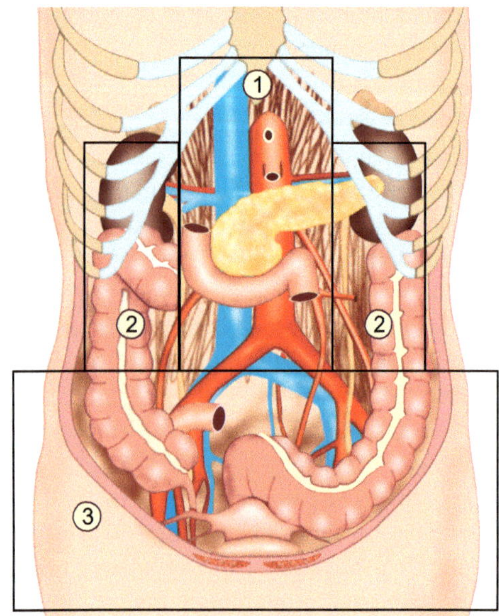

Figure 5: Zones for retroperitoneal and abdominal aortic injuries

Blunt aortic injury contributes to between 10% and 15% of deaths after MVC. Motor vehicle collisions actually account for greater than 70% of blunt aortic injuries and occur in 1.9% of all MVCs.[1] It has been found that ejection during an MVC results in a 2-fold increased risk of having a blunt aortic injury, but seat belts and restraints decrease this risk by a factor of four.[2] Most patients who sustain significant blunt aortic injury will die from massive hemorrhage at the scene and will not be evaluated by emergency teams. Of the patients who survive, 75% will initially be hemodynamically stable but 50% will die before a definitive repair. Almost all these patients will have associated injuries, and the aortic injury may be missed or deemed not as emergent as another injury that is present. The American Association for the Surgery of Trauma (AAST) found that 51% of patients with blunt aortic injury had a concomitant closed head injury, 46% had rib fractures, 38% had pulmonary contusions, and up to 35% had orthopedic injuries.[1]

The majority of these injuries involve the proximal descending thoracic aorta, distal to the take-off of the left subclavian artery. This accounts for 54% of blunt aortic injuries. Most blunt aortic injuries will also be full thickness tears and those patients that survive to the emergency department will likely have a contained rupture. The surrounding soft tissues or pleura will prevent rapid expansion and exsanguination. Partial thickness injuries are less common but will occur posteriorly and involve the intima and media of the vessel.

There are three major theories as to the pathophysiology of blunt aortic injury. The first explains why most injuries are seen at the aortic isthmus. The belief is that the aorta is relatively fixed here by the ligamentum arteriosum, the paired intercostal arteries and the left mainstem bronchus. The aortic isthmus is anatomically at the junction of the relatively mobile aortic arch and the fixed descending thoracic aorta. Deceleration forces during blunt trauma can allow the aorta to displace longitudinally enough to tear without a direct blow to the chest. The next major theory as to the physiology behind blunt aortic injury is based on the idea of the 'water-hammer effect.' This theory claims that the problem is more of hydraulics than of classic Newtonian mechanics. The aorta is considered a tube filled with a non-compressible fluid. This flow can be acutely obstructed at the level of the diaphragmatic hiatus, the level of thoracic vertebra twelve. This obstruction creates a high-pressure wave in the aorta that is transmitted up to the aortic arch. The curvature of the aortic arch then amplifies this pressure wave, thus resulting in injury to the aorta. The third major theory is known as the '*osseous pinch.*' This theory claims injury to the aorta occurs as it is sheared between the manubrium, sternum, clavicular heads, or first ribs anteriorly and the thoracic vertebrae posteriorly.[1]

A high index of suspicion is needed to diagnose a blunt aortic injury promptly and accurately. In patients who have been in an MVC, steering wheel and column deformity, ejection, and high-speed collision should all raise suspicion for possible aortic injury. Other mechanisms such as a fall from greater than 3 meters or a pedestrian struck at a high speed can also cause blunt aortic injury. On a physical exam, these patients may be hemodynamically stable or have signs of shock. They may have bony thoracic injury to structures like the sternum, manubrium, scapula, or multiple ribs. There may be a steering wheel imprint on their chest, or a new murmur may be found. Unequal extremity pulses or paraplegia can also be seen. A standard antero-posterior (AP) chest X-ray can have multiple findings suspicious for aortic injury and should be obtained in patients with an appropriate history. These findings include loss of the aortic silhouette, tracheal shift to the right, widened mediastinum, left sided apical cap, opacified aorto-pulmonary window, and multiple thoracic fractures. The gold standard diagnosis of blunt aortic injury was once aortography. This modality has a sensitivity and sensitivity of almost 100% but is operator dependent and can be quite time consuming. Computed tomography angiography (CTA) has now come to the forefront of diagnosis as it is now more readily available and fast to perform. The added benefit of CTA is the ability to identify other injuries, as noted earlier most patients with blunt aortic injury will have other associated injuries. TEE may have a role in the diagnosis of aortic injury but is limited to the distal aortic arch and proximal descending aorta, and it is also very operator dependent.

The approach to management of patients with blunt aortic injury is similar to all trauma patients because the airway should be secured, evacuation of a pneumothorax and hemothorax with a chest tube thoracostomy should be performed, and hemodynamics should be stabilized. If the patient is unstable and they need an emergent operation, hemorrhage control should be paramount. In a patient with a simultaneous intracranial injury with hemorrhage and associated mass effect or edema, they should be addressed urgently, and herniation prevented. Patients should be resuscitated appropriately to avoid end organ hypoperfusion and shock, and the use of short acting beta blockers have been shown to reduce in-hospital aortic rupture rates and do not adversely affect overall outcomes from associated injuries.[1] Beta blockade reduces wall stress on the aorta by reducing heart rate and blood pressure. Patients considered high risk for definitive aortic repair include those with significant TBI, those with significant pulmonary trauma who will not tolerate one lung ventilation, patients with pre-existing cardiac disease who need inotropic support, patients who are coagulopathic, and those with significant associated injuries that need stabilization and control prior to aortic repair. Patients considered high risk for definitive repair are recommended to continue beta blockade and delay aortic repair.

Open repair is still considered the gold standard operation for this injury. The ideal approach to a blunt aortic injury at the typical location, passed the aortic isthmus, is via a 4th intercostal space posterolateral thoracotomy. The clamp and sew technique for direct reconstruction involves dissecting the aorta proximal to the left subclavian artery, the distal aorta, and the left subclavian and then encircling all these areas with umbilical tape. Then, after alerting anesthesia, these areas are clamped, and the injured segment can be removed and replaced with an appropriately sized Dacron graft. This graft is sewn in using a 2-0 polypropylene suture in an end-to-end fashion. Following the operation, paraplegia is a possible complication. This has been associated with length of clamp time, perioperative hypotension, and ligation of multiple intercostal arteries. The incidence of paraplegia following aortic replacement surgery is about 10%.[1]

Another technique that has become popularized in the literature recently is thoracic endovascular aortic repair (TEVAR) otherwise known as aortic stent grafting. This is a relatively minimally invasive technique that allows for aortic repair with a flexible endograft. There have been a number of studies in the literature comparing TEVAR to open repair for the treatment of blunt aortic injury. These studies have found a reduction in mortality by up to 50% for TEVAR when compared to an open aortic repair. The risk of paraplegia is also minimal with TEVAR ranging from 0% to 5.6%.[2] There are no studies comparing the long-term outcomes of open repair and TEVAR, so even though there seems to be a lower rate of mortality and possibly a lower rate of paraplegia with TEVAR, it cannot be recommended as the gold standard repair at this time. Further studies comparing TEVAR to open repair with long term follow-up are needed.

Abdomen

Blunt abdominal trauma can be a complex and confusing problem for patients and care providers. The problem of hypotension in a patient with penetrating abdominal trauma is relatively straight-forward, these patients need a laparotomy. The same problem of hypotension in a patient with blunt trauma is more complicated because a laparotomy may not necessarily fix the situation. If the patient has overt signs of peritonitis, often not seen early in trauma presentation, they likely need a laparotomy; however, in a patient without this symptom, more information is needed. Adjuncts such as the Focused Assessment with Sonography for Trauma (FAST), diagnostic peritoneal lavage or aspirate (DPL/DPA) are useful in identifying the presence of free intra-abdominal fluid or blood, respectively. The FAST exam is a bedside, clinician performed ultrasound that has revolutionized management of trauma patients. The exam allows for the assessment of fluid within the pericardial and abdominal cavities. The FAST exam should be performed to visualize four areas: the pericardium, hepatorenal fossa (Morrison's pouch), splenorenal fossa, and bladder.

DPL should be considered in circumstances when the FAST exam is equivocal and a rapid assessment of the presence of intra-abdominal injury is needed. At the R Adams Cowley Shock Trauma Center, they encourage trainees to practice this skill in the cadaver lab to maintain proficiency. It is performed at the bedside by either a percutaneous or cut-down technique.

Management Approach

The approach to a patient with blunt abdominal trauma depends on whether the patient is able to be evaluated clinically. If the patient is alert and responsive and exhibits signs of peritonitis, emergent laparotomy should be considered. The FAST exam can provide additional information regarding the presence of fluid in the abdomen. The exam only assesses the presence of fluid in the abdomen. It does not localize its origin. Hypotensive patients with a positive abdominal FAST examination should be taken for emergent diagnostic and therapeutic laparotomy. Patients with these findings should ***not*** undergo further radiographic imaging such as CT scan as this delays management of potentially life-threatening injury. A hemodynamically stable patient with a positive FAST exam can undergo further imaging, such as CT scan of the abdomen and pelvis, which provides significantly more detailed anatomic information and can localize the source of the fluid. Specific Organ Injury Scales, as defined by the American Association for the Surgery of Trauma (AAST) are helpful in determining intervention strategies (i.e., observation, interventional radiology, surgery).

If the FAST exam is negative for free fluid and the patient is hemodynamically stable with no abdominal pain, management options can include a period of observation or discharge, provided there are no associated injuries. It is important to realize that radiographic and ultrasound studies provide a static image for a dynamic process. Interval or delayed repeat examinations can be beneficial.

Once the decision has been made to proceed to the operating room, the surgical team should have a clear plan for the management of the patient. Patients requiring massive transfusion should be considered for a *Damage Control* operation, first described by Rotondo et al. in the early 1990s, although the concept was used for several decades prior. The term Damage control originated from the merchant marine industry and is used to describe all actions performed to keep a damaged ship afloat. In the trauma setting, the goals of damage control are straightforward and performed to prevent the development of hypothermia, coagulopathy, and metabolic acidosis. The key steps are to stop arterial hemorrhage, pack venous bleeding, and control contamination and spillage. These goals should be met expeditiously. Bowels can be left in discontinuity and no attempts should be made at preforming definitive anastomosis. The initial damage control operation should take no longer than 90 minutes. The patient's abdomen should be left open using one of several open abdomen temporary closure devices. Management of the patient should then shift to the intensive care unit for continued resuscitation and rewarming. Acidosis, coagulopathy, and hypothermia should all be corrected. Once the patient's physiology is restored, in 24 to 48 hours, the patient is brought back to the operating room for a second look at laparotomy and unpacking. Definitive management of injuries and restoration of bowel continuity can now be performed.

Liver

The liver is the most commonly injured organ in blunt trauma. The liver is divided into two lobes, the left and right. These are divided by Cantlie's line, which is found on the posterior surface of the liver from the gallbladder fossa to the left of the inferior vena cava. The segmental anatomy of the liver is based on the branch points of the hepatic veins. The right hepatic vein is divided between the anterior segments V and VIII and the posterior segments VI and VII. The left hepatic vein is divided between anterior segments III and IV and posterior segment II. The caudate lobe or segment I drains directly into the inferior vena cava. The middle hepatic vein drains into the left hepatic vein in 90% of patients.

The celiac trunk comes off the aorta and gives off the common hepatic artery. This brings in 25% of the hepatic blood flow whereas the portal vein brings in the remaining 75%. The common hepatic artery branches into the gastroduodenal artery and the proper hepatic artery. The proper hepatic artery is found in the portal triad, which consists of the portal vein, the proper hepatic artery, and common bile duct. The artery is found anteriorly to the portal vein and to the left of the common bile duct. This artery then branches into right and left hepatic arteries as it enters the liver parenchyma.

The portal vein is the structure that lies most posteriorly in the portal triad and is formed when the splenic vein and superior mesenteric vein come together. This then divides into right and left portal veins extrahepatically, where the right is shorter than the left.

Liver injury is classified according to the grading system laid out by the AAST. A grade I liver injury is either a capsular tear with less than 1 cm parenchymal injury or a subcapsular hematoma that is less than 10 cm surface area. A grade II liver injury involves either a 1 to 3 cm parenchymal laceration, a subcapsular hematoma that is less than 50% surface area, or an intraparenchymal hematoma that is less than 10 cm in diameter. A grade III liver injury is defined as a laceration involving greater than 3 cm of the parenchyma or a subcapsular hematoma which is greater than 50% of the surface area, ruptured or with active bleeding. A grade III injury also can have a greater than 10 cm intraparenchymal hematoma. A grade IV liver injury involves a ruptured intraparenchymal hematoma with active bleeding or is a laceration involving up to 3 segments within a single lobe. A grade V liver injury involves either destruction of greater than 75% of a lobe of the liver or injury to the juxta-hepatic or retro-hepatic vena cava. A grade VI liver injury is hepatic avulsion.[1]

In the hemodynamically stable patient, CT scan has become the method of choice for staging liver injury after both blunt and penetrating injury. Non-operative management of liver injury in the hemodynamically stable patient is considered the standard of care at many major centers. A prospective study found that 89% of hemodynamically stable patients with all grades of liver injury and all volumes of hemoperitoneum could be managed non-operatively.[1]

Most blunt liver injury is due to hepatic venous bleeding which is a low-pressure system, and bleeding will stop once a clot forms. In high grade injuries, with CT scan evidence of active bleeding and pseudoaneurysm formation, non-operative management can be tried, but these patients have a higher risk of failure of non-operative therapy, and they may need adjunctive therapy such as angioembolization.

In patients who have major blunt liver injury and exhibit hemodynamic instability, operative management may be necessary. A midline laparotomy is the standard approach and allows adequate exposure to the liver and the rest of the abdominal viscera. Prior to entering the peritoneal cavity, the surgeon should alert the anesthesia team that they are about to lose the tamponade effect and that there may be a sharp blood pressure drop until hemostasis can be achieved. This allows the anesthesia team to try to resuscitate the patient up front in anticipation of hemorrhage. The first maneuver after evacuation of the hematoma and blood is manual compression of the liver. If there is still bleeding present, perihepatic packing with laparotomy pads should be performed. This requires pads to be tightly packed both anteriorly and posteriorly to the liver. Perihepatic packing requires mobilization of the liver by taking down the triangular and coronary ligaments as well as ligating the falciform ligament. This should be performed if there is no retro-hepatic venous injury or evidence of a retro-hepatic hematoma, as these maneuvers will release the beneficial tamponade that may be present. If there is still bleeding, then a Pringle maneuver to control hepatic inflow is recommended. This involves placing a vascular clamp across the portal vein and hepatic artery, and reports of up to 75 minutes of clamp time have been well tolerated. If bleeding is still coming from the liver after manual compression and a Pringle maneuver, then bleeding could be coming from the retro-hepatic veins and vena cava.

Other methods for controlling hemorrhage from liver bleeding include (1) finger fracture of a hepatic laceration down to the bleeding vessels so that they can either be directly ligated or repaired and (2) directly suturing larger lacerations of the liver with a 0 chromic suture with a blunt tipped needle to created tissue to tissue tamponade. This is typically performed in a horizontal mattress fashion and tied down gently so as to not tear the liver capsule. Omental packing has been described where the omentum is taken down off the colon and stomach, but a vascularized pedicle of the right gastroepiploic artery is maintained. Then this is placed tightly into a liver wound to create hemostasis. Nonanatomic hepatic resection has been shown to have a lower mortality than anatomic resections when performed for hemorrhage control. This can be performed with finger fracture and direct ligation method, electrocautery and Argon beam coagulation, or stapled resection using a vascular staple load. The key to the stapled method is to gently insert the stapler into the parenchyma without extending the wound, firing the stapler, and then ligating the bleeding vessels under direct visualization.

Both nonoperative and operative management of liver injuries have the potential for complications. Non-operative management has a 12% rate of complications for grade III to V injuries.[1] These injuries included bile leaks, abscesses, hemorrhage, haemobilia, and others such as portal hypertension. Bile leaks occur with a rate of 3% to 20% in these patients, and depending on the symptoms and laboratory abnormalities, may be observed or get percutaneous drainage of the bile. Occasionally endoscopic retrograde cholangiopancreatography (ERCP) with sphincterotomy or stent, needs to be performed to lower the resistance in the biliary tree. This provides a path of least resistance for bile to flow through, thus allowing the leak to heal. Abscesses are usually due to hepatic necrosis and can be managed with a CT-guided drain. These patients can present with fevers and have an elevated white blood cell count. Signs of sepsis can also be a presentation of hepatic abscess after non-operative management of blunt liver trauma. Hemorrhage is uncommon after non-operative management except in high grade injuries and injuries where there are signs of active bleeding. Delayed hemorrhage from lower grade injuries can usually be managed nonoperatively. Haemobilia is a very rare complication in non-operative management of liver trauma. This was typically seen after resection or operative ligation that resulted in pseudoaneurysm formation and rupture into the biliary system.

Complications after operative management of blunt liver injury include bleeding complications and fistulae formation. Bleeding is uncommon after operative intervention because presumably, the patient would not have left the operating room with bleeding that could be managed surgically. Postoperative bleeding is most often due to coagulopathy.

Haemobilia, as mentioned above, is sometimes seen after operative management when a pseudoaneurysm forms and ruptures into the biliary tree. These patients present with larger upper gastrointestinal bleeding and can have jaundice and worsened right upper quadrant pain. These patients may require angioembolization or further operative repair. Biliary fistula can be found in up to 22.5% of liver trauma that is managed operatively. They are defined as a bilious drainage from an injury of 50 mL or more per day. The majority of these can be managed by drain placement but ERCP and sphincterotomy or stent placement may be needed and, if this still does not stop the drainage, then a biliary bypass procedure may be required.

Spleen

The spleen is the second most commonly injured organ after blunt abdominal trauma, but it most commonly requires intervention for hemorrhage. An adult spleen typically has a mass of 100 to 250 grams. This organ is located in the left upper quadrant of the abdomen and located posteriorly. Posterior-laterally the spleen is attached to the diaphragm and abdominal wall by the spleno-phrenic ligament. Posterior-inferiorly the spleen is attached to the left kidney by the splenorenal ligament. Inferiorly the spleen is attached to the transverse colon and splenic flexure by the splenocolic ligament. The blood supply to the spleen is from the splenic artery which is a branch of the celiac trunk. Additional blood supply is from the short gastric arteries which come from the left gastroepiploic artery and run along the greater curvature of the stomach.

The approach to a patient with blunt splenic injury involves assessing and securing their airway, assessing breath sounds and checking hemodynamics. Listening to the prehospital provider's report of the accident is important. If this was a side impact collision MVC on the passenger side and the patient was a front seat passenger, spleen injury is a distinct possibility. If they have left sided tenderness or bruising and tender lower thoracic ribs on the left, again splenic injury is possible and warrants expeditious diagnosis. Presence of left shoulder pain could be a manifestation known as Kehr's sign, which signifies left subphrenic injury causing referred pain along the phrenic nerve.

Splenic injury is classified based on the AAST grading system. A grade I injury is either a capsular tear with less than 1 cm of parenchymal injury, or a subcapsular hematoma that is less than 10 cm of surface area. A grade II splenic injury involves either a 1 to 3 cm parenchymal laceration or a subcapsular hematoma that is less than 50% of the surface area or an intraparenchymal hematoma that is less than 5 cm in diameter. A grade III splenic injury is defined as a laceration involving greater than 3 cm of the parenchyma or a subcapsular hematoma which is greater than 50% of the surface area, ruptured or with active bleeding. A grade III injury can also have a greater than 5 cm intraparenchymal hematoma. A grade IV splenic injury involves laceration of the hilar vessels and major devascularization of the spleen. A grade V spleen injury is a completely shattered spleen or complete devascularization (Figure 6).

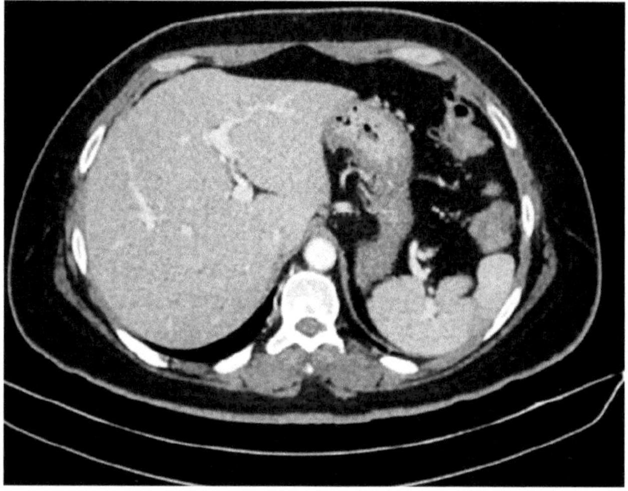

Figure 6: Wedge shaped hypodense area in spleen indication splenic infarction

If the patient arrives hemodynamically stable, a patient with suspected blunt splenic injury should be taken to the CT scanner. If a splenic injury is present and a contrast extravasation is seen, angiography and embolization should be considered. If there is no contrast extravasation, then evaluation of the splenic injury should take place in the context of the patient's other injuries. Non-operative management of a splenic injury with no contrast extravasation is a viable option, provided the ability to perform serial blood draws, hemodynamic monitoring and repeated physical exams are present. If these resources are not available, then splenectomy should be considered. In the hemodynamically unstable patient, a FAST exam should be performed with the physical examination and management as described above according to FAST findings.

Approximately 60% of patients with blunt splenic injury receive non-operative intervention. These patients are selected based on their hemodynamic stability, the absence of peritoneal signs, an unaltered mental status, and extent of their splenic injury. The reported success of non-operative management is approximately 80%, meaning that only 20% will end up needing operative intervention.[1] Patients who exhibit contrast blush or have a pseudoaneurysm on CT scan have a higher rate of failure of non-operative management and need operative intervention. The reported rate for need of operation in patients with presence of blush or pseudoaneurysm is 67% versus 6% in patients without these findings.[2] Failures of non-operative management will most often occur early in the admission. Up to 70% of failures occur by 48 hours after admission. Only 10% will occur after one-week post-injury.

If a patient with blunt splenic trauma is to be managed nonoperatively, there are several considerations. The patient should be admitted for serial abdominal examinations, continuous hemodynamic monitoring, and serial complete blood counts. Patients should typically be left nil per os (NPO) for at least the first 24 hours in case they need to be taken to the operating room for surgical intervention for failure of non-operative management or their other injuries. Early mobilization is associated with faster overall recovery, and hospital discharge and can help prevent morbidities associated with continued bed rest. There is no good evidence to show that early mobilization results in failure of non-operative management. Mobilization of the patient should be performed in the context of their concomitant injuries, if orthopedic or brain injuries preclude mobilization, this may prevent moving the patient out of bed. Patients should be started on deep venous thrombosis (DVT) prophylaxis shortly after operation, angioembolization, or observation. There have not been any randomized prospective trials looking at failure of non-operative management or rate of thromboembolic events in patients who received DVT prophylaxis after blunt splenic injury. There is currently no level I recommendations regarding the optimal timing of DVT prophylaxis initiation. In general, prophylaxis should be started as soon as the patient's other injuries permit.

Operative therapy for splenic injuries falls into two broad categories, splenectomy, or splenic preserving procedures. The procedure for a splenectomy involves dividing its peritoneal attachments and bringing the spleen to the midline. Once it is in the midline, the tail of the pancreas should also be up and visualized so it does not get injured. The hilar vessels are dissected free, clamped, and transected near the hilum, again to avoid pancreatic injury. Once the hilum is controlled, the short gastric arteries are identified, and suture ligated along the greater curvature of the stomach. These are varying numbers of short gastric arteries, usually between 6 and 8, and not identifying them can cause continued bleeding.

Splenic preserving procedures depend on the severity of the injury and whether or not it is actively bleeding. A splenorrhaphy is typically performed in Grade II and III splenic injuries. This can be performed by placing a hemostatic agent over the injury or using electrocautery or Argon beam coagulation to stop the bleeding. Suturing the spleen is more difficult than the liver as the tissue is softer and does not hold sutures well. Using a pledgeted monofilament suture can be helpful in reapproximating the wound. Partial splenectomy can be performed if the injury is isolated to a particular area of the spleen. Since there is segmental blood supply to the spleen, part of the hilar blood supply can be ligated, and the area of demarcation that develops on the spleen will show the surgeon where to perform the partial splenectomy. The raw edge can then be coagulated with electrocautery or Argon beam, and a hemostatic agent can be applied. Mesh wrapping the spleen can be performed with an absorbable mesh but should only be performed in patients with no other significant intra-abdominal injury and those who are hemodynamically stable as it can be time consuming. The other concern is that of the intense inflammatory reaction the patient will have in their left upper quadrant which can result in pain and a sympathetic pleural effusion that will be slow to resolve.

A feared complication of splenectomy is overwhelming post-splenectomy sepsis (OPSI). This is a very rare complication and estimated to have a 0.026 % lifetime risk of occurrence in adults who have had a splenectomy. The concern over this rare complication is due to its extremely high mortality. It is believed that the infection can be caused by encapsulated bacteria such as *Neisseria meningococcus, Strep pneumococcus,* and *Haemophilus influenzae*. The spleen functions to remove senescent erythrocytes from the circulation as well as forms antibodies to act against certain antigens found on bacteria. This second function is its immune function. The bacteria are captured in the red pulp of the spleen and the antigen on the bacterial wall is then presented to the adjacent white pulp. The white pulp has lymphocytic activity and is a source of immunoglobulin production in response to the antigen. Encapsulated bacteria are filtered by the spleen; thus, splenectomy removes this important immunologic function. The spleen also is a source of opsonins like tuftsin and properdin, as well as complement activation, needed for further immune function. It is standard of care to vaccinate patients with congenital hemolytic anemia requiring elective splenectomy two weeks prior to operation to optimize antibody production. In trauma patients who undergo splenectomy, vaccine immunizations should be given prior to discharge from the hospital. The necessity for routine immunization for patients undergoing splenic angioembolization is less clear. Newer literature from animal studies has shown that the embolized spleen retains immune function.

Duodenum and Pancreas

The duodenum and pancreas are intimately associated, sharing a common blood supply; therefore, when discussing injuries to one, the other must be included in the discussion. The duodenum is the first part of the small bowel, it has a length of approximately 30 cm and goes from the pylorus to the Ligament of Treitz. The duodenum is divided into four portions. The first portion is from the pylorus to the common bile duct and is called the superior portion. The second portion is from the common bile duct to the Ampulla of Vater and is called the descending portion. The third portion is known as the transverse portion and goes from the ampulla to the superior mesenteric vessels. The fourth portion goes from the superior mesenteric vessels to the left of the second lumbar vertebra and terminates at the Ligament of Treitz. The fourth portion is known as the ascending portion.

The pancreas is divided into four portions. These are the head and uncinate process, the neck, the body, and the tail. The head's vascular supply is from the superior pancreaticoduodenal artery which is a branch of the gastroduodenal artery, and the inferior pancreaticoduodenal artery which is a branch of the superior mesenteric artery. As the names imply, these arteries share a blood supply to the head of the pancreas and duodenum. Behind the neck of the pancreas, the superior mesenteric vessels are found. At the superior edge of the pancreas is the typical location of the splenic artery, and the inferior edge is where the splenic vein is typically found. The tail is often found in the lienorenal ligament and abuts the splenic hilum. The pancreas' body and tail are supplied by branches that enter its posterior surface directly from the splenic artery. Since this area is so richly vascularized and near so many sensitive structures, trauma to this part of the abdomen is not an area to enter lightly (Figure 7).

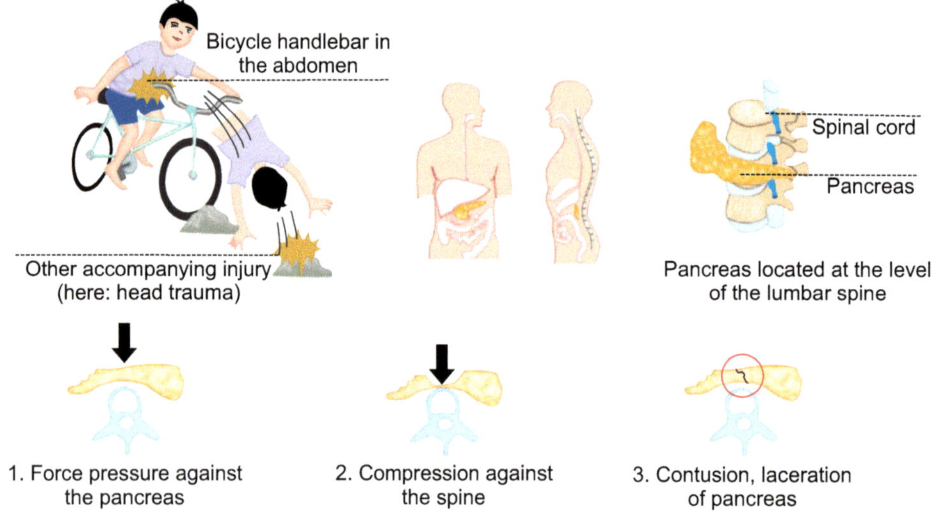

Figure 7: Handlebar injury causing pancreas fracture

Patients who arrive with a duodenal or pancreatic injury can manifest symptoms of significant abdominal pain in the epigastrium. The route of injury in blunt abdominal trauma is due to deceleration injuries with blunt force to the epigastrium. This causes the duodenum to become crushed between the vertebrae and the anterior abdominal wall. This may be difficult to diagnose because there may be no physical findings distinctly across the abdomen, the FAST exam may be negative for intra-abdominal free fluid, and plain X-ray films of the abdomen will rarely show signs of this injury. The signs on X-ray include presence of retroperitoneal air, loss of the right psoas shadow, and spine scoliosis in the lower thoracic and upper lumbar spine. As mentioned, these are all extremely rare findings. In the hemodynamically stable patient, a CT scan of the abdomen is very useful and, if duodenal trauma is suspected, then oral contrast medium is also very helpful.

CT scan findings of mesenteric stranding, retroperitoneal air or fluid, hemorrhage around the duodenum, and loss of tissue planes will need an operative exploration to confirm or rule out a duodenal injury. The associated morbidity of a missed duodenal or pancreatic injury is too high to allow simple observation for a possible injury.

Duodenal injury is graded based on a scale devised by the AAST. Grade I injuries are hematomas in a single portion of the duodenum or a partial thickness laceration. Grade II injuries are hematomas involving multiple portions or have less than 50% disruption of the duodenal wall. Grade III duodenal injuries involve 50% to 75% disruption of D2 or 50% to 100% disruption of D1, D3, or D4. Grade IV injuries results from greater than 75% disruption of D2 or injuries involving the distal common bile duct or ampulla of Vater. Grade V lacerations result in massive damage to the pancreas and duodenum or result in duodenal devascularization. Staging is important because it guides operative repair.

Grade I and II injuries require either nasogastric decompression and jejunal feeding or duodenotomy, evacuation of large hematomas and primary repair. Grade III injuries will either need a primary repair with pyloric exclusion, gastrojejunostomy and jejunal feeding, or a Roux-en-Y jejunoduodenostomy. Grade III injuries also need evaluation of the ampulla of Vater. Grade IV and V injuries are extremely complex and will require a damage control procedure, drainage of the common bile duct, drainage of the pancreas, and enteral bypass in the form of a pancreaticoduodenostomy.

Pancreatic injuries are also graded based on a AAST scale. Grade I injuries are superficial injuries that do not include duct damage. Grade II injuries are deeper injuries or significant contusions but there is still no ductal damage or tissue loss. Grade III injuries include distal transection of duct damage. Grade IV injuries to the pancreas involve injury to the head of the pancreas, right of the superior mesenteric vein. Grade V pancreatic injuries are massive damage to the pancreatic head.

The management of pancreatic injury is also based on the grade of injury. A grade I injury requires only observation, but a grade II injury will need closed suction drainage as there is a deeper laceration or injury. Grade III pancreatic injuries with ductal injury will necessitate a distal pancreatectomy, depending on where the injury occurred, splenic salvage may be possible. A jejunostomy feeding tube should be placed at the time of closure. A grade IV injury where there is significant pancreatic head injury but no injury to the common bile duct or pancreatic duct, requires wide drainage and post operative ERCP for evaluation of the ducts and possible stent placement. Another option when there is significant tissue damage to the head of the pancreas is to divide the pancreas at the neck. The proximal pancreas is oversewn and drained. The distal pancreas is preserved and drained via a Roux-en-Y pancreaticojejunostomy. A feeding jejunostomy tube should also be placed during the closure of this procedure. For grade V pancreatic injuries, a damage control procedure to control hemorrhage should be performed initially but definitive reconstruction will involve a pancreaticoduodenectomy and feeding jejunostomy tube placement. Reconstruction should be delayed until the patient is hemodynamically stable, out of shock, and preferably not requiring vasopressor support. Three tube drainage techniques for pancreatic or duodenal injuries involve placing a gastric drainage tube, a retrograde duodenostomy tube, and a distal feeding jejunostomy tube. This management strategy has been challenged in the literature. Most experts recommend primary repair, when possible, with wide drainage of the injured area.

Pancreatic fistulas will occur in up to 20% of patients after pancreatic trauma. This number increases in patients who have had combined pancreaticoduodenal trauma. All surgical interventions of the pancreas should have a drain left in place for that reason. It is arguable that a drain should be left for duodenal injuries or if the repair was tenuous. A minor pancreatic fistula has an output of less than 200 mL per day. These will typically resolve within several weeks if they are adequately drained. High output pancreatic fistulas will have an output of greater than 700 mL per day. These are difficult to manage and may need an ERCP with stent placement if it continues at such a high output for greater than 2 weeks. Octreotide administration may also result in decreased pancreatic fistula output and should be tried if there is persistent output. The caveat is, it will not result in earlier spontaneous closure of the pancreatic fistula, just possibly decrease the output.

Gastrointestinal Tract

The intra-abdominal gastrointestinal tract includes the stomach, the small bowel, and the colon. Injury to these organs can take the form of contusions, hematomas, partial and full thickness injuries and injuries to the mesentery and vasculature. Injuries to the gastrointestinal tract carry significant risk of intra-abdominal contamination and severe infectious complications.

Blunt injury to the stomach resulting in gastric rupture is uncommon, but it can lead to large amounts of intraperitoneal contamination and the possibility of developing intra-abdominal sepsis. The most frequent mechanism of blunt trauma resulting in gastric perforation and rupture is when a pedestrian is struck by a motor vehicle. The force required to rupture the stomach is very large because the stomach is such a compliant organ, and the force is dispersed to other parts of the victim's body. Therefore, associated injuries are very likely in a patient with gastric rupture from blunt trauma.

The most frequent cause of blunt small intestine ruptures are motor vehicle collisions. This is becoming a more recognized injury as a result of increased use of restraints such as seatbelts. Three-point restraints increase the risk of small bowel injury by 4.38 times and lap belts increase the risk by 10 times.1 These types of restraints are associated with a number of potential injuries. The presence of ecchymosis on the abdominal wall in the shape of a seat belt is known as a seat belt sign. The seat belt sign was found to have a significantly greater chance of abdominal injury and small bowel injury. One multi-institutional study found that if a seat belt sign was present, there was a 4.7% increase in small bowel perforation risk after an MVC.[1] The seat belt sign is also associated with transverse lumbar spine fractures which are known as Chance fractures. The significance of a Chance fracture is that they are also associated with hollow viscus injury, either small bowel or colon. Additionally, the presence of blunt small bowel injury is associated with other significant injury in the majority of patients.

The approach to a patient with suspected blunt gastrointestinal tract injury is similar to patients with any blunt abdominal trauma. A thorough report of the trauma should be obtained from the prehospital providers. The mechanism and site of impact are of utmost importance.

After securing the patient's airway, auscultating for breath sounds, and assessing hemodynamics, a physical exam should be conducted. Wounds should be noted, and the abdomen felt for signs of peritonitis. Peritonitis is an indication for an exploratory laparotomy. If the patient's abdomen is tender but not peritonitic, then adjunctive studies should be performed if the patient's hemodynamics allow. Abdominal ultrasound is useful to find free fluid but is not very sensitive in discovering hollow viscus injury. Therefore, a diagnostic peritoneal lavage (DPL) or CT scan is needed to make a diagnosis. A DLP is a sensitive test in identifying intra-abdominal injury but is not used often due to the adoption of the FAST exam. If on DPL, succus entericus, stool, vegetable, or other food matter is found, this is a sign of hollow viscus injury. If not, then checking alkaline phosphatase levels in the DPL fluid may be beneficial. An alkaline phosphatase level of greater than 10 international units was found to have a specificity of 99.8% and sensitivity of 94.7% for hollow viscus injury.[2] CT scan is used very often in patients with blunt trauma who are hemodynamically stable, due to its speed of acquisition at most institutions and the wealth of information that can be obtained about intra-abdominal injuries.

Findings such as bowel wall thickening, mesenteric stranding or hematoma, lack of bowel wall enhancement on a contrasted scan, pneumatosis, free intraperitoneal fluid, and pneumoperitoneum are all signs of possible hollow viscus injury. If oral or rectal contrast is given, and if there is contrast extravasation, this is also a sign of likely bowel injury.

If a patient has a suspected injury, they should be taken to the operating room. A midline laparotomy will allow greatest access to the intra-abdominal viscera. The entire gastrointestinal tract from the gastroesophageal junction to the rectum should be visualized and injuries identified. Blunt stomach injury is graded on am I to IV scale. Grade I stomach injuries are hematomas, contusions, or a partial thickness laceration. Grade II stomach injuries are lacerations <2 cm at the gastroesophageal (GE) junction or pylorus, <5 cm in the proximal one-third of the stomach, or <10 cm in the distal two-thirds of the stomach. Grade III stomach injuries are lacerations >2 cm at the GE junction or pylorus, >5 cm in the proximal one-third of the stomach, or >10 cm in the distal two-thirds of the stomach. Grade IV stomach injuries are when there is significant devascularization or tissue loss.

Stomach injuries should be repaired primarily if possible after devitalized tissue is debrided. Typically, the repair should be performed in two layers, the first being an absorbable suture in a continuous running locking fashion. The second layer should be interrupted 3-0 silk sutures taking imbricating seromuscular bites. Grade III injuries involving the greater curvature can be managed using the gastrointestinal anastomotic linear stapler. Injury to the pylorus may necessitate pyloroplasty. Grade IV stomach injuries, with total loss or devascularization of greater than 2/3 of the stomach, may require major resection with either gastroduodenostomy (Billroth I) or gastrojejunostomy (Billroth II) anastomoses. Grade V injuries are rare and may require total gastrectomy followed by Roux-en-Y esophagojejunostomy.

Small bowel injuries should be repaired primarily if the damage involves less than 50% of the bowel wall circumference. The injury should be repaired in a transverse fashion provided this can be performed tension free. This is done to prevent structuring of the small bowel by the repair. Larger wounds may not be able to be repaired transversely and can be repaired lengthwise, but care must be taken to not narrow the lumen. Single- and two-layer repairs have been shown to have similar efficacy. A multi-institutional trial currently underway by the AAST, Stapled vs Handsewn: A Prospective Emergency Surgery Study (SHAPES) is aimed at assessing superiority of either method. If a two-layer repair is chosen, the outer layer should be a 3-0 silk interrupted imbricating suture. If resection is performed, then the mesenteric defect should be closed primarily to prevent internal hernia formation. If there is only an intramural hematoma, repair is done using seromuscular sutures, but one must be careful to again not narrow the lumen. It is important to close potential mesenteric defects to prevent the development of internal hernias.

Colon and rectal injuries can also occur with blunt trauma. The colon can be injured when there is the creation of a closed loop and rupture due to increased intraluminal pressure. It can be damaged by shear injury due to tearing at the junction of the mobile and immobile colon, and there can be mesenteric avulsion injuries due to deceleration mechanisms. This leads to de-vascularized segments and delayed rupture.

Patients who have evidence of colonic or rectal injury on physical exam or on CT scan should be taken to the operating room for repair or drainage procedures. For colon injuries the major decisions to make will be to either primarily repair the injury, perform a resection and anastomosis, or to divert the patient with a colostomy. There have been numerous retrospective works looking at the decision to primarily repair versus performing a diverting colostomy for colon trauma, and the majority of them concluded that direct repair is acceptable in virtually all situations.[1]

Although blunt injury to the rectum is extremely rare, blunt injury resulting in pelvic fractures can cause a rectal injury. Physical exam, when a rectal injury is suspected, should involve a digital rectal exam. Blood is a cause for concern and can mean there is a possible rectal injury. The patient should be taken to the operating room after diagnostic work up is completed, and rigid proctosigmoidoscopy should be performed. This will likely reveal only intraluminal blood but occasionally an injury can be identified.

Rectal injury is treated as a colonic injury, with direct repair in patients with intraperitoneal rectal injuries. Extraperitoneal rectal injury is uncommon in blunt trauma, but the mainstay of treatment historically was presacral drainage, rectal washout, and diverting colostomy. The rectal washout has fallen out of favor due to potential for making the injury worse or introducing rectal contamination into the abdomen. Presacral drainage has also been shown to not reduce the incidence of infectious complications from extraperitoneal injury. These drains also do not adequately function for anterior rectal injuries.[1] Additionally, the decision of whether or not to repair an extraperitoneal rectal injury has also changed to not recommending primary repair and instead only performing a diverting colostomy.

Genitourinary Tract

The genitourinary tract goes from the kidneys to the urethra. This consists of bilateral kidneys and ureters, the urinary bladder, and the urethra. The kidneys are situated in the retroperitoneum, inferior to the liver on the right and inferior to the spleen on the left. In blunt trauma the liver and spleen are most often affected when there is blunt kidney injury on the ipsilateral side. The blood supply to the kidney is from the renal artery which is a branch off the aorta. The renal artery provides a segmental blood supply to the kidney, which is why one can perform a partial nephrectomy. The renal artery divides into apical, superior, middle, and inferior branches. Occasionally there are accessory renal arteries that come off the aorta. The ureters have a more delicate blood supply. The superior part of the ureter gets its blood supply from the renal artery. The middle part of the ureter gets its blood supply from branches off the aorta and the lower ureter receives arterial blood flow from the common iliac artery. The arterial supply comes in medially and is very fragile, which is why dissection should not be performed on the ureter itself, but in the periureteral tissue planes.

Injuries to the kidney are graded on an organ injury scale developed by the AAST Grade I renal injuries include contusions that result in hematuria or a subcapsular hematoma. Grade II renal injuries include retroperitoneal perirenal hematomas and are less than 1 cm lacerations into the parenchyma. Grade III renal injuries are lacerations greater than 1 cm in depth but do not involve the collecting system. Grade IV renal injuries include extension into the collecting system or injury to the major vein or artery with contained hemorrhage. Grade V injuries are a shattered kidney or avulsion of the kidney off its hilum and devascularization.

The majority of injuries to the kidneys are secondary to a blunt trauma. The most common blunt mechanisms include direct blows to the back from assault, falls, and deceleration injuries. These patients frequently have hematuria on presentation. Other physical exam findings that may be a sign of renal injury include abdominal or costovertebral angle tenderness, flank pain, a flank mass, and flank ecchymosis.

Radiographic imaging of renal injuries is most often performed with CT scan and intravenous contrast. This is because in blunt trauma, there may be multiple injuries in the abdomen and a CT scan can give more information than isolated studies. Although CT scan has become a mainstay in the diagnostic algorithm for blunt trauma, being able to interpret findings on an intravenous pyelogram (IVP) is still important, as this study may be necessary either preoperatively or intraoperatively. Findings suggesting renal injury on IVP include ipsilateral transverse process fracture, loss of the psoas shadow, mass effect pushing soft tissues to the contralateral side, vertical displacement of the kidney, loss of renal cortex outline, extravasation of contrast, poor opacification of some areas of the kidney but not others, and opacification defects in the collecting system. Of note IVP may be normal in up to 20% of patients with renal injury.

Non-operative management of kidney injuries has become more commonplace in management after blunt trauma. Some advocate for non-operative management, regardless of injury grade, as long as the patient is hemodynamically stable. The most common indications for operative intervention include hemodynamic instability, hemorrhage requiring significant transfusion, pulsatile or expanding hematoma, and avulsion of the kidney off its vascular pedicle.

Operative management of kidney injuries falls into two broad categories, nephrectomy, and renal salvage procedures. A nephrectomy is performed when the patient is hemodynamically unstable and the source of hemorrhage is felt to be the injured kidney, or when there is such extensive damage to the kidney that reconstruction is unlikely to be successful. For a nephrectomy obtaining vascular control first is preferable. This can be achieved by incising the peritoneum to the left of the aorta, under the inferior mesenteric vein. Developing this plane will allow access to the renal vessels and the vena cava. Once vessel loops are placed around the vessels supplying the injured kidney, the colon and kidney can be mobilized and inspected. Another technique is to mobilize the colon and kidney first, understanding that there may be more blood loss, and dissecting the renal vessels at the hilum from the posterior aspect. Either way, vascular control is an important initial concern. Gerota's fascia overlying the kidney is incised and the kidney is delivered into the field. Careful inspection should occur and if it looks as though there is no hope for renal salvage, the artery and vein should be ligated separately and overseed if there is concern for bleeding. If there is possible renal salvage, the damaged tissue should be sharply debrided and bleeding vessels identified and ligated with a 3-0 absorbable monofilament suture. The collecting system, if injured, should be repaired in a similar fashion. Hemostasis can be obtained by packing the parenchymal wound with an absorbable hemostatic agent or with vascularized omentum and closing the capsule over. Renal salvage should be performed by those who have experience with this surgery, because when performed by those who are inexperienced, there is a much higher rate of conversion to nephrectomy.

Ureter injury occurs in less than 1% of blunt trauma. On CT scan, an excretory phase run should be performed to identify a ureter injury with signs of contrast extravasation. As mentioned earlier, blunt injury to the ureter is very rare and when it happens most surgeons opt for operative repair. Operative planning and repair depend on the level of the injury. For blunt trauma, there is typically not a large amount of tissue loss, but the edges should be debrided, and devitalized tissue should be removed. A double J stent should be placed, and the repair should be performed around this stent. If possible, a primary end to end spatulated repair should be performed using 5-0 absorbable monofilament suture in an interrupted or running fashion. Avulsion of the ureter proximally off the renal pelvis is best managed in the same manner described above. In distal injuries that occur below the level of the pelvic brim and the iliac vessels, ureteral reimplantation into the bladder is the treatment of choice. The importance of a tension free repair cannot be stressed enough, as such maneuvers such as the psoas hitch may be necessary. This requires extensive mobilization of the bladder by taking down its anterior and lateral peritoneal attachments. Occasionally the bladder needs to be opened anteriorly to allow its wall to be attached to the psoas muscle with 2-0 absorbable suture. Then the ureter is reimplanted into the bladder using a tunneled anastomosis over a double J stent. The bladder is then closed in two layers and a drain left in place. A Boari flap can be used to give more length and aid in anastomosing the ureter to the bladder. This requires creating a tongue of appropriate length and width so it can be rolled on itself, and a tube created to attach to the ureter. Care must be taken not to reduce the volume of the bladder too greatly using this technique. If there is extensive ureteral tissue loss from trauma, kidney auto-transplantation may be necessary, placing it into the pelvis and anastomosing the remnant ureter to the bladder directly. This also means the renal artery and vein must be anastomosed to the iliac vessels.

Bladder injuries in blunt trauma are usually due to compressive forces on a full bladder that causes rupture (Figure 8). This rupture typically occurs at the dome of the bladder and is associated with gross hematuria. Diagnostic imaging for bladder rupture used to be a stress cystogram, now a CT cystogram scan is used. Both are performed in a similar fashion where a standard volume of contrast medium, about 400 mL, is instilled into the bladder and various films are obtained, starting with a full bladder and then incremental films are taken as it washes out. Contrast can either stay in the bladder, extravasate into the peritoneal cavity, extravasate into the extraperitoneal space, or extravasate into both areas. Extraperitoneal bladder injuries are typically treated with foley catheter drainage for about 2 weeks. After 2 weeks, a cystogram is performed to check for persistence of contrast leak. If there is none, the catheter can be removed. If the contrast leak persists, another 1 to 2 weeks of non-operative therapy and drainage will continue. If there is persistent leak of contrast, then cystoscopy should be performed to look at the laceration and remove any foreign bodies, such as boney fragments. Then operative repair may be needed. Intraperitoneal bladder injuries will typically require operative repair. This includes laparotomy to explore the abdomen and then either a one or two layered repair. We prefer a running continuous 0-0 or 2-0 absorbable monofilament suture. The second layer is typically a row of interrupted imbricating seromuscular sutures of 3-0 silk. Again, a catheter should remain in place for about 2 weeks and, prior to removal, a contrast cystogram should be performed to check for a leak. Leaving a drain over the repair is a good idea when there is a large or extensive injury that was repaired.

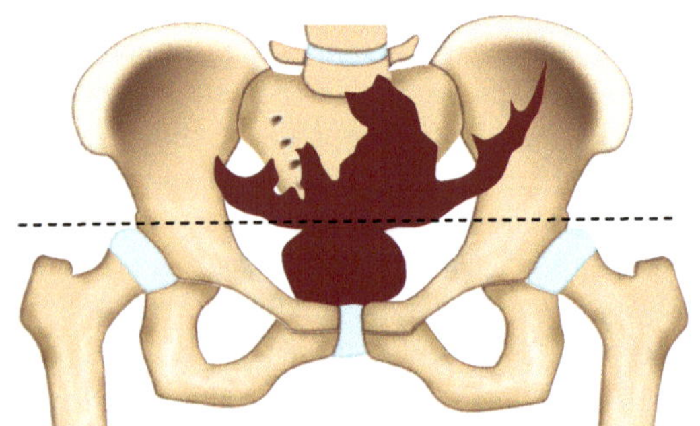
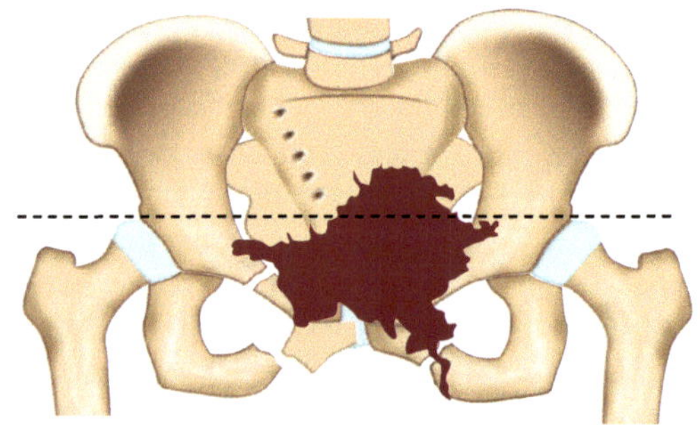

Figure 8: Intraperitoneal (left) and extraperitoneal (right) bladder trauma

SUMMARY

In this chapter we reviewed the pertinent principles of Newtonian physics as they relate to specific mechanisms of blunt trauma. We also reviewed the way to approach and work up a trauma patient after sustaining blunt injuries. Then the types of individual injuries and possible management options were discussed. This chapter serves as an overview to some of the most common problems facing the trauma team in evaluating and caring for patients after blunt trauma. It is important to emphasize the need for a systematic method for evaluation and triaging care of these patients, and it is also important to note that the information gathered from the scene by the prehospital providers is not just useful, but vital to patient care.

REFERENCES

1. Newton I. Philosophiae Naturalis Principia Mathematica. Motte A, trans. 1729. Reprint. New York: Prometheus Books, 1995.
2. Mackay M. Mechanisms of injury and biomechanics: vehicle design and crash performance. World J Surg. 1992;16:420.
3. Gongora E, Acosta JA, Wang DSY, et al. Analysis of motor vehicle ejection victims admitted to Level I trauma center. J Trauma. 2001;51:854.
4. Kanglois JA, Rutland-Brown W, Thomas KE. Traumatic brain injury in the United States: Emergency Department Visits, Hospitalizations, and Deaths. Centers for Disease Control and Prevention, National Center for Injury Prevention and Control. 2004.
5. Gennarelli TA, Champion HR, Copes WS, et al. Comparison of mortality, morbidity and severity of 59,713 head injured patients with 114,447 patients with extracranial injuries. J Trauma. 1994;37:962.
6. Kelly G. Appearances observed in the dissection of two individuals; death from cold and congestion of the brain. Trans Med Chir Sci Edinb. 1824;1: 84–169.
7. Lee RB, Bass SM, Morris JA Jr, et al. Three or more rib fractures as an indicator for transfer to a Level I trauma center: A population-based study. J Trauma. 1990;30:689.
8. Ziegler DW, Agrawal NN. The morbidity and mortality of rib fractures. J Trauma. 1994;37:975.
9. Tarlow MH, Hauser CJ. Prospective study of neutrophil chemokine responses in trauma patients at risk for pneumonia. Am J Resp Crit Care Med. 2005;171:753.
10. Parmley LF, Manion WC, Mattingly TW. Non penetrating traumatic injury of the heart. Circulation. 1958;18:371.
11. Biffl WL, Moore FA, Moore EE, et al. Cardiac enzymes are irrelevant in the patient with suspected myocardial contusion. Am J Surg. 1994;169:523.
12. Bertinchant JP, Polge A, Mohty D, et al. Evaluation of incidence, clinical significance, and prognostic value of circulating cardiac troponin I and T elevation in hemodynamically stable patients with suspected myocardial contusion after blunt chest trauma. J Trauma. 2000;48:924.
13. Pasquale M, Fabian TC. EAST Ad Hoc Committee on Practice Management Guideline Development. Practice management guidelines for trauma from the Eastern Association for the Surgery of Trauma. J Trauma. 1998;44:941.
14. Fitzharris M, Frankly M, Frampton R, et al. Thoracic aortic injury in motor vehicle crashes: the effect of impact direction, side of body struck, and seat belt use. J Trauma 2004;57:582–590.
15. Dischinger P, Cowley R, Shankar B. The incidence of ruptured aorta among vehicle fatalities. Proc Assoc Adv Automot Med Conf 1988;32:15.
16. Fabian T, Richardson J, Croce M, et al. Prospective study of blunt aortic injury: multicenter trial of the American Association for the Surgery of Trauma. J Trauma 1997;42(3):374–380.
17. Neschis DG, Scalea TM, Flinn WR, et al. Blunt aortic injury. N Engl J Med. 2008;359:1708-1716.
18. Fabian T, Davis K, Gavant M, et al. Prospective study of blunt aortic injury: helical CT is diagnostic and antihypertensive therapy reduces rupture. Ann Surg 1998;227:666–76.
19. Mattox KL. Fact or fiction about management of aortic transaction (editorial). Ann Thorac Surg. 1989;48:1-2.
20. Cook CC, Gleason TG. Great vessel and cardiac trauma. Surg Clin N Am. 2009;89:797–820.
21. Moore EE, Cogbill TH, Jurkovitch GJ, et al. Organ injury scaling-spleen, liver (1994 revision). J Trauma. 1995;38:323.
22. Croce MA, Fabian TC, Menke PG, et al. Non-operative management of blunt hepatic trauma is the treatment of choice for hemodynamically stable patients. Results of a prospective trial. Ann Surg. 1995;221:744.
23. Kozar RA, Moore FA, Cothren CC, et al. Hepatic-related morbidity associated with non-operative management of complex blunt hepatic injuries: AAST multicenter trial. Atlanta, Georgia: Sixty-Fourth Meeting of the American Association for the Surgery of Trauma;2005.
24. Dent D, Alsabrook G, Erickson BA, et al. Blunt splenic injuries: High management rate can be achieved with selective embolization. J Trauma. 2004;56:1063.

25. Schurr MJ, Fabian TC, Gavant M, et al. Management of blunt splenic trauma: Computed tomographic contrast blush predicts failure of non-operative management. J Trauma. 1995;39:507.
26. Anderson PA, Rivara FP, Maier RV, et al. The epidemiology of seatbelt associated injuries. J Trauma. 1991;31:60.
27. Watts D, Fakhry S, Scalea T, et al. Blunt hollow viscus injury (HVI) and small bowel injury (SBI): Prevalence, mortality, and morbidity results from a large multi-institutional study. J Trauma. 2001;51:1233.
28. Jaffin JH, Ochsner G, Cole FL, et al. Alkaline phosphatase levels in diagnostic peritoneal lavage fluid as a predictor of hollow visceral injury. J Trauma. 1993;34:829.
29. Murray JA, Demetriades D, Colson M, et al. Colonic resection in trauma: Colostomy versus anastomosis. J Trauma. 1999;46:250.
30. Navsaria PH, Shaw JM, Sellweger R, et al. Diagnostic laparoscopy and diverting sigmoid loop colostomy in the management of civilian extraperitoneal rectal gunshot injuries. BR J Surg. 2004;91:460.

49

CHAPTER

Penetrating Abdominal and Thoracic Trauma

Khanjan H. Nagarsheth, MD
Mayur Narayan, MD, MPH, MBA, FACS, FICS

INTRODUCTION

The study of penetrating trauma and its management has become increasingly more important over the last 25 years. In the 15–44-year-old age group, interpersonal violence and suicide were ranked as third and fourth in the world's leading causes of poor health and premature mortality. To keep this in perspective, war-related injuries and death ranked sixth.

Global estimates of small arms and weapons available fall in the realm of 875 million. Almost 75% or 650 million of these are in the hands of civilians. Although almost every nation has some form of legislation to minimize gun violence, this still accounts for about 525,000 deaths every year. This number is possibly a gross underestimation due to the lack of reliable global data. There are likely millions more people who survive these kinds of injuries that are left with permanent physical disabilities or mental health issues such as post-traumatic stress disorder.

Penetrating trauma and small weapons violence continue to be global problems. This problem extends beyond the morbidity and mortality associated with the trauma itself. Consider for example, that in the United States of America, this type of trauma relates to an economic burden of almost 100 billion dollars per year. This includes efforts to reduce crime and trauma associated with firearms and knives. This estimate also includes healthcare costs, rehabilitation costs, and loss of workforce. These are huge financial and social burdens for any nation to bear and become even more relevant in low to middle income countries.

With this background as to the toll that penetrating trauma and small weapon violence takes on population and economics it is now important to look at how these weapons cause the injuries they do and then look at site specific trauma.

BALLISTICS AND KINEMATICS

Ballistics is the study of energy transfer in firearms and projectiles. The field of ballistics owes a great debt to an unlikely scientist. Emile Theodor Kocher was a Swiss born surgeon who was Professor of Surgery at the University of Bern from 1872 to 1917. Kocher's name is synonymous with the subcostal incision, the maneuver to mobilize the duodenum and head of the pancreas, and hemostatic tissue clamps. He is also known for his work on thyroid physiology and meticulous anatomic dissection which was awarded the 1909 Nobel Prize in Medicine, and his contributions to the field of ballistics.

In 1875, Kocher published his examinations and experiments, which looked at the way bullets fired from a rifle cause tissue disruption. Before, the prevailing thought was that projectile melting and centrifugal forces were the primary forces responsible for tissue disruption. Kocher was able to show that instead tissue disruption from a fired projectile was more likely due to hydraulic pressures. He also felt that the melting of the projectile occurred when it came in contact with bone, and this resulted in transfer of kinetic energy into heat. Kocher proposed four main ways for kinetic energy from a projectile to be dissipated: generating heat, displacing the tissue radially outward from its path, directly crushing the tissue, and deforming the projectile.

The characteristics of projectiles as they enter tissue include penetration, fragmentation, temporary cavity, and permanent cavity. Penetration is the distance into the tissue from where the projectile enters. Fragmentation is based on the pattern the projectile makes as it breaks apart and disperses into the tissue. In Kocher's terms, this would be the energy of deformation of the projectile. Temporary cavity can be thought of as the pressure wave that passes out radially from the direct path of the projectile. This causes a certain amount of give in the tissue that is not directly related to the path of the projectile. The permanent cavity is due to the path of the projectile itself. This can be thought of as the tissue crushing energy transfer mentioned above.

The concepts of the temporary and permanent cavities are important in managing penetrating injuries from projectiles. As the projectile's velocity increases, the temporary cavity size will increase as well. Extension of this allows us to understand why the largest area of temporary cavity will be found on the tissue surface. The surface is where the projectile will have its maximum velocity, and, hence, maximum kinetic energy prior to both being decreased as tissue disruption occurs. The permanent cavity is caused by direct transfer of energy in the form of heat and tissue crushing, and this leaves a very tangible tract in the tissue. The projectile to tissue interface is affected by properties of the bullet itself. These properties include its deformability, ability to tumble through space and tissue, its ability to fragment, and its yaw. The deformability of the projectile causes an increase in surface area in contact with tissue thus creating a greater permanent cavity. The tumbling through tissue is around a fixed point of the projectile's center of mass, otherwise known as its barycenter. In thinking about the barycenter of a projectile it is important to accept that this is a fixed point but will not necessarily correspond to the geometric center given the conical shape of most modern bullets. This tumbling effectively increases the size of the permanent cavity. Fragmentation is when a projectile breaks up into pieces when it enters the tissue. This effectively increases its surface area and contact area with the tissue leading to a larger permanent cavity. The yaw of a bullet is its movement away from 0° on the y-axis. The projectile will increase the permanent cavity, but it has been noted that this is not as large a contribution as was one believed.

The importance of these concepts is involved in wound debridement. The permanent cavity should be cleared, and debridement conducted of all devitalized material, but the temporary cavity should not be violated as the tissue will typically not have significant damage.

APPROACH TO PATIENTS WITH PENETRATING INJURY

The basic principles of assessing and securing the airway, listening for breath sounds, and addressing hemodynamic instability remain paramount and primary. This constitutes the primary survey for any trauma patient. After addressing your primary and secondary surveys, if there is no clear indication for immediate operative intervention, adjunctive studies can be obtained to help in garnering more information and determining if an operation will be needed. It is important to remember the five major body cavities that can contain massive hemorrhage. These are the chest, the abdomen/pelvis, the retroperitoneum, the long bones, and externally. This simple rule can help practitioners determine what imaging modalities to obtain as well as guide surgical decision making. Local wound exploration has been shown to be beneficial in anterior abdominal stab wounds in allowing for earlier discharge from the emergency department (ED) without the need for laparotomy, but the authors did advocate for computed tomography (CT) scan or other abdominal imaging in cases where the patient is obese, or the wound is long and tangential. That being said, local wound exploration should not occur with suspected vascular injuries or indications for immediate operative exploration. In the hemodynamically non-labile patient, radiographic imaging may be helpful in determining missile trajectory. Exterior entry wounds should be marked with a radiopaque marker that can help delineate point of entry on either CXR or CT. If the patient is alert and awake, obtaining a proper history of injury is necessary as they may have suffered other blunt trauma in addition to the penetrating wound. A complete medical and surgical history can also prove very valuable. The basic operative plan will remain the same for any penetrating trauma case. This includes controlling arterial hemorrhage, packing of venous hemorrhage followed by definitive repair versus ligation, control of gross contamination, thorough exploration and assessment of wounds and damage control, and resuscitation of the patient.

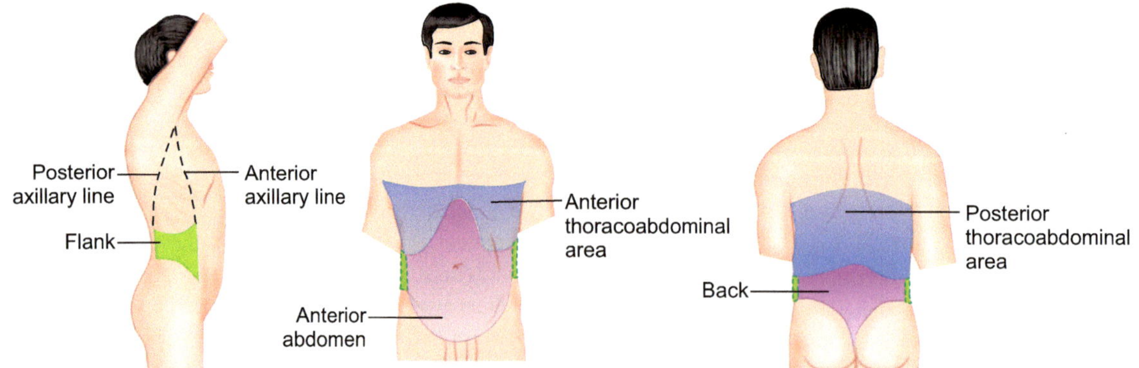

Figure 1: Different regions have an increased risk for specific injuries. Injury to the posterior abdomen and flank often results in retroperitoneal and solid organ injuries, injury to the thoracoabdominal region often results in diaphragm and anterior abdomen injuries, and this site has the highest risk for hollow viscus injuries.

SITE SPECIFIC INJURY

Neck

Classically, the neck is anatomically divided into three zones. Zone I is from the thoracic outlet to the level of the cricothyroid membrane. Zone II is from the cricothyroid membrane to the angle of the mandible. Zone III extends from the angle of the mandible to the base of the skull. As zones I and III are difficult to access surgically, their management is very different that a Zone II injury, where the primary diagnostic and therapeutic options involve surgery (Figure 2).

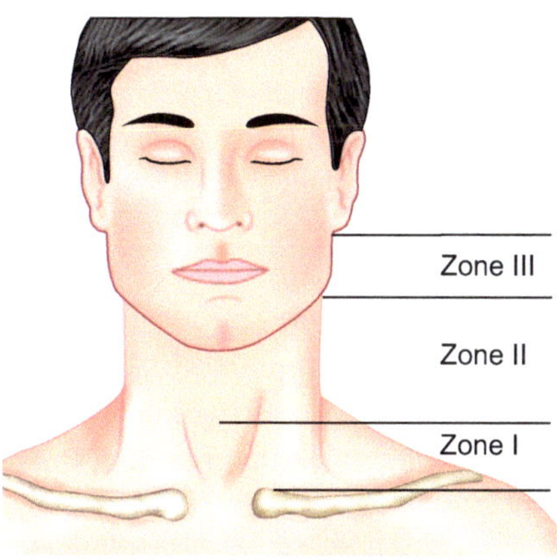

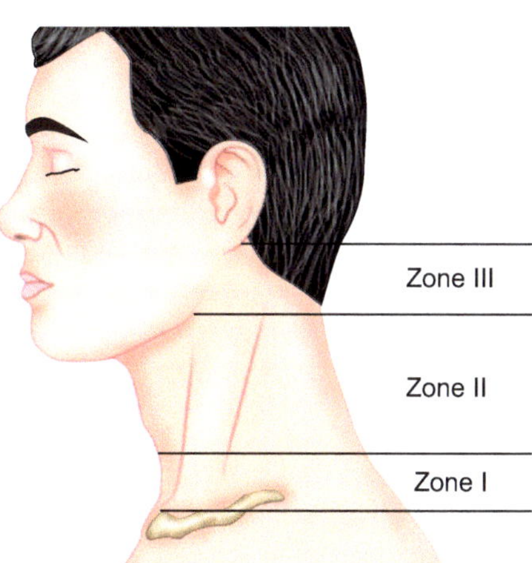

Figure 2: Zones of the neck

Hard and Soft Signs

After the airway is secured and primary survey is completed, the wound can be examined, and diagnostic and therapeutic plans can be made. When examining the wound, it is important to look for findings suggesting vascular or aero-digestive injury. These findings are divided by convention into hard signs and soft signs. Hard signs will require immediate operative exploration and control whereas soft signs may afford the opportunity to do further workup before operative intervention is required. Hard signs include airway compromise, pulsatile bleeding or hematoma, significant subcutaneous emphysema, or signs of shock. Soft signs include hemoptysis, changes in phonation and voice, complaints of dysphagia, and widened mediastinum on chest x-ray.

Clinical Practice Guidelines

The management of penetrating neck injuries has been long debated in the literature. Historically prior to and including World War I, these injuries were observed and had a very high mortality rate. In 1956, Fogelman and Stewart found a significantly decreased mortality when a mandatory exploration practice was implemented in penetrating neck injuries. This recommendation came from the observation that asymptomatic victims still harbored significant injuries. Over the next 50 years there have been a number of papers published advocating both for mandatory exploration of Zone II injuries and for selective exploration. In 2008 the Eastern Association for the Surgery of Trauma (EAST) developed clinical practice guidelines for Zone II penetrating neck injuries. These guidelines are based on extensive review of the available literature. The level I recommendation for exploration of Zone II penetrating neck injuries was for selective exploration to minimize unnecessary operations. The level II recommendation was for making CT angiography the diagnostic test of choice in determining vascular injury in these patients.

This clinical practice guideline also made level II recommendations for vascular and esophageal injuries. The group felt that CT angiography or arterial duplex ultrasound could effectively rule out a Zone II arterial injury. It was also felt that either contrast esophagography or esophagoscopy could be used to rule out esophageal injury that would require operative exploration and repair. The group did note that this work up should be performed within the first 24 hours as delay increases morbidity from a missed esophageal injury.[13] A newer "No Zone" approach is an evidence-based method eliminating neck zone differentiation during triage and management. Shiroff et al. concluded that a comprehensive physical exam with a CTA is enough to effectively triage in both identifying or excluding vascular and aerodigestive injury after penetrating neck trauma.[41] They also state that traditional zone-based algorithms can potentially lead to an increased reliance on diagnostic modalities and subsequently could lead to a higher incidence of non-therapeutic neck exploration.[41]

Operative Exposure

Operative exposure to Zone I injuries can be obtained by way of a supraclavicular incision with possible resection of the clavicular head or a 'trapdoor' type incision that uses a supraclavicular incision with a median sternotomy and an anterolateral chest wall incision. The pitfall of this approach is that it is time consuming and depending on the injuries the patient may not have that time to lose. Zone III injuries can be operatively approached by an extension of the anterior sternocleidomastoid incision towards the base of the skull and if necessary, disarticulation or resection of the mandible, resection of the styloid process, or a limited craniotomy. Surgical approaches to Zone II injuries are more straightforward and exposure can be obtained by way of a midline vertical incision, an anterior sternocleidomastoid incision, or a transverse collar incision. All of these incisions will allow access to the vital structures within the neck.

Laryngeal Trauma

In penetrating Zone II injuries, there is a 10% risk of the patient having sustained an esophageal or airway injury, meaning securing the airway is again of utmost importance. The airway of choice is an endotracheal intubation with direct laryngoscopy. If this is unsuccessful then a surgeon should be present to perform an emergent cricothyroidotomy for surgical airway control. The only situation where an emergency tracheostomy should be attempted should be if there is suspected injury to the larynx or junction of the larynx and trachea.

Laryngeal injuries are divided anatomically into supraglottic, glottic, and subglottic. Supraglottic injuries are usually associated with a fractured thyroid cartilage. Glottic injuries also can include a fractured thyroid cartilage, and the thyroarytenoid muscles are torn with tears extending to the true vocal cords. Subglottic injuries can lead to rapid respiratory compromise and require an emergency surgical procedure. Typically, however, if the cricoid cartilage is intact, this does not happen.

Thorax

Penetrating injuries to the thorax have been recorded as early as 3000 BC. There is a story of penetrating trauma to the sternum in the Edwin Smith Surgical Papyrus which is widely regarded as being the oldest known surgical text for trauma. Up until World War II the mortality from a penetrating thoracic injury remained in the realm of about 25 to 30%. It was only in World War II that guidelines were established for the treatment of penetrating thoracic injuries. The mortality fell to just over 5%. Around the time of the Vietnam War, Ashbaugh and his colleagues described a form of respiratory failure that was severe and refractory to current therapies. They described a series of patients who had acute onset of tachypnea, hypoxemia, pan-lobar infiltration on chest X-ray, and loss of lung compliance. They found that the use of positive end-expiratory pressure (PEEP) was beneficial in these patients. Our ability to help these patients and our ability to care for patients with thoracic trauma in general has improved with our better understanding of chest wall physiology and with advancements in supportive adjuncts like mechanical ventilation.

The following section will give an overview on management of chest wall trauma, injury to the heart and great vessels, tracheal and airway injuries, and pulmonary injuries

Chest Wall

The anatomy of the thorax is that of a rigid and non-collapsible frame that protects the thoracic organs and supports the upper part of the axial skeleton. There are 12 paired ribs, sternum, 2 clavicles, 12 thoracic vertebrae and multiple cartilages. The first 7 ribs are known as true ribs as they articulate with the sternum and the lower 5 ribs are known as false ribs as they do not directly connect to the sternum. Ribs 11 and 12 are known as floating ribs and only articulate with the thoracic vertebrae.

The sternum is a flat bone that ranges from 15 to 20 cm in length. This structure is divided into three portions, the manubrium superiorly, the body, and the xiphoid inferiorly. The clavicles articulate with the manubrium and the manubrium meets the body of the sternum at the angle of Louis, which is also the anterior part of the junction of the second rib.

The musculature of the thorax involves two groups of muscles, the primary and secondary muscles of respiration. The primary muscles of respiration are diaphragm and intercostal muscles. The intercostals are found in the intercostal spaces and are of three types. The outermost is the external intercostals, the next layer is the internal intercostals, and the innermost are known as the transverse intercostal muscles. The secondary muscles of respiration are the sternocleidomastoid, the serratus posterior, and the levatores costarum. A third group of muscles found on the thorax are those that help attach the upper extremities to the body. These include the pectoralis major and minor muscles, the trapezius, latissimus dorsi, serratus anterior, and the major and minor rhomboids.

About 20% of chest wall trauma is secondary to penetrating causes, either gunshot wounds or stabbings. Stab wounds in general offer a more favorable outcome than gunshot wounds, as there is typically a well delineated tract and less chance of multiple organ injury. Gun shots are again divided into low velocity handguns and high velocity rifles. The higher velocity injuries impart a greater kinetic energy and have greater tissue destruction.

Sucking Chest Wound

Penetrating thoracic injuries can result in what is known as a sucking chest wound. These wounds occur when there is disruption of the chest wall that causes equilibration between atmospheric and pleural pressure. This can present as an emergency as without negative intrathoracic pressure, normal respiration is not possible and respiratory failure can rapidly occur. Classical teaching describes using a three-sided dressing so that there is not complete occlusion and formation of a tension pneumothorax. This type of dressing can act as a one-way valve, allowing air to escape but not enter. Definitive care should include placement of a tube thoracostomy through a separate clean site, debridement, and closure of the chest defect. A bridge to the operative repair can be endotracheal intubation and positive pressure mechanical ventilation. This removes the need for negative intrathoracic pressure for spontaneous respiration.

Another issue that can arise with chest wall disruption from penetrating trauma includes massive bleeding that may require operative intervention in the form of a thoracotomy to control. This bleeding can be secondary to muscular bleeding or from a lacerated intercostal artery, which typically runs underneath the ribs. Lung hernias are a feared complication of chest wall injury, but this is not common in the acute setting. These are typically seen chronically and again from failure of healing or closing a chest wall defect. These wounds should be closed primarily, if possible, but use of a prosthetic material like mesh or tissue transfer like a muscle flap may be needed.

Pneumothorax and Hemothorax

Pneumothorax is the presence of air within the pleural space. This is therefore found extra-pulmonic but intra-thoracic. This is a known complication in penetrating trauma as there is often pleural violation and laceration to the pulmonary parenchyma. Pneumothoraces can be subdivided into three categories: simple, open, and tension. A simple pneumothorax is more likely to occur in blunt trauma when there is a closed chest wall and lung injury. An open pneumothorax is also known as a sucking chest wound and this is when there is disruption in the chest wall allowing air to enter the pleural space from the atmosphere. The concern with this wound is equilibration of intrapleural and atmospheric pressure, which is incompatible with effective spontaneous respiration. Tension pneumothorax occurs when there is a buildup of air in the pleural space without an outlet for its release. This can be seen in blunt injury where the lung injury that leads to a pneumothorax acts as a ball-valve and allows only escape of air from the airways into the pleural space. In penetrating trauma, this is most often seen when an occlusive dressing is placed over a sucking chest wound. This maneuver converts an open pneumothorax into a tension pneumothorax. Tension pneumothorax can lead to cardiac arrest because the increased intrathoracic pressure leads to not only decrease in preload coming back to the heart but also in a tamponade-like effect on the heart, compressing on the lower pressure right sided system.

Classically, it is taught that pneumothorax can be suspected based on clinical findings of breathlessness to auscultation on the affected side. In reality, when evaluating a patient in a busy and loud emergency department or trauma resuscitation bay, this may not always be possible. A simple chest radiograph may allow for rapid and definite diagnosis of pneumothorax. There is a lot of interest in the use of rapid and focused thoracic ultrasound to identify pneumothorax in the trauma patient. A recent study looking at the accuracy of pneumothorax detection by chest X-ray compared to ultrasound and CT scan found that chest X-ray was sensitive in 32% of cases whereas ultrasound was sensitive for detection of pneumothorax in 82% of patients. CT scan was considered the gold standard and was 100% sensitive.

A hemothorax is the presence of blood in the pleural space. In penetrating trauma, the blood can come from a chest wall source, a cardiac or great vessel injury, and intercostal artery laceration, or a primary lung laceration. Also, in the context of thoracoabdominal penetrating wounds, it is important to consider an intra-abdominal source of bleeding coming up through the diaphragm. Hemothorax can be suspected clinically based on diminished breath sounds, location of penetrating trauma, and hemodynamics of the patient. Chest radiograph or thoracic ultrasound can help to make a definitive diagnosis in these patients and would be the next step in the diagnostic and treatment algorithm. Typically, a hemothorax becomes evident on chest X-ray when there is 200 to 300 mL of blood in the chest. Hemothorax is defined as massive when there is greater than one liter in the pleural space or associated with signs of shock. Chest CT scan has been shown to be beneficial in determining tract of wound and injury pattern in penetrating injury, but the patient should only be transported to CT scan once it is established that they are stable in terms of airway and hemodynamics.

In the field, treatment for pneumothorax is usually reserved for suspected tension or an open pneumothorax. These treatments are typically needle decompression in the second intercostal space in the midclavicular line or three-sided dressing, respectively. Treatment in the hospital setting of symptomatic pneumothoraxes, large pneumothorax or hemothorax should be with tube thoracostomy drainage. This is placed typically in the fourth or fifth intercostal space and directed posteriorly and to the apex.

Hemothorax should be evacuated when it is clinically detected. As mentioned above, the majority of hemothorax can be evacuated with placement of a tube thoracostomy, very rarely will a thoracotomy be needed. Typically, if there is greater than 1500 mL of blood evacuated from the chest or ongoing bleeding from the chest, then a thoracotomy would be indicated for evaluation and hemorrhage control. If early (within 5 days) in the course of a patient's hospitalization, it is noted that there is a clot of retained hemothorax, it is beneficial to operatively remove the clot via a video assisted thoracoscopic surgery (VATS). This enables removal of the clot and hemothorax, evaluation of the chest wall and lung, as well as avoids the morbidity associated with a full thoracotomy. Again, the goal of this procedure is to evacuate the clot, stop the bleeding, and allow the lung to fully expand.

The concern with retained hemothorax and clot in a trauma patient is that the patient undergoes a systemic inflammatory response which can overwhelm the body's ability to absorb the hemothorax. The blood and chest wall injury create a local inflammatory state in the pleural space. This inflammatory reaction leads to an influx of neutrophils but also results in decreased phagocytic activity. This is a rich medium that can promote infection and bacterial growth.

Tracheal Injury

Penetrating injury to the trachea is mainly in the cervical trachea. As in any patient presenting to the trauma center, it is important to make certain that a secure airway is present or to obtain one. Penetrating neck injuries have a 3 to 6% incidence of tracheal injuries. Less than 1% of penetrating thoracic injury will include a tracheal injury. Of all penetrating chest trauma, only 1 to 2% will actually have tracheal or bronchial injury.

Penetrating tracheal injury will most often be caused by a knife stab wound, gunshot wound, impaling injuries, and slash injuries. Most knife stab wounds and bladed injuries will result in a linear laceration or perforation. Again, most often this is to the cervical trachea. Although gunshot wounds are more common in the cervical trachea, it is not uncommon to find intrathoracic injury to the trachea or mainstem bronchus from this mechanism.

Penetrating tracheal injuries are associated with various other injuries (Figure 3). Based on the literature, penetrating cervical tracheal injuries have been associated with esophageal injury in 28% of cases, hemopneumothorax in 24%, major vascular injury in 13%, recurrent laryngeal nerve injury in 8%, and spinal cord injury in 3%. This varies slightly from penetrating injuries to the intrathoracic trachea. These injuries are associated with esophageal injury in 11%, hemopneumothorax in 32%, major vascular injury in 18%, cardiac injury in 5%, spinal cord injury in 7%, and abdominal injury in 18% of cases.

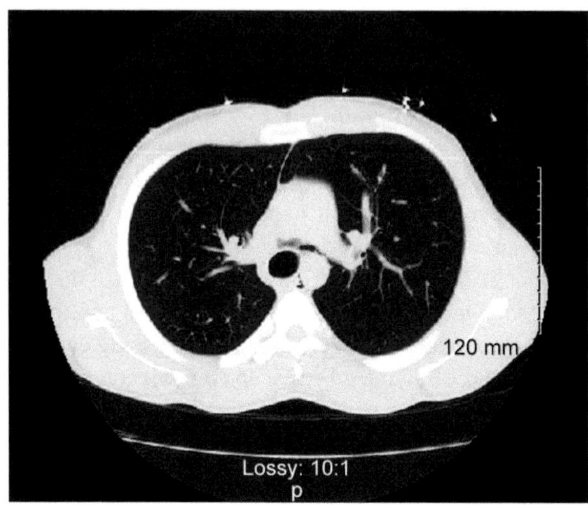

Figure 3: Pneumomediastinum from tracheal injury

As stated, early airway control is paramount. If there is significant concern of suspicion for a tracheal injury, blind intubation may not be preferable, especially if there is access to fiberoptic bronchoscopy. This affords the clinician the ability to directly visualize the airway as an endotracheal tube is passed over the end of the bronchoscope. Also, this maneuver allows for securing the airway without having to extend the neck in someone with a neck injury. If endotracheal intubation is not possible, the next emergency airway of choice is a surgical cricothyroidotomy. This is performed by finding the thyroid cartilage and making a vertical incision in the midline between the thyroid and cricoid cartilages. Next the cricothyroid membrane is identified and incised transversely. A cricothyroidostomy tube is placed through the incision and the patient is ventilated. This maneuver will allow one to bridge the patient to the operating room where a definitive procedure to secure the airway should be performed. If the patient has a cervical tracheal injury with air emanating from the wound, it is possible to directly intubate the patient through the wound to secure an airway until definitive airway management can be obtained.

If the patient is stable and there is no obvious cervical tracheal injury but still suspicion for an airway injury, then CT scan can provide a tremendous amount of data and help to locate the injury and identify extent of the injury. If the patient is not stable and there is concern for a distal airway injury, either intrathoracic trachea, carina, or mainstem bronchus, then fiber optic contralateral mainstem intubation is preferred over a double lumen endotracheal tube. The double lumen tubes are wider in diameter and more rigid and can make the injury worse.

Management of these injuries depends on extent of injury, presence of air leak, and amount of tissue loss. If there is injury to less than one third the circumference of the airway, no air leak, and minimal tissue loss, the patient may be a candidate for non-operative management. Surgical exposure is best achieved for the proximal half of the trachea by creating a cervical collar incision or a vertical midline incision. If access to the proximal intrathoracic trachea is needed then a partial sternotomy, splitting the manubrium to the second intercostal space will allow for better visualization. If the injury is in the distal third of the trachea, carina, right mainstem bronchus, or proximal left mainstem bronchus, a right sided posterolateral thoracotomy would be the approach of choice. If the injury is to the left mainstem bronchus, a left posterolateral thoracotomy should be used to gain access to this area.

Linear lacerations in the airway with a knife or blade can be repaired primarily as long as the edges are viable. This is typically performed with a 4-0 absorbable suture, either monofilament or braided. If there is devitalized tissue as will occur with a gunshot wound, this should be debrided to viable tissue and if necessary, a circumferential resection of the affected rings followed by a primary end to end anastomosis should be performed. Dissection should be performed only in the area of injury, as the blood supply to the trachea and bronchus is segmental and extensive dissection runs the risk of devascularizing the trachea. It is important to have a well vascularized and tension free repair. Injuries to the carina should be primarily repaired and resection avoided if possible. Some maneuvers that will give more length on the trachea include neck flexion, suprahyoid laryngeal release, and division of the pericardium from the inferior part of the hilum which will mobilize the distal airway.

Lung Injury

The pattern of injury to the lung after penetrating trauma is typically lung laceration and hemopneumothorax. In most cases a tube thoracostomy is sufficient to evacuate air and blood and the re-inflation of the lung will result in bleeding to stop. Thoracotomy and partial pneumonectomy are not typically needed, although a Western Trauma Association Multicenter study found that after tube thoracostomy was placed for penetrating injury, 40% of patients still required thoracotomy and some kind of partial pneumonectomy. This was a surprisingly large percentage of patients requiring partial pneumonectomy and the authors attributed this to possibly increase in high velocity weapon use or with the advances in trauma care, more badly injured patients were making it to the Level I centers in the study. It could be that the studies of the past that quoted rates as low as 15-20% of patients needing partial pneumonectomy were not seeing these badly injured patients because they were dying in the field. Another explanation could be that Level II and III trauma centers are now seeing a greater acuity of patients and this could be how some of the patients that could be managed with chest tube drainage and observation are being selected away from the Level I center. In this same study they did note that the majority of patients with lung injury who needed a thoracotomy could be managed with pulmonary tractotomy or stapled non-anatomic resections.

Stapled pulmonary tractotomy is a useful operative tool in hemorrhage control from lung injury (Figure 4). The tract of the knife or bullet is opened by placing an automatic stapling device into it and firing it. This can be repeated down the length of the tract. This will create hemostasis and close air leaks along the tract and allow visualization and identification of larger bleeding vessels that can then be suture ligated. It is important to note that merely closing the entry and exit sites in the lung tissue can lead to intraparenchymal hemorrhage and collection of blood. If this communicates with the airway, then can lead to difficulty with gas exchange. Therefore, it is not recommended to just close and oversew the wounds; rather it is better to either explore the tract safely or to perform a resection.

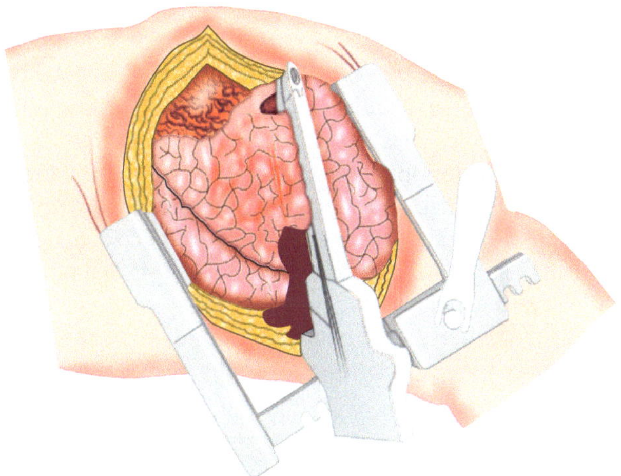

Figure 4: Tractotomy

When performing lung resections for trauma, it is important to try to preserve as much lung tissue as possible and only resect what is absolutely necessary. Lung resections fall into one of three broad categories: non-anatomic lung or wedge resections, anatomic resections or lobectomies, and complete pneumonectomies. Non-anatomic resections should minimize the lung tissue resected, and this should be performed for significant air leaks, hemorrhage control, or for serious blast injury. It has been shown in the literature that patients who require lobectomies are typically those who have sustained a high velocity gunshot wound, close range shotgun blast, hilar injury, or main bronchus injury. The patients that have a bronchial injury tend to have better outcomes than those who had a major vascular injury.

The mortality from a pneumonectomy for penetrating trauma has been shown to be anywhere from 50 to 100%.

Again, when this is performed for hemorrhage control, patients have a worse outcome. The prevailing theory as to why there is such a high mortality is that the sudden increase in pulmonary vascular resistance and decrease in vital capacity led to a sudden onset of congestive heart failure and respiratory failure that the patient may not be able to recover from. Additionally, it is believed that these procedures are done after significant blood loss and when the patient is in shock, again leading to a poor outcome. Options in this situation include placing a vascular clamp across the hilum or performing a hilum twist. The pulmonary hilum twist is described as division of the inferior pulmonary ligament and then anteriorly rotating the lower lobe over the upper lobe. This has successfully been used in a damage control setting where it physiologically acts as a pneumonectomy, and in a patient in severe shock this is expeditious and can allow time to resuscitate the patient and then bring them back to the operating room for a definitive resection.

Cardiac and Great Vessel Injury

Penetrating cardiac injury is a rare occurrence and most of these injuries are likely to be seen at large urban centers. The initial presentation of a patient with penetrating cardiac injury is highly variable. The patient may present normotensive and alert, in cardiac arrest, or anywhere in between. Patients may develop muffled heart tones, jugular venous distension, and hypotension, otherwise known as Beck's Triad, a sign of pericardial tamponade. The classical teaching is that patients with pericardial tamponade will have the components of Beck's Triad, but in the literature this constellation of signs is seen in about 10% of cases of cardiac injury.

Tamponade occurs because the intrapericardial pressure builds and this causes compression of the low-pressure right atrium and ventricle. Therefore, the right heart's ability to allow the systemic blood to return is impaired, and this results in the left heart not having the preload needed to effectively support the body's cardiac output needs. The pericardium is a fibrous layer that encases the heart. This material does not have the compliance needed to allow it to stretch acutely after injury to the heart. It has been noted, however, that it can stretch over an extended period of time. This is why patients who have long standing congestive heart failure or a slow leak from the ventricle from a misplaced pacer wire are able to accommodate almost a liter of fluid or blood into the pericardial sac without the hemodynamic changes associated with tamponade. There has been work to show that tamponade may have a beneficial effect in patients who have had a penetrating cardiac injury. The results of one study found that out of 100 patients with penetrating cardiac injury, 77 had tamponade on arrival to the emergency department. Of these, 31% were found to survive. They also found that patients with right heart injuries had a 79% survival rate, whereas patients with left heart injuries had only a 28% survival rate. This is likely secondary to the low-pressure right heart system.

The procedure of choice to relieve pericardial tamponade is a subxiphoid or transdiaphragmatic pericardial window. This has been shown in the literature over the last 35 years to be a safe and effective method of relieving tamponade and has largely replaced percutaneous pericardiocentesis as both a diagnostic and therapeutic tool.

Another diagnostic modality that has come to the forefront in trauma care has been bedside sonography. The use of this technique has been validated for penetrating cardiac injury in a multicenter study which looked at 209 patients and found ultrasound to be 100% sensitive and 97.3% specific for detection of pericardial fluid.

Once a cardiac injury has been diagnosed and a repair is warranted, the patient should be taken to the operating room and their chest and abdomen prepped for surgery. If the patient is in extremis in the resuscitation bays, then a left sided anterolateral thoracotomy is appropriate and can be extended across the sternum and bilateral, anterolateral, or 'clamshell' thoracotomy can be used to gain better visualization of the heart. The most versatile incision for cardiac repair is a median sternotomy, though this is best performed in the operating room.

Since the atrium has a thin wall, repair of a laceration or penetrating injury can be achieved by placing a Satinsky partial occlusion vascular clamp along the area of injury. This will control hemorrhage and allow cardiac repair. The cardiorrhaphy should be performed with a 2-0 permanent monofilament suture. Due to the fragile nature of the walls, a careful and meticulous repair is needed to prevent further damage. Ventricular injuries tend to bleed more and require digital occlusion while the repair is being performed. Due to the thick wall and dense myocardium of the ventricle, this is an area where pledgets are useful to reinforce the repair. Again, a 2-0 permanent monofilament suture should be used, and the repair should be performed using interrupted horizontal mattress sutures which are tied down against the pledgets. In patients who have had a penetrating cardiac injury with injury to a coronary artery, it is important to avoid further injury to the coronary arteries during the cardiorrhaphy. The sutures should be placed under the coronary artery, not over it. If the proximal portion of a coronary artery is injured this may require a bypass operation to revascularize the myocardium; if it is very distal, it can often be ligated.

Greater than 90% of thoracic great vessel injuries are secondary to penetrating injury by gunshot wounds, stab wounds, and sometimes shrapnel. Patients who have thoracic aortic injury, either blunt or penetrating, can be placed into one of three categories. They are dead at the scene of the injury, they are unstable during transport to the emergency department, or they are stable. The importance of this classification is that it points towards mortality and reason for death. In the first group, mortality is 100%, and the cause of death is going to be hemorrhage. The second group has greater than 96% mortality, and they die of multisystem trauma and exsanguination from multiple injuries. The third group has anywhere from 5 to 30% mortality, which is most often secondary to associated central nervous system injury.

On arrival to the emergency department or trauma resuscitation bay, patients with a suspected penetrating great vessel injury should have an airway secured, breathing confirmed, and hemodynamics assessed. A supine anteroposterior chest X-ray and markings of all penetrating wounds with a radiopaque marker are helpful. Penetrating wound findings on X-ray that are concerning for a great vessel injury include large hemothorax, foreign bodies near where the great vessels are, missing missile--which may indicate penetration into another body cavity, embolism, and unidentifiable trajectory. CT scan has been used to gather more information about missile trajectory and possible vascular injury. Only stable patients should be transported to CT scan; if they are unstable, urgent operation may be needed. For penetrating trauma and suspected great vessel injury, catheter directed angiography should be performed to identify lesions as well as possibly provide intervention and hemorrhage control. Localization of injury is important in planning operative repair if necessary. Patients who arrive stable with a suspected trans-mediastinal gunshot wound or knife stab wounds should go to CT scan to obtain more information about the tract of the missile and possible great vessel injuries. In patients that need immediate operative intervention, catheter directed angiography and echocardiography can help guide which incision will be needed.

Aortic injuries are divided into ascending aorta, transverse aortic arch, and descending thoracic aorta. Penetrating ascending aortic injuries are uncommon and have a 50% survival rate in patients that arrive at the emergency department with stable hemodynamics. Many of these injuries can be approached with a median sternotomy and repaired primarily. Transverse arch injuries have similar survival rates as ascending aortic injuries in patients that arrive in stable condition. Again, a median sternotomy with possible neck extension should be used to gain access and primary repair should be performed if possible. A descending thoracic aortic injury is best approached with a posterolateral fourth interspace thoracotomy. This will typically give enough visualization for repair. Primary repair for simple lacerations is preferred if possible but for extensive injuries, the current gold standard repair is the clamp and sew technique for direct reconstruction. This aorta proximal to the left subclavian artery, the distal aorta and the left subclavian are all dissected free and encircled with umbilical tapes. Then after alerting anesthesia, these areas are clamped, and the injured segment can be removed and replaced with an appropriately sized Dacron graft. This graft is sewn in using a 2-0 polypropylene suture in an end-to-end fashion. Paraplegia is a possible complication for this operation. This has been associated with length of clamp time, perioperative hypotension, and ligation of multiple intercostal arteries. The incidence of paraplegia following aortic replacement surgery is about 10%. Though thoracic aortic stent grafts are becoming more prevalent and are an attractive option, they are not considered the standard of care yet. There is still no prospective, randomized trial proving aortic stent grafts superiority to the clamp and sew technique. Also, there is no data available on the long-term complications associated with stent graft as the patient becomes older and the aorta naturally dilates. Therefore, this cannot yet be the recommended standard, though, if available, is still an option in caring for these injuries.

Subclavian artery injuries after penetrating trauma require different operative strategies depending on laterality and location. A right sided subclavian artery injury can be approached via a median sternotomy and a cervical extension if needed. Distal control can be obtained at the deltopectoral groove. A left sided subclavian artery injury is more complex and proximal control is classically taught as being obtained via a third interspace left sided anterolateral thoracotomy. This is a difficult and can be a time-consuming approach as there is a significant amount of muscle that must be divided to enter the chest. We advocate either clavicle head resection and sternotomy or a posterolateral fourth interspace thoracotomy. A bilateral fourth interspace anterolateral thoracotomy is also a useful and versatile incision that gives excellent exposure to both sides of the thorax and the mediastinum. Another technique for proximal control is catheter directed endovascular balloon occlusion. This is becoming a more attractive option for proximal control of the left subclavian artery to avoid exsanguination. Distal control is again obtained by the deltopectoral groove.

Intrapericardial pulmonary artery injury is a difficult injury to reach and carries a significant mortality, noted to be up to 70%. A median sternotomy is the incision of choice, and the main and proximal left pulmonary artery are both readily identified with minimal dissection, but the right pulmonary artery has to be dissected away from the aorta and superior vena cava. If there is an anterior injury, a primary repair can be performed, but gentle tissue handling, and meticulous hemostasis must be achieved due to the fragility of the vessel. Posterior injuries are difficult to repair without having the patient on cardiopulmonary bypass.

Emergency Department Resuscitative Thoracotomy

The role of emergency department (ED) thoracotomy in patients who sustained penetrating thoracic trauma was first promoted by the Ben Taub General Hospital in Houston, Texas. This was then adopted by many large trauma centers, but questions began to arise about the absolute indications for this heroic procedure. The decision to perform an ED thoracotomy is based on injury patterns, prehospital provider report and physiologic status at the time of arrival. The length of prehospital cardiopulmonary resuscitation (CPR) and cardiac rhythm at time of arrival play heavily into the decision to perform this procedure.

In a recent Western Trauma Association multicenter study on ED thoracotomy, it was identified that the most common injury was a stab wound to a ventricle. which was found in 30% of survivors, and the second most common injury was a gunshot wound to the lung which accounted for 16% of survivors. They also noted that two patients with isolated head trauma were also revived after abrupt physiologic decompensation and ED thoracotomy. In subgroup analysis, this study revealed that 34% of survivors received prehospital CPR. In the survivors who had stab wounds, they received between 2 and 10 minutes of CPR and in the gunshot wound group, they received CPR between 1 to 15 minutes in the field. Of note, both patients who received CPR for the longest time had evidence of cardiac tamponade on arrival. Based on their findings, blunt trauma itself was not an absolute contraindication for ED thoracotomy. The only exception to this was in patients with an overtly devastating head injury. They did find that duration of prehospital CPR was a predictor of futility. There were no survivors who underwent ED thoracotomy for blunt trauma who had more than 10 minutes of prehospital CPR. For penetrating trauma, there were no survivors who underwent ED thoracotomy after more than 15 minutes of prehospital CPR. The final finding in this group's study was the survival in 7 patients who arrived at the ED in asystole. There has been mention in the literature that patients who arrive without a discernible cardiac rhythm should not undergo heroic procedures. This group noted that all 7 of the survivors who presented in asystole had cardiac tamponade. Therefore, they concluded ED thoracotomy was not likely to result in survival if blunt trauma patients had greater than 10 minutes of prehospital CPR, if penetrating trauma patients had greater than 15 minutes of prehospital CPR, and if asystole patients did not have signs of cardiac tamponade.

Abdomen

Findings that necessitate immediate operative exploration include peritoneal signs, evisceration, uncontrollable hemorrhage from the wound, blood from a natural orifice, hemodynamic instability with penetrating injury, impaled objects, signs of intra-abdominal injury on radiographic studies, and high velocity missile injuries. The abdomen can be divided into four different anatomic sites. These include the thoracoabdomen, the anterior abdomen, the flank and back, and the retroperitoneum. Here we will briefly discuss each site.

Thoracoabdomen

Anatomically, this area is defined as being from the nipple line to the costal margin. There are a number of structures in this region which would need expeditious diagnosis and operative repair. The heart lies in the middle of the thoracoabdomen and injury into the cardiac box can be assessed by physical exam, ultrasound study, diagnostic pericardiocentesis, pericardial window, or sternotomy. First on a physical exam, one may encounter any or all of Beck's triad (muffled heart sounds, jugular venous distension, and hypotension), which are signs of pericardial tamponade. If the physical exam is not as clear, then ultrasound has a significant utility in this area. The Focused Assessment for the Sonographic Evaluation of the Trauma Patient examination (FAST) is very useful in identifying intra-abdominal free fluid or signs of pericardial fluid and tamponade. One will use the subxiphoid view with a phase array (square head) ultrasound probe to identify hypoechoic fluid in the pericardial sac. This, coupled with hypotension, is an indication for exploration within the pericardial window and possible sternotomy. Pericardiocentesis can be performed but should be performed in an operating room ready for possible sternotomy.

Another object in the thoracoabdomen that can have an occult injury is the diaphragm. Unfortunately, a diaphragmatic rent or laceration is not easily identified on physical exam or conventional imaging. A thoracoabdominal wound with ipsilateral hemothorax and intraperitoneal blood is very suggestive of a diaphragm injury. A prospective study including 50 patients at a large level 1 trauma center used CT scan to classify specific and non-specific findings for diaphragm injury. Specific findings for diaphragm injury were found in only 40% of patients. These specific findings included adjacent organ injury and herniation of intra-abdominal contents into the thorax. The non-specific findings included wound tract extending to the diaphragm, thickening of the diaphragm by blood or edema, and defect in the diaphragm without blood or hernia. The use of laparoscopy in the diagnosis of diaphragm injuries has also been proposed. One study found that laparoscopy revealed diaphragm injury in 32% of thoracoabdominal penetrating injury. This same study showed that on laparotomy they also found concomitant intra-abdominal injury in 89% of patients.

Anterior Abdomen

The anterior abdomen is defined anatomically as going from xiphoid to pubis and between the anterior axillary lines. The literature has long shown that only one half to three quarters of all anterior abdominal stab wounds will actually penetrate the abdomen, and of these patients only 50-75% will require operative repair of a stabbing induced injury. There has been significant work performed in determining who needs a laparotomy for anterior abdominal wall stabbings. This is evident when reviewing the Western Trauma Association's (WTA) guidelines for this type of penetrating trauma. The centers in the WTA's prospective study utilized modalities such as serial clinical assessment, diagnostic peritoneal lavage, aspirate (DPL/DPA), FAST exam, and CT scanning all to help identify patients who needed a laparotomy. Additionally, they also employed local wound exploration to look for fascial penetration. These were performed in patients who were hemodynamically stable. What this study found was only 36% of patients in their study with anterior abdominal stab wounds required laparotomy, and of those, 26% were non-therapeutic laparotomies. Another finding of this study was that after selecting outpatients who needed emergent laparotomy for the above stated reasons, only 22% or 61 out of 278 patients needed a therapeutic laparotomy. Therefore, if the resources are available to perform these adjuncts, not every anterior abdominal stab wound needs a laparotomy for exploration.

Gunshot wounds to the anterior abdomen have primarily been treated with operative exploration since the majority of these patients will have other intra-abdominal injury. There has been work showing that some patients may be candidates for non-operative therapy. The stable patient who does not exhibit peritoneal signs can potentially go through CT scan to obtain more information about projectile path and possible injuries. Some even say if there is an isolated solid organ injury after gunshot wound, the patient can be safely observed and operated on only if there is a clinical change.

The Flank and Back

The flank is defined as the region between the anterior and posterior axillary lines. This region can prove difficult to clinically evaluate and so diagnostic imaging with CT scan has been advocated. There is some evidence that oral and rectal contrast can help, but with today's multi-detector CT scans (MDCT), this has been called into question. It has been found that the flank and back can adequately be imaged without rectal contrast, and injuries still become evident. The most worrisome injuries in this region include damage to the vascular system, the kidney and urinary tract, and the colon.

Retroperitoneum

The retroperitoneum is divided into three zones where injury can occur. Zone I is central and includes the aorta, vena cava, renal and lumbar vessels. Zone II is perinephric or lateral. Zone III is in the pelvis. For penetrating traumatic injury, all retroperitoneal hematomas should be explored, even if non-expanding. When doing this type of exploration, it is important to realize that this is most often for a vascular injury, and the tenets of vascular surgery, namely obtaining proximal and distal control, should be observed.

Extremity

In penetrating extremity trauma, whether upper or lower extremity, three aspects must be evaluated at time of admission. The first is a full vascular exam, noting palpable pulses or doppler-able signals in all the major vessels of the extremity. These should be symmetric on both sides, and it is useful to check the uninjured side if there is one. The next examination should include a full motor and sensory neurologic exam of the extremity. Abnormalities in motor and sensation should be assessed and documented in the patient while they are awake. Next skeletal stability should be assessed to make sure there are no wounds communicating with a broken bone, making it an open fracture. Once these three aspects of the exam are completed adjunctive tests can be ordered to help with diagnosis.

On physical exam, if there are 'hard' signs of major vascular injury such as a large, pulsatile, or expanding hematoma, absent distal pulses, palpable thrill, or audible bruit over the wound, then the patient should go emergently to the operating room for exploration and repair. If there are signs of distal ischemia such as pulselessness, pallor, paralysis, paresthesias, pain, and poikilothermy then the patient may have a significant vascular injury and may need to go emergently to the operating room. 'Soft' signs such as small and stable hematomas, report of bleeding at the scene of injury, wound near a major nerve or vascular structure and hypotension have been shown to have no correlation with the presence of vascular injury and should not dictate operative approach. Even though the literature does not support making decisions based only on 'soft' signs, a penetrating wound that is in close proximity to a major vessel can be deceiving. It has been noted in the literature that the incidence of major vessel injury in these wounds can range from 5- 24%, as such this has caused many to advocate for exploration of these wounds to prevent late complications of ischemia.

In patients with 'hard' signs that do not necessarily localize the injury to a specific area or when a physical exam is questionable, adjunctive studies may be helpful. These include both contrast angiography and CT angiography. CT angiography is a rapid exam that could help to show the tract of the knife or missile and elucidate vascular injury. This can help in operative planning and is a useful tool, especially in patients who are being sent for CT scans of other body parts looking for injury. If the patient is exhibiting unstable hemodynamics, they should be taken to the operating room where an on-table contrast angiogram can be performed, and the injury visualized. This is helpful for operative planning and can be used for therapeutics for hemorrhage control also.

Repair for single lacerations can be performed with arteriorrhaphy as long as the edges are clean without devitalized tissue. These wounds are repaired using a 4-0 or 5-0 polypropylene suture in an interrupted fashion to prevent constriction at the repair. The majority of arterial injuries (85 to 90%) will require a segmental resection and either primary end to end anastomosis or a graft interposition with either autogenous vein or artificial graft material. For these repairs a 4-0 or 5-0 polypropylene suture will be used in a running fashion circumferentially around the anastomosis, taking care to make sure the knots are tied on the outside of the repair.

After an anastomosis or arteriorrhaphy is completed, an on-table angiogram is warranted to make sure there is distal flow and no evidence of thrombus or vasospasm. This is performed by placing a 22-gauge butterfly needle into the artery proximal to the repair and flushing the artery with a water-soluble contrast medium. This is done either under continuous fluoroscopy or with static X-ray images. In the event that thrombus is noted, performing a balloon embolectomy through the repair is a good idea. If there is evidence of possible vasospasm, then using an intraluminal injection of a calcium channel blocker may help.

In patients who are in profound shock and have significant acidosis, it may be necessary to get the patient off the operating room table and resuscitate them. After proximal and distal control is obtained, a shunt can be placed quickly and maintain blood flow to a threatened limb. A shunt can be as simple as sterile intravenous tubing or can be a commercially available shunt like a Pruitt-Inahara shunt (LeMaitre Vascular, Burlington, MA). This technique is also useful in patients with orthopedic injuries that have not been fully reduced as it can allow the boney reduction and fixation before a definitive repair of the vessel is performed. In some instances, it may be necessary to choose life over limb. This means that ligating the bleeding vessel, accepting the risk of ischemia to the limb to get the patient to a place where they can be resuscitated, and then coming back to the operating room to either complete an amputation or try a revascularization procedure may be necessary.

Compartment Syndrome

Extremity injury can result in increased upper or lower extremity compartment pressures. These pressures can be elevated beyond the capillary perfusion pressure needed to deliver blood to the tissue and can lead to nerve injury and myonecrosis. This is a limb threatening condition and must be treated when clinically suspected. The hallmark of compartment syndrome in the awake patient is pain in the passive range of motion. In many trauma patients this is difficult because they may have multiple injuries that necessitate sedation and mechanical ventilation. In these patients it is imperative to remember this disease process and check compartment pressures when clinically indicated. Patients will develop signs of ischemia which, as noted above include pain, pallor, pulselessness, paresthesias, paralysis, and poikilothermy.

To check a compartment pressure, one can hook an 18-gauge needle to an arterial monitor, insert the needle into the compartment, inject about 1-2 mL of saline into the compartment, and then measure the pressure. If a solid-state transducer device, otherwise known as a Stryker device (Stryker Surgical, Kalamazoo, MI), is available, this can rapidly give a read out of the compartment pressure after puncturing the compartment in question with a needle. Though there may be some difference of opinion as to the exact number for a pressure that constitutes compartment syndrome, a normal compartment pressure is between 0- and 5-mmHg. If the patient has clinical signs that are worrisome for compartment syndrome and a significantly elevated pressure, intervention may be warranted.

Intervention in the form of a fasciotomy is indicated for compartment syndrome. This is necessary before tissue damage occurs. The technique for fasciotomy is not within the scope of this chapter, but it varies based on area of concern. The basic tenets include dissection through skin and soft tissue until the fascial layer is identified. Then this fascial covering is incised fully, and the underlying tissue should be noted to bulge out. The tissue should be inspected for signs of ischemic compromise and necrosis as this may require further debridement. Fasciotomies can be limb saving and once a diagnosis of compartment syndrome is made, this procedure should be performed emergently.

SUMMARY

This chapter covered the broad topic of penetrating trauma and certain site-specific injuries and management options. In any penetrating injury, it is important to identify the type of weapon that caused the injury and the tract of the missile or blade. As with any patient, airway, breathing and hemodynamic assessment should take place first and then hemorrhage control. There is a role for damage control surgery in any trauma and if the center where the patient is brought cannot safely perform the definitive care needed, then damage control should be performed, and the patient then transferred after stabilization.

REFERENCES

1. Murray CL, Lopez AD (eds). The global burden of disease: a comprehensive assessment of mortality and disability from diseases, injuries and risk factors in 1990 and projected to 2020. Vol. 1. Boston, Harvard School of Public Health, 1996.
2. Small Arms Survey, Small Arms Survey 2007: Guns and the City (Cambridge, UK: Cambridge University Press, 2007), p. 39.
3. Geneva Declaration Secretariat, Global burden of armed violence: Lethal encounters (Geneva: Geneva Declaration Secretariat, 2011).
4. Krug E. Statement for the UN Conference on the Illicit Trade in Small Arms and Light Weapons in All its Aspects. (presentation at the UN Conference on the Illicit Trade in Small Arms and Light Weapons in All its Aspects, New York, July 9-20, 2001).
5. Cook PJ, Ludwig J. Gun violence: The real costs (Oxford: Oxford University Press, 2000); Miller TR, Cohen MA. Costs of gunshot and cut/stab wounds in the United States, with some Canadian comparisons. Accident Analysis and Prevention 29/3 (1997), pp. 329-341.
6. Fackler ML, Dougherty PJ. Theodor kocher and the scientific foundation of wound ballistics. Surg Gynecol Obstet. 1991;172:153-60.
7. Kocher T. Uber die Sprengwirkung der modernen Kleingewehr-Geschosse. Cor.-Br. Schweiz Aerzte, 1875;5:3-7;29-33;69-74.
8. Fackler ML, Bellamy RF, Malinkowski JA. Wounding mechanism of projectiles striking at more than 1.5km/sec. J Trauma 1986;26:250.
9. Fackler ML. Wound ballistics: a review of common misconceptions. JAMA. 1988;259;2730-2736.
10. Biffl WL, Kaups KL, Cothren CC, et al. Management of patients with anterior abdominal stab wounds: a western trauma association multicenter trial. J Trauma. 2009;66:1294-301.
11. Mocquot P. Plais des gros vaisseaus du cou. Rev de Chir. 1917;52:241.
12. Fogelman MJ, Stewart RD. Penetrating wounds of the neck. Am J Surg. 1956;91:581-596.
13. Tisherman SA, Bokhari F, Collier B, et al. Clinical practice guidelines: penetrating zone II neck trauma. J Trauma 2008;64:1392-1405.
14. Ascensio JA, Valenziano CP, Falcone RE, et al. Management of penetrating neck injuries: the controversy surrounding zone II injuries. Surg Clin North Am. 1991;71:267-296.
15. Allen JP. The Art of Medicine in Ancient Egypt. New York: The Metropolitan Museum of Art, 2005. Print.
16. Ashbaugh DG, Bigelow DB, Petty TL, Levine BE. Acute respiratory distress in adults. Lancet. 1967;2:319-323.
17. Nagarsheth K, Kurek S. Ultrasound detection of pneumothorax compared with chest x-ray and computed tomography scan. Am Surg. 2011;77:480-484.
18. Tarlow MH, Hauser CJ. Prospective study of neurtophil chemokine responses in trauma patients at risk for pneumonia. Am J Resp Crit Care Med. 2005;171:753.
19. Lee RB. Traumatic injury to the cervicothoracic trachea and major bronchi. Chest Surg Clin N Am. 1997;7:285-304.
20. Kelly JP, Webb WR, Moulder PV, et al. Management of airway trauma. I: tracheobronchial injuries. Ann Thorac Surg. 1985;40:551-555.
21. Karmy-Jones R, Jurkovich G, Shatz D, et al. Management of traumatic lung injury: a western trauma association multicenter review. J Trauma. 2001;51:1049.
22. Jones W, Mavroudis C, Richardson J, et al. Management of tracheobronchial disruption resulting from blast trauma. Surgery. 1984;95:319.
23. Wilson A, Wall MJ Jr, Maxson R, Mattox K. The pulmonary hilum twist as a thoracic damage control procedure. Am J Surg. 2003;186:49-52.
24. Asensio JA, Stewart BM, Murray JA, et al. Penetrating cardiac injuries. Surg Clin North Am. 1996;76:685-724.
25. Moreno C, Moore EE, Majure JA, et al. Pericardial tamponade: a critical determinant for survival following penetrating cardiac wounds. J Trauma. 1986;26:821-825.
26. Garrison RN, Richardson JD, Fry DE. Diagnostic transdiaphragmatic pericardiotomy in thoracoabdominal trauma. J Trauma. 1982;22:147-149.
27. Rozycki GS, Feliciano DV, Oschner MG, et al. The role of ultrasound in patients with possible penetrating cardiac wounds: a prospective multicenter study. J Trauma. 1999;46:543-551.
28. Mattox KL, Feliciano DV, Beall AC Jr, et al. Five thousand seven hundred sixty cardiovascular injuries in 4459 patients epidemiologic evolution 1958 – 1988. Ann Surg. 1989;209:698-705.
29. Mattox KL. Fact or fiction about management of aortic transaction (editorial). Ann Thorac Surg. 1989;48:1-2.
30. Beall AC Jr, Diethrich EB, Cooley DA, DeBakey ME. Surgical management of penetrating cardiovascular trauma. South Med J. 1967;60:698–704.

31. Moore EE, Knudson MM, Burlew CC, et al. Defining the limits of resuscitative emergency department thoracotomy: a contemporary western trauma association perspective. J Trauma. 2011;70:334-339.
32. Shanmuganathan K, Mirvis SE, Chiu WC, et al. Penetrating torso trauma: triple-contrast helical CT in peritoneal violation and organ injury: a prospective study in 200 patients. Radiology 2004; 231:775–784.
33. Uribe RA, Pachon CE, Frame SB, et al. A prospective evaluation of thoracoscopy for the diagnosis of penetrating thoracoabdominal trauma. J Trauma. 1994; 37:650–654.
34. Thompson JS, Moore EE, Van Duzer-Moore S, et al. The evolution of abdominal stab wound management. J Trauma 1980; 20:478–484.
35. Biffl WL, Kaups KL, Cothren CC, et al. Management of patients with anterior abdominal stab wounds: a Western Trauma Association Multicenter Trial. J Trauma 2009; 66:1294–1301.
36. Demetriades D, Hadjizacharia P, Constantinou C, et al. Selective nonoperative management of penetrating abdominal solid organ injuries. Ann Surg 2006; 244:620–628.
37. Ramirez RM, Cureton EL, Ereso AQ, et al. Single-contrast computed tomography for the triage of patients with penetrating torso trauma. J Trauma 2009;67:583–588.
38. Fykberg ER, Crump JM, Dennis JW, et al. Nonoperative observation of clinically occult arterial injuries: a prospective evaluation. Surgery. 1991;109:85-96.
39. Perry MO, Thal ER, Shires FT. Management of arterial injuries. Ann Surg. 1971;173:403-408.
40. Busquets AR, Acosta JA, Colon E, et al. Helical computed tomographic angiography in the diagnosis of injuries of the extremities. J Trauma. 2004;56:625-628.
41. Shiroff AM, Gale SC, Martin ND. Penetrating neck trauma: a review of management strategies and discussion of the 'No Zone' approach. Am Surg. 2013 Jan;79(1):23-9.

❑❑❑

50

CHAPTER

Head Trauma

Manjunath Markandaya, MBBS
Scott A Marshall, MD
Mayur Narayan, MD, MPH, MBA, FACS

INTRODUCTION

Trauma to the brain and spinal cord (neurotrauma) is a growing health problem and a leading cause of morbidity and mortality worldwide. Around 50% of all early trauma deaths are secondary to neurotrauma. Severe neurotrauma, when not fatal, is often a life altering event for patients and their families due to the resource intensive nature of the disease. Survivors are left with varying degrees of disability and disruptions to their lifestyles and livelihoods. In addition, family members and caregivers of patients with neurotrauma often face the onerous task of caring for them. While the most effective intervention for neurotrauma remains prevention, appropriate clinical management of the patient in order to prevent secondary injury to the nervous system is paramount.

Incidence, Prevalence, and Epidemiology

Traumatic brain injury (TBI) and spinal cord injuries (SCI) are on the rise in India.[1] India is experiencing rapid industrialization and economic progress associated with increased mobility of the masses. However, modernization of infrastructure, vehicular safety protocols, and behaviors (e.g., consistent use of helmets, lane discipline while riding and/or driving) has not kept pace, leading to a complex interaction between the environment and the individual resulting in an increase in incidence, severity, morbidity, and mortality associated with TBI.[1,2] Around 850,000 to 1,000,000 individuals are killed every year in India as a result of injuries[3] and perhaps even more concerning is the ratio of deaths to serious injuries to mild injuries is around 1:15:70. Estimates show that around 2,000,000 people are afflicted with TBI and around 200,000 die every year due to TBI.[1] In addition, it is estimated that around 1,000,000 persons would require rehabilitation services for TBI at any given time (point prevalence).[1]

Etiology

India has the highest numbers of fatalities from road traffic accidents (RTA) in the world. They are the leading cause of neurotrauma in India, accounting for anywhere from 44% to 61% of cases, see Table 1.[1] Falls account for around 11% to 35% of cases, and assault for 9% to 30% of cases. Compared to Western societies, two-wheeler occupants, pedestrians, and bicyclists represent the majority of cases from RTA's as opposed to car occupants.[1] The highest occurrence of neurotrauma was in the 20 to 39 age group.[1] Compared to RTAs, falls were more common in children and the elderly. Falls comprised of domestic falls (68%), falls on the road (12%), construction site falls (15%), and agricultural lands falls (6%). Injuries resulting from violence, especially those caused by blunt weapons are on the rise in India and have been attributed to political, communal, and interpersonal reasons.[1] Alcohol consumption appears to be a major risk factor for neurotrauma. About 16% of neurotrauma patients in the age group of 15 years and above were under the influence of alcohol, at the time of the injury. Also, the mortality in this group was around 15% as opposed to 9% in the non-alcohol use group.[1]

Table 1: Etiology of Neurotrauma in India[1]

Etiology	Percent
Road Traffic Accidents (two-wheeler occupants, pedestrians, and bicyclists)	44% to 61%
Falls	11% to 35%
Assault	9% to 30%

Pathophysiology (Primary and Secondary Injury)

The pathophysiology of neurotrauma is based on the concepts of primary injury and secondary injury. Primary injury occurs at the time of injury and is due to (1) blunt force trauma, (2) penetrating injury, and (3) a combination of blunt force trauma and penetrating injury such as that seen with blast injuries and explosive mechanisms. This mechanism accounts for a large portion of the immediate trauma deaths, as the apnea caused by TBI, and high SCI is rapidly fatal. Secondary injury is injury that afflicts the injured brain or spinal cord when systemic and external factors cause deleterious effects on the already vulnerable brain and spinal cord. Hypoxic-ischemic injuries, loss of autoregulation, decrease in cerebral perfusion (hypotension), increased intracranial and intrathecal pressures, neuronal excitotoxicity, free radical damage, ionic dysregulation, generation of inflammatory mediators, development of cerebral edema, hyperthermia, and immune mediated injury. Immune mediated injury occurs because the brain is an immunologically privileged organ, and damage to the blood brain barrier can lead to exposure of brain antigens to the immune system. The cornerstone treatment for TBIs and spinal cord injuries is the prevention and amelioration of secondary brain injury. As above, this secondary injury can come in many forms and, in some cases, is preventable. For example, even a single episode of hypotension (systolic blood pressure <90) doubles mortality, and the presence of both hypotension and hypoxia increase the mortality risk 3-fold and substantially increases the risk of a bad outcome.[4]

Risk Factors

A number of behavioral, environmental, and social factors serve as risk factors for neurotrauma detailed in Table 2.

Table 2: Risk Factors for Neurotrauma[1]

	Risk Factors for Neurotrauma in India
1.	Poor infrastructure (roads and highway construction)
2.	Rapid increases in type and number of vehicles
3.	Lack of vehicular safety standards
4.	Behavioral issues such as lack of lane discipline, aggressive driving, and failure to follow traffic laws and red light stops
5.	Overcrowding of roads
6.	Lack of pedestrian awareness
7.	Lack of seatbelt use
8.	Alcohol use
9.	Interpersonal violence
10.	Communal and religious disharmony
11.	Political disharmony

Nomenclature of Neurotrauma:

Neurotrauma can be classified in a number of ways as seen in Tables 3, 4, and 5 and Figure 1. TBI can be isolated, associated with relatively minor extracranial injuries, or occur in combination with severe systemic extracranial injuries. TBI is classified as mild (mild uncomplicated and mild complicated), moderate, and severe. Common classifications schemes are most often based on the presenting Glasgow Coma Scale (GCS) score after hemodynamic resuscitation of the trauma patient and in the absence of confounding factors such as drug intoxication, sedation, and use of paralytic medications.

Table 3: Types of Neurotrauma

Type	Injuries
Traumatic Brain Injury (Mild, Moderate and Severe)	Epidural Hemorrhage (EDH) Subdural Hemorrhage (SDH) Traumatic Subarachnoid Hemorrhage (tSAH) Intraparenchymal Hemorrhage (IPH) Hemorrhagic Contusions Intraventricular Hemorrhage (IVH) Cerebral Edema Mass Effect, Midline Shift Brain Herniation Diffuse Axonal Injury (DAI)
Traumatic Spinal Cord Injury	Cervical Spinal Cord Injury (SCI) Thoracic Spinal Cord Injury Lumbar and Sacral Cord Injury Conus Medullaris and Cauda Equina Syndromes
Traumatic Neuropathy	Injury to Nerve Roots Injury to Nerve Bundles Injury to Nerve Plexuses (Brachial Plexus and Lumbar Plexus) Injury to Peripheral Nerves
Traumatic Injury to Bony Structures	Skull Fractures Spinal Column (bony) injuries
Traumatic Injury to Surrounding Tissues	Scalp Injury/Laceration Injury to spinal Ligaments Neurovascular Trauma (blunt cerebrovascular injury; traumatic dural venous sinus injury with thrombosis)

Table 4: Types of Traumatic Brain Injury

Injury Type	Etiology	Clinical Features	Treatment
Epidural Hemorrhage (EDH)	Collection of blood between the bone (skull) and dura. Tear in middle meningeal artery (85%); middle meningeal vein or dural sinus (15%)	Classically associated with the "lucid interval"	Urgent neurosurgical evaluation and craniotomy or craniectomy. A small minority of EDHs can be clinically observed without need for surgery
Subdural Hemorrhage (SDH)	Collection of blood between the dural layers (pachymeninges and leptomeninges)	Can be acute, subacute, or chronic. Usually associated with significant underlying brain parenchymal injury/cerebral edema	Urgent neurosurgical evaluation and craniotomy, craniotomy, or placement of a drain with burr holes depending on chronicity and clinical presentation. A small minority of SDHs can be clinically observed without need for surgery
Traumatic Subarachnoid Hemorrhage (tSAH)	Blood in the subarachnoid space	Usually located over hemispheric surfaces	Medical management in most cases. Surgical management if there are associated lesions or development of hydrocephalus. May be associated with late vasospasm necessitating a combination of medical and surgical (endovascular) management
Intracerebral Hemorrhage (ICH) and Intraparenchymal Contusions	Blood clot/hematoma in brain parenchyma	Various neuro-deficits depending on location of bleeding. Most commonly over frontal gyrus, temporal tips, and occipital pole	Medical versus surgical management depending on clinical presentation, lesion location, size, associated cerebral edema and presence or absence of brain herniation.
Intraventricular Hemorrhage (IVH)	Blood in the ventricular system of the brain	Usually associated with IPH with extension into ventricles. Can lead to obstructive hydrocephalus	Neurosurgical placement of an external ventricular drain (EVD) to drain blood and CSF. Small IVHs with a good clinical exam can be medically managed
Diffuse Cerebral Edema	Secondary to trauma and breakdown of blood-brain barrier (BBB) leading to diffuse swelling of traumatized brain	More common in children and usually peaks around 2-3 days post-trauma. Can lead to brain herniation and death	Depending on extent of edema, medical or surgical management
Diffuse Axonal Injury (DAI)	Shear injury at gray-white matter junction. Usually identified by petechial hemorrhage or hypodense foci	Clinical presentation is very variable and dependent on extent and location of DAI	Medical management is the mainstay of therapy for DAI

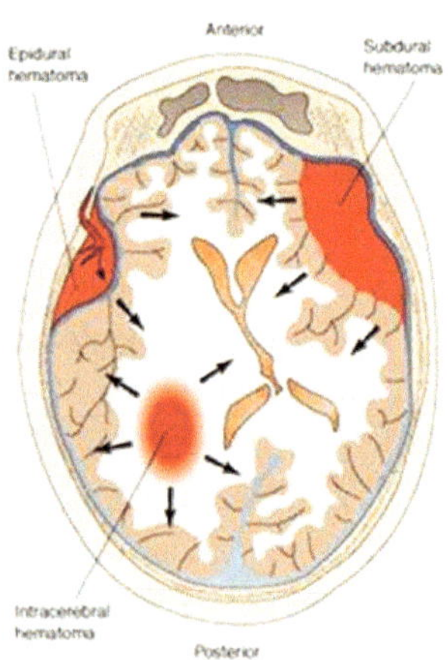

Figure 1: Types of Traumatic Brain Injury

Table 5: Mechanisms of Traumatic Brain Injury

Mechanism	
Blunt	Seen with high-speed collisions, direct blunt force trauma to head
Penetrating	Due to high or low velocity projectiles
Blast/Explosive	Injury occurs via transmitted forces from a concussive pressure wave

Mild TBI, also known as a concussion, is the most common subset of neurotrauma and accounts for around 80% of all TBIs. It is characterized by a GCS score of 13 to 15. Patients often suffer a brief loss of consciousness, amnesia surrounding the incident, and have varying degrees of nausea, vomiting, and headache. Most patients recover fully within a few hours to days, though a small subset can suffer from delayed symptoms such as headache, difficulty with concentrating on tasks, insomnia, dizziness, and mood disturbances. This is known as the post-concussive syndrome and if symptoms persist for more than a year, resolution is unlikely. For patients with sports related concussions, return to play should be judiciously considered; adequate time should be given for full recovery and avoidance of subsequent TBIs before full recovery. "Guidelines for Return to Play" published by the American Academy of Neurology can be used by clinicians in guiding patients to full activity.[5,7]

Mild TBI with any one of the following criteria is defined as mild complicated TBI: brain lesions on CT scan, moderate to severe multiple traumas, focal neurological findings, skull fracture, cerebrospinal fluid (CSF) leak, recent pre-injury history of psychiatric disorder, recent pre-injury substance abuse, prior brain injury, post-traumatic amnesia lasting more than 24 hours and development of seizures.

Second Impact Syndrome (SIS) is a syndrome that is most often seen in children and adolescents with TBI and can be fatal in around 50% of cases. It is seen after a second head injury during recovery from the initial TBI. There is an exponential worsening of clinical outcome. This may be related to impaired cerebral autoregulation and subsequent development of diffuse cerebral edema, intracranial hypertension, and brain herniation.

Moderate TBI is defined as a post-resuscitation GCS of 9 to 12 and can occur in around 10% of TBI patients. Moderate TBI is often associated with prolonged loss of consciousness and neurological deficits. These patients usually have abnormal Computed Tomography (CT) scans and/or Magnetic Resonance Imaging (MRI) of their brain, and they need in-patient hospitalization and neurosurgical intervention.

Severe TBI is defined as a post-resuscitation GCS of 8 or less and is also seen in around 10% of all TBI patients. They almost always show evidence of brain lesions on CT and/or MRI. These patients most often need Intensive Care Unit (ICU) care, with a secure airway, need for mechanical ventilation, neurosurgical evaluation, intervention, and consideration for monitoring of intracranial pressure.

Focal brain Injuries include epidural hematomas, subdural hematomas, intracerebral hemorrhage/hematoma, subarachnoid hemorrhage if it is localized to one area, and contusions. It is a contusion if it is located at the coup and contra-coup sites, common locations being anterior temporal lobes, orbitofrontal cortex, and the occipital cortex.

Diffuse brain injuries include diffuse axonal injury (DAI) and diffuse cerebral edema. DAI occurs due to shearing of the axons in the cerebral white matter. A higher incidence of DAI is seen with lateral impact mechanisms.

Clinical Evaluation and Management

The initial clinical evaluation and management of a patient with neurotrauma should follow the guidelines specified in the Advanced Trauma Life Support (ATLS) course developed by the American College of Surgeons and the Guidelines provided by the Brain Trauma Foundation (BTF).[4,7,8] It is paramount that one adheres to the ABCDE principles which stands for Airway with Cervical Spine precautions, Breathing, Circulation and control of Hemorrhage, Disability, and Exposure with avoidance of hypothermia. The ABCDE principle was created by the ATLS and should be performed as the primary and secondary surveys during the initial evaluation and management of a trauma patient.

Pre-Hospital Setting

The "Golden Hour" of trauma care is an extremely important concept in the initial care of a trauma victim. For head injury, survival benefits for admission to the trauma center may extend beyond this 60-minute period.[9] The safe and rapid transport of the patient to a capable healthcare facility should take priority. After ensuring safety of the scene, the first responder should assess the patency of the airway while maintaining cervical spine protection, ensuring adequacy of breathing, circulation, and a quick examination of patients' responses to stimuli. Placement of a cervical collar and a long spine board to protect a possible injured spinal column and/or cord should be undertaken to facilitate safe transport of the patient. Obtaining intravenous (IV) access and initiation of warm crystalloid solutions should be considered during transportation if possible. If there is a suspicion of neurotrauma, the choice of crystalloid solutions should be normal saline or hypertonic saline with the avoidance of low sodium IV fluids such as ringers' lactate. In cases of penetrating torso trauma, the concept of hypotensive resuscitation (systolic blood pressure around 90 mmHg) is usually advocated prior to hemorrhage control surgery. However, in the event of concomitant TBI a higher systolic blood pressure (100 to 110 mmHg) should probably be targeted.[10] In fact, a seminal study which showed the benefit of hypotensive resuscitation explicitly excluded patients with known head trauma.[11]

The location and time of the closest capable healthcare center, one able to provide care for a patient with polytrauma, should be factored in when deciding if a "scoop and run" approach as opposed to a "stay and play" approach is best. In most cases, getting the patient in a timely manner to a capable trauma hospital, the "Golden Hour", will serve the patient best. Unfortunately, the lack of a well-organized and systematic prehospital provider and transportation system, coupled with the majority of the populace living in a rural environment remote to adequate surgical capabilities, makes this a challenging proposition. More frequently, victims of trauma are transported by their family members to the closest healthcare facility, irrespective of the facility's capabilities.

Emergency Department/Accident and Emergency/ Trauma Bay Care

In the accident and emergency (A&E) department the care of the trauma victim should again focus on the principles of the primary and secondary survey of the ATLS. The primary survey and its adjuncts consist of:

- Assessment and securing of the airway while ensuring cervical spine protection: This may involve performance of endotracheal intubation for patients with decreased mental status (GCS 8 or less) to protect the airway.
- Ensuring adequacy of breathing: This is important in a patient with TBI, as hypoxia (oxygen saturation less than 90%), hypoventilation (hypercarbia), and hyperventilation (hypocarbia) can all result in detrimental outcomes.[4]
- Assessment of circulation and hemorrhage control: In patients with TBI, the avoidance of hypotension (SBP less than 90 mmHg) is paramount, as this is associated with a significant increase in mortality. In patients with high SCI, the occurrence of neurogenic shock characterized by relative bradycardia and hypotension should be recognized, and consideration for the use of fluids as well IV dopamine. Resuscitation fluids with lower sodium should be avoided, normal saline or hypertonic saline is often preferred.
- Assessment of neurological status: Evaluation of the GCS, pupillary symmetry, reaction to light, and presence of lateralizing signs should be carried out to determine the presence and severity of neurotrauma, including SCI. Early involvement of a neurosurgeon should be considered.
- Full exposure and subsequent protection from hypothermia should also be carried out: Adjuncts to the primary survey involve connecting the patient to cardiac, blood pressure and pulse oxygenation monitors, placement of oro/nasogastric tubes (no nasal tubes in the event of facial or basal skull fractures), urinary catheters and obtaining radiographs of the chest, pelvis and cervical spine.
- The secondary survey of the ATLS includes obtaining an AMPLE history: Allergies, Medications, Past medical/surgical history and Pregnancy, Last meal, and Environment/circumstance related to the traumatic event. Also, a thorough evaluation of the patient from head to toe to identify and treat injuries.

For patients with isolated mild TBI, monitoring in the A&E department and subsequent discharge home under supervision is reasonable. Please see the above section on mild uncomplicated and mild complicated TBI for management principles. The guidelines for the management of these patients have recently been updated by the American Academy of Neurology.[6]

Patients with moderate and severe TBI should be admitted to the hospital for further evaluation and management. Prompt CT scans of the head and spine, if indicated clinically, should be obtained and neurosurgical consultation and expertise should be sought for these patients. MRI of the brain and spine can be completed when patients are clinically stable. These studies may assist in lesion quantification and, to a certain extent, in prognosis.

Acute Care Hospital Management

Patients with moderate to severe TBI should be admitted to the hospital to an ICU setting. Those with emergent indications for neurosurgical intervention, seen in Table 6, need placement of an external ventricular drain (EVD) seen in Table 7, and a craniotomy and/or craniectomy for evacuation of a mass lesion. These procedures should be performed immediately or concurrent with initial damage control surgery to control life threatening hemorrhage in a multiple-injury trauma patient.

Table 6: Indications for Neurosurgical Intervention[4,7]

Type of Brain Lesion	Intervention
Epidural Hemorrhage (EDH) • Greater than 30 cm^3 with any GCS • Less than 30 $cm^3$and with more than 15 mm thickness and with more than 5mm midline shift • Acute EDH with GCS less than 9 with anisocoria	Hematoma evacuation via craniotomy or craniectomy
Subdural Hemorrhage (SDH) • Acute SDH with 10 mm or more thickness or with midline shift greater than 5mm regardless of GCS • SDH less than 10 mm thick and a midline shift less than 5 with GCS less than 9, if GCS drops by ≥2 points since admission and/or patient presents with asymmetric or fixed and dilated pupils and/or the ICP is >20 mmHg	Hematoma evacuation via craniotomy or craniectomy and duraplasty
Intraparenchymal Hemorrhage (IPH) • IPH and signs of progressive neurological deterioration referable to the lesion, medically refractory intracranial hypertension, signs of mass effect on CT • GCS 6 to 8, and there is a frontal or temporal contusions >20 cm^3 with a 5 mm midline shift and/or cisternal compression on CT scan, and with any lesion >50 cm^3	Craniotomy or craniectomy with evacuation of mass lesion
Diffuse medically refractory post-traumatic cerebral edema	Bifrontal decompressive craniectomy within 48 hours
Refractory Intracranial Hypertension and diffuse parenchymal injury • evidence of impending transtentorial brain herniation on both clinical and radiographic evidence	Decompressive procedures • subtemporal decompression • temporal lobectomy • hemispheric decompressive craniectomy
Patients with posterior fossa mass lesion • CT evidence of mass effect • Neurological dysfunction or deterioration	Suboccipital craniectomy and evacuation of mass lesion
Hydrocephalus	Placement of External Ventricular Drain (EVD)
Open (compound) Cranial Fractures • With depression greater than the thickness of cranium • With clinical or radiographic evidence of dural penetration, significant ICH, depression more than 1 cm, frontal sinus involvement, gross cosmetic deformity, wound infection, pneumocephalus, gross wound contamination	Elevation and debridement Antibiotic use
Spinal Column Injuries with or without cord injury/compression	Spinal decompression and stabilization procedures

Table7: Indications for Placement of an ICP Monitor[4,7]

Indications for Placement of an Intracranial Pressure Monitor
All patients who are salvageable and have a severe TBI and an abnormal CT scan Abnormal CT scan Contusions Hematomas Herniation Swelling Compressed basal cisterns
All patients with severe TBI and a normal CT scan if 2 or more of the following are noted on admission: Age >40 years Unilateral or bilateral motor posturing SBP less than 90 mmHg

The critical care of a TBI patient is guided by the principle of avoidance of secondary brain injury. This involves keeping the patient sedated with lightening of sedation for scheduled neurological assessments (i.e., monitoring of hourly GCS scores, pupillary size, and reactivity) to detect changes in exams that may warrant surgical attention and/or escalation of medical treatment options. Those patients with indications for Intracranial Pressure (ICP) monitoring should have one placed, seen in Table 7 and Table 8. However, recent data seems to suggest that placement of a monitor may have a limited role in determining outcome.[13] Other authors disagree, and the subject of invasive intracranial monitoring remains controversial.[14] Medical and/or surgical measures should be taken to keep ICP below 20 mmHg.[4] For all patients with severe TBI, and for most patients with moderate TBI and complicated mild TBI, a 7-day course of an antiseizure medication such as phenytoin is recommended to prevent early seizures.[4] Other evidence-based options exist for prophylaxis of early post-traumatic seizures, including levetiracetam.[15] However, this does not decrease the incidence of late post-traumatic epilepsy. Measures should be taken to keep the cerebral perfusion pressure (CPP) above 60 mmHg. It is imperative that hypotension (SBP less than 90) be avoided, as this can worsen mortality.[4]

Table 8: Other Multimodality Neuro-monitors[18]

Other types of brain monitors	Brief description
Brain Tissue Oxygen Tension (LICOX)	Intraparenchymal catheter that measures brain tissue oxygenation ($PbtO_2$). This is an indirect measure of perfusion and can be used to detect ischemia in at-risk brain tissue
Jugular Bulb Oxygenation	Used to assess global extraction of oxygen by the brain. Use is limited. Can be useful in tailoring hyperventilation therapy in refractory high intracranial pressure (ICP)
Regional Cerebral blood Flow (Hemedex, Bowman)	Intraparenchymal catheters that measure blood flow in a spherical volume of tissue surrounding the sensor
Cerebral Microdialysis	Intraparenchymal catheter that samples brain extracellular fluid and monitors dynamic changes in brain neurochemistry (glucose, lactate/pyruvate ratio, and glutamate). This provides information on brain energy supply and cellular metabolism
Continuous Electroencephalogram (cEEG)	Provides information on the electrical activity of the cerebral cortex. Useful in detecting subclinical seizures. Quantitative EEG (qEEG) provides information on delayed ischemia in patients with poor neurological exams and can be used in prognostication
Transcranial Doppler (TCD)	Uses Doppler Ultrasound to detect cerebral blood flow velocities and can be used to detect vasospasm. Using complex algorithms TCD in conjunction with Arterial line blood pressure measurement and the pulsatility index can estimate ICP or poor intracranial compliance in some situations[19,20,21,22,23]

Most patients with severe TBI are endotracheally intubated in order to protect the airway from aspiration complications. It is imperative that hypoxia (PaO2 <60 or oxygen saturation <90) be avoided, as this can also contribute to worse outcomes.[4] Adequate ventilation should be provided to maintain normal arterial carbon dioxide (PaCO2 35 to 40 mmHg) as abnormalities in these levels have been associated with poor outcomes. Low PaCO2 levels can promote cerebral ischemia by vasoconstriction. High PaCO2 levels with low pH can lead to cerebral vasodilation. For patients with loss of cerebral autoregulation where the cerebral perfusion pressure is linearly correlated to the mean arterial pressure and poor intracranial compliance, High PaCO2 levels can lead to high ICPs. Likewise, hyperoxemia has been shown to be detrimental to patients with brain injury, and an arterial blood partial pressures of oxygen (PaO2) >487 mmHg should be avoided.[16]

Provision of early adequate nutrition is also key to improving outcomes as evidenced by many studies in TBI patients. These patients are hypermetabolic and have increased caloric requirements. Thus, early consultation with a nutritionist is vital. Patients who are intubated should receive prophylaxis for stress gastritis with H2 blockers. Aggressive bowel care should be encouraged with the use of stool softeners and laxatives. In general, critically ill patients with constipation have increased ICU length of stay and increased days requiring mechanical ventilation.[17]

All patients should receive mechanical prophylaxis for the prevention of thromboembolic events. Chemical prophylaxis should be initiated as soon as (1) the risk for worsening of any intracranial or intraspinal hemorrhage is minimal and (2) there exists no other contraindications for its use. In many centers, patients are placed on chemical prophylaxis 48 to 72 hours after the injury.

For patients with severe TBI and poor neurological status (i.e., not following commands, unable to protect airway) should be considered for an early tracheostomy (3 to 7 days) and placement of percutaneous enteral feeding tubes. This will allow early liberation from the ventilator with decreased risk of ventilator associated pneumonia, and this will decrease the need for sedation allowing for easier pulmonary toileting.

Complications

Patients with TBI can have many complications affecting their clinical course Seen in Table 9.

Table 9: Complications of Neurotrauma

Complication	Clinical Features	Management
Blunt Cerebrovascular Injury Ischemic Strokes	Injury to the carotid and/or vertebral arteries	CT angiogram or catheter angiogram to diagnose and follow up progression of lesion. Use of anti-platelet and/or anticoagulation if not contraindicated due to TBI
Post-traumatic Vasospasm	Spasm of cerebral arteries leading to ischemic complications and persistent altered mental status. Increasingly recognized in TBI especially in those with blast injuries.	Use of Nimodipine or intra-arterial therapies (angioplasty, IA Verapamil) in severe cases. May perform surveillance with TCD or CT Angiogram [24,25]
Diencephalic Storms (Sympathetic Storms)	Paroxysms of fever, tachycardia, hypertension, tachypnea, pupillary dilation, and sweating	Use of propranolol, clonidine, IV dexmedetomidine, fentanyl, bromocriptine
CSF leaks	Leakage of CSF from skull fracture sites, or EVD burr holes. Places patient at high risk of infection	CSF diversion procedure (either EVD or Lumbar drain – if no risk of herniation) along with operative repair of dural defect
Meningitis/Ventriculitis	Bacterial and/or fungal infection of meninges or ventricular lining and CSF secondary to traumatic contamination, due to CSF leak, post-surgical complication, or due to the presence of an EVD	Antibiotics (or antifungals) with CNS penetration used intravenously. Usually Vancomycin and Cefepime (to cover pseudomonas) Refractory cases can be treated with intrathecal antibiotics
Aspiration Pneumonia and Ventilator Associated Pneumonia (VAP)	Pneumonia secondary to aspiration or as a risk of being on mechanical ventilation	Antibiotics for aspiration – clindamycin or extended spectrum B-lactams Antibiotics for VAP – empiric coverage with Vancomycin and Zosyn and tailor therapy based on clinical response and culture data
Venous Thrombo-embolic Complications – Deep Venous Thrombosis (DVT) and Pulmonary Embolisms (PE)	Associated with extremity swelling PEs can be fatal, asymptomatic or lead to severe hypoxia, tachycardia, and signs of right ventricular strain	Prophylaxis with mechanical devices (Sequential compression devices SCD or Compression Stockings) Chemical Prophylaxis with Low molecular weight heparin or unfractionated heparin when risk of hematoma expansion is minimal Therapy for DVTs – Therapeutic anticoagulation if no contraindication exists, use of inferior vena cava filter is controversial, thrombectomy may be considered in severe cases Therapy for PEs – Supplemental oxygen, therapeutic anticoagulation, thrombolytics in PEs associated with cardiac arrest of severe RV failure, pulmonary thrombectomy in severe cases of PE with refractory hypoxemia and RV failure

Complication	Clinical Features	Management
Pressure sores/Skin Breakdown	Due to immobility and/or coma	Frequent turning and attention to skin hygiene Local wound care in established cases Antibiotics and surgery in severe cases
Varying degrees of motor and weakness	Hemiplegia/paresis Quadriplegia/paresis	Rehabilitation
Psychiatric/Personality changes	Varying degrees of change in personality, mood, attention span, ability to hold gainful employment	TBI rehab Psychiatric consultation
Persistent Vegetative State/Minimally Conscious State	Some patients with severe TBI progress to these states and lack meaningful interaction with internal or external stimuli	Total care of the patent in a nursing home or home with dedicated caregivers
Death		

Rehabilitation

Early and continued involvement of a multi-disciplinary care team, including physical therapists, occupational therapists, speech and language pathologists, social workers, and case managers is essential to the care of these patients. While in the hospital, physical therapists can provide a range of motion exercises and teach family members the exercises and maneuvers that they can perform to benefit the patient. They can also provide assessments that can place patients in appropriate rehabilitation facilities upon discharge from an acute care hospital. Occupational therapists can provide casts and/or boots for the upper and lower extremities to maintain the joints of weak and/or paralyzed limbs in anatomic congruity. They can also provide assessment of functional ability of patients (i.e., ability to perform activities of daily living) and recommendations on home accommodations. Sleep and language pathologists provide assessments of swallowing ability with recommendations on diet consistency (i.e., regular, mechanical soft, pureed, liquid). They can also provide assessment of speech and aphasias, and a provision of speech therapies as part of a comprehensive cognitive evaluation.

Brain Death and Organ Donation

A small subset of patients with severe neurotrauma can progress to cessation of all brain function and, in many countries such as the United States, with appropriate testing the patient can be declared dead (death by neurological criteria). In India and the United Kingdom, the irreversible damage to the brainstem, with all functions of the brainstem being absent along with apnea, can be used as criteria to declare a person dead. Patients who are declared dead by neurological criteria and who themselves or their families have consented for organ donation, should be considered for organ and tissue donation. The details of this process are beyond the scope of this chapter.

Long Term/Nursing Home Care

Several patients with severe neurotrauma may require extended periods of time for recovery of neurological function. They are often discharged from the acute care hospital to a long-term care facility with or without chronic ventilator capabilities. Some of these centers offer coma stimulation programs and other therapies to help improve functional outcomes. Unfortunately, some of these patients will remain with a poor neurological exam and, after a period of 4 weeks, they are diagnosed as being in a vegetative state (VS) or minimally conscious state (MCS). Guidelines for the classification of these patients have been recently published.[26] Transition to awareness of patients in VS for long periods of time have been observed with functional MRI and EEG analysis, but the methodology of some of this work has been recently questioned.[27,28,29]

Prognosis

Prognosticating of neurotrauma is an inherently difficult proposition. Multiple studies have been done in an attempt to identify prognostic indicators and determine what outcomes patients might have.[30,31,32] The outcome can be quantified in multiple ways: (1) mortality, (2) Glasgow Outcome Scale because it can indicate good recovery and mild disability versus severe disability, vegetative state, and mortality, (3) health-related quality of life, (4) neuroimaging, and (5) neuropsychological assessment.[33] A complex interaction between a number of factors such as patient characteristics, admission variables, and clinical course determine outcome, seen in Table 10. A web-based resource based on the MRC-CRASH Trial[32] is available and provides risk estimates of 14-day mortality and risk of unfavorable outcomes (i.e., death and severe disability) at 6 months.[34] This model dichotomizes country of origin into high-income vs low/middle income countries and uses age, GCS (within 8 hours of injury), pupil reactivity, and presence of extracranial injuries. CT scan information can be incorporated if available.

Table 10: Prognostic Factors:[33]

Patient Characteristics	Admission Variables	Clinical Course
Biological Constitution Genotype	**Injury Details** Type (Closed, Penetrating, Etiology)	**Biological Response to Injury** Metabolomics
Demographic Factors Age Sex Ethnic Origin	**Clinical Severity** Intracranial (GCS/Pupils) Extracranial Injuries (AIS/ISS)	**Change in Admission Variables** Clinical severity Biomarkers CT changes Laboratory Values (Hypercarbia or Hypocarbia, Hyper or Hypoglycemia, Coagulation Values)
Socioeconomic Status and Level of Education	**Secondary Insults** Systemic (hypoxia, hypothermia, hypotension) Intracranial (seizures, neuro-worsening)	**Other Predictors** Secondary Insults Clinical Monitoring (brain tissue PO_2, ICP, evoked potentials)
Medical History (comorbid conditions)	**Computed Tomography (CT) characteristics**	**Neuroimaging** MRI Brain (Diffusion Tensor Imaging)

AIS: Abbreviated Injury Score ISS: Injury Severity Score

Spinal Cord Injury

Traumatic SCIs can occur with or without concomitant TBI. The cervical spinal cord is most commonly injured (54.1%).[35] Bell reported a high incidence of cervical spine injuries in his serial of combat-related head trauma.[24] Clinical signs of SCI include partial or complete muscular weakness, sensory loss, or both. This can be at and below the level of the lesion.[37] Quadriplegia and/or paresis occur in patients with cervical or thoracic spinal cord injuries. Around 21% of patients with spinal cord injuries can have one of the classic syndromes seen in Table 11 and Figure 2.[38] Plain X-rays (limited value), CT of the spine (diagnosis of bony injuries), MRI (diagnosis of ligament and cord pathology), and conventional CT myelography (diagnosis of spinal canal compromise and cord impingement in patients unable to undergo MRI) are some of the diagnostic modalities employed in evaluating traumatic SCI. Acute treatment for patients with spinal cord injuries focus on stabilizing the spinal column in order to prevent further traumatic cord injury and to provide good supportive management. This is used in the ICU or on the trauma wards to prevent secondary injury and early, sustained efforts at rehabilitation.[37] The use of IV steroids (methylprednisolone) is controversial. The protocol, as outlined in the NASCIS III study reported in 1997, consists of a bolus of 30 mg/kg of methylprednisolone, followed by an infusion of 5.4 mg/kg/hour for 24 hours.[41] Interestingly, the US military no longer recommends the use of high dose corticosteroids for non-penetrating SCI (USAISR 2012). The life-expectancy for SCI patients is increasing, but it still remains much shorter than that for age-matched patients without SCIs. Pneumonia, pulmonary thromboembolism, septicemia, and renal failure are leading causes of mortality.[39,40]

Table 11: Syndromes of Spinal Cord Injury[38]

Syndrome	Clinical Features
Anterior Cord Syndrome	Characterized by complete paralysis with hyperesthesia and hypoalgesia below the level of the lesion, together with preservation of touch, position, 2-point discrimination, and vibratory sense. The mechanism of injury may either be traumatic or vascular, the latter due to interruption of flow from the anterior spinal artery. Prognosis is generally poor for recovery to ambulation.

Syndrome	Clinical Features
Central Cord Syndrome	Likely the most common of the spinal cord syndromes, this manifests as a disproportionately larger degree of motor impairment of upper versus lower extremities, bladder dysfunction (generally urinary retention), and varying degrees of sensory loss below lesion. Classically associated with older age and pre-existing spinal stenosis with concomitant hyperextension injury of the neck. Prognosis is often favorable, although older age carries a worsened prognosis for ambulation
Brown-Sequard Syndrome (Cord Hemi-section syndrome)	Ipsilateral motor and proprioceptive loss and contralateral loss pain and temperature sensation below the level of the lesion. Minority of spinal cord syndromes but generally has a good prognosis, including regaining ambulation
Posterior Cord Syndrome	Selective posterior column lesion resulting in a loss of vibration and proprioceptive sense below the level of injury, but preserved temperature, muscle strength, and pain sensation. Uncommon and with multiple etiologies for its cause including vascular causes, trauma, and nutritional deficiency.
Conus Medullaris Syndrome (injury of the sacral cord (conus) and lumbar nerve roots within the spinal canal)	Saddle anesthesia, areflexic bladder and bowel, and variable degrees of lower extremity weakness. May clinically show upper and lower motor neuron signs, and a variable degree of pain
Cauda Equina Syndrome (injury to the lumbosacral nerve roots within the neural canal)	Not a true spinal cord injury, damage to the proximal nerve roots in the spinal canal result in saddle anesthesia, bladder and bowel dysfunction, and variable lower extremity involvement with absence of upper motor neuron signs, and asymmetric lower extremity weakness. This syndrome is often associated with a great deal of neuropathic pain

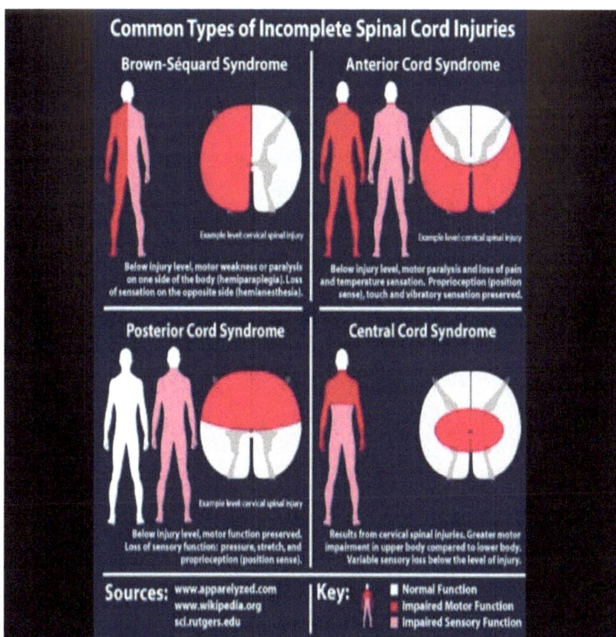

Figure 2: Types of Spinal Cord Injuries

Preventive Care (Department of Community Medicine)

While a certain proportion of accidents leading to neurotrauma are inadvertent and unavoidable, a large number are preventable. Accidents can be better prevented with better education of the populace, improved vehicular safety features (i.e., improved infrastructure and roads, laws to severely prevent driving under the influence of alcohol and drugs, laws to improve safety features of vehicles and infrastructure, laws to enforce helmet use for motorcycle riders, and laws to improve safety in the workplace), and promotion of communal harmony among others will go a long way in decreasing the incidence and severity of neurotrauma. In addition, the development of nation-state trauma systems with quick access to qualified pre-hospital care providers and transport systems, and the establishment of trauma centers (Levels 3 to 1) fully staffed with trained professionals will serve to improve outcomes from traumatic illnesses, including neurotrauma. The use of established training systems such as the Advanced Trauma Life Support (ATLS) offered by the American College of Surgeons should be used in the training of healthcare personnel involved in trauma care. In India, the Departments of Community and Preventive Medicine should be adequately funded and supported in their endeavor to educate and promote healthy lifestyles.

REFERENCES

1. Gururaj G. Epidemiology of traumatic brain injuries: Indian scenario. Neurol Res. 2002 Jan;24(1):24-8.
2. Hyder AA, Wunderlich CA, Puvanachandra P, Gururaj G, Kobusingye OC. The impact of traumatic brain injuries: a globalperspective. NeuroRehabilitation. 2007;22(5):341-53.
3. G Gururaj. Injuries in India: A national Perspective Burden of Disease in India, National Commission on Macroeconomics & Health, Ministry of Health and Family Welfare, Government of India (ed), 2005 325-327.
4. Bratton SL, Chestnut RM, Ghajar J, et al. (2007). "Guidelines for the management of severe traumatic brain injury." J Neurotrauma 24(supl 1): S21-S25.
5. American Academy of Neurology Guidelines on Concussion. http://www.aan.com/professionals/practice/guidelines/pda/Concussion_sports.pdf. Accessed on January 10, 2013.
6. Giza C, Kutcher JS, Ashwal S, Barth J, Getchius TS, Gioia GA, Gronseth GS, Guskiewicz K, Mandel S, Manley G, McKeag DB, Thurman DJ, Zafonte R. Summary of evidence-based guideline update: Evaluation and management of concussion in sports: Report of the Guideline Development Subcommittee of the American Academy of Neurology. 2013. Neurology.
7. Brain Trauma Foundation Guidelines. https://www.braintrauma.org/coma-guidelines/searchable-guidelines. Accessed on February 2nd, 2013.
8. ACS, A. C. o. S. 2004. Advanced Trauma Life Support, Program for Doctors. Chicago.
9. Dinh M, Bein K, Roncal S, Byrne CM, Petchell J, Brennan J. Redefining the golden hour for severe head injury in an urban setting: The effect of prehospital arrival times on patient outcomes. 2013. Injury.
10. Eastridge BJ, Salinas J, Wade CE, Blackbourne LH. Hypotension is 100 mm Hg on the battlefield. Am J Surg. 2011 Oct;202(4):404-8.
11. Morrison CA, Carrick MM, Norman MA, Scott BG, Welsh FJ, Tsai P, Liscum KR, Wall MJ Jr, Mattox KL. Hypotensive resuscitation strategy reduces transfusion requirements and severe postoperative coagulopathy in trauma patients with hemorrhagic shock: preliminary results of a randomized controlled trial. 2011. J Trauma 70: 652-663.
12. Brain Trauma Foundation: Guidelines for the Management of Severe Traumatic Brain Injury, 3rd edition. www.braintrauma.org/pdf/protected/Guidelines_Management_2007w_bookmarks.pdf. Accessed on February 2nd, 2013.
13. Chesnut R, Temkin N, Carney N, Dikmen S, Rondina C, Videtta W, Petroni G, Lujan S, Pridgeon J, Barber J, Machamer J, Chaddock K, Celix JM, Cherner M, Hendrix T. A Trial of Intracranial-Pressure Monitoring in Traumatic Brain Injury.2012. N Engl J Med 367(26): 2471-2481.
14. Farahvar A, Gerber LM, Chiu YL, Carney N, Härtl R, Ghajar J. Increased mortality in patients with severe traumatic brain injury treated without intracranial pressure monitoring. 2012. J neurosurg 117(4): 729-734.
15. Szaflarski JP, Sangha KS, Shutter LA. Prospective, randomized, single-blinded comparative trial of intravenous levetiracetam versus phenytoin for seizure prophylaxis. 2010. Neurocrit Care 12(2): 165-172.
16. David DP, Meade W, Sise MJ, et al. Both hypoxemia and extreme hyperoxemia may be detrimental in patients with severe traumatic brain injury. 2009. Journal of Neurotrauma 26: 2217-2223.
17. Mostafa S, Bhandari S, Ritchie G, Gatton N, Wenstone R. Constipation and its implications in the critically ill patient.2003. Br J Anaesth 91(6): 815-819.
18. Oddo M, Villa F, Citerio G. Brain multimodality monitoring: an update. Curr Opin Crit Care. 2012 Apr;18(2):111-8.
19. Bellner J, Romner B, Reinstrup P, Kristiansson KA, Ryding E, Brandt L. Transcranial Doppler sonography pulsatility index (PI) reflects intracranial pressure (ICP). 2004. Surg Neurol 62(1): 45-51.
20. Voulgaris S, Partheni M, Kaliora H, Haftouras N, Pessach IS, Polyzoidis KS. Early cerebral monitoring using the transcranial Doppler pulsatility index in patients with severe brain trauma. 2005. Medical Science Monitor 11(2): 49-52.
21. Razumovsky A, Armonda RA. We still do not have a reliable and validated noninvasive technique that can provide an accurate quantitative measurement of intracranial pressure (ICP) that could replace invasive quantitative measurements of ICP. 2011. Neurosurgery 68(1): E289-292.
22. de Riva N, Budohoski KP, Smielewski P, Kasprowicz M, Zweifel C, Steiner LA, Reinhard M, Fábregas N, Pickard JD, Czosnyka M. Transcranial Doppler pulsatility index: what it is and what it isn't. 2012.

Neurocrit Care 17(58-66).

23. Zweifel C, Czosnyka M, Carrera E, De Riva N, Pickard JD, Smielewski P. Reliability of the Blood Flow Velocity Pulsatility Index for Assessment of Intracranial and Cerebral Perfusion Pressures in Head Injured Patients. 2012. Neurosurgery.
24. Armonda RA, Bell RS, Vo AH, et al. Wartime traumatic cerebral vasospasm: recent review of combat casualties. 2006. Neurosurgery 59: 1215-1225.
25. Razumovsky A, Tigno T, Hochheimer SM, Stephens FL, Bell R, Vo AH, Severson MA, Marshall SA, Oppenheimer SM, Ecker R, Armonda RA. Cerebral hemodynamic changes after wartime traumatic brain injury. 2013. Acta Neurochir Suppl 115: 87-90.
26. Seel R, Sherer M, Whyte J, Katz DI, Giacino JT, Rosenbaum AM, Hammond FM, Kalmar K, Pape TL, Zafonte R, Biester RC, Kaelin D, Kean J, Zasler N. Assessment scales for disorders of consciousness: evidence-based recommendations for clinical practice and research. 2010. Arch Phys Med Rehabil 91(12): 1795-1813.
27. Cruse D, Chennu S, Chatelle C, Bekinschtein TA, Fernández-Espejo D, Pickard JD, Laureys S, Owen AM. Bedside detection of awareness in the vegetative state: a cohort study. 2011. Lancet 378(9809): 2088-2094.
28. Bardin J, Schiff ND, Voss HU. Pattern classification of volitional functional magnetic resonance imaging responses in patients with severe brain injury. 2012. Arch Neurol 69(2): 176-181.
29. Dyer C. Researchers challenge findings of team that showed awareness in three patients in vegetative state. 2013. BMJ.
30. Hukkelhoven CW, Steyerberg EW, Habbema JD, Farace E, Marmarou A, Murray GD, Marshall LF, Maas AI. Predicting outcome after traumatic brain injury: development and validation of a prognostic score based on admission characteristics. J Neurotrauma. 2005 Oct;22(10):1025-39.
31. Steyerberg E, Mushkudiani N, Perel P, Butcher I, Lu J, McHugh GS, Murray GD, Marmarou A, Roberts I, Habbema JD, Maas A. Predicting outcome after traumatic brain injury: development and international validation of prognostic scores based on admission characteristics. 2008. PLoS Med 5(8): e165.
32. MRCCRASH Trial Collaborators, Perel P, Arango M, Clayton T, Edwards P, Komolafe E, Poccock S, Roberts I, Shakur H, Steyerberg E, Yutthakasemsunt S. Predicting outcome after traumatic brain injury: practical prognostic models based on large cohort of international patients. BMJ. 2008 Feb 23;336(7641):425-9.
33. Lingsma HF, Roozenbeek B, Steyerberg EW, Murray GD, Maas AI. Early prognosis in traumatic brain injury: from prophecies to predictions. Lancet Neurol. 2010 May;9(5):543-54.
34. Edwards P, Arango M, Balica L, et al. CRASH trial collaborators (2005). Final results of MRC CRASH, a randomised placebo-controlled trial of intravenous corticosteroid in adults with head injury-outcomes at 6 months. Lancet 365(9475): 1957-1959.
35. Jackson AB, Dijkers M, DeVivo MJ, Poczatek RB. A demographic profile of new traumatic spinal cord injuries: Change and stability over 30 years. Arch Phys Med Rehabil. 2004 Nov;85(11):1740-8.
36. Steyerberg E, Mushkudiani N, Perel P, Butcher I, Lu J, McHugh GS, Murray GD, Marmarou A, Roberts I, Habbema JD, Maas A. Predicting outcome after traumatic brain injury: development and international validation of prognostic scores based on admission characteristics. 2008. PLoS Med 5(8): e165.
37. Markandaya M, Stein DM, Menaker J. Acute Treatment Options for Spinal Cord Injury. Curr Treat Options Neurol. 2012 Feb 3.
38. McKinley W, Santos K, Meade M, Brooke K. Incidence and Outcomes of Spinal Cord Injury Clinical Syndromes J Spinal Cord Med. 2007; 30(3): 215–224.
39. Spinal Cord Injury Facts. http://www.fscip.org/facts.htm Accessed January 21st, 2013.
40. DeVivo MJ, Kartus PL, Stover SL, Rutt RD, Fine PR. Cause of death for patients with spinal cord injuries. Arch Intern Med. 1989;149(8):1761.
41. Bracken MB, Shepard MJ, Holford TR, et al. Administration of methylprednisolone for 24 or 48 hours or tirilazad mesylate for 48 hours in the treatment of acute spinal cord injury. Results of the Third National Acute Spinal Cord Injury Randomized Controlled Trial. National Acute Spinal Cord Injury Study. JAMA. 1997 May 28;277(20):1597-604. PMID: 9168289.

❑❑❑

51

CHAPTER

Penetrating Neck and Thoracic Trauma

Mayur Narayan, MD

INTRODUCTION

The initial evaluation of the patient with a penetrating thoracic injury is relatively straightforward and should follow the standard ATLS trauma algorithm. However, patients with vascular injuries in the thoracic cavity are likely to be unstable and require immediate intervention. In the case of injury to the great vessels or their major branches, exsanguinating hemorrhage into the thoracic cavity is commonplace; each hemithorax can accommodate more than half of a patient's normal circulating volume.[1] In hemodynamically unstable patients, exploratory thoracotomy should be performed in the operating room as soon as possible. For those with stable vital signs, chest radiography should be obtained to identify a hemothorax, and a tube thoracostomy performed to evacuate any blood. Approximately 150-200 mL of blood needs to be present in the chest cavity in order to appear on chest x-ray.[2] Generally agreed-upon indications for thoracotomy are immediate drainage of greater than 1500 mL, or ongoing bleeding greater than 250 mL/hr.[3] For these patients, operative planning should be based on the suspected site of injury. For example, a left-sided thoracotomy may provide better exposure of the descending aorta and left subclavian vessels, while a median sternotomy may be required to adequately visualize the proximal arch, innominate vessel, and aortic root injuries.

Emergency Department Thoracotomy

Vascular injuries often necessitate an emergency department thoracotomy (EDT) to obtain control over the hemorrhage. The American College of Surgeons (ACS) has published guidelines regarding the use of EDT, and it is prudent to briefly outline their application here. With regard to penetrating chest wounds, the ACS recommends EDT for patients with witnessed loss of vital signs shortly before arrival or in the trauma unit. The goals of the procedure are to release pericardial tamponade, control intrathoracic or intracardiac hemorrhage, occlude the descending thoracic aorta in order to maximize cerebral and coronary blood flow, and to perform open cardiac massage.[4] To perform an EDT, the patient is positioned supine. An anterolateral thoracotomy is made in the 5th intercostal space and the chest cavity is entered. This incision is advantageous as it does not require a saw, and can easily be extended in a clam-shell fashion for access to the right hemithorax if needed.[5] Once the pericardium is identified, pericardiotomy should be made longitudinally, parallel with and anterior to the left phrenic nerve. Repair of cardiac injuries is covered below. Bleeding from the central lung area can be controlled with the placement of a large Satinsky clamp or by twisting the hilum around its axis.[4] In order to clamp the descending thoracic aorta, the lung is first mobilized superiorly by incising the inferior pulmonary ligament. The ligament ends proximally at the inferior pulmonary vein, so care should be taken not to transect this structure during the maneuver.[4] Once the lung is retracted, the aorta is identified posterior to the esophagus, which should be intubated with a nasogastric tube to aid in identification. The mediastinal pleura is either incised under direct vision or finger dissected free of the aorta, and a clamp placed across, avoiding any intercostal arteries arising posteriorly. If these maneuvers are successful in restoring vital signs, the patient should then be transported to the operating room for definitive management.

PENETRATING CARDIAC INJURIES

Cardiac injuries have been found to represent approximately 6% of all penetrating thoracic traumas.[6] Not unexpectedly, penetrating trauma involving the heart portends a grave prognosis, with overall mortality approaching 80%.[7] Of these patients, over half generally die at the scene of the incident.[8] Of those who do make it to a trauma center, factors associated with improved likelihood of survival include stab wounds (versus gunshot wounds), hemodynamic stability on presentation, and the presence of pericardial tamponade.[9] Improved survival seen in patients with tamponade is controversial, but most likely reflects the fact that penetrating cardiac injuries generally present with either tamponade or exsanguinating hemorrhage, with the former being by definition contained.

Cardiac Tamponade

Cardiac injury should be suspected with any penetrating injury to the so-called "cardiac box," defined as the area bordered superiorly by the clavicles, laterally by the nipples, and inferiorly by the costal margins. Physical examination may reveal distended jugular veins, muffled heart tones, dyspnea, and pulsus paradoxus, although none of these findings are overly specific. Tamponade may acutely prove beneficial, as increased pericardial pressure may slow bleeding from the injured heart chamber. However, this quickly leads to depression of cardiac output, cardiogenic shock, and arrest.[3] Along the same lines, opening the pericardium will immediately relieve the tamponade, but the surgeon should be prepared to expeditiously repair the underlying injury. If pericardial blood or a clot is encountered, the next step should be to proceed to either sternotomy or thoracotomy.[7]

In hemodynamically stable patients with cardiac box injuries, echocardiography should be obtained expediently to evaluate for abnormal pericardial fluid. This may be obtained in the emergency department by use of the subxiphoid window of the FAST (Focused Abdominal Sonography for Trauma) exam. Echocardiography is an excellent diagnostic tool for hemopericardium, with sensitivity of 90-100% reported.[10,11] If ultrasound is not readily available, a subxiphoid pericardial window may be performed for diagnosis as well as evacuation of pericardial blood. This should be done in the operating room, as opening the pericardium may lead to massive hemorrhage which can be difficult to control. An incision should be made in the midline at the level of the xiphoid process. The sternum is elevated and retracted anteriorly, and blunt dissection used to separate the diaphragm from the pericardium. The pericardium can then be grasped with an instrument such as an Allis clamp and incised sharply.

Cardiac Repair

Once the pericardium has been opened (either in a controlled setting or during EDT), attention should be turned to the identification of the cardiac defect. Temporary control can be obtained by simply placing a finger over the hole, or by inserting a Foley catheter and inflating the balloon. One advantage of the latter is that fluid and medications can be administered through the lumen,[3] but the balloon can expand the hole if too much traction is used. Immediate closure can also be obtained with a skin stapler, especially in the setting of an emergency resuscitative thoracotomy. These measures will allow some time for fluid resuscitation and internal cardiac massage, should it be necessary. Sutures placed in the heart should ideally be placed by an experienced cardiac surgeon, and should be small caliber, pledgeted monofilament sutures (such as polypropylene). Care should be taken to avoid coronary vessels running along the myocardium, specifically the left anterior descending artery in cases of left ventricular injury.

BLUNT CARDIAC INJURY

Blunt cardiac injury (BCI) is a common clinical entity, occurring in 20-76% of patients with blunt thoracic trauma.[1] In simpler cases of minor bruising to the myocardium, diagnosis is difficult and BCI may go unnoticed without consequence. Severe cases may include cardiac free wall rupture and death.[1] Any patient with blunt trauma to the chest should have an ECG performed to evaluate for arrhythmia, ST abnormalities and heart block, as well as a troponin-I drawn.[12] If both of these are normal, BCI can essentially be ruled out.[12] Evidence of valvular dysfunction (i.e. murmur) or CHF on physical exam, arrhythmia or hypotension should prompt echocardiographic evaluation.

BLUNT AORTIC INJURIES

Blunt aortic injury (BAI) yields a very low survival rate, with 75-90% of patients dying on-scene, and only approximately 8% surviving more than 4 hours.[13] BAI usually occurs with rapid deceleration, leading to extreme shearing force on the vessel. The aortic isthmus, just distal to the takeoff of the left subclavian artery, is at particular risk as it is fixed in place relative to the more mobile arch.[1] Identification of BAI requires a high index of suspicion, and information from the scene can often help identify those patients at risk. Factors associated with blunt aortic injury in motor vehicle crashes include head-on collisions, changes in velocity of greater than 20 mph, impacts on the victim's side of the car, and intrusions of greater than 15 cm.[14] As these generally involve high impact forces, they are associated with other significant injuries in up to 90% of cases, up to a quarter of which require intervention prior to aortic repair.[15] Injuries associated with a concomitant blunt aortic injury include closed head injuries, multiple rib fractures, pulmonary contusions, and orthopedic injuries.[16]

Plain radiography can often yield clues to an underlying aortic injury. A widened mediastinum to greater than 8 cm or 25% of the chest width at the level of the aortic arch should prompt further evaluation.[17] More specific findings suggestive of BAI, although uncommon, include opacification of the aortopulmonary window and irregularity of the aortic knob, tracheal and esophageal deviation to the right, left apical capping, and depression of the left mainstem bronchus.[18] The gold standard for the diagnosis of BAI is aortography, but as a non-invasive alternative computed tomography angiography (CTA) is an excellent diagnostic modality and should be used whenever BAI is suspected. A mediastinal hematoma is a sensitive finding but may be present in up to 20% of scans performed for trauma without a BAI.[18] Direct signs of injury including intimal tear, dissection (Figure 1 and 2), intramural hematoma, pseudoaneurysm, or active extravasation of contrast.

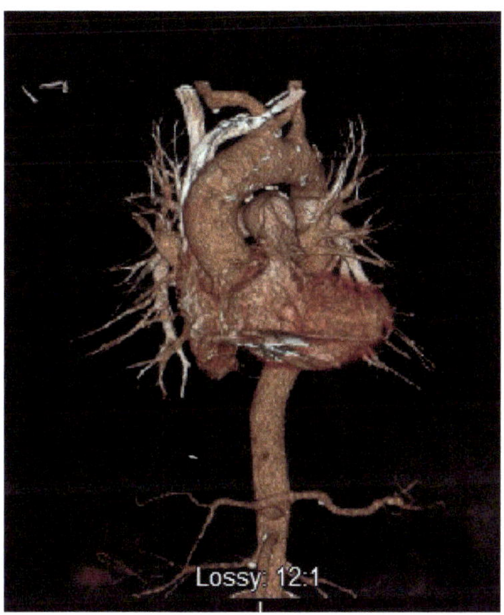

Figure 1: Normal CT angiogram for aortic dissection

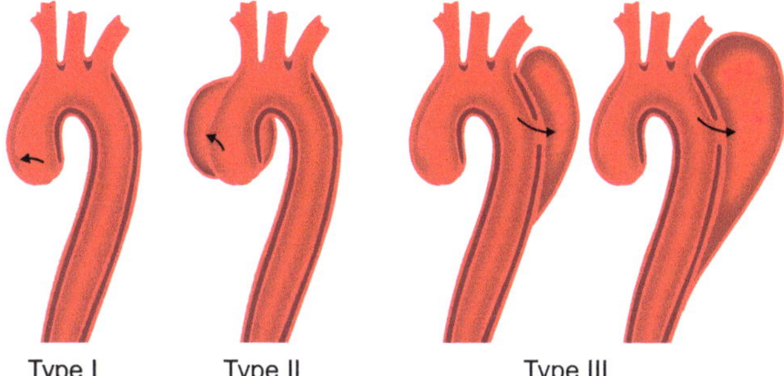

Figure 2: Aortic dissection classification

With regard to the degree of injury, transection of the aorta is almost uniformly lethal at the scene.[19] The remainder of patients are graded based on the severity of the injury: grade I involves intimal tear, grade II involves intramural hematoma, grade III involves pseudoaneurysm, and grade IV involves frank rupture.[20] For those with grade I and select grade II injuries, non-operative management with strict blood pressure control and serial imaging studies to evaluate for progression is reasonable and associated with resolution in the majority of patients.[21,22] For those with higher grade injuries, open or endovascular repair is indicated.

Open repair

Traditionally, thoracic aortic injuries have been treated similarly to aneurysmal disease. Circumferential control is obtained proximal and distal to the injury, the aorta is cross-clamped, and an interposition graft is used to replace the damaged segment. This is the tried-and-true method of repair, and the standard to which other methods should be compared. Mortality from open repair is approximately 12%.[23] However, cross-clamping the aorta leads to a significant rate of paralysis secondary to spinal cord ischemia (on the order of 2-8%)[24-26] and other morbidities including stroke and recurrent laryngeal nerve injury.[27] Most series demonstrate the durability of open repair, with most patients not needing to readdress their thoracic aorta.[28]

Endovascular Repair (TEVAR)

Endovascular therapy for thoracic aortic injuries has largely replaced open repair in areas where this technology is readily available (Figure 3). Interest in applying endovascular techniques to traumatic injuries largely came about because of the well-described high morbidity and mortality associated with traditional open repair, and the success with which non-emergent thoracic and abdominal aortic aneurysms have been repaired using this method. Many studies have shown the superiority of TEVAR, and meta-analysis has demonstrated decreased mortality, improved paraplegia and stroke rates, and decreased hospital stay.[27,29,30] A large, prospective, multi-center study again demonstrated lower mortality as well as a smaller transfusion requirement, but did express some concerns for device-related complications such as endoleak.[26] Although this technique appears to be a good alternative to open repair, TEVAR is not without its disadvantages. Injury to the access vessel (iliac or femoral) is common.[26] Coverage of the left subclavian artery can lead to a vertebral-basilar stroke and arm ischemia requiring revascularization procedures,[31] and endoleak can necessitate either endovascular re-intervention or a conversion to open repair.[26] Given these concerns, TEVAR in the traumatic setting should be limited to those centers with extensive expertise and a large endovascular case volume.

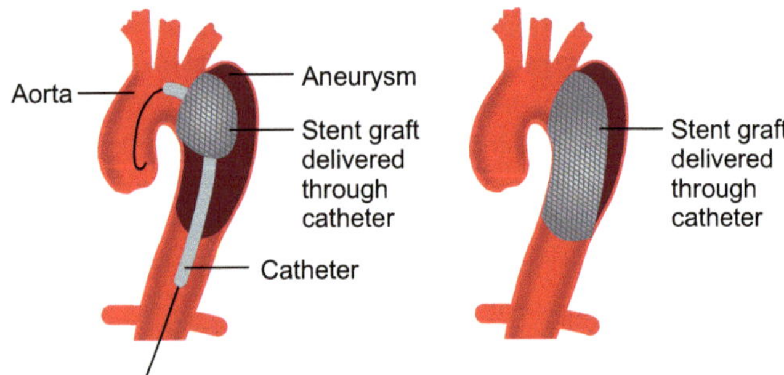

Figure 3: TEVAR Procedure

BLUNT VASCULAR NECK INJURY

Blunt injury to the great vessels of the neck and thoracic outlet are difficult to diagnose, and potentially catastrophic, with high rates of stroke and injury-specific mortality.[32,33] Therefore, identification and screening of those blunt trauma patients at highest risk is of critical importance. A careful and thorough physical exam should be the standard, although this is a poorly sensitive tool. Factors associated with higher risk and which justify screening include patients presenting with neurologic deficit (GCS ≤8) unexplained by another injury, arterial epistaxis, petrous bone fracture, diffuse axonal injury, cervical spine fractures (specifically C1-C3 or through the transverse foramen, or with subluxation or rotational component), or Lefort-II or -III midface fractures.[34] These patients may be screened with either multislice computed tomographic angiography (CTA) or magnetic resonance angiography (MRA), when available. These modalities have shown similar sensitivity in diagnosis and are more cost-effective and less invasive than traditional angiography.[35,36] However, CT angiogram can be compromised by poorly timed contrast administration, motion artifact, and body habitus so negative studies should be taken with caution in the setting of high clinical suspicion.[37] Additionally, when non-invasive screening is not possible, angiographic evaluation of the neck is warranted and remains the gold-standard.

Blunt injuries to the arteries of the neck are generally graded as follows: (1) intimal irregularity with <25% luminal compromise, (2) dissection or intramural hematoma with >25% compromise, (3) pseudoaneurysm, (4) vessel occlusion, and (5) transection with contrast extravasation.[38] Management should be based on the consensus guidelines from the Eastern Association for the Surgery of Trauma (EAST):[34] grade I and II injuries should be managed with anti-thrombotic therapy including heparin or aspirin, although the use of these agents is often precluded by the presence of associated injuries. Follow-up angiograms may be considered at 7 days, to evaluate for resolution or progression of these low severity injuries. These patients should be subsequently treated for 3-6 months with oral anticoagulation. Injuries of grade III and higher warrant intervention, either via open repair or endovascular intervention where feasible. Endovascular stenting may be particularly suited to internal carotid injuries not easily accessible through a cervical incision.[39] Also, any carotid or vertebral injury with an associated neurologic deficit should be intervened on in order to restore cerebral blood flow.

PENETRATING VASCULAR NECK INJURY

As is the case with blunt injury, penetrating wounds often lead to devastating injuries of the neck vasculature. These wounds are classified into three anatomic zones, based on the potentially injured structures in each and organized by simple physical landmarks.[40] Zone I represents the area from the thoracic inlet inferiorly to the cricothyroid membrane superiorly. Zone II includes the area from the cricothyroid membrane to the angle of the mandible, and Zone III above the angle of the mandible. Zone I trauma is generally managed as thoracic injuries, with the vascular structures most at risk being the proximal branches of the aortic arch and the arch itself. Zone III injuries are generally treated as head traumas. The major vessel in jeopardy in this area is the internal carotid artery (ICA). Access to, and control of the ICA above the mandible is challenging, and assistance from otorhinolaryngology or neurosurgery may be prudent. Zone II injuries represent the bulk of penetrating vascular neck injuries, and put the common, internal, and external carotid arteries at risk, as well as the superior thyroid artery and other smaller branches. Venous structures including the internal jugular and common facial veins may also be injured. Therefore, management of Zone II injuries shall be the main focus of this section.

Many patients with penetrating Zone II neck injuries are asymptomatic at presentation but may still have significant underlying injuries.[41] However, most patients with vascular injuries will be symptomatic in some way,[42] and the physical exam is extremely sensitive in detecting major arterial injury.[43] Therefore, it has been proposed that asymptomatic patients be initially managed non-operatively and undergo angiography, esophagoscopy, and bronchoscopy. From a vascular standpoint this is reasonable given the low likelihood of major vascular injuries in this population. Where possible, CT angiogram or duplex ultrasound are safe, non-invasive alternatives.[40] Regarding symptomatic patients, those with hard signs (active hemorrhage, expanding hematoma) should undergo immediate neck exploration. In patients with soft signs only (bruit, non-expanding hematoma, pulse deficit), angiogram or an appropriate non-invasive diagnostic test should be used.

In cases of carotid injury, it is safe to observe non-occlusive intimal injuries.[40] For higher grade injuries, exposure is obtained via a longitudinal incision along the medial border of the sternocleidomastoid muscle. Proximal and distal control should be obtained, which may require extension of the incision to either an anterior thoracotomy or median sternotomy. Any identified injuries should be repaired (when possible) either primarily or patch angioplasty when there is concern for luminal narrowing. An interposition graft may also be used if there is significant loss of arterial length. Injuries to the internal carotid artery should always be repaired if possible, even in the presence of a significant neurologic deficit,[40] as arteriorrhaphy provides better long term neurologic outcomes when compared to simple ligation.[44] Vertebral arterial injuries represent a distinct challenge due to their anatomic location which makes exposure and control difficult; distal control may require a suboccipital craniectomy.[45] Angiographic embolization can be safely used in cases of complex pseudoaneurysms and arteriovenous fistulae.[46] Operative repair should therefore be reserved for major, uncontrolled hemorrhage from these vessels.[40] In cases of venous injury, simple ligation of the major branches such as the internal jugular or subclavian vein is safe, especially in the setting of hemodynamic instability.[47]

REFERENCES

1. Bernardin B, Troquet JM. Initial management and resuscitation of severe chest trauma. *Emerg Med Clin N Am.* 2011:377-400.
2. Miller L. Chest wall, lung and pleural space trauma. *Radiol Clin North Am.* 2006;44:213.
3. Bastos R, Baisden CE, Harker L, Calhoon JH. Penetrating thoracic trauma. *Semin Thorac Cardiovasc Surg.* 2008;20:19-25.
4. Mejia J, Stewart RM, Cohn SM. Emergency department thoracotomy. *Semin Thorac Cardiovasc Surg.* 2008;20(1):13-18.
5. McGonigle N, McManus K. Penetrating thoracic trauma. *Surgery (Oxford).* 2011;29(5):227-230.
6. Mandal A, Sanusi M. Penetrating chest wounds: 24 years experience. *World J Surg.* 2001;25(9):1145-1149.
7. O'Connor J, Ditillo M, Scalea T. Penetrating cardiac injury. *JR Army Med Corps.* 2009;155(3):185-190.
8. Naughton M, Brissie RM, Bessey PQ, McEachern MM, Donald JM, Law HL. Demography of penetrating cardiac trauma. *Ann Surg.* 1989;209(6):676-681.
9. Tyburski J, Astra L, Wilson RF, Dente C, Steffes C. Factors affecting prognosis with penetrating wounds of the heart. *J Trauma.* 2000;48(4):587-590.
10. Rozycki G, Feliciano DV, Oschner MG, Knudson MM, Hoyt D, Davis F, Hammerman D, Figueredo V, Harviel JD, Han DC, Schmidt JA. The role of ultrasound in patients with possible penetrating cardiac wounds: a prospective multicenter study. *J Trauma.* 1999;46(4):543-551.
11. Jimenez E, Martin M, Krukenkamp I, Barrett J. Subxyphoid window versus echocardiography: a prospective evaluation of the diagnosis of occult penetrating cardiac injury. *Surgery.* 1990;108(4):676-679.
12. Clancy K, Velopulos C, Bilaniuk JW, Collier B, Crowley W, Kurek S, Lui F, Nayduch D, Sangosanya A, Tucker B, Haut E. Screening for blunt cardiac injury: an Eastern Association for the Surgery of Trauma practice management guideline. *J Trauma Acute Care Surg.* 2012;73(5):S301-S306.
13. Cook C, Gleason TG. Great vessel and cardiac trauma. *Surg Clin N Am.* 2009;89:797-820.
14. Neschis D, Scalea TM, Flinn WR, Griffith BP. Blunt aortic injury. *N Eng J Med.* 2008;359:1708-1716.
15. Pate J, Fabian TC, Walker W. Traumatic rupture of the aortic isthmus: an emergency? *World J Surg.* 1995;19:119-126.
16. Fabian T, Richardson JD, Croce MA, et al. Prospective study of blunt aortic injury: Multicenter Trial of the American Association for the Surgery of Trauma. *J Trauma.* 1997;42(3):374-380.
17. Steenburg S, Ravenel JG, Ikonomidis JS, Schönholz C, Reeves S. Acute traumatic aortic injury: imaging evaluation and management. *Radiology.* 2008;248(3):748-762.
18. de Gracia M, Artigas Martin JM, Soto JA. Evaluation of thoracic vascular trauma with multidetector computed tomography. *Semin Roentgenol.* 2012;47(4):342-351.
19. Smith R, Chang FC. Traumatic rupture of the aorta: still a lethal injury. *Am J Surg.* 1986;152:660-663.
20. Lee W, Matsumura JS, Mitchell RS, Farber MA, Greenberg RK, Azizzadeh A, Murad MH, Fairman RM. Endovascular repair of traumatic thoracic aortic injury: clinical practice guidelines of the Society for Vascular Surgery. *J Vasc Surg.* 2011;53(1):187-192.
21. Kidane B, Abramowitz D, Harris JR, Derose G, Forbes TL. Natural history of minimal aortic injury following blunt thoracic aortic trauma. *Can J Surg.* 2012;55(6):377-381.
22. Paul J, Neideen T, Tutton S, Milia D, Tolat P, Foley D, Brasel K. Minimal aortic injury after blunt trauma: selective nonoperative management is safe. *J Trauma.* 2011;71(6):1519-1523.
23. Cannon R, Trivedi JR, Pagni S, Dwivedi A, Bland JN, Slaughter MS, Ross CB, Richardson JD, Williams ML. Open repair of blunt thoracic aortic injury remains relevant in the endovascular era. *J Am Coll Surg.* 2012;214(6):943-949.
24. Cindy M, Sabrina H, Kim D, Geert M, Inge F. Traumatic aortic rupture: 30 years experience. *Ann Vasc Surg.* 2011;25(4):474-480.

25. Celis R, Park SC, Shukla AJ, Zenati MS, Chaer RA, Rhee RY, Makaroun MS, Cho JS. Evolution of treatment for traumatic thoracic aortic injuries. *J Vasc Surg.* 2012;56(1):74-80.
26. Demetriades D, Velmahos GC, Scalea TM, et al. Operative repair or endovascular stent graft in blunt traumatic thoracic aortic injuries: results of an American Association for the Surgery of Trauma Multicenter Study. *J Trauma.* 2008;64(3):561-570.
27. Tang G, Tehrani HY, Usman A, Katariya K, Otero C, Perez E, Eskandari MK. Reduced mortality, paraplegia, and stroke with stent graft repair of blunt aortic transections: a modern meta-analysis. *J Vasc Surg.* 2008;47(3):671-675.
28. Patel H, Hemmila MR, Williams DM, Diener AC, Deeb GM. Late outcomes following open and endovascular repair of blunt thoracic aortic injury. *J Vasc Surg.* 2011;53(3):615-620.
29. Xenos E, Abedi NN, Davenport DL, Minion DJ, Hamdallah O, Sorial EE, Endean ED. Meta-analysis of endovascular vs open repair for traumatic descending thoracic aortic rupture. *J Vasc Surg.* 2008;48(5):1343-1351.
30. Patel H, Williams DM, Upchurch GR Jr, Dasika NL, Deeb GM. A comparative analysis of open and endovascular repair for the ruptured descending thoracic aorta. *J Vasc Surg.* 2009;50(6):1265-1270.
31. Mitchell M, Rushton FW Jr, Boland AB, Byrd TC, Baldwin ZK. Emergency procedures on the descending thoracic aorta in the endovascular era. *J Vasc Surg.* 2011;54(5):1298-1302.
32. Schneidereit N, Simons R, Nicolaou S, Graeb D, Brown DR, Kirkpatrick A, Redekop G, McKevitt EC, Neyestani A. Utility of screening for blunt vascular neck injuries with computed tomographic angiography. *J Trauma.* 2006;60(1):209-215.
33. McKevitt E, Kirkpatrick AW, Vertesi L, Granger R, Simons RK. Blunt vascular neck injuries: diagnosis and outcomes of extracranial vessel injury. *J Trauma.* 2002;53(3):472-476.
34. Bromberg W, Collier BC, Diebel LN, Dwyer KM, Holevar MR, Jacobs DG, Kurek SJ, Schreiber MA, Shapiro ML, Vogel TR. Blunt cerebrovascular injury practice management guidelines: the Eastern Association for the Surgery of Trauma. *J Trauma.* 2010;68(2):471-477.
35. Wang A, Charters MA, Thawani JP, Than KD, Sullivan SE, Graziano GP. Evaluating the use and utility of noninvasive angiography in diagnosing traumatic blunt cerebrovascular injury. *J Trauma Acute Care Surg.* 2012;72(6):1601-1610.
36. Eastman A, Chason DP, Perez CL, McAnulty AL, Minei JP. Computed tomographic angiography for the diagnosis of blunt cervical vascular injury: is it ready for primetime? *J Trauma.* 2006;60(5):925-929.
37. Malhotra A, Camacho M, Ivatury RR, et al. Computed tomographic angiography for the diagnosis of blunt carotid/vertebral artery injury: a note of caution. *Ann Surg.* 2007;246(4):632-642.
38. Biffl W, Moore EE, Offner PJ, Brega KE, Francoise RJ, Burch JM. Blunt carotid arterial injuries: implications of a new grading scale. *J Trauma.* 1999;47:845-853.
39. Seth R, Obuchowski AM, Zoarski GH. Endovascular Repair of Traumatic Cervical Internal Carotid Artery Injuries: A Safe and Effective Treatment Option. *Am J Neuroradiol.* 2012;Epub.
40. Tisherman S, Bokhari F, Collier B, Cumming J, Ebert J, Holevar M, Kurek S, Leon S, Rhee P. Clinical practice guideline: penetrating zone II neck trauma. *J Trauma.* 2008;64(5):1392-1405.
41. Markey J, Hines JL, Nance FC. Penetrating neck wounds: A review of 218 cases. *Am Surg.* 1975;41:77-83.
42. Nason R, Assuras GN, Gray PR, Lipschitz J, Burns CM. Penetrating neck injuries: analysis of experience from a Canadian trauma centre. *Can J Surg.* 2001;44(2):122-126.
43. Demetriades D, Theodorou D, Cornwell E 3rd, Weaver F, Yellin A, Velmahos G, Berne TV. Penetrating injuries of the neck in patients in stable condition. Physical examination, angiography, or color flow Doppler imaging. *Arch Surg.* 1995;130(9):971-975.
44. Weaver F, Yellin AE, Wagner WH, Brooks SH, Weaver AA, Milford MA. The role of arterial reconstruction in penetrating carotid injuries. *Arch Surg.* 1988;123(9):1106-1111.
45. Demetriades D, Theodorou D, Asensio J, Golshani S, Belzberg H, Yellin A, Weaver F, Berne TV. Management options in vertebral artery injuries. *Br J Surg.* 1996;83(1):83-86.
46. Albuquerque F, Javedan SP, McDougall CG. Endovascular management of penetrating vertebral artery injuries. *J Trauma Inj Infect Crit Care.* 2002;53:574-580.
47. Nair R, Robbs JV, Muckart DJ. Management of penetrating cervicomediastinal venous trauma. *Eur J Vasc Endovasc Surg.* 2000;19(1):65-69.

❑❑❑

52

CHAPTER

Vascular Trauma

Morgan McMonagle, MD, FRCSI
S Rai, FRCS
Rajiv Vohra, Ph.D., FRCSEd, FRCSEng

Mechanism of Vascular Injury

The mechanism of injury in vascular trauma may be blunt, penetrating (high vs. low velocity), or iatrogenic. For both blunt and penetrating injuries, the force is directed from the external environment, passing through the surrounding tissues, and therefore carries a high risk of associated injury patterns to other organs and tissue planes (with added bleeding), in addition to the vascular injury itself. The injured vessel will almost always have evidence of surrounding hematoma or traumatic streaking of the adventitia, even if very small. On the other hand, iatrogenic injury typically results from injury during an endovascular procedure. Thus, unless the vessel wall is traversed completely by the instrument, these injuries may not have the surrounding hematoma and inflammation as described above and may only be confined to a small intimal tear or irregularity.

Epidemiology

Overall, significant arterial injuries account for less than 10% of injuries. However, when present, these injuries represent a very challenging subgroup of patients at risk of rapid exsanguination, but at the same time, many are amenable to a complete repair with successful outcomes, if there is survival upon arrival to the hospital. Massive hemorrhage followed by a spiraling combination of hypothermia, coagulopathy, and acidosis ('Triad of Death'), representing metabolic and physiologic exhaustion, leads to the demise of the trauma patient. Expedient hemorrhage control and reversal of this triad is, therefore, key to survival after major vascular injury.

Decision Making

Decision making in trauma, especially when active hemorrhage is present, is based on patient physiology. Physiologically unwell patients, often referred to rather misleadingly as 'unstable,' mandate immediate surgical management. Patients who are physiologically within normal limits can be afforded time to undergo further investigations, as indicated. CT scanning for the trauma patient is now a well-established investigation in western healthcare, enabling the treating physician to identify life-threatening injury earlier. However, it is important for the examining physician to appreciate that any patient presenting with "hard" signs of vascular injury should undergo immediate surgical management, or occasionally endovascular management, without the need for further diagnostic work-up (save for an on-table angiogram as indicated) (Table 1).

Table 1: Hard vs. soft signs of vascular injury

Signs of Vascular Injury	
Hard Signs **(High sensitivity and specificity)**	**Soft Signs** **(Low sensitivity and specificity)**
• Active arterial hemorrhage • Expanding/pulsatile hematoma • Bruit/thrill over hematoma • Loss of distal pulses	• History of bleeding • Injury in close proximity to a vessel • Non-pulsatile hematoma • Non-pulsatile bleeding • Neurological deficit • Unexplained hypotension • Diminished (but not absent) pulse

Hard versus Soft Signs of Vascular Injury

Hard signs of vascular injury are clinical signs representing either arterial bleeding or arterial ischemia, and if present, mandate further operative exploration and management without the need for diagnostic investigations (Table 1). Hard signs include active hemorrhage, pulsatile hematoma, audible bruit/palpable thrill over a hematoma, or an absence of distal pulses and the classic signs of acute limb ischemia. Such signs are highly predictive of significant arterial injury.[1]

Soft signs are anything else associated with injury that may alert the examining physician to the possibility of vascular injury, but they have a low sensitivity and specificity for significant arterial trauma. Soft signs include injury or trajectory in close proximity to a vessel, history of bleeding on scene, non-pulsatile bleeding, non-pulsatile hematoma, nerve deficit, and unexplained hypotension. In the absence of hard signs of vascular injury, significant arterial injury is unlikely, although 'minimal vascular injury' may still be present (Table 1).

It should also be remembered that the hard and soft signs are best applied to the extremities, and obviously do not predict vascular injury in the chest or abdominal-pelvic cavity, i.e., the non-compressible cavities. In addition, carotid injury may display classic hard signs, but detecting the loss of distal pulses in this situation is difficult. A high index of suspicion is needed for these potentially challenging injuries.

Minimal Vascular Injury (MVI)

Minimal vascular injury (MVI) is a term used to describe minor vessel trauma that does not lead to hard signs and is usually picked up incidentally during investigations: CT angiogram, catheter-directed angiography, or Duplex scanning. Additionally, the injury is often confined to the intimal layer.[2,3] There are four recognized subtypes: focal segmental narrowing, intimal flap/irregularity, small pseudoaneurysms, and small arterio-venous (AV) fistulas (Table 2). The important characteristic of MVI is that there is no active bleeding outside the vessel, and there is preservation of antegrade flow with no distal ischemia (i.e., hard signs are absent).

Table 2: Minimal vascular injury

Minimal Vascular Injury	
Type	**Characteristics**
1. Focal segmental narrowing	Smooth, regular narrowing with no constriction to flow. It may be caused by external compression, vessel wall hematoma or reactive spasm
2. Intimal flap or irregularity	Small tear in intima protruding into lumen. The flap may be raised with either an antegrade or retrograde orientation, but there is no obstruction to luminal flow
3. Pseudoaneurysm	Incomplete laceration of vessel with contained bleeding into a small volume of surrounding tissue, probably <1.5 cm
4. AV fistula	Simultaneous lacerations in adjacent and juxtaposed artery and vein that actively communicate without passing through the capillary bed, probably <1.5 cm

The natural history of untreated MVI is well-described in the literature, and simple observation appears to be the management of choice as the vast majority heal spontaneously.[4-7] About 10% of cases will develop symptoms which can be managed effectively, without any associated increase in either mortality or morbidity. Although more likely to develop symptoms, those with small pseudoaneurysms (<2 cm) can be safely observed. However, 40% of larger pseudoaneurysms will eventually require treatment; harm to the patient is unlikely.

Emergency Department Management of Vascular Injuries

All trauma patients should be examined and managed *as per* the Advanced Trauma Life Support (ATLS®) guidelines of the American College of Surgeons. The trauma team should maintain a high index of suspicion for vascular injuries due to the potential for rapid exsanguination, especially with injuries to a non-compressible cavity. Always consider the mechanism of injury (e.g., trans-abdominal gunshot wound, open-book pelvic fracture, etc.). In addition, any patient presenting with hard signs of vascular injury mandates immediate surgical exploration.

Vascular injuries do not require large amounts of fluid resuscitation. It is better for actively bleeding patients to become relatively hypotensive ('permissive hypotension' or 'resuscitative hypotension') as a 'bridge' to definitive hemostasis and further surgical management.[8] The actively bleeding poly-trauma patient only requires a survivable blood pressure (SBP 80-90 mmHg), and not a normal blood pressure. It is the "time to hemostasis" that is the single most important determinant of survival in active hemorrhage in the absence of a significant head injury. Hypotensive resuscitation minimizes blood loss prior to surgical hemorrhage control.[9]

Higher pressures, when artificially created with fluids and vasoconstrictors or inotropic agents, run the risk of dislodging the already vital but unstable thrombus at the site of bleeding ('pop the clot' syndrome), thereby encouraging further hemorrhage. In addition, fluids especially crystalloid and colloids, will further contribute to a dilutional coagulopathy as well as worsening hypothermia. Any fluid used should be in the form of blood and clotting factors and administered through a warming device.

The surgeon must also decide the order of priority for other 'competing' injuries, especially in the presence of head trauma at the time of entering the operating room. However, in general, significant vascular injury will take highest priority.

General Approach to Operative Management

The operating room should be well equipped with both major vascular and general surgery instruments for both the chest and abdomen. The operating room temperature should be set at 30°C to avoid hypothermia, which itself is an independent predictor of mortality. The blood cell-saver should be primed and ready for use. A blood-fluid warmer used for cold blood or room-temperature fluids should never be administered to bleeding patients as it will worsen the coagulopathy and hypothermia (Figure 1).

Rapid Infuser

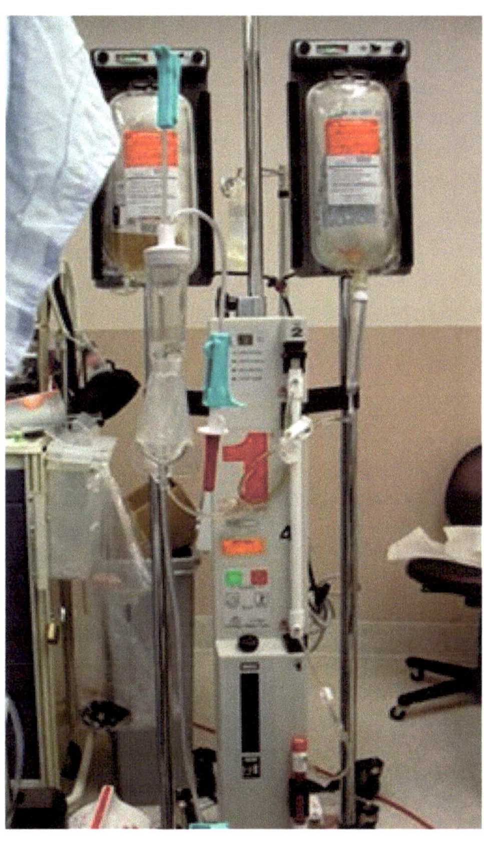

Cell Saver

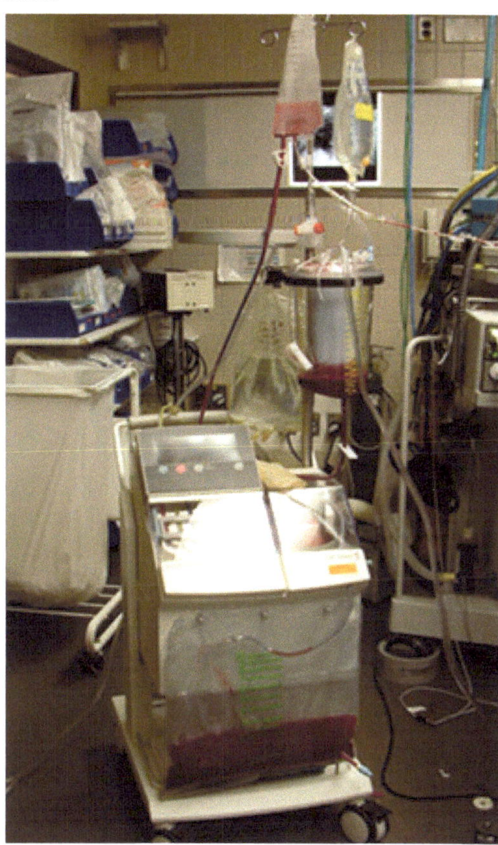

Figure 1: Rapid fluid infuser, which also warms fluids to body temperature, and cell saver (auto-transfuser) used in surgery where there is a high risk of rapid exsanguination

Individual staff members should be assigned tasks by the lead trauma surgeon (*e.g.,* blood checking and administration, anesthetic support, circulating for equipment, etc.). Close communication with anesthetic staff is paramount, especially at critical times, such as simultaneous intubation and initiation of surgery. If not already intubated, induction of anesthesia in the bleeding patient is a coordinated effort between the anesthetist and surgeon. Use of a reduced dose of induction agent to avoid further worsening of the hypotension, and the rapid sequence intubation (RSI) should occur at the same time, and in-parallel with the 'first cut' of surgery. This is particularly important for major cavity bleeding, where hemorrhage is non-compressible, *i.e.*, chest, abdomen, and pelvis. The first surgical incision is made as the anesthetist views the endotracheal tube pass through the vocal cords. Further communication between the anesthesiologist and surgeon is a continuous exercise, and the surgeon should be kept up-to-date at regular intervals with regard to the patient's vital signs, but also with regard to the measurable parameters in the 'Triad of Death' (pH, bicarbonate levels, base excess, coagulation profile a temperature). These parameters may determine if the surgery should be abbreviated.

The patient should be prepared from the base of the neck to the knees, so that all body cavities can be accessed, and the long saphenous vein in the thighs is readily accessible for use in bypass procedures. Additionally, both arms should extend outwards in the 'crucifix' position so that intravenous and arterial lines may be accessed (Figure 2). Warming devices over the patient are cumbersome and unnecessary, if the ambient temperature is maintained at 30°C, although a thermal warmer below the patient may be used in addition. In the physiologically unwell patient, direct rapid opening of the bleeding cavity, with sharp dissection is the preferred approach; slower dissection with diathermy homeostasis only increases the time before hemostasis can be safely achieved.

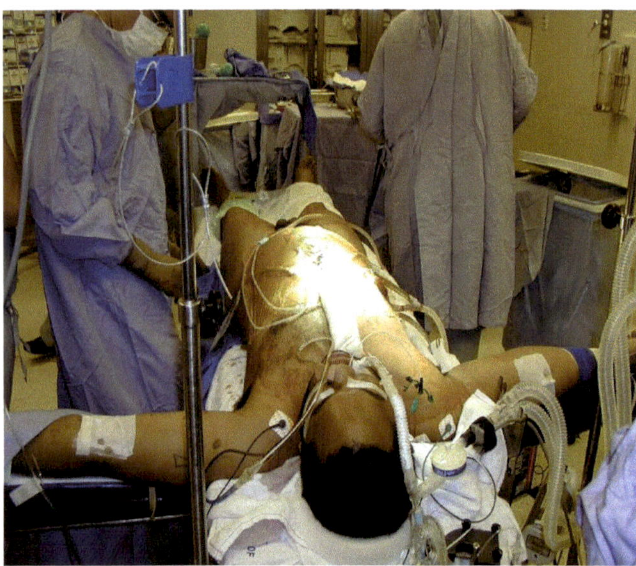

Figure 2: Patient in 'crucifix' position for full access to all body regions, especially the chest-abdomen-pelvis

Managing Vascular Injuries

The approach to emergency operative control of vascular injuries follows the same pattern as in elective surgery, but with a more progressive and rapid time-motion continuum. The surgeon should first control the vessel proximal to the injury by looping it with a vascular sling, so that it may be elevated by an assistant prior to clamping (Figure 3). If there is active hemorrhage, then a vascular clamp may be applied at this stage whilst pressure is applied over the site of bleeding.

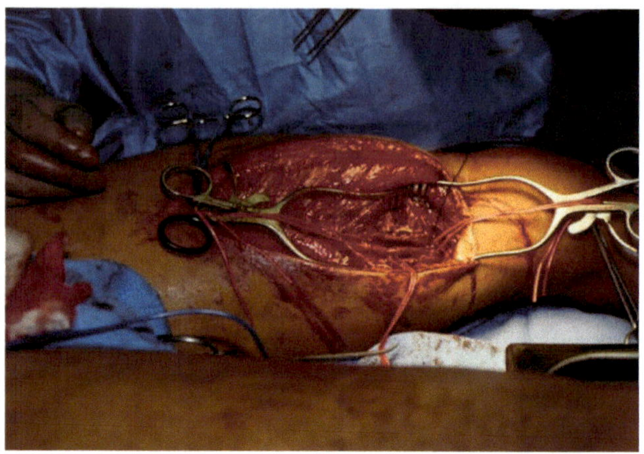

Figure 3: Dissection of left SFA with looping of vessel to control artery

Distal vessel dissection and slinging should then follow below the site of injury. Following control and clamping proximally and distally, the hematoma is then opened directly to expose the site of injury. Often the normal dissection planes are distorted by a combination of tissue injury and hematoma, but typically a dissection plane leading to the injury is readily discernible, often with digital dissection alone as hematomas often separate the tissue planes. Heparin should be avoided in the bleeding patient as many of these patients are already coagulopathic. Major venous injuries may be approached in the same way with control, although direct dissection, without proximal and distal control, is also acceptable as venous bleeding may be readily controlled with direct pressure alone.

The injured ends of arteries should be inspected and surgically trimmed, taking care to avoid further traumatizing the intimal layer; in young patients this layer is prone to recoil back into the vessel, creating a dissection flap, if it is not recognized. Small single injuries to the vessel wall may be sutured directly or repaired with a vein patch, but typically the vessel will have to be mobilized and partly resected. If a tension-free repair can be achieved, then direct anastomosis of the vessel ends may be performed. More typically, a grafting procedure will be necessary, either with interposition grafting or ligation, and bypass. Venous injuries may be ligated, especially if *in extremis*. However, many advocate venous repair in the injured limb and IVC, where possible, to reduce post-ligation side effects.

The choice of material for grafting may be either an autologous vein, such as a long saphenous vein, or synthetic. This will depend on the physiologic state of the patient and associated concurrent injuries which contribute to the decision whether to abbreviate the operation (due to worsening physiology). Although vein grafting is associated with better resistance to infection in elective vascular practice, it has not been well-supported in the trauma literature. Similar infection rates with vein and prosthetic vascular grafts are reported in trauma patients (<2%). Infected venous grafts, however, are more prone to autodigestion and rapid bleeding from a 'blow-out', compared with synthetic grafts which tend to form pseudoaneurysms. Provision of good muscle and tissue cover over a vascular repair is of utmost importance for reducing infection risk.

Shunting Vascular Injuries

Shunts may be inserted into any vessel including the carotid, aorta, iliac arteries, mesenteric arteries, IVC; the technique is particularly useful in peripheral vascular injury, especially in the presence of co-existing and extensive skeletal and soft tissue injury where rapid reperfusion is desirable (Figure 4).[10,11] The shunt may be fixed *in situ* with ligatures and left until skeletal fixation is achieved, and subsequently removed for definitive vascular repair. Alternatively, in the exsanguinating patient, a shunt may be inserted and firmly tied *in situ* as a damage control measure. Although it is desirable to remove the shunt within 24 hours, this decision is determined by patient physiology and metabolic derangement.[12,13] Shunts have reportedly been left *in situ* for up to 72 hours, without anticoagulation whilst awaiting reversal of the 'triad of death,' with no increase in mortality or morbidity.[14] In general, if an injured limb is shunted as part of the damage control sequence, then fasciotomies should also be undertaken. A venous injury may also be shunted, which aids in the reduction of swelling and on-going vascular ooze that is commonly seen with venous hypertension that follows acute ligation.

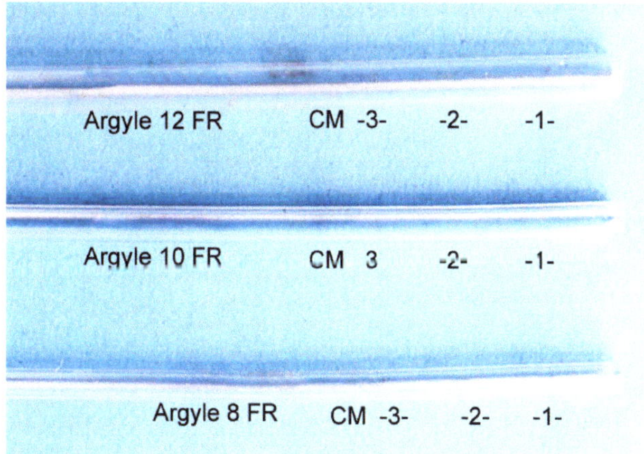

Figure 4: Selection of 'Argyle' shunts for use in vascular surgery

Trauma to the Neck and Thoracic Outlet

Carotid and subclavian vascular injuries account for less than 2% of vascular trauma, but carry a very high mortality and morbidity, including stroke.[15,16] Injuries may be blunt or penetrating, but management is more dependent on the region of the neck that is injured, which is divided into three distinct anatomical zones (Figure 5). Physical examination will alert the trauma surgeon to the injured zone, but it should also be remembered that injuries often involve more than one zone, especially with penetrating injuries where the trajectory may cross zones and even body cavities.

Zones of the Neck

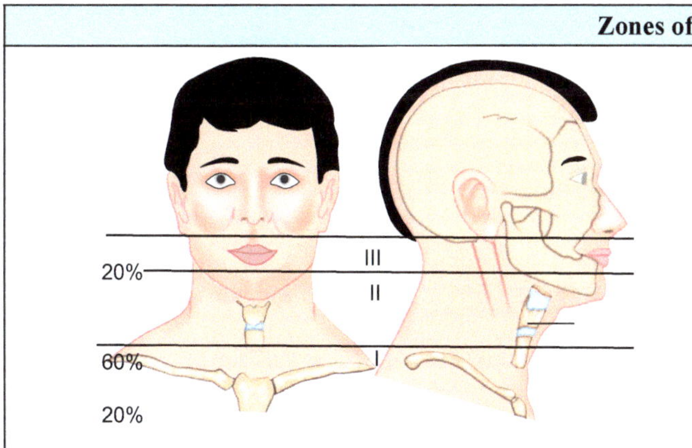

Zones of the Neck
Zone III: From the angle of the mandible up to the base of the skull. Contains the internal carotid artery along with V3 of the vertebral artery
Zone II: From the cricoid cartilage to the angle of the mandible. Contains the common carotid artery and its bifurcation into the internal and external along with the internal jugular vein and vagus nerves along with V2 of the vertebral artery
Zone I: From the level of the clavicle to the cricoid cartilage. Contains the subclavian vessels and common carotid artery and V1 of the vertebral artery

Figure 5: Anatomical zones of the neck

Blunt Carotid Injury

Blunt carotid injuries carry a high mortality and stroke rate.[15] Unfortunately, many patients also have a concomitant significant head injury, accounting for the high mortality and poor neurological outcomes. In addition, patients often present with multiple other competing injuries including chest, abdominal, and pelvis, contributing to the poor overall outcomes. If the patient is physiologically well enough with no immediate indication for surgery, then an arterial and venous phase contrast CT scan, from the head to the pelvis, is the diagnostic test of choice in blunt neck trauma.[16-19] Table 3 outlines the described grade of vessel injury and its associated mortality and stroke rate.[20]

Table 3: Carotid and vertebral artery injury grade and associated stroke rate and mortality (adapted from Biffl et al, J Trauma 1999;228:462-479)

Injury Grade	Abbreviated Injury Score (AIS)		Stroke Rate (%)		Mortality (%)		Description
	Intracranial	Extracranial	Carotid	Vertebral	Carotid	Vertebral	
I	3	3	3	19	11	31	Intimal tear or dissection <25% luminal narrowing
II	3	3	11	40	11	0	Intimal tear, dissection, wall hematoma or luminal thrombus >25% luminal narrowing
III	3	3	33	13	11	13	Pseudoaneurysm
IV	4	3	44	33	22	11	Occlusion
V	5	4	100		100		Transection with free hemorrhage

Unfortunately, irreversible neurological damage often occurs at the time of initial injury from either associated head injury, or embolic stroke from vessel injury.[21] Operative interventions have not been shown to alter outcomes in these patients for either mortality or neurological recovery. The only treatment demonstrating improvement in survival or stroke is anticoagulation.[22,23] However, anticoagulation is often contraindicated in polytrauma, especially when an intracranial bleed is present.

Free hemorrhage mandates immediate operative management, but often will not change the outcome. Endovascular intervention, as an alternative to surgery, may have a role in selective cases, but this has not been well-scrutinized to date in the trauma literature. A post-hanging injury, although by definition 'blunt,' should be repaired if described as grade II or greater, especially in the absence of neurological symptoms. A grade I injury may be managed with simple observation and an antiplatelet agent such as aspirin.

Penetrating Carotid Injury

Operative management has a much greater role to play in penetrating neck injury, and most decisions can be made on clinical grounds alone; however, a preoperative CT angiogram can also yield useful information if patient physiology allows. Patients who require surgery should have the thorax prepared within the operative field in case proximal control needs to be achieved from inside the chest.[24]

Zone I Injury

Zone I injuries cannot be controlled safely through a neck dissection alone, and therefore proximal control is obtained from within the chest either *via* median sternotomy or clamshell thoracotomy for patients *in extremis*.[25,26] The proximal brachiocephalic (innominate), left common carotid artery (CCA) and left subclavian artery (SCA) can then be safely controlled inside the chest cavity, although access to the left SCA is often difficult *via* median sternotomy due to the deep posterior position of its origin along the aortic arch (orientated anterior to posterior). The left SCA is often easier to control through a 5th intercostal space left lateral thoracotomy, or even a high left lateral thoracotomy *via* the 2nd or 3rd intercostal space. If the patient is *in extremis* in the trauma bay, then a clamshell thoracotomy is an appropriate approach, which allows for excellent exposure of the heart, aorta, and its great branches (Figure 6).

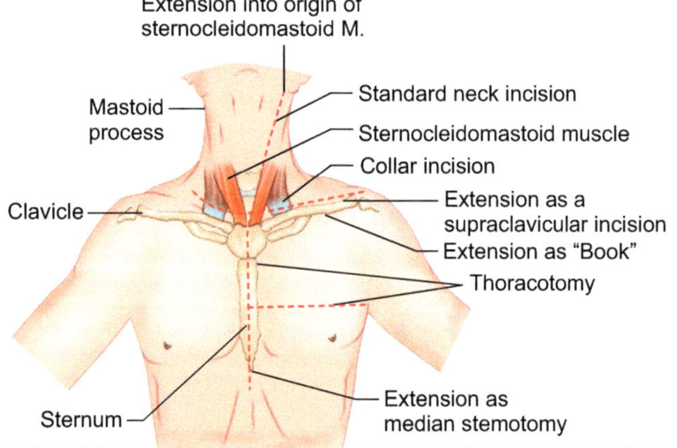

Figure 6: Approaches for Control of the Neck Vessels

If a median sternotomy has been performed, the incision may be extended further cephalad, along the anterior border of the sternocleidomastoid muscle to gain control of the vessel in zone 2, or along the superior border of the clavicle (collar incision) to gain access to the SCA, or both as necessary (Figure 2). The old fashioned 'trap-door' incision consisting of a supraclavicular dissection, upper median sternotomy, and high anterior anterolateral thoracotomy on the same side, to allow the anterior chest to be partially opened, is a cumbersome technique to perform. It can leave a morbid wound and offers no exposure advantage over the approaches described above.

Zone II Injury

Zone II injuries should be approached *via* the standard carotid surgery exposure incision, along the anterior border of the sternocleidomastoid muscle, retracting the muscle and internal jugular vein posteriorly. This should occur after ligation and division of the facial vein, which overlies the approximate level of the carotid bifurcation. If injury is present, adventitial hematoma, it is important to inspect the inside of the vessel for an intimal tear and repair this as appropriate. The carotid artery is amenable to direct end-to-end anastomotic repair if it is tension-free. Otherwise, an interposition graft (vein or synthetic) may be used. If only the anterior wall is injured, then a patch graft repair may be performed. Alternatively, for the patient *in extremis*, the vessel may be ligated, which carries an acute stroke rate of about 15%.

Zone III Injury

Zone III injuries are challenging as this distal segment of internal carotid artery is often inaccessible for rapid control; it is a narrow, funnel-shaped corridor leading to the base of the skull. However, the surgical approach is the same as for zone II, although extended more cephalad. If distal bleeding is still problematic there are numerous techniques described to aid surgical exposure, many of which are cumbersome to achieve and time-consuming, especially in the presence of active bleeding. Adjunctive techniques for exposure include resecting the mastoid bone (mastoidectomy), dislocating the mandible forward, carrying the incision behind the ear to bring the ear forward, resecting the styloid bone, resecting the mandibular ramus, and dividing the jugulo-digastric muscle which overrides the distal ICA. A more practical solution to control bleeding from a high zone III injury is occlusion of the internal carotid artery using a Fogarty balloon catheter. For the patient *in extremis*, the Fogarty catheter may be clipped to keep the balloon inflated, and then cut to leave the balloon *in situ*, followed by ligation of the vessel and closure of the wound.

Vertebral Artery Injuries

Trauma to the vertebral arteries is rare, with rates slightly higher for penetrating over blunt trauma.[27] Due to the relative inaccessibility of these vessels, endovascular management is now considered the first line in management with open repair reserved for failed endovascular repair with persistent active hemorrhage. The endovascular approach involves both antegrade, from the subclavian artery, and retrograde, crossing the basilar artery from the contralateral side, access to the vessel followed by coiling. Intraoperatively, a V_1 injury (vertebral artery as it ascends from the subclavian artery, before entering the bony canal at the level of C6) should be ligated.[28,29]

If a V_2 injury is suspected (active bleeding coming from within the vertebral canal) then bone wax can be firmly molded into the bony injury to create a tamponading effect. Failure to achieve homeostasis will mandate direct surgical exposure of V_2 by dissecting and sweeping the carotid artery posteriorly to gain access to the anterior midline cervical vertebrae. The overlying cervical fascia is dissected off the cervical vertebrae and swept backwards to expose the vertebral canal laterally (within the cervical transverse processes). Bone wax hemostasis may then be re-attempted. Otherwise, a 'bone nibbler' should be used to open the vertebral canal directly, followed by ligation of the bleeding vessel. However, this is a difficult technique and best avoided if other measures are available

Thoracic Aortic Injuries

The majority of thoracic aortic trauma is blunt, comprising 10-15% of road traffic fatalities, necessitates traumatic aortic transection (TAT). Rapid deceleration (falls >10 ft and road crash >30 mph) leads to tearing at relatively 'fixed' points along the aorta which is summarized in Table 4.[30,31]

Table 4: Location of Thoracic Aortic Transection

Fixed Points along the Thoracic Aorta where Transection Occurs
1. Ascending aorta due to the relatively fixed large branches (15%)
2. Descending aorta, just distal to the origin of the left subclavian artery, and the location of ligamentum arteriosum fixation (75%)
3. Junction of the thoracic and abdominal aorta as it passes through the diaphragm (10%)

The majority of these patients die at the scene (70-90%), usually from free-rupture and rapid exsanguination in combination with other fatal injuries, especially head and chest injuries.[32] Those who arrive to hospital alive have a contained hematoma surrounding the transection; the hematoma is contained by the aortic adventitia and mediastinal parietal pleura. These patients do not present with hypotension as there is no free hemorrhage. Conversely, many will be hypertensive in the absence of any hemorrhage, secondary to the baroreceptor stretch reflex that is stimulated by aortic wall injury.

Other clinical findings may include a measurable discrepancy in systolic blood pressure between the two upper limbs (>20 mmHg) or decreased femoral pulses ('pseudo-coarctation'). However, these findings are unreliable and often not present. In addition, patients with TAT typically have multi-system trauma, including chest, abdomen, pelvis, head, and spine injuries, that should be triaged accordingly for further management.

Investigations

Specific investigations may be delayed due to the presence of other life-threatening injuries in need of more emergent treatment. Screening for blunt thoracic aortic injury includes a chest x-ray, preferably an erect PA film, which is rarely possible after a blunt multisystem injury. The findings on chest x-ray (CXR) consistent with an aortic transection due to a mediastinal hematoma are described in Figure 7. Overall, a normal upright CXR has a negative predictive value of 95-98%.[33] However, these are neither sensitive nor specific for an aortic injury. In addition, the majority of trauma CXRs are supine antero-posterior views which tend to exaggerate the mediastinal contour. Conversely, 10-15% of patients with a thoracic aortic transaction will have a reported normal CXR.[34]

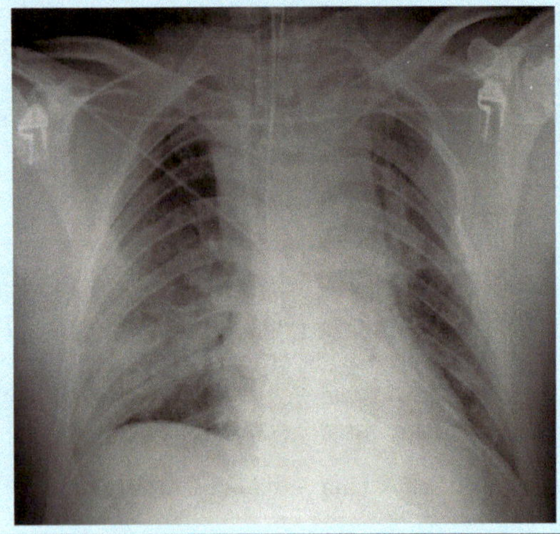

CXR Findings of Thoracic Aorta Transaction

- Widened mediastinum (>8 cm on an erect PA film)
- Loss of the aortic knuckle contour
- Obliteration of the aorto-pulmonary window
- 'Splitting' of calcium in aortic arch wall
- Left apical capping (blood tracking above the left lung)
- Left main stem bronchus pushed inferior
- Trachea pushed to the right chest
- Development of a paravertebral stripe (blood tracking posterior)
- Left hemothorax
- Oro-gastric tube displaced to the right

Figure 7: CXR findings suggestive of a Thoracic Aortic Transection

The best screening modality for TAT is a multiline CT angiogram with reconstructed images, which can identify an aortic wall injury with peri-aortic hematoma. The outline of the aorta at the level of transection will be irregular and slightly dilated; active contrast extravasation or a pseudoaneurysm is rarely seen. Catheter directed angiography is still the gold-standard test (Figure 2), but CT angiogram is a very sensitive screening tool that can effectively rule-out an aortic injury, reserving catheter-directed angiography for patients with positive CT findings undergoing further endovascular treatment. CT scanning also helps visualize other associated injuries and is the most widely accepted and ubiquitous test employed in trauma cases.[35,36]

A transesophageal echocardiogram is also a useful screening modality but is more invasive than CT scanning and is probably best suited for intraoperative use if a CT has not been performed prior to emergency surgery.[37] However, a transthoracic echocardiogram is not considered sensitive enough to rule-out an aortic injury.

Management

All patients should be managed according to ATLS® principles and the most life-threatening injuries managed in order of priority, with the primary goal being hemorrhage control. Fluid resuscitation should not be vigorous, so as to avoid escalating the bleeding; any fluids administered, should be in the form of warmed blood and blood products titrated to effect, whilst allowing the patient to remain relatively hypotensive (SBP 80-100 mmHg) until definitive hemorrhage control has been achieved.

Medical management

Medical management should take place in a critical care setting with full monitoring capabilities. Systolic blood pressure should be kept at <120 mmHg or even as low as 100mmHg, with a combination of an intravenous nitrate with beta-blockade (HR<60 bpm) to reduce aortic wall shear stress (pulsatile pressure per unit of heartbeat time).[38,39] Of note, parameters may change in accordance with the patient's condition, but prerenal acute kidney injury from hypotension should be avoided. However, most aortic transections may be safely managed medically overnight whilst other injuries take priority (e.g., head injury). Emergent surgery or endovascular management is rarely needed.

Open Surgery versus Endovascular management

Historically, >60% of patients with an aortic transection, managed nonoperatively, died; older data seems to suggest that for every hour a transection remains untreated, the mortality doubles.[40] However, this probably represents the high incidence of other more life-threatening injuries, and a poor understanding of the effectiveness of medical management. Now in the era of ubiquitous CT scanning, many smaller aortic injuries are being diagnosed early, the majority of which can undergo delayed management, especially when other, more life-threatening injuries are present. Therefore, in selected cases, patients may undergo safe, delayed repair of a TAT.[41,42]

Open repair is performed *via* a posterolateral thoracotomy ('taxi-hailing' position) with either direct anastomosis (unlikely) or interposition grafting (more likely) (Figure 8). Open surgery is associated with a mortality of almost 20%, and a significant morbidity (from high aortic cross clamping), including mesenteric ischemia, acute kidney injury (8%) and spinal ischemia with paraplegia (10%). Endovascular repair is now the recommended treatment of choice and is associated with a lower mortality (9%), less spinal cord ischemia (3%), and lower incidence of acute kidney injury (3%). Stroke rates are similar (3%) between both open and endovascular repair (Table 5). These long-term outcomes for thoracic stenting remain to be fully defined; however, the overwhelming better outcomes associated with stenting than with surgery, make it the preferred standard of care (Figure 9). Nonetheless, all patients will require life-long follow-up for stent complications (i.e., slippage, leak, fracturing, etc.) and currently there is a growing trend towards re-intervention in this population for such complications.[43-46]

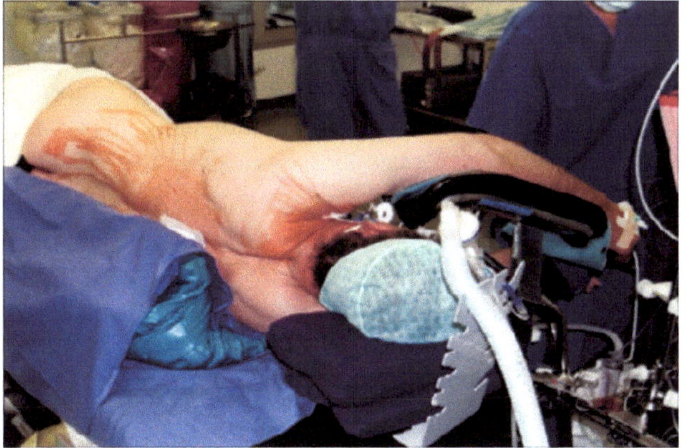

Figure 8: Typical position for left posterolateral thoracotomy ('Taxi-Hailing' position) for surgical repair of thoracicaorta

1

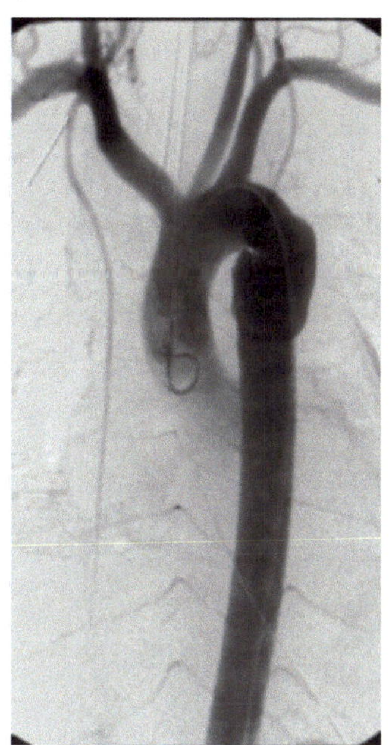

2

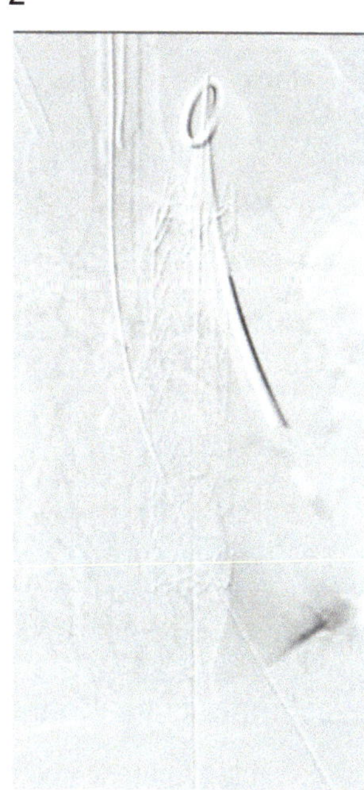

Figure 9: (1) Catheter-directed angiogram (digital subtraction) displaying thoracic aortic transection just distal to the origin of the left subclavian artery. Note the flush catheter within the ascending aorta. (2) Deployed thoracic stent in thoracic aorta

Table 5: Complication rates for both open surgery and endovascular repair of traumatic aortic transection

Complication Rates after Blunt Aortic Injury Repair[43,44]		
	Open Surgery	Endovascular
Mortality	20%	9%
Acute Kidney Injury	8%	3%
Paraplegia	10%	3%
Stroke Rate	3%	3%

Abdominal Vessels Injuries

Injuries to the large abdominal vessels are time-critical, carrying a very high mortality for both blunt and penetrating trauma.[47-49] These vessels are relatively well-protected within the retroperitoneal space and include the aorta and its branches, the inferior vena cava and its tributaries, and the portal venous system. The retroperitoneum is divided into three distinct anatomical zones, and management is dependent on the zone involved (Figure 10).

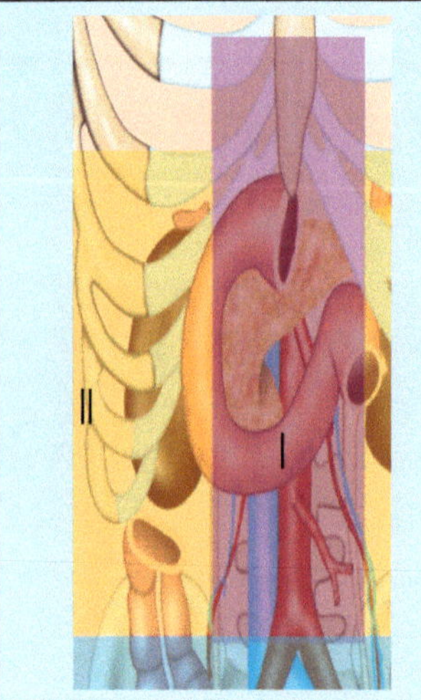

Zones of the Retroperitoneum
Zone I: The central portion containing the great vessels (aorta and IVC), pancreas and lesser sac and D2-D4 of the duodenum. Operative exploration is mandatory for injuries in this zone
Zone II: This is lateral to Zone I and contains the kidneys and their vessels, ureters, and psoas muscle. Most Zone II blunt injuries can be managed nonoperatively, unless there are signs of arterial bleeding (expanding / pulsatile hematoma, contrast extravasation on CT). All penetrating injuries here should be explored
Zone III: This is the pelvic complex, containing the bladder, rectum, and iliac vessels. Most pelvic hematomas should be managed nonoperatively (80% venous) unless the patient is physiologically unstable with a high suspicion for on-going bleeding. A combination of endovascular treatment and pelvic packing may be used. Penetrating injuries carry a high morbidity and should be operatively explored

Figure 10: Anatomical zones of the retroperitoneum and their contents

Investigation and Management

The decision to immediately manage these injuries emergently, or to investigate further is dependent on patient physiology at the time of presentation. In general, all physiologically unwell patients should be managed operatively, as the mortality from on-going hemorrhage is high and further investigations offer little value in the decision-making process; hemorrhage control should take priority.[47,49] Bedside abdominal ultrasound may be useful in diagnosing intra-abdominal free fluid but is limited at excluding it. However, if patients are physiologically well, and emergent operative intervention is not immediately required, then a contrast-enhanced CT scan with reconstructed images (arterial and portal venous phases) is the most sensitive and specific investigation.

Bleeding patients should be managed with permissive hypotension, and fluids should be kept to a minimum.[50] Upon entering the abdomen, blood should be suctioned with a cell-saver, for reuse, and the abdomen should be packed tightly for acute, rapid hemorrhage control. Once this is achieved, further resuscitation with warmed blood and blood products may continue. Other injured organs may also need to be operatively managed (e.g., packing of the injured liver, splenectomy for the injured spleen, etc.), after which the retroperitoneum may be exposed directly.

Trauma to Retroperitoneal Zone 1

Zone 1 contains the abdominal aorta, IVC, portal system and other organs such as the duodenum and pancreas which are also prone to injury and bleeding and make dissection difficult for the operating surgeon. Any hematoma in zone 1 adjacent to the great vessels, whether seen on CT scanning or intra-operatively, mandates further exploration.

Abdominal Aortic Trauma

Injuries to the abdominal aorta carry a high mortality, with most patients dying before reaching hospital.[47,49] An injury in this zone surviving to hospital mandates immediate operative management. The safest and fastest approach is to control and clamp the aorta supraceliac. This is best performed by retracting the stomach downwards and opening the lesser omentum to gain direct access to the aorta. The right (and perhaps left) diaphragmatic crus may need to be divided, and the lower esophagus swept to the left to aid safe clamping. If the patient is *in extremis,* then a left lateral thoracotomy or clamshell thoracotomy should be performed with clamping of the descending thoracic aorta. Once hemorrhage control is achieved, the aorta may be adequately exposed either transperitoneally or with a left lateral visceral rotation, and the aortic clamp transferred to the infrarenal aortic segment. In general, a supraceliac aortic clamp left *in situ* for longer than 60 minutes in the setting of trauma carries a mortality close to 100%. Therefore, an aortic injury should be repaired rapidly, and the clamp removed or transferred to below the visceral vessels.

Small aortic sidewall tears may be sutured directly for rapid hemostasis. However, typically if an aortic injury survives to the operating theater, an interposition graft will more than likely be required. Smaller injuries, seen on CT scanning may be amenable to stent grafting, although this scenario is unusual as patients are usually hemodynamically unwell. Smaller intimal tears are unusual but can be managed expectantly (±antiplatelet agents).

Trauma to the visceral branches is also associated with a high mortality ranging between 33-67%.[51] Inferior mesenteric artery ligation carries a risk of sigmoid ischemia of about 1% in elective surgery, but the incidence is variable in trauma depending on the degree of shock. Therefore, a relook laparotomy within 24-48 hours should be undertaken. The coeliac or superior mesenteric artery (SMA) may be ligated as long as one or the other remains intact (preferably the SMA), but again the high risk of gut ischemia makes a relook laparotomy mandatory. An alternative approach is to insert a shunt into the injured vessel and come back later for more definitive repair when the patient's condition allows (aim for 24-48 hours). If the injury is close to its aortic origin, then ligation and bypass is the better option. If there is injury to the renal artery, then a nephrectomy and ligation of the vessel is the safest choice as long as the other kidney is intact. Otherwise, a renal artery repair or bypass will be necessary.

Inferior Vena Cava (IVC)

Due to the relatively well-protected position of the IVC it takes a significant amount of force to injure it. Up to 30% of patients with IVC injuries will die before reaching hospital; IVC injury carries a high mortality of 50-90%, with a high incidence of concomitant associated injuries, in particular liver injury.[52,53] Conversely, 15% of liver injuries will also have an IVC injury.[54]

The IVC has four anatomical divisions: infrarenal, suprarenal/subhepatic, retrohepatic and suprahepatic with abdominal and thoracic segments. Retrohepatic and suprahepatic IVC injuries are more commonly associated with blunt trauma due to their relatively fixed position within the retroperitoneal space, but they also carry the highest mortality. Even if patients survive upon arriving at the operating theater, the injuries still carry a high mortality due to a combination of massive hemorrhage and difficult, hazardous surgical access with free exsanguination once the tamponade is released. Patients who have survived to theater, have usually, at least temporarily, self-tamponaded. Access to the infrarenal portion may be transperitoneal or *via* a right medial visceral rotation with a Kocher maneuver, as necessary.[54-56]

The IVC cannot be safely mobilized forward, and vascular clamping runs the risk of tearing its thin wall. Therefore, hemostasis should be achieved above and below the injury by applying direct pressure to the vessel itself using a sponge-forceps, (e.g., swap on a stick) (Figure 11). Posterior wounds should be approached through the anterior wall, either by extending an anterior wound, if present, or by making a new anterior venotomy. Posterior wounds are sutured directly, before repairing the anterior wall. If *in extremis,* the IVC may be ligated, although bilateral, post-operative massive lower limb edema with acute venous hypertension is a morbid side effect, mandating lower limb fasciotomies.

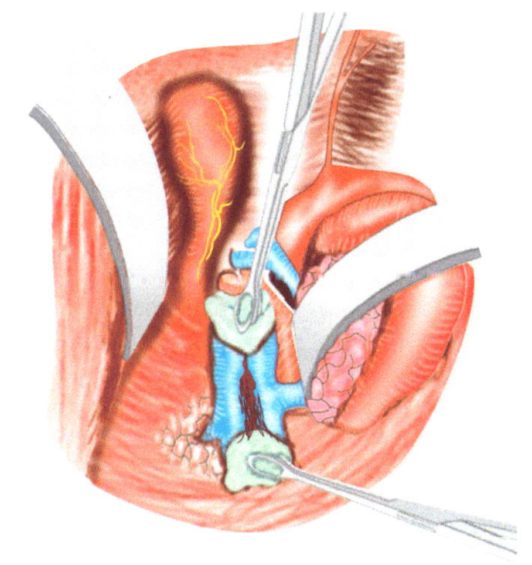

Figure 11: Exposure and Control of the IVC using Sponge-forceps above and below Site of Injury

Supra-hepatic IVC injuries should be managed in combination with a right-sided thoracotomy, or a clamshell thoracotomy, although access for rapid clamping may also be achieved through a left lateral thoracotomy (if this has already been done). The right diaphragm may also be divided to aid exposure, and for rapid repair of the injury. Unfortunately, suprahepatic IVC injuries are associated with a mortality greater than 90%.[57,58]

The retrohepatic IVC is challenging to dissect and control due to the overlying position of the liver, which must be mobilized forward by dividing both the left and right triangular ligaments. This runs the risk of destabilizing the contained hematoma leading to rapid exsanguination. Therefore, if a retrohepatic hematoma is discovered intra-operatively, it is best to leave it undisturbed, pack it for damage control with a planned re-look in 24-48 hours when the patient is physiologically improved. Veno-venous bypass with the help of a specialized liver team may be necessary.[59] The utility of an atrio-caval shunt (Schrock shunt) has been described (large bore tube, e.g., size 32 chest drain); it is placed inside the IVC, from the infra-renal segment to the right atrium of the heart, as an effective temporizing measure, which acts as a stent whilst maintaining cardiac return. However, this technique is technically challenging, time-consuming and is associated with a very high mortality, making it an almost obsolete maneuver except for those who are rigorously trained.

When a retrohepatic IVC injury must be repaired, advice from a specialized liver surgeon is recommended. Total hepatic isolation (Heany maneuver) may be achieved by controlling the sub-hepatic IVC, supra-hepatic IVC and portal vein-hepatic artery pairing within the free edge of the lesser omentum (Pringle's maneuver). After the hepatic ligaments are divided, the liver is mobilized forward. The individual large hepatic veins that drain directly into the IVC may also be controlled, but these are easily injured in the process of dissection. It is better not to disturb them, unless also injured, but instead to allow some back bleeding (recovered in the autotransfuser), and to repair the IVC injury with a rapid running suture before returning the organ to its anatomical location and restoring perfusion. In general, the liver can withstand up to 60 minutes of ischemia in the elective setting, although this figure is likely to be much lower in the shocked, bleeding, and coagulopathic patient.

Portal Vein Injuries

Portal vein injuries are associated with a mortality of about 50% and are usually associated with other sources of bleeding (coeliac artery and SMA). Where possible, the portal vein should be repaired (e.g., direct anastomosis, patch grafting, interposition grafting) except for patients *in extremis,* for whom ligation should be performed.[60] If safe access to the portal vein behind the pancreatic head is proving difficult, then the pancreas may be divided at the pancreatic neck, immediately to the left of the superior mesenteric vessels, using a GIA stapler to gain wide exposure. A distal pancreatectomy becomes necessary, but this can be temporarily drained, and the resection can be postponed until the patient been rewarmed, and has had their coagulopathy corrected (24 to 48hrs).[61]

After portal vein ligation, massive, small bowel oedema (portal venous congestion and hypertension) is an unavoidable and morbid side effect. This may be offset somewhat by the relative hypotension for a number of hours and may not be immediately appreciated in the shocked patient. However, there is a risk of mesenteric venous ischemia (±infarction) with a high incidence of abdominal compartment syndrome (ACS). Therefore, the abdomen should be left open with a temporary cover and a relook laparotomy, planned in 24-48hrs time, to inspect the bowel. Primary closure of the abdomen may be achievable in the second laparotomy, but it is more likely for there to be a delayed staged closure.

Trauma in Zone 2

Zone 2 of the retroperitoneum contains the kidneys, ureters, and lumbar vessels. Since the renal complex is surrounded by Gerota's fascia, this usually offers a hemostatic renal layer capable of arresting venous (low pressure) hemorrhage. A contained hematoma in this region should be left undisturbed unless it is expanding or pulsatile (suggesting arterial hemorrhage). A contrast extravasation blush seen on a CT angiogram is also a sign of arterial bleeding, equivalent to an expanding hematoma, and therefore merits surgical exploration.

Arterial bleeding from the kidney can usually be repaired, leaving the organ intact or partially resected and repaired using a mesh. A bleeding renal artery is difficult to repair and often requires nephrectomy, but the surgeon should ensure that the contralateral kidney is present and intact. If the contralateral kidney is not present or is also injured, then an attempt should be made to save one kidney (e.g., direct renal artery repair or bypass). Rarely, bilateral nephrectomies may need to be performed to save a life for the patient *in extremis*. However, this is not a decision that should be taken lightly as the patient will be rendered completely anuric and dialysis-dependent (independent predictor of mortality); it is recommended to try and save at least one kidney. In contrast, an injured renal vein should be ligated, and carries little clinical consequence.

Trauma in Zone 3

Zone 3 of the retroperitoneum is essentially the pelvic complex; the management of injuries in this region is more difficult. Considerations include unstable pelvic ring fracture, vascular injuries, including the large pelvic venous complex, urological injuries (bladder and ureter), and damage to various other pelvic organs (uterus, fallopian tubes, ovaries, etc.) (Figure 12).

Eighty percent of significant pelvic bleeding is venous in origin, and hemostasis is best achieved with pressure through a combination of closure and stabilization of the fractured pelvic ring with pelvic packing. The fractured pelvic ring may be closed using an external pelvic binder such as the T-POD™ device (Figure 13) and/or pelvic fixation (internal or external), which reduces the volume inside the pelvis for bleeding. Packing of the pelvis, which creates a tamponading effect, may be performed *via* extraperitoneal exposure (lower midline incision and sweeping the peritoneum upwards and backwards to open the pelvic cavity) with abdominal swabs to fill the pelvic space, without disturbing the hematoma. Alternatively, it may be performed *via* intraperitoneal exposure, if a laparotomy is already in progress, but there is a higher risk of free exsanguination.

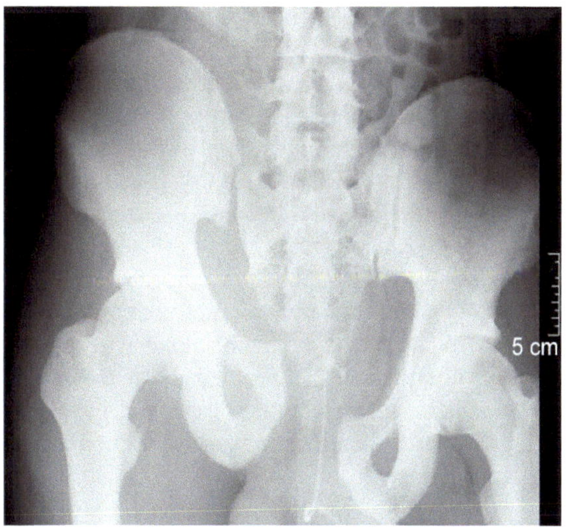

Figure 12: 'Open-book' pelvic fracture showing widened symphysis pubis, and hence increase in pelvic volume, and widening at the right sacro-iliac joint where the pelvic vessels are torn

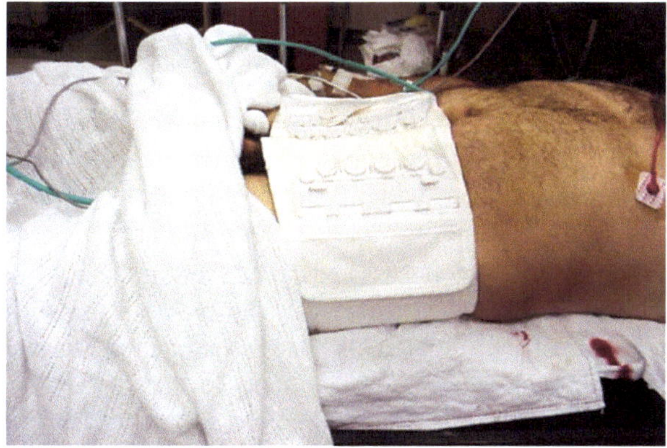

Figure 13: T-POD applied

Twenty percent of pelvic bleeding is arterial in origin (e.g., contrast extravasation blush on CT scanning), which in the absence of an immediate indication for surgery should be managed endovascularly (coiling or embolizing actively bleeding vessels) as long as the patients' physiology allows. Failure to control the hemorrhage by endovascular mandates surgical control. However, the mortality is high in this patient subgroup, especially after blunt injury, with an unstable open-book pelvic fracture. Close co-operation with the orthopedic team is absolutely necessary, using a combination of pelvic packing by the vascular/trauma surgeon, with bony fixation by the orthopedic team to stabilize the injury and control the hemorrhage. A trip to the endovascular suite is still an option after gross, open surgical control. Large arterial injuries may be shunted as part of the damage control sequence until the patient is physiologically fit for more definitive surgery. If the patient is already in the angiography suite, stenting a large arterial injury with a covered stent can be performed, but the surgeon should have a high index of suspicion for on-going venous bleeding, (i.e., bleeding that cannot be managed with endovascular techniques).

Peripheral Vascular Injury

Peripheral vascular injury is the most common of the vascular trauma subgroups, comprising greater than 80% of vascular trauma.[62] The etiology is summarized in Table 6. Table 7 summarizes classic trauma-vascular associations after blunt injury; a high index of suspicion is needed when patients present with one or more of the findings in Figure 7.

Table 6: Etiology of peripheral vascular injury

Causes of Peripheral Vascular Injury	
Penetrating	Gunshot, shotgun, stabbings, intravenous drug abuse
Blunt	Direct blunt injury (contusion), bony fracture, joint displacement
Iatrogenic	Arteriography, cardiac catheterization, balloon angioplasty, inadvertent arterial puncture, aortic balloon pump

Table 7: Typical patterns of ortho-vascular trauma[63]

Vascular Injury Patterns	
Injury Mechanism	**Artery Injury**
Posterior knee dislocation	Popliteal artery
Femur fracture	Superficial femoral artery
Supracondylar fractures	Brachial artery
Elbow dislocation	Brachial artery
Clavicular fracture	Subclavian artery
Anterior shoulder dislocation	Axillary artery

Physical Examination

Most decision making can be made on physical examination alone. This includes a detailed examination of the vascular, neurological, skeletal, and soft tissues. Physical examination for arterial injury has been shown to be very reliable with a high degree of sensitivity (98%). The examination is tailored towards the hard signs of injury (Figure 7), which effectively examines for evidence of either active arterial hemorrhage and/or arterial ischemia. In the presence of hard signs, immediate surgical exploration, without any further diagnostic work-up, is mandatory.[64,65]

In the absence of hard signs, significant vascular injury is unlikely, and therefore operative exploration is unnecessary-unless other injuries requiring surgery are present. Further diagnostic work-up is generally also unnecessary due to the very low incidence of significant arterial injuries in this group. All pulses must be palpated, both proximal and distal to the injury, and comparison should be made with the contralateral, uninjured limb. The approach to peripheral vascular injury is summarized in Figure 14.

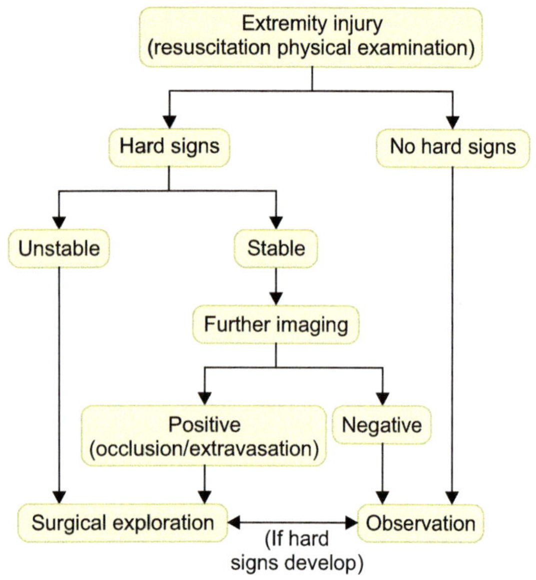

Figure 14: Approach to limb trauma at risk of vascular injury

Diagnostic Studies

The presence of flow on a hand-held Doppler device, when used in isolation, is not a reliable test of either the absence of vascular injury or adequate limb perfusion. A handheld Doppler is only useful if the Ankle Brachial Pressure Index (ABPI) is also measured. The ABPI may be measured in the injured limb and compared with the contralateral, uninjured limb. It is not reliable in the assessment of upper limb perfusion due to the more ischemia-resistant qualities of the arm. The normal ABPI is 0.9 - 1.1, which if present rules out a significant arterial injury with a very high negative predictive value. If ABPI <0.9, then a vascular injury is more likely. However, in the absence of hard signs, ABPI measurements offer little information in the assessment over physical examination alone. Therefore, if the ABPI is <0.9, but hard signs are absent, then these injuries can still be managed expectantly, as any missed arterial injury is likely to be self-limiting (i.e., minimal vascular injury). Of course, this situation may evolve later into a complete arterial occlusion, which mandates surgical management; however, hard signs will be present at this stage. Thus, the key to a successful non-operative management, in suspected peripheral vascular injury, is serial physical examination, preferably by the same surgeon.

Vascular duplex is an accurate diagnostic test but is often unavailable out of normal working hours. A diagnostic angiogram, with or without digital subtraction, is still considered the gold standard diagnostic test in all vascular disease. However, it is only available in specialist centers, and unless the vascular injury is isolated and the patient physiologically well enough for transportation to the angiography suite, its use should be reserved for on-table angiography as an adjunct to operative management. Furthermore, as stated above, angiography has not been shown to be superior to physical examination alone in the assessment for significant arterial injury. In addition, due to the now almost ubiquitous and frequent use and CT scanning in trauma, the CT angiogram has now almost replaced traditional catheter-directed arteriography. It is a highly accurate diagnostic test, although minimal vascular injuries are also picked up frequently that do not require further treatment.[66-68]

Operative Management

In the absence of hard signs, patients may undergo further diagnostic work-up or may be managed expectantly (non-operatively). The key to non-operative management is repeated and frequent physical examination such that, should the situation evolve (e.g., a non-occlusive injury progresses to an occlusive one) then surgical intervention will become necessary, but without any demonstrable increase in morbidity.[1]

When surgery is necessary, immediate transfer to the operating suite should take place. The massive transfusion protocol should be initiated, as once the contained hematoma is opened, massive hemorrhage may occur. As with all vascular operations, proximal and distal control of the vessel is mandatory to minimize blood loss (Table 8). An on-table angiogram may be performed proximal to the injury if accurate location of the damaged segment is warranted, but this is usually unnecessary, and reserved for post-repair imaging.

The segment of injured vessel may be resected, and an interposition graft can be placed, or it may be ligated followed by bypass, using either a vein or synthetic graft. The recommended conduit of choice is the native, autologous vein (preferably LSV) as many of these patients are young and fit, and the longevity of a venous graft is better than synthetic. However, a synthetic graft may also be used to expedite limb reperfusion and earlier termination of surgery (Figure 15). If an autologous vein is used, then it is recommended to harvest from the contralateral, uninjured limb. This is based on the premise that if the deep veins of the injured limb are also injured, then the limb will be reliant on its superficial venous drainage alone, and therefore its LSV should be preserved. However, it is recommended that in such a situation, the deep vein should also be repaired. In addition, as long as the profunda vein remains intact, venous drainage should be adequate. Good tissue coverage, especially healthy muscle, is mandatory to avoid infection and graft 'blow-out'.

Table 8: Standard operative approach in peripheral vascular injury

Operative Approach to Management of Peripheral Vascular Injury
1. Control the hemorrhage
a. Proximal control first
b. Distal control
c. Open the hematoma and visualize the injury
2. Manage ischemia
a. Shunt the vessel across the injury if physiologically unwell or there are multiple competing injuries
b, More definitive repair if physiology / time allows
Vein graft from the contralateral (uninjured) limb
Synthetic graft
3. Perform a Fasciotomy

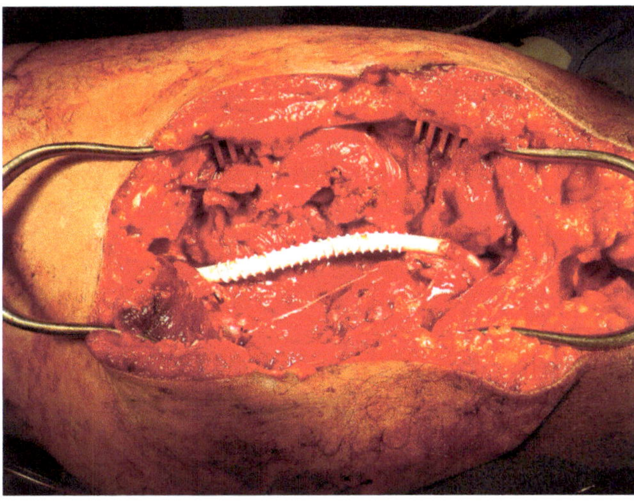

Figure 15: Repair of SFA using reinforced PTFE after GSW to thigh

The insertion of a vascular shunt (e.g., Pruitt-Inahara™, Javid™, Argyle™) is a useful adjunct, especially if one is hemodynamically unwell. The shunt is inserted to maintain vessel continuity and prograde limb perfusion (Figure 16). The ends of the shunt should be fixed in place inside the vessel using a braided suture and a material such as silk. These ligated vessel ends need to be trimmed later at the time of definitive repair. If there is a combined orthopedic-vascular injury, it is important to establish adequate vascular perfusion before any other injuries are managed. A shunt is useful in this situation, as during skeletal manipulation there is a high propensity for a vascular repair to become disrupted and thrombosis to occur. Shunt insertion will re-establish flow allowing the other injuries to be managed before removing and performing a definitive repair. A shunt may be left in place for 24-48 hrs safely, provided serial physical examinations are carried out.[10-13] Anticoagulation is usually unnecessary.[14]

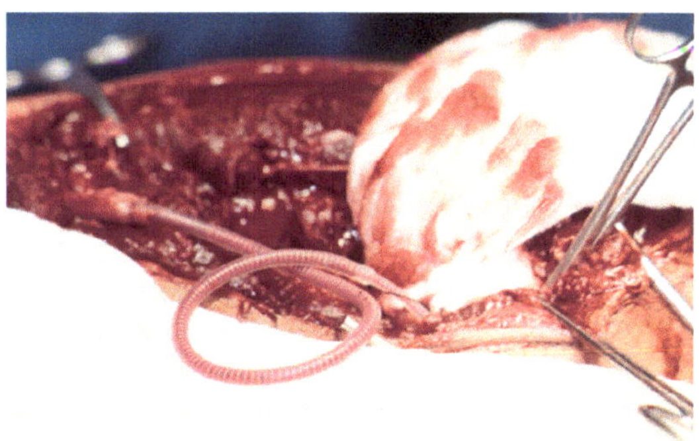

Figure 16: Vascular shunt in SFA

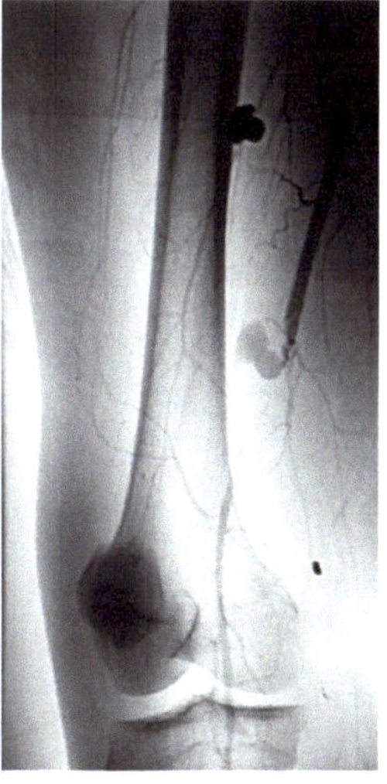

Figure 17: Angiogram of right lower limb post-GSW demonstrating occlusion of distal SFA with active bleeding

Venous Injury

The combination of arterial and venous injury in a shocked patient increases the amputation rate, as well as decreasing the functional outcome for the limb. The management of venous injuries is somewhat controversial, especially in the presence of concomitant arterial injury. Injured deep veins may be either ligated or repaired. Opponents to venous repair claim that up to 20-60% of repaired veins thrombose within days to weeks following repair, and that venous ligation carries little consequence.[70,71,72] However, where possible, venous flow should be preserved (either via shunt or repair) to reduce the venous hypertension and swelling that accompanies deep vein ligation.[73] This will minimize bleeding and the on-going ooze that is seen after reperfusion, by reducing venous hypertension, especially if fasciotomies have also been performed.

Although up to 30-60% of venous repairs will occlude after about 2 weeks, the reduction in the acute venous hypertension in the first few days is important for numerous reasons. Preservation of venous outflow from the limb will reduce venous ooze and swelling, and thus reduce blood loss, and the frequency of compartment syndrome; this will also result in earlier closure of fasciotomy wounds with enhanced recovery, earlier ambulation, and reduced hospital stay. By keeping the venous pressure close to normal, limb loss rates after arterial repair reduce. Additionally, through reducing the risk of venous ischemia and ischemia related reperfusion injury, functional outcomes can.[74]

Furthermore, greater than 50% of occluded venous repairs may recanalize over time (with good long-term patency rates), reducing chronic ambulatory venous hypertension, and its long-term consequences.[75] Thus, venous repair should be undertaken, if possible, especially in the presence of a concomitant arterial-venous trauma, prolonged ischemic time, and significant blood loss with shock. This is especially important for popliteal arterial-venous injuries which are associated with a much higher rate of limb loss (Table 9).[76,77] The vein may also be repaired directly, often unlikely, or with an interposition graft (non-reversed vein or synthetic). In the acute setting, both arterial and venous shunting should be performed, pending definitive repair. Of course, if *in extremis*, then a venous injury may be ligated, although shunting and repair is still preferable if physiology allows.

Table 9: Factors associated with high rates of limb loss in peripheral vascular injury[69]

Factors Associated with Higher Rates of Limb Loss
1. Treatment delay (>6hours)
2. Shock
3. Blunt mechanism of injury
4. Lower extremity > upper extremity
5. Associated injuries
a. Nerve (most predictive of amputation)
b. Bone
c. Vein
d. Soft tissue
6. High velocity gunshot wound
7. Pre-existing disease (esp. Peripheral Arterial Disease)
8. Failure / delay in performing fasciotomy

Compartment Syndrome

Compartment syndrome represents an elevated and sustained tissue pressure within a fascial compartment. The relatively inelastic fascia lacks the necessary compliance to accommodate tissue swelling after an ischemia-reperfusion injury, resulting in a rise in the absolute pressure.[78,79] Potential compartments involved include the calf (most common), thigh, buttocks (rare), forearm, and hands and feet (very rare). Etiologies of compartment syndrome are detailed in Table 10.

Table 10: Etiology of compartment syndrome

Causes of Compartment Syndrome
Vascular (ischemia-reperfusion injury)
Trauma and crush injury
Fractures (50% of Compartment Syndrome, e.g.: tibial plateau)
Hemorrhage into a compartment
Shock and over-resuscitation (swelling of a compartment)
Drug injection into a limb
Prolonged compression (e.g.: during surgery)

Clinical Signs of Compartment Syndrome

All the P's associated with an acute ischemia of a limb may be present, but the dominant early symptom is pain. The pain is typically confined to the affected muscle group and is often described as 'out of proportion' to the clinical findings which are often unreliable. Patients invariably complain of pain on passive stretch of the muscle compartment by the examiner (e.g., flexing the great toe can cause stretch and pain within the calf compartment). Patients will also experience pain on active movement of the muscle. Further, tender muscle upon palpation is a sign of muscle ischemia.

Diagnosis of Compartment Syndrome

Compartment pressures may be measured directly using a Stryker™ needle attached to a pressure gauge (Figure 18). This needle is inserted directly into the individual compartments, and an absolute pressure reading is measured. Most clinicians consider a pressure greater than 30 mmHg as diagnostic, mandating decompression; however, lower pressures in a symptomatic patient may also be diagnostic.[80] However, compartment pressure measurement can be cumbersome to perform, and only provides a static pressure measurement. It is also prone to both false negative and positive results, adding little to the clinical examination, and a high index of suspicion. In addition, inserting a needle may convert a 'closed fracture' to an 'open fracture,' with higher rate of infections.[81]

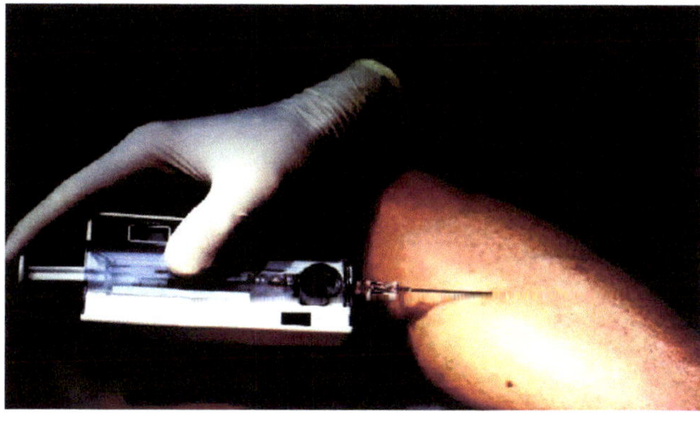

Figure 18: Stryker™ needle in use

Complications of Compartment Syndrome

The complications of untreated compartment syndrome are summarized in Table 11 and include local complications (confined to the limb itself) and systemic side effects.

Table 11: Potential complications of limb compartment syndrome

Compartment Syndrome	
Limb Complications	**Systemic Complications**
• Limb ischemia	• Rhabdomyolysis
• Neuropathy	• Myoglobinuria
• Painful neuritis	• Acute renal failure
• Loss of limb function	• Hyperkalemia
• Need for amputation	• Acidosis
	• Acute cardiac arrhythmia

Local Complications of Compartment Syndrome

Limb Ischemia directly results from a rise in compartment pressure, giving rise to venous and capillary congestion, which in turn leads to tissue ischemia. An absence of pulses is a very late, and often irreversible sign. Additionally, neuropathy may result from a combination of raised compartment pressure compressing the peripheral nerves, and prolonged ischemia. Often a sensory deficit is the earliest sign, eventually progressing to a motor neuropathy and/or a chronic painful neuritis. Complete paralysis is a late and usually irreversible finding. Compartment syndrome carries a significant limb loss rate.

Systemic Complications of Compartment Syndrome

Ischemia leads to muscle necrosis and breakdown, or rhabdomyolysis. Creatinine kinase (CK) levels, although not toxic in itself, serve as a useful biomarker for ongoing rhabdomyolysis. As the ischemic muscle breaks down, its intracellular cations (H^+ and K^+) are released into the bloodstream leading to acidemia and hyperkalemia respectively, and a significant risk of cardiac arrhythmia and sudden death.

Additionally, myoglobin is released from the ischemic muscle. It is filtered by the kidneys, and gives rise to myoglobinuria, which is toxic to the renal tubules as it precipitates out in the acidic environment of urine. This in turn causes acute kidney injury, which worsens the acidosis and hyperkalemia.

Management of Compartment Syndrome

This includes treatment of the underlying cause (e.g., correct ischemia, correction of coagulopathy, etc.). Direct management of ischemia may include embolectomy with revascularization, venous repair, fixation of fractures and evacuation of hematoma. Systemic management includes optimization of coagulation and fluid resuscitation (taking care not to over-resuscitate which may exacerbate the compartment syndrome). Surgical management includes fasciotomy of all compartments. A fasciotomy is best done as a prophylactic procedure in the high-risk patient. Finally, management of any systemic complications including rhabdomyolysis and its systemic effects is vital, preferably in a critical care setting (Table 12).

Table 12: Treatment of compartment syndrome and its complications

Management of Compartment Syndrome
Treat the underlying cause
Optimize fluid resuscitation (do not over-resuscitate)
Correct coagulopathy
Perform fasciotomy
Treat the rhabdomyolysis and acute renal failure
Treat hyperkalemia
Manage acidosis

Fasciotomy

A fasciotomy involves widely opening the fascia enveloping all compartments to decompress and normalize tissue pressures (and to accommodate any further tissue swelling), thereby restoring perfusion and reducing the venous and capillary ischemia (or preventing this in the case of a prophylactic procedure). Often the swollen muscle is seen to 'bulge' from the wound after decompression.

Typically, a limb has a 4-6 hour 'ischemic window' before irreversible necrosis occurs. However, this mantra is very variable and depends on a number of factors including collateral blood supply, presence or absence of shock, acuity of the ischemia and amount of tissue trauma. In the setting of trauma, this 4-6hr rule is not reliable as the 'ischemic window' is greatly shortened if there is accompanying shock, thereby reducing the associated 'ischemic window' for limb loss closer to 2 hrs. Furthermore, the 4-6hr window is a guide for the risk of limb loss only and not the functional outcome for the limb, which may be as short as 1hr if ischemia with shock present *in unison.*

Calf Fasciotomy

There are three anatomical (but four functional) calf compartments: (1). anterior compartment (anterior tibial vessels, deep peroneal nerve, and anterior muscle group), (2). lateral compartment (superficial peroneal nerve and peroneal muscle group) (3). posterior deep compartment (posterior tibial vessels and nerve, peroneal vessels, and soleus muscle) and (4). posterior superficial compartment (gastrocnemius muscle group). All four compartments must be decompressed for adequate and complete decompression.

Two longitudinal incisions are made:

1. Medial (access to the deep and superficial posterior compartments)
2. Lateral (access to the anterior and lateral compartments)

The lateral incision is made approximately halfway between the anterior spine of the tibia and the fibula bone in the muscle groove. Care must be taken not to injure the deep or superficial peroneal nerve (foot drop). The incision is deepened down to fascia and skin flaps are raised over the compartments which are then opened by two separate parallel longitudinal incisions. A 'T'-shaped incision is then created across the dividing septum (Figures 19 and 20).

The medial longitudinal incision is made about a finger breaths width below the medial edge of the tibia taking care not to injure the LSV. Flaps are raised and the fascia opened longitudinally. This effectively decompresses the superficial compartment. The soleus muscle is then detached from the medial aspect of the tibia posteriorly (relatively avascular plane) to decompress the deep compartment.

Viable muscles will contract on stimulation (pinching/ diathermy). Only frankly necrotic muscle should be debrided at this stage. However, if muscle viability is unclear then a planned re-look in 24-48 hrs should be undertaken.

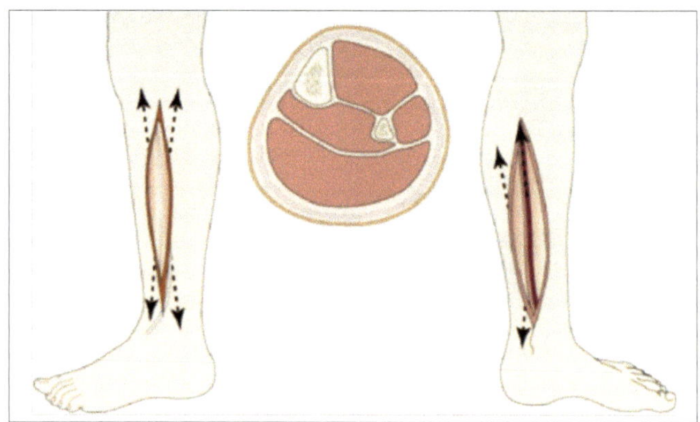

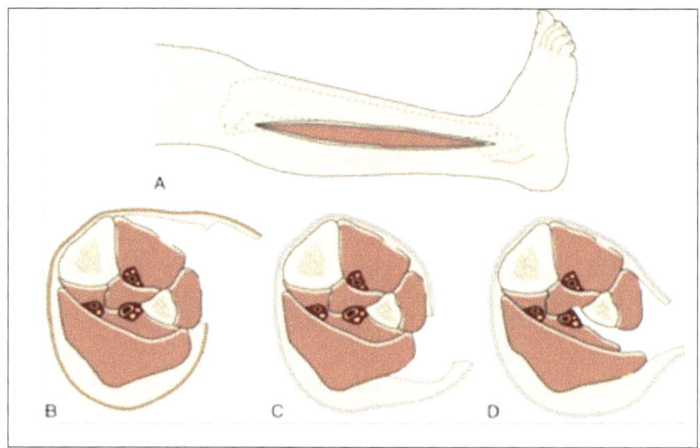

Figure 19: Calf Fasciotomies

Lateral Claf Fasciotomy

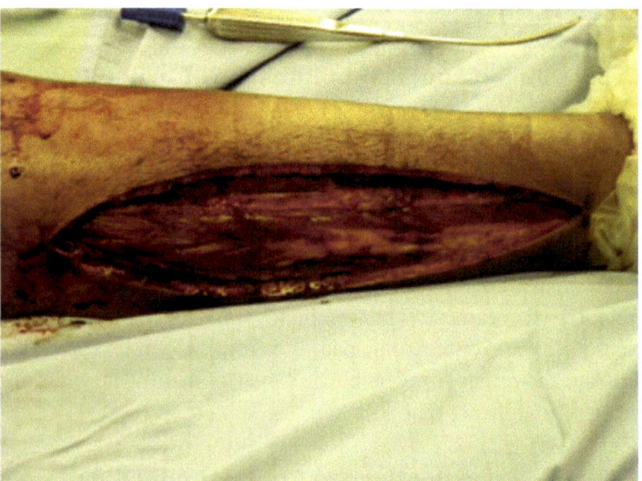

Medical Calf Fasciotomy

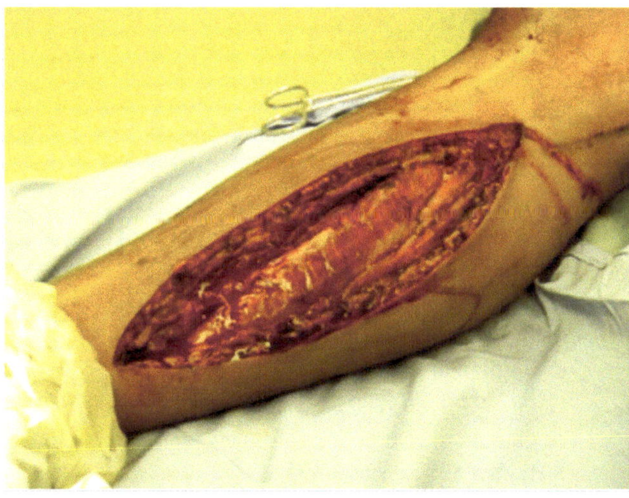

Figure 20: Example of calf fasciotomy with bulging muscle (after GSW to thigh)

Closure of Fasciotomy Wounds

Once soft tissue swelling has subsided, fasciotomy wounds should be closed to reduce the incidence of infection with improved rates of ambulation and rehabilitation. If skin flaps were raised at the initial operation, then often the edges may be closed primarily with a running suture. Failing this, a staged closure is associated with a high success rate, where a 'shoelace' technique is employed. We would advocate using a vascular rubber sling to approximate the skin edges together, which can be tightened every few days as the skin stretches and primary closure re-tried. Failing successful closure with this technique, skin grafting may be used or if only a narrow segment of uncovered tissue remains, healing by secondary intention may occur.[82, 83]

Thigh Fasciotomy

The thigh contains three compartments: (1) medial (adductor) compartment, (2) anterior (quadriceps) compartment, and (3) posterior (hamstring) compartment. Typically, only the anterior and posterior compartments need to be decompressed and this is performed via a longitudinal incision on the lateral aspect of the thigh (Figure 21). The underlying fascia is opened via two separate parallel incisions under raised skin flaps to release the anterior and lateral compartments. Then a 'T'-shaped incision is created across the dividing septum (tensor fascia lata). If necessary, a separate medial incision can be made to decompress the medial compartment (but this is rarely necessary).

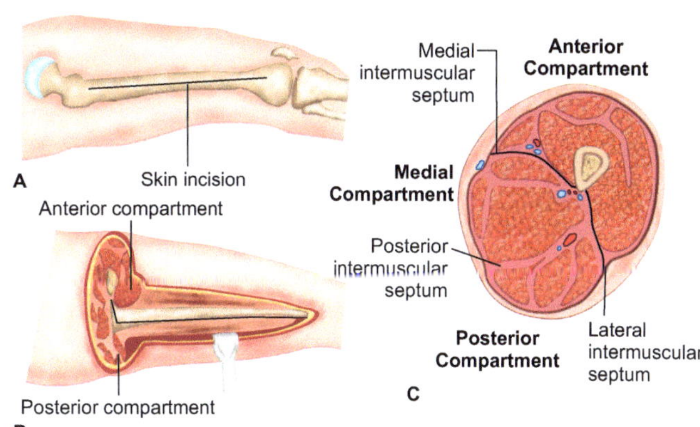

Figure 21: Thigh Fasciotomy

Upper Limb Trauma

The upper limb is more resistant to acute ischemia in comparison with the lower limb, (especially if the injury is distal to the profunda brachii artery origin). Upper limb amputation after an ischemic insult is rare. However, the long-term consequences of upper limb ischemia can be very morbid especially arm claudication of an ischemic contracture (e.g., Volkmann's ischemic contracture) in the dominant arm and therefore, upper limb trauma with hard signs should be managed aggressively.[84] Common injury sites include brachial artery (e.g., penetrating injury from putting arm through glass) and axillary artery (severely displaced fracture of the head of humerus). The radial or ulnar vessels may be ligated as long as one or other remains intact to perfuse the hand. Proximal injuries (e.g., subclavian artery) may be stented if the patient is physiologically well and facilities are available, otherwise operative exposure and repair will be necessary (median sternotomy may be required for safe proximal control).

Forearm Fasciotomy

Upper limb fasciotomy is performed *via* two incisions, one on the volar aspect of the forearm and the other on the dorsum. The flexor compartment (anterior/volar) compartment contains the most muscle as well as two arteries (radial and ulnar) and two nerves (median and ulnar). Also, this compartment crosses two joints (elbow and wrist). This is decompressed using a 'lazy-S' incision beginning on the medial aspect of the distal humerus and carried across the elbow joint from medial to lateral in a 'lazy S' configuration (to prevent joint contracture) followed by a loose wavy pattern across the volar aspect of the forearm coming back to the midline at the center of the wrist and then crossing the wrist joint (Figure 22). The fascia is opened including the flexor retinaculum (wrist) and extended into the palmar fascia for about 2 cm (beware median nerve).

The dorsal incision is a simple single semilunar incision and does not cross any joints.

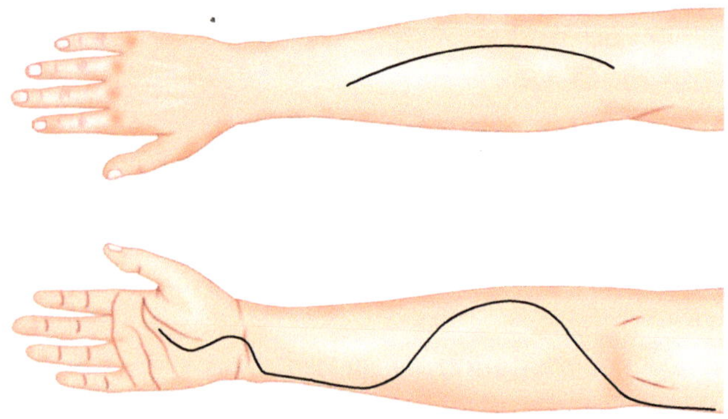

Figure 22: Forearm fasciotomy

Treatment of Rhabdomyolysis

Hyperkalemia-associated cardiac irritability should be treated with calcium infusion (e.g., calcium gluconate or calcium chloride) to stabilize the myocardium. K^+ ions can be 'driven' back intracellularly using β-agonists (nebulized or occasionally IV), sodium bicarbonate ($NaHCO_3$) infusion or an insulin-dextrose IV regimen as well as preventing further K^+ absorption using oral and rectal resonium. Renal replacement therapy can be used to manage life-threatening hyperkalemia and acidosis, resistant to the medical management.

Myoglobinuria may be treated with aggressive fluid resuscitation to encourage diuresis (although this can worsen compartment syndrome, including abdominal compartment syndrome). Alkalinization of the urine (to keep urine pH >6.5) by administering intravenous $NaHCO_3$ has also been advocated but does not offer greater benefit over hydration alone. In addition, urine alkalinization is cumbersome to achieve and requires regular urinary pH measurements. Furthermore, intravenous $NaHCO_3$ carries added side effects including venous thrombosis and intracellular alkalosis as well as running the risk of systemic alkalemia which is difficult to manage. The use of diuretics (e.g., mannitol) is controversial and probably offers little benefit over fluids alone but may be tried in difficult cases where optimum hydration has been achieved. The advice of a renal physician should be sought.

REFERENCES

1. Dennis JW, Frykberg ER, Veldenz HC, et al. Validation of nonoperative management of occult vascular injuries and accuracy of physical examination alone in penetrating extremity trauma: 5 to 10 year follow-up. J Trauma 1998;44:243-253.
2. Stain SC, Yellin AE, Weaver FA, et al. Selective management of non-occlusive arterial injuries. Arch Surg 1989;124:1136-1141.
3. Panetta TF, Sales CM, Marin ML, et al. Natural history, duplex characteristics and histopathologic correlation of arterial injuries in a canine model. J Vasc Surg 1992;16:867-876.
4. Frykberg ER, Vines FS, Alexander RH. The natural history of clinically occult arterial injuries: a prospective evaluation. J Trauma 1989;29:577-583.
5. Frykberg ER, Crump JM, Dennis JW, et al. Non-operative observation of arterial intimal injuries in an experimental model. J Trauma 1991;31:669-675.
6. Neville RF, Hobson RW, Watanabe B, et al. A prospective evaluation of arterial injuries in an experimental model. J Trauma 1991;31:669-675.
7. Hoffer EK, Sclafani SJ, Herkowitz MM, Scalea TM. Natural history of arterial injuries diagnosed with arteriography. J Vasc Interv Radiol 1997;8:43-53.
8. Morrison CA, Carrick MM, Norman MA, Scott BG, Welsh FJ, Tsai P, Liscum KR, Wall MJ Jr, Mattox KL. Hypotensive resuscitation strategy reduces transfusion requirements and severe postoperative coagulopathy in trauma patients with hemorrhagic shock: preliminary results of a randomized controlled trial. J Trauma 2011;70:652-63.
9. Shapiro MB, Jenkins DH, Schwab CW, et al. Damage control: Collective review. J Trauma 2000;49:969-978.
10. Subramanian A, Vercruysse G, Dente C, Wyrzykowski A, King E, Feliciano DV. A decades experience with temporary intravascular shunts at a civilian level I trauma center. J trauma 2008;65:316-26.
11. Taller J, Kamder JP, Greene JA, Morgan RA, Blankenship CL, Dabrowski P, et al. Temporary vascular shunts as initial treatment of proximal extremity vascular injuries during combat operations: the new standard of care at echelon II facilities? J trauma 2008;65:595-603.
12. Rasmusen TE, Clouse WD, Jenkins DH, et al. The use of temporary vascular shunts as a damage control adjunct in the management of wartime vascular injury. J Trauma 2006;61:8-15.
13. Chambers LW, Green DJ, sample K, Gillingham BL, Rhe P, Brown C, et al. Tactical surgical intervention with temporary shunting of peripheral vascular trauma sustained during operation Iraqi freedom: one unit's experience. J Trauma 2006;61:824-30.
14. Granchi T, Schmittling Z, Vasquez J, Schreiber M, Wall M. Prolonged use of intraluminal arterial shunts without systemic anticoagulation. Am J Surg. 2000;180:493-7.

15. Biffl WL, Moore EE, Ellicott JP, et al. The devastating potential of blunt vertebral arterial injuries.AnnSurg 2000;231:672-681.
16. Biffl WL, Moore EE, Offner PJ, et al. Optimizing screening for blunt cerebrovascular injuries. Am J Surg 1999;178:517-522.
17. Biffl WL, Ray CE, Moore EE, et al. Noninvasive diagnosis of blunt cerebrovascular injuries: A preliminary report. J Trauma 2002;53:850-856.
18. Miller PR, Fabian TC, Croce MA, et al. Prospective screening for blunt cerebrovascular injuries. Analysis of diagnostic modalities and outcomes. Ann Surg 2002;236:386-395.
19. Rogers FB, Baker EF, Osler TM, et al. Computed tomographic angiography as a screening modality for blunt cervical arterial injuries: Preliminary results. J Trauma 1999;46:380-385.
20. Biffl WL, Moore EE, Offner PJ, et al. Blunt carotid arterial injuries: Implications of a new grading scale. J Trauma 1999;47:845-853.
21. Carrillo EH, Osborne DL, Spain DA, et al. Blunt carotid artery injuries: Difficulties with the diagnosis prior to neurologic event. J Trauma 1999;46:1120-1125.
22. Biffl WL, Moore EE, Ryu RK, et al. The unrecognized epidemic of blunt carotid arterial injuries: Early diagnosis improves neurologic outcome. Ann Surg 1998;228:462-470.
23. Fabian TC, Patton JH Jr, Croce MA, et al. Blunt carotid injury: Importance of early diagnosis and anticoagulant therapy. Ann Surg 1996;223:513-525.
24. Clouse WD, Rasmussen TE, Peck MA, Eliason JL, Cox MW, Bowser AM, et al. In-theatre management of vascular injury: 2 years of the Balad vascular registry. J Am Coll Surg 2007;204:625-32.
25. Demetriades D, Rabinowitz B, Pezikis A, et al. Subclavian vascular injuries. Br J Surg 1987;74:1001-1003.
26. Lin PH, Koffron AJ, Guske PJ, Lujan HJ, Heilizer TJ, Yario RF, et al. Penetrating injuries of the subclavian artery. Am J Surg 2003;185:580-4.
27. Risgaard O, Sugrue M, D'Amours S, Christey G, Smith K, Caldwell E, Lariviere C. Blunt cerebrovascular injury: An evaluation from a major trauma centre. ANZ J Surg 2007;77:686-689.
28. Mwipatayi BP, Jeffery P, Beningfield SJ, Motale P, Tunnicliffe J, Navsaria PH. Management of extracranial vertebral artery injuries. Eur J Vasc Endovasc Surg 2004;27:157-162.
29. Giacobetti FB, Vaccaro AR, Bos-Giacobetti MA, et al. Vertebral artery occlusion associated with cervical spine trauma: A prospective analysis. Spine 1997;22:188-192.
30. Williams JS, Graff JA, Uku JM, et al. Aortic injury in vehicular trauma. Ann Thorac Surg 1994;57:726-730.
31. Feczko J, Lynch L, Pless J, et al. An autopsy case review of 142 nonpenetrating (blunt) injuries of the aorta. J Trauma 1992;33:846-849.
32. Mattox K, Feliciano D, Beal A. Five thousand seven hundred and sixty cardiovascular injuries in 4459 patients. Epidemiologic evolution 1958-1988. Ann Surg 1989;209:698-705.
33. Mirvis S, Bidwell J, Buddemeyer E, et al. Value of chest radiography in excluding traumatic aortic rupture. Radiology 1987;163:487-493.
34. Ho R, Blackmore C, Bloch R. Can we rely on mediastinal widening on chest radiography to identify subjects with aortic injury? Emerg Radiol 2002;9:183-187.
35. Mirvis S, Shanmugathan K, Miller B. Traumatic aortic injury: diagnosis with contrast enhanced CT-five-year experience at a major trauma center. Radiology 1996;200:413-422.
36. Dyer D, Moore E, Mestek M. Can chest CT be used to exclude aortic injury? Radiology 1999;213:195-202.
37. Chirillo F, Totis O, Cavarzerani A. Usefulness of transthoracic and transesophageal echocardiography in recognition and management of cardiovascular injuries after blunt trauma. Heart 1996;75:301-306.
38. Pate J, Gavant M, Weiman D, Fabian T. Traumatic rupture of the aortic isthmus: program of selective management. World J Surg 1999;23:59-63.
39. Fabian T, Devis K, Gavant M, et al. Prospective study of blunt aortic injury. Helical CT is diagnostic and antihypertensive therapy reduces rupture. Ann Surg 1998;227:666-677.
40. Parmley L, Mattingly T, Manion T. Nonpenetrating traumatic injury of the aorta. Circulation 1958;17:1086-1101.
41. Caffarelli AD, Mallidi HR, Maggio PM, Spain DA, Miller DC, Mitchell RS. Early outcomes of deliberate nonoperative management for blunt thoracic aortic injuries in trauma. J Thor Cardiovasc Surg 2010;140:598-605.
42. Lebl DR, Dicker RA, Spain DA, Brundage SI. Dramatic shift in the primary management of traumatic thoracic aortic rupture. Arch Surg 2006;177-180.
43. Murad MH, Rizvi AZ, Malgor R, Carey J, Alkatib AA, Erwin PJ, Lee A, Fairman RM. Comparative

effectiveness of the treatments for thoracic aortic transection. J Vasc Surg 2011;53:193-199.

44. Lee WA, Matsumura JS, Mitchell RS, Farber MA, Greenberg RK, Azizzadeh A, Murad MH, Fairman RM. Endovascular repair of traumatic thoracic aortic injury: Clinical practice guidelines of the society for vascular surgery. J Vasc Surg 2011;53:187-192.
45. Demetriades D, Velmahos GC, Scalea TM, Jurkovich GJ, Karmy-Jones R, Teixeira PG, Hemmila MR, O'Connor JV, McKenney MO, Moore FO, London J, Singh MJ, Lineen E, Spaniolas K, Keel M, Sugrue M, Wahl WL, Hill J, Wall MJ, Moore EE, Marguiles D, Malka V, Chan LS. Operative repair or endovascular stent graft in blunt traumatic thoracic aortic injuries: Results of an American Association for the Surgery of Trauma Multicenter Study. J Trauma 2008;64:561-571.
46. Demetriades D, Velmahos GC, Scalea TM, Jurkovich GJ, Karmy-Jones R, Teixeira PG, Hemmila MR, O'Connor JV, McKenney MO, Moore FO, London J, Singh MJ, Lineen E, Spaniolas K, Keel M, Sugrue M, Wahl WL, Hill J, Wall MJ, Moore EE, Marguiles D, Malka V, Chan LS. Diagnosis and treatment of blunt aortic injuries: Changing perspectives. J Trauma 2008;64:1415-1419.
47. De Mestral C, Dueck AD, Gomez D, Haas B, Nathens AB. Associated injuries, management and outcomes of blunt abdominal injury. J Vasc Surg 2012;56:656-660.
48. Loh SA, Rockman CB, Chung C, Maldonado TS, Adelman MA, Cayne MS, Pachter L, Mussa FF. Existing trauma and critical care scoring systems underestimate mortality among vascular trauma patients. J Vasc Surg 2011;53:359-366.
49. Shalhub S, Starnes BW, Tran NT, Hatsukami TS, Lundgren RS, Davis CW, Quade S, Gunn M. Blunt abdominal aortic injury. J Vasc Surg 2012;55:1277-1285.
50. Dutton RP, Mackenzie CF, Scalea TM. Hypotensive resuscitation during active hemorrhage: Impact on in-hospital mortality. *J Trauma.* 2002;52:1141-1146.
51. Asensio JA, Britt LD, Borzotta A, Peitzman A, Miller FB, Mackersie RC, Pasquale RC, Pachter HL, Hoyt DB, Rodriguez JL, Falcone R, Davis K, Anderson JT, Ali J, Chan L. Multiinstitutional experience with the management of superior mesenteric artery injuries. J Am Coll Surg 2001;193:354-65.
52. Rosengart M, Smith DR, et al. Prognostic factors in patients with inferior vena cava injuries. Am Surg. 1999;65:849-856.
53. Hansen CJ, Bernadas C, West MA, et al. Abdominal vena caval injuries: outcomes remain dismal. *Surgery.* 2000;128: 572-578.
54. Buckman RF, Pathak AS, Badellino MM, et al. Injuries of the inferior vena cava. *Surg Clin North Am.* 2001;81: 1431-1447.
55. Stewart MK, Stone HH. Injuries of the inferior vena cava. *Am Surg.* 1986; 51: 9-13.
56. Burch JM, Feliciano DV, Mattox KL, et al. Injuries of the inferior vena cava. *Am J Surg.* 1988; 156: 548-552.
57. Davis TP, Feliciano DV, Rozycki GS, et al. Results with abdominal vascular trauma in the modern era. *Am Surg.*. 2001;67:565-570.
58. Asensio JA, Chahwan S, Hanpeter D, et al. Operative management and outcome of 302 abdominal vascular injuries. *Am J Surg.*. 2000;180:528-533.
59. Cogbill TH, Moore EE, Jurkovich GJ, et al. Severe hepatic trauma: a multi-center experience with 1,335 liver injuries. *J Trauma.* 1988;28:1433-1438.
60. Stone HH, Fabian TC, Turkleson ML. Wounds of the portal venous system. World J Surg 1982;6:335-41.
61. Buckman RF, Pathak AS, Badellino MM, Bradley KM. Injuries of the inferior vena cava. Surg Clin North Am 2001;81:1431-1447.
62. Rich NM. Surgeons response to battlefield vascular trauma. Am J Surg 1993;166:91-6.
63. Attebery LR, Dennis JW, Russo-Alesi F, et al. Changing patterns of arterial injuries associated with fractures and dislocations. J Am Coll Surg 1996;183:377-383.
64. Frykberg ER, Crump JM, Dennis JW, et al. Nonoperative observation of clinically occult arterial injuries: A prospective evaluation. Surgery 1991;109:85-91.
65. Frykberg ER, Dennis JW, Bishop K, et al. The reliability of physical examination in the evaluation of penetrating extremity trauma for vascular injury. : Results at one year. J Trauma 1991;31:502-511.
66. Applebaum R, Yellin AE, Weaver FA, et al. Role of routine arteriography in blunt lower extremity trauma. Am J Surg 1990;160:221-225.
67. Gillespie DL, Woodson J, Kaufman J, et al. Role of arteriography for blunt or penetrating injuries in proximity to major vascular structures: An evolution in management. Ann Vasc Surg 1993;7:145-149.
68. Schwartz MR, Weaver FA, Bauer M, Siegel A, Yellin AE. Refining the indications for arteriography in penetrating extremity trauma: a prospective analysis. J Vasc Surg 1993;17:116.
69. Hafez HM, et al. Lower extremity arterial injury: Results of 550 cases and review of risk factors associated with limb loss. J Vasc Surg 2001;33:1212-1219.
70. Meyer J, Walsh J, Schuler J, et al. The early fate of venous repair after civilian vascular trauma: a clinical,

hemodynamic and venographic assessment. Ann Surg 1987;206:458.

71. Hobson RW, Yeager RA, Lynch TG, et al. Femoral venous trauma: Techniques for surgical management and early results. Am J Surg 1983;146:220.
72. Agarwal N, Shah PM, Class RH, et al. Experience with 115 civilian venous injuries. J Trauma 1982;22:827.
73. Rich NM, Hobson RW, Collins GJ, et al. The effect of acute popliteal venous interruption. Ann Surg 1976;183:365.
74. Rich NM. Principles and indications for primary venous repair. Surgery 1982;91:492.
75. Nypaver TJ, Schuler JJ, McDonnel P, et al. Long-term results of venous reconstruction after vascular trauma. J Vasc Surg 1992;16:762.
76. Lim LT, Michuda MS, Flanagan P, et al. Popliteal artery trauma: 31 consecutive cases. Arch Surg 1980;115:1307-1313.
77. Miranda FE, Dennis JW, Veldenz HC, et al. Confirmation of the safety and accuracy of physical examination in the evaluation of knee dislocation for popliteal artery injury: A prospective study. J Trauma 2000;49:375.
78. Kostler W, Strohm PC, Sudkamp NP. Acute compartment syndrome of the limb. Injury 2004;35:1221-1227.
79. Gulli B, Templeman D. Compartment syndrome of the lower extremity. Orthop Clin North Am 1994;25:677-684.
80. Hargens AR, Schmidt DA, Evans KL, et al. Quantitation of skeletal-muscle necrosis in a model compartment syndrome. J Bone Joint Surg Am 1981;63:631-636.
81. Boody AR, Wongworawat MD. Accuracy in the measurement of compartment pressures: a comparison of three commonly used devices. J Bone Joint Surg Am 2005;87:2415-2422.
82. Zorilla P, Marin A, Gomez LA, Salido JA. Shoelace technique for gradual closure of fasciotomy wounds. J Trauma 2005;59:1515-1517.
83. Berman SS, Schilling JD, McIntyre KE, et al. Shoelace technique for delayed primary closure of fasciotomies. Am J Surg 1994;167:435-436.
84. McCready RA. Upper-extremity vascular injuries. Surg Clin North Am 1988;68:725-740.

53
CHAPTER

Burns

Silvy Celine Akrawe, MD
Apram Jyot, MD
Vijay Mittal, MD

NTRODUCTION

Burn injuries tend to be associated with significant morbidity and mortality and are often underappreciated. Severe burns are often accompanied by a significant inflammatory response, changes in body metabolism, and hypotension related to shock in a distributive nature. This poses management challenges for healthcare providers and can eventually lead to multiple organ failure. Overall, burns affect not only the physical health, but also the quality of life and mental health of the patient. Profound alterations are caused that last long term, which need to be addressed for an optimum quality of life. Providers are faced with significant challenges including critical care management and the acute phase, followed by long term rehabilitation.

Burn related injuries are highly variable with respect to different sources (i.e., flame, electrical, scald, and chemical burns). Morbidity increases with burn severity and surface area.[2,3]

Classification

There are multiple factors that determine the severity of burns. The main factors include location of the burn on the body, temperature, and duration of exposure. There is no synergism between the exposure time and degree of temperature contributing to the severity of burn.[3]

It is essential to classify a burn accurately because it guides initial management and determines outcome including morbidity and mortality.

Some classifications include differentiating the extent of the basis of depth and differentiating between minor versus major injuries which is mostly dictated by total burn surface area.

Burn Depth Classification

- First degree burns: these are superficial burns, involving only the epidermis. They tend to be painful, erythematous, and blanch when touched. No blistering is usually noted (e.g., sunburn).
- Second degree burns: these are partial thickness burns involving the epidermis and dermis. The dermis depth can vary, superficial versus deep dermis. These tend to be erythematous, blistered, painful, and blanch when touched (e.g., scald burns).
- Third degree burns: these full thickness burns extend through the epidermis, dermis, and into the subcutaneous fat or involve deeper layers. The appearance tends to be brown, charred, pale, feels firm and leathery to palpation, no blanching is noted, and there is minimal pain.[1]

Only consider partial and full thickness burns when calculating the extent of the burn. Superficial burns are excluded.[1]

Table 1: Characteristics of burns by depth

Burn Thickness	Deepest Skin Structure Involved	Appearance	Pain	Prognosis (Without Surgical Intervention)
Superficial (First-degree)	Epidermis	Dry, balancing erythema	Painful	Heals without scarring, 5-10 days
Superficial partial-thickness (second-degree)	Upper dermis	Blister; wet, blanching erythema	Painful	Heals without scarring, < 3 weeks
Deep partial-thickness (second-degree)	Lower dermis	Yellow or white, dry, nonblanching	Decreased sensation	Heals in -8 weeks; likely to scar if healing > 3 weeks
Full-thickness (third-degree)	Subcutaneous structures	White or black/brown, nonblanching	Decreased sensation	Heals by contracture > 8 weeks; will scar

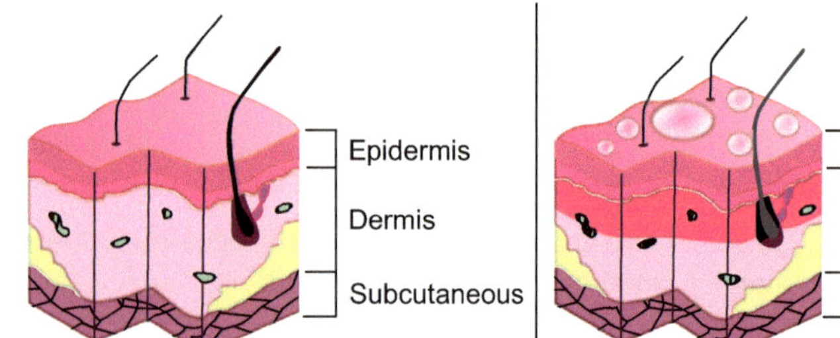

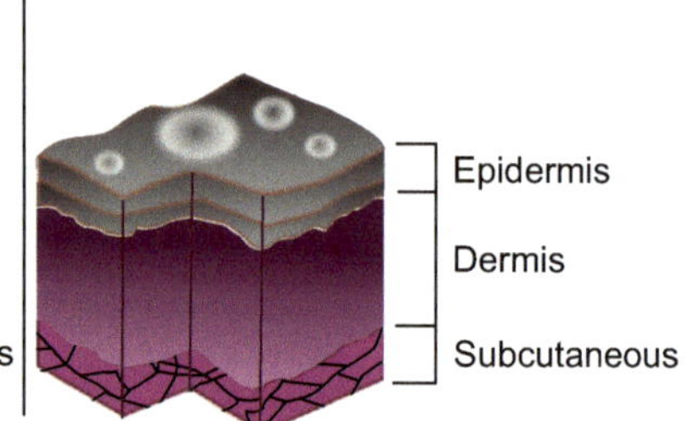

Figure 1: Diagram of burn degrees

Minor Vs Major Burn Injury

Classification for burn severity is determined by the patient's age, total body surface area burned, the depth of burn, type of burn, and the involved body parts.

A minor burn is usually less than 10% of the total body surface area, with mostly superficial burns being the predominant type.

Major or severe burns fall under the following categories:

- Greater than 20% TBSA in adults
- High voltage and electrical burns
- Significant/severe burns to your face, ears, eyes, joints or genitalia[4]

Assessment

Extent of the Burn

Multiple methods are available for estimating the total body surface area burned.

Rule of nines: as depicted in Figure 2, the head represents 9%, each arm represents 9%, the anterior chest and abdomen are 18%, the posterior chest and back are 18%, the perineum is 1%, and each leg is 18%. The rule of nines is different for children, where the head is 18% and the legs are 13.5% each. Other methods used more commonly in children can be found in the Lund and Browder chart.

Another commonly used method that can be used to calculate the extent of burns on the body for small burns is: the surface area of the patient's hand represents approximately 1%.[1]

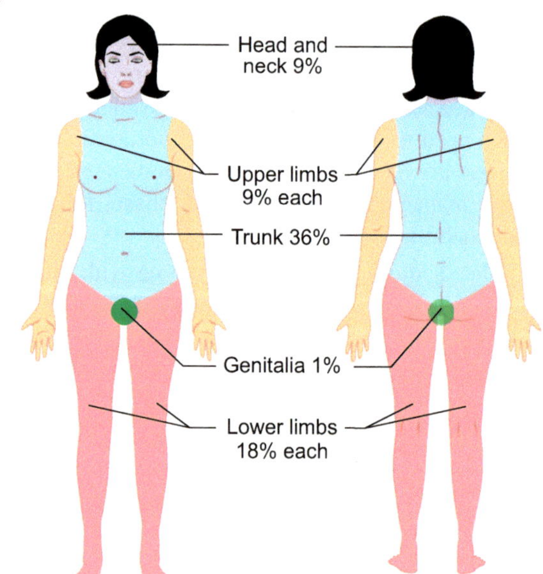

Figure 2: Wallace Rule of Nine for determining percent of burned body surface area

Management: Initial Assessment and Resuscitation

Initial Assessment

When doing the initial assessment for a burn patient, it is important to keep in mind that the ABCs should not be ignored. Burns can often be dramatic and can draw attention away from more immediate life-threatening problems.

More specific to burn patients, the initial step should be to terminate the burning process and break the contact between the skin and the burning item. Primary trauma survey with the ABCDE comes next. Special attention should be paid to the airway of a burn patient who has been exposed to inhalation/smoke injury. With severe exposure, early intubation is key.

On the other hand, for minor burns, the "4C" burn care can be used to approach and treat these patients.

- Cooling: cooling of the affected areas using saline soaked gauze or irrigation to prevent burn progression.
- Cleaning: often saline irrigation or mild soap with water and with or without antibacterial wash is adequate. Smaller sized blisters involving the palms or souls are left intact, and bigger blisters are debriding.
- Covering: topical hydrophilic ointments or creams with absorbent dressings or burn-specific dressing materials can be used.
- Comfort: multimodal pain control including over the counter non-narcotic pain medications, when possible, should be used. In some selected cases, splints can provide comfort and support to the burn areas.[1]

Resuscitation

After the initial survey is completed, the next step is a secondary survey with a complete physical exam. This involves continuing fluid resuscitation and immediate intervention for any other known life threats. Evaluation and treatment of burns are a part of secondary survey.

It is important to document under the physical exam findings the full extent of burns. These should be noted as percentage total body surface area burned (%TBSA) and severity/depth of the burns, documented as first degree, second degree, or third-degree burns.[4]

As discussed above, greater than 20% total body surface burns should be managed with aggressive IV fluid resuscitation to prevent the distributive shock that is often seen in these scenarios. Multiple formulas can be used to calculate the amount of fluid to be used for resuscitation based upon total body surface area burned. The most common formula used is called the Parkland formula. This gives us an estimate of the amount of fluid to be given in the first 24 hours.[4]

Total amount of fluids to be administered in the first 24 hours = 4 X %TBSA burned X patient's weight in kgs

Half of this fluid needs to be administered in the first eight hours, and the other half over the next 16 hours. For pediatric patients, normal maintenance fluids are added to the fluids calculated via the Parkland formula.

End Points

It is very essential to keep in mind that the amount of fluid calculated using these formulas is just a guideline. Decisions should be made on a case-to-case basis taking into account the patient's hemodynamics, peripheral perfusion, mentation, and urine output. These factors should be assessed and reassessed in a dynamic manner, and the fluid rates should be adjusted accordingly. A urine output of 0.5 CC per kilo per hour for children less than 30 kgs, and 0.5 CC per kilo per hour for adults is a good marker for adequate resuscitation. Although adequate resuscitation is key in decreasing morbidity and mortality of these patients, it is important to have high vigilance for side effects of over resuscitation.[4]

Other Considerations

Strict hemodynamic monitoring in the intensive care setting, telemetry and pulse oximetry when indicated, Foley catheter for accurate urine output management, and, if indicated, a nasogastric tube for patients with ileus or needing enteral tube feeding is essential.

Adequate pain control can be tough in patients with severe burns, hence multimodal pain control should be pursued to decrease opiate use. Tetanus prophylaxis should be administered if not given within the last five years. Always have a high index of suspicion for carbon monoxide or cyanide poisoning in patients with associated signs of inhalational injury.[4]

The American Burn Association recommendations for burn center referrals should be known so that there is timely and adequate referral to a local burn center. Following other recommendations for transfer:

- Any percentage of full thickness burns
- Greater than 10% total body surface area involving partial thickness burns
- Face, hands, feet, genitalia, or joints in Wildwood burns
- Electrical, lightning strike related injuries, and chemical burns
- Severe inhalational injuries
- Burn patients with multiple medical comorbidities
- Burn patients with associated traumatic injuries[1]

Nutrition

Adequate nutritional support is key in the management of patients with moderate and severe burn injuries. After significant burn injuries, due to hypermetabolism, distinctive demands are placed upon the body leading to an overwhelming hypermetabolic response.

Nutritional support is especially challenging because of the significant metabolic derangements that happen in severe burns. The metabolic rates are approximately twice the normal level. Failure to fulfill these requirements can lead to increased life-threatening protein calorie malnutrition, susceptibility to infection, issues with wound healing, and potentially organ dysfunction.[9]

Target Groups

While there is limited evidence to support the decision-making process and the timing of the initiation of nutrition support in the critical care setting, the combined Society of Critical Care Medicine (SCCM) and American Society for Parenteral and Enteral Nutrition (ASPEN) guidelines suggest, based on expert consensus, that very early initiation of enteral feeds should be targeted in patients with burn injuries:

- Moderate-to-severe burns: burn patients who are not expected to initiate an oral diet within 6 to 12 hours of sustaining the burn injury are started on nutrition support. Metabolic rate increases proportionally with burn size. A minimum of 15 to 25% total body surface area (TBSA) burn injury can initiate a catabolic response that includes impaired immunity and fluid shifts. Patients with burns greater than 40% TBSA consistently experience hypermetabolism.
- Inhalational injury: patients who have sustained inhalation injury or who have extensive facial burns, both of which are likely to result in a prolonged ventilator course, usually meet criteria for nutritional support.
- Failure to maintain weight: failure to maintain lean body mass (LBM) and body weight (i.e., dry body weight or weight on postburn day five) with oral intake, is an accepted indication for nutrition support in burn patients. Patients with burns that involve 20 to 40% of TBSA may not be able to consume sufficient calories to maintain LBM and weight. Similarly, patients who require extensive surgery, develop complications of their injury, or have a known nutritional deficiency at the time of admission may not consume adequate calories.
- Selected patients with less severe burns: nutrition support is used selectively in patients with less extensive burn injuries (<20%). Patient groups that may benefit include children, older adults, and patients with obesity.[6]

Timing

Initiation: the safety and efficacy of initiating enteral feedings in burn patients has been established, since it shows a trend toward decreasing infection rates and decreasing calorie deficits; however, the optimal timing of initiating nutrition support is debated. Early enteral nutrition may help to attenuate the hypermetabolic response to burn injury. In the hemodynamically stable patient with moderate-to-severe burn injury (>20% total body surface area [TBSA]), we suggest initiating nutrition support in the form of enteral feeding as early as possible.

Guidelines from the Society of Critical Care Medicine (SCCM) and American Society for Parenteral and Enteral Nutrition (ASPEN) support early enteral nutrition initiation, within four to six hours of injury for all critically ill burn patients, if possible. The recommendations from the European Society for Clinical Nutrition and Metabolism (ESPEN) recommend early enteral nutrition for moderate-to-severe burn patients who will not or cannot initiate oral nutrition within 6 to 12 hours of injury. Consultation with a dietitian experienced in the nutritional care of burn patients can prove exceptionally helpful in all aspects of the nutritional care of these patients.[7]

For hemodynamically unstable patients, nutrition support should be started as soon as the perfusion of the intestine is thought to be adequate. Care must be taken when delivering full feeds in the setting of marked hemodynamic instability or with high vasopressor requirements due to the risk of causing nonocclusive mesenteric ischemia. In spite of this, the use of enteral nutrition in patients on low or decreasing doses of vasopressors can be safely accomplished.[9]

Cessation: there has been little research into the optimal diet for patients in the acute postburn phase; however, it is suggested that they continue to receive adequate nutrition following discharge. It is known that the hypermetabolic state of burn injury can persist for over a year and that in addition to therapies that attenuate the hypermetabolic response, patients may benefit from increased caloric intake and increased consumption of protein during this time period. Patients should monitor their weight closely, and those who are not able to maintain their weight with their normal diet may benefit from supplementation.[6,8]

Delivery

Enteral nutrition, rather than parenteral nutrition, is generally preferred in burn patients who require nutrition support. Early enteral nutrition has been associated with improved functioning of the gastrointestinal tract, less ischemia/reperfusion injury, and reduced intestinal permeability in burn patients receiving enteral nutrition compared with a parenteral route. Enteral nutrition support can be delivered into the stomach or small intestine. In many burn centers, postpyloric feeding is preferred over gastric feeding and may be recommended if a patient has a particularly high risk for aspiration or has demonstrated intolerance for gastric nutrition support.

The effectiveness of gastric versus postpyloric nutrition support remains an area of controversy in burn care. Many burn centers safely and successfully use only gastric feedings or use a combination of gastric and enteric feedings. While placement of a postpyloric tube is technically more difficult than the placement of a gastric tube, and there is a greater risk of dislodgement with the intestinal tube, the minimally lower risk of pneumonia with postpyloric feedings and the ability to continue using them during patient repositioning, wound care, and even through operative procedures provides a slight advantage over gastric feeding in severe burns.

Parenteral nutrition is appropriate only in those burn patients who have persistent intolerance to enteral feeds and who are unable to attain adequate protein and calorie intake on enteral nutrition or those who suffer with burns or other injuries that limit access to the stomach or small intestines. Feeding intolerance is identified by abdominal distention, ileus, high gastric residuals, or intractable diarrhea following initiation of enteral nutrition. Our threshold for initiating parenteral nutrition in burn patients is persistent feeding intolerance for more than 48 to 72 hours.[6,10]

Nutritional Formulas

Various formulations and equations (e.g., Harris Benedict, Curreri) and other methods (e.g., indirect calorimetry) have been developed to estimate the energy requirements of adult and pediatric burn patients. Indirect calorimetry remains the standard for estimating energy expenditure in patients who are critically ill. The Curreri formula is widely used for estimating the total caloric needs of the burn patient. The two factors used in this formula, percent TBSA and body weight prior to the burn, estimate the energy requirements by linear regression analysis based on the number of calories required to prevent weight loss during the first few weeks postburn. The formula was based on nine adult patients. It does not take into account sex, age, activity, or ventilatory status. The Curreri formula overestimates the caloric needs of burn patients when compared to metabolic expenditure measured by calorimetry. High-fat feeding may increase complications including hyperlipidemia, hypoxemia, fatty liver infiltration, higher incidence of infection, and higher postoperative mortality.[6,8]

Burn Wound Management

Topical Treatment

Multimodal therapies with antimicrobial properties are typically used. One of the most widely used topical therapies is silver sulfadiazine. It is used as prophylaxis against infection rather than a treatment for an existing infection. It is inexpensive and easily applied with limited systemic absorption. Side effects include neutropenia, although this could be attributed to the migration of neutrophils as part of the burn inflammatory response. A true allergic reaction to sulfa is rare and can be avoided by using the patch test in patients with a suspected sulfa allergy. Silver sulfadiazine is also contraindicated on skin grafts as it causes destruction of newly grafted areas.

Mafenide acetate is another topical antimicrobial that is effective as both prophylaxis and treatment of an existing infection. It can also penetrate eschar. Unlike silver sulfadiazine, it can be used on fresh skin grafts. The side effects include metabolic acidosis. Its use can be limited by pain at the application site when used on partial thickness burn areas.

Silver nitrate is inexpensive and has broad spectrum antimicrobial activity. However, it can cause black stains, and prolonged application can lead to hyponatremia. Another rare side effect is methemoglobinemia.[12]

Dakin's solution (0.5% sodium hypochlorite) is an extensive topical antimicrobial, although there is no definitive evidence regarding its use in the burn population.

Topical ointments such as bacitracin, neomycin, and polymyxin B can be used for smaller burns, nearly healed large burns, or superficial partial-thickness facial burns. Another application for these topical agents includes nearly healed meshed skin grafts, where it is typically covered with greasy gauze for moisture retainment. Side effects include nephrotoxicity limiting their use in larger burns.

For patients with known risk factors for methicillin-resistant Staphylococcus aureus (MRSA) or those with positive wound culture for MRSA, mupirocin can be used. Silver-impregnated dressings are being widely used for donor sites, skin grafts, and partial thickness burns as they allow for less frequent dressing changes, although their use may limit serial wound examinations (Table 2).[17]

Table 2: Topical antimicrobial agents used in burns

Antimicrobial agents	Clinical indications	Effectiveness	Contraindications	Adverse effects
Silver sulfadiazine (1% cream with or without cerium	Small, medium and large surface area burns	Decreased colonization of wounds Alleviates pain Broad spectrum No evidence to support improvved wound healing or reduction in bacterial wound infections[3]	Burns near eyes Pregnancy Breastfeeding newborns <2 months Allergic to sulfonamides signs of reepithelialization	Skin hypersensitivity neutropenia (usually transient) Leukopenia (usually transient) methemoglobinemia

Antimicrobial agents	Clinical indications	Effectiveness	Contraindications	Adverse effects
Silver containing dressings (eg. Acticoat, Aquacel Ag)	Small, medium, and large surface area burns	Stronger antimicrobia activity, longer duration of action than silver sulfadiazine, some evidence for reduced wound infection rates[3]	Burns near eyes Pregnancy Allergic to silver	Systemic silver uptake, temporary staining of the skin, argyrosis-argyria* [4,5]
Bacitracin ointment 500 units/gram	Small surface area burns Face Ears Perinuem Graft sites Alternative if allergic to sulfonamides	Ease of application and of removal Painless Frequent dressing changes	Bacterial resistance Signs of reepithelialization	Yeast colonization Skin hypersensitivity
Combination antibiotic ointment (eg. Bacitracin, neomycin, and polymyxin B)	Small surface area burns Face Ears Perineum Fraft sites Alternative if allergic to sulfonamides	Ease of application and of removal Painless Frequent dressing changes	Bacterial resistance Allergic reaction Sings of reepithelialization	Yeast colonization Skin hypersensitiviy Ototoxicity and nephrotoxicity with neomycin-containing ointments (eg. Neosporin)
Mupirocin ointment/ cream 2%	Small, medium surface area burns Face Ears Nose Perineum Alternative if allergic to sulfonamides	Gram-positive coverage includes methicilin-resistant stophylococcus Aureus (MRSA) Ease of application and of removal Painless Frequent dressing changes	Bacterial resistance Allergic reaction Sings of reepithelialization	Yeast colonization Skin hypersensitivity
Mafenide (8.5Z% cream, 5% solution)	Ears Nose Dense bacterial proliferation	Excellent eschar penetration Penetrates cartilage Gram-negative coverage indudes Pseudomonos	Burns >40% total body surface area Allergic to sulfonamides	Metabolic acidosis (inhibits carbonic anhydrase) Painful Inhibits epithelial regeneration

Surgical Management

Wound Excision

Early excision and grafting in burn patients are key components to improving survival outcomes related to mortality, reconstruction surgery, hospital length of stay, and cost. Excision should be considered immediately following the initial resuscitation phase when the patient is hemodynamically stable, ideally within the first few days. Serial excisions are usually necessary for larger burns. Excision is usually accomplished using the Watson or Goulian blade in repeated tangential slices until viable, diffusely bleeding tissue is encountered. Healthy dermis that appears white with punctate bleeding can be left intact. However, in deeper burns, excision to fat or fascia may be necessary. Tangential excision is associated with high blood loss, which can be mitigated using certain techniques that contributed to the significant decrease in the number of blood transfusions in this population. Examples include the installation of an epinephrine tumescence solution beneath the burned area, the use of pneumatic tourniquets in extremity burns, and the application of compresses soaked in a dilute epinephrine solution. The use of fibrinogen and thrombin spray sealant (Tisseel Fibrin Sealant) has the added benefit of graft adherence to the wound bed, in addition to hemostasis. Facial excision can be employed in patients with deep burns with a concern for excessive blood loss, although the cosmetic outcomes are inferior due to the loss of subcutaneous tissue. A pressurized water dissector can offer a more precise excision of burns in difficult anatomic areas, such as the face or hands.[11,12]

Compartment syndrome occurs with circumferential full thickness burns. The rigid eschar can have a tourniquet effect with the progression of edema, leading to initial venous outflow followed by arterial inflow compromise. When indicated, escharotomies are usually performed at bedside, preferentially using electrocautery to minimize loss of blood. Incisions of the extremity are created on the medial and lateral parts of the limbs in an anatomic position. These incisions can extend onto the thenar and hypothenar eminences of the hand. Digital escharotomies are not recommended since they do not have any meaningful salvaging of functional tissue. Fasciotomy may be indicated when there is inadequate perfusion despite proper escharotomies, although it should not be performed routinely with the eschar release. Thoracic escharotomies are made along the anterior axillary lines with bilateral subclavicular and subcostal extensions. The anterior axillary incision can extend down the lateral abdomen, generally allowing adequate release of abdominal eschar (Figure 3).[12,16]

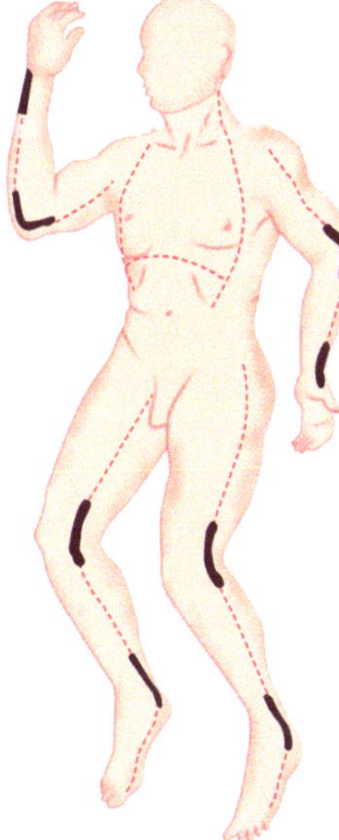

Figure 3: Escharotomy Incisions

Wound Coverage

Many options exist for wound coverage. Skin grafts are generally classified into split-thickness and full-thickness grafts. Split-thickness grafts include only a portion of the dermis, while full-thickness grafts contain the entire dermis. The likelihood of survival and the level of contracture is determined by the amount of dermis in the graft.[15] Split-thickness autografts are suitable for most wounds as they are durable and have acceptable cosmetic outcomes. They have the ability to survive in environments with less vascularity, but the likelihood of contracture is greater. They are usually harvested with a power dermatome and can be meshed to provide coverage for larger burn wounds. Meshing has an added benefit of allowing drainage of blood and serous fluids that can lead to the formation of hematoma and seroma, respectively, and potential graft loss. Non-meshed grafts are used in certain areas of cosmetic significance such as the face, neck, and hands (Figure 4). In contrast, full-thickness grafts need a better vascular bed to survive but have less contracture. They are harvested using the scalpel and include all the dermis with as little subcutaneous fat as possible. Donor site is closed primarily (Figure 5).[12,14]

Temporary wound coverage can be achieved using skin substitutes to help with protection from mechanical trauma, act as a physical barrier to bacteria, and create a moist wound environment.

Temporary wound coverage can be achieved using human cadaveric allografts. They initially incorporate into the wound but must be replaced as they are eventually rejected by the immune system. Xenograft is a considerably less expensive option that functions as well as allograft for temporary wound coverage. Synthetic skin substitutes are another option for patients with massive burns and limited donor sites. Examples include integra, Alloderm, and NovoSorb Biodegradable Temporizing Matrix. They are used with split-thickness skin grafts for final wound coverage at approximately two weeks from the synthetic graft placement.

Thighs are the preferred option for donor sites because harvesting is easy and generally hidden from an esthetic standpoint. In older patients, the skin from the back is useful because it is thicker than elsewhere which results in easier healing of donor sites. For infants and toddlers, the buttock is a great donor site. One should apply silver sulfadiazine to the donor site and cover it with a diaper. Another excellent donor site is the scalp since it allows rapid healing due to the thick skin and many hair follicles, additionally, the site will be completely hidden after the regrowth of hair. During harvesting of the scalp, epinephrine tumescence is required for hemostasis of this hypervascular area and to make a smooth contoured surface that helps with harvesting. The choice of donor site dressing is largely institution dependent, and little data supports a clear advantage of using one treatment plan over another. Options include simple transparent films to hydrocolloids, silver-impregnated dressings, and petrolatum gauzes. When a donor site is near a fresh graft, it may be dressed with a porous nonadherent gauze. Additionally, both the grafts and donors are soaked with an antimicrobial solution.[12,18]

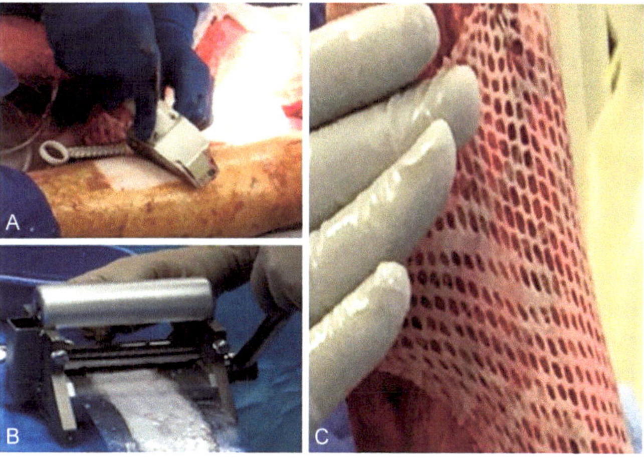

Figure 4: Autologous skin grafting: (A) Partial-thickness skin graft from the healthy donor site. (B) Skin graft is meshed, increasing the surface area (C) Application of skin graft on the wound bed.

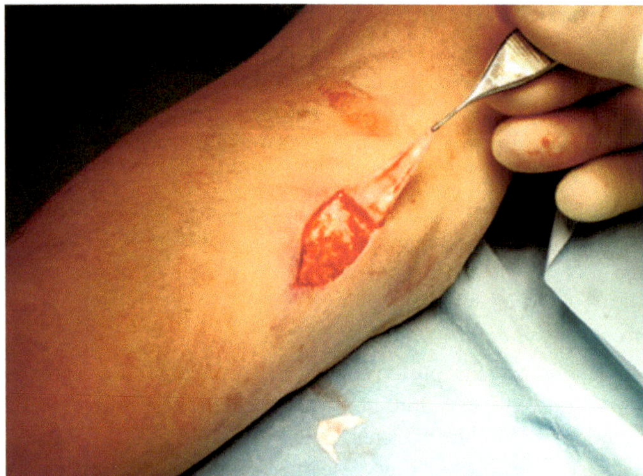

Figure 5: Full-thickness skin graft harvest from the medial forearm donor area. Note the shiny undersurface of the graft dermis

Late Complications: Contractures

Following recovery from the acute burn phase, many patients face hypertrophic scar-related morbidity, which include erythema, pruritus, pain, thickened skin, and contractures. Nonsurgical therapy is usually sufficient and includes compression garments, silicone gel sheets, massage and physical therapy, and steroids. Laser therapy provides an additional treatment option for the symptomatic patients. Examples include pulsed dye laser (PDL) and the ablative carbon dioxide (CO_2) laser. These are outpatient and office-based procedures that are well tolerated by the patients. Literature supports starting these treatments at six to twelve months from the insult and offering three treatment sessions. Surgical options such as excision and scar revision might be necessary for functional and esthetic recovery. Contracture represents another dreaded long-term complication with significant morbidity to burn patients that limits range of motion of the affected joints. Depth of the burn influences contracture development. Other factors include activation of dermal fibroblasts, myofibroblasts, fibrocytes, and helper T cells. They develop in as many as one-third of the burn patients. The shoulder is the most affected joint, followed by the elbow, wrist, ankle, and knee. Treatment of contractures includes both nonsurgical options which include pressure garments, splints, and laser therapy and surgical options with excisions and scar revisions. Heterotopic ossification is another long-term morbidity, although less common, with an incidence of 1 to 3% in burn patients. This involves the pathologic development of lamellar bone in peripheral tissues resulting in decreased range of motion and pain of the affected joint. It can be visualized on plain X-rays. Treatment includes aggressive physiotherapy, NSAIDs, bisphosphonates, radiation therapy, and rarely surgical excision.[12,13,18]

REFERENCES

1. Schaefer TJ, Szymanski KD. Burn Evaluation And Management. [Updated 2021 Dec 9]. In: StatPearls [Internet]. Treasure Island (FL): StatPearls Publishing; 2022 Jan. Available from: https://www.ncbi.nlm.nih.gov/books/NBK430741/.
2. Jeschke MG, van Baar ME, Choudhry MA, Chung KK, Gibran NS, Logsetty S. Burn injury. Nat Rev Dis Primers. 2020 Feb 13;6(1):11. doi: 10.1038/s41572-020-0145-5. PMID: 32054846; PMCID: PMC7224101.
3. Warby R, Maani CV. Burn Classification. [Updated 2021 Sep 5]. In: StatPearls [Internet]. Treasure Island (FL): StatPearls Publishing; 2022 Jan. Available from: https://www.ncbi.nlm.nih.gov/books/NBK539773/.
4. Schaefer TJ, Nunez Lopez O. Burn Resuscitation And Management. [Updated 2022 Jan 31]. In: StatPearls [Internet]. Treasure Island (FL): StatPearls Publishing; 2022 Jan. Available from: https://www.ncbi.nlm.nih.gov/books/NBK430795/.
5. Papini R. Management of burn injuries of various depths. BMJ. 2004 Jul 17;329(7458):158-60. doi: 10.1136/bmj.329.7458.158. PMID: 15258073; PMCID: PMC478230.
6. Romanowski K. Overview of nutrition support in burn patients. UpToDate. 2021 Jul 23.
7. Taylor BE, McClave SA, Martindale RG, et al. Guidelines for the Provision and Assessment of Nutrition Support Therapy in the Adult Critically Ill Patient: Society of Critical Care Medicine (SCCM) and American Society for Parenteral and Enteral Nutrition (A.S.P.E.N.). Crit Care Med 2016; 44:390.
8. Rousseau AF, Losser MR, Ichai C, Berger MM. ESPEN endorsed recommendations: nutritional therapy in major burns. Clin Nutr 2013; 32:497.
9. Pereira CT, Herndon DN. The pharmacologic modulation of the hypermetabolic response to burns. Adv Surg 2005; 39:245.
10. Flynn MB. Nutritional support for the burn-injured patient. Crit Care Nurs Clin North Am 2004; 16:139.
11. Browning JA, Cindass R. Burn Debridement, Grafting, and Reconstruction. [Updated 2022 Jun 5]. In: StatPearls [Internet]. Treasure Island (FL): StatPearls Publishing; 2022 Jan. Available from: https://www.ncbi.nlm.nih.gov/books/NBK551717/.
12. Brunicardi FC. Schwartz's principles of surgery (Eleventh edition). New York: McGraw-Hill. 2019.

13. van Baar ME, Essink-Bot ML, Oen IMMH, Dokter J, Boxma H, van Beeck EF. Functional outcome after burns: A review, Burns, Volume 32, Issue 1, 2006, Pages 1-9, ISSN 0305-4179, https://doi.org/10.1016/j.burns.2005.08.007.
14. Ray S, Rao K. Full Thickness Skin Grafts. In (Ed.), Skin Grafts - Indications, Applications and Current Research. IntechOpen. 2011. https://doi.org/10.5772/22385.
15. Shimizu R, Kishi K. Skin graft. Plast Surg Int. 2012;2012:563493. doi: 10.1155/2012/563493. Epub 2012 Feb 6. PMID: 22570780; PMCID: PMC3335647.
16. Burn 7. Wound Care, Size Estimate, Escharotomy, Infection. UK Trauma Protocol Manual. http://uktraumaprotocol.blogspot.com/2014/03/burn-7-wound-care-burn-size-estimate.html.
17. Tenenhaus M, Rennekampff HO. Topical agents and dressings for local burn wound care. UpToDate. 2021 Oct 15.
18. Wang Y, Beekman J, Hew J, Jackson S, Issler-Fisher AC, Parungao R, Lajevardi SS, Li Z, Maitz PKM. Burn injury: Challenges and advances in burn wound healing, infection, pain and scarring, Advanced Drug Delivery Reviews, Volume 123, 2018, Pages 3-17, ISSN 0169-409X, https://doi.org/10.1016/j.addr.2017.09.018.

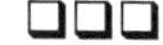

SECTION 6: ONCOLOGY AND ENDOCRINOLOGY

54

CHAPTER

Thyroid

Francisco Igor Macedo, MD
Edsa Negussie, MD
Barry Herschman, MD
Kayla K. Umemoto, BA
Vijay K. Mittal, MD

HISTORY AND EVOLUTION OF THYROID SURGERY

The thyroid gland was first described by Vesalius (1543) as *Glandulare laryngis*... The first reports of thyroid surgery were described at the School of Salerno in the thirteenth century. To complete the surgery, they were limited to using Setons and hot irons, and then they applied asphodel powder to the remnant.[1] Technical improvements did not occur until the middle of the 19th century. The operation by Pierre Joseph Desault in 1791 was the first thyroidectomy and was similar to the procedure performed nowadays. The most notable thyroid surgeons were Emil Kocher (1841 -1917) and Theodorus Billroth (1829-1894). Kocher performed hundreds of thyroid operations, refining the technique and anatomical dissection. He is considered the Father of thyroid surgery and, in recognition of his work on the thyroid gland, won the Nobel Prize in Medicine in 1909. Billroth also gave enormous contributions to the study of thyroid surgery. In particular, he advanced the understanding of the postoperative complications associated with thyroid surgery, including tetany and injury to the recurrent laryngeal nerve.[2]

W. S. Halsted began his experiments with thyroid transplants in dogs in 1887. This work resulted in the discovery of histological changes such as hyperplasia, and the accurate histological description of an exophthalmic goiter. He was the first to administer iodine to prevent post-operative or recurrent hyperplasia. Overtime, the subtotal thyroidectomy became the worldwide standard procedure for bilateral benign thyroid disease. More recently, the reports from Mayo Clinic have been an important milestone in disseminating and understanding the surgical technique and operative complications, greatly improving the thyroid surgery.[3]

ANATOMY

The thyroid gland lies below the larynx, weighing about 20 g. It is made up of two lateral lobes with an isthmus joining the lobes. The lower lobe border lies at the level of the 4th or 5th tracheal ring. The thyroid lobes are surrounded by the esophagus and trachea medially, and the carotid sheath posteriorly and laterally. Anteriorly, lie the sternocleidomastoid and strap muscles (i.e., sternohyoid, sternothyroid, and superior belly of the omohyoid).

The blood supply of the superior pole of the gland derives from the superior thyroid artery (STA), which derives from the external carotid artery. The inferior thyroid artery (ITA) arises from the thyrocervical trunk and supplies the upper and middle third of the gland. The ITA is strongly associated with the recurrent laryngeal nerve (RLN), generally having a path that intersects the RLN as it branches and terminates into the thyroid gland.

The venous drainage includes the superior thyroid veins (adjacent to the STA), inferior thyroid veins, and the middle thyroid vein(s). These veins travel laterally for direct drainage into the internal jugular vein.

One branch of the vagus nerve is the superior laryngeal nerve which further branches into external and internal branches. The external branch of the superior laryngeal nerve (EBSLN) provides motor innervation to the cricothyroid muscle which is responsible for vocal cord tensing. Due to its close association with the STA, injury to the EBSLN may occur.[4] The internal branch of the superior laryngeal nerve provides sensory innervation to the mucosal lining of the supraglottic larynx.

The left RLN branches off the vagus nerve and crosses the arch of the aorta. Then it loops around the aorta and ascends posterior to the thyroid gland within the tracheoesophageal groove. The right RLN branches off the vagus nerve and crosses anterior to the right subclavian artery. Many variations of the RLN exist in relation to the ligament of Berry and the inferior thyroid artery.[6] As the RLNs ascend toward the middle of the thyroid gland, they are intimately associated with the inferior thyroid artery. The RLN can be encountered where it enters the larynx just behind the inferior cornu of the thyroid cartilage.[7]

The RLN provides motor innervation to all of the intrinsic muscles of the larynx (except the cricothyroid muscle) and sensory innervation to the proximal trachea and subglottic area. Damage to the RLN results in a mixed pathology. The most significant is paralysis of the ipsilateral vocal cord, leading to the cord remaining in a paramedian position. If there is injury to the RLN bilaterally, both vocal cords will be fixed in the adducted position, resulting in severe airway obstruction, which may require a tracheostomy.

PHYSIOLOGY

The thyroid gland produces triiodothyronine (T_3), thyroxine (T_4), and the calcium-regulating hormone calcitonin. Iodine is essential for normal thyroid function. Thyroid-stimulating hormone (TSH) regulates the transport of iodide into follicular cells. Iodide is then oxidized into organic iodide when coupled to tyrosine moieties on thyroglobulin forming monoiodotyrosine (MIT) or diiodotyrosine (DIT). Thyroid peroxidase is the intracellular agent that catalyzes these reactions. This is a fundamental step in the organification and storage of inorganic iodide. Coupling of MIT and DIT forms the two biologically active thyroid hormones (T_3 and T_4).

At this point, T_3 and T_4 lie within vesicles. Then when lysosomal hydrolysis takes place, disulfide bonds between the hormones and thyroglobulin are reduced releasing T_3 and T_4. The hormones then freely pass the basement membrane and are absorbed into the circulation, 99% of which are bound to serum proteins. The half-life of T_3 and T_4 is about 8 to 12 hours and 7 days, respectively.[9]

BIOCHEMICAL TESTS

The work-up of thyroid nodules is done through the biochemical assessment of the thyroid.[10] In most cases, normal levels of TSH is sufficient to discontinue additional testing. Thyroid antigens (e.g., thyroid-stimulating immunoglobulin, antimicrosomal antibodies) are made in autoimmune thyroid disorders such as Hashimoto's thyroiditis and Graves' disease. To diagnose these autoimmune disorders, tests for antibodies against thyroid-specific antigens, thyroglobulin (Tg), TSH receptors (TSH-R), and antithyroid peroxidase (TPO) are performed. TSH-R antibodies against thyroid follicular cells are commonly seen in Graves' disease. The antibodies' value in diagnosis and prognosis is decreased by differences in the sensitivity and specificity of current methods. About 95% of Hashimoto's thyroiditis patients and 80% of Grave's disease patients have detectable levels of antimicrosomal antibodies.

In patients with thyroid masses and, in whom multiple endocrine neoplasia type 2 (MEN 2) syndrome or isolated medullary carcinoma is suspected, a baseline calcitonin level is required. Pentagastrin- or calcium-stimulated calcitonin evaluation can be performed when there is doubt about the diagnosis.

DISEASES OF THE THYROID

GOITER

A *goiter* is the enlargement of the thyroid gland usually due to an iodine deficiency. An endemic goiter is secondary to iodine deficiency and, in certain geographic areas, affects over 10% of the population. Euthyroid multinodular goiter (MNG) is the enlargement of the thyroid gland but has no thyroid dysfunction seen clinically or through laboratory studies. A toxic nodule goiter (TNG) is the enlargement of the thyroid gland with hyperthyroidism.

The thyroid can also be enlarged in chronic Hashimoto's thyroiditis, Graves'disease, or in a neoplasia. If nontoxic, the clinical manifestations of the goiter are due to mass effects including breathing difficulties and dysphagia. The differential diagnosis consists of a benign nodular goiter, diffuse goiter, follicular adenoma, carcinoma, and Hashimoto's thyroiditis. An anaplastic or lymphomatous malignancy should be suspected if the goiter is rapidly enlarging, appearing within weeks to months.

The goals of goiter treatment are relief of local compressive symptoms, preventing further enlargement of the thyroid, cosmetic deformity, removal of a potential coexistent thyroid cancer, and treatment of any associated thyroid dysfunction. The treatment options include observation, levothyroxine (T4) suppression, radioactive iodine, and surgical resection.

Surgery is indicated in MNG patients if the goiter extends into the thoracic cavity, the patient has compressive symptoms, cancer is suspected, the patient has symptoms of hyperthyroidism, and the patient wants to improve their cosmetic appearance. Subtotal thyroidectomy is the procedure of choice due to its presumed lower complication rate if patients have bilateral MNG. However, many surgeons also perform total thyroidectomies to prevent recurrence, where an incomplete resection could potentially grow later and require a second thyroid operation. Surgeons try to avoid additional thyroid operations since the procedure has a higher risk of injuring the RLN and the parathyroid glands resulting in hypoparathyroidism. A sternotomy is indicated for patients with a low-lying carcinoma involving the lymph node, recurrent intrathoracic goiter, and any unsuccessful cervical delivery of a large goiter.

HYPERTHYROIDISM

Hyperthyroidism is when the thyroid gland overproduces hormones. Thyrotoxicosis is the physiologic syndrome of excess thyroid hormone.

Graves' disease is a hyperthyroid disease due to circulating IgG autoantibodies which stimulate TSH-R, a G-protein-coupled receptor. The prevalence of Graves' disease is about 0.5% of the population which is the majority (50% to 80%) of hyperthyroidism cases. There is a 5:1 to 10:1 female to male ratio of Graves with the peak incidence being 40 and 60 years old. The clinical presentation of Graves depends on the amount of excess hormone, thus the symptoms, duration of disease, and presence of comorbidities can be variable. Common complaints include restlessness, nervousness or anxiety, palpitations, sensitivity to heat, and weight loss. Common clinical findings include warm skin, moist skin, tachycardia, and mild tremor. Additionally, due to an increase in sympathetic activity, patients may have "lid lag," a delay of the eyelid when following the eye when looking downward. Other specific findings on physical exam are pretibial myxedema, exophthalmos, and acropachy (finger and toe clubbing). Patients may have incidences of thyrotoxicosis which is a potentially life-threatening condition known as a thyroid storm. Patients will present with fever, severe tachycardia, congestive heart failure, arrhythmias, psychosis, agitation, and coma.

The initial treatment for Graves' disease patients most often includes antithyroid drugs. The most frequently used medications are thioamides (i.e., methimazole and propylthiouracil). Thyrotoxicosis symptoms (i.e., tachycardia, tremor, sweating, and palpitations) occur during the 3 to 4 weeks of starting therapy, and interim, prompt treatment with β-adrenergic blocking agents is initiated to address these symptoms. These symptoms typically reduce significantly in 3 to 4 weeks. The goal of treatment is to tailor antithyroid medication dosages to obtain normalized levels of serum T3 and T4, and eventually TSH. Thirty to fifty percent of Graves' patients treated with antithyroid medications achieve remission, which is defined as a normal range of TSH while not receiving therapy. However, over 50% will relapse.

Another initial treatment includes RAI therapy with iodine-131, which can also be used after medical therapy. RAI therapy induces hypothyroidism, thus preventing recurrence of Graves. It has a roughly 80% success rate. If after initial RAI therapy the patient's hyperthyroidism is persistent, they will require another ablation in about 6 months. The recurrence rate of hyperthyroidism is about 3% each year, thus patients should be continuously monitored. This therapy is contraindicated during pregnancy; thus, women of childbearing age must obtain a pregnancy test prior to any therapy.

Surgery is reserved for selected patients, such as those who are pregnant or nursing, have complications or side effects due to the medication therapy, have suspicious nodules or large goiters, refuse radioactive therapy, and desire a short and definitive treatment. The surgery performed is usually a subtotal thyroidectomy, with an attempt to leave about 2 g of tissue which overlay the RLNs. Total thyroidectomy is becoming more common because it decreases the 2-20% of hyperthyroidism recurrences seen with subtotal resection. If undergoing a total thyroidectomy, patients should take a saturated potassium iodide solution (SSKI) 7 to 10 days prior to surgery. This pretreatment decreases the size and vascularity of the gland, thus enabling a less difficult surgery to perform.

Toxic Nodular Goiter

Toxic nodular goiter refers to a condition in which a nodule in a multinodular goiter becomes autonomous and secretes large amounts of thyroid hormones, also referred to as Plummer's disease. Physical exam may reveal an enlarged thyroid which can be multinodular in nature. Thyroid hormone levels are elevated with suppressed TSH. Ultrasound confirms a multinodular goiter which may have retrosternal extension. An I-131 scan reveals focal area(s) of increased function with suppression of the rest of the gland.

The choice of treatment of a toxic nodular goiter is radioiodine therapy. Surgery involves a lobectomy in the case of a single adenoma, or near total thyroidectomy in the case of a toxic multinodular goiter.

MANAGEMENT OF A THYROID NODULE

Thyroid nodules are a common clinical problem, especially in women and the elderly. From a group of randomly selected individuals, 19-67% had thyroid nodules detected on high-resolution ultrasound (US).[10] In high-risk cases (Table 1), it is important to exclude thyroid cancer which is seen in 5-15% of thyroid nodules; factors include age, sex, family history, radiation exposure history, and other factors.[10] Important findings on examination suggestive of malignancy include fixation of the nodule to surrounding tissues, vocal cord paralysis, and lateral cervical lymphadenopathy.

Table 1: Clinical characteristics suspicious of thyroid nodules[10]

High Risk	• Rapid growth of the nodule, especially with levothyroxine therapy • Family history of thyroid cancer or multiple endocrine neoplasia syndrome • History of irradiation to the head or neck • Nodule is firm or hard • Nodule is fixed to adjacent structures • Cervical lymphadenopathy
Moderate Risk	• Age <20 or > 60 years • Male • Size of nodule is >4 cm • Complex cystic nodule • Symptoms of mass effect: cough, dysphagia, dyspnea, voice change

The same risk of malignancy is seen in both nonpalpable and palpable nodules of the same size. Only nodules greater than 1 cm are generally evaluated because they pose a higher risk of being a clinically significant cancer. Occasionally, nodules less than 1 cm need further evaluation due to suspicious findings on US, and a history that includes irradiation to the head and neck, associated lymphadenopathy, or a family history of thyroid cancer in at least one first-degree relative and 18FDG-PET-positive thyroid nodules.

Diagnostic thyroid US should be performed in all patients with a suspected thyroid nodule, nodular goiter, or radiographic abnormality. Various sonographic characteristics of a thyroid nodule have been associated with a higher likelihood of malignancy, including nodule hypoechogenicity, increased intranodular vascularity, a cystic nodule with a large solid component and irregular infiltrative margins, microcalcifications, and an absent halo. In patients who have a known thyroid cancer, using preoperative ultrasonography to diagnosis locally advanced or metastatic disease has shown to change the planned operative procedure and guide the extent of lymphadenectomy through the identification of suspicious cervical lymphadenopathy.[11] Cervical US should be performed at 6 to 12 months and then periodically, depending on the patient's risk for recurrent disease and their thyroglobulin status.[12]

Radionuclide scanning is an important test when working up a patient with hyperthyroidism or thyrotoxicosis because it determines if a nodule is autonomously functioning. The malignancy incidence in cold (hypofunctional) nodules is about 15% versus in warm (normal function) nodules it is about 9%, and in 'hot' (hyperfunctional) nodules it is about 5%. In cases of a hot nodule, the risk for malignancy is extremely low and further investigation is no longer recommended. In patients who have thyroid cancer, radioiodine is also used during a whole-body scan radiotracer to assess surgical resection completeness, to diagnose metastatic disease, or to detect recurrence.

It is not recommended to use other imaging studies (CT, MRI, and PET) preoperatively. These imaging modalities may be useful in assessing the involvement of extrathyroidal tissues of large, rapidly growing, retrosternal, or invasive tumors. MRI generally has specific indications for its use, such as evaluating substernal goiters and their relation to other structures, assessing the local extent of thyroid carcinomas, and localizing the site of thyroid neoplasia recurrence. For thyroid nodule evaluation, fine needle aspiration (FNA) is the most common modality because it is accurate and cost-effective. It can be performed as an outpatient procedure, is relatively inexpensive, and is only associated with rare complications. Traditionally, the results of a FNA biopsy are separated into the four categories of nondiagnostic, benign, intermediate or suspicious for neoplasm, and malignant (risk of malignancy at surgery is >95%). Additional immediate diagnostic tests are not required routinely if the nodule is found to be benign on cytology. However, these nodules should be followed up 6-18 months after initial FNA with serial US exams. A nodule is considered stable if (1) there is <50% volume change or (2) there is a <20% increase in dimensions of two or more nodules either the solid nodules or the solid portion of mixed cystic-solid nodules. If a nodule is stable, the clinical exam or US follow-up interval can be longer (e.g., every 3-5 years). A nodule is considered growing if there is >50% volume change or there is a 20% increase in at least two dimensions of the nodule. If a nodule shows evidence of growth by either palpation or sonograph, a repeat FNA should be performed, preferably with US guidance. If there is suspicion of a Hurthle cell neoplasm or papillary carcinoma, the patient does not need a radionuclide scan and, depending on the size of the lesion and other risk factors, is recommended to undergo either a lobectomy or total thyroidectomy.

There is increasing push to perform a routine laryngoscopy for both benign and malignant diseases prior to thyroid surgery. A flexible laryngoscopy with topical nasal anesthetics and a fiberoptic scope is an easy procedure to perform in the office. It is extremely important to determine the vocal cord status before surgery if a pre-existing voice changes or if there is a suspected thyroid cancer.

THYROID CANCER

Thyroid cancer is relatively rare, consisting of 2% of all cancers, however among endocrine malignancies it is the most common, and the incidence has been steadily increasing over the past 15 to 20 years, especially in patients >30 years old.

Risk factors

Ionizing radiation is the most important environmental risk factor leading to thyroid cancer.[14] Studies have shown there to be a 30-40% increase in risk after ionizing radiation exposure. Additionally, estrogen is a stimulus for genomic instability, exerting a mutagenic effect on the thyroid. A history of thyroid carcinoma in the family can increase one's risk. There is a 3-fold increase in risk when a parent has thyroid carcinoma and up to a 6-fold increase in risk when a sibling has thyroid carcinoma. Additionally, thyroid cancer is associated with several germline mutation syndromes including familial adenomatous polyposis or Gardner syndrome, Carney syndrome, Werner Syndrome, and Cowden disease. However, only a few of these patients will eventually develop thyroid carcinoma. Mutations associated with nearly 70% of thyroid carcinomas involve RET, BRAF, NTRK1, PPARg, and kRAS. Mutations seen in follicular carcinoma include PPARg (rarely found in papillary thyroid cancer), AKT pathways, and kRAS.

Prognostic factors

There is an overall 7% mortality rate in patients with thyroid cancer. Most patients are either cured or live with recurrent disease for years. Up to 11% of patients will have recurrent disease, of which up to 50% will ultimately die due to the disease. In patients with papillary thyroid cancer, recurrence after the initial surgical treatment can occur up to four decades later, whereas in patients with follicular thyroid cancer, recurrence after the initial treatment almost always occur within 14 years. The most important prognostic factors uniformly are an age of <40 years (good prognostic factor), size of the tumor, and presence of extrathyroidal extension of the tumor. Extrathyroidal tumor extension is associated with an increased incidence of recurrent disease and mortality.

PAPILLARY THYROID CARCINOMA

Papillary thyroid cancer (PTC) is the most common histologic type of thyroid cancer. It occurs in about 80% of cases. There are several variants of PTC including a follicular variant which has a follicular pattern of growth and several other variants that are more aggressive (e.g., tall cell, insular, columnar cell, and diffuse sclerosing). Genetic and environmental factors increase one's chance of developing PTC and roughly 3% are familial. PTC is more common in women than men by a ratio of 3:1. Patients with PTC are generally asymptomatic, presenting with either a solitary thyroid nodule or a palpable cervical lymph node. Occasionally, symptoms that increase the worry of an aggressive or invasive cancer will present. These include dysphagia, hemoptysis, or hoarseness. Even in these cases, distant metastases are uncommon. If US detects a suspicious-appearing lymph node (Figure 1), FNA biopsy is recommended. Some professionals recommend a selective preoperative laryngoscopy to be performed only on patients who are symptomatic or have previously had a cervical operation.

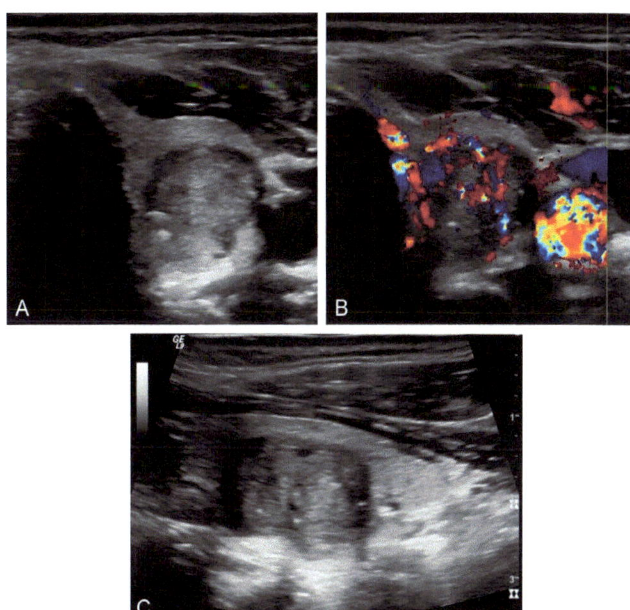

Figure 1: Papillary thyroid carcinoma. (A) Transverse view exhibits calcifications within the upper nodule which are better seen in this view using a proprietary image enhancement scheme. (B) Color doppler flow shows an increase in the peripheral vascularity of the nodule in the upper lobe. The mid-pole nodule shows no increased vascularity. (C) Sagittal image of the thyroid demonstrates clumps of calcification within a poorly marginated lesion.

Treatment options include surgery, ablation with adjunctive RAI, and in some cases, TSH suppression, and surveillance. Resection options include thyroid lobectomy and near-total thyroidectomy or total thyroidectomy. The extent of thyroidectomy is controversial, especially for PTCs that are small, low risk, intrathyroidal, and well-differentiated (Figure 2). Some studies demonstrate a lack of survival benefit with more extensive thyroidectomy, and a lower complication rate with lobectomy (e.g., RLN injury, permanent hypoparathyroidism). On the other hand, other studies demonstrate lower rates of recurrence and higher rates of survival with more extensive thyroidectomy compared with lobectomy. The two procedures have comparable complication rates. Up to 80% of PTCs are multifocal and up to 60% are bilateral, thus total thyroidectomy allows (1) postoperative RAI to be used to remove the residual microscopic or metastatic disease and (2) serum thyroglobulin (Tg) to be used postoperatively as a sensitive marker for disease recurrence.

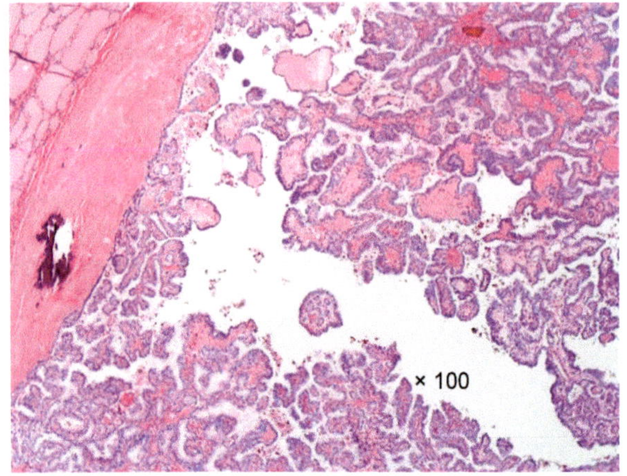

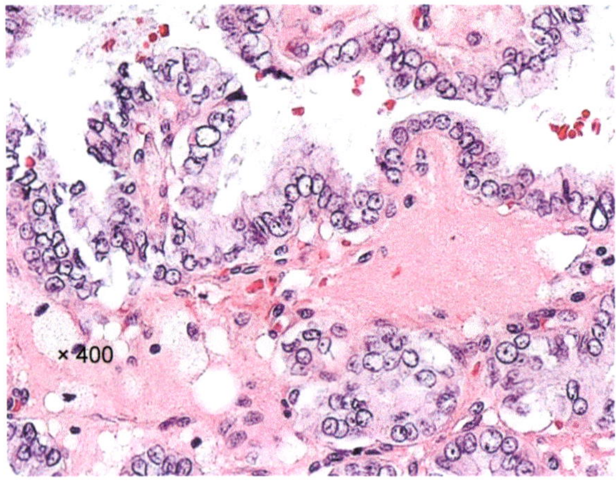

Figure 2: Microscopic image of papillary thyroid carcinoma. These indolent tumors have a long survival. The local lymph node located in the neck is the most common site for metastasis and a nodal metastasis is sometimes the first sign of the cancer. Microscopically, psammoma bodies and cells with clear nuclei are characteristic features of papillary thyroid carcinoma.

The preferred initial treatment of PTC, according to consensus guidelines, is a total or near-total thyroidectomy, with absolute indications such as radiation exposure history, family history of thyroid cancer, tumor size >4 cm, cervical lymph node, known extrathyroidal extension, distant metastasis, or histology demonstrating an aggressive PTC variant. The role of prophylactic lymphadenectomy in treating PTC is controversial. Opponents of routine prophylactic central neck dissection argue that no impact on overall survival is achieved and is even associated with higher complications, including transient vocal cord paralysis (2-7%), transient hypoparathyroidism (14-60%), and permanent hypoparathyroidism (2-5%). In patients with a known cervical nodal metastasis, a therapeutic compartment-oriented lymph node dissection is indicated.

FOLLICULAR CANCER

Of cancers originating from thyroid follicular cells, follicular thyroid carcinomas (FTC) make up 10-15%, and oncocytic (Hurthle) cell carcinomas (HCCs) make up 3-5%. FTC is more common in regions that are iodine deficient and are up to 25-40% of the thyroid carcinomas. Follicular thyroid carcinoma is approximately two-fold more common in women than men. Follicular thyroid cancer cytology generally demonstrates benign features and often includes minimal capsule or capsular blood vessel invasion. It is more difficult to diagnose FTC on FNA and generally is read as a follicular lesion or neoplasm, most are benign. FTC is oftentimes diagnosed with a diagnostic lobectomy and thus is the basis for further treatment decisions. Malignancy is when there is either capsular or vascular invasion.

As opposed to PTC, follicular carcinomas have a tendency to invade blood vessels, thus metastasizing hematogenously. At initial presentation, it is uncommon to see lymph node metastases (2-13%), but, fairly common to see distant metastases (5–33%). Regardless of capsular invasion extent, signs of angioinvasion show a tendency for metastasis relative to lesions with only capsular invasion. Tumors that are low risk, with capsular invasion (no angioinvasion), only need lobectomy and isthmectomy for management. However, one may consider completion thyroidectomy for the facilitation of long-term follow-up, similar to total thyroidectomy in the treatment of PTC. The surgical treatment of choice for invasive tumors is a total thyroidectomy/completion thyroidectomy. It is not advised to perform routine lymphadenectomy of the central compartment.

HURTHLE CELL CARCINOMA (HCC)

Hurthle cell carcinoma (HCC) is often classified as a more aggressive variant of FTC, presenting at a mean age of around 55 years. Histologically, FTC is made of large cells with abundant eosinophilic (pink) cytoplasm and a large nucleus. HCC is less iodine avid, making it different from other thyroid carcinomas. Compared with FTC, HCC is more often an advanced tumor at presentation, and has a higher risk for recurrence locally (24% versus 3%), and metastasis regionally, with a 25% versus 15% 10-year mortality. This cancer requires an aggressive surgery of total thyroidectomy, ipsilateral central compartment lymphadenectomy, and lateral neck dissection.

ANAPLASTIC THYROID CANCER

Anaplastic cancer is rare (<2% of all thyroid cancers) but extremely aggressive (40% of deaths related to thyroid cancer). The median survival rate is estimated to be 4-6 months. Modest survival improvement is seen in a multimodal approach consisting of neoadjuvant chemoradiation followed by surgery. Surgery is reserved for patients showing an initial response to treatment and for whom R0 resection is feasible, which is extremely unlikely. For patients who have progressive compromise of the airway, palliation is achieved with tracheal stents.

Table 2: Thyroid carcinoma TNM Staging for Papillary, Follicular, Poorly Differentiated, Hurthle Cell, Medullary, and Anaplastic Thyroid Carcinomas. Adapted from AJCC UICC 8th Edition

Primary Tumor (T)	Regional Lymph Nodes (N)	Distant Metastasis (M)
TX: Cannot assess primary tumor	NX: Cannot assess regional lymph nodes	M0: There is no distant metastasis
T0: There is no evidence of a primary tumor	N0: N0a: 1+ benign lymph node(s) confirmed histologically or cytologically N0b: Lymph node metastasis is not evident radiologically or clinically	M1: There is distant metastasis
T1: T1a: Greatest dimension is ≤1 cm, limited to thyroid T1b: Greatest dimension is >1 cm, ≤2 cm, limited to thyroid	N1: N1a: Lymph nodes show level VI or VII metastasis (pre/paratracheal, prelaryngealDelphian, upper mediastinal). Unilateral or bilateral N1b: Lymph nodes are retropharyngeal or uni/bi/contralateral lateral neck levels I, II, III, IV, or V metastasis	
T2: Greatest dimension is >2 cm, ≤4 cm, limited to thyroid		
T3: T3a: Greatest dimension is >4 cm, limited to thyroid T3b: Tumor of any size, invades strap muscles only grossly		
T4: T4a: Tumor of any size, invades subcutaneous soft tissues, trachea, larynx, RLN, esophagus T4b: Tumor of any size, invades prevertebral fascia or encasing the mediastinal vessels or carotid artery		
Subdivide categories into solitary tumors (s), multifocal tumors (m). Classification is based on the largest tumor		

MEDULLARY THYROID CANCER

A relatively rare malignant neuroendocrine tumor is medullary thyroid carcinoma (MTC). This is a tumor of parafollicular cells which produce calcitonin. The parafollicular cells originate from neuroectodermal cells and belong to the amine precursor uptake decarboxylation cell family (Figure 3). Five to ten percent of thyroid cancers are MTC; most commonly arising sporadically (75%) and less commonly related to a familial predisposition (25%). However, the *RET* mutation is seen in up to 70% of sporadic MTC tumors. *RET* is a 21-exon proto-oncogene located on chromosome 10q11.2. This gene encodes receptor tyrosine kinase (RET), functioning as a signal transducer that regulates cell growth and survival. Germline *RET* mutations may lead to multiple endocrine neoplasia type 2 (MEN2), an inherited autosomal dominant syndrome.

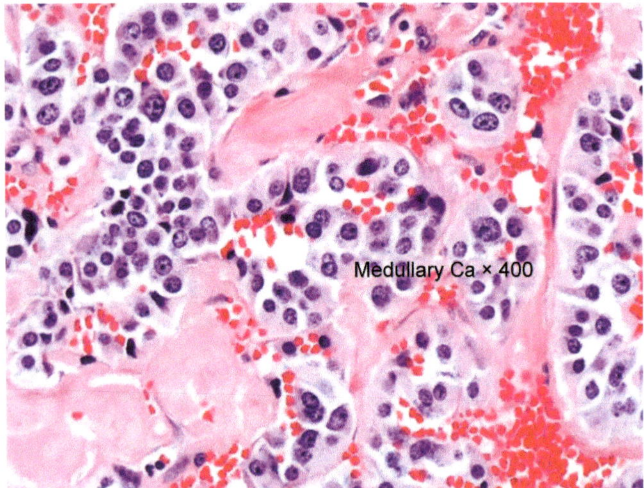

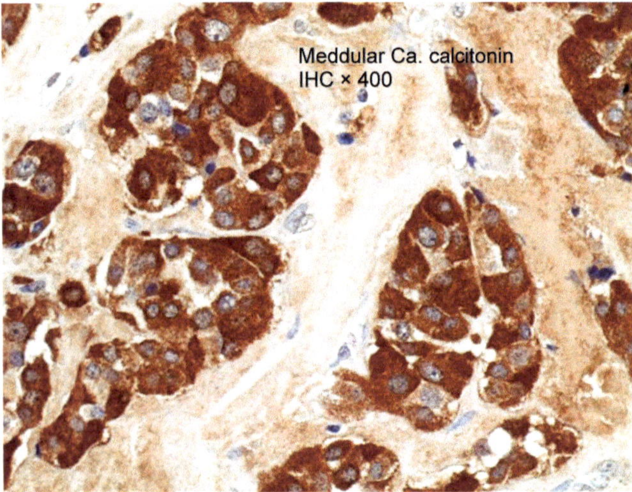

Figure 3: Medullary thyroid cancer. (A) Microscopic appearance shows pink hyaline material that looks like amyloid. This is a neoplasm of the thyroid "C" cells and, thus has neuroendocrine features including calcitonin secretion. (B) Congo red stained amyloid stroma of the medullary thyroid carcinoma.

Sporadic medullary thyroid carcinoma

Sporadic MTC is generally unicentric and occurs equally in both men and women in their forties. Additionally, MTC is not often associated with the germline mutation in the RET proto-oncogene, C-cell hyperplasia, or a family history that would suggest either a pheochromocytoma or MTC.[14]

Hereditary medullary thyroid carcinoma

Hereditary MTC is often an activating germline mutation of the RET proto-oncogene. This carcinoma is multifocal with diffuse, simple, and nodular C-cell hyperplasia. This carcinoma can occur at various ages but is normally seen in patients <20 years old. Additionally, patients generally have a family history that suggests a pheochromocytoma or MTC. Similar to a sporadic MTC, these carcinomas have the ability to spread to the neck, mediastinal lymph nodes, bones, liver, and lungs.

Hereditary MTC is a component of MEN2. The most common hereditary MTC is seen in MEN2A or Sipple's syndrome and the carcinoma is in about 80% of MEN2 cases. Ninety percent of gene carriers have bilateral, multicentric MTC; 50% have bilateral or unilateral pheochromocytomas, and 10-20% have primary hyperparathyroidism. MEN type 2B (MEN2B) is rarer, consisting of roughly 20% of all MEN2 patients. All patients have MTC; 50% have pheochromocytomas; 90% have mucosal ganglioneuromas in the gastrointestinal tract, eyelids, and distal tongue; and nearly all patients have a marfanoid habitus. It is extremely important to identify MTC early in patients with MEN2B since metastases are described to occur during the first year of life.[15]

The diagnosis of Hereditary MTC is through biopsy with fine-needle aspiration, but it can be difficult to diagnose through thyroid cytopathology, and occasionally is mistaken for a carcinoma that is poorly differentiated and of unknown etiology, or even a parathyroid tumor. Elevated levels of calcitonin confirm a MTC diagnosis. Since carcinoembryonic antigen (CEA) is also secreted by MTC tumors, CEA levels are used in adjunct with calcitonin levels to determine disease extent. Additionally, a neck ultrasonography is obtained and is important in evaluating the tumor or tumors and the compartments of the central and lateral cervical lymph nodes. A direct or indirect laryngoscopy is done to identify RLN involvement of a locally invasive tumor.

All patients who present with MTC should have genetic counseling with *RET* proto-oncogene mutation testing. The standard biochemical tests used for screening a pheochromocytoma are 24-hour urine metanephrine/normetanephrine levels or plasma-free metanephrine levels. If a patient's levels are elevated, they should undergo a dedicated adrenal-protocol CT or MRI abdominal scan. Additionally, patients with MEN2A should undergo a primary hyperparathyroidism screening prior to neck operation of the MTC. If patients have hyperparathyroidism, the surgeon can address the parathyroid glands during the initial cervical operation. MTC patients and carriers should have a total extra capsular thyroidectomy to treat the disease and prevent future MTC development respectively. However, depending on if the thyroidectomy is for treatment or prophylactic measures, the extent of cervical lymph node dissection will vary. MTC patients are classified into three groups for surgical purposes. Sporadic MTC patients undergoing therapeutic thyroidectomy, who have a thyroid nodule but US do not demonstrate cervical lymph node metastases, should also have a bilateral central neck dissection.[16] Lateral neck dissection should be performed only if there is central or lateral node disease, visible with high-quality imaging. A rare exception to following these guidelines is when a patient has high serum calcitonin levels and distant metastases is not detectable. These patients may consider having an ipsilateral lateral neck dissection. Cases of either sporadic or hereditary MTC with lymph node metastases in any cervical compartment have a high chance of having coexisting metastases in another compartment. Such patients may require central and bilateral lateral neck dissection. If there is no surgical cure for a patient, they may undergo a total thyroidectomy with resection of other identifiable disease for airway protection.

The penetrance of hereditary MTC is nearly 100%. All individual carriers of a RET mutation should be evaluated and treated for MTC. Carriers of mutations are total thyroidectomy candidates with central node dissection and should undergo the procedure promptly after identification of the phenotype, usually in the first month of life. Experts recommend prophylactic thyroidectomy amongst carriers by 5 or 10 years of age. During the prophylactic thyroidectomy of a child $\leq$5 years old with MEN2A, or FMTC patients who have both normal levels of serum calcitonin and US findings, cervical LN dissection is not generally needed. However, if a patient has elevated serum calcitonin levels or preoperative cervical US findings that suggest a higher chance of invasive cancer, they should consider a bilateral central neck dissection.

Follow-up and Surveillance

It usually takes about 72 hours for calcitonin levels to stabilize after surgery, but they may continue to decrease after. Patients undergoing thyroidectomy for MTC should have baseline calcitonin and CEA levels measured and US of the neck should be performed 2 to 3 months after the procedure and then once a year. Hereditary MTC patients should also have annual hyperparathyroid and pheochromocytoma screenings. Serum calcitonin levels are helpful because increased levels may mean an MTC that is either microscopically persistent or recurrent. Calcitonin levels can detect MTC long before conventional imaging can visualize a regional lymph node or distant metastases. Patients who have elevated postoperative calcitonin levels and had inadequate cervical lymph node clearance during thyroidectomy, should have standard management which consists of high-quality imaging and serial observation until there is a detectable lymph node metastasis, at this time reoperation is now indicated.

Treating patients with locally advanced or metastatic MTC with chemotherapy has had disappointing results. However, advancements in understanding MTC molecular oncogenesis have enabled the development of novel molecular targets for treatment. Most of these current targeted molecular therapies are tyrosine kinase inhibitors (TKIs).[17] One therapy is a novel anilinoquinazoline compound called Vandetanib (ZD6474), which is a selective RET tyrosine kinase, endothelial growth factor receptor, and vascular endothelial growth factor receptor inhibitor.[17]

SURGICAL TECHNIQUE: THYROIDECTOMY

General anesthesia, endotracheal intubation, and muscle relaxation is given to the patient. They are positioned supine on the operating table with the head tilted upwards. A pillow or sandbag is placed in the interscapular region to enable extension of the neck and access to the thyroid.

For the procedure, the surgeon must expose the thyroid gland, dissect the upper pole and superior laryngeal nerve, then dissect the lateral aspect of the thyroid lobe, while making sure to preserve the parathyroid glands and RLN. More specifically are the following steps:

1. A curvilinear skin incision is placed 3-4 cm above the sternum and extends laterally to the sternomastoid muscle.
2. The incision is deepened to the platysma, then the upper and lower skin flaps are raised with both blunt and sharp dissection in the plane anterior to the anterior jugular vessels.
3. A midline incision is made through the fascia over the thyroid. If there is a need for more exposure for safer access to an enlarged or vascular goiter, the strap muscles may be divided, but this is not routinely performed
4. The index finger is inserted between the thyroid lobe and strap muscles to deliver the thyroid lobe forward.
5. If the middle thyroid vein is apparent at this point, it should be ligated and divided.
6. Blunt and sharp dissection is used to divide any adhesions lateral to the thyroid lobe.
7. The superior suspensory ligament and its vessels is divided to dissect the upper border of the isthmus off the trachea, and the midline is identified.
8. To mobilize the upper lobe, an avascular plane is created between the cricothyroid muscle and the medial border of the thyroid lobe upper pole by retracting the lobe laterally.[18]
9. Then the superior thyroid vessels located at the upper pole are ligated and divided, enabling full mobilization of the thyroid lobe. Access to these vessels is gained by blunt dissection oriented in the plane behind the vessels. This breaks down any adhesions. Then there is gentle traction downward on the thyroid.

10. The superior thyroid artery and vein branches must be tied individually using absorbable ligatures. It must be close to the thyroid gland to avoid damaging the superior laryngeal nerve external branch. Twenty percent of the time, the nerve passes between the vessel branches and can be damaged if mass ligation is carried out.
11. The thyroid lobe is retracted medially and elevated out of the wound.
12. Tertiary branches of the vessels that lie on top of the thyroid capsule are ligated and divided individually, moving posteriorly toward the region containing the inferior thyroid artery and the RLN.
13. At this point, the parathyroid glands should be identified and, when in their most usual positions, one can locate the inferior gland near the lower pole of the thyroid anterior to the RLN.
14. The superior gland is normally right above the inferior thyroid artery, and in >90% of people, it is within a 1-cm radius of the junction created by the inferior thyroid artery and the RLN.
15. One should dissect near the gland capsule when removing the thyroid and the individual branches of the inferior thyroid artery should be ligated and divided to preserve the branches supplying the parathyroid glands.
16. Then there should be mobilization and reflection of the superior and inferior parathyroid glands postero-laterally along with their vascular pedicle.
17. The dissection continues medially, dividing the thyroid capsule.
18. The RLN is normally deep to the inferior thyroid artery but may become vulnerable by anterior fixation in a fork made by the artery's glandular branches.
19. One must be cautious when the RLN passes superficially to the inferior thyroid artery, appears to be pulsating, and therefore potentially mistaken for a vessel and then ligated.
20. Around its point of entry into the larynx and passing through Berry's ligament, the nerve is in its most dangerous position. It oftentimes loops before entering the larynx.
21. At this point, it is important to carefully clip and ligate the small vessels close to the nerve, for fear of bleeding which can obscure the nerve's entry point to the larynx.
22. Once the nerve is free from any overlying thyroidal tissue, it can then fall into the tracheoesophageal grove from the area which it was dissected off of.
23. The ligament of Berry and its surrounding terminal branches from the inferior thyroid artery can then be divided from the tracheal surface.
24. Due to their location, sometimes it is not possible to save the blood supply to all of the parathyroid glands, and it may become ischemic after dissecting its vascular pedicle.[19]
25. If in doubt of preserving enough parathyroid tissue, it must be autotransplanted immediately into a bloodless pocket in the ipsilateral sternocleidomastoid muscle and the site marked with a permanent clip or suture.
26. Strap muscles divided at the beginning of the procedure should be re-approximated using absorbable sutures.
27. Finally, a subcuticular suture will be used to close the skin.

Intraoperative nerve monitoring

Nerve monitors were introduced to help identify and preserve the RLN. Some studies demonstrated benefit to nerve monitors being used routinely. They to improve nerve identification and decrease nerve injury. However, other studies did not show prognostic benefit. Nerve monitoring has potential benefit during thyroid reoperations or procedures treating locally advanced disease.

To identifying the EBSLN, it is important to develop the avascular plane between the medial border of the upper pole of the thyroid lobe and the cricothyroid muscle, this maneuver is facilitated by laterally retracting the lobe. Superior laryngeal nerve injury may result in voice changes after surgery that are often subtle, going unnoticed unless the patient is a professional singers or public speaker. After injury, patients will be unable to project their voices, reach high pitches, or will have easy vocal fatiguability after prolonged speech.

The most common complications of thyroidectomy are listed in Table 3. Assessing ESLN external branch damage is difficult since changes are often subtle and therefore overlooked easily. Indirect laryngoscopic changes of lesions of the ESLN are less obvious compared to changes seen in recurrent laryngeal nerve palsy. However, disability can lead to changes in range, voice pitch, fatigability, and especially the quality of the singing voice.

Table 3: Complications of thyroid surgery

Complications of thyroid surgery
Injury to the recurrent laryngeal nerve
Injury to the external branch of superior laryngeal nerve
Laryngeal edema-airway obstruction
Hypoparathyroidism
Bleeding hematoma
Hyperthyroidism
Hypothyroidism
Infection of the wound
Suture granuloma
Keloid scar

To avoid permanent hypoparathyroidism, carefully identifying the parathyroid glands and preserving their delicate arterial blood supply is crucial. The worst and potentially life-threatening thyroidectomy complication is post-operation airway obstruction as a result of subglottic or laryngeal edema. Generally, this occurs due to postoperative bleeding associated with a wound hematoma. Luckily, this complication is very uncommon, and the risk can be minimized through careful attention to hemostasis and avoiding larynx manipulation during the procedure. Another complication that is now rare is thyroid crisis or storm due to adequate preoperative preparation to bring the patient into a euthyroid state.

Follow-up care

Four to twelve weeks post-surgery, RAI ablation is administered to destroy remaining thyroid tissue and to treat occult or known metastatic disease. All patients who have PTC should undergo RAI ablation except select patients who have a low risk for recurrence (stage I disease). Additionally, this procedure should be avoided if the patient has a negative whole-body RAI scan, Tg levels <1 ng/mL, and negative anti-Tg antibodies with TSH stimulation. RAI is contraindicated during pregnancy and lactation.

Thyroid cancer that is well differentiated, expresses cell membrane TSH receptors which respond to TSH stimulation. The cancer can be TSH stimulated though increased thyroid-specific protein expression (i.e., the sodium-iodide symporter and Tg). Using supra-physiologic doses of thyroxine to suppress TSH is a common way to treat thyroid cancer and a way to attempt decreasing recurrence risk. Recurrence of thyroid cancer is common, occurring in around 30% of patients. Recurrence generally happens locally and within 10 years of the initial surgery. Age <15 and >45 years old, a family history, male sex, tumor size >4 cm, disease that is bilateral, presence of vascular invasion, and an unfavorable histology are risk factors for recurrence. Recurrence is found on US and should undergo surgical resection if possible. Compartment oriented resection is indicated when the compartment is not formally cleared. When recurrence occurs in a field that has undergone compartment-oriented dissection previously, image-guided wire placements and intraoperative US can aid in defining non-palpable disease, serving as a guidance for resection. Recurrence found through elevated thyroglobulin but cannot be found through high-resolution sonography may require whole-body radioiodine scanning for identification. In addition to the radioiodine scan, a CT or even thyrotropin-stimulated PET/CT may also be used to identify the disease's anatomic location. Surgical resection while minimizing patient morbidity is the mainstay treatment; however, if this cannot be done, radioiodine ablation can be used.

REVISION OR REDO THYROID SURGERY

Indications for revision thyroidectomy include completion thyroidectomy after ipsilateral thyroid lobectomy with a final diagnosis of thyroid cancer.[20]

Determining when to complete a thyroidectomy is dependent on findings and scarring from the initial surgery. One should consider early surgical intervention, during the 5 to 7 days where there is no inflammation of the tissues. When the central compartment has a considerable amount of induration and scarring, postponement of the surgery is indicated until there is a reduction in the induration, which will take roughly 2 to 3 months. Considerable scarring of the central compartment makes exploration difficult, thus one should consider a lateral approach.[20] This dissection is performed medial to the sternomastoid muscle to expose the thyroid's lateral portion, where the tracheoesophageal grove is then dissected. Here, the RLN must be identified and dissected. It may be necessary to sacrifice the strap muscles if they are strongly adherent to the thyroid gland. Though nerve monitoring during thyroid surgery is of unknown benefit, use during re-operative thyroid surgery can prove helpful when there is intense scarring that makes identifying the RLN difficult. The parathyroid glands should be carefully identified, dissected, and preserved during re-operative thyroid surgery. Devascularization of the parathyroid glands may occur due to retraction, surface hematoma, and manipulation.

Certain complications come with re-operative thyroid surgery, and these complication rates have a high incidence. A major complication is when the tumor is strongly adherent to the trachea resulting in potential tracheal perforation during tumor resection. If this complication occurs, one must consider an immediate tracheostomy or appropriately resecting the tracheal wall. If there is a minor tracheal tear, it may be simply sutured. If there is a minor esophageal mucosal tear, the tear must undergo repair, a drain should be placed, and the patient should be closely observed postoperatively. A life-threatening emergency is bilateral RLN injury that may occur when the patient is extubated in the recovery room. These patients must be closely observed, and if concern of their airway exists, they must be reintubated and the physician must consider appropriate airway stabilization (tracheostomy). If the patient has a neck dissection performed during the procedure, a major complication that can occur is a persistent chyle leak which may require extended hospitalization. Additional complications exist such as injury to the superior laryngeal nerve, phrenic nerve, vagus nerve, and jugular veins.

MINIMALLY INVASIVE THYROID SURGERY

During a minimally invasive thyroid surgery, small single central incisions are made, using advanced energy devices to maintain hemostasis in a small space. Additionally, guidance using endoscopy enables management of the vasculature of the thyroid gland and to identify and preserve the parathyroid glands and RLNs.[21] When comparing minimally invasive video-assisted thyroidectomy to conventional surgery, patients who underwent minimally invasive surgery reported more satisfaction in regards to scarring and pain levels.[22] Thorough thyroid removal with endoscopy was confirmed with postoperative serum thyroglobulin levels and radioactive iodine uptake compared with conventional thyroidectomy.[23] Numerous reports have been made of remote access thyroidectomy using surgical ports placed in several locations (e.g., anterior chest wall, axillary region, or subclavicular region). In thyroid surgery, to facilitate ease of remote access and avoid needing insufflation, robotics were introduced. Patients can now undergo minimally invasive and endoscopic thyroidectomy and parathyroidectomy and benefit from less dissection and smaller incisions associated with these approaches. Though proven to provide cosmetic, quality of life, and functional benefits, a better understanding of the procedure and its indications will continue to develop even as the technique itself evolves, and as new approaches emerge.

REFERENCES

1. Casper F, Hegner A. History of thyroid surgery. Ann Surg 1932; (95):481-492.
2. Billroth TH. Clinical surgery: extracts from the reports of surgical practice between the years of 1860–1876 London: The New Sydenham 1881; 638-640.
3. Stevane RJ, Kaufman GL. A Historical Perspective on Surgery of the Thyroid and Parathyroid Glands. Otolaryngol Clin N Am 2008;4 1:1059–1067.
4. Cernea CR, Ferraz AR, Nishio S, et al. Surgical anatomy of the external branch of the superior laryngeal nerve. Head Neck 1992;14: 380.
5. Pelizzo MR, Toniato A, Gemo G. Zuckerkandl's tuberculum: an arrow pointing to the recurrent laryngeal nerve (constant anatomical landmark). J Am Coll Surg 1998; 187:333.
6. Bliss RD, Gauger PG, Delbridge LW. Surgeon's Approach to the Thyroid Gland: Surgical Anatomy and the Importance of Technique. World J Surg 2000; 24:891–897.
7. Gray SW, Skandalakis JE, Akin JT. Embryological considerations of thyroid surgery: developmental anatomy of the thyroid, parathyroids and the recurrent laryngeal nerve. Am Surg 1976; 42(9):621–8.
8. Fancy T, Gallagher III D, Hornig JD. Surgical Anatomy of the Thyroid and Parathyroid Glands, Otolaryngol Clin N Am 2010; 43:221–227.
9. Hanks JB, Salomone LJ. Thyroid. Sabiston Text Book of Surgery 36; 917-954.
10. Hegedius L. The Thyroid Nodule. N Eng J Med. 2004; 351:1764-71.
11. Vazquez BJ, Richards ML. Imaging of the Thyroid and Parathyroid Glands. Surg Clin N Am. 2011; 91:15–32.
12. Cooper DS, Doherty GM, Haugen BR, et al. Revised American Thyroid Association Management Guidelines for Patients with Thyroid Nodules and Differentiated Thyroid Cancer The American Thyroid Association (ATA) Guidelines Taskforce on Thyroid Nodules and Differentiated Thyroid Cancer. Thyroid 2009; 19(11): 1167-1214.
13. Suliburk J, Delbridge L. Surgical Management of Well –Differentiated Thyroid Cancer: State of the Art, Surg Clin N Am 2009; 89: 1171–1191.
14. Moley JF, Fialkowski EA. Evidence-based approach to the management of sporadic medullary thyroid carcinoma. World J Surg 2007; 31(5):946–56.
15. Brandi ML, Gagel RF, Angeli A, et al. Guidelines for diagnosis and therapy of MEN type 1and type 2. J Clin Endocrinol Metab 2001; 86(12):5658–71.
16. Kloos RT, Eng C, Evans DB, et al. Medullary thyroid cancer: management guidelines of the American Thyroid Association. Thyroid 2009; 19:565–612.
17. Chau NG, Haddad RI. Vandetanib for the treatment of medullary thyroid cancer. Clin Cancer Res 2013; 19(3):524-9.
18. Sabet A, Kim M. Postoperative Management of Differentiated Thyroid Cancer. Otolaryngol Clin N Am 2010:43: 329–351.
19. Delbridge L. Total thyroidectomy: The evolution of surgical technique ANZ J. Surg. 2003;73: 761–768.
20. Shaha AR. Revision Thyroid Surgery. Technical Considerations. Otolaryngol Clin N Am 2008; (41):1169–118.
21. Miccoli P, Bellantone R, Mourad M, et al. Minimally invasive video-assisted thyroidectomy: multi-institutional experience. World J Surg 2002; 26(8):972-5.
22. Lu JH, Materazzi G, Miccoli M, et al. Minimally invasive video assisted thyroidectomy versus endoscopic thyroidectomy via the areola approach: a retrospective analysis of safety, postoperative recovery and patient satisfaction. Minerva Chir 2012; 67(1):31-7.
23. Terris DJ, Anderson SK, Watts TL, et al. Laryngeal nerve monitoring and minimally invasive thyroid surgery: complementary technologies. Arch Otolaryngol Head Neck Surg 2007; 133(12):1254-7.

❑❑❑

55

CHAPTER

Parathyroid

Francisco Igor Macedo, MD
Edsa Negussie, MD
Barry Herschman, MD
Vijay K. Mittal, MD

INTRODUCTION

In 1879, Anton Wolfler recognized tetany in a patient operated for total parathyroidectomy by Theodor Billroth. The association between hypocalcemia and the parathyroid glands was made much later, in 1909, after it became possible to measure blood calcium levels. The first successful parathyroidectomy was completed by Felix Mandl in 1925 on a patient with osteitis fibrosa cystica.[1]

The parathyroid glands are located at the level of the cricoid cartilage, dorsal to recurrent laryngeal nerves (RLN) and on the posterior aspect of the thyroid gland. They can appear in different shapes, measuring 5-7 mm in size, and weighing 40-50 mg each. The superior gland usually lies on the postero-lateral aspect in the tracheo-esophageal groove, above the RLN and inferior thyroid artery (ITA) intersection. However, the position of the parathyroid glands can be unusual, including the intrathyroid, posterior neck above the upper thyroid pole and the retropharyngeal space. The inferior parathyroid glands can be found in the postero-lateral part of the lower pole of the thyroid gland, dorsal to the ITA.[2] They also can be in the superior mediastinum within the thymus. Each of the parathyroid glands generally have their own arterial supply, most often originating from the ITA, although sometimes the superior parathyroid gland can be supplied by a superior thyroid artery branch.

The parathyroid glands produce parathyroid hormone (PTH) which regulates calcium metabolism. Extracellular calcium (1% of total calcium stores) is essential for excitation-contraction coupling in the muscle, coagulation, hormone regulation, and synaptic transmission. Intracellular calcium mainly acts as a second messenger. The inorganic form of calcium is absorbed in the small bowel, but when in the serum, it is either found in its ionized form (active, 50%), albumin bound (40%), or as an anions (10%) such as citrate or phosphate.[3] The parathyroid glands regulate PTH secretion by sensing levels of extracellular calcium through calcium-sensing receptor (CASR), but can also be stimulated by numerous other factors including vitamin D, catecholamines, and low magnesium levels.

PTH increases extracellular calcium at three levels: bone, kidney, and small bowel. In the bone, PTH increases resorption by stimulating osteoclasts; in the kidney, PTH limits calcium excretion at the distal convoluted tubule and inhibit phosphate reabsorption; and in the small bowel, PTH indirectly increases intestinal calcium absorption.

Calcitonin, which is made by *C cells* of the thyroid, has antagonist effects, causing hypocalcemia, by increasing renal phosphate excretion and inhibiting osteoclasts. Vitamin D stimulates small bowel absorption of calcium and phosphate and bone reabsorption of calcium.

Diseases of Parathyroid

Hyperparathyroidism (HPT) is the hyper-regulation of the parathyroid glands. It is classified as primary, secondary and tertiary. It leads ultimately to increased calcium levels and its associated with symptoms including *"kidney stones, painful bones, abdominal groans, psych moans, and fatigue overtones."* Occasionally, calcium may reach extremely high levels, known as a hypercalcemic crisis, which can be life-threatening. In hypothyroidism, secretion or action of PTH is deficient, resulting in hypocalcemia and hyperphosphatemia.

Primary Hyperparathyroidism

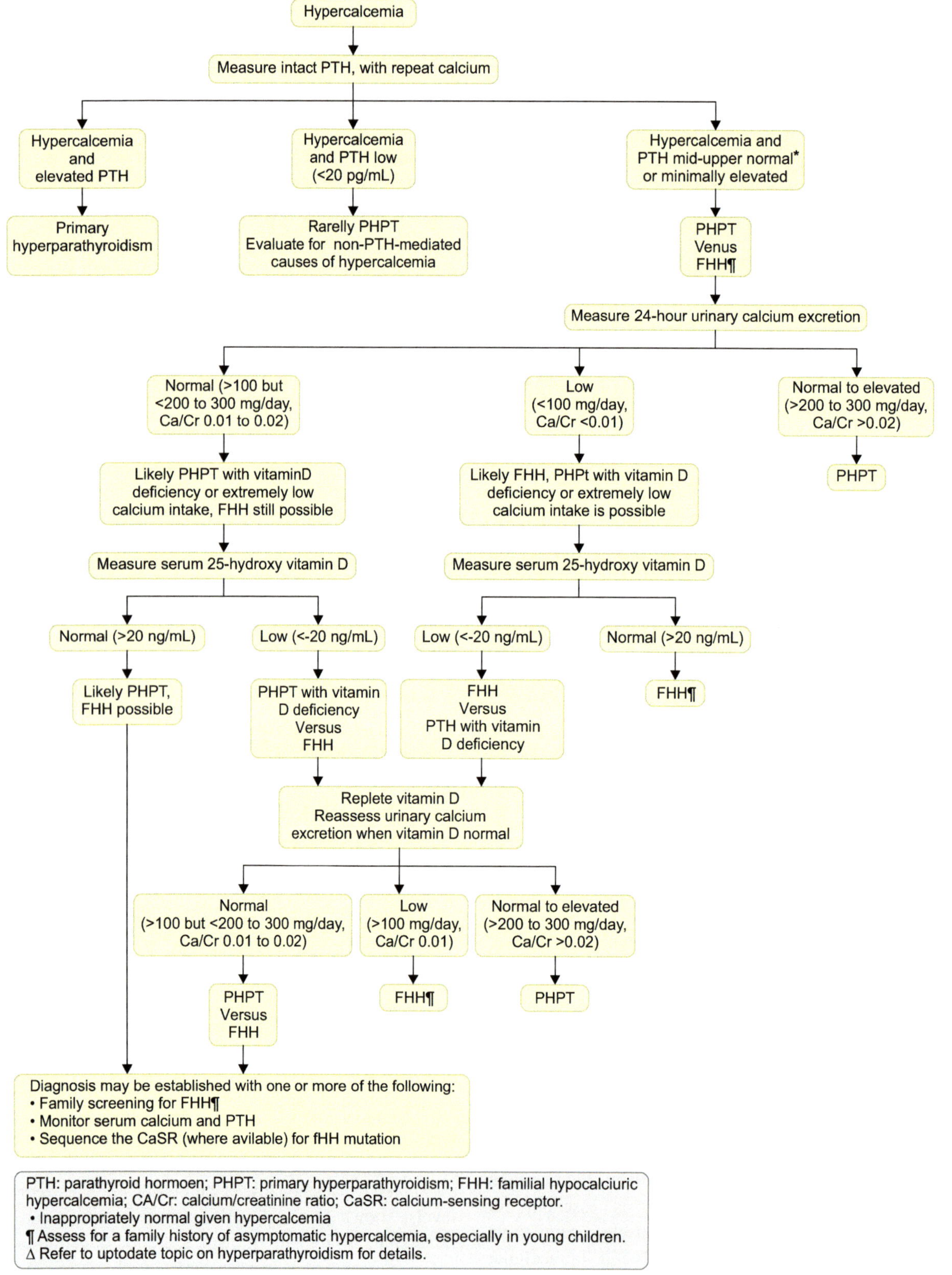

Figure 1: Algorithm for the diagnosis of primary hyperparathyroidism

The third most common endocrine disorder is primary hyperparathyroidism (pHPT), affecting over 100,000 individuals annually in the United States. It usually affects middle-aged women and is characterized by the hypersecretion of PTH from abnormal parathyroid glands. Although ionizing radiation and a genetic predisposition have been related, the exact etiology is yet unknown. Most cases of pHPT are sporadic, however it may occur with multiple endocrine neoplasia (MEN 1 and MEN 2A), and in isolated familial HPT. In MEN 1, pHPT is the most common clinical presentation and has been shown to be secondary to the germline MEN1 gene mutation, located on chromosome 11q12-13.[4] HPT occurs in nearly 20% of patients with MEN2A, due to a RET proto-oncogene germline mutation on chromosome 10.

Clinical signs include weakness, polyuria, bone pain, constipation, fatigue, polydipsia, nausea, heartburn, decreased appetite, pruritus, depression, and memory loss. In 80% of cases, patients have some degree of renal dysfunction with nephrolithiasis found in 20-25%. Chronic hypercalcemia may lead to impaired renal function, resulting in polyuria, polydipsia and nocturia. Bone disease may involve a constellation of signs including osteopenia, osteoporosis, and osteitis fibrosa cystica which, together, corresponds to 15% of cases. In the physical exam, a palpable neck mass is usually either a thyroid mass or parathyroid carcinoma. Adenomas or hyperplasia will most likely be palpable only with profound hypercalcemia and are otherwise seldom palpable (Figure 2 and 3).

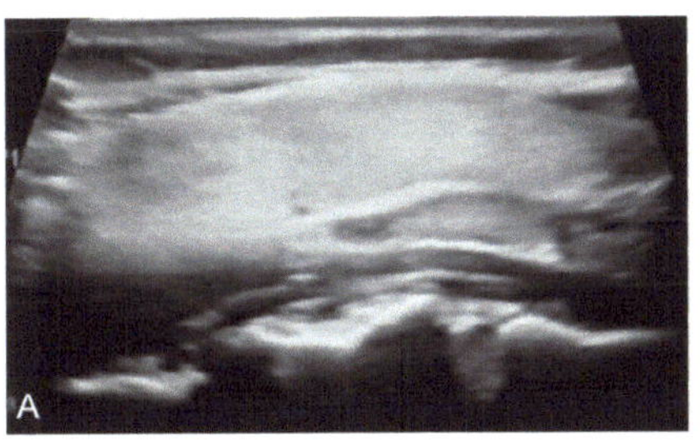

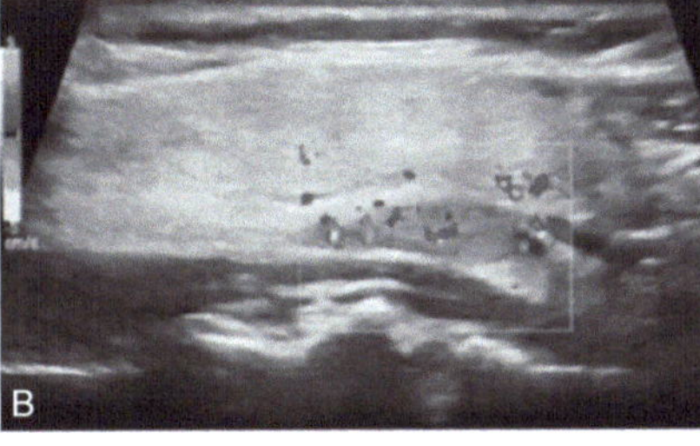

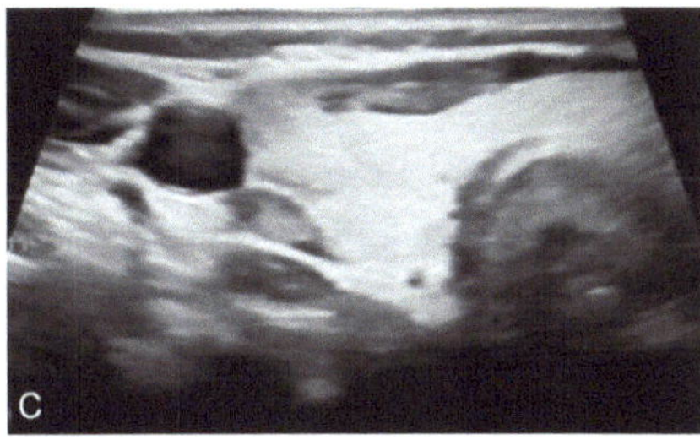

Figure 2: Ultrasound of the neck revealing a parathyroid adenoma. A: Sagittal view showing the thyroid gland with multiple nodules within the gland. The nodule appears to be just outside the gland and has a demarcating capsule. B: Color Doppler view showing an arc of prominent vessels surrounding and leading into the nodule is demonstrated. C: Transverse view demonstrating the nodule in the region adjacent to the thyroid bed, with an echogenic curvilinear capsule seen anteriorly.

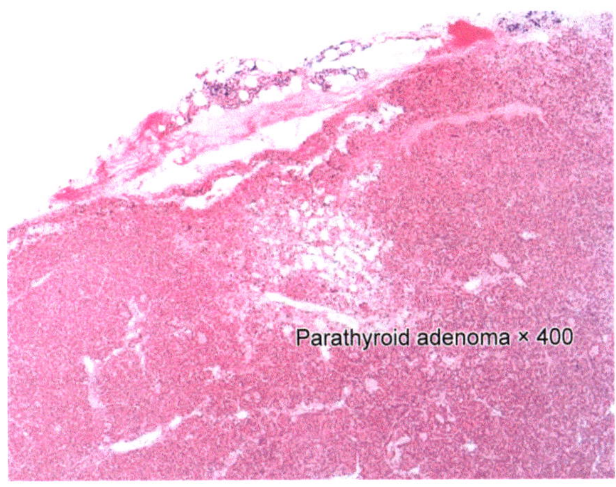

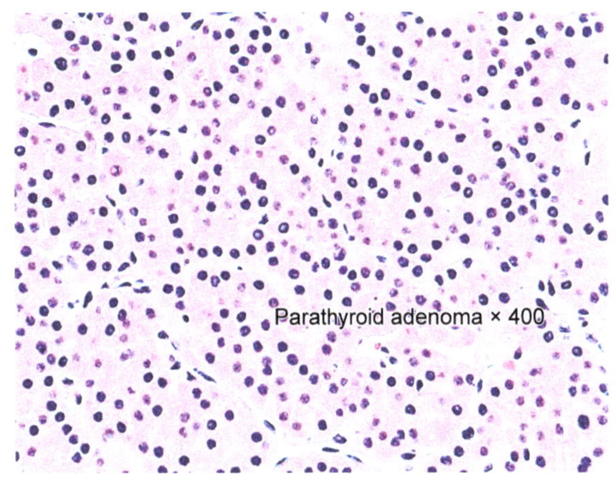

Figure 3: Parathyroid adenoma: The most common cause for primary hyperparathyroidism. Histology shows a rim of normal parathyroid tissue mixed with adipose tissue cells compressed to the left and upper edge of the adenoma.

Diagnosis is established when serum calcium levels are elevated with an intact PTH level, or with elevated two-site PTH levels. In cases of metastatic cancer and hypercalcemia, a concurrent primary HPT can be determined with an intact PTH level. Other laboratory tests include elevated concentrations of 24-hour urinary calcium or decreased levels of serum phosphate. Ten percent of patients with pHPT have an elevated alkaline phosphatase, indicating a high-turnover bone disease. During work-up, X-rays of the hand and skull can determine the extent of osteitis fibrosa cystica, however X-rays are only routinely performed in patients with elevated levels of alkaline phosphatase. Abdominal ultrasound may reveal renal stones, and radiologic localization studies are becoming more accepted with the introduction of minimally invasive parathyroid surgery. Compared to sestamibi scans (Figure 4), CT and MRI are less sensitive, but they can help localize mediastinal glands. Nowadays, it is common to obtain an intraoperative parathyroid hormone level to determine the adequacy of resection. Surgery is terminated with a >50% decrease in PTH level compared with either pre-incision or levels prior to gland excision.

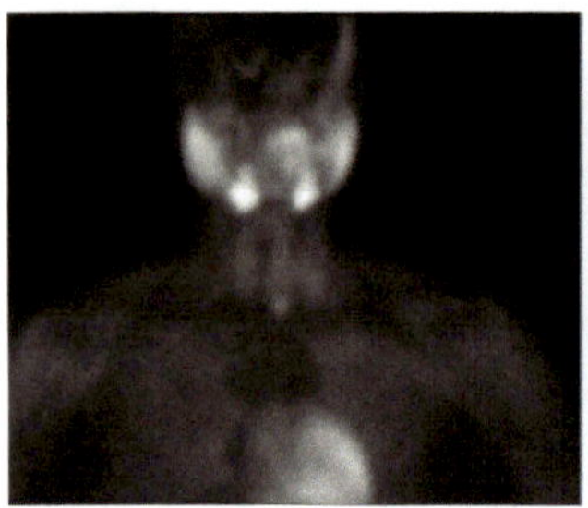

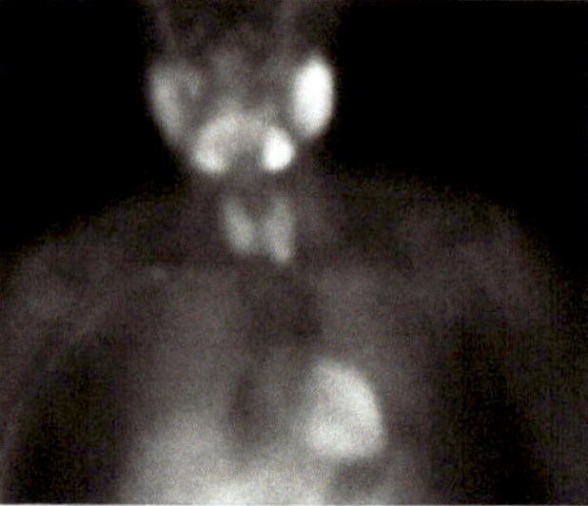

Figure 4: A technetium-99 sestamibi parathyroid scan. Early images (A) are followed by delayed images at 2 hours (B). There is residual activity on the delayed images at the inferior aspect of the left lobe of the thyroid (arrow), consistent with a parathyroid adenoma.

Secondary Hyperparathyroidism

Secondary HPT is classically seen in patients with long-standing renal failure. It is usually managed medically with diet changes, phosphate binders, and vitamin D supplementation. Surgical management is indicated when calcium levels are >11 mg/dL in addition to an elevated PTH, calciphylaxis, soft-tissue calcification, and progressive renal osteodystrophy.

Calciphylaxis is rare and is characterized by painful limb lesions which can progress to non-healing ulcers, sepsis, and death. The surgical approach is usually a bilateral neck exploration, and an abnormal parathyroid gland will be enlarged and asymmetric with nodular hyperplasia. Resection options may include subtotal resection or total parathyroidectomy with autotransplantation into the brachioradialis muscle to the nondominant forearm. Parathyroidectomy improves survival, mineral density, and sexual function in secondary HPT patients.[5]

Tertiary Hyperparathyroidism

Tertiary HPT occurs in patients with long-standing renal failure following kidney transplantation. It is postulated that parathyroid glands become autonomous after transplantation. Additional factors that can contribute to HPT in this population include glucocorticoids, cyclosporine, thiazides, or glomerular alterations from rejection episodes. The spectrum of symptoms resembles those of pHPT, including bone fractures, nephrolithiasis, peptic ulcer disease, pancreatitis, and mental illness. Surgical resection, which may include subtotal or total parathyroidectomy with autotransplantation, is indicated if symptoms persist or if PTH levels increase for more than 1 year after renal transplantation and if there is acute hypercalcemia (calcium levels >12.5 mg/dL) in the immediate post-transplantation period.[6]

Hypercalcemic Crisis

This condition occurs with severe hypercalcemia (may range from 16-20 mg/dL) and concurrent uncontrolled PTH secretion that leads to hemodynamic instability, dehydration, and varying degrees of renal failure. Patients usually present with nausea, vomiting, fatigue, weakness, confusion, disorientation, and coma. It occurs more commonly in patients with parathyroid carcinoma or familial HPT. Initial management is based on restoring intravascular volume with normal saline infusions to keep urine output greater than 100 mL/h, followed by furosemide after adequate urine output is achieved. In refractory cases, especially in unstable patients, hemodialysis may be implemented.

Hypoparathyroidism

The most common cause of hypoparathyroidism is having a previous thyroid surgery. Clinical manifestations include a tingling sensation in the fingers, perioral numbness, confusion, and anxiety. Late signs may result in tetany, convulsions, or laryngospasm, and, although rare, can be potentially fatal. Inherited forms of hypocalcemia include DiGeorge syndrome (abnormal third/fourth branchial pouches), hemochromatosis, Wilson's disease, sarcoidosis, tuberculosis, or amyloidosis. Hypocalcemia is usually managed medically with oral calcium and vitamin D supplements.

Parathyroid Carcinoma

Parathyroid carcinoma is a rare condition with no prevalence with gender, in contrast to female preponderance with adenomas. Patients usually have considerably higher calcium levels (usually >14mg/dL) and increased associated complications (Figure 5). Special caution should be taken in a patient with extreme hypercalcemia, a palpable neck mass, and significant uptake on sestamibi scan or with concurrent lymphadenopathy on ultrasound.[7] Adverse prognostic factors include simple parathyroidectomy alone, nodal or distant metastases, local recurrence, nonfunctional tumor status, and a higher index Ki-67 antigen >10%.

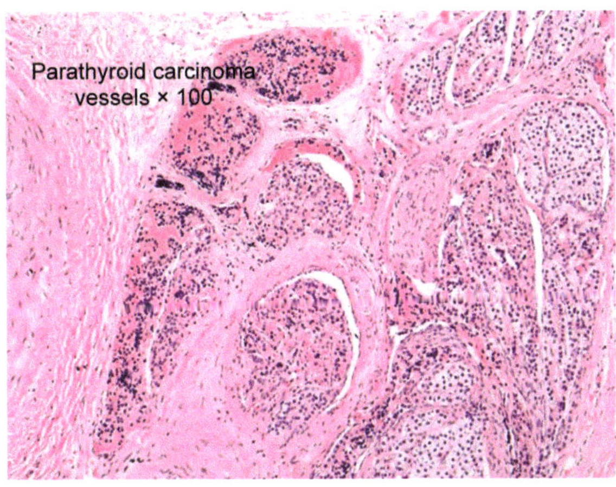

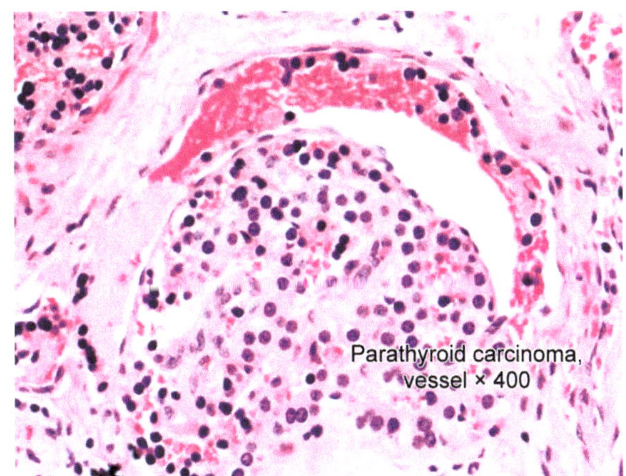

Figure 5: Parathyroid carcinoma. The nests of neoplastic cells that are not very pleomorphic. Bands of fibrous tissue between the nests. Parathyroid carcinomas infiltrate surrounding structures in the neck.

Table 1: TNM Staging for Parathyroid Carcinoma. Adapted from AJCC UICC 8th Edition

Primary Tumor (T)	Regional Lymph Nodes (N)	Distant Metastasis (M)
TX: Cannot assess primary tumor	NX: Cannot assess regional lymph nodes	M0: There is no distant metastasis
T0: There is no evidence of a primary tumor	N0: There is no metastasis to the regional lymph nodes	M1: There is distant metastasis
Tis: Atypical parathyroid neoplasm (uncertain malignant potential)	N1: N1a: Level VI lymph node metastasis (pre/paratracheal, prelaryngeal/Delphian) or level VII lymph nodes (superior mediastinal) N1b: Retropharyngeal lymph node metastasis or level I, II, III, IV, or V uni/bi/contralateral cervical lymph node metastasis	
T1: Tumor is localized to parathyroid gland, extension only to soft tissue		
T2: Tumor directly invades thyroid gland		
T3: Tumor directly invades RLN, trachea, skeletal muscle, esophagus, thymus, adjacent lymph nodes		
T4: Tumor invades spine or major blood vessels		

In parathyroid carcinoma, surgery involves en bloc tumor resection, ipsilateral thyroid lobectomy, and adjacent soft tissue resection. A frozen section biopsy is contraindicated due to risk of capsular rupture. Recurrence occurs in approximately 40% of cases and overall survival rate is around 89%.[8] There is no effective chemotherapeutic regimen to date. In high-risk patients, radiation may slightly increase survival; however, results are still contradictory.

Technical Aspects: Parathyroid Surgery

Bilateral neck exploration

For bilateral neck exploration, a 3-4 cm incision is performed inferior to the cricoid cartilage, strap muscles are separated in the midline, and dissection is undertaken lateral to the thyroid gland to facilitate parathyroid gland visualization. The middle thyroid veins are ligated and divided and the RLN is identified after blunt dissection superior from the cricoid cartilage and inferior from the thymus. Usually, the parathyroid glands are located around the lower thyroid pole, within 1 cm of the inferior thyroid artery and RLN junction. Careful attention is taken to differentiate parathyroid glands from fatty tissue, lymph nodes, and an ectopic thymus. A normal parathyroid gland is light beige, a little darker than fat tissue. In 80% of patients with pHPT, a single adenoma is the only abnormal intraoperative finding. In these cases, the adenoma is dissected immediately adjacent to the mass by both blunt and sharp dissection followed by clamping, ligation, and division of the vascular pedicle. In about 15% of cases, parathyroid hyperplasia is encountered with all parathyroid enlarged, which are treated with subtotal parathyroidectomy or total parathyroidectomy with autotransplantation. The latter is associated with less recurrence rates in the neck, whereas the former is preferred by some surgeons due to avoiding failure of autotransplanted tissue (approximately 5% of cases).

The resected parathyroid tissue should be confirmed immediately by frozen section or PTH assay. In cases of autotransplantation, a horizontal skin incision is made above the brachioradialis muscle of the nondominant forearm, inferior to the antecubital fossa, and 12 to 14 tissue pieces that are 1-mm each are inserted into the belly of the muscle.

Minimally invasive parathyroidectomy

After the introduction of intraoperative PTH monitoring and preoperative localization imaging studies, different modalities of minimally invasive parathyroidectomy have been described, including endoscopic parathyroidectomy, video-assisted parathyroidectomy with lateral approach, and open minimally invasive parathyroid surgery by central or lateral approach.[9] Potential benefits include less early postoperative hypocalcemia, better cosmesis, less postoperative pain, and a shorter operative times in the minimally invasive approach when compared to the conventional bilateral neck exploration.[10-14]

Postoperative Care

After hospital discharge, follow-up is usually performed 2 weeks postoperatively with calcium, phosphate, and PTH measurements. Then, additional follow-up is completed annually. Recurrence rates are uncommon (<1%), usually secondary from unrecognized hyperplasia, ectopic or supernumerary parathyroid glands, parathyroid carcinoma, or suboptimal resection. Complications associated with parathyroid surgery include hypocalcemia, transient or permanent vocal cord palsy, and hypoparathyroidism usually secondary from bilateral neck exploration or failure of autotransplanted tissue. Symptomatic hypocalcemia (calcium <8 mg/dL) is medically managed with oral calcium supplementation and vitamin D.

REFERENCES

1. Giddings CE, Rimmer J, Weir N. History of parathyroid gland surgery: an historical case series. J Laryngol Otol. 2009;123(10):1075-81.
2. Akerstrom G, Malmaeus J, Bergstrom R. Surgical anatomy of human parathyroid glands. Surgery 1984; 95:14.
3. Carling T. Molecular pathology of parathyroid tumors. Trends Endocrinol Metab 2001; 12:53.
4. Skogseid B. Multiple endocrine neoplasia type 1. Br J Surg 2003; 90:383-5.
5. Llach F, Velasquez Forero F. Secondary hyperparathyroidism in chronic renal failure: pathogenic and clinical aspects. Am J Kidney Dis. 2001; 38:S20.
6. Townsend CM, Beauchamp RD, Evers RM, et al. Sabiston Textbook of Surgery: The Biological Basis of Modern Surgical Practice. 19th edition. Philadelphia, PA: Elsevier Inc., 2012: 924-41.
7. DeLellis RA. Parathyroid carcinoma: an overview. Adv Anat Pathol 2005; 12:53-61.
8. Iihara M, Okamoto T, Suzuki R, et al. Functional parathyroid carcinoma: Long-term treatment outcome and risk factor analysis. Surgery 2007; 142:936-43.
9. Hessman O, Westerdahl J, Al-Suliman N, et al. Randomized clinical trial comparing open with video-assisted minimally invasive parathyroid surgery for primary hyperparathyroidism. Br J Surg 2010; 97:177-84.
10. Gagner M. Endoscopic subtotal parathyroidectomy in patients with primary hyperparathyroidism. Br J Surg 1996; 83:875.
11. Miccoli P, Pinchera A, Ceccini G, et al. Minimally invasive, video-assisted parathyroid surgery for primary hyperparathyroidism. J Endocrinol Invest 1997; 20:429-30.
12. Henry JF, Defechereux T, Gramatica L, et al. Minimally invasive videoscopic parathyroidectomy by lateral approach. Langenbecks Arch Surg 1999; 384:298-301.
13. Miccoli P, Berti P, Materazzi G, et al. Endoscopic bilateral neck exploration versus quick intraoperative parathormone assay (qPTHa) during endoscopic parathyroidectomy: A prospective randomized trial. Surg Endosc. 2008;22(2): 398-400.
14. Gupta A, Unawane A, Subhas G, et al. Parathyroidectomies using intraoperative parathormone monitoring: when should we stop measuring intraoperative parathormone levels. Am Surg 2012: 78:844-50.

56

CHAPTER

Adrenal

Francisco Igor Macedo, MD
Edsa Negussie, MD
Binit Katwal
Vijay K. Mittal, MD

INTRODUCTION

The first anatomical description of the adrenal gland was given by Eustauchius in 1563. Much later in 1805, Cuvier recognized the division of the adrenal gland into a cortex and medulla, which made possible the correlation of many clinical entities.[1] Histologically, the adrenal cortex can be distinguished into three separate zones: *zona glomerulosa*, the site of mineralocorticoid and aldosterone hormone synthesis; *zona fasciculata*, the site involved in the production of glucocorticoids; and *zona reticularis*, the site of androgen synthesis. The adrenal medulla is responsible for the synthesis of the catecholamine hormones, epinephrine, and norepinephrine. Anatomically, the adrenal glands are retroperitoneal and lie along the superomedial aspect of the two kidneys. The right adrenal is partially covered by the liver and right triangular ligament, and medially lies adjacent to the inferior vena cava (IVC). The left adrenal is covered anteriorly by the spleen and tail of the pancreas, and inferiorly it lies over the left kidney. The arterial supply is similar bilaterally and is derived from the small branches of the inferior phrenic artery, right renal artery, and aorta. Each adrenal gland is drained by a single central vein; the left adrenal vein (enters left renal vein) is longer than the right adrenal vein (drains into the IVC).

Adrenal Disorders

Adrenal tumors include a wide spectrum of pathological entities, varying from a benign non-secretory adrenal adenoma to a secretory adrenocortical carcinoma (ACC). Diagnosis usually occurs after symptoms arise, the most common being hypertension;[2] however, they may appear incidentally as an adrenal enlargement on abdominal imaging, namely an adrenal incidentaloma or in the context of hereditary diseases (multiple endocrine neoplasia, MEN 1 and MEN 2), Von-Hippel-Lindau (VHL) disease, type 1 neurofibromatosis (NF1) and others.

Disorders of Adrenal Cortex

Hyperaldosteronism (Conn's syndrome)

Hyperaldosteronism can be primary (PHA) or secondary, commonly due to renal artery stenosis or low-flow states such as congestive heart failure and cirrhosis which stimulate the renin-angiotensin system. PHA results from the autonomous hypersecretion of aldosterone, leading to low serum renin levels. Clinically, patients present with long-standing refractory hypertension and hypokalemia despite potassium replacement and increased cardiovascular morbidity. The most common causes are solitary functioning adrenal adenoma (70%) or bilateral hyperplasia (30%) but may occur in ACC or hereditary disorders (< 1%) such as 11 β-hydroxylase deficiency. Diagnostic work-up includes biochemical (plasma aldosterone concentration to plasma renin activity ratio of 25:1 to 30:1) and imaging studies (Table 1). In equivocal cases or when a tumor cannot be localized, selective venous catheterization may be used for the measurement of aldosterone to cortisol ratios between the adrenal veins. A four-fold difference indicates a unilateral tumor.[3]

Table 1: Staging Systems for Adrenal carcinoma

AJCC Stage	TNM Staging	Description
I	T1N0M0	The tumor remains within the adrenal gland and is at or under 5 cm (approximately 2 in). The tumor has not metastasized to proximal lymph nodes (N0) or further locations (M0).
II	T2N0M0	The tumor is larger than 5 cm (2 in) but remains within the adrenal gland (T2). The tumor has not metastasized to proximal lymph nodes (N0) or further locations (M0).
III	T1N1M0	The tumor remains within the adrenal gland and is at or under 5 cm (approximately 2 in). The tumor has metastasized to the proximal lymph nodes (N1) but not to further locations (M0).
Or	T3N0	
	T2N1M0	The tumor is larger than 5 cm (2 in) but remains within the adrenal gland (T2). The tumor has metastasized to the proximal lymph nodes (N1) but not to further locations (M0).
IV	Any T Any N M1	The tumor has metastasized to further locations such as the liver or lungs (M1). The tumor size does not matter (Any T), and it might have metastasized to the proximal tissues (Any T) or lymph nodes (Any N).
Or	T3N1, T4	

(AJCC- American Joint Committee on Cancer)

A unilateral aldosteronoma is usually cured with an adrenalectomy, either laparoscopic (preferred) or via a posterior open approach, with postoperative normalization of hypertension and hypokalemia. On the other hand, surgery has not proved effective for bilateral hyperplasia which should be medically treated with spironolactone, amiloride, or triamterene.[2]

Cushing's syndrome

Cushing's syndrome consists of complicated symptoms and presentations secondary to the hypersecretion of cortisol, whereas Cushing's disease refers to a pituitary tumor, causing bilateral adrenal hyperplasia and hypercortisolism. Women are affected more frequently than men (male to female ratio is 1:8). Most cases of hypercortisolism are due to exogenous steroid use. In patients with endogenous Cushing's syndrome, the most common causes are ACTH-secreting pituitary tumors (70%), adrenal carcinoma or adenoma (20%), ectopic ACTH-secreting carcinoid tumor (10%), MEN1, or bronchial adenoma. The clinical presentation may vary but includes progressive truncal obesity (most common symptom), peripheral muscle wasting, purple striae, fat deposition in the posterior neck region ('buffalo-hump'), moon facies, subcutaneous tissue thinning, and hair changes.

Diagnostic work-up includes an overnight low-dose dexamethasone suppression test (1 mg dexamethasone given at 11:00PM and plasma cortisol measured at 8:00AM) with levels greater than 3 *μg/dL* suggesting Cushing's syndrome. A 24-hour cortisol measurement is an alternative modality (<100 *μg/dL rules out hypercortisolism). Following this step,* the measurement of plasma ACTH (immunoradiometric assay) is used to differentiate between a cortisol-secreting adrenal tumors (levels suppressed, <5 pg/mL), adrenal hyperplasia, (mildly elevated, 15-500 pg/mL), and ectopic sources of ACTH (> 1000 pg/mL). A high-dose dexamethasone suppression test (overnight 8 mg dexamethasone or 2 mg given every 6 hours for 2 days, followed by 24-hour urinary cortisol) is also used to differentiate ACTH-dependent causes such as pituitary (suppression of cortisol) versus ectopic (failure to suppress cortisol by 50%). CT (computed tomography) or MRI (magnetic resonance imaging) scans are essential for localizing the adrenal tumor, differentiating between an adenoma versus a carcinoma (Table 1), and defining the surgical plan.

In the absence of radiological findings suggestive of ACC (Table 2), a laparoscopic adrenalectomy is the preferred treatment. Patients undergoing this treatment are at a greater risk for postoperative infection, bleeds, and a more difficult dissection due to obesity, which increases the conversion rate to open laparotomy (0-15%) and morbidity (up to 25%).[4] If there is doubt preoperatively about the diagnosis or in large tumors, the treatment plan should be changed to that for a malignancy. Postoperatively, all patients should receive 100 mg of IV hydrocortisone every 12 hours for 3 days, starting during the surgery to avoid adrenal insufficiency. Bilateral adrenalectomy is sometimes indicated in patients with Cushing's disease following unsuccessful hypophysectomy and ectopic secretion of ACTH.[5] Most symptoms resolve within 6 to 9 months after adrenalectomy with a significant improvement in the quality of life.

Table 2: Radiological Findings of Adrenal Tumors

Adrenal Adenoma	• Unilateral, 0.5-2 cm tumor • Normal contralateral gland • Study of choice: CT scan without contrast (Hounsfield unit <10) or with contrast (15 min washout >60%) • MRI used in pregnancy, and atypical CT findings with low suspicion for carcinoma
Adrenocortical Carcinoma	• Tumor with heterogenous texture • Abnormal contour • Foci of hemorrhage or necrosis • Most are larger than 5 cm • Usually associated with peritumoral lymphadenopathy, metastasis (lung, liver, bone, or peritoneum)
Adrenal Metastasis	• Usually, bilateral • Vascular kinetics on CT/MRI scans

CT: computed tomography; MRI: magnetic resonance imaging

Congenital Adrenal Hyperplasia

Congenital adrenal hyperplasia consists of a group of enzymatic disorders involved in adrenal steroidogenesis. The most common enzyme deficiency is 21 β-hydroxylase (90%), which is characterized by diminished production of glucocorticoids and aldosterone, leading to raised ACTH and adrenal androgens levels, such as 17-hydroxyprogesterone. In peripheral tissues, these androgens are converted to testosterone, thereby leading to virilizing features. Diagnosis involves measuring the steroid content of both urine and plasma, as well as analyzing a karyotype. Standard management is medical therapy with cortisol and mineralocorticoid replacement; however, bilateral laparoscopic adrenalectomy has been proposed in some small series of patients with satisfactory results.[6] Further evidence is needed to recommend this modality for widespread use.

Disorders of Adrenal Medulla

Pheochromocytoma

Pheochromocytomas are rare tumors which arise from chromaffin cells in the adrenal medulla and, in extra-adrenal locations (paragangliomas). It is commonly seen in familial syndromes (MEN 2, VHL, NF1, tuberous sclerosis or Sturge-Weber syndrome). The classic triad includes headache (most common), palpitations, and diaphoresis. However, other non-specific symptoms such as anxiety, paresthesia, flushing, nausea, and vomiting may be present. Diagnosis involves 24-hour urine metanephrines, fractionated epinephrine and norepinephrine, vanillylmandelic acid (VMA), plasma metanephrines and chromogranin A (protein stored in the adrenal medulla and released with catecholamine hormones). Imaging tests (CT, MRI scans, and functional MIBG scintigraphy) are used to localize the tumor and metastasis. The imaging tests should depict from the diaphragm to the aortic bifurcation in order to visualize the organ of Zuckerkandl.[7] CT scans should be done without contrast to decrease the chance of hypertensive crisis. MRI has slightly increased sensitivity and specificity compared to CT since these tumors are characterized by a unique appearance on T2-weighted images or after gadolinium.[7]

Laparoscopic adrenalectomy is feasible and yields good results.[8] Kercher et al.[9] showed no conversion rates and no excess of catecholamine excess at 24-month follow-up in a series of 80 pheochromocytoma patients undergoing laparoscopic adrenalectomy. It is important to avoid excessive pneumoperitoneum pressure and tumor manipulation as it can increase the likelihood of hypertensive crises during the operation or capsular rupture with tumor dissemination.[9] An open anterior approach is recommended in bilateral tumors or extra-adrenal lesions. Intraoperative medications include nitroprusside, nitroglycerin, and phentolamine; arrhythmias can be managed with fast-acting beta-blockers, such as esmolol. Large tumors (>5 cm) are often cystic, fragile, and at an increased risk for rupture, so the surgeon should judge whether or not converting to an open surgery is necessary to assure quality resection.[10,11] A postoperative course may be remarkable for hypotension requiring medical management and large volume resuscitation.

Adrenal Insufficiency

Adrenal insufficiency can be primary and arise from an intrinsic adrenal disorder (autoimmune disorder, infection, and metastatic adrenal disease), or secondary due to ACTH deficiency (exogenous corticosteroids after discontinuation, trauma, severe stress, systemic infections, and coagulopathies).[12] Clinical signs usually mimic sepsis with severe hypotension in a stressed patient. Hyponatremia, hyperkalemia, eosinophilia, mild azotemia, and reactive hypoglycemia are common findings in laboratory studies. An ACTH stimulation test (measurement of cortisol levels at 0, 20, and 60 minutes after intravenous ACTH administration; diagnostic peak levels > 20 μg/dL) is used for diagnosis. Management involves volume resuscitation (2-3 L normal saline) and intravenous dexamethasone or hydrocortisone. Mineralocorticoids (fludrocortisone 0.05-0.1 mg daily) might be necessary after saline infusions are terminated.[7]

Adrenocortical carcinoma (ACC)

ACC is rare with an incidence between only 1-2 patients per million annually.[2] Most tumors are non-functioning (50%), however hormonal hypersecretion may occur: cortisol (30%), androgens (20%), and estrogens (10%).[13] Rapid onset Cushing's syndrome accompanied by virilizing features can often be a sign of a functioning tumor. Approximately 70% of these patients present at stage III or IV (Table 1). Diagnosis is usually made by imaging studies, either CT or MRI scans (Table 2). ACC is an aggressive disease and surgery remains the most effective therapy. Adequacy of resection is still the prime predictive factor with regards to patient survival. Overall, 5-year survival rates are 32-48% for patients who undergo complete resection, whereas median survival in those with incomplete removal is under 1 year.[14] En-bloc removal of the lesion via an open approach should allow for wide exposure, decreased likelihood of rupturing the capsule and causing the tumor to spill, and permit vascular control of major vessels (aorta, inferior vena cava, and renal vessels). The magnitude of lymphadenectomy is yet to be precisely defined.[4] Mitotane is a derivative of DTT, an insecticide, and it has previously been used in the adjuvant treatment of unresectable or metastatic disease.[15] Although, external beam radiation therapy is not effective in ACC, it may be used in palliation of bone metastasis.

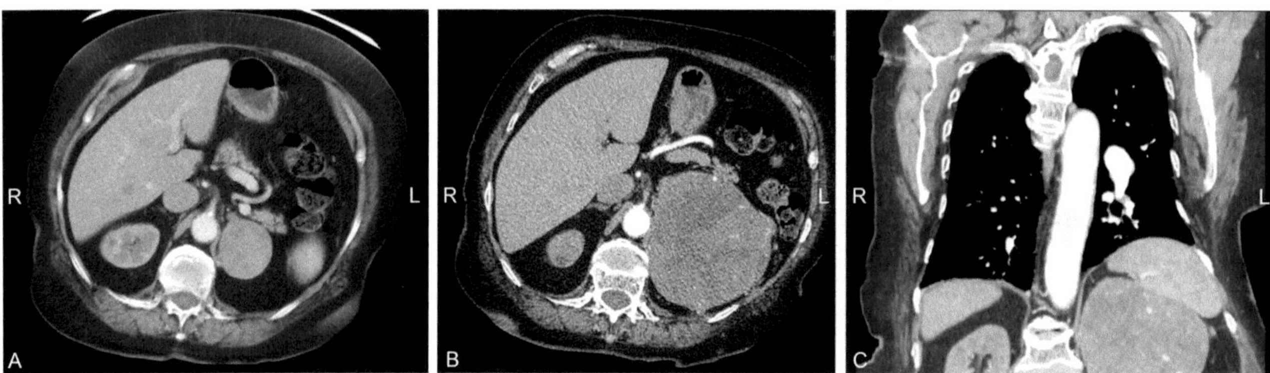

Figure 1: Axial contrast enhanced CT depicts an enhancing left adrenal mass (A). Six months later, the mass has markedly been consistent with adrenal cortical carcinoma (B and C).

Adrenal Metastasis

If the patient presents with an adrenal mass (>2 cm) and a past history of cancer (most commonly from lung, colon, breast, kidney, and melanoma), adrenal metastasis should be suspected. In cases of isolated adrenal metastasis without evidence of locoregional invasion, adrenalectomy is advised to improve survival rates and decrease local symptoms.[16] The median survival after adrenalectomy is still poor, ranging from 3-30 months.[16] The size of metastasis and site of primary tumor (renal cell cancer is associated with better survival) are predictive factors and should be taken into account in the surgical plan.

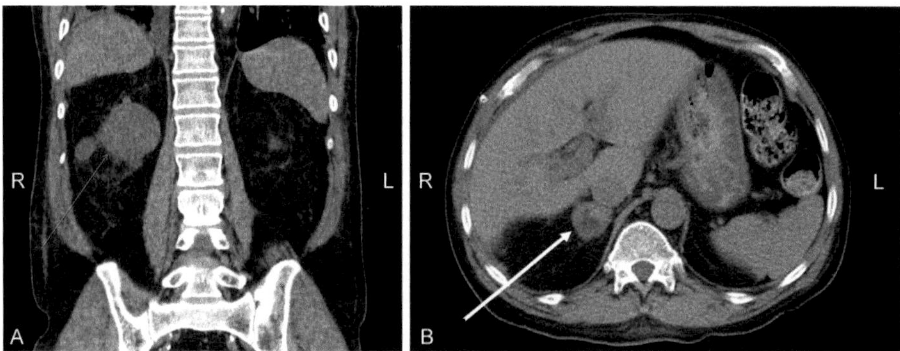

Figure 2: Coronal (A) and axial (B) reformatted non-contrast enhanced CT images demonstrate a heterogenous right adrenal mass in a patient with known primary bronchogenic carcinoma.

Adrenal Incidentaloma

Adrenal incidentaloma is defined as an adrenal tumor discovered unintentionally during body imaging for other reasons. Due to the rising number of CT scans, the incidence of adrenal incidentaloma is increasing (0.3-4.4% of CT scans). Most tumors are benign non-secretory (70%); however, in 3-5% of cases ACC is encountered.[17] The probability of malignancy is indicated by the size of the tumor (>6 cm), and CT results atypical for adenoma as described in Table 2. On the other hand, on MRI, signal loss on the out of phase T1 sequences when compared to in-phase sequence is predictable of a benign adenoma composed primarily of fat.[18] Sodium, urinary or plasma metanephrines, cortisol level, free urinary cortisol, and sometimes dexamethasone suppression tests should all be included as the minimum for laboratory studies.[7] Most adrenal incidentalomas may just be monitored, however surgical resection is indicated in hormone-secreting tumors, ACC, or potentially malignant tumors.[19] The threshold for adrenalectomy is lowered to about 3 to 4 cm for younger patient without comorbidity, whereas the 5 cm threshold is maintained for older patients with significant co morbidities.[4] Laparoscopy is usually the approach of choice, however alternate options may be used in large incidentalomas or those with high suspicion for malignancy. For those with no surgical indications, surveillance consists of CT scan at 6-month intervals in the first 2-5 years.[4] Lesions that grow during follow-up should be elected for adrenalectomy.

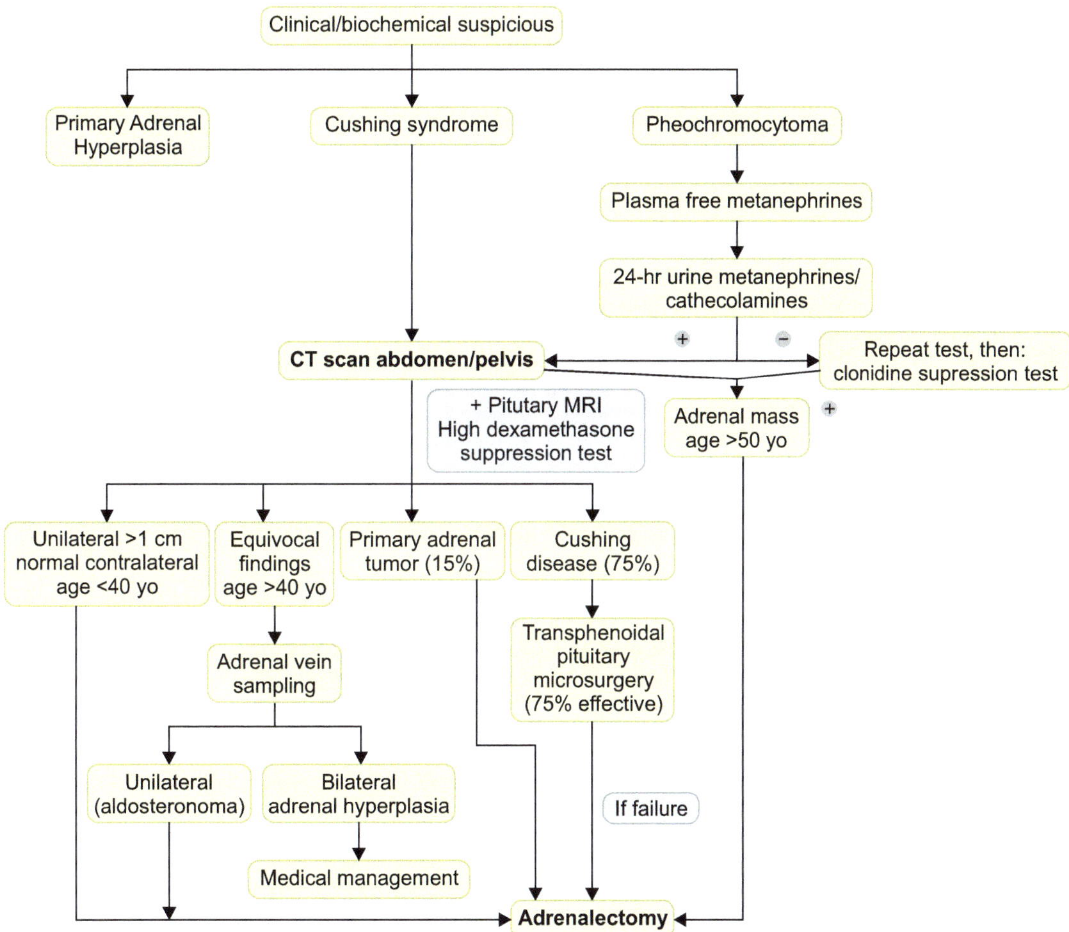

Figure 3: Workup for an adrenal mass

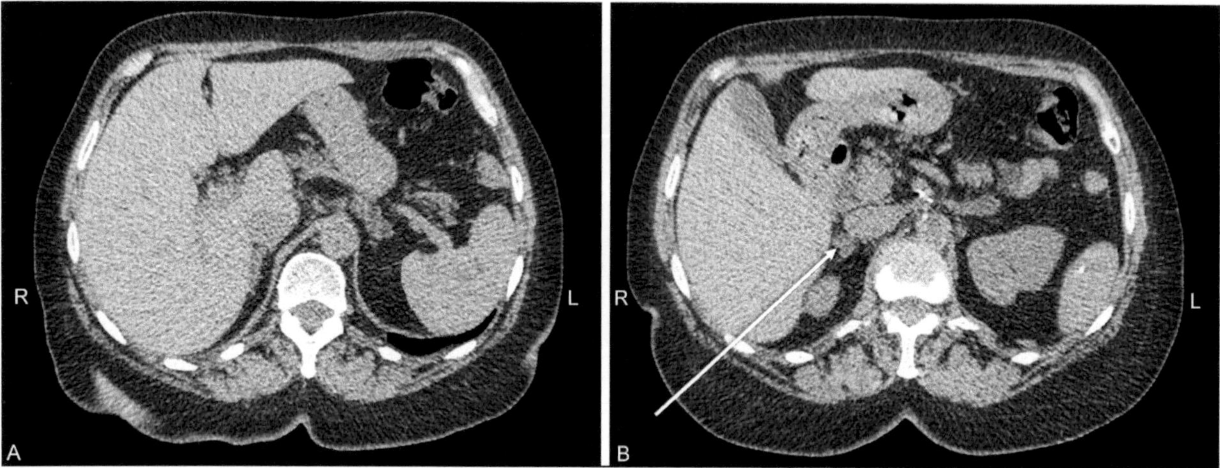

Figure 4: Multiple non-contrast enhanced axial CT images demonstrate bilateral adrenal nodules with low density (Hounsfield unit measurements).

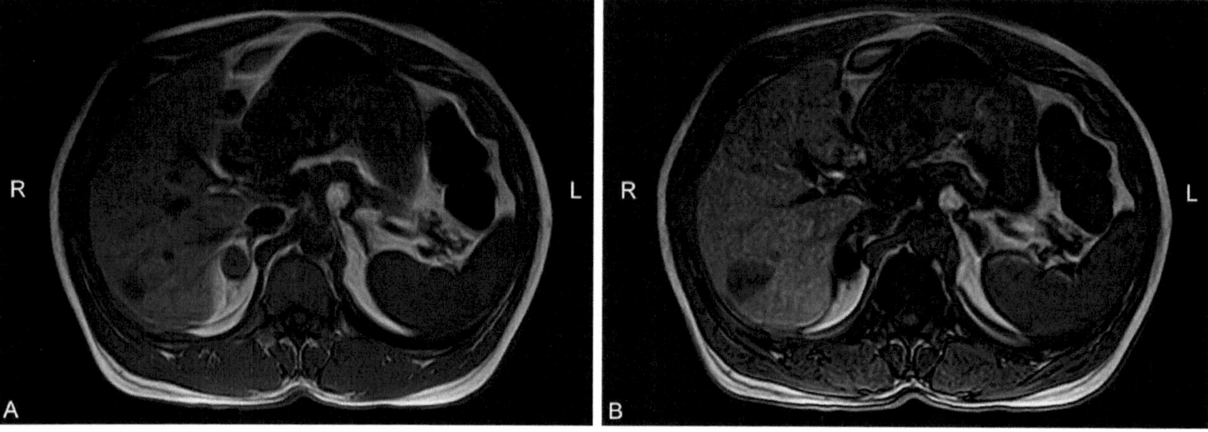

Figure 5: Axial in-phase (A) and out-of-phase (B) T1 sequences performed for liver lesions demonstrate signal drop out in an incidental right adrenal nodule consistent with a lipid rich benign adrenal cortical adenoma.

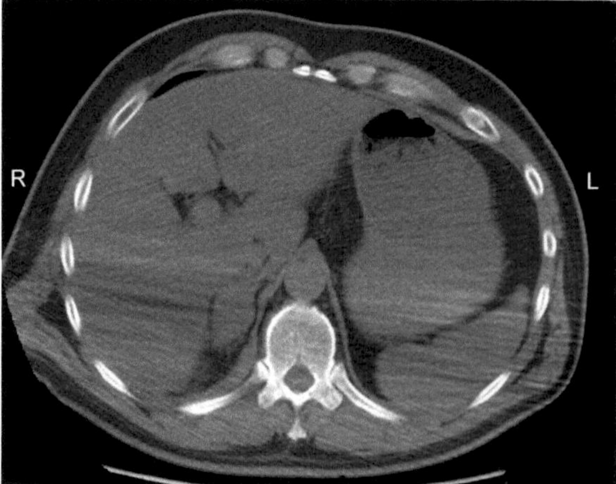

Figure 6: Axial non-contrast CT images in a patient who sustained blunt abdominal trauma demonstrates an elliptical shaped right adrenal gland which became a normal shape on follow-up studies consistent with hemorrhage.

Adrenal surgery

The first successful adrenalectomies were performed in 1926 by César Roux, in Switzerland and Charles Mayo in the United States.[1] Adrenal surgery can be done through an open, laparoscopic, or robotic method. Regardless of whichever option chosen, the gland can be assessed anteriorly, laterally, or posteriorly based on the size and nature of the lesion and the surgeon's preference.

Open Adrenalectomy

This procedure requires the patient to be under general anesthesia, which is recommended to be delivered through a nasogastric tube, Foley catheter, or sequential compression devices. An anterior open approach consists of a midline incision or bilateral subcostal incision. For right side approaches, the hepatic flexure of the colon is moved inferiorly, the triangular ligament is incised for liver retraction, and the Kocher maneuver is employed for anterior mobilization of the duodenum and exposure of the adrenal gland. Gerota's fascia is then incised, and the lateral and superior surfaces of the gland are freed. Then, the right adrenal vein is ligated and divided, and the gland is removed after medial dissection. On the left, the adrenal is localized lateral to the aorta and distal to the tail of the pancreas, which is mobilized superiorly. The gland is removed via the same method as described on the right side.

The most frequent complications after an adrenalectomy include deep vein thrombosis, wound and urinary tract infections, and injury to adjacent organs during pneumoperitoneum. Postoperative hemodynamic instability may occur after removal of the pheochromocytoma, and adrenal insufficiency after bilateral adrenalectomy. Patients with Cushing's syndrome are at an increased risk for postoperative infection, particularly incisional and intra-abdominal abscess.

Laparoscopic Adrenalectomy

Gagner et al. conducted the first laparoscopic adrenalectomy in 1992.[20] It is now the recommended approach for the removal of nearly all benign-appearing adrenal tumors, even though only a few randomized studies have compared it to an open approach. The advantages include less postoperative pain, shorter stay in the hospital, quicker return to usual activities, and fewer complications (e.g., blood loss, wound infection, and incisional hernia).[21,22] The most common laparoscopic approaches are lateral transperitoneal and posterior retroperitoneal (Table 3).[4] The former offers good exposure due to effect of gravity, being suitable for tumors up to 8-15 cm. The latter provides direct access, which is especially important in patients with adhesions secondary to previous abdominal surgeries and in bilateral adrenalectomies without the need for repositioning the patient.[23] However, because the amount of working space is restricted, exposure is more difficult, thereby making it unsuitable for large (>5 cm) tumors and obese patients. Table 2 describes technical aspects of different approaches in laparoscopic adrenalectomy. Contraindications include the presence of a breach or rupture risk of the tumor capsule, an incomplete tumor resection (invasion of adjacent structures), severe obesity, and tumors greater than 8-15 cm.[4,24]

Table 3: Different Approaches in Laparoscopic Adrenalectomy[7]

Lateral transabdominal
• The patient is set in a lateral decubitus position. • After pneumoperitoneum is created, four 10 mm trocars are set (mid-clavicular line - medially, to anterior axillary line - laterally), 1-2 fingerbreadths below the right costal margin. A 30-degree laparoscope is then introduced via the 2nd port. • The right triangular ligament is dissected, and the liver rotated medially. The adrenal gland is appreciated on the superomedial side of the kidney. • By using hook cautery, Gerota's fascia is incised. • The right adrenal vein is visualized at its junction and ligated with clips. The arterial branches can be electro-coagulated or clipped and divided. • For left adrenalectomy, lateral anchors to the spleen and tail of the pancreas are separated by electrocautery. The remainder of the dissection proceeds similar to that of the right adrenal. • Note: For a right adrenalectomy, a fan retractor is inserted via medial port to retract the liver. For the left, a retractor is used to retract the spleen. • Drain is rarely necessary.
Posterior Retroperitoneal
• The patient is placed in the prone-jackknife position and the twelfth rib is then palpated. Ultrasound may be used to determine the underlying kidney and adrenal. • A 1.5 cm incision is done 2 cm inferior to the 12th rib. Under direct vision, a 12 mm trocar with a zero-degree laparoscope is inserted through the posterior abdominal wall up to Gerota's fascia. • A 12 mm trocar is then inserted into this space and CO_2 is insufflated to 12-15 mmHg and the zero-degree is replaced by a 45-degree laparoscope. • 2 trocars (5 and 10 mm) are placed on each side of the first port. Dissection proceeds from superior to lateral and inferior aspects. • Medially, vessels ligated, clipped, and divided as described above.

Recent interest has increased worldwide after the introduction of the single-port laparoscopic adrenalectomy.[25,26] For the procedure, multi-instrument access ports allow three laparoscopic tools to be wielded simultaneously through separate trocars located in the port. A 3 cm incision is opened under the 12th rib, in the retroperitoneal area. The cut is made deeper to allow entry into the retroperitoneum. The SILS™ (Covidien®, Hamshire, UK) port is placed, and gas insufflation is initiated until a pressure of 15-18 mmHg is reached. A 5 mm 30-degree Endoeye™ (Olympus Medical®, Tokyo, Japan) is incorporated. Further technical details including dissection are then performed similarly to the conventional laparoscopic technique. Studies to date are limited to safety and feasibility reports of the technique. A prospective, randomized controlled trial is warranted to look at the efficacy of this novel approach and compare it with that of a standard laparoscopy for adrenalectomy.

The role of laparoscopic adrenalectomy in ACC is still controversial. Traditionally, en bloc excision of the tumor via an open approach with a subcostal incision or a right thoracoabdominal excision has been recommended. Concerns for laparoscopic adrenalectomy include a greater risk of capsular rupture, peritoneal seeding, metastases at the trocar site, and suboptimal resection. However, Choh et al. showed similar outcomes of the laparoscopic versus open approach with rates of local recurrence at 26%, rates of peritoneal metastases at 32%, and rates of distant metastases at 29% at 6-60 months follow-up.[27] Similarly, a recent multicenter study confirmed analogous oncologic results regarding the two types of surgery.[28] The laparoscopic method may be acceptable for treating an adrenal carcinoma in small tumors (diameter <8 cm) and when conducted within specialized centers with extensive experience in adrenal surgery with regards to a randomized prospective study.

Robotic Adrenalectomy

The first robotic adrenalectomy performed on a human was described in 2001 by Horgan and Vanun.[29] Steps are the same as those used for a lateral transperitoneal laparoscopic adrenalectomy. Few studies have compared laparoscopic to robotic adrenalectomies (Table 4), however more consistent data is still lacking for standardization of the best surgical approach.

Table 4: Studies of Robotic versus Laparoscopic Adrenalectomies

Study	Design	Sample Size		Results	
		LA	RA	Clinical	Others
Brunaud[32] 2004 France	Prospective non-randomized	14	19	Similar perioperative quality of life	
Morino[33] 2004 Italy	Prospective randomized controlled	10	10	RA: Increased total/skin-to-skin operative time. Increased total cost	• No conversion to open approach • RA: 40% converted to laparoscopic Similar LOS
Brunaud[34] 2008 France	Prospective non-randomized	59	50	RA: Less blood loss Longer operative times	• No difference in operative times after first 20 cases. Tumor size/BMI >30 kg/m2: no effect in RA while increased operative times in LA group.
Wu[35] 2008 China	Prospective randomized controlled	5	7	RA: Increased operative time Improved surgical technique	• No mortality. Similar outcomes at 1-yr follow-up
Pineda-Solis[36] 2012 USA	Retrospective	30	30	RA: Increased operative time (190 vs. 160 min). Less blood loss	• No mortality Similar morbidity and LOS.
Agcaoglu[37] 2012 USA	Prospective non-randomized	38	24	For large tumors (>5cm), RA: shorter operative time, less conversion rate, shorter LOS	
Agcaoglu[38] 2012 USA	Prospective non-randomized	31	31	Similar operative times (skin-to-skin) and blood loss	• No mortality. Similar morbidity RA: Lower pain score

LA: laparoscopic adrenalectomy; RA: robotic adrenalectomy; LOS: length of hospital stay; BMI: body mass index

SUMMARY

Adrenal masses have a broad-spectrum of potential diseases, therefore management should focus on tumor localization, differentiation between secreting and non-secreting lesions, benign versus malignant process, and adequacy for resectability. Prognosis may vary widely based on tumor staging, tumor size, and patient's comorbidities. Recent surgical advancements, including robotic and single-port adrenalectomy are matters of further investigation and substantial data is still lacking for recommendation of widespread use.

REFERENCES

1. Welbourn RB. The adrenal glands. In the History of Endocrine Surgery. Edited by Welbourn RB. New York: Praeger; 1990; 147-216.
2. Shen W, Sturgeon C, Duh QY. From incidentaloma to adrenocortical carcinoma: the surgical management of adrenal tumors. J Surg Oncol 2005; 89:186-92.
3. McKenzie T, Lillegard JL, Young WF, et al. Aldosteronomas – state of the art. Surg Clin North Am 2009; 89:1241-53.
4. Germain A, Klein M, Brunaud L. Surgical management of adrenal tumors. J Visc Surg 2011:148:e250-61.
5. Takata MC, Kebebew E, Clark OH, et al. Laparoscopic bilateral adrenalectomy: results for 30 consecutive cases. Surg Endosc 2008; 22:202-7.
6. Gmyrek GA, New MI, Sosa RE, et al. Bilateral laparoscopic adrenalectomy as a treatment for classic congenital adrenal hyperplasia attributable to 21-hydroxylase deficiency. Pediatrics 2002; 109:E28.
7. Brunicardi FC, Andersen DK, Billiar TR, et al. (Eds) In: Schwartz's Principles of Surgery. 8th ed. New York, NY: McGraw Hill 2005; p. 1465-1468.
8. Walz MK, Alesina PF, Wenger F, et al. Laparoscopic and retroperitoneoscopic treatment of pheochromocytomas and retroperitonteal paragliomas: results of 161 tumors in 126 patients. World J Surg 2006; 30:899-908.
9. Kercher K, Novitsky YW, Park A, et al. Laparoscopic curative resection of pheochromocytomas. Ann Surg 2005; 241:926-8.
10. Li M, Fitzgerald P, Price D, et al. Iatrogenic pheochromocytomatosis: a previously unreported result of laparoscopic adrenalectomy. Surgery 2001; 130:1072-7.
11. Shen W, Sturgeon C, Clark OH, et al. Should pheochromocytoma size influence surgical approach? A comparison of 90 malignant and 60 benign pheochromocytomas. Surgery 2004; 136:1129-37.
12. Bornstein SR. Predisposing factors for adrenal insufficiency. N Engl J Med 2009; 360:2328-39.
13. Ng L, Libertino JM. Adrenocortical carcinoma: diagnosis, evaluation and treatment. J Urol 2003; 169:5.
14. Bilimoria K, Shen W, Elaraj D, et al. Adrenocortical carcinoma in the United States. Cancer 2008; 113:3130-6.
15. Baudin E, Leboulleux S, Al Ghuzian A, et al. Therapeutic management of advanced Adrenocortical carcinoma: what do we know in 2011? Horm Canc 2011; 2:363-71.
16. Lam KY, Lo CY. Metastatic tumours of the adrenal glands: a 30-year experience in a teching hospital. Clin Endocrinol 2002; 56:95-101.
17. Conzo G, Tricarico A, Belli G, et al. Adrenal incidentalomas in the laparoscopic era and the role of correct surgical indication. Can J Surg 2009; 52: E281-5.
18. Taffel M, Haji-Momenian S, Nikolaidis P, et al. Adrenal imaging: a comprehensive review. Radiol Clin N Am 2012:50:219-43.
19. Alves A, Scatton O, Dousset B. Diagnostic and therapeutic strategy for an incidental finding of an adrenal mass. J Chir (Paris) 2002; 139:205-13.
20. Gagner M, Lacroix A, Bolté E. Laparoscopic adrenalectomy in Cushing's syndrome and pheochromoctoma. N Engl J Med 1992; 327:1033.
21. Gumbs AA, Gagner M. Laparoscopic adrenalectomy. Best Pract Res Clin Endocrinol Metab 2006; 20:483-99.
22. Ariyan C, Strong V. The current status of laparoscopic adrenalectomy. Adv Surg 2007; 41:133-53.
23. Lombardi CP, Raffaelli M, De Crea C, et al. Endoscopic adrenalectomy: is there na optimal operative approach? Results of a single-center case-control study. Surgery 2008; 144:1014-5.
24. Sturgeon CK. Laparoscopic adrenalectomy for malignancy. Surg Clin North Am 2004; 84-755-74.
25. Goo TT, Agarwal A, Goel R, et al. Single-port access adrenalectomy: our initial experience. J Laparoendosc Adv Surg Tech A. 2011;21(9):815-9.
26. Kwak HN, Kim JH, Yun JS, et al. Conventional laparoscopic adrenalectomy versus laparoscopic adrenalectomy through mono port. Surg Laparosc Endosc Percutan Tech. 2011 Dec;21(6):439-42.
27. Choh M, Madura J. The role of minimally invasive treatments in surgical oncology Surg Clin North Am 2009; 89:53-77.

28. Brix D, Allolio B, Fenske W, et al. German Adrenocortical Carcinoma Registry Rroup. Laparoscopic versus open adrenalectomy for adrenocortical carcinoma: surgical and oncologic outcome in 152 patients Eur J Endocrinol 2010; 58(4):609-15.
29. Horgan S, Vanuno D. Robots in laparoscopic surgery. J Laparoendosc Adv Surg Rech A 2001; 11:415-9.
30. Sung GT, Gill IS. Robotic laparoscopic surgery: a comparison of the da Vinci and Zeus systems. Urology 2001; 58:893-898.
31. Brunaud L, Germain A, Zarnegar R, et al. Robot-assisted adrenalectomy. Surg Laparosc Endosc Percutan Tech 2011; 21(4):248-54.
32. Brunaud L, Bresler L, Zarnegar R, et al. Does robotic adrenalectomy improve patient quality of life when compared to laparoscopic adrenalectomy? World J Surg 2004; 28:1180-5.
33. Morino M, Beninca G, Giraudo G, et al. Robot-assisted vs. laparoscopic adrenalectomy: a prospective randomized controlled trial. Surg Endosc 2004; 18:1742-46.
34. Brunaud L, Bresler L, Ayab A, et al. Robotic-assisted adrenalectomy: what advantages compared to lateral transperitoneal laparoscopic adrenalectomy? Am J Surg 2008; 195:433-8.
35. Wu JC, Wu S, Linc MS, et al. Comparison of robot-laparoscopic adrenalectomy with traditional laparoscopic adrenalectomy: 1-year follow-up. Surg Endosc 2008; 22463-66.
36. Pineda-Solis K, Medina-Franco H, Hestlin MJ. Robotic versus laparoscopic adrenalectomy: a comparative study in a high-volume center. Surg Endosc 2012 (in press).
37. Agcaoglu O, Aliyev S, K, Karabulut K, et al. Robotic vs laparoscopic posterior retroperitoneal adrenalectomy. Arch Surg 2012; 147(3):272-5.
38. Agcaoglu O, Aliyev S, Karabulut K, et al. Robotic versus laparoscopic resection of large adrenal tumors. Ann Surg Oncol 2012; 19:2288-94.

57

CHAPTER

Peritoneal Surface Malignancy

William Yoon, MD
Richard Berri, MD

INTRODUCTION

Peritoneal surface malignancies (PSM) refer to a wide variety of tumors that can manifest with extensive peritoneal dissemination. Patients with PSM often suffer from direct consequences of expansive tumor progression in the peritoneal cavity, such as intestinal obstruction, and typically progress to death in less than a year. Hence, peritoneal dissemination has been regarded as a manifestation of the terminal phase. With limited treatment options, PSM has traditionally been treated with systemic chemotherapy along with palliative surgery. However, in the last two decades, the medical community has come to recognize that this disease can remain confined to the peritoneal cavity during most of its natural history. With this point of interest shift in PSM from disease stage to disease site, a new combined modality of cytoreductive surgery (CRS) plus hyperthermic intraperitoneal chemotherapy (HIPEC) has emerged as a potentially curative treatment option for PSM.

This chapter presents the definitions, anatomy, pathophysiology, epidemiology, clinical manifestations, diagnostic evaluation, and current treatment options of PSM. The malignancy conditions to be discussed include appendix cancer and pseudomyxoma peritonei, colorectal peritoneal carcinomatosis, gastric peritoneal carcinomatosis, ovarian peritoneal carcinomatosis, abdominal sarcomatosis, and peritoneal mesothelioma.

DEFINITIONS

A peritoneal surface malignancy can result from carcinomatosis, sarcomatosis, lymphomatosis, and primary peritoneal tumors.[1,2] Among these, peritoneal carcinomatosis (PC) is the most well-known and commonly encountered peritoneal surface malignancy condition. PC is defined as extensive metastasis and implantation of tumor cells in the peritoneal cavity, resulting in malignant tissue deposits onto the parietal and visceral peritoneum. This may develop as a part of the natural history of gastrointestinal (GI) or gynecologic cancers, or from primary peritoneal neoplasms. Peritoneal sarcomatosis is defined as the disseminated intraperitoneal spread of sarcoma in the absence of a significant extra-abdominal site of origin.[2] Primary peritoneal tumors are defined as tumors with a primary manifestation in the peritoneum, and without a visceral site of origin.[1] These primary malignancies can stem from the mesothelial or sub-mesothelial layers of the peritoneum, and include malignant mesothelioma, multi-cystic mesothelioma, primary peritoneal serous carcinoma (papillary serous cancer), leiomyomatosis peritonealis disseminate, and desmoplastic small round cell tumor.[1]

ANATOMY OF THE PERITONEUM

The peritoneum is a thin, translucent serosal membrane that lays over the surface of the abdominopelvic cavities and is made up of a single layer of mesothelial cells supported by a sub-mesothelial connective tissue layer. Mesothelial cells have surface microvilli which entrap hyaluronate. The resulting thin layer of hyaluronate that coats the peritoneal surface reduces friction as the viscera moves over the peritoneum.[1] Vascular and lymphatic capillary networks are contained in the sub-mesothelial connective tissue layer. The basal lamina underlying the mesothelial layer serves as a peritoneal-plasma barrier that acts as a passive semipermeable membrane, preventing the transport of large molecules and cellular material across it.[3,4] Consequently, only small amounts of systemic drugs can penetrate this barrier into the peritoneal cavity. The resultant systemic drug resistance has brought about a change in route of drug administration in treating patients with PSM; chemotherapy is given intraperitoneally in a new combined approach.

The peritoneum can be divided into two components: visceral and parietal. Intraperitoneal organs are covered by the visceral peritoneum (i.e., stomach, proximal first segment of duodenum, jejunum, ileum, transverse colon, sigmoid colon, liver, spleen). Two layers of visceral peritoneum form the peritoneal ligaments (i.e., coronary, falciform, gastro-hepatic, hepatoduodenal, splenorenal, gastrocolic, phrenicocolic) and mesenteries (i.e., small bowel mesentery, transverse mesocolon, sigmoid mesentery). The intraperitoneal organs are suspended within the peritoneal cavity by peritoneal ligaments and mesenteries. The parietal peritoneum lines the undersurface of the diaphragm, the abdominal walls, the anterior surface of the retroperitoneal viscera, and the pelvis. Notably, the parietal peritoneum is sensitive to pain, whereas the visceral peritoneum is insensitive.

The visceral peritoneum turns into the parietal peritoneum at the peritoneal reflections, and the spaces formed by the reflections are called parietal recesses. In the pelvis, the rectovaginal pouch (pouch of Douglas) in the female, and the retro-vesical pouch in the male are the most caudal and dependent peritoneal recesses.

The peritoneum is continuous in the male pelvis, whereas the peritoneum is discontinuous at the ostia of the oviducts in the female. Through these openings, communication can take place between the peritoneal cavity and pelvic extraperitoneal spaces.[3]

PHYSIOLOGY OF THE PERITONEAL FLUID

The peritoneal cavity, a space between the visceral and parietal peritoneum, contains a small amount of fluid. This peritoneal fluid arises from the filtration or transudation of blood through capillary walls so that it contains almost all the protein constituents of the plasma. In addition to its function as a lubricator, it has anti-inflammatory properties.[5]

The peritoneal fluid continuously circulates. This circulatory movement is generated by the movement of the diaphragm, peristalsis of the bowel, as well as gravity. It predominantly flows up toward the undersurface of the diaphragm, especially through the right paracolic gutter because it is deeper and wider than the left.[5]

The peritoneal fluid absorption is believed to occur throughout the peritoneum. However, because large molecules like proteins and cellular materials cannot pass through the peritoneal-plasma barrier, they are absorbed via lymphatic channels.[3] The densest lymphatic network is found in the muscular portion of the right diaphragm. The majority of peritoneal lymph from the subphrenic lymphatics is carried via retrosternal lymphatic channels to anterior mediastinal nodes, and then proceeds to the right lymphatic duct. Consequently, contrary to the abdominal viscera which has the thoracic duct as the main lymph collecting trunk, lymphatic absorption in the peritoneal cavity occurs through the right lymphatic duct.[5]

This unique peritoneal fluid dynamics dictates the dissemination of peritoneal malignancies. The most common seeding sites are the right lower quadrant, the right diaphragm and hepatoduodenal ligament, the omentum, and the pelvic peritoneum.[5] Furthermore, Hagiwara et al. reported the presence of "milky spots" which appear to function as lymphatic and immunologic filters, thereby serving as a tumor cell trapping area. According to the report, these "milky spots" are concentrated in the omentum, hepatoduodenal ligament, mesentery base, pouch of Douglas, and epiploic appendices.[6] The presence of peritoneal tumor masses that block these clearing routes may hinder the peritoneal fluid reabsorption, resulting in malignant ascites. The protein-rich ascites further promotes cancer growth.[7]

MECHANISMS OF TUMOR CELL DISSEMINATION IN THE PERITONEAL CAVITY

There are two distinctive mechanisms that give primary GI tumors access to the peritoneal cavity. These mechanisms correlate to the type of primary tumor. First, low-grade, well-differentiated tumors such as mucinous tumors of the appendix and ovary tumors grow slowly and then rupture due to sheer pressure built up by the increased tumor mass, releasing tumor cells into the peritoneal cavity (pressure-burst phenomenon). Second, high-grade, poorly differentiated tumors disseminate via primary organ invasion with subsequent spilling of tumor cells.[3]

Several factors dictate the dissemination of tumor cells in the peritoneal cavity. First of all, the physiologic flow of peritoneal fluid renders the undersurface of the right hemidiaphragm as the most favorable site for tumor cell implants because free tumor cells are pulled into the right subphrenic lymphatics.[1,5,7,8] The second driving force is gravity. Because the rectovaginal and retro-vesical spaces are situated in the most dependent portions of the peritoneal cavity, peritoneal malignancies commonly seed in these areas.[3,7,8] The next important factor is the phagocytic activity of the omentum and the appendices epiploicae, described by Hagiwara et al. as "milky spots." Infiltration and implantation of tumor cells in the greater omentum is known as "omental cake".[7] Finally, surgical intervention contributes to tumor cell implantation, which is known as the "tumor cell entrapment" hypothesis. According to the hypothesis, surgical resection of large primary lesions can release tumor cells into the peritoneal cavity. The inflammatory response ensued by surgical trauma entraps these free tumor cells in a fibrin exudate, protecting them from the immune system clearance.[8-10] Additionally, growth factors involved in the wound healing process further promote the progression of entrapped tumor cells. Moreover, the implantation efficiency on raw surgical surfaces is high, thus even a small number of spilled tumor cells can result in cancer recurrence on peritoneal surfaces.[10]

HISTOPATHOLOGY OF PERITONIEAL SURFACE MULIGNANCIES

Primary peritoneal malignancies originate from mesothelial cells, sub-mesothelial mesenchymal cells, or uncommitted stem cells of the peritoneum, including malignant mesothelioma, multicystic mesothelioma, primary peritoneal (serous) carcinoma, leiomyomatosis peritonealis disseminata, and desmoplastic small round cell tumors.[1] Secondary peritoneal malignancies result from invasion or metastasis of tumor cells into the peritoneum from other organs, most commonly GI or gynecologic organs.

Mucin

Mucins are a family of glycoproteins that comprise more than 50% of carbohydrate and mucin peptides. There are two forms of mucin, an extracellular form from epithelial cells and an intracellular form known as signet ring cells. The intracellular form is less common than the extracellular form, and it carries a poor prognosis.[11]

Mucin production is the hallmark of adenocarcinomas. Mucin in normal tissues function as a lubricator of the GI epithelial lining and as a barrier to harmful chemicals or pathogens in the intestinal lumen.

Mucinous tumors account for approximately 60% of all appendix tumors, 15% of colorectal tumors, and 36% of epithelial ovarian tumors.[11] These mucinous adenocarcinomas have a strong propensity for spreading to peritoneal surfaces, but they spare the small intestine in low-grade mucinous peritoneal dissemination.[12]

Appendiceal tumors with peritoneal dissemination

Epithelial malignancies of the appendix have a broad spectrum of aggressiveness, from benign adenomas to low-grade mucinous adenocarcinomas, and to poorly differentiated mucinous adenocarcinomas. Nonetheless, these mucinous appendiceal tumors spread to the peritoneal surface in all levels of aggressiveness, often referred to as pseudomyxoma peritonei (PMP) syndrome.[3]

PMP is the term often used to describe a pathologic finding which is characterized by copious, gelatinous intraperitoneal mucin. The most common cause of PMP is a perforated mucinous appendiceal tumor. However, because PMP can be caused by both benign and malignant GI tumors as well as primary peritoneal tumors, there is much confusion when diagnosing it. In fact, consensus on the appropriate nomenclature for the appendiceal tumors and their peritoneal tumors has not yet been formed. The center of the debate is whether PMP represents proliferation of adenomatous epithelium or carcinomatous epithelium.[13]

In 1995, Ronnett et al. studied 109 cases of PMP and classified them into three groups.[14] When the primary appendiceal tumor was an adenoma, a peritoneal neoplasm was associated with mucin containing simple to focally proliferative mucinous epithelium with low-grade cytology. Ronnett et al. named this low-grade group as diffuse peritoneal adenomatosis (DPAM). When the primary appendiceal tumor was a mucinous adenocarcinoma, a peritoneal neoplasm was associated with high-grade cytology involving more proliferative epithelium, glands, or individual cells such as signet ring cells (i.e., complex architectural features). This group was then designated as peritoneal mucinous carcinoma (PMCA). The third group existing between DPAM and PMCA mostly has features of DPAM, but with focal well-differentiated mucinous adenocarcinoma. This group was named as PMCA-intermediate (PMCA-I). The authors also found a significant difference in survival between these three groups; higher 5-year survival rate was observed in the DPAM group and low survival rate was observed in the PMCA group.[14] In a follow-up study in 1997, Ronnett et al. reported that the PMCA-I group behaved similar to PMCA, and therefore suggested to incorporate the PMCA-I group into the PMCA group.[15]

Another recommendation was presented in 2003 by Misdraji et al. after studying 107 low-grade appendiceal mucinous tumors.[16] Because there was no difference between appendiceal tumors that were confined to the appendix and those that disseminated to the peritoneal cavity, Misdraji et al. suggested the term "low-grade appendiceal mucinous neoplasm (LAMN)" for all low-grade noninvasive mucinous tumors of the appendix. When the appendiceal tumor expresses high-grade cytology or invasion, they made a diagnosis of adenocarcinoma.[16]

Later in 2006, Bradley et al. reviewed 101 patients with peritoneal mucinous tumors. In the study, they classified peritoneal mucinous tumors as DPAM, PMCA-I, and PMCA according to the Ronnett et al. criteria. At the end of the study, they confirmed better survival rates among low-grade groups and took the view that PMP represents low-grade mucinous carcinomatosis. Based on this view, they proposed that all peritoneal mucinous tumors be classified as mucinous carcinoma peritonei.[17]

In summary, pathologists agree that PMP is a low-grade neoplastic process regardless of which terminology one employs to describe it, and higher-grade proliferation results in a worse prognosis.[13] They further agree that peritoneal disease classification should be based on the origin and pathologic characteristics of the primary tumor. For this reason, they also argue PMP should never be used as a diagnosis but used to describe the clinical findings of abundant extracellular mucin release into the peritoneal cavity, malignant cells may or may not be present.[3,18]

Colorectal peritoneal carcinomatosis

Peritoneal carcinomatosis is a frequent mode of spread from primary adenocarcinoma of the colon and rectum.[3] There are two mechanisms of colorectal peritoneal carcinomatosis (CRPC). One mechanism is direct cancer cell invasion through the full thickness of the bowel wall, followed by cancer cell implantation and proliferation in the peritoneal cavity.[19] This transmural invasion of cancer cells may occur without any evidence of lymphatic or hematogenous metastasis.[20] Another mechanism of peritoneal seeding is a result of surgical manipulation as discussed in the previous section. In approximately 25% of patients with colorectal cancer recurrence, the recurrence is confined to the peritoneal cavity.[19]

Ovarian peritoneal carcinomatosis

Papillary serous ovarian carcinoma is the most common type of ovarian epithelial cancer. Since the ovarian epithelial layer and the peritoneum both originate from the coelomic epithelium,[1] papillary serous ovarian carcinoma is histologically indistinguishable from papillary serous carcinoma of the peritoneum, which is a primary tumor of the peritoneum. While papillary serous carcinoma of the peritoneum spares the ovaries,[21] a majority of patients with papillary serous ovarian cancer have peritoneal dissemination.[22]

Peritoneal Mesothelioma

Peritoneal mesothelioma arises from mesothelial or multipotential sub-mesothelial mesenchymal cells lining the peritoneal cavity. It has traditionally been categorized by microscopic appearance and prognosis into three groups: benign, borderline, and malignant. Benign mesothelioma, the least common of the three groups, includes adenomatoid and localized fibrous mesothelioma.[3] Borderline mesothelioma includes multi-cystic and well-differentiated papillary peritoneal mesothelioma.[3] Peritoneal malignant mesotheliomas are further subclassified into diffuse and localized subtypes. Diffuse malignant mesotheliomas are highly aggressive, whereas localized malignant mesotheliomas usually have a good prognosis after complete excision.[1]

Multiple, firm, and whitish nodules that are scattered over the peritoneum is the characteristic finding of diffuse peritoneal malignant mesotheliomas. Hence, diffuse peritoneal malignant mesotheliomas may present grossly similar to peritoneal carcinomatosis. As the disease advances, the small bowel may become encased by the spreading tumor masses, rendering it fixed, rigid, and immobile. On the other hand, a localized peritoneal malignant mesothelioma forms a focal solid mass and may invade adjacent organs.[1]

Histologically, malignant mesothelioma can be classified into three groups: epithelial, sarcomatous, and mixed. Among them, the epithelial type is the most common. Epithelial malignant mesothelioma is composed of cells that look like normal mesothelial cell; thereby, it carries the best prognosis.[1] The sarcomatoid and mixed tumors are more rapidly growing, invasive tumors.[3]

Peritoneal Sarcomatosis

Peritoneal sarcomatosis refers to disseminated intraperitoneal spread of a soft tissue sarcoma in the absence of any extra-abdominal dissemination. The source of peritoneal sarcomatosis includes retroperitoneal soft tissue sarcomas, liposarcomas, pelvic tumors such as uterine leiomyosarcomas, GI stromal tumors (GISTs), and rarely the desmoplastic small round cell abdominal tumor of young adults or adolescents. When considering therapeutic options, all histologic subtypes of sarcomas may be regarded together; treatment options are dictated by tumor grade, size, and location of the disease.[23]

EPIDEMIOLOGY

Peritoneal carcinomatosis

With the traditional palliative treatment approach, the reported median survival of peritoneal carcinomatosis (PC) used to be about 6 months.[24] Since the introduction of CRS and HIPEC, there has been an improvement in survival rates for PC in selected patients.

Appendix tumors are unusual, accounting for 0.4% of GI tract malignancies; PMP is rare, with an incidence of about one per million per year.[25] In 1995, Ronnett et al. reported an 84% 5-year survival rate in patients with DPAM and an 6.7% 5-year survival rate in patients with PMCA. PMCA-I had intermediate survival.[14] Follow-up studies showed a 10-year survival rate of 70% in the DPAM group, and a 10-year survival rate of less than 5% in the PMCA group.[15]

In western countries, colorectal cancer is the second leading cause of cancer-related deaths. About 25% of colorectal cancer patients present with metastatic disease. While the liver is the most common metastatic site,[27] about 8% of these patients present with isolated peritoneal dissemination at the time of diagnosis.[19,28,29] In recurrent disease, disease is confined to the peritoneal cavity in 25% of patients.[19] The median survival has been traditionally reported as less than six months.[30,31] However, mounting evidence suggests, when all grossly apparent colorectal peritoneal disease could be eradicated surgically, the median survival could be improved.[32] In fact in 2009, Elias et al. compared survival rates in patients with resectable PC from colorectal cancer treated with oxaliplatin (or irinotecan) or by CRS and HIPEC.[33] The median survival was 63 months in the group treated by CRS and HIPEC, compared to 24 months in the group treated by systemic chemotherapy alone.[33]

Worldwide, stomach adenocarcinoma is the fourth leading cause of cancer-related deaths. In the United States, annually, the incidence of gastric cancer is about 22,400 and the incidence is decreasing.[34] Based on a previously published series, about 20% to 30% of gastric patients who were thought to have resectable disease, were found to actually have peritoneal dissemination at the time of exploratory surgery.[30] The median survival reported in patients with gastric PC is 7 months after diagnosis and best-supportive care.[4]

Epithelial ovarian cancer accounts for 80% to 90% of all ovarian malignancies. Ovarian peritoneal carcinomatosis is the leading cause of death for all gynecological tumors.[30] According to Yan et al., the median survival after CRS and HIPEC is 46 months.[35]

Primary Peritoneal Malignancies

Primary peritoneal malignancies are rare, and peritoneal mesothelioma is much less common than pleural mesothelioma.[24] The incidence of peritoneal mesothelioma is approximately 1 per 1,000,000, representing one-fourth of all mesotheliomas,[22,36,37] and the incidence is increasing.[3]

Primary peritoneal malignancies also have a poor prognosis; the median survival reported was uniformly about one year after palliative surgeries and systemic chemotherapy.[19,37] In general, primary peritoneal carcinoma shows a predominance in women. Two exceptions are malignant mesothelioma and desmoplastic small round cell tumors (DSRCT). Malignant mesothelioma, which has a strong association with asbestos exposure, occurs exclusively in older men and DSRCT occurs most often in young men.[1]

Peritoneal sarcomatosis

Sarcomas account for 1% of adult solid tumors, and 19% of sarcomas occur in the trunk.[38] Visceral sarcomas frequently present with peritoneal sarcomatosis and carries a poor prognosis. After reviewing 13 patients with peritoneal sarcomatosis who underwent CRS and HIPEC, one study reported a median disease-free survival of 11 months and an overall survival of 12 months.[39]

NATURAL HISTORY OF PERITONEAL MALIGNANCIES

Appendiceal Malignancies and Pseudomyxoma Peritonei

In a majority of patients, appendiceal tumors present with peritoneal dissemination.[30] It has a characteristic finding of abundant mucin produced by adenomatous tumor cells along with mucous ascites within the peritoneal cavity.[40] It has been termed as pseudomyxoma peritonei (PMP).[40]

Most often PMP arises from a mucinous appendiceal tumor that initially obstructs the lumen of the appendix. The resultant pressure built up inside the narrow appendiceal lumen causes rupture and perforation, allowing the adenomatous tumor cells to access the peritoneal cavity. Eventually, free tumor cells and a large volume of mucin accumulates and implants at the peritoneal fluid absorption sites such as the undersurface of the right hemidiaphragm, the greater omentum, and within dependent areas.[41,42] However, due to continuous peristaltic motion, the small intestine is most often spared from tumor implantation. In contrast, tumor implantation occurs invariably on the surfaces of the stomach and large intestine. Moreover, mucinous appendiceal tumors rarely metastasize to lymph nodes or the liver.[30] Despite a near absence of lymph node and liver metastases, the extensive peritoneal implantation of tumor cells results in a failure of intestinal function, causing extreme pain and suffering as the disease advances, eventually leading to death.

Colorectal Peritoneal Carcinomatosis

About 10% to 15% of patients with colorectal cancer present with peritoneal dissemination at the time of diagnosis,[22,29,30] and 25% of patients with recurrence have disease confined to the peritoneal cavity.[19] With few patients surviving beyond 6 months, colorectal peritoneal carcinomatosis carries a poor prognosis.[19,32] Newer chemotherapeutic regimens have shown improved survival rates. For example, the systemic therapy regimen, including fluorouracil and leucovorin combined with oxaliplatin or irinotecan, has demonstrated a median survival of 20 months for advanced colorectal cancer.[32,43]

Gastric Peritoneal Carcinomatosis

About 10% to 20% of gastric cancer patients present with peritoneal carcinomatosis at the time of initial surgery. About 40% to 50% of these patients experience recurrent disease after one to three years after their initial cytoreductive surgery. However, the peritoneum is the only site of recurrence.[9,44] This high incidence of isolated peritoneal carcinomatosis from gastric cancer suggests that CRS plus HIPEC, in selected patients, could improve survival.[30]

Ovarian Peritoneal Carcinomatosis

Most ovarian cancers arise from the epithelium of the ovary, and epithelial ovarian cancer is the source of the most deaths amongst all gynecological tumors.[45] The peritoneum is most often the first site of ovarian tumor dissemination that is frequently confined to the peritoneal cavity.[22] The disease recurrence is common, and the peritoneum is often the only site of recurrence.[46]

Malignant Peritoneal Mesothelioma

Peritoneal mesothelioma arises from the serosal membrane of the abdominal and pelvic cavities, and it involves both the parietal and visceral peritoneum. Asbestos is one factor known to cause malignant peritoneal mesothelioma, with a reported association ranging from 50% to 83%.[47] But, the association between asbestos and peritoneal mesothelioma is less compared to the observed association with pleural mesothelioma.[3]

Malignant peritoneal mesothelioma is commonly present with ascites. This neoplasm is characterized by numerous whitish tumor nodules of variable size which may coalesce to entirely cover the peritoneal surface, but it stays localized in the peritoneal cavity. Compared to mucinous carcinomatosis from appendiceal cancer, the peritoneal nodular implants do not spare the small bowel and its mesentery.[48] Hence, although the disease is predominantly confined within the peritoneal cavity, complete resection of these tumors is often not possible.[3] Death is usually caused by intestinal obstruction, fistula formation, and resulting starvation.[22]

Peritoneal Sarcomatosis

Peritoneal sarcomatosis is rare and occurs most commonly due to a GI stromal tumor (GIST), liposarcoma, and leiomyosarcoma.[49] Spillage of tumor cells during a prior sarcoma resection can cause recurrent peritoneal sarcomatosis. Recurrence rates after an initial debulking surgery range between 25% and 85%.[50,51] Recently, adjuvant therapy with imatinib has been shown to affect the natural history of GIST but has no value for other sarcomas.[52]

CLINICAL MANIFESTATIONS

Pseudomyxoma peritonei syndrome

In a series of 217 cases of PMP, Esquivel and Sugarbaker found that suspected acute appendicitis is the most common presentation overall (27%); it was the most common presentation in males (34%) and the second most common presentation in females (20%). For females, the most common presentation was an ovarian mass (39%), more commonly the right ovary. The second most common presentation overall was increasing abdominal girth (23%). Additionally, 14% of patients presented with a new onset hernia, mostly an inguinal hernia especially in males. In 4% of cases, ascites was the initial presenting symptom.[53] PMP was an incidental finding more commonly in females than males, often associated with gynecological complaints or infertility investigations.[8,54]

Colorectal Peritoneal Carcinomatosis

Symptoms are related to the impact of tumor burden on bowel function. Common complaints include bleeding, obstruction, perforation, and intractable pain.

Malignant Peritoneal Mesothelioma

Due to diffuse thickening of the peritoneal surfaces, ascites is a common manifestation.[1] Accordingly, a majority of patients present with abdominal pain or discomfort, abdominal distension, or increasing abdominal girth due to tumor volume and ascitic fluid. As the disease advances, GI complications such as intestinal obstruction may occur.[1,19]

Peritoneal Sarcomatosis

The presenting symptoms of all sarcomas are nonspecific. The presence of ascites is variable. Peritoneal implants from sarcomas are often vascular and therefore associated with minimal ascites. Additionally, bowel obstruction is not a common finding in peritoneal sarcomatosis.[49]

DIAGNOSTIC EVALUATION

Imaging

Owing to similar gross pathologic appearances, peritoneal malignancies share similar radiologic features.[49] Seeding of tumor cells occurs along the peritoneum and omentum, assuming the normal contours of the intraperitoneal structures. As a result, it is difficult to quantify these malignancies accurately by traditional radiologic modalities (i.e., ultrasound, CT, and MRI). The detection of peritoneal implants on the small bowel surface is particularly limited.[7,55] For both CT and ultrasound, the reported detection rate is about 25% for peritoneal implants one cm or less.[56] Accordingly, the staging of peritoneal diseases by these radiologic modalities is limited.

Nonetheless, ultrasound, CT, and MRI are sensitive for the detection of omental implants or indirect evidence of a tumor such as the presence of ascites or extracellular mucin, mesenteric thickening, or matting of bowel loops. Sonography is particularly useful in detecting ascitic fluid.[1]

CT scan offers some advantages in planning treatments in patients with mucinous adenocarcinoma. First, a CT scan of the chest is effective in ruling out systemic spread into the pleural surface, which would indicate an advanced stage. Next, a CT scan of the abdomen and pelvis is useful in quantifying copious mucin produced by these tumors, which is readily distinguishable from normal structures both by shape and density.[57] Lastly, an abdominal CT scan is effective in detecting small bowel involvement; the presence of obstructed segments in the small bowel, and the presence of tumor nodules >5 cm in diameter on the small bowel surface or directly adjacent to the small bowel mesentery, suggesting a non-resectable disease.[57]

In practice, MRI is a less commonly used modality for diagnosing suspected PC compared to CT. CT is easier to obtain, has a lower incidence of movement artifacts, and is preferred by patients.[3] Consequently, CT is the most widely used imaging modality for the detection of PC.[4] However, MRI is a primary modality for patients in whom intravenous contrast-enhanced CT is contraindicated.[1] Recently, some centers have suggested that an MRI protocol imaging study may have more value in the detection of peritoneal metastases and is particularly useful in surveillance scans after surgery.

Peritoneal Cytology

Peritoneal cytology has been used in patients with new-onset ascites to identify or exclude a possibility of malignancy.[3] It has been also utilized to identify patients with an increased risk for developing local recurrence after surgery. The presence of tumor cells in peritoneal washings obtained at the time of surgical resection is correlated with increased local recurrence.[58]

Tumor Markers

More than 20 tumor markers are currently in use. Among them, the tumor markers Carbohydrate Antigen 19-9 (CA 19-9), Carcinoembryonic Antigen (CEA), and CA-125 are the most often used in the management of PSM. CA 19-9 was discovered in patients with colon cancer and pancreatic cancer in 1981,[59] and has been used primarily in the management of pancreatic cancer. CEA is normally produced during the development of a fetus and has been used in monitoring patients with colorectal cancer. CA-125 is a marker commonly found elevated in ovarian cancer patients.

CA 19-9, CEA, and CA-125 are the three tumor markers commonly used in the management of PMP. High CEA levels or an elevation in any two of the three tumor markers prior to surgery is a predictor of early recurrence even after complete cytoreduction.[54] The tumor markers most often elevated in advanced colorectal cancer are CEA and CA 19-9. Multiple studies report that preoperative CEA levels are of limited value in predicting prognosis following curative resection for colorectal carcinoma, but serial CEA monitoring is valuable in the detection of residual or recurrent cancer.[60,61] In general, while a progressive rise indicates progressive disease, changes in tumor marker levels cannot be used to assess treatment response.[11]

Cytoreduction Surgery (CRS) and Hyperthermic Intraperitoneal Chemotherapy (HIPEC)

Rationale

Surgery is a mainstay of treatment in most cases with localized disease. In PSM, localization of the tumor within the peritoneal cavity in the absence of systemic metastasis makes regional surgical resection a logical treatment option.

Nonetheless, surgery alone cannot achieve significant survival improvement. For microscopic disease that remains even after complete cytoreduction, surgery is unavoidable. These residual tumor cells become entrapped in intraperitoneal adhesions following surgery, thereby becoming extremely difficult to eradicate by systemic chemotherapy.[63] In this context, direct and early intraperitoneal chemotherapy has emerged as a better method for exposing the residual tumor cells before adhesions encase and protect them. In addition, peritoneal surface malignancies are notoriously resistant to systemic chemotherapy, largely due to the peritoneal-plasma barrier. This barrier can be overcome by administering drugs intraperitoneally.[24,62]

However, there is a limit to the depth of penetration that intraperitoneally administered antineoplastic drugs can diffuse into the tumor. Theoretically, optimal intraperitoneal chemotherapy can penetrate through a 2.5 mm tumor nodule.[64] Hence, it is imperative to remove all gross disease to promote maximum drug penetration. Sugarbaker et al. introduced the new concept of cytoreduction surgery along with a new staging system known as the Peritoneal Cancer Index (PCI) and a scoring system to define the completeness of cytoreduction.[11,65]

Peritoneal Cancer Index

To obtain a concise and clinically relevant evaluation of the sites of PC, a scoring system of cancer extent, peritoneal cancer index (PCI), was created by Jacquet and Sugarbaker.[11] PCI is an integration of both peritoneal implant size and distribution of PSM, described in Figure 1.

The size of intraperitoneal nodules in each region is assessed using the lesion size (LS) score: LS-0 to LS-3. In scoring, the number of nodules is not scored; instead, only the size of the largest nodule is scored. An LS-0 means an absence of malignant deposits in a particular region. An LS-1 indicates that tumor nodules <0.5 cm in diameter are present. An LS-2 means that tumor nodules between 0.5 cm and 5.0 cm are present. Finally, an LS-3 means that tumor nodules >5.0 cm are present. If an organ is covered by a mat of tumor, then the region is scored as LS-3.[11]

To assess the distribution of PSM, the abdominopelvic region is divided into nine regions using two transverse planes and two sagittal planes (AR-0 to AR-8). The upper transverse plane is the lowest aspect of the costal margin; the lower transverse plane is the anterior superior iliac spine; the sagittal planes divide the abdomen into three equal sectors. The regions are numbered 0 to 8, starting at the umbilical region, and proceeding in a clockwise manner, AR-0: central, AR-1: right upper, AR-2: epigastrium, AR-3: left upper, AR-4: left flank, AR-5: left lower, AR-6: pelvis, AR-7: right lower, and AR-8: right flank. It should be noted that the small bowel is assessed as a separate entity and that the large bowel is evaluated along with the abdominal region. The small bowel is designated AR-9 to AR-12; AR-9 includes the upper jejunum, AR-10 is the lower jejunum, AR-11 is the upper ileum, and AR-12 is the lower ileum.[11]

The LS scores in each of the 13 abdominopelvic regions (AR-0 to AR-12) are determined and added. The resultant summation is the PCI. A maximum possible score is 39 (13 x 3).

There are two important points that need to be addressed. First, non-invasive tumors may be completely resectable even though extensive tumor dissemination has already occurred, accumulating a large volume of tumor cell deposits on the peritoneal surface. Examples include pseudomyxoma peritonei, grade I sarcoma, and minimally invasive peritoneal mesothelioma. Second, when tumor nodules are implanted at crucial anatomic sites, a complete cytoreduction may not be achievable. For example, if the small bowel mesentery has evidence of tumor implantation with several segmental sites of partial obstruction, there is no surgical option to remove all gross disease. The prognosis for this example is poor even if the PCI score was low.[66]

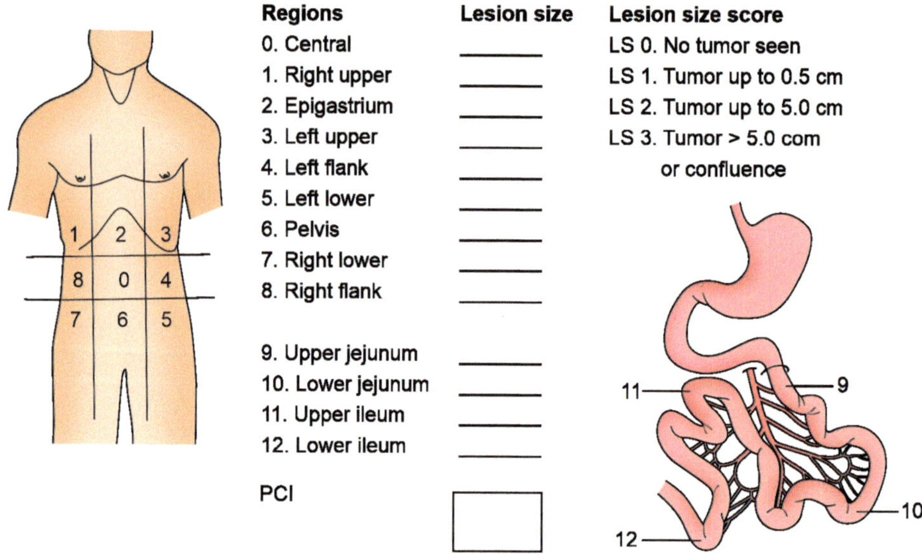

Figure 1: Peritoneal Carcinomatosis Index (PCI) staging system for peritoneal carcinomatosis

Peritoneal Surface Disease Severity Score

In an attempt to identify predictive criteria for the outcome of CRPC patients treated with CRS and HIPEC, Pelz et al. recently developed a new scoring system known as the Peritoneal Surface Disease Severity Score (PSDSS). This score incorporates three clinicopathological variables: clinical symptoms, extent of carcinomatosis, and primary tumor histopathology detailed in Table 1. Each of these categories was divided into three subcategories with specific points based on the severity: none (0 points), mild (1 point), and severe (6 points) subcategories in the 'clinical symptom' category. PCI score <10 (1 point), PCI score 10 to 20 (3 points), and PCI score >20 (7 points) subcategories in the 'extent of carcinomatosis' category. Well or moderately differentiated and N0 (1 point), moderately differentiated and N1 or N2 (3 points), and poorly differentiated or signet ring (9 points) subcategories in the 'primary tumor pathology' category. Patients were then staged according to the sum of the points: Stage I has a sum <4; Stage II has a sum of 4 to 7; Stage III has a sum of 8 to 10; Stage

IV has a sum of >10.[67] Further, an analysis on the impact of PSDSS on survival showed that PSDSS Stages I and II had better survival rates compared to Stages III and IV, thereby suggesting PSDSS may be instrumental in patient selection and a portent of outcome.[68]

Table 1: Estimated Severity of Peritoneal Surface Disease in Patients with Colorectal Cancer Peritoneal Carcinomatosis

Severity Score: Peritoneal Surface disease for Colorectal Cancer		
Clinical Symptoms	**Carcinomatosis Extent (PCI)**	**Pathology of the Primary Tumor**
None 0 points	Less than 10 1 point	Well to Moderately Differentiated Tumor (N0) 1 point
Mild 1 point	10 to 20 3 points	Moderately Differentiated Tumor (N1 or N2) 3 points
Severe 6 points	Greater than 20 7 points	Poorly Differentiated Tumor (Signet Ring) 9 points

Completeness of Cytoreduction

The goal of cytoreduction surgery is to remove all gross disease, so that only minimal microscopic residual tumor remains.[24,65] During CRS, lysis of adhesions is performed simultaneously. Macroscopic complete cytoreduction (CCR) and complete lysis of adhesions are to ensure maximal contact and penetration of chemotherapy into the residual tumor.

Pioneered and introduced by Sugarbaker, peritonectomy is necessary for CCR, and involves six peritoneal striping procedures to be performed at the initial surgery to remove all gross disease. These procedures are (1) greater omentectomy and splenectomy, (2) left upper quadrant peritonectomy, (3) right upper quadrant peritonectomy, (4) lesser omentum with cholecystectomy, (5) pelvic peritonectomy with rectosigmoid resection, and (6) partial or total gastrectomy.[21] When visceral peritoneum invasion by large tumor nodules is present, resection of a portion of the stomach, small intestine, colon, or rectum is required. Patients usually do not require all six procedures. Sugarbaker et al. reported a mean of 3.4 procedures per patient from their own experience.[65,66]

The resection status of patients after CRS is assessed using the CCR scoring system shown in Table 2. A CCR-0 indicates a patient in whom no tumor is visualized. The CCR-1 status means that tumor nodules <2.5 mm in diameter are left behind after CRS. The CCR-2 status is assigned when residual tumors are between 2.5 mm and 2.5 cm in diameter. The CCR-3 resection indicates that tumors >2.5 cm in diameter remain. Of note, patients with CCR-0 or CCR-1 are usually considered to have a complete resection.[11]

Table 2: Completeness of Cytoreduction Score

CCR Score	Amount of Tumor remaining after cytoreduction (resection)
0	There is no visible residual tumor
1	The residual tumor is < 2.5 mm
2	The residual tumor is 2.5 mm to 2.5 cm (25 mm)
3	The residual tumor is > 2.5

Variables associated with an increased chance of having a CCR include (1) ECOG performance status <2, (2) extra-abdominal disease is not evident, (3) ≤3 small, resectable parenchymal hepatic metastases, (4) biliary obstruction is not evident, (5) ureteral obstruction is not evident, (6) intestinal obstruction at more than one site is not evident, (7) gross disease in the small bowel mesentery with several segmental sites of partial obstruction is not evident, and (8) no or small volume disease in the gastro-hepatic ligament.[70]

Hyperthermic Intraperitoneal Chemotherapy

Peritonectomy is followed by intraoperative hyperthermic intraperitoneal chemotherapy (HIPEC). An intraoperative chemotherapy administered immediately after CRS has several advantages. Firstly, after aggressive cytoreduction surgery, not only are all adhesions lysed, but also all peritoneal surfaces are exposed. Moreover, there is no healing within the peritoneal cavity yet. Consequently, better drug distribution is expected when compared to a postoperative procedure. Secondly, by administering chemotherapy directly into the peritoneal cavity, it is possible to achieve higher drug levels than which can be obtained with systemic administration, thereby overcoming relative intrinsic drug resistance. Additionally, the single intraoperative dose administration eliminates the need for postoperative administration of several cycles of treatment.[10,24]

The effect of a chemotherapeutic agent depends on drug concentration and the amount of time there is drug contact with the malignant cells. Because of the peritoneal-plasma barrier, intraperitoneally administered drugs have late clearance, limiting systemic absorption.[24] The pharmacokinetic advantage of intraperitoneal perfusion can be shown by the area-under-the-curve (AUC) ratios. The AUC ratios of intraperitoneal concentration to plasma concentration indicate the amount of chemotherapy agent that is sequestered in the peritoneal cavity to how much of it is cleared into the systemic circulation. Therefore, the effective agents have high AUC ratios. For this reason, cytotoxic agents with hydrophilic properties and high molecular weights are chosen for intraperitoneal chemotherapy.[10,30] For example, mitomycin C (334 DA) has an AUC ratio of 75:1.

The rationale for hyperthermia is based on laboratory studies. The results have shown that the addition of hyperthermia (42°C to 43°C) affects cell membranes, cytoskeletons, synthesis of macromolecules, and DNA repair mechanisms.[72,73] In other words, heat itself is toxic to cancerous tissue. More importantly, hyperthermia results in synergy with certain cytotoxic drugs.[24] For instance, the synergy between Mitomycin C and hyperthermia occurs independent of the cell cycle, allowing for major anti-neoplastic activity with brief exposures.[24,74] Furthermore, hyperthermia increases the drug penetration into tissue.

One important drawback is that the cytotoxic effect of hyperthermia can happen at temperatures that will irreversibly damage normal cells. This obstacle has been shown to be technically feasible.[75] Near the completion of CRS, patients are passively cooled to a core temperature of approximately 34°C to 35°C. The chemotherapy is then instilled in a large volume of fluid. This ensures wide drug distribution and provides sufficient dilution.[10]

There are two different technologies for hyperthermic intraperitoneal chemotherapy, which are (1) the closed abdomen technique and (2) the open abdomen manually distributed technique. Both techniques have pros and cons. The advantages for an open technique include (1) it allows continued cytoreduction, (2) uniform distribution of heat and chemotherapy solutions, (3) allows pharmacokinetic monitoring of tumor and normal tissue, and (4) when the peritonectomy procedure has incurred diaphragm perforation, seeding of the pleural space can be prevented by treatment with HIPEC. With a closed technique in which the diaphragm is closed prior to HIPEC, the pleural space cannot be treated. In addition, when using a closed technique, no surgery is possible during chemotherapy and tissue uptake of chemotherapy cannot be determined. However, a closed technique may result in increased intraabdominal pressure, which, in turn, increases chemotherapy penetration into tissue. Furthermore, there is an increasing concern over the presumed safety hazard that may occur with an open abdomen, where aerosols produced during heated chemotherapy may contaminate the operating environment.[62]

According to published data, CRS combined with HIPEC carries a morbidity rate of 20% to 50% and mortality rate of 1% to 10% in general.[76] In light of current standards for management of GI cancer, these ranges of morbidity and mortality rates may be acceptable, but can be reduced with improved patient selection, technical skills, and postoperative care.[19]

In summary, the synergistic cytotoxic effect of hyperthermia and antineoplastic agents can result in the effective eradication of residual disease up to 2.5 mm remaining in the peritoneal cavity after CCR 0-1. Therefore, the efficacy of HIPEC depends on the CCR, and optimal therapeutic benefit can be attained when HIPEC is performed immediately following CCR.

CURRENT MANAGEMENT

Patients with Disseminated Appendiceal Mucinous Tumors and the Pseudomyxoma Peritonei Syndrome

The treatment of patients with peritoneal dissemination from an appendiceal tumor is not standardized.[13] Historically, PMP was treated with serial debulking surgeries until resultant postoperative adhesions prevented additional procedures.[8,13]

The appendix is a narrow tube, so that even small tumor masses occurring in this tiny space can result in obstruction, leading to appendix perforation. This incurs tumor cell spillage into the peritoneal cavity. As a result, peritoneal seeding takes place before lymph nodes or liver metastasis. Additionally, dissemination is usually confined to the peritoneal cavity with relative sparing of the small bowel. These unique clinical features make CCR achievable in this group of patients using peritonectomy procedures. Hence, despite a great tumor burden, low-grade minimally invasive mucinous disease can be completely resected using peritonectomy procedures.

Localization of a tumor within the peritoneal cavity renders an intraperitoneal route of drug administration more effective in eradicating the residual tumor after attaining CCR, compared to systemic administration. Furthermore, the mucinous character of the implants facilitates drug penetration administered intraperitoneally. For all these reasons, PMP has been considered the classic indication for CRS and HIPEC.[7,8,77]

A favorable outcome after CRS and HIPEC treatment is highly correlated with CCR.[77] Another important prognostic factor includes pathologic characteristics.[24] Patients with low-grade mucinous appendiceal malignancies experience better clinical outcomes. Using CRS and HIPEC, Sugarbaker et al. attained 5-year survival rates of 86% with CCR in patients with DPAM, and survival rates of 50% with complete resection in patients with PMCA or PMCA-I. Therefore, low-grade histopathology is critical in selecting patients who will benefit from this treatment approach.[77]

Colorectal Peritoneal Carcinomatosis

Peritoneal dissemination is a common mode of disease progression in patients with colorectal cancer. In the past, colorectal peritoneal carcinomatosis (CRPC) was considered a form of systemic metastasis; hence, CRPC was treated with systemic chemotherapy, and surgery was offered for palliative purposes only.[19] However, CRPC is due to direct invasion of the primary cancer or intraperitoneal seeding during surgical manipulation.[20] In this context, CRPC should be regarded as a locoregional extension of disease rather than as a manifestation of systemic metastasis.

In a phase III randomized clinical trial by Verwaal et al., palliative surgery with chemotherapy (i.e., 5FU-Leucovorin) was compared to CRS and HIPEC with the same systemic chemotherapy in patients with peritoneal dissemination of colorectal cancer. This randomized trial found a doubling of survival rates for the group treated with CRS and HIPEC (22.3 months versus 12.6 months).[32,78]

In 2006, a Consensus Statement on the treatment of patients with recurrent and/or metastatic colon cancer with peritoneal involvement was presented after the first International Symposium on Regional Cancer Therapies and the subsequent Society of Surgical Oncology annual meeting. In the Consensus Statement, it was acknowledged that systemic treatment alone is no longer appropriate for patients with limited peritoneal dissemination from a primary or recurrent colon cancer.[70]

In accordance with the Consensus Statement, Esquivel et al. created a clinical pathway for the management of peritoneal surface malignancies of colorectal origin. According to the guidelines, the management should start with a rigorous diagnostic work-up to evaluate the extent of peritoneal dissemination. The recommended work-up includes a complete colonoscopy evaluation; a CT scan of the chest, abdomen, and pelvis with maximum oral and IV contrast; and a PET scan if extra-abdominal disease is suspected. If a patient has only peritoneal carcinomatosis without distant disease, CCR assessment should be followed. If a patient has other distant metastasis in addition to peritoneal carcinomatosis and is in good performance status, Esquivel et al. recommend the best systemic therapy. If it is determined that a CCR is possible, then CRS is offered. If a CCR score of 0 or 1 is achieved, then HIPEC can be performed with mitomycin C (15 to 35 mg/m^2) with a target intraperitoneal temperature of 39°C to 42°C for 60 to 120 minutes. The choice of the chemotherapeutic perfusion method (i.e., open or closed) and the use of early post-operative intraperitoneal chemotherapy (EPIC) are left to the discretion of surgeons. Additionally, for patients with intractable ascites in whom an adequate cytoreduction could not be achieved, the authors suggest surgeons to offer HIPEC for palliative purposes.[70]

There has been a recent substantial improvement in chemotherapy such as irinotecan, oxaliplatin and bevacizumab, and 5-FU alone. Since 5-FU was the dominant chemotherapeutic agent in the previous randomized trial, demonstrating an advantage to CRS and HIPEC, Barlett et al. recently evaluated the contribution of CRS and HIPEC to survival in patients receiving contemporary systemic therapy.[43] This included 5-FU and leucovorin combined with oxaliplatin or irinotecan with or without biologic agents (i.e., targeted antibody therapy utilizing Bevacizumab or Detuximab).[43] From the time of diagnosis of peritoneal disease, they reported a median survival longer with CRS and HIPEC (34.7 months versus 16.8 months). After comparing these results to Verwaal's data, Barlett et al. concluded that (1) contemporary chemotherapy is associated with prolonged survival as compared with historical controls (i.e., 5-FU) and (2) the addition of CRS and HIPEC to modern chemotherapy regimens may significantly prolong survival.[79]

Gastric Peritoneal Carcinomatosis

As discussed previously, peritoneal dissemination is a common manifestation in gastric adenocarcinoma. Hence, it was expected that most gastric PC patients may benefit from intraperitoneal therapy. However, when Yu et al. randomized 248 patients with stage II or III gastric cancer to surgical resection alone versus resection plus intraperitoneal chemotherapy, increased survival was seen only in the subset of patients with stage III cancer.[80] Other series of similar patients using intraperitoneal chemotherapy also did not show statistically significant improvements in survival, except in patients with serosal invasion by tumors.[4,81]

Recently, Yonemura et al. proposed a therapy called neoadjuvant intraperitoneal-systemic chemotherapy protocol (NIPS) for treatment of patients with peritoneal carcinomatosis from gastric cancer. In Yonemura's protocol, intraperitoneal chemotherapy and systemic chemotherapy are given simultaneously before cytoreductive surgery. This bidirectional approach is to attack PC from both sides of the peritoneum, aiming to reduce tumor burden before cytoreductive surgery. Then, after performing cytoreductive surgery and HIPEC, early postoperative intraperitoneal chemotherapy (EPIC) is also given.[4,82] With regards to the safety and efficacy of NIPS, further validation is needed.

Ovarian Peritoneal Carcinomatosis

Treatment of ovarian cancer differs depending on the stage of disease, but most ovarian cancer cases are discovered at an advanced stage. For stage III and IV ovarian cancer, the current frontline treatment consists of cytoreductive surgery followed by systemic chemotherapy combining platinum and taxens (i.e., cisplatin and paclitaxel), as ovarian cancer is usually very sensitive to chemotherapy.[83] However, owing to residual tumor cells after primary debulking surgery, disease recurrence is common within 5 years and it is often resistant to additional systemic chemotherapy.[63,84] Locoregional (lymph node) and peritoneal dissemination are the two most common recurrence patterns. In addition, the disease remains confined to the peritoneal cavity during most of its course.[46] As a result, a potential role for CRS and HIPEC for advanced primary and recurrent epithelial ovarian cancers has been suspected and investigated. A number of studies reported their experiences with treating patients with recurrent epithelial ovarian carcinoma with CRS followed by HIPEC. These studies used cisplatin at varying doses from 25 to 150 mg/m^2 and achieved morbidity rates of 0% to 17% and mortality rates of 0% to 4%, thereby showing that the CRS and HIPEC treatment regimen is feasible with acceptable toxicity.[85,86]

Peritoneal Mesothelioma

The previously reported median survival of peritoneal mesothelioma is 12 to 17 months.[87,88] Traditionally, peritoneal mesothelioma was managed with systemic chemotherapy along with palliative surgery. However, in a majority of patients with peritoneal mesothelioma, metastases to other sites do not occur and disease remains confined to the peritoneal cavity.[22,24] Hence, CRS combined with HIPEC has a strong rationale for treating peritoneal mesothelioma.

According to the reports by Sugarbaker et al., their treatment regimen for malignant peritoneal mesothelioma (MPM) includes HIPEC with cisplatin (50 mg/m^2) and doxorubicin (15 mg/m^2) given at 42°C in 1.5 L/m^2 of 1.5% dextrose peritoneal dialysis solution for 90 minutes.[22, 89] The morbidity and mortality rates of 68 diffuse MPM patients who underwent this treatment were 24% and 7% respectively.[89] In the following study, Sugarbaker et al. investigated 100 consecutive patients with peritoneal mesothelioma who underwent HIPEC treatment and reported a median survival of 50 months.[37] Additionally, previously published studies have shown that the HIPEC treatment can produce relief from ascites, a common manifestation of malignant mesothelioma, in the range of 86% to 99%.[89,90] This data suggests that peritoneal mesothelioma can be an excellent indication for CRS and HIPEC. In a study by Feldman et al., they analyzed factors associated with outcome in patients with MPM undergoing CRS and intraperitoneal chemotherapy. The factors associated with improved survival included previous debulking surgery, absence of deep tissue invasion, and maximum cytoreduction before the age of 60.[91]

Peritoneal Sarcomatosis

Rossi et al. evaluated the utility of CRS and HIPEC for the treatment of peritoneal sarcomatosis in 60 consecutive patients. In this study, the median overall survival was 34 months.[92] In a recent study by Salti et al., 13 patients with peritoneal sarcomatosis underwent CRS and HIPEC with cisplatin and doxorubicin between 2007 and 2010. During review, the authors found that CCR was an important prognostic indicator. When a score of CCR-0 was achieved, the mean disease-free survival and overall survival were 27.25+5.71 months and 35.25+4.75 months, respectively. On the other hand, when a CCR score of greater than 1 was attained, both median disease-free survival time and overall survival time were 4 months. PCI was another factor that influenced survival.[39] This published data suggests a possible benefit of CRS and HIPEC in patients with peritoneal sarcomatosis with complete CRS and low PCI.

SUMMARY

Multiple studies on the natural history of PSM uniformly report dismal prognosis with a median survival of less than a year. Patients with PSM were traditionally treated with systemic chemotherapy and surgery to treat tumor-related complications. Over the past two decades, the management of PSM has changed from palliative only to attempts for a cure. With better insight into the natural history of PSM, the combined approach of CRS and HIPEC has emerged and has demonstrated an improved survival in selected patients. CRS and HIPEC is currently the only treatment with the potential to cure these patients. However, this combined treatment is not for all patients. Unresectable disease represents a therapeutic challenge. Meanwhile, there has been impressive progress with modern systemic chemotherapy. Biological agents have been introduced and new targeted therapeutic options are being actively explored with the aim of advancing the treatment of PSM. In this regard, the addition of contemporary chemotherapy to the CRS combined with HIPEC treatment approach may lead to better oncologic and surgical results.

REFERENCES

1. Levy AD, Arnáiz F, Shaw FC, et al. Primary peritoneal tumors: imaging freatures with pathologic correlation. RadioGraphics 2008;28:583-607.
2. Oei TN, Jagannathan JP, Ramaiya N, et al. Peritoneal sarcomatosis versus peritoneal carcinomatosis: Imaging findings at MDCT. AJR 2010;195:W229-W235.
3. Pingpank JF. Diagnosis and treatment of peritoneal carcinomatosis. In: DeVita VT, Lawrence TS, Rosenberg SA, editors. Cancer: Principles and Practice of Oncology. Baltimore: Lippincott Williams & Wilkins; 2008. Pp. 2389-2400.
4. Yonemura Y, Elnemr A, Endou Y, et al. Multidisciplinary therapy for treatment of patients with peritoneal carcinomatosis from gastric cancer. World J Gastrointest Oncol 2010;15:85-97.
5. Feldman GB, Knapp RC. Lymphatic drainage of the peritoneal cavity and its significance in ovarian cancer. Am J Obstet Gynecol 1974;119:991-994.

6. Hagiwara A, Rakanhashi T, Sawai K, et al. Milky spots at the implantation site for malignant cells in peritoneal dissemination in mice. Cancer Res 1993;53:687-692.
7. Esquivel J. Cytoreductive surgery for peritoneal malignancies-development of standards of care for the community. Surg Oncol Clin N Am 2007;16:653-666.
8. Sugarbaker PH. Disseminated appendiceal mucinous tumors and the pseudomyxoma peritonei syndrome. J Gynecol Oncol 2003;8:204-211.
9. Sugarbaker PH, Yu W, Yonemura Y. Gastrectomy, peritonectomy and perioperative intraperitoneal chemotherapy: evolution of treatment strategies for advanced gastric cancer. Semin Surg Oncol 2003;21:233-248.
10. Sugarbaker PH, Cunliffe WJ, Belliveau J, et al. Rationale for integrating early postoperative intraperitoneal chemotherapy into the surgical treatment of gastrointestinal cancer. Semin Oncol 1989;16:83-97.
11. Jacquet P, Sugarbaker PH. Current methodologies for clinical assessment of patients with peritoneal carcinomatosis. J Exp Clin Cancer Res 1996;15:49-58.
12. Sugarbaker PH. Pseudomyxoma peritonei. A cancer whose biology is characterized by a redistribution phenomenon. Ann Surg 1994;219:109-111.
13. Misdraji J. Appendiceal mucinous neoplasm controversial issues. Arch Pathol Lab Med. 2010;134:864-870.
14. Ronnett BM, Zahn CM, Kurman RJ, et al. Disseminated peritoneal adenomucinosis and peritoneal mucinous carcinomatosis. A clinicopathologic analysis of 109 cases with emphasis on distinguishing pathologic features, site of origin, prognosis, and relationship to "pseudomyxoma peritonei" Am J Surg Pathol 1995; 19: 1390–408.
15. Ronnett BM, Shmookler BM, Sugarbaker PH, et al. Pseudomyxoma peritonei: new concepts in diagnosis, origin, nomenclature, and relationship to mucinous borderline (low malignant potential) tumors of the ovary. Anat Pathol 1997;2:197-226.
16. Misdraji J, Yantiss RK, Graeme-Cook FM, et al. Appendiceal mucinous neoplasms: a clinicopathologic analysis of 107 cases. Am J Surg Pathol 2003;27:1089.
17. Bradley RF, Stewart JH the 4th, Russell GB, et al. Pseudomyxoma peritonei of appendiceal origin: a clinicopathologic analysis of 101 patients uniformly treated at a single institution, with literature review. Am J Surg Pathol. 2006;30(5):551-559.
18. Ronnett BM, Yan H, Kurman RJ, et al. Patients with pseudomyxoma peritonei associated with disseminated peritoneal adenomucinosis have a significantly more favorable prognosis than patients with peritoneal mucinous carcinomatosis. Cancer 2001;92(1):85-91.
19. Yan TD, Black D, Sugarbaker PH, Zhu J, Yonemura Y, Petrou G, et al. A Systematic review and meta-analysis of the randomized controlled trials on adjuvant intraperitoneal chemotherapy for resectable gastric cancer. Ann Surg Oncol 2007;14:2702-13.
20. Glehen O, Osinsky D, Beaujard AC, et al. Natural history of peritoneal carcinomatosis from nongynecologic malignancies. Surg Oncol Clin N Am 2003;12:729-739.
21. Morita H, Aoki J, Taketomi A, et al. Serous surface papillary carcinoma of the peritoneum: clinical, radiologic, and pathologic findings in 11 patients. AJR 2004;183:923-928.
22. Sugarbaker PH, Yair IZ, Gonzalez-Moreno S, et al. Diagnosis and treatment of peritoneal mesothelioma: The Washington Cancer Institute experience. Semin Oncol 2002;29:51-61.
23. Rossi CR, Casali P, Kusamura S, et al. The consensus statement on the locoregional treatment of abdominal sarcomatosis. J Surg Oncol 2008;98:291-294.
24. Levine EA, Stewart IV JH, Russell GB, Geisinger KR, Loggie BL, Shen P. Cytoreductive surgery and intraperitoneal hyperthermic chemotherapy for peritoneal surface malignancy: Experience with 501 procedures. J Am Coll Surg 2007;204:943-53.
25. Moran BJ, Cecil TD. The etiology, clinical presentation, and management of pseudomyxoma peritonei. Surg Oncol Cin N Am 2003; 12: 585-603.
26. Siegel R, Ward E, Brawley O, et al. Cancer Statistics, 2011. Ca Cancer J Clin 2011;61:212-236.
27. Bartlett DL, Chu E. Can metastatic colorectal cancer be cured? Oncol 2012;26(3):266-275.
28. Sugarbaker PH, Graves T, deBruijn EA, et al. Rationale for early postoperative intraperitoneal chemotherapy (EPIC) in patients with advanced gastrointestinal cancer. Cancer Res 1990;50:5790-5794.
29. Chang GJ, Lambert LA. Hidden opportunities for peritoneal carcinomatosis of colorectal origin. Ann Surg Oncol 2008; 15:2993-95.
30. Yan TD, Stuart OA, Yoo D, et al. Perioperative intraperitoneal chemotherapy for peritoneal surface malignancy. J Translational Med 2006;4:17.
31. Sadeghi B, Arvieux C, Glehen O, et al. Peritoneal carcinomatosis from non-gynecologic malignancies: results of the EVOCAPE I multicentric prospective study. Cancer 2000;88:358-363.
32. Esquivel J, Nissan A, Stojadinovic A. Cytoreductive

surgery and heated intraperitoneal chemotherapy in the treatment of peritoneal carcinomatosis of colorectal origin: the need for practice altering data. J Surg Oncol 2008;98:397-8.

33. Elias D, Lefevre JH, Chevalier J, Brouquet A, Marchal F, Classe JM, et al. Complete cytoreductive surgery plus intraperitoneal chemohyperthermia with oxaliplatin for peritoneal carcinomatosis of colorectal origin. J Clin Oncol 2009:27:681-5.
34. Crew KD, Neugut AL. Epidemiology of gastric cancer. World J Gastroenterol 2006;12:354-62.
35. Look M, Chang D, Sugarbaker PH. Long-term results of cytoreductive surgery for advanced and recurrent epithelial ovarian cancers and papillary serous carcinoma of the peritoneum. Int Gynecol Cancer 2004;14:35-41.
36. Price B. Analysis of current trends in the United States mesothelioma incidence. Am J Epidemil 1997;145:211-218.
37. Sugarbaker PH, Yan TD, Stuart OA, et al. Comprehensive management of diffuse malignant peritoneal mesothelioma. J Cancer Surgery 2006;32:686-691.
38. Sondak VK, Economou JS, Eilber FR. Soft tissue sarcomas of the extremity and retroperitoneum: advances in management. Adv Surg 1991;24P:333-59.
39. Salti GI, Ailabouni L, Undevia S. Cytoreductive surgery and hyperthermic intraperitoneal chemotherapy for the treatment of peritoneal sarcomatosis. Ann Surg Oncol 2012;19:1410-1415.
40. Sugarbaker PH. cytoreductive surgery and perioperative intraperitoneal chemotherapy as a curtative approach to pseudomyxoma peritonei syndrome. Eur J Surg Oncol 2001;27:239-243.
41. Sugarbaker PH. The natural history, gross pathology and histopathology of appendiceal epithelial neoplasms. Eur J Surg Oncol 2006;32(6):644-7.
42. Teo M. Peritoneal-based malignancies and their treatment. Ann Acad Med Singapore 2010;39:54-7.
43. Kabbinavar FF, Schulz J, McCleod M, et al. Addition of bevacizumab to bolus fluorouracil and leucovorin in first-line metastatic colorectal cancer: Results of a randomized phase II trial. J Clin Oncol 2005;23:3697-3705.
44. Hammed al-Shammaa HA, Li Y, Yonemura Y. Current status and future strategies of cytoreductive surgery plus intraperitoneal hyperthermic chemotherapy for peritoneal carcinomatosis. World J Gastroenterol 2008;14:1159-66.
45. Yancik R. Ovarian cancer: age contrasts in incidence, histology, disease stage at diagnosis and mortality. Cancer 1993;71:517-523.
46. Everett EN, French AE, Stone RL, Pastore LM, Jazaeri AA, Andersen WA, et al. Initial chemotherapy followed by surgical cytoreduction for the treatment of stage III/IV epithelial ovarian cancer. Am J Obstet Gynecol 2006;195:568-76.
47. Manavoglu M, Orhan B, Evrensel T, et al. Malignant peritoneal mesothelioma following asbestos exposure. J Environ Pathol Toxicol Oncol 1996;15:191-194.
48. Sugarbaker PH, Yan TD, Stuart OA, Yoo D. Progress in management of diffuse malignant peritoneal mesotheliama. Eur J Surg Oncol 2006;32(6):686-92.
49. Oei TN, Jagannathan JP, Ramaiya N, et al. Peritoneal sarcomatosis versus peritoneal carcinomatosis: imaging findings at MDCT. AJR 2010;195:W229-W235.
50. Berther B, Sugarbaker TA, Chang D, et al. Quantitative methodologies for selection of patients with recurrent abdominopelvic sarcoma for treatment. Eur J Cancer 1999;35:413-9.
51. Stewart JH, Shen P, Levine EA. Intraperitoneal hyperthermic chemotherapy for peritoneal surface malignancy: current status and future directions. Ann Surg Oncol 2005:12:765-77.
52. H. Joensuu, M. Eriksson, J. Hatrmann, et al. Twelve versus 36 months of adjuvant imatinib (IM) as treatment of operable GIST with a high risk of recurrence: Final results of a randomized trial (SSGXVIII/AIO). J Clin Oncol 29: 2011 (suppl; abstr LBA1).
53. Esquivel J, Sugarbaker PH. Clinical presentation of the pseudomyxoma peritonei syndrome. Br J Surg 2000;87:1414-1418.
54. Mukherjee A, Moran BJ. Pseudomyxoma peritonei – symptoms, signs and clinical differential diagnosis. J Gynecol Oncol 2003;8:199-203.
55. Archer AG, Sugarbaker PH, Jelinek JS. Radiology of peritoneal carcinomatosis. Cancer Treat Res 1996;82:263-288.
56. Sugarbaker PH. Comprehensive management of peritoneal surface malignancy using cytoreductive surgery and perioperative intraperitoneal chemotherapy: the Washington Cancer Institute approach. Expert Opin Pharmacother 2009;10(12):1965-1977.
57. Jacquet P, Jelinek JS, Chang D, Koslowe P, Sugarbaker PH. Abdominal computed tomographic scan in the selection of patients with mucinous peritoneal carcinomatosis for cytoreductive surgery. J Am Coll Surg. 1995;181:530–8.
58. Kamellos I, Demetriades H, Zintzaras E, et al. Incidence

and prognostic value of positive peritoneal cytology in colorectal cancer. Dis Colon Rectum 2003;46:535-539.
59. Koprowski H, Herlyn M, Steplewski Z, et al. Specific antigen in serum of patients with colon carcinoma. Science. 1981;212:53–55.
60. Lewi H, Blumgart LH, Carter CR, et al. Pre-operative carcino-embryonic antigen and survival in patients with colorectal cancer. Br J Surg 2005;92:206-208.
61. Cooper MJ, Mackie CR, Skinner DB, et al. A reappraisal of the carcinoembryonic antigen in the management of patients with various neoplasms. Br J Surgery 2005;92:120-123.
62. Dedrick RL, Flessner MF. Pharmacokinetic problems in peritoneal drug administration: tissue penetration and surface exposure. J Natl Cancer Inst 1997;89:480-7.
63. Stewart JH, Shen P, Levine EA. Intraperitoneal hyperthermic chemotherapy for peritoneal surface malignancy: current status and future directions. Ann Surg Oncol 2005:12:765-77.
64. Los G, McVie JG. Experimental and clinical status of intraperitoneal chemotherapy. Eur J Cancer 1990;26:755-762.
65. Sugarbaker PH. Peritonectomy procedures. Annals of Surgery 1995;221(1):29-42.
66. Sugarbaker PH. Review of a personal experience in the management of carcinomatosis and sarcomatosis. Jpn J Clin Oncol 2001;31:573-583.
67. Pelz JO, Stojadinovic A, Nissan A, et al. Evaluation of a peritoneal surface disease severity score in patients with colon cancer with peritoneal calcinomatosis. Journal of Surgical Oncology 2009;99:9-15.
68. Chua TC, Morris DL, Esquivel J. Impact of the Peritoneal Surface Disease Severity score on survival in patients with colorectal cancer peritoneal carcinomatosis undergoing a complete cytoreduction and hyperthermic intraperitoneal chemotherapy. Annals of Surgical Oncology 2010;17(5):1330-6.
69. Sugarbaker PH. Management of peritoneal surface malignancy: a short history. Cancer Res 2007;169:1-9.
70. Esquivel J, Sticca R, Sugarbaker P, et al. Cytoreductive surgery and hyperthermic intraperitoneal chemotherapy in the management of peritoneal surface malignancies of colonic origin: a consensus statement. Annals of Surgical Oncology 2007;14(1):128-133.
71. Sugarbaker PH, Cunliffe WJ, Belliveau J, et al. Rationale for integrating early postoperative intraperitoneal chemotherapy into the surgical treatment of gastrointestinal cancer. Semin Oncol 1989;16:83-97.
72. Los G, Sminia P, Wondergem J, et al. Optimization of intraperitoenal cisplatin therapy with regional hyperthermia in rats. Eur J Cancer 1991;27:472-477.
73. Dikomey E, Franzke J. Effect of heat on induction and repair of DNA strand breaks in X-rated CHO cells. Int J Radiat Biol 1992;61:221-233.
74. Van Ruth S, Verwaal VJ, Zoetmulder FAN. Pharmacokinetics of intraperitoneal mitomycin C. Surg Oncol Clin N Am 2003;12:771-780.
75. Spratt JS, Adcock RA, Muskovin M, et al. Clinical delivery system for intraperitoneal hyperthermic chemotherapy. Cancer Res 1980;40:256-60.
76. Stephens AD, Alderman R, Chang D, et al. Morbidity and mortality of 200 treatments with cytoreductive surgery and hyperthermic intraoperative intraperitoneal chemotherapy using the Coliseum technique. Ann Surg Oncol 1999;6(8):790-6.
77. Sugarbaker PH, Chang D. Results of treatment of 385 patients with peritoneal surface spread of appendiceal malignancy. Ann Surg Oncol 1999;727-31.
78. Verwall VJ, Ruth SV, Bree ED. Randomized trial of cytoreduction and hyperthermic intraperitoneal chemotherapy versus systemic chemotherapy and palliative surgery in patients with peritoneal carcinomatosis of colorectal cancer. J Clin Oncol 2003;21:3737-3743.
79. Franko J, Ibrahim Z, Gusani NJ, et al. Cytoreductive surgery and hyperthermic intraperitoneal chemoperfusion versus systemic chemotherapy alone for colorectal peritoneal carcinomatosis. Cancer 2010;116:3756-62.
80. Yu W, Whang I, Young C, et al. Indications for early postoperative intraperitoneal chemotherapy of advanced gastric cancer: results of a prospective randomized trial. World J Surg 2001;25(8):985-90.
81. Sugarbaker PH, Yonemura Y. Clinical pathway for the management of resectable gastric cancer with peritoneal seeding: best palliation with a ray of hope for cure. Oncology 2000;58:96-107.
82. Yonemura Y, Endou Y, Shinbo M, et al. Safety and efficacy of bidirectional chemotherapy for treatment of patients with peritoneal dissemination from gastric cancer: selection for cytoreductive surgery. J Surg Oncol 2009;100:311-316.
83. McGuire WP, Hoskins WJ, Brady MF, et al. Cyclophosphamide and displatin compared with paclitaxel and cisplatin in patients with stage III and stage IV ovarian cancer. N Engl J Med 1996;334:1-6.
84. Ozols RF, Bundy BN, Greer BE, et al. Gynecologic oncology group. Phase III trial of carboplatin and

paclitaxel compared with cisplatin and paclitaxel in patients with optimally resected stage III ovarian cancer. J Clin Oncol 2003;21:3194-200.

85. Deraco M, Rossi CR, Pennacchioli E, et al. Cytoreductive surgery followed by intraperitoneal hyperthermic perfusion in the treatment of recurrent epithelial ovarian cancer: a phase II clinical study. Tumori 2001;87:120-126.
86. Van der Vange N, van Goethem AR, Zoetmulder FA, et al. Extensive cytoreductive surgery combined with intraoperative perfusion with cisplatin under hyperthermic conditions in patients with recurrent ovarian cancer: a feasibility pilot. Eur J Surg Oncol 2000;26:663-668.
87. Chan PS, Balfour TW, Bourke JB, et al. Peritoneal mesothelioma. Br J Surg 1975;62:576-80.
88. Brenner J, Sordillo PP, Magill GB, et al. Malignant peritoneal mesothelioma: review of 25 patients. Am J Gastroenterol 1981;75:311-3.
89. Sugarbaker PH, Welch LS, Mohamed F, et al. A review of peritoneal mesothelioma at the Washington Cancer Institute. Surg Oncol Clin N Am 2003;12:605-621.
90. Loggie BW, Fleming RA, McQuellon RP, et al. Prospective trial for the treatment of malignant peritoneal mesothelioma. Am Surg 2001;67:999-1003.
91. Feldman AL, Libutti SK, Pingpank JF, et al. Analysis of factors associate outcome in patients with malignant peritoneal mesothelioma undergoing surgical debulking and intraperitoneal chemotherapy. J Clin Oncol 2003;21:4560-7.
92. Rossi CR, Deraco M, De Simone M, et al. Hyperthermic intraoperative chemotherapy after cytoreductive surgery for the treatment of abdominal sarcomatosis: clinical outcome and prognostic factors in 60 consecutive patients. Cancer 2004;100:1943-50.

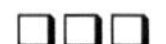

58

CHAPTER

Chemotherapy Agents

Peter Kurniali MD
Anas Al-Janadi MD

HISTORY

One of the first applications of modern chemotherapy was the use of nitrogen mustard. During World War I, when the chemical warfare agent, mustard gas, was employed, it was incidentally found to be a potent suppressor of hematopoiesis. The cytotoxic effects of nitrogen mustards were studied and used in 1942 to treat several patients with advanced lymphomas and showed significant temporary improvement of the disease. It was learnt that this agent which damaged the rapidly growing white blood cells might be a potential anti-neoplastic agent.[1,2] This discovery was followed by the development of other agents such as chlorambucil, cyclophosphamide, procarbazine, vinblastine, and vincristine.[2,3] At that time, most of these drugs were used as a single agent. In 1967, Dr. DeVita et al. introduced combination chemotherapy, with four drug combinations, as a treatment for Hodgkin lymphoma. In his original study, the combination use of nitrogen mustard, oncovin (vincristine), procarbazine, and prednisone (later known as the MOPP regimen), was found to have more efficacy against Hodgkin lymphoma compared to the use of a single agent, without a significant increase in toxicities. To date, multiple newer antineoplastic agents have successfully changed the course of some cancers into chronic diseases. However, the journey to fight cancer continues. Some people contrast classic cytotoxic chemotherapy with other newer agents such as targeted therapy, and immunotherapy; the latter is often referred to as a biologic agent. The introduction of these biological therapies has marked the start of the personalized cancer therapy era.

Types of Antineoplastic Agents

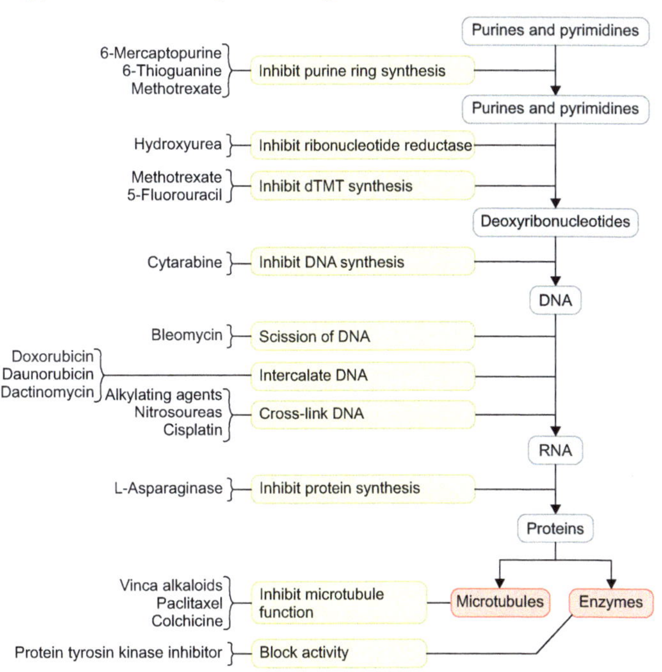

Alkylating Agents

General Information

The first antineoplastic molecules developed were alkylating agents. Through interacting with the DNA, alkylating agents inhibit DNA replication and cell division, thus producing their characteristic cytotoxic effects.[4,5] Furthermore, alkylating agents are effective regardless of the cell cycle stage. The pharmacokinetics of these molecules depends on the individual agent and is highly variable across the class. However, they share the common features of a high reactivity and a short half-life.

Use and Class

Alkylating agents are used to treat leukemia, lymphoma, Hodgkin disease, multiple myeloma, sarcoma, as well as lung, breast, and ovarian cancers. The family contains several major classes: nitrogen mustards (such as mechlorethamine or nitrogen mustard, chlorambucil, cyclophosphamide, ifosfamide, and melphalan), aziridines sulfonates (such as thiotepa and altretamine), alkyl sulfonates (such as busulfan), nitrosoureas (such as streptozocin, carmustine, and lomustine), and triazine compounds (such as dacarbazine and temozolomide).

Side Effects and Toxicities

Because these drugs damage DNA, a vast majority of alkylating agents lead to dose-limiting toxicities affecting hematopoietic cells in the bone marrow, causing pancytopenia.[5] Myeloid growth factors, such as granulocyte colony-stimulating factor (G-CSF), which stimulate the differentiation and proliferation of hematopoietic precursors can be used following treatment with most of the agents, as indicated, to enhance bone marrow recovery.[6,7] In rare cases, treatment with alkylating agents can precipitate myelodysplastic syndrome and acute leukemia. The risk of leukemia after receiving an alkylating agent is dependent on dose and is highest approximately 5 to 10 years after treatment.[7,8]

Platinum Analogs

General Information

The first platinum antineoplastic compound was discovered in the 1970s at Michigan State University. While examining the relationship between an exogenous electrical current and bacterial growth, Rosenberg and colleagues observed growth inhibition by a platinum complex of ammonia and chloride. They later found these compounds possess anti-tumor capabilities against murine tumors in vivo.[9,10] Platinum-based antineoplastic agents inhibit DNA repair and/or DNA synthesis in cancer cells through the crosslinking of DNA as a monoadduct, interstrand crosslinks, intrastrand crosslinks, or DNA protein crosslinks.[11,12] These agents are sometimes described as "alkylating-like" due to similar effects as alkylating antineoplastic agent by forming strong chemical bonds with thiol sulfurs and amino nitrogens in proteins and nucleic acids, although they do not have an alkyl group.[5]

Use and Class

Either by itself or along with other drugs, cisplatin, carboplatin, and oxaliplatin are the current staples for the systemic therapy for lung cancer, gastrointestinal malignancies, gynecologic malignancies, breast cancer, non-Hodgkin lymphoma, and genitourinary malignancies.

Side Effects

Renal toxicity is the most severe and usually dose-limiting toxicity of cisplatin. Kidney function must be monitored during the treatment course with this agent. Increasing the volume of fluid intake with forced diuresis can abate the incidence and severity of the renal toxicity.[13-15] Ototoxicity and gastrointestinal toxicity are also a known side effect of Cisplatin.[15,16] Dopamine antagonist, metoclopramide, and steroids have been used prior to and during cisplatin administration to help control the nausea and vomiting.[17,18] The primary toxicity of carboplatin is hematopoietic suppression.[19] Platinum-based chemotherapies, particularly oxaliplatin, also produce neurotoxicity as a side effect, which is usually the main dose-limiting toxicity. Many patients treated with oxaliplatin develop persistent peripheral neuropathy that may be alleviated by avoiding cold environments.[20,21]

Antimetabolites

General Information

Antimetabolites exert their antineoplastic effects by interfering with DNA and RNA growth by replacing the physiologic precursors of RNA and DNA. This class of drug damages cells specifically during the S phase and works as cytostatics.[22] This class of drugs target several metabolic pathways. Two major subcategories of this class are folate antagonists and nucleoside analogues. Folate antagonists function via multiple mechanisms. They compete with folates for cellular entry, inhibit the synthesis of folate coenzymes, and prevent chemical reactions mediated by said folate coenzymes.[23] Nucleoside analogues (including purine and pyrimidine analogs) function by outcompeting nucleosides in one or more normal cell pathways because of their chemical similarity to endogenous reactants.[22]

Use and Class

Folate Antagonist

In 1947, Aminopterin (AMT) was the first antimetabolite to show clinical efficacy treating children with acute leukemia.[24] In the early 1950s, because the toxicity caused by AMT was greater and less predictable, Methotrexate (MTX), a dihydrofolate reductase inhibitor, replaced the use of AMT. MTX remains to be one of the most commonly used antineoplastic agents.[25] The latest generation of folate antagonists is a multi-targeted folate antagonist, Pemutrexed, which was FDA approved in 2004.[26]

Nucleoside Analogues

Pyrimidine analogs include 5-fluorouracil (5-FU), cytarabine, 5-azacytidine, gemcitabine, and capecitabine (an oral 5-FU prodrug). Purine analogs include 6-mercaptopurine (6-MP), fludarabine, cladribine, hydroxyurea, and clofarabine, which is a newer generation purine nucleoside. They are frequently employed as a therapeutic for leukemias, as well as breast, ovary, lung, and gastrointestinal tract malignancies.

Side Effects and Toxicities

Like most other anti-metabolites, this class of drugs causes toxicity to cells that are rapidly dividing. Accordingly, myelosuppression and mucositis are common side effects, but they are generally reversible upon cessation of chemotherapy. The treatment can begin again once levels have returned to baseline.[22,27] Folate antagonists are generally teratogenic and have been shown to cause spontaneous abortions in animal studies.[28]

Antitumor Antibiotics

General Information

The anti-tumor antibiotics are a diverse class of antineoplastic therapeutics that all originate as products of fermentation from microbial cultures.[29] The mechanism of action of this class is the interference of enzymes involved in DNA replication, which prevents DNA synthesis and DNA-dependent RNA synthesis.[29] This class of drugs works in all cell cycles.

Use and Class

Anthracyclines are the most widely used agents in this class and include daunorubicin, doxorubicin, epirubicin, and idarubicin. Other non-anthracycline antitumor antibiotics comprise of actinomycin-D, bleomycin, mitomycin-C, and mitoxantrone. Mitoxantrone, an antitumor antibiotic that shares many similarities with doxorubicin, is also a topoisomerase II inhibitor (see separate section below) and can cause treatment-related leukemia. Anthracyclines are indicated to treat prostate cancer, breast cancer, gastrointestinal cancer, testicular cancer, gynecological cancer, sarcoma, lymphoma, and leukemia.

Side Effects and Toxicities

Cardiac toxicities are the main dose limiting toxicities for anthracyclines, especially doxorubicin and daunorubicin by which toxicities are usually observed with doses greater than 300 mg/m^2. It is important for patients to get a proper measurement of cardiac function prior to administration of this drug.[30,31] Bleomycin can also cause cumulative dose-related interstitial pulmonary disease, which may be progressive and fatal.[32] Another main toxicity includes myelosuppression.[29]

Topoisomerase Inhibitors

General Information

DNA topoisomerases are enzymes that regulate the geometry of the DNA double helix during DNA replication or RNA transcription.[33] Topoisomerase inhibitors interfere with this process by inhibiting either topoisomerase I or II.[34] Topoisomerase I jumpstarts the cleavage of a single strand of DNA, whereas topoisomerase II cleaves both DNA strands. These processes help double-helical DNA to be separated, which is a process required for DNA replication, transcription, and recombination. Inhibiting this DNA replication mechanism in any manner causes an accumulation of stable, cleavable complexes, which build up to toxic levels, and thus resulting in cell death.[33-35]

Use and Class

Topoisomerase inhibitors are categorized according to the types of enzymes they inhibit. Topoisomerase I inhibitors include irinotecan, topotecan, and camptothecin which target type IB topoisomerases. Examples of topoisomerase II inhibitors include etoposide (VP-16), doxorubicin, daunorubicin, and mitoxantrone. They are commonly used as a therapeutic for certain leukemias, lung, ovarian, and gastrointestinal malignancies.

Side Effects and Toxicities

The main toxicities of irinotecan are acute cholinergic-like syndrome, delayed onset diarrhea, nausea, and vomiting. These symptoms can be overcome by giving pre-medications including anti-emetic and atropine.[36] Other common side effects of this class include alopecia and myelosuppression, especially in topotecan. A side effect of topoisomerase II inhibitors is the increased risk for acute myelogenous leukemia (AML), which can arise as soon as 2-3 years after initiating the drug.[37]

Mitotic Inhibitors

General Information

Microtubules are created by the polymerization of alpha and beta tubulin, are formed during physiologic cell functions, and are disassembled when the cell has no further need for them. Therefore, microtubules are crucial players in the process of cell division, directional transport of vesicles and organelles, signaling, cell shape, and polarity. An antimicrotubule agent or mitotic inhibitor interferes with the polymerization and depolymerization of tubulin monomers into microtubule polymers causing irregular spindle formation, chromosome misalignment, and the induction of a prolonged mitotic arrest which leads to mitotic cell death.[38,39] Drugs targeted at microtubules, damage the cell at any point in the cell cycle, but specifically exert their effects during the M phase.

Use and Class

Taxanes (paclitaxel and docetaxel), epothilones (ixabepilone), and vinca alkaloids (vinblastine, vincristine, vinorelbine, and estramustine) are all examples of mitotic inhibitors. They are widely utilized for a variety of cancers, mainly breast, lung, and genitourinary malignancies, as well as myelomas, lymphomas, and leukemias. Other antineoplastic agents that are also categorized into this group are anthracyclines, which are antitumor antibiotics that also interfere with enzymes involved in DNA replication (see section on antitumor antibiotics above).

Side effects and Toxicities

Taxanes and vinca alkaloids can cause significant peripheral nerve damage, which can be a dose-limiting side effect.[40-42] These drugs can also cause myelosuppression.[43]

Corticosteroids

Steroids are natural hormones and hormone-like drugs. They are commonly used prior to chemotherapy for pre-medication to reduce the likelihood of allergic reactions and vomiting. Corticosteroids have been shown to be efficacious in lymphoma and multiple myeloma, and they are a part of most treatment regimens. Furthermore, corticosteroids can function as *antiemetics*, and they are frequently used to help prevent the nausea and vomiting caused by chemotherapy. If used prior to chemotherapy, corticosteroids also prevent severe hypersensitivity reactions. Examples of steroids include prednisone, methylprednisolone, and dexamethasone.

Targeted Therapies

General Information

Targeted therapies are a form of cancer medications that are directed against cancer-specific molecules and signaling pathways and have a high specificity toward tumor cells. Because targeted therapy can effectively discriminate between rapidly dividing healthy cells such as differentiating between gastrointestinal tract cells and cancerous cells, they provide a broader therapeutic window with more limited, nonspecific toxicities compared to conventional chemotherapies. The two primary forms of targeted therapy include monoclonal antibodies and small molecule inhibitors.[44] One of the earliest targeted therapies are monoclonal antibodies, which target specific cell surface markers displayed on lymphoma and leukemia cells, cluster of differentiation (CD20, CD33, and CD52). The anticancer mechanisms behind monoclonal antibodies are diverse and varied. They recruit host immunologic pathways (i.e., natural killer cells and the complement cascade) to activate against the target cell and bind to ligands or receptors, thereby disrupting necessary tumor cell functions and carrying radioisotope or toxins to the target cell (i.e., conjugated monoclonal antibodies).[44,45] Small molecule inhibitors, on the other hand, usually interfere with cellular processes by disrupting the intracellular signaling of tyrosine kinases such as EGFR, HER2/neu, and VEGF receptors. Tyrosine kinases are a prime target because of their important role in the regulation of growth factor signaling in normal and malignant tissues and are a common mechanism of tumor genesis.[44]

Use and Class

FDA approved monoclonal antibodies include rituximab, bevacizumab, cetuximab, panitumumab, trastuzumab, and alemtuzumab. There are several types of small molecule inhibitors of tyrosine kinases including tyrosine kinase inhibitors (TKI) which inhibit the nonreceptor tyrosine kinases BCR-ABL and KIT (imatinib, dasatinib), receptor TKI which are directed at epidermal growth factor receptor (EGFR) (ErbB/HER) and related receptors (gefitinib, erlotinib, lapatinib), vascular endothelial growth factor receptors (VEGFR) (sunitinib, sorafenib), and platelet-derived growth factor receptors (PDGFR) (leflunomide).

Side Effects and Toxicities

For EGFR inhibitors (e.g. cetuximab and erlotinib), the most common observed dose-dependent side effect is folliculitis, also commonly known as an acneiform eruption or an acne-like rash, which can take place in the majority of patients.[46,47] Diarrhea is an additional dose-limiting toxicity (DLT) for most small molecule EGFR TKIs.[48] Transtuzumab can cause cardiomyopathy characterized by a lowering of left ventricular ejection fraction.[49] Hypertension and venous thromboembolism are the most significant adverse events of anti-VEGF bevacizumab.[50,51] Most anti-angiogenesis agents may also impair wound healing and should be held prior to major surgical procedures and chronic wounds.[52] Multi-targeted kinase inhibitors, sorafenib and sunitinib, may cause hand-foot skin toxicities.[51]

Immunotherapy

General Information

Improved understanding of the underlying principles of tumor biology and immunology have brought immunotherapy into the next level of modern cancer treatment. The primary principle of cancer immunotherapy is inducing the inherent immune system to target the pathogenic malignant tumor cells. Because these drugs are characterized by a distinct mechanism of treatment, they are often classified separately from chemotherapy.[53]

Use and Class

Immunotherapy agents used to treat cancer include interferons (interferon-alpha) and other cytokines (interleukin-2), immunomodulating drugs such as thalidomide and lenalidomide (Revlimid®), T-cell therapy, and vaccine therapies such as BCG and Provenge®. Monoclonal antibodies are often categorized as immunotherapy and used in conjunction with immunotherapy. Cancer immunotherapy has been used to treat malignant melanoma, lymphoma, renal cell carcinoma, leukemia, and prostate cancer.[53,54]

Side Effects and Toxicities

In general, immunotherapy agents can cause hypersensitivity reactions. Interleukin-2 may cause capillary leak syndrome.[55] Interferon therapy is known to cause flu-like symptoms.[56]

Hormonal Therapy

General Information

The principle of hormonal therapy in cancer treatment is the manipulation of the endocrine system through the administration of specific exogenous hormones that negatively affect cancer growth by inhibiting hormone synthesis, acting as an antagonist to the hormone receptor, or acting as a hormone supplementation. Inhibitors of hormone synthesis such as aromatase inhibitors and gonadotropin-releasing hormone (GnRH) analogs also known as luteinizing hormone-releasing hormone (LHRH) agonists, work by inhibiting the production of hormones that promote cancer growth.[57-59] Hormone receptor antagonists such as selective estrogen receptor modulators (SERM's) and anti-androgens, competitively bind to the hormone receptor and prevent its activation which will decrease its production.[60] Some hormonal therapies are actually hormone supplements that may inhibit tumor growth or may function like hormone antagonists by providing negative feedback for the production of other hormones. Hormone supplementations include estrogen, progesterone, androgens, and somatostatin analogs.

Use and Class

They are used to slow the growth of cancers that are derived from hormonal responsive tissues such as breast, prostate, and endometrial (uterine) cancers which normally grow in response to natural hormones in the body. Examples include anti-estrogens (i.e., fulvestrant, tamoxifen, and toremifene), aromatase inhibitors (i.e., anastrozole, exemestane, and letrozole), anti-androgens (i.e., bicalutamide, flutamide, and nilutamide), GnRH or LHRH analogs (i.e., leuprolide and goserelin), and somatostatin analogs (i.e., octreotide).

Side Effects and Toxicities

Aromatase inhibitors and anti-estrogen therapy may increase the risk of osteoporosis. For this reason, bisphosphonates are often prescribed in conjunction with these treatments.[59,61,62] GnRH or LHRH analogs and anti-androgens may cause osteoporosis, hot flashes, gynecomastia, and reduce sexual interest.[57,63] Somatostatin analogs may cause cholelithiasis; therefore, patients treated with this agent require a routine abdominal ultrasound.[64]

Adjuvant and Neoadjuvant Therapy for Cancers

Adjuvant therapy, also referred to as adjuvant care, is any additional treatment other than the primary, main, or initial treatment to eliminate undetected cancer cells after surgical removal of the tumor. The principle of adjuvant therapy arises from the nature of cancer cells to micro metastasize to lymph nodes and further locations despite the resection of the tumor, leading to locoregional and distant recurrences.[65,66] Neoadjuvant therapy, in contrast to adjuvant therapy, is given before the main treatment to reduce the size or tumor burden prior to surgical resection.[66,67] Neoadjuvant therapy will improve local and distant control and is an organ-sparing treatment, therefore it will reduce post-surgical complications, decrease radiation therapy fields, and reduce the risk of tumor seeding due to surgical handling.[68,69] In the past, adjuvant and neoadjuvant therapies were defined as systemic therapies and were administered prior to local treatment. However, this concept has been extended to include radiation therapy before surgery.[69] Neoadjuvant therapy has been widely applied toward rectal, breast, and head and neck cancers. Multiple clinical studies are currently being conducted to identify more cancers that may benefit from this treatment. Adjuvant therapy is much more commonly used for malignancies with locally advanced disease. Several molecular markers have been used to predict the risk of recurrence and whether or not adjuvant therapy should be given, such as in the early stages of breast and colorectal cancer.

The Use of Chemotherapy in Developing Countries with Limited Resources

Many of the antineoplastic agents have been used for years and are available in generic forms. However, the rapid development and advancement of cancer therapies might be a great challenge in developing countries with limited resources. Combination therapies have been proven to improve survival; however, this may lead to increases in treatment costs. For this reason, the treatment regimens are often simplified by using cheaper agents. Using simpler or cheaper therapies, even if this means sacrificing some quality of results, can improve population health and increase survival rates through making treatment more readily available as well as potentially decreasing toxicity.[70] As discussed above, the newer targeted therapies have brought cancer treatments to a higher level. However, the cost of these agents might be unaffordable for the majority of patients in developing countries. For example, the cost of erlotinib, an FDA approved medication for non-small cell lung cancer treatment, is approximately $3,000 per month. On top of this, since several targeted therapies are proven to be more beneficial in certain conditions, additional testing is often required. Erlotinib specifically targets the epidermal growth factor receptor (EGFR) tyrosine kinase. For this reason, the ideal patient must have an EGFR mutation.[71] However, pathologic diagnostics that are used to check the status of EGFR mutations in developing countries might be logistically challenging. Oftentimes, treatment is given without checking the EGFR status. To overcome this issue, clinical research has to be intensified to identify effective and affordable treatment regimens.

Special Consideration: Stopping ongoing chemotherapy before surgical procedure?

Many cancer patients require surgical procedures while they are treated with chemotherapy. For emergent surgical procedures, the options are limited. Any scheduled chemotherapy will usually be put on hold until the acute disease is resolved. For elective or semi-urgent conditions, procedures can be arranged in between chemotherapy cycles if the patient does not have complications from the chemotherapy, such as pancytopenia. Except for the anti-angiogenesis class (see section on targeted therapy) that may impair wound healing, other classes of chemotherapy are generally tolerable with standard surgical procedures.

CAR T-Cell Therapy

General Information

Chimeric antigen receptor (CAR) T-cell therapy is part of the adoptive cell transfer (ACT), a treatment that collects, genetically modifies, then uses the patient's inherent immune cells to treat their cancer. This treatment customizes the patients' own T-lymphocytes to be directed against the cancer cell. The cells are reengineered in a laboratory and transduced with a gene that encodes a CAR.

Use and Class

The autologous T-cell that is altered to express a CAR toward CD19, has been effective in patients with refractory B-cell hematologic malignancy.[73]

In 2017, the Food Drug Administration (FDA) approved the CAR T-Cell therapy, tisagenlecleucel, a genetically modified autologous T-cell immunotherapy targeting CD19 to treat children diagnosed with acute lymphoblastic leukemia (ALL) and adults with advanced lymphoma. In 2021, brexucabtagene, a CD19 CAR T-cell therapy was also approved as a treatment for relapsed or refractory B-ALL in adults.[74,75]

Side Effects and Toxicities

The most common side effects of CAR T-cell therapy are cytokine release syndromes (CRS), neurological toxicities, and B-cell aplasia.[73] CRS is a systemic inflammatory response syndrome involving increased proinflammatory cytokines and T-cell activation expansion. After CAR T-cell inclusion, patients may present with clinical features that may include fevers, myalgias, and malaise. More serious CRS can present with capillary leak syndrome implicated with hypoxia, hypotension, and sometimes renal dysfunction and coagulopathy.[73] This syndrome can be treated with anti-cytokine therapy, corticosteroids, or tocilizumab the IL-6 receptor inhibitor. B-cell aplasia caused by CAR T-cell or other B-cell depleting therapies (such as anti-CD20 immunotherapy) can cause significant morbidities in the era of the COVID-19 pandemic due to an impaired ability of the natural antibody response to fight the COVID-19 infection.[77] Effective ramifications of B-cell aplasia can be rescinded, at least partially, through administering intravenous immuneglobulin.[73,76]

Future Use

The research and application of CAR T-cells have continued to grow in hematological malignancies. The majority of the studies conducted thus far have used CD19-targeted CAR

T-cells. Multiple studies have aimed to use CAR T-cells for solid tumors. Some of the challenges include identifying unique antigens accessible on the surface of solid tumors and assessing tumor response due to pseudoprogression.[78,79]

REFERENCES

1. Goodman LS, Wintrobe MM, Dameshek W, Goodman MJ, Gilman A, McLennan MT. Landmark article Sept. 21, 1946: Nitrogen mustard therapy. Use of methyl-bis(beta-chloroethyl) amine hydrochloride and tris(beta-chloroethyl) amine hydrochloride for Hodgkin's disease, lymphosarcoma, leukemia and certain allied and miscellaneous disorders. JAMA. 1984 May 4;251(17):2255-61.
2. Papac RJ. Origins of cancer therapy. Yale J Biol Med. 2001 Nov-Dec;74(6):391-8.
3. Burchenal JH. The historical development of cancer chemotherapy. Semin Oncol. 1977 Jun;4(2):135-46.
4. Lawley PD, Brookes P. The Action of Alkylating Agents on Deoxyribonucleic Acid in Relation to Biological Effects of the Alkylating Agents. Exp Cell Res. 1963;24:SUPPL9:512-20.
5. Colvin DM. Alkylating Agents and Platinum Antitumor Compounds. In: Bast RCJ, Kufe, D.W., Pollock, R.E., et al., editor. Holland-Frei Cancer Medicine Hamilton (ON): BC: Decker; 2000.
6. Talmadge JE, Tribble H, Pennington R, Bowersox O, Schneider MA, Castelli P, et al. Protective, restorative, and therapeutic properties of recombinant colony-stimulating factors. Blood. 1989 Jun;73(8):2093-103.
7. Brandt SJ, Peters WP, Atwater SK, Kurtzberg J, Borowitz MJ, Jones RB, et al. Effect of recombinant human granulocyte-macrophage colony-stimulating factor on hematopoietic reconstitution after high-dose chemotherapy and autologous bone marrow transplantation. N Engl J Med. 1988 Apr 7;318(14):869-76.
8. Dorr FA, Coltman CA Jr. Second cancers following antineoplastic therapy. Curr Probl Cancer. 1985 Feb;9(2):1-43.
9. Rosenberg B, VanCamp L, Trosko JE, Mansour VH. Platinum compounds: a new class of potent antitumour agents. Nature. 1969 Apr 26;222(5191):385-6.
10. Rosenberg B, Vancamp L, Krigas T. Inhibition of Cell Division in Escherichia Coli by Electrolysis Products from a Platinum Electrode. Nature. 1965 Feb 13;205:698-9.
11. Poklar N, Pilch DS, Lippard SJ, Redding EA, Dunham SU, Breslauer KJ. Influence of cisplatin intrastrand crosslinking on the conformation, thermal stability, and energetics of a 20-mer DNA duplex. Proc Natl Acad Sci U S A. 1996 Jul 23;93(15):7606-11.
12. Rudd GN, Hartley JA, Souhami RL. Persistence of cisplatin-induced DNA interstrand crosslinking in peripheral blood mononuclear cells from elderly and young individuals. Cancer Chemother Pharmacol. 1995;35(4):323-6.
13. Gottlieb JA, Drewinko B. Review of the current clinical status of platinum coordination complexes in cancer chemotherapy. Cancer Chemother Rep. 1975 May-Jun;59(3):621-8.
14. Chary KK, Higby DJ, Henderson ES, Swinerton KD. Phase I study of high-dose cis-dichlorodiammineplatinum(II) with forced diuresis. Cancer Treat Rep. 1977 May-Jun;61(3):367-70.
15. Piel IJ, Perlia CP. Phase II study of cis-dichlorodiammineplatinum(II) (NSC-119875) in combination with cyclophosphamide (NSC-26271) in the treatment of human malignancies. Cancer Chemother Rep. 1975 Sep-Oct;59(5):995-9.
16. Skinner R, Pearson AD, Amineddine HA, Mathias DB, Craft AW. Ototoxicity of cisplatinum in children and adolescents. Br J Cancer. 1990 Jun;61(6):927-31.
17. Gralla RJ, Itri LM, Pisko SE, Squillante AE, Kelsen DP, Braun DW Jr., et al. Antiemetic efficacy of high-dose metoclopramide: randomized trials with placebo and prochlorperazine in patients with chemotherapy-induced nausea and vomiting. N Engl J Med. 1981 Oct 15;305(16):905-9.
18. Aapro MS, Plezia PM, Alberts DS, Graham V, Jones SE, Surwit EA, et al. Double-blind crossover study of the antiemetic efficacy of high-dose dexamethasone versus high-dose metoclopramide. J Clin Oncol. 1984 May;2(5):466-71.
19. Schmitt A, Gladieff L, Laffont CM, Evrard A, Boyer JC, Lansiaux A, et al. Factors for hematopoietic toxicity of carboplatin: refining the targeting of carboplatin systemic exposure. J Clin Oncol. 2010 Oct 20;28(30):4568-74.
20. Kurniali PC, Luo LG, Weitberg AB. Role of calcium/magnesium infusion in oxaliplatin-based chemotherapy for colorectal cancer patients. Oncology (Williston Park). 2010 Mar;24(3):289-92.
21. Wilson RH, Lehky T, Thomas RR, Quinn MG, Floeter MK, Grem JL. Acute oxaliplatin-induced peripheral nerve hyperexcitability. J Clin Oncol. 2002 Apr 1;20(7):1767-74.
22. Kaye SB. New antimetabolites in cancer chemotherapy and their clinical impact. Br J Cancer. 1998;78 Suppl 3:1-7.

23. Fridland A. Effect of methotrexate on deoxyribonucleotide pools and DNA synthesis in human lymphocytic cells. Cancer Res. 1974 Aug;34(8):1883-8.
24. Farber S, Diamond LK. Temporary remissions in acute leukemia in children produced by folic acid antagonist, 4-aminopteroyl-glutamic acid. N Engl J Med. 1948 Jun 3;238(23):787-93.
25. Jolivet J, Cowan KH, Curt GA, Clendeninn NJ, Chabner BA. The pharmacology and clinical use of methotrexate. N Engl J Med. 1983 Nov 3;309(18):1094-104.
26. Manegold C. Pemetrexed (Alimta, MTA, multitargeted antifolate, LY231514) for malignant pleural mesothelioma. Semin Oncol. 2003 Aug;30(4 Suppl 10):32-6.
27. Pinedo HM, Zaharko DS, Bull JM, Chabner BA. The reversal of methotrexate cytotoxicity to mouse bone marrow cells by leucovorin and nucleosides. Cancer Res. 1976 Dec;36(12):4418-24.
28. Hausknecht RU. Methotrexate and misoprostol to terminate early pregnancy. N Engl J Med. 1995 Aug 31;333(9):537-40.
29. Davis HL Jr., von Hoff DD, Henney JE, Rozencweig M. The role of antitumor antibiotics in current oncologic practice. Cancer Chemother Pharmacol. 1978;1(2):83-90.
30. Chlebowski RT. Adriamycin (doxorubicin) cardiotoxicity: a review. West J Med. 1979 Nov;131(5):364-8.
31. Gharib MI, Burnett AK. Chemotherapy-induced cardiotoxicity: current practice and prospects of prophylaxis. Eur J Heart Fail. 2002 Jun;4(3):235-42.
32. Hay J, Shahzeidi S, Laurent G. Mechanisms of bleomycin-induced lung damage. Arch Toxicol. 1991;65(2):81-94.
33. Ewesuedo RB, Ratain MJ. Topoisomerase I Inhibitors. Oncologist. 1997;2(6):359-64.
34. Chen AY, Liu LF. DNA topoisomerases: essential enzymes and lethal targets. Annu Rev Pharmacol Toxicol. 1994;34:191-218.
35. Binaschi M, Zunino F, Capranico G. Mechanism of action of DNA topoisomerase inhibitors. Stem Cells. 1995 Jul;13(4):369-79.
36. Rothenberg ML. Topoisomerase I inhibitors: review and update. Ann Oncol. 1997 Sep;8(9):837-55.
37. Ezoe S. Secondary leukemia associated with the anti-cancer agent, etoposide, a topoisomerase II inhibitor. Int J Environ Res Public Health. 2012 Jul;9(7):2444-53.
38. Chan KS, Koh CG, Li HY. Mitosis-targeted anti-cancer therapies: where they stand. Cell Death Dis. 2012;3:e411.
39. Weaver BA, Cleveland DW. Decoding the links between mitosis, cancer, and chemotherapy: The mitotic checkpoint, adaptation, and cell death. Cancer Cell. 2005 Jul;8(1):7-12.
40. Cella D, Peterman A, Hudgens S, Webster K, Socinski MA. Measuring the side effects of taxane therapy in oncology: the functional assesment of cancer therapy-taxane (FACT-taxane). Cancer. 2003 Aug 15;98(4):822-31.
41. Roca E, Bruera E, Politi PM, Barugel M, Cedaro L, Carraro S, et al. Vinca alkaloid-induced cardiovascular autonomic neuropathy. Cancer Treat Rep. 1985 Feb;69(2):149-51.
42. Swain SM, Arezzo JC. Neuropathy associated with microtubule inhibitors: diagnosis, incidence, and management. Clin Adv Hematol Oncol. 2008 Jun;6(6):455-67.
43. Vaishampayan U, Parchment RE, Jasti BR, Hussain M. Taxanes: an overview of the pharmacokinetics and pharmacodynamics. Urology. 1999 Dec;54(6A Suppl):22-9.
44. Gerber DE. Targeted therapies: a new generation of cancer treatments. Am Fam Physician. 2008 Feb 1;77(3):311-9.
45. Adams GP, Weiner LM. Monoclonal antibody therapy of cancer. Nat Biotechnol. 2005 Sep;23(9):1147-57.
46. Cunningham D, Humblet Y, Siena S, Khayat D, Bleiberg H, Santoro A, et al. Cetuximab monotherapy and cetuximab plus irinotecan in irinotecan-refractory metastatic colorectal cancer. N Engl J Med. 2004 Jul 22;351(4):337-45.
47. Soulieres D, Senzer NN, Vokes EE, Hidalgo M, Agarwala SS, Siu LL. Multicenter phase II study of erlotinib, an oral epidermal growth factor receptor tyrosine kinase inhibitor, in patients with recurrent or metastatic squamous cell cancer of the head and neck. J Clin Oncol. 2004 Jan 1;22(1):77-85.
48. Widakowich C, de Castro G Jr., de Azambuja E, Dinh P, Awada A. Review: side effects of approved molecular targeted therapies in solid cancers. Oncologist. 2007 Dec;12(12):1443-55.
49. Seidman A, Hudis C, Pierri MK, Shak S, Paton V, Ashby M, et al. Cardiac dysfunction in the trastuzumab

clinical trials experience. J Clin Oncol. 2002 Mar 1;20(5):1215-21.

50. Kilickap S, Abali H, Celik I. Bevacizumab, bleeding, thrombosis, and warfarin. J Clin Oncol. 2003 Sep 15;21(18):3542; author reply 3.
51. Robert C, Soria JC, Spatz A, Le Cesne A, Malka D, Pautier P, et al. Cutaneous side-effects of kinase inhibitors and blocking antibodies. Lancet Oncol. 2005 Jul;6(7):491-500.
52. Saltz LB, Douillard JY, Pirotta N, Alakl M, Gruia G, Awad L, et al. Irinotecan plus fluorouracil/leucovorin for metastatic colorectal cancer: a new survival standard. Oncologist. 2001;6(1):81-91.
53. Kirkwood JM, Butterfield LH, Tarhini AA, Zarour H, Kalinski P, Ferrone S. Immunotherapy of cancer in 2012. CA Cancer J Clin. 2012 Sep-Oct;62(5):309-35.
54. Weiner LM. Cancer immunotherapy--the endgame begins. N Engl J Med. 2008 Jun 19;358(25):2664-5.
55. Siegel JP, Puri RK. Interleukin-2 toxicity. J Clin Oncol. 1991 Apr;9(4):694-704.
56. Jonasch E, Haluska FG. Interferon in oncological practice: review of interferon biology, clinical applications, and toxicities. Oncologist. 2001;6(1):34-55.
57. Brawer MK. Hormonal therapy for prostate cancer. Rev Urol. 2006;8 Suppl 2:S35-47.
58. Simpson ER. Sources of estrogen and their importance. J Steroid Biochem Mol Biol. 2003 Sep;86(3-5):225-30.
59. Mokbel K. The evolving role of aromatase inhibitors in breast cancer. Int J Clin Oncol. 2002 Oct;7(5):279-83.
60. Osborne CK, Zhao H, Fuqua SA. Selective estrogen receptor modulators: structure, function, and clinical use. J Clin Oncol. 2000 Sep;18(17):3172-86.
61. Mouridsen HT, Lonning P, Beckmann MW, Blackwell K, Doughty J, Gligorov J, et al. Use of aromatase inhibitors and bisphosphonates as an anticancer therapy in postmenopausal breast cancer. Expert Rev Anticancer Ther. 2010 Nov;10(11):1825-36.
62. Delmas PD, Balena R, Confravreux E, Hardouin C, Hardy P, Bremond A. Bisphosphonate risedronate prevents bone loss in women with artificial menopause due to chemotherapy of breast cancer: a double-blind, placebo-controlled study. J Clin Oncol. 1997 Mar;15(3):955-62.
63. Smith JA Jr. Management of hot flushes due to endocrine therapy for prostate carcinoma. Oncology (Williston Park). 1996 Sep;10(9):1319-22; discussion 24.
64. Redfern JS, Fortuner WJ the 2nd. Octreotide-associated biliary tract dysfunction and gallstone formation: pathophysiology and management. Am J Gastroenterol. 1995 Jul;90(7):1042-52.
65. Moser L, Ritz JP, Hinkelbein W, Hocht S. Adjuvant and neoadjuvant chemoradiation or radiotherapy in rectal cancer--a review focusing on open questions. Int J Colorectal Dis. 2008 Mar;23(3):227-36.
66. Ringborg U. Adjuvant chemotherapy. A discussion of some basic principles. Acta Oncol. 1991;30(2):251-3.
67. Goldie JH. Scientific basis for adjuvant and primary (neoadjuvant) chemotherapy. Semin Oncol. 1987 Mar;14(1):1-7.
68. Tonelli F, Asteria CR, Marcucci T. The rational principles of neo-adjuvant therapy for rectal cancer. Acta Biomed. 2003;74 Suppl 2:96-102.
69. Trimble EL, Ungerleider RS, Abrams JA, Kaplan RS, Feigal EG, Smith MA, et al. Neoadjuvant therapy in cancer treatment. Cancer. 1993 Dec 1;72(11 Suppl):3515-24.
70. Magrath I. Chemotherapy in developing countries--is less better? Eur J Cancer. 2003 Jul;39(11):1497-500.
71. Rosell R, Carcereny E, Gervais R, Vergnenegre A, Massuti B, Felip E, et al. Erlotinib versus standard chemotherapy as first-line treatment for European patients with advanced EGFR mutation-positive non-small-cell lung cancer (EURTAC): a multicentre, open-label, randomised phase 3 trial. Lancet Oncol. 2012 Mar;13(3):239-46.
72. Tsao AS, Tang XM, Sabloff B, Xiao L, Shigematsu H, Roth J, et al. Clinicopathologic characteristics of the EGFR gene mutation in non-small cell lung cancer. J Thorac Oncol. 2006 Mar;1(3):231-9.
73. Park JH, CD19-targeted CAR T-cell therapeutics for hematologic malignancies: interpreting clinical outcomes to date, Blood (2016) 127 (26): 3312–3320. PMID: 27207800.
74. Mian A, Hill BT. Brexucabtagene autoleucel for the treatment of relapsed/refractory mantle cell lymphoma. Expert Opin Biol Ther. 2021 Apr;21(4):435-441. doi: 10.1080/14712598.2021.1889510. Epub 2021 Mar 11. PMID: 33566715.
75. Reagan PM, Friedberg JW. Axicabtagene ciloleucel and brexucabtagene autoleucel in relapsed and refractory diffuse large B-cell and mantle cell lymphomas. Future Oncol. 2021 Apr;17(11):1269-1283. doi: 10.2217/fon-2020-0291. Epub 2021 Jan 15. PMID: 33448873.

76. Porter DL, Hwang WT, Frey NV. Chimeric antigen receptor T cells persist and induce sustained remissions in relapsed refractory chronic lymphocytic leukemia. Sci Transl Med. 2015 Sep 2;7(303):303ra139. doi: 10.1126/scitranslmed.aac5415. PMID: 26333935; PMCID: PMC5909068.
77. Hueso T, Pouderoux C, Péré H, Beaumont AL, Convalescent plasma therapy for B-cell-depleted patients with protracted COVID-19. Blood. 2020 Nov 12;136(20):2290-2295. doi: 10.1182/blood.2020008423. PMID: 32959052; PMCID: PMC7702482.
78. Salter AI, Pont MJ, Riddell SR. Chimeric antigen receptor-modified T cells: CD19 and the road beyond. Blood. 2018 Jun 14;131(24):2621-2629. doi: 10.1182/blood-2018-01-785840. Epub 2018 May 4. PMID: 29728402; PMCID: PMC6032892.
79. Chai LF, Prince E, Pillarisetty VG, Katz SC. Challenges in assessing solid tumor responses to immunotherapy. Cancer Gene Ther. 2020 Aug;27(7-8):528-538. doi: 10.1038/s41417-019-0155-1. Epub 2019 Dec 11. PMID: 31822814.

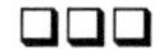

SECTION 7: CARDIOTHORACIC AND TRANSPLANT

59 CHAPTER

Chest Wall, Pleura, and Mediastinum

Wickii T. Vigneswaran, MD, FACS, FCCP

CHEST WALL DEFORMITIES AND TUMORS

The most common chest wall deformities are Pectus Excavatum, Pectus Carinatum, and Scoliosis. Other deformities are cleft sternum, and deformities associated with Poland Syndrome. The pectus deformities are most commonly encountered by thoracic surgeons in their practice.

Pectus Deformities

Surgical intervention of pectus deformities is for cosmetic reasons and to prevent cardiopulmonary compromise or postural abnormalities. Generally, the timing of the operation is pre-pubertal unless there is concern for cardiopulmonary compromise. The classic open procedure, was described by Ravitch. Increasingly, the minimally invasive procedure described by Nuss is being performed, often assisted by the video thoracoscopic technique.

Early complications associated with the Nuss procedure are pneumothorax (60%) with only a small percentage requiring chest tube (4%), Horner's syndrome (17%), and drug reactions (4%). Late complications are bar displacement (6%), infection (1%), over correction (3%), and bar allergy (3%).[1]

However, a recent meta-analysis comparing the Nuss and Ravitch procedures shows no difference in patient satisfaction, complications, or hospital length-of-stay. Re-operation, pneumothorax, and hemothorax occur more frequently with the Nuss procedure; however, the duration of surgery is longer for the Ravitch procedure.[2]

Chest Wall Tumors

Primary chest wall tumors are uncommon. Patients present with pain or swelling, generally over a long period since these tumors are slow growing. The age of the patient can provide diagnostic clues; Osteogenic and Ewing's sarcomas are common in younger age groups, while plasmacytomas are common in older age groups. The most common chest wall tumor is a fibrosarcoma, followed by chondrosarcomas and plasmacytomas. There are smaller numbers of Osteogenic sarcoma, Ewing's sarcoma, and rhabdomyosarcoma.

Diagnosis

On physical examination, bone and soft tissue involvement should be assessed. Radiographic studies include standard chest X-rays (CXR), CT scans, MRIs, and PET scans; these studies help evaluate the extent and nature of the tumor. Additionally, histological confirmation is imperative for management; open biopsy is the method of choice and adequate tissue must be obtained from the tumor's non-necrotic area. Core needle biopsy can also provide adequate tissue for diagnosis. If a lesion is localized and small, excision *in toto* is possible and resection with clear margins is the definitive procedure.

Benign Tumors

Superficial benign tumors can be either a lipoma, lymphangioma, or hemangioma. In contrast, when benign tumors are deep, they can be either a fibroma, neurofibroma, desmoid, or rhabdomyoma. However, benign tumors that involve bone can be either a fibrous dysplasia, chondroma, or osteochondroma. The treatment is excision with clear margins to confirm diagnosis and malignant transformation, and repair or reconstruction of the lesion as indicated.

Malignant Tumors

The soft tissue malignancies can present as a melanoma, liposarcoma, lymphangiosarcoma, malignant fibrous histiocytoma, basal cell carcinoma, rhabdomyosarcoma, or neurofibrosarcoma. When there is bone involvement, the tumors can present as a chondrosarcoma, osteogenic sarcoma, Ewing's sarcoma, or myeloma. Carcinoma of lung with local extension and metastatic tumors to the chest wall are not uncommon.

Presence or absence of metastatic disease needs to be evaluated in patients with malignant tumors. If the disease is metastatic and the patient presents with pain, consideration should be given to local radiation therapy for the relief of pain. Solitary metastasis may be considered for resection if clear margins can be obtained. Systemic chemotherapy should be considered for metastatic disease, with the choice of chemotherapy depending on the cell type. In Ewing's sarcoma, chemotherapy is often times the sole treatment, except in a few cases where salvage resection may be required. Fibrosarcoma is treated pre-operatively with chemotherapy, with or without radiation, and surgical resection. Plasmacytomas are treated with chemotherapy and surgery should be considered when unresponsive. The goal of surgical treatment is to obtain wide (4 cm) margins.

Generally, chest wall reconstruction is required if the defect is greater than 5 cm or involves 4 or more ribs. Special consideration is needed if the defect is close to the tip of the scapula to prevent trapping. Reconstruction is not required if it involves the apex of the chest or if the defect is completely covered by the scapula. If the tumor involves non-vital structures, en-bloc resection with clear margins is required.

The risk factors associated with resection include age, concomitant lung resection, and the size of the defect.[3] Complication rates range from 46 to 69%, with respiratory complications (24%) being the most common. Other complications include wound infection and cardiac arrhythmia.[4-6]

Pleura

Pleural diseases can be divided into three broad categories: pneumothorax, empyema, and malignancy.

Pneumothorax

Pneumothoraces are either due to trauma or are spontaneous in nature; the most frequent pneumothorax is iatrogenic in the hospital setting. A spontaneous pneumothorax is categorized as primary when the underlying lung is relatively normal, or secondary when the underlying lung is significantly diseased. Among the traumatic pneumothorax, iatrogenic remains the most common type.

Surgical treatment is considered when the pneumothorax is recurrent. Such treatment should also be considered in patients having their first pneumothorax, if there is concern for continued air leak, or when the occupation or hobbies of the patient would render them vulnerable due to lack of immediate medical help. The surgical procedure of choice is a video assisted thoracoscopic surgical (VATS) resection of the bleb or potential source of air leak and pleurodesis. The technique of pleurodesis is mechanical pleural abrasion for younger populations, or chemical pleurodesis which involves medical talc insufflation.

Empyema

Infection of the pleural space is called empyema. Empyema is caused by the spread of infection from adjacent organs or structures. The pleural space can also become infected by (1) spread along the fascial planes of the abdomen and neck into the mediastinum and the pleural space or (2) direct implantation by injury or intervention.

When empyema is in the early stage, it is effusive and adequate drainage is possible with a chest tube alone. When in the sub-acute phase, the empyema tends to be loculated and a video assisted thoracoscopic (VATS) approach is used to allow breakdown of the loculi for drainage and decortication to re-expand the lung. Fibrinolytic agents have also been used selectively in this stage and have achieved satisfactory outcomes. In the chronic stage of empyema, a thick fibrous 'peel' is often formed on the parietal and visceral pleura trapping the lung. An open decortication is necessary to adequately remove the thick 'peel' from the lung and the chest wall to allow lung re-expansion and relieve the chest wall restriction.

Malignant Pleural effusion

The most common cause of malignant pleural effusion is secondary pleural metastasis of advanced malignancies from other primary sites. Primary malignancy of the pleura is a less common cause of pleural effusion.

Symptom control is best achieved by fluid drainage and preventing recurrent effusions. Talc pleurodesis and indwelling pleural catheters are effective first line therapies, however, it is necessary to establish the lung's ability to re-expand following drainage of the pleural effusion to achieve a pleurodesis. Definitive diagnosis of primary pleural malignancy requires pleural biopsy as treatment will be determined by etiology.

Primary Malignancy of the Pleura

Primary malignancy of the pleura is rare compared to metastatic disease. Patients usually present with non-specific symptoms such as shortness of breath, chest pain, or weight loss. Malignant pleural mesothelioma and pleural adenocarcinoma are common primary tumors of the pleura. Primary malignant pleural mesothelioma is a rare, but lethal cancer that has been associated with asbestos exposure in about 80% of cases. Other suspected etiologies include (1) exposure to Eronite, a mineral that is mined in several parts of the world, (2) previous radiation to the chest, or (3) past exposure to Simian Virus 40 (SV40). The incidence of mesothelioma has been increasing around the world and is expected to have a major economic impact in developing countries where asbestos is still widely used. The median survival in untreated patients is reported to be between 4 to 9 months, while less than 10% have a 5-year survival.

Complete surgical removal, if possible, is the preferred treatment, but is only possible in a small percentage of patients with an early-stage tumor. In others, maximal cyto-reductive surgery (extended pleurectomy and decortication) has been associated with good symptom relief, improved quality of life, and prolonged survival. Patients must be carefully selected for surgery as it carries substantial morbidity and mortality. Predictors of favorable outcomes include epithelioid histology, stage of cancer, and surgical resection followed by adjuvant therapy. Purely sarcomatoid cell types appear to have little benefit from cyto-reductive surgery.

Mediastinum

Mediastinitis

Acute mediastinitis is rare and usually results from perforations of adjacent organs, either spontaneous or secondary to instrumentation (Figure 1). This can also result from descending or ascending infection along the fascial planes from the neck or abdomen. Acute mediastinitis following cardiac surgery has been reported to occur in 1 to 6% of cases. Early diagnosis is assisted by careful clinical history, examination, and radiological investigations (i.e., CT or MRI). Aggressive treatment is important as patients can rapidly develop septicemia and muti-organ failure. Treatment includes surgical drainage and debridement of necrotic tissue with appropriate antibiotic treatment.

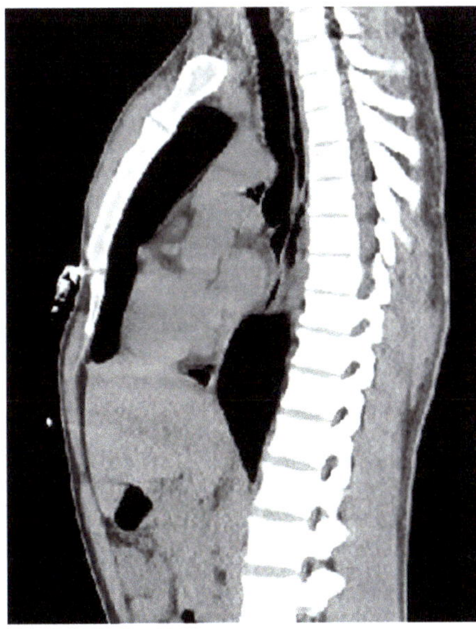

Figure 1: Pneumomediastinum

The etiology of chronic mediastinitis is thought to be poorly treated acute mediastinitis or granulomatous infection related to fungus or tuberculosis. A hypersensitivity response to fungus (e.g., histoplasma, coccidiomycosis) or tuberculous infection can result in an invasive proliferation of fibrous tissue in the mediastinum resulting in fibrosing mediastinitis. The process can result in compression and strictures of vital structures, causing substantial morbidity and mortality. Symptoms are due to involvement of major airway, vascular structures, and the esophagus. Limited success has been achieved by anti-inflammatory and antifungal agents, but the mainstay of treatment is aimed at relieving symptoms using interventional techniques or surgery.[14]

Tumors and Cysts

Tumors and cysts of the mediastinum are generally classified based on their anatomical location; anterior, middle, and posterior mediastinal pathology. More than half of patients do not have any symptoms and tumors and cysts are incidental findings. The other half of patients present with non-specific symptoms, or symptoms that are produced by compression or obstruction of adjacent structures. Generally, when symptoms are present there is an increased chance that the lesion is malignant. The most common mediastinal tumors are related to the thymus gland. Other mediastinal tumors are lymphomas, germ cell tumors, tumors related to the thyroid gland, and neurogenic tumors.

Physical examination may reveal superior vena cava obstruction or cervical lymph node involvement. CXR and PET scan (Figure 2 and 3) may give clues, but a CT scan with intravenous contrast is invaluable in delineating the extent and nature of the mediastinal mass. Blood should be tested for biomarkers of germ cell origin. Biopsies should be obtained if the lesion is suspicious for lymphoma, or the lesion is not resectable. A solitary lesion that is resectable should be excised to establish diagnosis and treatment. Asymptomatic masses, where a benign etiology can be established with certainty, are appropriately observed with serial studies. Examples are non-obstructing foregut cysts, pericardial cysts, and small euthyroid intrathoracic goiters.

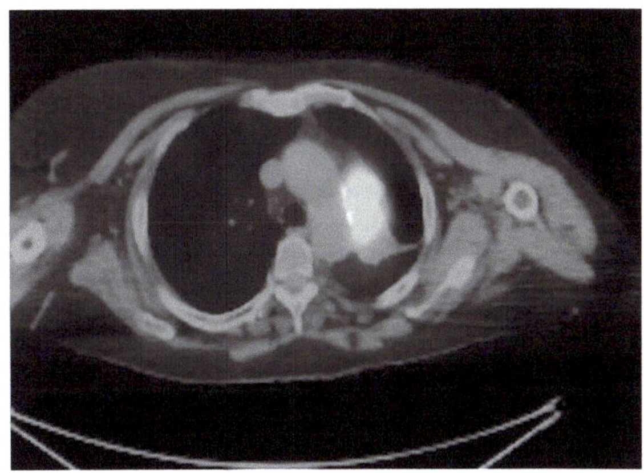

Figure 2: PET scan of a mediastinal tumor

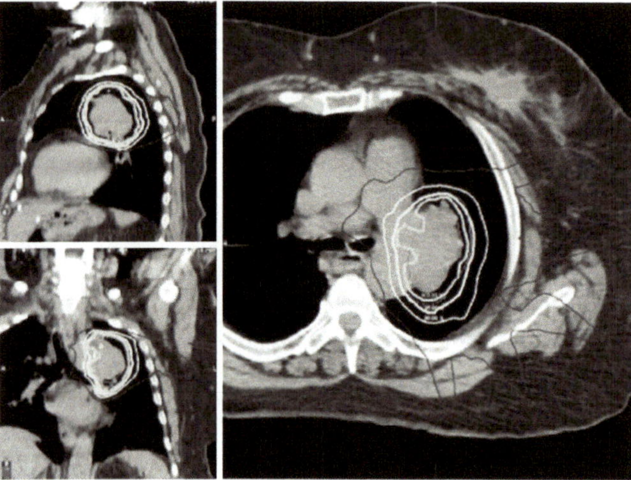

Figure 3: Mediastinal mass

The choice of approach for surgical resection is usually determined by the size and location of the tumor. Video assisted thoracoscopic surgery (VATS) and robotic resections are increasingly being used for small tumors. A lateral thoracotomy for middle and posterior masses, and a partial or full median sternotomy for large anterior mediastinal tumors provide excellent exposure; they were the traditional approaches and should be the choice of therapy for the resection of large tumors.

Thymoma

Thymomas arise from epithelial cells in the thymus gland and are associated with a variable degree of T-cell proliferation. The World Health Organization (WHO) histologic classification and Masaoka clinical staging are widely used.[11] Treatment depends on the clinical stage of the disease. When the tumor is confined within the capsule (Masaoka I) complete resection alone is recommended, when it invades the capsule or adjacent tissue (Masaoka II) or when it invades neighboring organs (Masaoka III) complete en-bloc resection is recommended with adjuvant radiation therapy. If deemed unresectable due to organ involvement or Pleural /pericardial dissemination (Masaoka IV a), neoadjuvant therapy and surgery or chemotherapy with or without radiation is recommended. In patients with hematogenous or lymphogenous metastatic disease (Masaoka IVb), chemotherapy alone is recommended.[12,13]

In patients with lymphomas, the surgical goal is to obtain adequate tissue for diagnosis. Ninety percent of lymphomas in the mediastinum are of the nodular sclerosing Hodgkin's type. However, 50% of the mediastinal diseases are associated with diseases in the neck. The definitive treatment is non-surgical; radiation therapy, chemotherapy, or a combination of both.[14,15]

Germ cell tumors of the mediastinum are benign teratomas, seminomas, or non-seminomatous malignant germ cell tumors. Elevated levels of beta-HCG, alpha FP, or both are seen in patients with non-seminomatous germ cell tumors. Chemotherapy and radiation are used to treat these patients and any residual mass in the mediastinum is subsequently resected.[14]

Neurogenic tumors are the most common tumors in the posterior mediastinum. These tumors arise from neural crest derived cells (i.e., nerve sheath, paraganglionic tissue, and autonomic ganglion cells). Nerve sheath tumors or Schwannomas are the most common tumor of neurogenic origin in the mediastinum. Tumors arising from autonomic nerve cells, the most common being a neuroblastoma, can secrete various vasoactive substances, but less often ganglioneuroma and ganglioneuroblastomas also produce such substances. The primary treatment of tumors of neurogenic origin is surgical resection.[15]

REFERENCES

1. Nuss D, Kelly RE Jr. Minimally invasive surgical correction of chest wall deformities in children (Nuss procedure) Adv Pediatr 55; 2008; 395-410.
2. Nasr A, Fecteau A, Wales PW. Comparison of the Nuss and Ravitich procedure for pectus excavatum repair: a meta-analysis. J Pediatr Surg 45; 2010; 880-86.
3. WeyantMJ, Bains MS, Venkatraman E, Downey RJ, Park BJ, Flores RM, Rizk N, Rusch VW. Results of chest wall resection and reconstruction with and without rigid prosthesis. Ann Thorac Surg 81; 2006 279-85.
4. Mansur KA Thourani VH, Losken A et al. Chest wall resection and reconstruction: A 25 year experience. Ann Thorac Surg 73; 2002; 1720-6.
5. Deschamps C, Tirnaksiz BM, Darbandi R et al. Early and long term results of prosthetic chest wall reconstruction. J Thorac Cardiovasc Surg 117; 1999; 588-92.
6. Miller DL, Force SD, Pickens A, Fernandez FG, Luu T, Mansur KA. Chest wall reconstruction using biomaterials. Ann Thorac Surg 95; 2013: 1050-6.
7. Lans TE, van der Pol C, Wouters MW, Schmitz PI, van Geel AN . J Thorac Oncol Complications in wound healing after chest wall resection in cancer patients. A multivariate analysis of 220 patients. J Thorac Oncol 4; 2009;639-43.
8. Davies HE, Lee YC. Management of malignant pleural effusions: questions that need answers. Curr Opin Pulm Med. 2013 May 13. [Epub ahead of print].
9. Rusch VW, Giroux D, Kennedy C, Ruffini E, Cangir AK, Rice D, Pass H, Asamura H, Waller D, Edwards J, Weder W, Hoffmann H, van Meerbeeck JP; IASLC

Staging Committee. Initial analysis of the international association for the study of lung cancer mesothelioma database. . J Thorac Oncol. 2012 Nov;7(11):1631-9.

10. Peikert T, Colby TV, Midthun DE, Pairolero PC, Edell ES, Schroeder DR, Specks U. Fibrosing Mediastinitis. Clinical presentation, therapeutic outcomes and adaptive immune response. Medicine 90; 2011; 412-23.
11. Japanese Association for Research on the Thymus (JART) General rules for study of mediastinal tumors. Tokyo; Kanehara Publishing, 2009.
12. Fujii Y. Published guidelines for management of thymoma. Thoracic Surg Clin 2011; 21(1): 125-29.
13. Detterbeck FC, Zeeshan A. Thymoma: current diagnosis and treatment. Chin Med J 126; 2013; 2186-91.
14. van Besien K, Kelta M, Bahaguna P. Primary mediastinal B-cell lymphoma: a review of pathology and management J Clin Oncol. 2001; 15;19(6):1855-64.
15. Gobbi PG, Ferreri AJ, Ponzoni M, Levis A Hodgkin lymphoma Crit Rev Oncol Hematol. 2013 Feb;85(2):216-37.
16. Kang CH, Kim YT, Jheon SH, Sung SW, Kim JH. Surgical treatment of malignant mediastinal nonseminomatous germ cell tumor. Ann Thorac Surg. 2008 ;85(2):379-84.
17. Reeder LB. Neurogenic tumors of the mediastinum Semin Thorac Cardiovasc Surg. 2000 ;12(4):261-7.

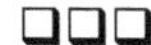

60

CHAPTER

Trachea and Lung

Wickii T. Vigneswaran, MD, FACS, FCCP

TRACHEA

Tumors of the Trachea

The majority of the primary tracheal tumors are malignant with a few benign conditions. Almost half of the malignant tumors are squamous cell carcinoma, while a third are adenoid cystic tumors. The remaining malignant tumors include carcinoid tumors, mucoepidermoid carcinoma, adenocarcinoma, and a small number of unusual primaries such as melanoma. Benign tumors include squamous papilloma, pleomorphic adenoma and mucus gland adenoma, granular cell tumors, and lipoma. Metastatic tumors of the trachea are mostly a result of direct invasion of cancer from adjacent organs including the larynx, thyroid, esophagus, mediastinum, and the lung.

Patients with tracheal tumors present with cough, hemoptysis, exertional dyspnea, wheezing, and stridor. Physical examination reveals presence of inspiratory and expiratory wheezing. Examination should include rigid and flexible bronchoscopy by an experienced endoscopist; the rigid bronchoscope will help to establish airway and enables detailed examination. The proximal and distal extent of the tumor needs to be confirmed during the endoscopy for planning the surgical resection. CT scans of the neck help localize the tumor, and the paratracheal extension and lymphadenopathy. Biopsy is necessary to determine tumor cell type, and plan therapy.

About a half of the tracheal tumors are amenable to primary resection and reconstruction. The other half present with remote metastasis and require long lengths of the tracheal resection that would lead to excessive tension or tumors that invade the mediastinal structures and are thus not resectable. Adjuvant radiotherapy is recommended following resection. An overall survival of over 50% at 5 years has been reported in the largest series of tracheal tumor resections, with squamous cell cancer performing the worst.[7]

Tracheal Stenosis

The most prevalent cause of benign tracheal stenosis is secondary to endotracheal intubation, or secondary to tracheostomy. The stenosis occurs more commonly at the site of the balloon, and less commonly in the case of tracheostomy at the stoma or tip of the tube. Blunt or penetrating injury and granulomatous infection such as tuberculosis or fungus with fibrosing mediastinitis can lead to stricture. Tracheomalacia can result in dynamic airway obstruction, and evaluation should be performed while the patient is spontaneously breathing. Bronchoscopic evaluation for surgical resection should also help determine the presence or absence of infection.

Fistula

Tracheal fistula to the innominate artery or to the esophagus is usually a catastrophic complication. In the case of tracheo-innominate fistula, the patient may present with signal bleeding. Presence of an anterior ulcer in the tracheal wall on bronchoscopic examination without bleeding should lead to angiographic confirmation and urgent repair. If there is bleeding, proceed to surgical repair without an angiogram.

Repair is accomplished through a median sternotomy. The artery is transected with proximal and distal control; the trachea is repaired and reinforced using vascularized soft tissue. The innominate vessel may or may not be reconstructed.

Patients with tracheo-esophageal fistulas present with episodes of coughing that coincide with ingestion of food or fluid due to the connection between the trachea and esophagus as seen in Figure 1. Endoscopy of both the esophagus and tracheobronchial tree coupled with esophagography will establish the diagnosis. If the etiology of the fistula is benign, and if the patient's general condition is good, the fistula can often be repaired with interposition of the vascularized pedicle tissue (either muscle or fat pad). Covered stents can be used in a patient who is a high-risk candidate for surgical repair and when the fistula is small. In malignant tracheo-esophageal fistulas where the life expectancy is less than 6 months, covered stents are the choice for management. If the life expectancy related to the malignancy is more than six months and if there is no current evidence of disease, surgical repair should be considered.

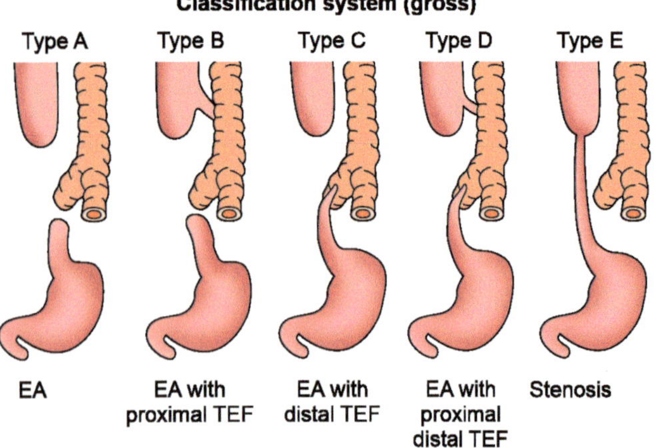

Figure 1: Classification of tracheo-esophageal fistulas

Tracheal and Carinal resection

The upper and mid tracheal resections are best approached anteriorly with partial division of the sternum and working behind the great vessels. The lower trachea and carina are best approached trans-thoracically, where a hilar mobilization may be required. A close collaboration needs to exist between the anesthesiologist and the surgeon in securing the airway, and proper conduct of the ventilation during the operative procedure. Intra-operative intubation across the surgical field is invariably required to maintain ventilation during resection and reconstruction. Reconstruction of the trachea is performed with absorbable sutures. Minimal de-vascularization and meticulous tension-free suturing of the ends is necessary for successful outcomes. Vascularized pedicle tissue wrap of the area of anastomosis protects and assists with healing.

LUNG CANCER

Cigarette smoking remains the predominant risk factor for lung cancer. Although the incidence of lung cancer related deaths in the United States has been decreasing starting around the year 2000, lung cancer is still forecasted to persist as the predominant reason for cancer deaths for the next several decades. In the developing world, deaths from lung cancer are predicted to have a marked increase due to the current prevalence of smoking endemic in these areas. There will be significant social and economic impacts in these countries due to cigarette smoking. There have been very few advances in the treatment of lung cancer. The five-year survival for all non-small cell lung cancer patients has increased by only 4% over the past 25 years (overall 5-yr survival of 18%). The five-year survival for all small cell lung cancer patients has increased from 3.4% to 7.1% during the same period.

Earlier detection of lung cancer and effective therapy is desperately needed. Attempts to develop a lung cancer screening had been unsuccessful. Recently, major progress has been made in understanding low dose CT scans (LDCT) for screening in high-risk populations (Figure 2).[2] LDCT scans identify small nodules in screened individuals; the overwhelming majority are benign. However, LDCT scans can detect early lung cancer, with the harm of LDCT being low. For a patient with an undetermined nodule on an LDCT scan showing clear evidence of growth on serial images (features suggestive of malignancy) or is hyper metabolic on a PET scan, non-surgical biopsy or surgical resection is recommended. Several randomized studies have shown that the current practice of chemoprevention is not effective in lung cancer.

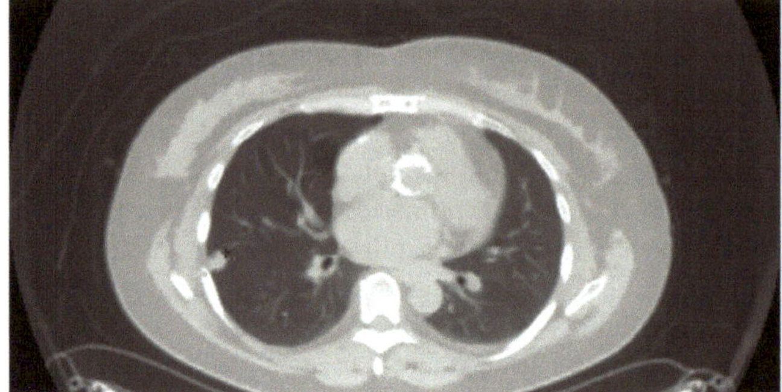

Figure 2: Chest CT showing right lung nodule

The American College of Chest Physicians have developed evidence-based management guidelines for lung cancer.[5] Diagnosing lung cancer requires histologic confirmation accompanied with confirmation of stage to develop a treatment plan. Histologically, lung cancer is broadly divided into small cell and non-small cell types. Non-small cell lung cancers (NSCLC) account for 80% of all lung cancers, while the small cell type account for the remaining 20%. The non-small cell type is further divided into three major histologic types: adenocarcinomas (50%), squamous cell carcinoma (30%), and large cell or undifferentiated carcinomas (20%). Some of the tumors can demonstrate a mixed type of these histologies.

The small cell and non-small cell lung cancers behave differently, resulting in different treatment approaches. Small cell lung cancer is treated primarily non-surgically, whereas non-small cell lung cancer is treated primarily by resection. A majority of the NSCLC are present in an advanced stage of the disease and therefore require a combined modality treatment. Recently, molecular markers that predict tumor behavior have been identified in patients with non-small cell lung cancer. Chemotherapeutic agents are currently available to target specific molecules that can predict outcomes. Relevant testing of molecular markers in tumor tissue is therefore needed to develop a strategy of targeted therapy. Obtaining adequate tissue is crucial at present, not only for defining the histologic subtype of lung cancer, but also for molecular subtyping.

Non-small Cell Lung Cancer

Staging: The TNM staging and the lymph node map described by the International Association for the Study of Lung Cancer (IASLC) are currently widely adopted for staging lung cancer.[3] The TNM stage guide therapy for NSCLC, CT scans, and PET imaging are non-invasive modalities used for clinical staging. However, in most situations, a biopsy is necessary to certify positive CT or PET findings. Ultrasound guided trans-bronchial or trans-esophageal examination can access most of the mediastinal lymph node stations, and needle aspiration can offer tissue for staging. Mediastinoscopy and video assisted thoracoscopic surgery may be necessary to complete the staging when adequate tissue cannot be obtained using bronchoscopic or esophagoscopy techniques. The current TNM descriptors and staging groups for NSCLC are shown in Table 1. Stages 1, 2, and 3 are divided into 'a' and 'b' based on the T and N findings. Any metastasis is classified as stage IV.

Table I: Lung Cancer TNM Descriptors[3,4]

T descriptors	
TX	Cannot assess the primary tumor or Malignant cells are present in bronchial washings or sputum, but tumor is not visualized via bronchoscopy or imaging
T0	There is no evidence of a primary tumor
Tis	Carcinoma *in situ*
T1	Tumor's greatest dimension is ≤3 cm. It is surrounded by lung or visceral pleura, there is no evidence of invasion more proximal than the main bronchus via bronchoscopy*
T1a	Tumor's greatest dimension is ≤2 cm
T1b	Tumor's greatest dimension is >2 cm but ≤3 cm
T2	Tumor's greatest dimension is >3 cm but ≤7 cm or Tumor with any of the following features (T2 tumors with these features are classified T2A if ≤5 cm)
T2a	Tumor's greatest dimension is >3 cm but ≤5 cm
T2b	Tumor's greatest dimension is >5 cm but ≤7 cm
T3	Tumor's greatest dimension is >7 cm or Tumor directly invades the chest wall (also includes superior sulcus tumors), diaphragm, phrenic nerve, parietal pericardium, or mediastinal pleura or Tumor is located in the main bronchus and is <2 cm distal to the carina‡, (no carina involvement) or Tumor is associated with obstructive pneumonitis or atelectasis of the entire lung or there is a separate tumor nodule(s) in the same lobe
T4	Tumor of any size and it invades the mediastinum, heart, trachea, carina, great vessels, recurrent laryngeal nerve, esophagus, or vertebral body or The tumor is a separate tumor nodule(s) in a different ipsilateral lobe
N descriptors	
NX	Cannot assess the regional lymph nodes
N0	There is no metastasis to any regional lymph node
N1	There is metastasis. It can be ipsilateral peribronchial, and/or ipsilateral hilar lymph nodes, and intrapulmonary nodes (this includes involvement by direct extension)
N2	There is ipsilateral mediastinal and/or subcarinal lymph node metastasis
N3	There is contralateral mediastinal, hilar, or scalene metastasis or There is ipsilateral, supraclavicular lymph node metastasis
M descriptors	
MX	Cannot assess distant metastasis
M0	No distant metastasis
M1	Distant metastasis
M1a	There are separate tumor nodule(s) in a contralateral lobe; tumor with pleural nodules or malignant pleural (or pericardial) effusion*
M1b	Distant metastases

NSCLC, TNM Staging[4]

T/M	Subgroup	N0	N1	N2	N3
T1	T1a	Ia	IIa	IIIa	IIIb
	T1b	Ia	IIa	IIa	IIb
T2	T2a	Ib	IIa	IIIa	IIIb
	T2b	IIa	IIb	IIIa	IIIb
T3	$T3_{>7}$	IIb	IIIa	IIIa	IIIb
	$T3_{Inv}$	IIb	IIIa	IIIa	IIIb
	$T3_{Satell}$	IIb	IIIa	IIIa	IIIb
T4	$T4_{Inv}$	IIIa	IIIa	IIIb	IIIb
	$T4_{Ipsi\ Nod}$	IIIa	IIIa	IIIb	IIIb
M1	$MIa_{Contra\ Nod}$	IV	IV	IV	IV
	$Mia_{Pl\ Disem}$	IV	IV	IV	IV
	MIb	IV	IV	IV	IV

Treatment of non-small cell lung Cancer

Surgery endures as the backbone of treatment for early-stage non-small cell lung cancer.[5] Evaluation of a patient's tolerance to lung resection is vital. The assessment should include the patient's cardiopulmonary reserve: post-operative predicted diffusion capacity and spirometry expressed as percentage of normal.[6,7] A simple cardiac risk assessment should be performed on the patient with further investigation required if there is a suggestion of risk. Formal exercise testing prior to surgical consideration should be performed for moderately impaired patients.[8] The prospect of thoracoscopic resection, sublobar resection, alternative (nonsurgical) treatments, preoperative pulmonary rehabilitation, and benefit from smoking cessation need to be taken into account when deciding to undertake surgery.

Treatment of patients with NSCLC is guided by the stage.[5] Patients presenting with stage 1 and stage II undergo anatomical resection with lymph node dissection, or sampling. Lobectomy is the choice of resection in patients with adequate pulmonary reserve and if a complete resection is possible. A bronchoplastic lobar resection or sleeve is recommended for treatment over a pneumonectomy. Sublobar resection is recommended instead of nonsurgical therapy for patients with a reduction in pulmonary function or comorbid disease who do not qualify for lobar resection, but operative intervention can be performed.

Treatment of Stage III NSCLC is controversial and confusing due to its extensive spectrum of disease burden. In individuals with infiltrative stage III (N2,3) NSCLC and performance status 0-1, who are being gauged for curative-intent treatment, the recommendation is combination radiotherapy (60-66 Gy) and platinum-based chemotherapy. In patients with discrete N2 involvement by NSCLC, identified preoperatively (IIIa), the current recommendation is definitive chemo-radiation therapy, or induction therapy with subsequent surgery in lieu of either radiation or surgery alone. In patients with NSCLC who have incidental (occult) N2 disease (IIIa) discovered at surgical resection, despite thorough preoperative staging, and where complete resection of the primary tumor and lymph nodes is possible, completing the planned mediastinal lymphadenectomy and lung resection followed by adjuvant platinum-based chemotherapy is recommended.

Adjuvant therapy

For individuals with fully resected pathologic stage IIa, IIb(N1) NSCLC, and a satisfactory performance status, the recommendation is postoperative platinum-based chemotherapy. For patients with stage I and II NSCLC and a positive bronchial margin (R1 resection), current evidence suggests radiation therapy postoperatively. The recommended treatment based on current evidence is summarized in Table 2.

Table 2: Recommended Treatment for NSCLC

Stage	Treatment
I	Surgery
II	Surgery and Adjuvant Chemotherapy
IIIa	Definitive Chemoradiation/ Neoadjuvant Chemoradiation and Surgery
IIIb	Definitive Chemoradiation
IV	Chemotherapy

To-date, clinical staging of lung cancer remains inaccurate, and the 5-year survival for lung cancer patients still remains low.

Certain abnormalities in the tumors can be found through biomarker testing. These changes are in the tumor DNA and can be mutations, additions, deletions or rearrangements. Some of these mutations can "targeted". Targeted treatments often cause fewer side effects because they focus on targeting what is exactly wrong with the cancer cell, instead of killing normal, healthy cells too. Many molecular targets are observed in non-small cell lung cancers but only a few of these mutations can be targeted at present. Another promising recent development in lung cancer is immunotherapy. Immunotherapy uses one's immune system to fight cancer. The body's disease-fighting immune system may not attack cancer because the cancer cells produce proteins that help them hide from the immune system cells. Immunotherapy works by interfering with that process. Immunotherapy treatments are currently used for people with locally advanced non-small cell lung cancer, to improve progression free survival in these patients.

Treatment of small cell lung cancer

When patients are diagnosed with small cell lung cancer (SCLC) they are in an advanced stage. Clinical stage I SCLC is rare and usually an incidental finding. There is anecdotal evidence suggesting surgical resection can offer a survival advantage in these individuals.[5] Therefore, patients with stage I who are suitable for lung resection should be considered for surgical resection with curative intent following invasive mediastinal staging and extra-thoracic imaging (head MRI/ CT and PET or abdominal CT plus bone scan) to confirm the stage. These patients undergoing surgical resection with intent to cure should be administered platinum-based adjuvant chemotherapy. Patients who are not stage I otherwise with limited disease to the ipsilateral chest, should receive chemoradiation and prophylactic cranial radiation. All patients with stage IV disease are candidates for chemotherapy if they are of satisfactory performance status or should be considered for palliative supportive therapy alone.

Infections of the lung

Lung Abscess

Lung abscesses result from suppurative infections of the pulmonary parenchyma; modern antibiotics have reduced the incidence significantly. The leading cause of lung abscess is aspiration. In particular, a lung abscess can develop from staphylococcus caused necrotizing pneumonia. Patients typically present with fevers, and radiological examination often demonstrates a cavity with an air fluid level. Effective treatment requires identification of the organism and administration of the appropriate intravenous antibiotic therapy. Bronchoscopy is useful to ensure that there is no airway obstruction due to foreign bodies or endobronchial lesions, and to obtain samples for cultures. If this is considered, precautions are necessary to prevent contamination of the unaffected lung during the procedure. When cultured organisms are absent, empiric intravenous therapy with broad coverage of gram-positive and gram-negative is appropriate.

Adequate drainage of the abscess facilitates resolution. If an abscess is peripheral, percutaneous drainage can be performed. This has been shown to be highly effective in the pediatric population. Bronchoscopy is frequently useful to open an occluded bronchus, but extra care should be exercised to avoid any contamination of the unaffected lung. Chest physiotherapy is an adjunct to the above measures to facilitate drainage.

Surgery is indicated for patients with severe hemoptysis and with no response for an extended period (generally two weeks) of intravenous antibiotic therapy and drainage. During surgery, every effort should be made to minimize parenchymal loss. This can be achieved by debridement and resection of necrotic material, or through performing a sub-lobar resection. Rarely, lobectomy is necessary to remove the abscess and necrotic lung.[9,10]

Bronchiectasis

Bronchiectasis are bronchi associated with chronic suppuration that are irreversibly dilated and damaged. Over the past several decades, bronchiectasis has had a low incidence rate due to effective antibiotics and widespread immunization. Bronchiectasis is primarily treated with medical management which consists of a prolonged course of appropriate antibiotics, chest physiotherapy, and postural drainage.

Surgery is indicated for localized bronchiectasis with indolent, recurrent infection and hemoptysis. The guiding principle of surgical treatment is preservation of as much of the lung parenchyma as possible. Generally, this consists of resection of the localized bronchiectatic segment.

Mycobacterium Infections

Tuberculous Mycobacterium Infection: Since appropriate drug regimens have developed, surgical procedures performed for pulmonary tuberculosis have changed. Chemotherapy is the mainstay of treatment; however, surgery has been reported to be an effective adjunctive therapy in selected cases. Other indications for surgical intervention are when patients have TB complications or sequelae like aspergillomas, bronchial stenosis, massive hemoptysis, destroyed lung, empyema, and bronchopleural fistula. For patients with resistance to almost all antibiotics, surgery should be optimally performed within 1–2 months following the initiation of the best available therapy. It is important that no grossly diseased lung is left remaining after resecting all cavitary disease and destroyed lung. A muscle pedicle flap is recommended if there is positive sputum at the time of surgery, pre-existing bronchopleural fistula, polymicrobial contamination of the thoracic cavity, or anticipated space problems after lobectomy.[11]

Non-tuberculous mycobacterium infection: Non-tuberculous mycobacteria (NTM) are opportunistic infections. NTM affect patients with lungs that are structurally damaged or with impaired cellular immunity. There are over 120 different species of NTM that are broadly disseminated in the environment. NTM pulmonary disease has three general patterns: fibro-cavitary form, nodular bronchiectatic type, and infiltrative hypersensitivity pneumonitis type. Host-and pathogen-related elements influence the greatly varying natural history of NTM disease. Each patient needs individually tailored treatment decisions which must prioritize three considerations: surgery, antibiotic therapy, and managing the underlying disease. Drawn out therapy with poorly tolerated antibiotics is detrimental to successful treatment.[12,13]

Surgery can be paramount in managing patients with cavitary and bronchiectatic types who have sufficient cardiopulmonary reserve. For patients failing chemotherapy and who are at elevated risk of failing treatment (i.e., infection with drug-resistant Mycobacterium or MAC abscesses), resection should be taken into consideration. Surgically managing NTM lung disease is linked with significant risks. According to the largest reported case series spanning from 1983 to 2006 of 236 patients who received treatment, operative mortality and morbidity was 2.6% and 18.5%, respectively; one-third of right pneumonectomies were complicated by bronchopleural fistulae.[14]

Fungal infections

The three major mycotic infections of the lung are histoplasmosis, coccidioidomycosis, and blastomycosis. Most often, they present like a mild flu and are of no clinical significance. Surgery is indicated to rule out malignancy, drain an abscess cavity, or attend to a complication secondary to the infection, such as hemoptysis or broncho-pleural fistula. Other unusual infections include nocardiosis, actinomycosis, and cryptococcosis. Aspergillus can cause infections in patients who are immunocompromised, presenting as bronchitis, aspergilloma, or invasive aspergillosis. Aspergilloma is due to colonization of the pre-existing cavity in the lung parenchyma by the aspergillus organism. It does not require treatment unless hemoptysis is present; if hemoptysis is present, the aspergilloma should be resected if the patient can tolerate lung resection.

REFERENCES

1. Gaissert HA, Grillo HC, Schadmehr MB Long term survival after resection of primary ACC and SC of the trachea and carina. J Thorac Cardiovasc Surg 2004; 78: 1889-1897.
2. Aberle DR, Adams AM, Berg CD, Black WC, Clapp JD, Fagerstrom RM, et al, National Lung Screening Trial Research Team. Reduced lung-cancer mortality with low-dose computed tomographic screening. N Engl J Med. 2011; 365:395-409.
3. Rusch VW, Asamura H, Watanabe H; et al. The IASLC Lung Cancer Staging Project: a proposal for a new international lymph node map in the forthcoming 7th edition of the TNM Classification for Lung Cancer, J Thorac Oncol 2009; 4 568-577.
4. Goldstraw P, Crowley J, Chansky K; et al. The IASLC Lung Cancer Staging Project: proposals for the revision of the TNM stage groupings in the forthcoming (seventh) edition of the TNM Classification of malignant tumours, J Thorac Oncol 2007; 2 706-714.
5. Clinical Practice Guidelines. Chest 143(5_suppl); 2013.
6. Ferguson MK, Little L, Rizzo L et al. Diffusing capacity predicts morbidity and mortality following pulmonary resection. J thoraccardiovasc Surg 1988; 96 894-900.
7. Ferguson MK, Watson S, Johnson E, Vigneswaran WT. Predicted postoperative lung function in associated with all-cause long term mortality after major lung resection. Eur J Cardiothorac Surg, 2013.
8. Ferguson MK, Lehman AG, Bolliger CT, Brunelli A. The role of diffusing capacity and exercise tests. Thorac Surg Clin 2008; 18: 9-18.
9. Merritt RE, Shrager JB Indications for surgery in patients with localized pulmonary infection. Thorac Surg Clin. 2012; (3):325-32.
10. Vigneswaran WT. Lung Abscess. Current Therapy in Thoracic and Cardiovascular Surgery. (Eds) Steven C. Yang and Duke E Cameron. Mosby, Philadelphia, PA (USA) 225-6, 2004.
11. Pomerantz BJ, Cleveland J, Olsen H, Pomerantz M.Pulmonary resection for multidrug resistant tuberculosis. J Thorac Cardiovasc Surg 2001;121:448-53.
12. Griffith DE, Aksamit T, Brown-Elliott BA, Catanzaro A, Daley C, Gordin F, Holland SM, Horsburgh R, Huitt G, Iademarco MF, Iseman M, Olivier K, Ruoss S, von Reyn CF, Wallace RJ, Jr, Winthrop K. An official ATS/IDSA statement: diagnosis, treatment, and prevention of nontuberculous mycobacterial diseases. Am J Respir Crit Care Med. 2007.
13. Glassroth J. Pulmonary disease due to nontuberculous mycobacteria. Chest. 2008;133:243–51. Glassroth J. Pulmonary disease due to nontuberculous mycobacteria. Chest. 2008;133:243–51.
14. Mitchell JD, Bishop A, Cafaro A, Weyant MJ, Pomerantz M. Anatomic lung resection for nontuberculous mycobacterial disease. Ann Thorac Surg. 2008;85:1887–93.

❑❑❑

61

CHAPTER

Heart Diseases in Children

Wickii T. Vigneswaran, MD, FACS, FCCP

INTRODUCTION

The specialty of heart surgery in children has advanced remarkably in the last 2 decades. This is mainly due to excellent teamwork between surgeons, pediatric cardiologists, and anesthesiologists, as well as advances in echocardiography, MRI, and post-operative intensive care. Much of the symptomatic heart disease in the world is treated during infancy due to availability of sophisticated facilities. Neonatal intensive care and cardio-pulmonary support including extra-corporeal membrane oxygenation (ECMO) are readily available and there are no financial constraints.

Many developing countries the situation is remarkably different. Children suffer from congenital heart disease as well as acquired diseases such as rheumatic and infectious diseases.[1] They frequently present in late stages and the disease is complicated by a lack of resources and malnutrition. The surgical procedures and their timing may have to be modified based on the resources available.[2] It may also be necessary to concentrate on debilitating heart diseases that can be cured in one stage, such as valve diseases and septal defects. On the other hand, complex diseases that can be treated by total correction in one stage during the neonatal period such as tetralogy of Fallot may have to be treated in stages when neonatal intensive care services are not available. Multi-stage palliative procedures such as Norwood's procedure for a hypoplastic left ventricle may have to be considered on the basis of cost-benefit analysis. Older operations such as atrial switch for transposition of the great arteries (TGA) are considered obsolete in the western world, but may still have a place in developing nations.

The incidence of congenital heart disease (CHD) varies from 6 to 75 per 1000 live births depending on the inclusion criteria. Moderate to severe diseases are about 6 per 1000. No statistical data is available in the developing nations, but several million children wait for surgery at any moment. In the past, developing countries could afford to take care of only a small fraction of these patients. Recently, due to globalization there has been a significant improvement in the economic status, nutrition, and knowledge, leading to a reduction in mortality due to infectious disease by prevention and treatment. The attention is now directed towards cardiovascular diseases.[3] International humanitarian efforts and surgeons with well-developed skills in collaboration with have resulted in more resources being allocated towards treating pediatric cardiovascular disease.[4]

In general, congenital heart defects are cyanotic or non-cyanotic on clinical presentation, and the onset and severity of symptoms is variable based on the failure of complete development, presence of obstructive valvular lesions, and size of the defects between left and right sides of the heart. It is important to understand the morphology and natural history of congenital cardiac lesions to plan the appropriate surgical procedure and its timing.[5] Detailed knowledge of physiology, natural history and treatment of common congenital defects, and an understanding of rare anomalies are essential.

ATRIAL SEPTAL DEFECT (ASD):

ASD represents about 10% of congenital heart defects.[6] There are four types: secundum, primum, sinus venosus, and unroofed coronary sinus (Figure 1). The secundum type is the most common and easily treatable. In some cases, a slit-like opening exists, known as a patent foramen ovale (PFO), which is fairly common in the general population[7] and does not usually require treatment.

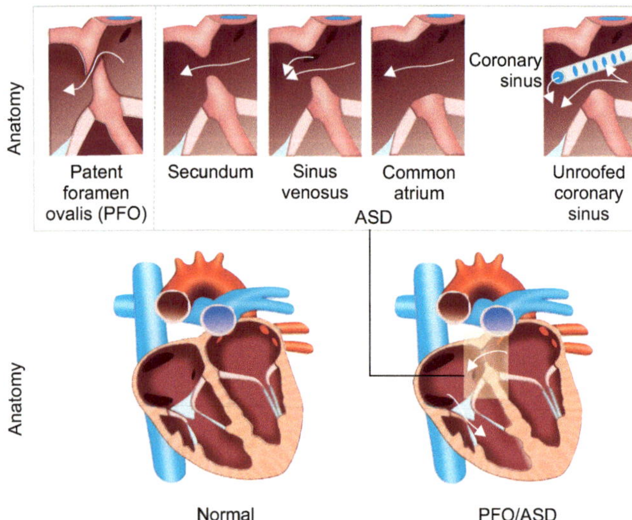

Figure 1: Types of atrial septal defects

Clinical features

Patients have fixed split second sound and systolic murmur due to increased right ventricular (RV) volume and pulmonary flow. Chest radiograph shows typical pulmonary plethora, right atrial enlargement, and RV enlargement. The clinical presentation is bimodal with children presenting with frequent respiratory tract infections, and adults presenting late with atrial arrhythmias and right heart failure.

Diagnosis is easily made by echocardiography. It is essential to have a congenital cardiologist to be involved as it is very easy to miss the type of ASD and its associated lesions. The shunt is calculated as a ratio between pulmonary and systemic blood flow (Qp/Qs). Symptomatic patients and the ones with a ratio greater than 1.5 will need surgery.

Anatomical features and surgical techniques of correction

The secundum defect is present in the middle of the septum in the fossa ovalis. It is corrected either by catheter-based techniques, deploying an occluder device,[8,9] or by open-heart surgery to close the defect with a patch of artificial material or pericardium. The procedure can be done by sternotomy or by several minimally invasive thoracic approaches.[10,11]

The sinus venosus type is located in the upper part of the septum. Frequently a partial anomalous, pulmonary venous drainage is close to the SVC opening. The patching technique involves redirecting the pulmonary venous flow to the left atrium.[12]

The primum defect is part of the endocardial cushion defect. It is located at the lower part of the septum and is frequently associated with the cleft mitral valve. It is important to identify the atrio-ventricular valves and coronary sinus opening while patching this defect.

An unroofed coronary sinus is seen at the lower part of the septum. A coronary sinus opening is seen straddling both atria. Patching involves redirecting the coronary sinus venous return. Careful technique is important to avoid A-V block because suturing at the margin of the coronary sinus or septal leaflet of the tricuspid valve at the lower end of the atrial septum is close to the conduction system.[13] Adults with atrial fibrillation may need additional Maze procedures that involve multiple incisions and ablations of the right and left atrial walls to block re-entry pathways causing atrial fibrillation.[14] The only contraindication to ASD closure is significant pulmonary vascular resistance in excess of 10 to 12 Woods units. Early surgery is advocated for all symptomatic children. Surgery is curative with no residual complications.

VENTRICULAR SEPTAL DEFECT (VSD)

The ventricular septum has three regions, which consist of the atrio-ventricular part, closely associated with the A-V valves, the lower muscular part, and the upper infundibular septum separating the outflow tracts. The distally located membranous septum, is closely related to the central fibrous body near the aortic, tricuspid, and mitral valves.

VSD is the second most common congenital abnormality next to bicuspid aortic valves. It occurs in 4 out of 1000 births and represents 40% of all heart defects. The treatment of isolated symptomatic VSD before the development of complications is very cost effective for a large population of children in the developing world as the surgery is curative. VSDs with associated abnormalities require complex surgery.

The natural history and clinical features depend on the size of the VSD. A large number of restrictive VSDs close spontaneously in the first year of life. Occasionally these VSDs can close late. The VSD is considered large or non-restrictive if the size of the VSD is larger than or equal to the aortic valve orifice. The left to right shunt with a Qp/Qs ratio >1.5 is considered significant and causes increased pulmonary blood flow leading to pulmonary hypertension and right heart failure.

Clinical findings include a loud systolic murmur in the left parasternal area. The murmur is louder in small defects with high velocity. Occasionally in sick children, it may be difficult to detect any murmur due to severe heart failure and tachycardia. Signs of heart failure in an infant include incessant crying, tachypnea, feeding difficulties, and failure to thrive. Chest radiography will show increased pulmonary vascularity and cardiomegaly. The diagnosis is confirmed by echocardiography.[15] It is important to identify associated lesions such as aortic regurgitation, aortic coarctation, and additional defects.

Cardiac catheterization may be needed in older patients to accurately assess operability based on the pulmonary vascular resistance (PVR) less than 8 to10 Woods units. It is important to determine whether the PVR is fixed or reactive to nitric oxide or 100% oxygen.

VSD closure is one of the most rewarding and curative operations in childhood. The decision to perform surgery depends on the size, location (Figure 2), shunt volume, and symptoms related to VSD. Small VSDs with a shunt fraction less than 1.5 do not need surgical closure. They will need follow up and endocarditis prophylaxis. Moderate VSD with controllable symptoms can wait until school age. Large VSD and intractable symptoms need early surgery. Patients with subaortic VSD may need early closure to avoid aortic regurgitation. Surgical closure has a mortality rate of less than 1%.

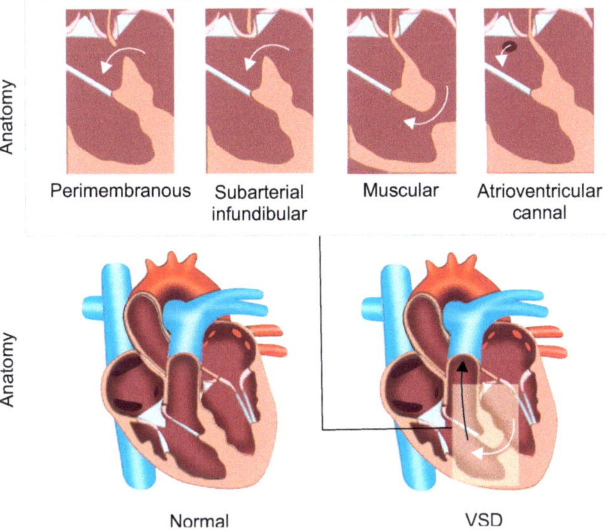

Figure 2: Types and locations of ventricular septal defects

The conduction system is closely associated with the inferior margin of the VSD, and suturing techniques are designed to avoid injury;[16-18] note that AV blocks occur in less than 1% of patients. Other associated lesions such as PDA, aortic coarctation, ASD, or pulmonary stenosis are frequently corrected at the time of surgery for VSD.

In the last few years, trans-catheter closure devices have become available and are mainly useful in muscular VSDs.[19] Incidence of AV conduction defects is high in perimembranous defects. Many VSDs can be closed via right sub-mammary incisions and thoracotomies to provide better cosmetic appearance, and therefore surgical closure is preferable in the majority of patients.

ATRIOVENTRICULAR SEPTAL DEFECT (AVSD)

AVSD is a more complex septal defect that occurs due to a developmental defect of the endocardial cushions, which is also responsible for the structural origin of atrio-ventricular valves. The defect therefore is associated with significant mitral and tricuspid valve abnormalities and is classified into three types based on complexity (Table 1).[20] Ostium primum ASD is an incomplete AVSD without the ventricular component.

Table 1. *Rastelli classification of AVSD*

Type	Structural Abnormality
A	The anterior bridging leaflet that is common to both valves is divided and chordae are attached to septum
B	The anterior bridging leaflet is attached to a large papillary muscle in the RV by multiple chordae
C	The anterior bridging leaflet floats free and has no attachment by chordae

AVSD is further complicated by many associated congenital cardiac anomalies such as patent ductus arteriosus (PDA), Tetralogy of Fallot (ToF), parachute mitral valve with one large papillary muscle, persistent left superior vena cava, unroofed coronary sinus, transposition of the great arteries (TGA), and very rarely Double Outlet Right Ventricle (DORV).[21] Left ventricular outflow obstruction can also occur.

The patients with typical AVSD frequently present early in heart failure. High-pitched systolic murmur from AV valve regurgitation and mid-diastolic murmur are heard on auscultation. When pulmonary vascular resistance is elevated one can hear a split first sound. Chest radiograph shows pulmonary plethora and cardiomegaly. Some features of ECG such as biventricular hypertrophy, atrial enlargement, left axis deviation, and sometimes long P-R interval are fairly constant. Echocardiography shows the location of the shunt, specific AV valvular abnormalities, and associated lesions. Because of large L-R shunts, pulmonary hypertension develops early, and cardiac catheterization is needed for children over a year old. If present, the reversibility should be assessed using nitric oxide or 100% oxygen. Fixed pulmonary resistance greater than 10 Woods units is considered inoperable. Surgery is usually performed before 6 months of age.[22] In a complicated AVSD and in places lacking excellent neonatal care, PA banding is allowed until the child is larger, despite the risk of two operations.

In the western world, most of the patients undergo operations at an early age. The surgery involves either a single patch or the two-patch technique to close the defect and repair the AV valves. The mitral valve is repaired very carefully by finding the line of separation and closing the cleft on the valve to achieve competence. In the presence of a single papillary muscle, the cleft is left open to avoid stenosis. The sutures to close the defect are placed on the right side using the interrupted technique to avoid injury to the conduction system that is very closely associated with the defect.[23] Perioperative echocardiography is a must in all these complex pediatric procedures. Any significant residual valve leak should be corrected before the patient leaves the operating theater. The mortality in the presence of significant mitral regurgitation is greater than 10%. Late recurrence of AV valve regurgitation necessitates repeat surgery.

TOTAL ANOMALOUS PULMONARY VENOUS DRAINAGE (TAPVD)

TAPVD occurs in about 1.5 to 3% of congenital heart defects. The pulmonary veins are connected to the systemic circulation. The three primary types are supra-cardiac, cardiac, and infracardiac.[24] Patients who survive with a large ASD can have an operation at a later stage in some cases. However, oftentimes, this condition is a surgical emergency and is complex.[25]

The supra and infra cardiac types are repaired by anastomosing the pulmonary venous confluence to the back of the left atrium and ligating the communicating channels. Placing an intracardiac baffle at the level of the ASD repairs the cardiac type.

TETRALOGY OF FALLOT (TOF)

ToF is a common cyanotic congenital defect. Pioneering efforts have been undertaken since the 1930s to treat this condition and it is one of the great success stories in congenital heart surgery. The defect occurs in about 5% of all congenital heart defects.[6]

The morphology consists of four interrelated components originating from a mal-aligned, developing infundibular septum.[26] The four components also depicted in Figure 3 are VSD, overriding aorta, pulmonary stenosis, and right ventricular hypertrophy. Though the abnormalities are constant, there is significant variation in severity and morphology of the lesions, and there may be many associated lesions such as an ASD, pulmonary atresia, AVSD, PDA, other VSD, and a right aortic arch. Coronary artery anomalies, with the left anterior descending artery arising from the right coronary trunk in some cases, are very important to establish to plan the operation.

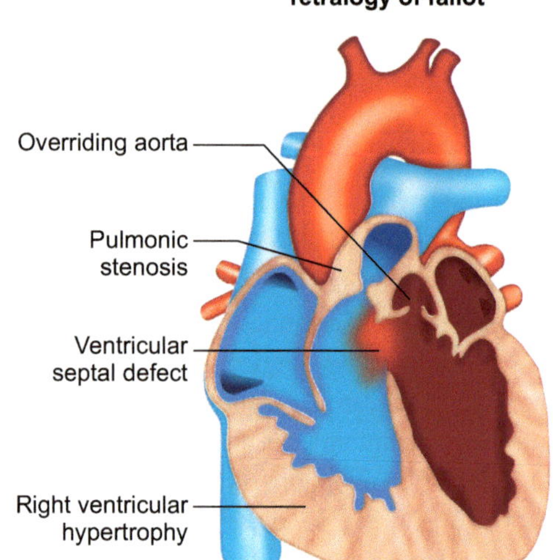

Figure 3: The four components of Tetralogy of Fallot

The severity of cyanosis varies depending on the pulmonary obstruction and it may be associated with cyanotic spells. Older children develop digital clubbing. Auscultation reveals a single second sound and systolic ejection murmur. Chest radiograph shows a typical boot shaped heart and pulmonary oligemia, while ECGs show right ventricular hypertrophy. However, echocardiography is diagnostic.

Surgery involves total correction in a majority of patients and is usually done between 4 to 6 months of age. It can also be completed earlier and is the procedure of choice in uncomplicated patients.[27] The procedure can be performed on cardio-pulmonary bypass using either a trans-atrial or a trans-pulmonary approach. The VSD is closed, followed by a pulmonary valvotomy or trans-annular patch over the pulmonary infundibulum. In the absence of a sophisticated neonatal intensive care unit, the procedure can be completed in two stages. The first stage involves creating a systemic pulmonary shunt usually between the left subclavian to the left pulmonary artery, known as the Blalock-Taussig shunt.[28,29] This adjusts pulmonary flow and relieves cyanosis. The second stage involves taking down the shunt, placing a patch closure of the VSD, and relieving the infundibular and pulmonary obstruction. These steps can be seen in Figure 4.

If placing a patch across the infundibulum is not possible due to abnormal coronary anatomy, homograft replacement of the pulmonary trunk may be needed. The mortality is low in typical ToF. Long-term complications include pulmonary stenosis or regurgitation, which can be corrected by repeat surgery or catheter based pulmonary valve replacement.[30] Regular follow up is necessary in all patients into adulthood, as the long-term survival is excellent.

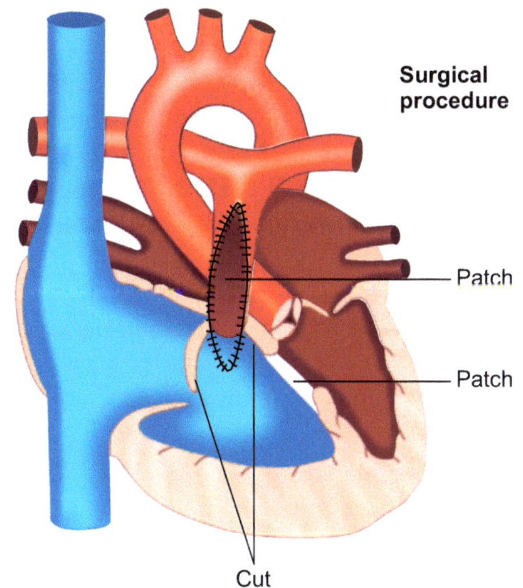

Figure 4: Surgical steps to treat Tetralogy of Fallot

ABNORMAL ORIGIN AND COURSE OF CORONARIES

These are rare conditions but are discussed here as they are correctable by prompt diagnosis and skilled management in one stage. These conditions vary in extent and therefore in presentation.[31]

The most dramatic abnormality is an anomalous left coronary artery arising from the pulmonary artery (ALCAPA). Patients present with ischemic left heart failure and occasionally a myocardial stunning between the 2nd and 3rd months of life. Echocardiogram and cardiac catheterization are necessary to make the diagnosis and discern the coronary anatomy. Various surgical techniques involving reimplantation of the left coronary artery to the aorta have been described. The procedures commonly use the tunnel of the pulmonary artery to provide additional length to reach the aorta.[32]

Other abnormalities are the left coronary artery arising from the right sinus or the right coronary artery arising from the left. In general, the abnormal arteries must course between the major arterial trunks, resulting in compression and ischemic symptoms and warranting surgery. Treatment is reimplantation or an arterial bypass in older patients. Occasionally, the intramural course of coronaries leads to compression and ischemia that can be treated by myotomy. All of these patients complain of dyspnea or a crunching sensation in the chest due to ischemia; a high index of suspicion is needed to make a diagnosis as it is very difficult to elicit symptoms. Dramatic improvement occurs after the surgical procedure.

TRANSPOSITION OF THE GREAT ARTERIES (TGA)

TGA accounts for 10% of all congenital cardiac defects and presents with cyanosis depending on the amount of blood mixing between the systemic and pulmonary flow. In simple terms, the aorta arises anteriorly from the right ventricle and the pulmonary artery arises posteriorly from the left ventricle. However, there are significant variations in morphology. The two circulations exist in parallel and mixing of blood at the atrial level is necessary to supply the body with some oxygenated blood. Children with VSD, although less cyanotic, develop heart failure due to increased pulmonary flow from left to right shunting early in life. The time of onset and severity of symptoms therefore varies based on the extent of mixing and shunting.

Children present with tachypnea, dyspnea, and various levels of cyanosis. There are overt signs of heart failure and pansystolic and mid-diastolic murmurs. The P2 is loud, and the ECG may be normal or may show right ventricular hypertrophy. Chest radiographs are not usually diagnostic, while echocardiography clearly demonstrates abnormal ventriculo-arterial connection and positions of the aorta and pulmonary trunk. Associated conditions including VSD, left ventricular outflow obstruction, ASD, and coarctation are diagnosed readily. Occasionally, cardiac catheterization is necessary to precisely demonstrate the anatomical features and if there is inadequate mixing, an atrial septal defect can be created by balloon septostomy at that time.

Prompt diagnosis and treatment is imperative in a sick TGA patient.[33] The mortality rate is 30% in the first week, 50% in the first month, 70% in 6 months, and 90% in one year. An infant born with cyanosis and TGA may have to go through several phases of treatment. Firstly, it is important to make sure there is adequate mixing. The ductus arteriosus is kept open by infusing prostaglandin E1 (PGE1) or the restrictive ASD is enlarged by balloon septostomy, known as Rashkind's procedure, while awaiting definitive surgery.

The surgery for TGA and the basic concepts have changed remarkably in the last decade. The most recent and advanced operation is known as an arterial switch. It is a logical solution to the problem where the ventriculo-arterial concordance is restored.[34,35] The aorta is transected and anastomosed to the left (systemic) ventricle. The coronary ostia is isolated and anastomosed to the new aorta, and the pulmonary trunk is connected to the anatomical right (pulmonary) ventricle. The defects in the pulmonary trunk caused by removing the coronary ostia are patched, usually with pericardium or gortex. This procedure must be performed within the first 2 weeks of life, before the systemic ventricle gets accustomed to the low resistance pulmonary circulation. In patients presenting with TGA later in life, placing a pulmonary band lead to some hypertrophy and can prepare the LV to face the systemic pressure for later corrective surgery. Patients with VSD are more stable, but the results are better with early surgery in this group as well. The patients with left ventricular outflow tract obstruction are the only patients who are not candidates for arterial switch. These patients usually have a large VSD, and the procedure involves redirecting the flow to the aorta from the LV through the VSD using a patch. Palliation with a systemic/pulmonary shunt early in life is rarely an option.

Historically, operations named after Mustard and Senning were used to treat the TGA. These involved operations at the atrial level, using a Dacron patch as a gusset to redirect the blood flow at the atrial level. Here, the oxygenated pulmonary venous blood is directed to the aorta and the systemic venous blood flows into the pulmonary artery. The discordant arterial connection remains. There are many late problems involving obstruction to the systemic and pulmonary venous drainage necessitating reoperations. Atrial dysrhythmias are also common. The most serious problem is the late dysfunction of the right ventricle, due to its inability to cope with systemic pressures. Though the results are suboptimal compared to arterial switches, many of these cyanotic patients undergo surgery later in their life, using less than optimal myocardial protection techniques which may have contributed to ventricular dysfunction. Therefore, there are no true comparisons available between the two procedures.[36] In developing nations the atrial switch repair still has a role as many children still present late in life, and neonatal intensive care units for arterial switch patients may not be optimal.

AORTIC STENOSIS

Congenital aortic stenosis is a completely different disease from the adult valve disease in terms of pathophysiology, morphology, and treatment.[37] It occurs in 4% of all congenital heart diseases. Left ventricular outflow tract obstruction may present itself in one of three forms: aortic valvar stenosis, sub-valvar stenosis, and supra-valvar stenosis.

Valvar stenosis is usually characterized by a significantly deformed valve in unicuspid or bicuspid morphology. Occasionally, it is the tricuspid valve that is affected. The annulus itself is small in about 20% of cases and may be associated with VSD, mitral stenosis, coarctation of the aorta, and PDA.

The clinical presentation depends on the severity of the stenosis. Systemic blood flow is maintained by ductus flow during intrauterine life. When the ductus closes after birth severe, systemic hypoperfusion occurs leading to acidosis and shock. The child is frequently in extremis and immediate echocardiogram is necessary to make the diagnosis. Emergency ventilation, resuscitations, and treatment is needed to save the child's life. The choice of therapy depends on valve morphology, the left ventricle, and associated anomalies. In patients with adequate sized ventricles, AS can be relieved by balloon aortic valvuloplasty, surgical valvotomy, or rarely valve replacement.[38] In spite of the high recurrence due to a badly diseased valve, the immediate results of valvotomy or valvuloplasty are dramatic. If valve replacement is necessary, the Ross procedure is the operation of choice. In this procedure, the pulmonary autograft is used to replace the aortic valve and the pulmonary trunk is replaced with a pulmonary homograft.[39] The pulmonary autograft has a potential for growth and a large homograft on the pulmonary side can last for a few years.[40] Fetal echocardiography in the future may facilitate earlier diagnosis and possibly treatment.

Subvalvular AS is treated by removal of the membrane if present, or by septal muscle resection. In extreme cases of muscular obstruction of the outflow tract, the Konno procedure to resect the ventricular septum is needed. In the case of outflow obstruction and valvar stenosis, the combined Ross-Konno procedure is performed.[41,42] If the LV is hypoplastic, the surgery is eventually directed towards achieving single ventricle physiology. However, older children do better with surgery.

Supra-valvar AS occurs due to thickening and fibrosis of the aorta above the sino-tubular junction. It may be a part of William's syndrome which is associated with intellectual disability and "elfin" facies.[43] The surgery involves enlargement with an elliptical patch or three separate triangular patches after cutting into the sinuses of the aorta. Overall, the results are excellent in the presence of normal cardiac chambers.

COARCTATION OF THE AORTA

Coarctation occurs in about 5% of all congenital defects and is usually characterized by thickening and narrowing of the aorta distal to the left subclavian artery. Coarctation may occur in isolation or in combination with VSD, AS, or PDA. It may be a part of Shone's complex along with mitral membrane, parachute mitral valve, and subaortic stenosis.

The clinical presentation depends on the severity and associated lesions. Some newborns present with acidosis and shock similar to critical AS due to systemic hypoperfusion once the ductus closes.

Older children and many adults may remain asymptomatic for several years. Frequently, the diagnosis is made after observing systemic hypertension and pressure differences between the arms and the legs. Severe complications of uncontrolled hypertension may bring attention to its presence.

Infants in extremis should undergo emergency surgery after initial resuscitation, maintaining ductus patency with prostaglandin. The surgery is done via a left thoracotomy. The choices of operations include resection and end-to-end anastomosis, left subclavian aortoplasty, or an extended aortoplasty depending on the extent of the disease.[44] Care is taken to avoid injury to the left recurrent laryngeal nerve.

Prosthetic material is rarely used to preserve further growth of the remaining aorta. In older patients graft replacement can be performed. It is important to be cognizant of spinal cord ischemia in older patients without adequate collaterals, partial left heart bypass is used in these cases. The incidence of paraplegia is less than 1%. However, post-operative control of hypertension is very important to avoid left heart failure and mesenteric arteritis.[45]

Trans-catheter aortoplasty with or without a stent is performed with good technical success, but has a significant recurrence rate in children and adults as the diseased aorta is not removed.[46,47] The procedure has significantly higher complication rates. Recurrent coarctation after surgery due to scarring is more amenable to balloon dilatation.

INTERRUPTED AORTIC ARCH

This is a severe form of aortic arch obstructive disease that occurs in less than 1% of congenital heart diseases. There are three types (Figure 5):

1. Type A – The arch vessels arise from the ascending aorta and the descending aorta is a continuation of the ductus
2. Type B – Interruption is between the left carotid and left subclavian arteries. There is a frequent occurrence of an aberrant right subclavian artery from the descending aorta
3. Type C – Interruption between the right innominate artery and the left common carotid artery.

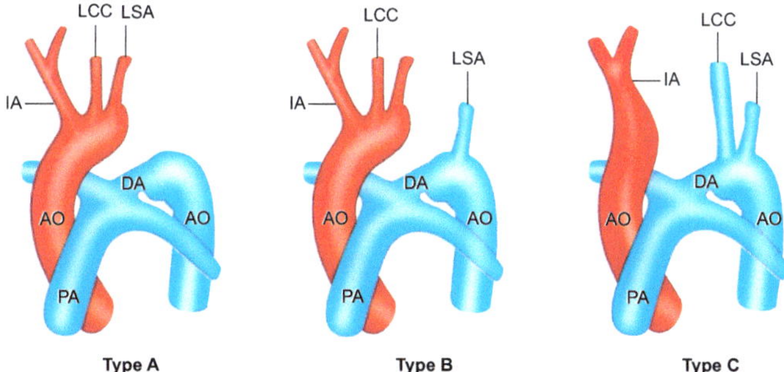

Figure 5: Types of interrupted aortic arch

There is always a large VSD. However, the surgery can be done in stages involving reconstruction of the arch, ligation of the PDA, and the late closure of the VSD.[48,49] The patients need pulmonary banding to prevent pulmonary hypertension from the shunt. Staged procedures allow for children to grow. Total correction in one stage is possible in centers with sophisticated neonatal post-operative care; the mortality is similar.

PATENT DUCTUS ARTERIOSUS

In fetuses, the ductus arteriosus connects the left pulmonary artery to the distal arch of the aorta. Once a child is born and starts breathing, the pulmonary vascular resistance drops leading to blood flow into the pulmonary circulation. Closure of the ductus occurs due to low flow and contraction of the predominantly muscle fibers within its media. The closure is mediated by higher oxygen tension and decreased levels of prostaglandin. Ductus closure usually occurs within 24 hours.[50] A patent ductus occurs in about 7% of all congenital heart diseases. As discussed in previous sections, PDA can occur in association with many complex heart diseases and maintenance of patency is imperative to sustain life in certain cyanotic heart diseases. However, it also occurs in isolation (Figure 6).

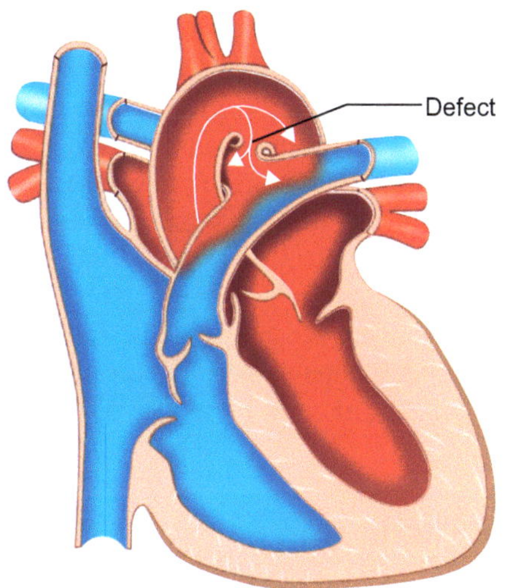

Figure 6: Patent ductus arteriosus

There is significant left to right shunting during both systole and diastole due to the fact the pulmonary vascular resistance is always lower. Since the shunt is distal, the effect of the shunt is due to increased venous return to the left side of the heart, leading to left heart failure. In later stages, the increased flow leads to pulmonary hypertension and right heart failure. The uncorrected shunt may reverse in direction leading to lower body cyanosis due to the right to left shunt. Endocarditis is another complication due to turbulent flow. Patients with associated defects are symptomatic early due to other defects. Isolated PDA causes symptoms if the shunt volume is large. Older children show signs of slowly progressive heart failure leading to failure to thrive and recurrent respiratory infection. Clinical diagnosis is easy to make by the presence of a continuous systolic and diastolic murmur, otherwise known as a "machinery," murmur.

Chest radiograph shows plethoric lung fields and left heart enlargement, while echocardiography is diagnostic.

Similar to other left to right shunts, cardiac catheterization is necessary in older adults and in patients where the murmur is not continuous which is suggestive of early reversal of shunt due to pulmonary hypertension. Reversibility of pulmonary vascular resistance is assessed by using vasodilators and 100% oxygen before considering operability.

Choice of treatment is based on the timing of presentation and how sick the patient is due to heart failure. Medical, open surgical, and trans-catheter are the three methods available to close a patent ductus. Medical treatment to close the ductus is used in premature infants. The drugs commonly used are cyclooxygenase inhibitors, such as indomethacin and ibuprofen.[51] They have significant contraindications due to renal toxicity and bleeding.

Surgery is performed through a left thoracotomy, and the duct is ligated with thick silk or a clip. This procedure can also be done thoracoscopically.[52] Important points in the surgery include (1) exposure of the area under the arch, (2) correct identification of the pulmonary artery, aorta, and the ductus, (3) avoidance of injury to the recurrent laryngeal nerve, and (4) minimal dissection around the friable PDA. Trans catheter deployment of occluder devices is possible in older and more stable children and adults.[53] Closure of the ductus by any method is a safe procedure and the mortality is usually due to prematurity and other complications. Complex PDAs in adults may need cardiopulmonary bypass and patch closure through the aorta or pulmonary artery, as simple ligation may not be possible

VASCULAR RINGS

This is an interesting developmental anomaly involving the aortic arch and its branches. The course of the arteries around the patient's trachea and esophagus lead to obstructive symptoms pertaining to those organs.[54,55] Vascular rings can occur in isolation or in association with other congenital heart defects such as tetralogy of Fallot, ASD, VSD, pulmonary arterial stenosis, aortic abnormalities, and right-sided aortic arch. The ligamentum arteriosum (the fibrous remnant of the ductus) contributes to the obstructive symptoms of the vascular ring. The time of onset and severity of symptoms depend on whether the ring is complete or partial. Late onset symptoms may be related to associated disorders such as atherosclerosis or aneurysmal disease of abnormal arteries.

Some children with complete rings present with respiratory obstruction in the form of stridor or upper respiratory infections. Dysphagia for solids occurs at a later stage. Pulmonary artery slings cause earlier respiratory symptoms and may be associated with tracheal stenosis due to long-standing compression. It is very difficult to diagnose vascular rings as the symptoms are nonspecific and mimic common respiratory problems in childhood. Usually, the patient arrives after going through multiple specialties or after incidental diagnosis made by specific investigations. The tests to confirm diagnosis are chest radiograph, barium esophagogram, CT, MRI, and bronchoscopy. Echocardiography is necessary, mainly to look for associated anomalies. In children it is easy to correlate the symptoms, but in adults it is important to make sure the symptoms are related to compression.

All vascular rings can be approached surgically by a left postero-lateral thoracotomy. Recurrent laryngeal nerves should always be identified. In the case of a double aortic arch, the ligamentum and the non-dominant aortic arch are divided. This is a difficult area to operate even for experienced surgeons. It is a good idea to monitor bilateral blood pressure and to identify changes when the artery in question is clamped before actually transecting it. The scar tissue around the trachea and esophagus is also lysed to ensure good outcomes. The procedure is similar in the right aortic arch. Innominate artery compression rarely occurs when this artery arises from the left side of the midline. Surgery is needed only when the symptoms do not resolve as the child grows. The aberrant right subclavian artery arises low down from the descending aorta. The surgery involves simple division. Pulmonary artery slings are repaired by transection and reimplantation of the left pulmonary artery in front of the trachea. Very rarely is tracheal reconstruction necessary. Recently, minimally invasive trans-thoracic techniques are available. It is extremely important to understand the anatomy while performing these surgical procedures.

TRUNCUS ARTERIOSUS

Patients have a single great vessel arising from the ventricle that has coronary arteries and all the arch vessels as well as pulmonary arteries. The VSD allows mixing of blood. But they do have two ventricles. The surgery involves complex reconstruction of the right ventricular outflow tract and pulmonary arteries after patch closure of large VSDs.[56]

DOUBLE (DOUBLE OUTLET RIGHT VENTRICLE)

In this condition, both great arteries arise from the same ventricle which is usually morphologically the right ventricle. There is a large VSD. There are variants of this disease that resemble the morphology of tetralogy of Fallot or transposition of the great arteries with VSD. The surgery is planned according to the morphology, especially the size and location of the VSD.[57,58]

COMPLEX RARE ANOMALIES

The following congenital and childhood cardiac anomalies occur rarely, but present in a dramatic fashion. These three conditions have a severe developmental abnormality of the ventricles resulting mainly in a single functioning ventricle, though many variations can occur.

There is a need for immediate, sometimes prenatal diagnosis, and treatment is soon after birth. Many patients need multiple, complex procedures and long-term follow up for complications. Enormous resources have to be dedicated for taking care of these infants in the neonatal period and later in life. If diagnosed prenatally, some of these conditions should lead to discussion and counseling. If the child is born and in extremis, the value of multiple palliative operations at high risk and cost needs to be addressed, especially in the developing world. Therefore, they are only briefly discussed.

HYPOPLASTIC LEFT HEART SYNDROME

This is a constellation of many defects, along with hypoplastic left ventricles and atretic aortas. Blood passes retrogradely into a tiny aorta and coronary arteries. The distal circulation is through the PDA. The abnormality is very complex, and treatment is either through a multi-stage reconstructive Norwood's procedure or cardiac transplantation in the neonatal period.[59,60] The procedure carries high mortality and morbidity and is performed in many stages.

TRICUSPID ATRESIA

The communication between the RA and RV is absent in these patients resulting in a small right ventricle

PULMONARY ATRESIA WITH INTACT VENTRICULAR SEPTUM

These patients may also frequently have a small RV that may not be adequate to support circulation. The level of development of the pulmonary arteries is variable.[61]

The common final pathway for a majority of these patients with the above conditions is to create a single ventricle physiology that supports the systemic circulation and a direct connection of venous return to pulmonary circulation. In simple terms, a ventricle is considered necessary to sustain high resistant systemic circulation. The pulmonary circulation is created by a procedure known as a modified Fontan's procedure, wherein the vena caval blood is directly diverted by anastomoses and conduits to the pulmonary arteries in multiple stages.[60]

EBSTEIN'S MALFORMATION

Ebstein's malformation of the tricuspid valve is a unique disease that is worth a separate mention. It is a congenital abnormality of variable morphology and severity, affecting the tricuspid valve and the right ventricle. The disease affects the leaflets, chordal attachment, and the leaflet position, which is attached low leading to what is known as atrialization of the ventricle. Many patients may remain asymptomatic and live through adulthood even in the presence of severe tricuspid regurgitation and a dilated right ventricle. Some patients have associated supraventricular tachyarrhythmias in the form of the Wolff-Parkinson-White syndrome that can be treated by catheter ablation. Children may present with cyanosis and heart failure, whereas adults, if they are symptomatic, may present with tiredness and dyspnea. The malformation is corrected by complex tricuspid valve repair or replacement in symptomatic patients.[62]

OLDER PATIENTS WITH CONGENITAL HEART DISEASE

The treatment of older and adult patients with congenital heart diseases has now become an important specialty. Patients with VSD, PDA, ASD, and other congenital shunts can present late and they can still undergo operation if they are symptomatic with reversible pulmonary hypertension.[63,64] There are also many patients with corrected, partially corrected, and uncorrected congenital cardiac disease who live to adulthood.[65,66] Palliative, supportive and surgical management of these patients requires specialists in congenital and adult cardiac disease.[67,68] The following situations are examples of important considerations:

1. Definitive operation for cyanotic patients who were palliated with systemic to pulmonary artery shunts should be planned. The surgery usually depends on the malformation. Usually, it is either a total correction of conditions (i.e., TOF)[69-72] or conversion to a single ventricle physiology utilizing Fontan's procedure.
2. Removal of pulmonary artery banding and closure of defects causing large left to right shunt, usually a VSD. The surgery usually requires reconstruction of the pulmonary artery after removal of the band.
3. Definitive aortic valve procedure after initial valvotomy leading to valve replacement or the Ross procedure.
4. ASD presenting in adulthood requiring patch or device closure, depending on whether it is ostium primum or a secundum defect.
5. Residual or newly diagnosed coarctation needing reconstruction.
6. Follow up of small VSDs to make sure that the patients do not develop right heart volume overload and pulmonary hypertension. Many of them do not need closure but they need antibiotic prophylaxis.
7. Residual atrio-ventricular valve disease in repaired AV canal defects requiring follow up and repeat repair of valve leaks.

8. Development of pulmonary regurgitation in patients with previously corrected ToF needing valve replacement.
9. Treatment of persistent pulmonary hypertension.[73,74]
10. Treatment of heart failure caused by ventricular dysfunction.[75,76]

It is also important for healthcare professionals to be aware of congenital heart diseases with residual issues that may increase the risk of other treatments and non-cardiac surgery. High-risk patients are the ones with pulmonary hypertension, cyanotic heart disease, cardiac symptoms, ventricular dysfunction, and left-sided obstructive lesions. Moderate risk patients are the ones with prosthetic valves or conduits and moderate levels of the above-mentioned lesions. It is also important to consider endocarditis prophylaxis[77] in patients with residual heart disease, lesions with turbulence, and artificial prosthesis. The patients are also prone to arrhythmias that need to be treated.[78] Overall, it is important to consult cardiologists who specialize in adult congenital heart disease for symptoms and in special circumstances.[79]

Reoperation is also required simply due to the growth of the patient.[80] Many patients who have had correction of a congenital heart disease need careful follow up for long-term complications inherent to the procedures.

REFERENCES

1. Suresh G Rao. Pediatric cardiac surgery in Developing countries. Pediatr Cardiol (2007) 28:144-148.
2. Larrazabal LA, Jenkins KJ, Gauvreau K, et al. Improvement in congenital heart surgery in a developing country: The Guatemalan experience. Circulation. 2007;116:1882-1887.
3. Stolf NAG. Congenital heart surgery in a developing country: A few men for a great challenge. Circulation. 2007;116:1874-75.
4. The development of cardiac surgery in an emerging country. Tex Heart Inst. J. 2008;35(3):301-6.
5. Kirklin JW, Barratt-Boyes BG. Cardiac surgery, Morphology, Diagnostic criteria, Natural history, Techniques, results and Indications. Churchill Livingstone, 3rd Edition.
6. Hoffman JI, Kaplan S. The incidence of congenital heart disease. J Am Coll Cardiol 2002;39(12):1890-900.
7. Incidence and size of patent foramen ovale during the first 10 decades of life. Mayo Clin Proc. 1984;59(1):17-20.
8. Everett AD, Jennings J, Siblinga, et al. Community use of Amplatzer Atrial septal defect occluder: results of the multi-center MAGIC atrial septal defect study. Pediatr Cardiol. 2008;30(3):240-47.
9. Correa R, Zahn E, Khan D. Mid-term outcomes of the Helex septal occluder for percutaneous closure of Secundum atrial septal defects. Congenit heart Dis. 2013 Mar 1.
10. Gil-Jaurena JM, Castillo R, Zabala JI, et al. Axillary approach to surgical closure of atrial septal defect. (Article in Spanish) Ann Pediatr (Barc) 2013 Feb 22. Pii: S16951-4033(13).
11. Poffo R, Cellulare AL, Pope RB, Toschi AP. Robotically assisted minimally invasive surgery for atrial septal defect correction. Rev Bras Cir Cardiovasc. 2012 Jul-Sep;27(3):488-90.
12. Bajwa G, Dostanic-Larson I, Krasuski RA, Pettersson GB. Lateral caval flap repair of adult sinus venosus atrial septal defect: a natural novel approach. J Thorac Cardiovasc Surg. 2012;144:984-5.
13. Xie MX, Yang YL, Cheng TO, et al. Coronary sinus septal defect (unroofed coronary sinus): Echocardiographic diagnosis and surgical treatment. Int J
14. Cardiol. 2012 Dec 22pii:S0167-5273(12).

Im YM, Kim JB, Yun SC, et al. Arrhythmia surgery for atrial fibrillation associated with atrial septal defect: right sided maze versus biatrial maze. J Thorac Cardiovasc Surg. 2013 Mar;145(5):648-54.
15. Spicer DE, Anderson RH, Backer CL. Clarifying the surgical morphology of inlet ventricular septal defects. Ann Thorac Surg. 2013 Jan;95(1):236-41.
16. Aydemir NA, Harmandar B, Karaci AR, et al. Results for surgical closure of isolated ventricular septal defects in patients under one year of age. J Card Surg. 2013 Mar;28(2):174-9.
17. Anderson PR, Stevens KN, Nicolson SC, et al. Contemporary outcomes of surgical ventricular septal defect closure. J Thorac Cardiovasc Surg. 2013 Mar;145(3):641-7.
18. Lopez-Ruiz N, Ramirez-Gil l, Escobar-Quijano C, et al. Ventricular septal defects in adults: 15 years of surgical experience in a single Colombian cardiovascular center. (Article in Spanish). Arch Cardiol Mex. 2013 Jan-Mar;83(1):24-30.
19. Liu S, Chen F, Ding X, et al. Comparison of results and economic analysis of surgical and transcatheter closure of peri-membranous ventricular septal defect. Eur J Cardiothorac Surg. 2012 Dec;42(6):e157-62.
20. Rastelli G, Kirklin J,W, Titus JL. Anatomic observations on complete form of persistent common

atrio-ventricular canal with special reference to atrio-ventricular valves. Mayo Clin Proc 1966;41(5):296-308.

21. Bharati S, Kirklin JW, McAllister HA Jr, et al. The surgical anatomy of common atrio-ventricular orifice associated with tetralogy of Fallot, double outlet right ventricle and complete regular transposition. Circulation 1980;61(6):1142-1149.
22. Suzuki T, Bove EL, Devaney EJ, et al. Results of definitive repair of complete atrio-ventricular septal defect in neonates and infants. Ann Thorac Surg2008;86(2):596-602.
23. Tagliari AP, Schroder DA, Teixeira Filho G, et al. Results of simplified single patch repair for complete atrioventricular septal defect. Ann Bras Cardiol. 2013 Mar;100(3):288-293.
24. Seale AN, Uemura H, Webber SA, et al. Total anomalous pulmonary venous connection: morphology and outcome from an international population study. Circulation. 2010 Dec 21;122(25):2718-26.
25. Jian XH, Huang J, Ding Y, et al. Surgical outcome of isolated total anomalous pulmonary venous connection in adults: a 14-year experience. J Card Surg. 2012 Nov;27(6):736-9.
26. Van Praagh R, Van Praagh S, Nebesar RA, et al. Tetralogy of Fallot: underdevelopment of the pulmonary infundibulum and its sequelae. Am J Cardiol. 1970;26(1)25-33.
27. Tamesberger MI, Lechner E, Mair R, et al. Early primary repair of tetralogy of Fallot in neonates and infants less than four months of age. Ann Thorac Sur. 2008;86(^): 1928-1935.
28. Dirks V, Pretre R, Knirsch W, et al. Modified Blalock-Taussig shunt: a not-so-simple palliative procedure. Eur J Cardiovasc Surg. 2013 Mar 28.
29. Arenz C, Laumeier A, Lutter S, et al. Is there any need for a shunt in the treatment of tetralogy of fallot with one source of pulmonary blood flow? Eur J Cardiothorac Surg. 2013 Mar 12.
30. Hill G. Repair and follow-up of tetralogy of Fallot with pulmonary stenosis. Congenit Heart Dis. 2013 Mar 1.
31. Dodge-khatami A, Mavroudis C, Backer CL. Congenital heart surgery nomenclature and database project: anomalies of the coronary arteries. Ann Thorac Surg 2002;69(4 suppl):S270-S297.
32. Ando M, Mee RB, Duncan BW, et al. Creation of a dual-coronary system for anomalous origin of the left coronary artery from the pulmonary artery utilizing the trapdoor flap method. Eur J Cardiothorac Surg 2002;22(4):576-581.
33. Hong SJ, Choi HJ, Kim YH, et al. Clinical features and outcomes of complete transposition of the great arteries. Korean J Pediatr. 2012 Oct;55(10):377-82.
34. Qamar ZA, Golberg CS, Devaney EJ, et al. Current risk factors and outcomes for the arterial switch operation. Ann Thorac Surg 2007;84(3):871-878; discussion 878-879.
35. Dodge-Khatami A, Mavroudis C, Mavroudis CD, Jacobs JP. Past, present and future of the arterial switch operation: historical review. Cardiol Young. 2012 Dec;22(6):724-31.
36. Junge C, Westhoff-Bleck M, Schoof S, et al. Comparison of late results of arterial switch versus atrial switch (Mustard procedure) operation for transposition of the great arteries. Am J Cardiol. 2013 Feb 19. Pii: S0002-9149(13)00403-7.
37. Anagnostopoulos PV, Johnson NC, Robertson L, Sapru A, Azakie A. Surgical management of left ventricular outflow tract obstruction. J Card Surg. 2012 Jan;27(1):103-11.
38. McCrindle BW, Blackstone EH, Williams WG, et al. Are outcomes of surgical versus transcatheter balloon valvotomy equivalent in neonatal critical aortic stenosis? Circulation 2001;104(12)(suppl 1):I152-I158.
39. Berdajs D. Ross procedure for everyone. Swiss Med Wkly. 2012 Jul 23;142:w13641.
40. Charitos EL, Takkenberg JJ, Hanke T, et al. Reoperations on the pulmonary autograft and pulmonary homograft after the Ross procedure: An update on the German Dutch Ross Registry. J Thorac Cardiovasc Surg. 2012 Oct;144(4):813-21.
41. Aszyk P, Thiel C, Sinzobahamvya N, et al. Ross-Konno procedure in infants: mid-term results. Eur J Cardiothorac Surg. 2012 Oct;42(4):687-94.
42. Talwar S, Malankar D, Garg S, et al. Aortic valve replacement with biological substitutes in children. Asian Cardiovasc Thorac Ann. 2012 Oct;20(5):518-24.
43. Ergul Y, Nisli K, Kayserili H, et al. Cardiovascular abnormalities of Williams syndrome: 20 years' experience in Istanbul. Acta Cardiol. 2012 Dec;67(6):649-55.
44. Ungerleider RM, Pasquali SK, Welke KF, et al. Contemporary patterns of surgery and outcomes for aortic coarctation: an analysis of the Society of Thoracic Surgeons Congenital Cardiac Surgery Database. J Thorac Cardiovasc Surg. 2013 Jan;145(1):150-7.
45. Morgan GJ, Lee KJ, Chaturvedi R et al. Systemic blood pressure after stent management for arch coarctation implications for clinical care. JACC Cardiovasc Interv. 2013 Feb;6(2):192-201.

46. Mollaei A, Merajie M, Mortezaeian H, et al. Complications of aortic stenting in patients below 20 years old: Immediate and intermediate follow-up. J Tehran Heart Cent. 2011 Nov;6(4):202-5.
47. Canniffe C, Ou P, Walsh K et al. Hypertension after repair of aortic coarctation – A systematic review. Int J Cardiol. 2012 Oct 4. Pii:S0167-5173(12)01190-4.
48. Shinkawa T, Jaquiss RD, Imamura M. Single institutional experience of interrupted aortic arch repair over 28 years. Interact Cardiovasc Thorac Surg. 2012 May;14(5):551-5.
49. Mishra PK. Management strategies for interrupted aortic arch with associated anomalies. Eur J Cardiothorac Surg. 2009 Apr;35(4):569-76.
50. Campbell M. Natural history of persistent ductus arteriosus. Br Heart J 1968;30(1):4-13.
51. Sekar KC, Corff KE. Treatment of patent ductus arteriosus:" indomethacin or ibuprofen? J Perinatol. 2008;28(suppl 1):S60-S62.
52. Burke RP, Jacobs JP, Cheng W, et al. Video assisted thoracoscopic surgery for patent ductus arteriosus in low birth weight neonates and infants. Pediatrics 1999;104(2 Pt 1):227-230.
53. Matter M, Almarsafawey H, Hafez M, et al. Patent ductus arteriosus stenting in complex congenital heart disease: Early and midterm results for a single-center experience at Children Hospital, Mansoura, Egypt. Pediatr Cardiol. 2012 Dec 13.
54. Backer CL, Mavroudis C, Rigsby CK, et al. Trends in vascular ring surgery. J Thorac Cardiovasc Surg. 2005;1299601339-1347.
55. Bai S, Li XF, Peng Y, et al. Surgical treatment for vascular anomalies and tracheoesophageal compression. Cin Med J (Engl) 2012 Apr;125(8):1504-7.
56. Qiu LS, Sun YJ, Liu JF, Zhu LM, Xu ZW. Surgical repair of truncus arteriosus in children: early results and long-term outcomes. Zhonghua Wai Ke Za Zhi. 2012 Sep;50(9):827-30.
57. Pshparajah K, Barlow A, Tran VH, et al. A systematic three-dimensional echocardiographic approach to assist surgical planning in double outlet right ventricle. Echocardiography. 2013 Feb;30(2):234-8.
58. Serraf A, Nakamura T, Lacour-Gayet F, et al. Surgical approaches for double-outlet right ventricle or transposition of the great arteries with straddling atrioventricular valves. J Thorac Cardiovasc Surg. 1996 Mar;111(3):527-35.
59. Ghanayem NS, Allen KR, Tabbutt S, et al. Interstage mortality after the Norwood procedure: results of the multicenter Single Ventricle reconstruction trial. J Thorac Cardiovasc surg. 2012 Oct; 144(4):896-906.
60. Rogers LS, Glatz AC, Ravishankar C, et al. 18 years of the Fontan operation at a single institution: results from 771 consecutive patients. J Am Coll Cardiol. 2012 Sep 11;60(11):1018-25.
61. Hoashi T, Kagisaki K, Kitano M, et al. Late clinical features of patients with pulmonary atresia or critical pulmonary stenosis with intact ventricular septum after biventricular repair. Ann Thorac Surg. 2012 Sep;94(3):833-41.
62. Yu JJ, Yun TJ, Won HS, et al. Outcome of neonates with Ebstein's Anomaly in the current era. Pediatr Cardiol. 2013 Mar 14.
63. Gurvitz M, Valente AM, Broberg C, et al. Prevalence and predictors of gaps in care among adult congenital cardiac disease patients (The health, education and access research trial: HEART-ACHD) J AM Coll Cardiol 2013 Mar 28.
64. Mello GA, Carvalho JL, Baucia JA, Magalhaes Filho J. Adults with congenital heart disease undergoing first surgery: prevalence and outcome at a tertiary hospital. Rev Bras Cir Cardiovasc. 2012 Dec;27(4):529-34.
65. Fteropoulli T, Stygall J, Cullen S, Deanfield J, Newman SP. Quality of life of adult congenital heart disease patients: a systematic review of the literature. Cardiol Young. 2013 Feb 6: 1-13.
66. Warnes CA, Williams RG, Bashore TM, et al. ACC/AHA 2008 Guidelines for the management of adults with congenital heart disease. Circulation. 2008;118:e714-e833.
67. Aboulhosn JA, Lluri G, Gurvitz MZ, et al. Left and right ventricular diastolic function in adults with surgically repaired tetralogy of Fallot: A multi-institutional study. Can J Cardiol. 2013 Jan 28.
68. Lopes AA. Is surgical treatment the cure for patients with congenital heart disease? Pulm Circ. 2012 Jul-Sep;2(3)273-274.
69. Hunter RM, Isaac M, Frigiola A et al. Lifetime costs and outcome of repair of tetralogy of Fallot compared to natural progression of the disease: great ormond street hospital cohort. PLoS One. 2013;8(#):e59734.
70. Jian X, Huang J, Zhuang J, et al. Surgical correction of tetralogy of Fallot in adults over 40 years of age (article in Chinese) Nan Fnag Yi Ke Da Xue Xue Bao. 2012 Dec;32(12):1808-11.
71. Bakhtiary F, Dahnert I, Leontyev S, et al. Outcome and incidence of re-intervention after surgical repair of tetralogy of Fallot. J Card Surg. 2013 Jan;28(1):59-63.

72. Sarris GE, Comas JV, Tobota Z, Maruszewski B. Results of reparative surgery for teralogy of Fallot: data from the European Association for Cardio-Thoracic Surgery Congenital Database. Eur J Cardiothoracic Surg. 2012 Nov;42(5):766-74.

73. Stamm JA, Risbano MG, Mathier MA. Overview of current therapeutic approaches for pulmonary hypertension. Pulm Circ. 2011;1:138-59.

74. Beghetti M, Galie N, Bonnet D. Can "inoperable" congenital heart defects become operable in patients with pulmonary arterial hypertension? Dream or reality? Congenit Heart Dis. 2012;7:3-11.

75. Dinardo JA. Heart failure associated with adult congenital heart disease. Seminars Cardiothorac Vasc Anesth. 2013 Mar;17(1):44-54.

76. Guihaire J, Haddad F, Mercier O, et al. The right heart in congenital heart disease, mechanisms and recent advances. J Clin Exp Cardiolog. 2012 Jun 15;8(10):1-11.

77. Fortun J, Centela T, Martin-Davila P, et al. Infective endocarditis in congenital heart disease: a frequent community acquired complication. Infection. 2013 Feb;41(1):167-74.

78. Mondesert B, Abadir S, Khairy P. Arrhythmias in adult congenital heart disease: the year in review. Curr Opin Cardiol. 2013 Mar 17.

79. Child JS, Perloff JK, Kogg B. Management of pregnancy and contraception in congenital heart disease. In. Congenital Heart Disease in Adults, 3rd Ed. 2009. Saunders Elsevier, pp 194-220.

80. Holst KA, Dearani JA, Burkhart HM, et al. Reoperative multi-valve surgery in adult congenital heart disease. Ann Thorac Surg. 2013 Apr;95(4):1383-9.

❑❑❑

62

CHAPTER

Valvular and Thoracic Aortic Disease

Wickii T. Vigneswaran, MD, FACS, FCCP

Pasala Ravichandran, MD

VALVULAR HEART DISEASE

Structural and Functional Anatomy

The heart has four valves (Figure 1). The basic structure of the valves is a combination of connective tissue and endocardium. They have a completely or partially developed fibrous skeleton. The fibrous annuli of the aortic and mitral valves are in continuity forming the central fibrous body. The skeleton gives some support to the valves, and they electrically isolate the atria and ventricles. Diseases of connective tissue affect the fibrous annulus and the leaflets.

The aortic valve usually consists of three semilunar cusps. The spaces between the cusps and the aorta are called the sinuses. The coronary ostia are present in the right and left sinuses. The third is a non-coronary sinus. The aortic valve is closely related to the mitral valve, membranous ventricular septum, and bundle of His. The aortic valve is barely visible on echocardiogram when it opens, and the flow is streamlined. It opens and closes passively due to a pressure gradient between the left ventricle (LV) and the aorta. The vortex created in the aortic sinuses during diastole also helps with perfect closure.

The mitral valve is more complex. It has anterior and posterior leaflets shaped like sails. The anterior leaflet occupies one-third of the circumference and two-thirds of the area. The posterior leaflet occupies the reverse. The posterior leaflet is also called the mural leaflet, as it is associated with the posterior-basal LV muscle. The circumflex artery and the coronary sinus are in close proximity to the posterior annulus. The anterior leaflet is attached to the fibrous trigone and closely related to the aortic valve. The leaflets are anchored to the papillary muscles by chordae tendineae. There are primary, secondary, and tertiary chordae. The primary chordae are near the free edge, and they are most important for apposition of the leaflets. The closure of the valve is again due to pressure changes, but the mechanism is governed in a complex fashion by the ventricle, papillary muscles, chordae, annulus, and atrial muscle. The height of apposition during closure is important to prevent valve leak and it depends on the complex interplay between annulus diameter and ventricular muscle. The pulmonary valve is similar to the aortic valve with a thinner fibrous skeleton. The tricuspid is similar to the mitral valve, but with three leaflets. The septal leaflet is closely related to the conducting system and the coronary sinus opening.

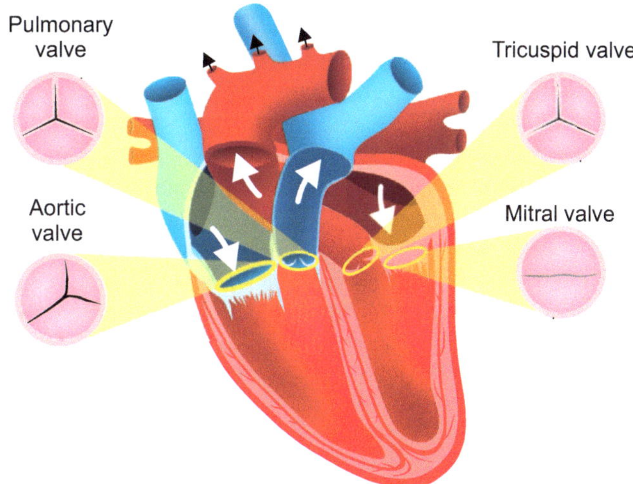

Figure 1: The heart valves

Etiology and Pathophysiology of Common Valvular Diseases

Aortic Stenosis

There are three major causes of aortic stenosis (AS). They are rheumatic, bicuspid, and degenerative.

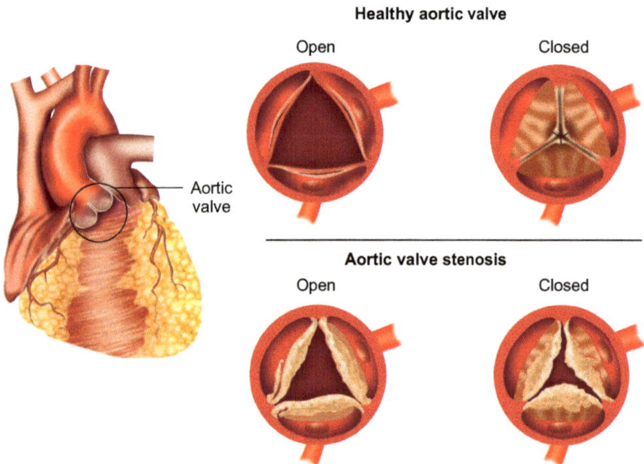

Figure 2: Aortic stenosis

Rheumatic AS is still the most frequent valvular disease in developing countries. Usually, the lesions cause mixed AS and regurgitation. Multivalvar disease is also common.[1] A bicuspid aortic valve is present in 2% of the normal population and it is the most common cause of AS before the age of 65 due to early degeneration. Occasionally regurgitation is a primary problem. Degenerative diseases are more common in western countries, and they are diseases of old age.[2] Frequently, the patients have associated coronary artery disease (CAD) because of common risk factors. The lesions usually seen include severe calcifications on both the aortic and the ventricular sides of the valve leaflets. Calcific deposits frequently burrow into the ventricular septum, LV muscle and mitral valve anterior leaflet.

The final pathological pathway to stenosis is similar in all causes.[3] The patient develops significant symptoms, usually when the valve area reaches around 1cm^2/m^2 from its normal size of 3 to 4 cm^2/m^2. LV hypertrophy occurs due to pressure overload. This results in relative ischemia and diastolic dysfunction. Endocardial fibrosis can occur causing arrhythmias. Systolic dysfunction occurs late, and it is a sign of end stage disease.

Clinical features

Three cardinal symptoms of significant AS are angina, syncope, and dyspnea.

Angina occurs in the absence of CAD due to relative ischemia of increased LV myocardial mass. Since degenerative AS is a disease of old age, a majority of the patients also have CAD. On the whole, this is an early symptom.

Syncope occurs due to reduced cerebral perfusion. It is frequently induced by vasodilation or exercise. It is an indication of a progressive disease and warrants urgent surgery.

Occasionally, patients with severe AS develop gastrointestinal bleeding due to angiodysplasias that are very difficult to treat. This is due to shear stress, induced platelet aggregation, and acquired von Willebrand syndrome.

Dyspnea due to heart failure is a late symptom. Occasionally, a change in rhythm like atrial fibrillation can tip the balance in an otherwise stable patient with minimal symptoms. Congestive biventricular heart failure is a sign of impending death. These patients need urgent surgery soon after the cardiac investigations and optimization of heart failure. The survival of patients decreases as symptoms progress, thus early surgery is preferable.[4,5]

Physical examination shows a small volume pulse and an ejection systolic murmur frequently radiating to the carotids.[6] Therefore, older patients will need carotid studies to assess significant disease.

Clinical tests

Electrocardiogram (ECG) usually shows LV hypertrophy and may also show ST segment depression as a sign of systolic strain. Echocardiography is the investigation of choice for assessing the severity and progression of AS. The echocardiography gives a picture of valve mobility, fibrosis, and calcification. Frequently, it is also possible to discern whether the valve is bicuspid or tricuspid, though it is very difficult in severely calcified valves. Doppler measurement calculates the velocity and the gradient of blood flow, aortic valve area, and the dimensionless index (DI). The DI takes into consideration additional factors for accurate diagnosis. A valve area index less than 1.0cm^2/m^2 is considered severe stenosis as described in Table 1.[7] The DI gives the relative valve size in relation to the LV outflow area, a ratio of 0.25 is considered severe.

Table 1: Aortic stenosis classification

Indicator	Mild	Moderate	Severe
Velocity of jet (m/sec)	<3.0	3.0 to 4.0	>4.0
Mean gradient (mm of Hg)	<25	25 to 40	>40
Area of valve (cm^2)	>1.5	1.0 to 1.5	<1.0
Valve area index (cm^2/m^2)			<0.6

Further assessment of other valves, especially the mitral valve, LV hypertrophy, diastolic function, and systolic function are all important to calculate the risk of surgery. In patients with a severely diseased valve and low gradient mostly likely due to impaired LV function, dobutamine echocardiography unmasks the gradient and gives an indication of LV function recovery after surgery. Cardiac catheterization is performed to assess the coronary arteries and, in specialized centers, to measure right heart hemodynamics accurately.[7]

Surgical treatment

Aortic valve replacement (AVR) is the only therapy for symptomatic AS, and surgery has shown to have excellent results.[8] AVR is also considered in cases of (1) if the patient has severe stenosis with non-specific symptoms and is undergoing a high-risk non-cardiac surgery, (2) if the patient has associated severe CAD and needs treatment, or (3) if the patient has LV dysfunction or dilation. Significant improvement in the quality of life occurs even in elderly patients.[9,10]

There are only a few choices available for AVR depending on the patient's age and their lifestyle, as well as the expertise of the surgeon. A mechanical prosthesis lasts one's lifetime but requires life-long anticoagulation. Recent advances in prosthesis have significantly reduced the required level of anticoagulation without increasing the risk of thrombosis and bleeding.[11-14] They are an appropriate choice for patients below 65 years old, and in some cases 70 years old in the absence of other concomitant disease.[15] The younger patients, especially below the age of 50, who are very active and dislike anticoagulation may choose the Ross procedure in which the patient's own pulmonary trunk with the valve (autograft) is used to replace the aortic valve.[16] The pulmonary trunk is replaced with a homograft. At least 20% will need reoperation in 10 years. The valve function is as good as a normal aortic valve and there are no associated thrombo-embolic or infective complications. On the other end of the spectrum, patients older than 70 years, and slightly younger patients who need concomitant CABG or have a reduced life expectancy can do well with a tissue valve.[17] The mechanical valves available are bi-leaflet disc valves made of pyrolite carbon, and the tissue valves are either porcine or bovine pericardial valves. Homografts have similar longevity as other tissue valves and are frequently used in atrioventricular endocarditis with annular abscesses.

Recent advances in AVR

Percutaneous transfemoral or transapical AVRs are new advances. The recently completed PARTNER trial (Placement of Aortic Transcatheter Valve) showed the feasibility and safety of the procedure leading to FDA approval.[18] At present, it is available for calcific tricuspid valve AS patients who are high risk by standard techniques due to comorbidities or surgical difficulties. The procedure is not approved for bicuspid valve and aortic regurgitation. The procedure has acceptable survival rates with higher stroke risks. The results are improving as surgeons become more experienced. Percutaneous balloon aortic valvotomy (PBAV) is performed very rarely for re-compensation of a decompensated heart before the definitive procedure of a conventional or transcatheter AVR (Figure 3).[19]

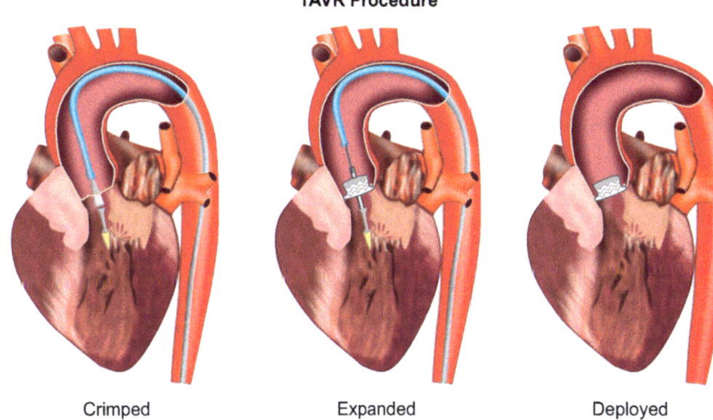

Figure 3: TAVR Procedure

Aortic Regurgitation

Aortic regurgitation (AR) occurs due to scarring and contraction of the valve leaflets or due to aortic annular dilation.[1,2] The causes of AR are rheumatic heart disease, bicuspid aortic valve, endocarditis, and aorto-annular ectasia both in isolation or as a part of a connective tissue disorder (e.g., Marfan's syndrome, Ehlers Danlos syndrome, rheumatoid arthritis, or aortic dissection). The natural history and operative survival depend on symptoms and etiology.[20]

The disease progresses with decreasing coaptation of valve leaflets and progressive regurgitation. The LV end-diastolic volume and pressure increase. At later stages, the ventricular systolic function deteriorates leading to severe heart failure and pulmonary hypertension.

Clinical features

Preservation of systolic function, in spite of ventricular enlargement, leads to an absence of symptoms in chronic AR. This sometimes lasts for several years, even in the presence of severe leakage. In acute onset regurgitation due to aortic dissection or endocarditis, there is no time for compensation and patients frequently present in cardiogenic shock and pulmonary edema. The main symptoms in chronic AR include gradual dyspnea and tiredness. Symptoms of syncope and angina may occur due to severe aortic run-off. Congestive heart failure is a late development.

Wide pulse pressure and a bounding pulse are characteristic of AR. The main auscultatory finding is a long, decrescendo diastolic murmur at the right sternal border and left second intercostal space. The severity of AR is assessed by color Doppler by measuring the regurgitant volume and width. Coronary angiography is performed in high-risk patients with a relevant history. Reassessment of volume on a regular basis is imperative in asymptomatic patients so that surgery can be offered in a timely manner before the development of LV dysfunction.[21,22] More accurate measurements of ventricular and regurgitant volumes and follow-up can also be performed using cardiac magnetic resonance imaging (MRI).[23]

Surgical treatment

AR patients who are symptomatic are referred for valve surgery and those who are asymptomatic, but with severe AR, are frequently treated with vasodilators and occasionally nifedipine.[24,25] This medication reduces the regurgitant volume and preserves systolic function for a while. In the absence of reliable follow-up, it is better to advise surgery before LV dysfunction develops insidiously. In the presence of normal or repairable valve leaflets, valve preservation is possible. Therefore, early referral to surgery is the best option. Severe AR with a LV diameter greater than 55 mm or a LV ejection fraction less than 50 are indications for surgery in patients with reliable follow-up. Mechanical AVRs are recommended in patients younger than 70 years old and tissue valves are recommended in patients older than 70 years. Younger patients can have tissue valve implantation if there is contraindication for Coumadin, if they have concomitant disease, or if they have comorbid factors that may reduce their survival.

AV repair should be considered should be considered in all patients with reasonably preserved leaflet tissue.[26] This is usually possible in the majority of patients with aorto-annular ectasia, aortic root aneurysm, aortic valve perforation, and valve prolapse. It is possible to replace the ascending aorta and preserve the aortic valve in patients with mild to moderate AR.[27-29] The Ross procedure is another option, especially in young patients, but it is a complex procedure involving two valves. It can be performed in selected patients with AR in centers with expertise and good follow-up care. It is important for healthy people who are less than 70-year-old and receiving tissue valves to be aware of the possibility of reoperation in the future. The patient's input is very important in the selection of the valve type, irrespective of age. Patients with a bicuspid aortic valve and with aortic root dilation represents a specific surgical challenge, many of whom require valvular surgery to replace or repair the aortic root.[30-32]

Mitral Stenosis

Mitral stenosis (MS) is the most common heart valve disease in developing countries due to the prevalence of rheumatic valvular disease. Rheumatic inflammation leads to significant scarring of mitral leaflets, subvalvular chordae, and papillary muscles.[33] This results in an almost tubular stenosis of the mitral apparatus and a small LV due to scarring and in some cases calcification. Other causes of MS are degenerative diseases, annular calcification, congenital malformations, carcinoid syndrome, left atrial myxoma, or thrombus mimicking valve obstruction.

Pathophysiology, disease progress, and complications

There is negligible or no gradient across the mitral valve between the left atrium and the LV during diastole in normal people. When the mitral valve orifice narrows approximately 50% from the normal of 4-5cm^2 to 2.5 cm^2, it is still considered a clinically mild stenosis and there are no symptoms.[7] This is further elaborated in Table 2.[7]

Table 2: Grading severity of MV stenosis

Indicator	Mild	Moderate	Severe
Mean gradient (mm of Hg)	<5	5 to 10	>10
Pulmonary artery systolic pressure (mm of Hg)	<30	30 to 50	>50
Area of valve (cm^2)	>1.5	1.0 to 1.5	<1.0

Progression of stenosis leads to increased left atrial pressure and pulmonary venous hypertension. This is followed eventually by pulmonary arterial hypertension and right heart failure. Functional tricuspid regurgitation occurs. Other complications are atrial fibrillation due to scarring and left atrial thrombus formation leading to systemic embolization.

Diagnosis

Patients develop classic symptoms due to high left atrial pressure, pulmonary venous congestion, and pulmonary edema. These symptoms are dyspnea, paroxysmal nocturnal dyspnea, and orthopnea. In severe cases, multiple syndromes occur such as hoarseness and dysphagia due to left atrial and pulmonary artery dilation compressing the recurrent laryngeal nerve and the esophagus. Hemoptysis may occur due to pulmonary hypertension and right heart failure. Ultimately, in late stages the patients develop severe congestive heart failure characterized by pulmonary as well as peripheral edema.

In otherwise asymptomatic patients, the compensatory mechanisms get overwhelmed in situations of stress, exertion, infection, pregnancy, and the onset of atrial tachyarrhythmias leading to severe acute symptoms of heart failure. MS in pregnant patients is an extremely difficult situation to treat and its occurrence is fairly common in developing countries.[34,35]

Physical signs of MS are classic.[36] The LV is small. There are signs of right ventricular hypertrophy. On auscultation, there is low-pitched, mid-late diastolic murmur with presystolic accentuation and an opening snap. In extreme cases, there may only be a few signs due to severely reduced flow. Congestive heart failure leads to signs of peripheral edema, hepatomegaly, and jugular venous pressure elevation.

Investigations

There are characteristic findings on chest radiograph showing an enlarged left atrium as a ball shaped shadow within the shadow of the heart, and large pulmonary artery leading to a straight left border known as mitralization. The large left atrium may also displace the left main bronchus and esophagus. Calcification of the mitral valve can be seen, especially in the lateral view.

Echocardiography with Doppler is the best tool for assessment and decision making in MS.[37] The presence of calcification, leaflet mobility, subvalvular fusion of chords, appearance of commissures, and left atrial thrombi are important morphological characters to be identified before deciding to perform catheter based or open surgical management of MS. Other factors that are assessed include the nature of the tricuspid valve and the severity of pulmonary hypertension.

Treatment

Patients with mitral valve disease and mild MS require careful, yearly follow-up with clinical examination and tests. Younger patients are advised to receive prophylaxis for rheumatic fever and infective endocarditis. Symptomatic patients with moderate or severe MS should be considered for a surgical procedure. Occasionally, it may be necessary to provoke signs and symptoms by exercise or using dobutamine if there is no correlation between severity of symptoms and stenosis. Valvuloplasty is indicated if there is an elevated mitral gradient of >15 mmHg, pulmonary systolic pressure >60 mmHg, and wedge pressure of >25 mmHg.[38]

Percutaneous Balloon Valvuloplasty (PMBV):[39]

Surgically closed mitral valvotomy was one of the most common and successful operations performed for MS. This was done through left thoracotomy and the mitral valve was dilated using a Tubb's dilator through the LV apex. The procedure is now replaced with percutaneous procedures using catheters.

This is a catheter-based single or double balloon technique. The usual approach is by perforating the atrial septum to move from the right atrium to the left side. The balloon is positioned at the mitral valve using echocardiographic imaging and then it is dilated forcibly (Figure 4).[40] The valve is expected to split along the commissures. The valve leaflets need to be mobile, non-calcified, and commissural fusion must be minimal to achieve good success without producing mitral regurgitation. It is important to make sure that there is no thrombus in the left atrium by either transthoracic or transesophageal echocardiogram. Mild mitral regurgitation is not a contraindication for valvuloplasty.[41] Overall, success of the procedure is 80% to 95% with a mortality of 1% to 2 %.[42,43] Long-term success depends on careful selection.[42,43]

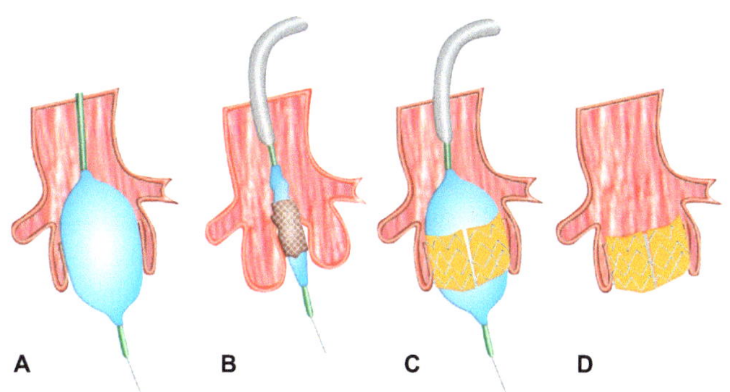

Figure 4: Balloon valvuloplasty treating mitral stenosis

Open mitral commissurotomy

Patients who are not perfect candidates for balloon valvuloplasty are referred for open mitral valvotomy and repair procedures. The surgery is performed using total cardiopulmonary bypass through midline sternotomy and left atriotomy exposure. The right thoracotomy approach with minimal incision also provides good exposure and is more cosmetic. The valve is carefully examined. Valvotomy in rheumatic MS is done by debriding any calcium, identifying the commissures by analyzing the attachment of the chordae, and dividing it with a sharp scalpel. It is also possible to release the subvalvar fusion. The left atrial appendage is removed, and an additional MAZE procedure can be performed if the patient is in atrial fibrillation.[44] The results of open surgery are better in severe valvular diseases and in older patients. Multiple techniques may be necessary including annuloplasty, leaflet extension, and chordal extension resulting in longer durability in open procedures.[45-49]

Mitral valve replacement

Mitral valve replacement (MVR) is necessary in many cases with severe calcific mitral valve disease with subvalvular fusion and/or moderate MR. Degeneration of tissue prosthesis is more rapid in mitral position, thus the mechanical valve is the prosthesis of choice in patients less than 70 years old and in otherwise good health, especially if they need anticoagulation for chronic atrial fibrillation with no contraindication. The mechanical mitral valve requires higher levels of anticoagulation than the aortic valve. Older patients can have tissue prosthesis. It is important to preserve the chordal apparatus and the posterior leaflet to prevent late LV dilation during valve replacement. This may not be possible in some rheumatic cases due to severe fibrosis of the chordal apparatus that must be released. Artificial chords with 4'0' Gortex are the best option in these cases to prevent LV dilation in the long-term.

Mitral Regurgitation

Etiology and pathophysiology

Mitral valve leaflet coaptation occurs due to a complex interplay of ventricular muscle, chordae, annulus, and leaflets. Problems with any one of these components will cause the valve to leak. Mitral regurgitation (MR) is more common than MS in the western world due to it having multiple etiologies. Common causes of MR include myxomatous disease, degenerative valve disease, rheumatic disease, endocarditis, collagen vascular disease, and drugs.[50-52] These diseases affect the valve leaflets and the annulus. MR is also caused by LV and annular dilation resulting from ischemic and non-ischemic cardiomyopathy. Acute severe MR may occur due to rupture of a papillary muscle due to ischemia as well as due to endocarditis and late myxomatous disease. LV diastolic volume increases eventually leading to systolic dysfunction and finally heart failure. In acute MR, the LV preload and pressure increase dramatically with reduced forward stroke volume leading to low output heart failure.

Clinical features and diagnosis

Acute MR leads to pulmonary edema and cardiogenic shock. Otherwise, MR is usually a chronic disease with slow progression of left heart failure symptoms that is medically manageable. Patients will have signs of an enlarged LV and a pansystolic murmur that radiates to the axilla.

Echocardiography is used to assess the severity of MR, mobility of each leaflet, restriction or prolapse of leaflet segments, and size of the annulus and LV.[53,54] A doppler study calculates the regurgitant volume and shows the direction of the flow. It may be necessary to perform transesophageal echocardiogram to pinpoint the nature of the lesion, as it is very important to know for sure whether the valve is repairable and to plan the technique.

Treatment

Patients with moderate MR remain asymptomatic unless associated with concomitant problems. Patients with severe MR may also remain asymptomatic with proper medical treatment with vasodilators for a long time, but eventually all the patients with severe MR will need surgery.[55] Earlier surgery in this group of patients may improve chances of repair and may prevent further complications.[56] Regular follow-up measuring the LV diameter and function is needed to catch issues before deterioration occurs.

Assessment of MR severity is performed by echocardiography and Doppler measurements as shown in Table 3.[7]

Table 3: Mitral regurgitation grading

Indicator	Mild	Moderate	Severe
Grade of angiograph	1+	2+	3 to 4+
Size of jet			Wall impinging jet of any size
Area of jet/area of left atria (%)	<20	20 to 40	>40
Volume of regurgitant (ml/beat)	<30	30 to 59	>60
Fraction of regurgitant (%)	<30	30 to 49	>50
Area of requrgitant orifice (cm^2)	<0.20	0.20 to 0.39	>0.40

Surgery

Mitral valve repair offers both short- and long-term benefits for patients with any type of MR, and it is possible in about 90% of patients. In rheumatic valve disease combined with fibrosis, the procedure requires a complex technique and there is less durability. Preservation of chordal attachment to papillary muscles leads to good LV function and normal LV size. This must be done even in valve replacements.

Repair techniques are based on the surgical classification of types of regurgitation as described in Table 4.

Table 4: Carpentier classification of types of MR and treatment principles

Type	Pathology	Repair procedure
Type 1	Normal leaflet motion Annular dilation or perforation	Restrictive full annuloplasty Patch closure of perforation
Type II	Excess leaflet motion Chordal or papillary muscle lengthening or rupture Leaflet prolapse	Chordal shortening Chordal transfer Artificial chords Leaflet resection Annuloplasty
Type III	Restricted leaflet motion due to rheumatic and ischemic restricted opening and closure Sub-vulvar scarring	Leaflet enlargement by patch Chordal release or transposition Specially shaped semi-rigid annuloplasty

The most common lesion in degenerative MR is posterior leaflet prolapse. This can be corrected by resection, plication, or neo-chords with Gortex sutures followed by partial or complete annuloplasty.[58] Similar procedures can be performed on the anterior leaflet as well. The mortality rate of repair is less than 1% with excellent, event-free survival long-term. A majority of the patients with ischemic MR are treated with complete annuloplasty.[59,60] Patients with severe LV dysfunction and symptoms can be treated with mitral annuloplasty and aggressive medical management of heart failure.[61]

MV replacement with a mechanical valve is done in patients younger than 70 years of age and replacement with a tissue valve for older patients. Again, the selection of the valve is based on patient preference and expected survival based on comorbid factors. Tissue valve replacement is usually done with bovine pericardial or porcine valves. In cases of ischemic MR, mitral valve repair has a high recurrence rate, and it may be prudent in difficult cases to replace the valves by preserving all the chordae.[62] The tissue valve in mitral position is less durable than aortic valves. One of the additional surgical techniques devised to improve success of repair was to place an edge-to-edge suture between anterior and posterior leaflets to provide added strength.[63] At present, the same concept is being applied in a percutaneous approach to fix the mitral valve. In this case, clips are used to bring the edges together in the middle of the orifice. Patients who are not candidates for surgery can be selected for this procedure.[64,65] A multidisciplinary approach to treating MR will be needed in the future for making the right choice of treatment in some cases.[66]

Tricuspid Valve Disease

The most common problem of TV is annular dilation and regurgitation caused by pulmonary hypertension and RV dilation from severe mitral or aortic valve disease.[67] In developing countries tricuspid disease is also caused by direct involvement by rheumatic disease leading to stenosis and regurgitation. Carcinoid syndrome and some collagen vascular diseases also affect it. Echocardiography and the decision to repair the valve must be done before surgery under normal loading conditions as the perioperative vasodilation may lead to under-estimation of valve leak. Mild to moderate regurgitation, with minimal pulmonary hypertension will resolve after left sided valve surgery. Infective endocarditis in intravenous drug users can be treated by tricuspid valvulectomy if the valve is beyond repair. It is always preferable to repair and conserve the tricuspid valve, as the morbidity is very low.[68] Repair is frequently achieved by annuloplasty. This is done after placing circumferential sutures. No sutures placed in the area of the septal leaflet near the coronary sinus to avoid injury to the conduction system. This area is known as Triangle of Koch. In case of irreparable valve, replacement with either mechanical or tissue valve leads to good long-term survival.[69] There are many Ebstein's tricuspid valve malformations that can be corrected by repair.[70]

THORACIC AORTIC DISEASE

The most common surgical diseases of the ascending and descending thoracic aorta are aortic dissections and aortic aneurysms. There are some rare forms of aortitis such as Takayasu's disease, which usually leads to occlusion of arch vessels.

There are two types of aortic dissection. A (Type A) involves the ascending aorta and the arch of the aorta. B (Type B) involves the descending thoracic aorta. Type I is a surgical emergency. It leads to dissection into the sinuses involving the coronary ostia and the aortic valve. The dissection frequently extends into the entire aorta and arch vessels. Death usually occurs in 24 hours due to rupture of the aorta into the pericardium, or coronary dissection and ischemia. Severe acute AR can also occur.[71]

Patients usually arrive at the emergency room with tearing chest pain radiating to the back, frequently mimicking a myocardial infarction. A contrast chest CT is the best diagnostic investigation for these patients. Occasionally, transesophageal echocardiogram can be used. Patients must be rushed to the operating room after initial management of blood pressure and resuscitation. The majority of patients have an ascending aorta replacement with a prosthetic graft and resuspension of the aortic valve. The distal open anastomosis is usually done under hypothermic circulatory arrest. Right subclavian or axillary cannulation is frequently used for continuing cerebral perfusion during hypothermia because it gives additional time for complex repair of the arch if needed.

Type II descending thoracic dissections are usually treated medically by reducing blood pressure and heart rate with beta-blockers. Surgery is warranted in patients with visceral ischemia, dilation, or rupture.

Aortic aneurysm of the ascending aorta can occur without any valve involvement, or it can be associated with a bicuspid valve or Marfan's syndrome. The usual procedures performed include aortic replacement with or without concomitant valve repair or replacement.[72,73] The diameter of >5 cm is an indication for surgery. In patients with suspected medial or connective tissue disease, 4.5 cm is the cut-off, especially when the patient needs aortic valve surgery.

A composite aortic root replacement is performed when there is also an aortic sinus dilation with valved conduits, either mechanical or tissue. The coronary ostia are anastomosed to the conduit and the distal anastomosis of the aortic graft is performed by either an open or closed technique depending on the extent of the aneurysm. Axillary cannulation or selective cerebral perfusion is needed if the circulatory arrest is expected to exceed 30 minutes. Debranching replacement of arch vessels and complete stenting of the aorta is possible with or without cardiopulmonary bypass depending on the extent of the disease.[74] Otherwise, the proximal arch anastomosis can be performed during circulatory arrest of 15 to 20 minutes and the graft can be re-cannulated to restart circulation.

In cases of aortic root destruction due to endocarditis or abscesses, aortic root replacement with either a homograft or a porcine root is required.

A unique condition known as aneurysm of sinus of valsalva occurs rarely in the west, but more common in the eastern hemisphere.[75,76] It commonly involves the non-coronary sinus. This can be congenital or acquired. The complications include free rupture, rupture into the right atrium or right ventricle causing acute left to right shunt and severe heart failure, infection, and AR. Treatment is usually resection and patch, or total replacement of the sinus(s) or root of the aorta. The valves can be preserved if the leaflets appear normal; otherwise, composite root replacement must be performed.

Descending thoracic aneurysmal disease can be treated with open surgery with or without cardiopulmonary bypass support. Recently, many of these cases are being treated with intravascular stents. Important considerations with these procedures are (1) protecting the spinal cord as many of the spinal arteries arise from the intercostal arteries and (2) that the blood supply to the spinal cord is segmental.

Infective endocarditis:

Infective endocarditis is a complex disease that is very difficult to treat, thus an interdisciplinary approach is needed to make decisions regarding appropriate medical treatment and timing of surgery. The decision frequently involves cardiologists, microbiologists, surgeons, neurologists, radiologists, and infectious disease specialists. Prevention of endocarditis is important during invasive procedures especially in patients with underlying cardiac disease.[77] Complex and extensive surgical procedures are described to treat infected valves and associated complications.[78-81]

REFERENCES

1. Zhang W, Mondo C, Okello E, et al. Presenting features of newly diagnosed rheumatic heart disease patients in Mulago hospital: a pilot study. Cardiovasc J afr. 2013 Mar;24(2):28-33.
2. Sun J, Meng DM, Jiang N, Wang LQ. Zhonghua Yi Xue Za Zhi. Histopathological features of degenerative aortic valve and its mechanisms. 2013 Jan 22;93(4):280-4. (Chinese).
3. Martin M, Munoz JP, Pichel IA, et al. Aortic stenosis: A complex, atherosclerosis-like, multifactorial disease. Int J Cardiol. 2013 Apr 17. (Epub ahead of print).
4. Carabello BA. The symptom of aortic stenosis: a step closer to understanding the cause. JACC Cardiovasc Imaging. 2013 Feb;6(2):147-9.
5. Marumoto A, Nakamura Y, Kishimoto Y, Saiki M, Nishimura M. The optimal timing of aortic valve replacement in elderly patients with severe aortic stenosis. Surg Today. 2013 Feb 6 (Epub ahead of print).
6. Helms AS, Bach DS. Heart valve disease. Prim care. 2013 Mar;40(1):91-108.
7. Bonow RO, Carabello BA, Chatterjee K, et al. 2008 focused update of ACC/AHA 2006 guidelines for the management of patients with valvular heart disease. J Am Coll Cardiol 2008;52 (13):e1-e142.
8. Shahian DM, He X, Jacobs JP, et al. The society of thoracic surgeons isolated aortic valve replacement (AVR) composite score: a report of the STS quality measurement task force. Ann Thorac Surg. 2012 Dec;94(6):2166-71.
9. Lancellotti P, Magne J, Donal E, et al. Clinical outcomes in symptomatic aortic stenosis. J Am Coll Cardiol. 2012;59:235-43.
10. Shan L, Saxena A, MaMahon R, Wilson A, Newcomb A. A systematic review on the quality of life benefits after aortic valve replacement in the elderly. J Thorac Cardiovasc Surg. 2013 May;145(5):1173-89.
11. Puskas J, Nichols D, Gerdisch M, et al. Reduced anticoagulation after mechanical aortic valve replacement: Interim results from the PROACT randomized FDA IDE trial. Presented AATS May 6, 2013.
12. Van Nooten GJ, Caes F, Francois K, et al. Twenty years' single center experience with mechanical heart valves: a critical review of anticoagulation policy. J Heart Valve Dis. 2012 Jan;21(1):88-98.
13. Chambers JB, Pomar JL, Mestres CA, Palatianos GM. Clinical event rates with the ON-X bileaflet mechanical heart valve: a multicenter experience with follow-up to 12 years. J Thorac Cardiovasc Surg. 2013 Feb;145(2):420-4.
14. Bourguignon T, Bergoend E, Mirza A, et al. Risk factors for valve-related complications after mechanical heart valve replacement in 505 patients with long-term follow up. J Heart Valve Dis. 2011 Nov;20(6):673-80.
15. Weber A, Noureddine H, Englberger L, et al. Ten-

year comparison of pericardial tissue valves versus mechanical prostheses for aortic valve replacement in patients younger than 60 years of age. J Thorac Cardiovasc Surg. 2012 Nov;144(5):1075-83.

16. Charitos EI, Takkenberg JJ, Hanke T, et al. Reoperations on the pulmonary autograft and pulmonary homograft after the Ross procedure: An update on the German Dutch Ross Registry. J Thorac Cardiovasc Surg. 2012 Oct;144(4):813-21.
17. Yap KH, Murphy R, Devbhandari M, Venkateswaran R. Aortic valve replacement: is porcine or bovine valve better? Interact Cardiovasc Thorac Surg. 2013 Mar;16(3)361-73.
18. Bohula May EA, Faxon D. Transcatheter aortic valve replacement: History and current status. Trends Cardiovasc Med. 2013 Jan 30. Pii: S1050-1738(12)00441-0.
19. Saia F, Marrozzini C, Moretti C, et al. The role of percutaneous balloon aortic valvuloplasty as a bridge for transcatheter aortic valve implantation. Eurintervention. 2011 Oct 30;7(6):723-9.
20. Honda S, Kitai T, Okada Y, et al. Impact of aortic regurgitation on the prognosis of severe aortic stenosis. Heart. 2012 Nov;98(21):1591-4.
21. Rahimatoola SH. The year in valvular heart disease. J Am Coll Cardiol. 2012 Jul 10;60(2):85=95.
22. Ren X, Banki NM. Classic hemodynamic findings of severe aortic regurgitation. Circulation. 2012 Jul 17;126(3):e28-9.
23. Myerson SG, d'Arcy J, Mohiaddin R, et al. Aortic regurgitation quantification using cardiovascular magnetic resonance: association with clinical outcome. Circulation. 2012 Sep 18;126(12):1452-60.
24. Scheuble A, Vahanian A. Aortic insufficiency: defining the role of pharmacotherapy. Am j Cardiovasc Drugs. 2005:5(2):113-20.
25. Taniguchi K, Sawa Y. Contemporary reviews by surgeon: timing of operation for chronic aortic regurgitation. Gen Thorac Cardiovasc Surg. 2012 Nov;60(11):735-43.
26. David TE. Aortic valve sparing operations: a review. Korean J Thorac Cardiovasc Surg. 2012 Aug;45(4):205-12.
27. Beyersdorf F, Rylski B. Current state of the reimplantation technique (DAVID operation): surgical details and results. HSR Poc Intensive Care Cardiovasc Anesth. 2012;4(2): 73-6.
28. Kari FA, Liang DH, Escobar Kvitting JP, et al. Tirone David valve-sparing aortic root replacement and cusp repair for bicuspid aortic valve disease. J Thorac Cardiovasc Surg. 2013 Mar;145(3 supp):S35-40.
29. Siyamek N. Management of bicuspid aortic valve with or without involvement of ascending aorta and aortic root. J Cardiovasc Surg (Torino). 2012 Nov 8.
30. Siyamek N. Management of bicuspid aortic valve with or without involvement of ascending aorta and aortic root. J Cardiovasc Surg. 2012 Nov 8. (Epub ahead of print).
31. Balistreri CR, Pisano C, Candore G, et al. Focus on the unique mechanisms involved in thoracic aortic aneurysm formation in bicuspid aortic valve vs tricuspid aortic valve patients: clinical implications of a pilot study. Eur J Cardiovasc Surg. 2012 Dec 17 (Epub ahead of print).
32. Opotowsky AR, Perlstein T, Landzberg MJ, et al. A shifting approach to management of the thoracic aorta in bicuspid aortic valve. J Thorac Cardiovasc Surg. 2012 Nov 9 pii: S0022-5223(12)01333-5.
33. Remenyi B, Wilson N, Steer A, et al. World heart federation criteria for echocardiographic diagnosis of rheumatic heart disease—an evidence based guideline. Nat Rev Cardiol. 2012 Feb 28;9(5):297-309.
34. Subbaiah M, Sharma V, Kumar S, et al. Heart disease in pregnancy: Cardiac and obstetric outcomes. Arch Gynecol Obstet. 2013 Feb 2.
35. Kannan M, Vijayanand B. Mitral stenosis and pregnancy: Current concepts in anesthetic practice. Indian J Anaesth. 2010 Sep;54(5):439-44.
36. Glancy DL. Mitral stenosis: I. Anatomical, physiological, and clinical considerations. J La State Med Soc. 2003 Mar-Apr;155(2):91-5.
37. Mirabel M, Celermajer DS, Ferreira B, et al. Screening for rheumatic heart disease: evaluation of a simplified echocardiography based approach. Eur Heart J Cardiovasc Imaging. 2012 Dec;13(12):1024-8.
38. Picano E, Pibarot P, Lancellotti P, Monin JL, Bonow RO. The emerging role of exercise testing and stress echocardiography in valvular heart disease. J AM Coll Cardiol. 2009 Dec 8;54(24):2251-60.
39. Cubeddu RJ, Palacios IF. Percutaneous techniques for mitral valve disease. Cardiol Clin. 2010 Feb;28(1):139-53.
40. Das P, Prendergast B. Imaging in mitral stenosis: assessment before, during and after percutaneous balloon mitral valvuloplasty. Expert Rev Cardiovasc Ther. 2003 Nov;1(4):549-57.
41. Turgeman Y, Feldman A, Suleiman K, et al. Mild rheumatic mitral regurgitation in the presence of

dominant stenotic pliable valve: an echocardiographic structural valve analysis in patients undergoing balloon vavuloplasty. Isr Med Assoc J. 2012 Oct 14(10):629-32.

42. Reichart DT, Sodian R, Zenker R, et al. Long-term (<50 years) results of patients after mitral valve commissurotomy—a single center experience. J Thorac Cardiovasc Surg. 2012 Apr;143(4 suppl):S96-8.
43. Anadolu Kardiyol Derg. Acute and long-term follow-up results of percutaneous mitral balloon valvuloplasty: a single center study. 2011 Sep;11(6):515-20.
44. Kim GS, Lee CH, Kim JB et al. Echocardiographic evaluation of mitral durability following valve repair in rheumatic valve disease: Impact of Maze procedure. J Thorac Cardiovasc Surg. 2012 Nov 20 pii S0022-5223912001247-0.
45. Severino ES, Petrucci O, Vilarinho KA, et al. Late outcomes of mitral repair in rheumatic patients. Rev Bras Cir Cardiovasc 2011 Oct-Dec;26(4):559-64.
46. Chotivatanapong T, Lerdsomboon P, Sungkahapong V. Rheumatic mitral valve repair: experience of 221 cases from Central Chest Institute of Thailand. J Med Assoc Thai. 2012 Aug;95 Suppl 8:S51-7.
47. Geldenhuys A, Koshy JJ, Human PA, et al. Rheumatic mitral repair versus replacement in a threshold country: the impact of commissural fusion. J Heart Valve Dis. 2012 Jul21(4):424-32.
48. Kalangos A. The rheumatic mitral valve and repair techniques in children. Semi Thorac Cardiovasc Surg Pediatr Card Surg Annu. 2012. 15(1) 80-7.
49. Dillon J, Yakub MA, Nordin MN. Leaflet reconstruction in rheumatic mitral valve reconstruction. Eur J Cardiothorac Surg. 2013 Feb 13.
50. Nishimura RA, Carabello BA, Faxon DP, et al. ACC/AHA 2008 guideline update on valvular heart disease: focused update on infective endocarditis. Catheter Cardiovasc Interv. 2008 Sep 1;72(3):E1-12.
51. Boudoulas H. Etiology of valvular heart disease. Expert Rev Cardiovasc Ther. 20033 Nov;1(4):523-32.
52. Chockalingam A, Gnanavelu G, Elangovan S, Chochalingam V. Clinical spectrum of chronic rheumatic heart disease in India. J Heart Valve Dis. 2003 Sep;12(5):577-81.
53. Silbiger JJ. Anatomy, mechanics, and pathophysiology of the mitral annulus. Am Heart J. 2012 Aug;164(2):163-76.
54. Castillo JG, Solis J, Gonzalez-Pinto A, Adams DH. Surgical echocardiography of the mitral valve. Rev Esp Cardiol. 2011;64(12):1169-1181.
55. Bonow RO. Chronic mitral regurgitation and aortic regurgitation: have indications for surgery changed? J Am Coll Cardiol. 2013 Feb 19;61(7):693-701.
56. De Bonis M, Bolling SF. Mitral valve surgery: wait and see vs. early operation. Eur Heart J. 2013 Jan;34(1):13-19a.
57. Park KJ, Woo JS, Yi JH, Park JY. Outcomes of mitral valve repair: Quandrangular resection versus chordal replacement. Korean J Thorac Cardiovasc Surg. 2013 May-Jun;70(3):318-25.
58. Kshettry VR, Aranki SF. Current trends in mitral valve repair techniques in North America. J Heart Valve Dis. 2012 Nov;21(6):690-5.
59. Chan KM, Punjabi PP, Flather M, et al. Coronary artery bypass surgery with or without mitral valve annuloplasty in moderate functional regurgitation: final results of the Randomized Ischemic Mitral Evaluation (RIME) trial. Circulation 2012 Nov 20;126(21):2502-10.
60. Timek TA, Miller DC. Another multidisciplinary look at ischemic mitral regurgitation. Semin Thorac Cardiovasc Surg. 2011 Autumn,23(3):220-31.
61. Parker JA, Kenes LN, Ruckert J, Dahm M, Vahl CE. Outcome after mitral valve operations with depressed left ventricular function. Asian Cardiovasc Thorac Ann. 2012 Jun 20(3): 292-8.
62. Mitral valve replacement combined with coronary artery bypass graft surgery in patients with moderate-to-severe ischemic mitral regurgitation. Rev Port cardiol 2013 Feb;32(2): 131-7.
63. Maisano F, LaCanna G, Colombo A, Alfieri O. The evolution from surgery to percutaneous mitral valve interventions. J AM Coll Cardiol. 2011;58:2174-82.
64. De Bonis M, Lapenna E, Buzzatti N, et al. Can the edge-to-edge technique provide durable results when used to rescue patients with sub-optimal conventional mitral repair? Eur J Cardiothorac Surg. 2013 Feb 13 (Epub ahead of print).
65. Conradi L, Treede H, Rudolph V, et al. Surgical or percutaneous mitral valve repair for secondary mitral regurgitation: comparison of patient characteristics and clinical outcomes. Eur J Cardiothorac Surg. 2013 Feb 10 (Epub ahead of print).
66. Boronyak SM, Merryman WD. The once and future state of percutaneous mitral valve repair. Future Cardiol. 2012 Sep;8(5):779-93. Review.
67. Ariyoshi T, Hashizume K, Taniguchi S et al. Which type of secondary tricuspid regurgitation accompanying mitral valve disease should be surgically treated? Ann Thorac Cardiovasc Surg 2013 Jan 31.

68. Taylor JT, Chidsey G, Disalvo TG, Byrne JG, Maltais S. Contemporary management of tricuspid regurgitation: an updated clinical review. Cardiol rev. 2013 Feb 21.

69. Morimoto N, Matsushima S, Aoki M et al. Long-term results of bioprosthetic tricuspid valve replacement: an analysis of 25 years of experience. Gen Thorac Cardiovasc Surg. 2012 Dec 6.

70. Said SM, Burkhart HM, Dearani JA. Surgical management of congenital (non-Ebstein) tricuspid valve regurgitation. Semin Thorac cardiovasc Surg Pediatr Card Surg Annu. 2012;15(1):46-60.

71. Tolenaar JL, van Bogerijen GH, Eagle KA, Trimarchi S. Update in the management of aortic dissection. Curr Treat Options Cardiovasc Med. 2013 Jan 10.

72. Kallenbach K, Kojic D, Oezsoez M, et al. Treatment of ascending aortic aneurysms using different surgical techniques: A single-center experience with 548 patients. Eur J Cardiothorac Surg. 2013 Jan 7. (Epub ahead of print).

73. Etz CD, von Aspern K, Girrbach FF, et al. Long-term survival after composite mechanical aortic root replacement: A consecutive series of 448 cases. J Thorac Cardiovasc Surg. 2013 Mar; 1¢5(3 suppl):S41-7.

74. Urbanski PP, Raad M, Lenos A. Open aortic arch replacement in the era of endovascular techniques. Eur J Cardiothorac Surg. 2013 Feb 20.

75. Xin-Jin L, Xuan L, Bo P, et al. Modified Sakakibara classification system for ruptured sinus of Valsalva aneurysm. J Thorac Cardiovasc Surg. 2013 Jan 10 pii: S0022-5223(12)01643-1.

76. Guo HW, Xiong H, Xu JP, Wang XQ, Hu SS. A new and simple classification for sinus of Valsalva aneurysms and the corresponding surgical procedure. Eur J cardiothorac Surg. 2013 Jan 4.

77. Radfar L, Settle S, Movaffagh Y, Masood F. Antibiotic prophylaxis: a literature review. Compend Contin Educ Dent. 2013 Mar;34(3):E33-7.

78. Hoen B, Duval X. Clinical practice. Infective endocarditis. N Engl J Med. 2013 Apr 11;368(15):1425-33.

79. Sabe MA, Shrestha NK, Menon V. Contemporary drug treatment of infective endocarditis. A J Cardiovasc Drugs. 2013 May 3. (Epub ahead of print).

80. Byrne JG, Rezai K, Sanchez JA, et al. Surgical management of endocarditis: the society of thoracic surgeons clinical practice guideline.

81. Kabbani SS, Sabbagh NA, Kudsi AY, Nabhani F, Jamil H. Update on the mitral pulmonary autograft. Asian Cardiovasc Thorac Ann. 2011 Jun;19(3-4):253-9.

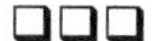

63

CHAPTER

Ischemic Heart Disease

Wickii T. Vigneswaran, MD, FACS, FCCP

ANATOMY OF CORONARY CIRCULATION

The number of branches, distribution, and size of coronary arteries is variable. The main right and left coronary arteries arise above the aortic cusps. The left ostium is located posteriorly, and the right ostium is located anteriorly. The left coronary artery supplies the anterior and anterolateral myocardium by the left anterior descending artery (LAD) and its diagonal branches. The left coronary artery also supplies the lateral and posterior-lateral myocardium by the circumflex artery and its obtuse marginal branches. The right coronary artery (RCA) supplies the right ventricular free wall, and the inferior and posterior-inferior left ventricular (LV) myocardium. Both arteries supply the septum. The atrioventricular node is supplied by the right coronary artery in the majority of cases. In general, the LAD is the most important artery, carrying nearly 50% of the blood flow to the heart. The main coronary arteries can have anomalous origins. The coronaries are mostly located on the epicardium and in some cases intra-myocardial. Coronary artery anomalies, frequently seen in adults, include branches of the left coronary artery arising from a separate ostium, a right main artery arising with the left, and a circumflex artery arising from the right. The arterial branches may course deep in the myocardium and can have just a bridge of myocardium over them. Coronary arteriovenous communications may occur.

The coronary veins have a more constant distribution. The posterior, middle, and great cardiac veins join the coronary sinus and drain into the right atrium. Very rarely will the patient have a superior vena cava (SVC) that communicates with the coronary sinus to drain into the right atrium.

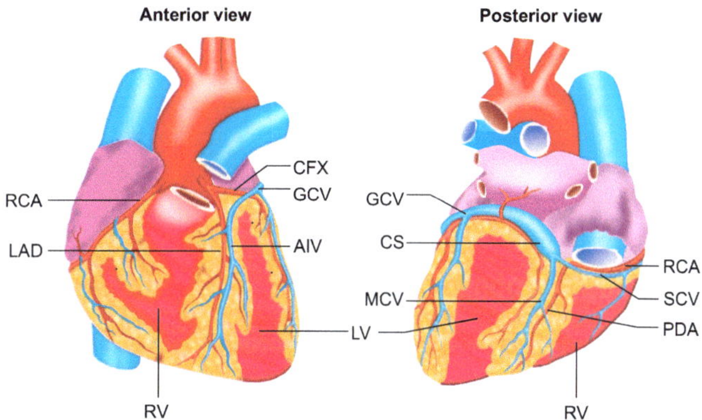

Figure 1: Anatomy of the coronary circulation

Clinical importance of coronary anatomy

The epicardial location of the coronary arteries make them amenable for surgery, but identification of the course is important. It is sometimes necessary to analyze the cause of symptoms when rare anomalies and disease co-exist. The region and the extent of myocardium supplied by an artery are also important, as they are all end-arteries. The LAD, circumflex, and RCA form the three main regions. The clinical pictures such as the size of infarction, presence of heart failure, A-V block, and mitral regurgitation can be interpreted by correlating the distribution of coronary arteries. It is also useful for prognosis.

The location of the coronary sinus opening in the right atrium is constant. Therefore, it can be easily cannulated for providing cardioplegia for myocardial protection and implantation of biventricular pacemakers for cardiac resynchronization therapy (CRT) in heart failure.

Physiology of coronary blood flow

Coronary filling occurs during diastole and is therefore dependent on aortic pressure and diastolic filling time.[1,2] Coronary circulation is extremely sensitive to endogenous and exogenous vasodilators and myocardial metabolism. Blood flow can increase to nearly 10-fold in response to exercise where oxygen extraction becomes very efficient.[3] Any reduction of blood flow significantly affects myocardial function regionally and globally. Significant vasodilation occurs in response to adenosine and nitric oxide.

Clinical importance of physiology

The sensitive nature of coronary physiology and blood flow is important, even in disease states. This property is utilized in testing for provocable ischemia using exercise or dipyridamole, and then measuring the fractional flow reserve (FFR) using adenosine. [4,5] This measurement unmasks the severity of stenosis by increasing the blood flow.[4,5] It also forms the basis for medical treatment of coronary artery disease (CAD) where reduced oxygen demand leads to symptom relief.

Pathology of obstructive CAD

Atherosclerosis is the most frequent coronary pathology. It is a diffuse endothelial disease and is progressive. Other infrequent causes of CAD in the developing world are syphilitic aortitis causing left main stenosis, Kawasaki disease causing diffuse CAD,[6,7] and coronary aneurysms.[8]

The severity of the disease in coronary arteries varies, it affects multiple areas and is more pronounced in proximal epicardial arteries. The etiology is multifactorial and frequently related to age, genetics, diabetes, hypertension, smoking, dyslipidemia, and is partly mediated by inflammation. Histopathology involves smooth muscle proliferation and lipid deposition in the endothelium. These early changes are reversible by modification of risk-factors. Late-stage atherosclerosis is characterized by calcification and stenosis. The stages and progression of an atherosclerotic plaque can be identified by noninvasive techniques.[9,10] The severity of luminal narrowing and speed of progression is variable. The signs and symptoms are therefore different. Slow progression of stenosis results in ischemia and stable angina. There is time for development of collaterals that can preserve myocardial viability. This may result in regional wall motion abnormality, myocardial stunning, or hibernation, even in the presence of complete occlusion without myocardial damage. Rapid progression and acute occlusion due to plaque rupture and thrombosis result in clinical syndromes of unstable angina, non-ST segment elevation myocardial infarction (NSTEMI), or ST elevation myocardial infarction (STEMI) depending on the extent of damage.[11,12] Ischemia is aggravated by increased oxygen demand due to tachycardia and hypertension. Left main disease is usually calcific and it can just affect the ostium or the level of branches, and it can present as global myocardial dysfunction and severe heart failure. Diabetics and women may also develop microvascular disease.

Clinical features

Chronic stable angina is common and is characterized by chest pain on exertion. The presentation may also involve pain or pressure of the chest, jaw, arms, or shoulders. Other symptoms include dizziness, tiredness, and shortness of breath. Atypical pain or asymptomatic ischemia is also common in diabetics and women. Unstable angina means there is a rapid acceleration of symptoms and angina at rest. This may progress to arterial occlusion leading to NSTEMI or STEMI, necessitating urgent intervention. Right coronary occlusion may lead to complete heart block with severe symptoms or right heart failure which is very difficult to diagnose in a patient who looks extremely sick. Left main stem stenosis causes global heart dysfunction and can present as flash pulmonary edema or sudden death in an asymptomatic patient. Patients may also present in heart failure due to complications of an acute myocardial infarction (MI) such as cardiogenic shock, post-infarction ventricular septal defect with left to right shunt, papillary muscle rupture with acute mitral regurgitation, ventricular free wall rupture, and tamponade. It is important to suspect these complications in a patient recovering from an acute MI by the appearance of sudden deterioration and new murmurs on auscultation. In late stages, a LV aneurysm may develop either anteriorly or inferiorly. These complications have become infrequent in developed countries due to the speed of revascularization known as door-to-balloon time (D2B), better intensive care, and better medical management.

Diagnosis

Diagnosis of ischemic heart disease starts with ECG showing ST changes at rest and/or with exercise in patients with typical stable angina. Difficult diagnostic cases need demonstration of ischemia by single photon emission computed tomography (SPECT) imaging or by dipyridamole thallium scan to demonstrate a reversible defect. Echocardiography, after increasing oxygen demand by using exercise or dobutamine, reveals myocardial dysfunction due to induced ischemia. Cardiac catheterization and coronary angiogram are definitive tests for demonstrating stenosis. New tests such as intravascular ultrasound and fractional flow reserve measurement (FFR) are frequently used additional modalities to guide treatment.[4,5] LV function can be assessed by LV angiogram or by an echocardiogram. If the patient has significant LV dysfunction, and no ischemic symptoms, studies to assess the myocardial viability using cardiac MRI with Gadolinium may be required. Poor LV function rarely improves unless the myocardium is viable and there are coronary arteries that can be grafted. Failure of intensive medical management in patients with stable angina, severe ischemia, and acute coronary syndrome are indications for revascularization. It is useful to measure pressures in the heart chambers and assess ventricular function during the catheterization study in high-risk patients with heart failure.

Medical management

Aggressive treatment is based on lifestyle changes and reducing myocardial oxygen demand to relieve symptoms. It is the mainstay treatment of patients with stable angina.[13] These include smoking cessation, weight loss, and diet along with medications such as aspirin or clopidogrel, beta-blockers, calcium channel blockers, ACE inhibitors, lipid lowering agents, and nitrates. Newer drugs such as ranolazine and noninvasive treatments such as external counter-pulsation are also available for patients with refractory angina who are not candidates for revascularization.[14,15] Patients with ischemic heart failure will need additional heart failure management. Maximal medical therapy to achieve adequate control of pulse, blood pressure, and lipids is necessary before resorting to invasive treatment strategies.[16,17]

Coronary revascularization strategies

The application of various strategies of invasive treatment for CAD is dependent on the clinical presentation, severity, number of vessels affected, feasibility, and patient related factors.[18,19] If a patient is in severe ischemic cardiogenic IABP (intra-aortic balloon pump) or if available shock, a temporizing measure such as the implementation of an Impella device is useful (Figure 2).

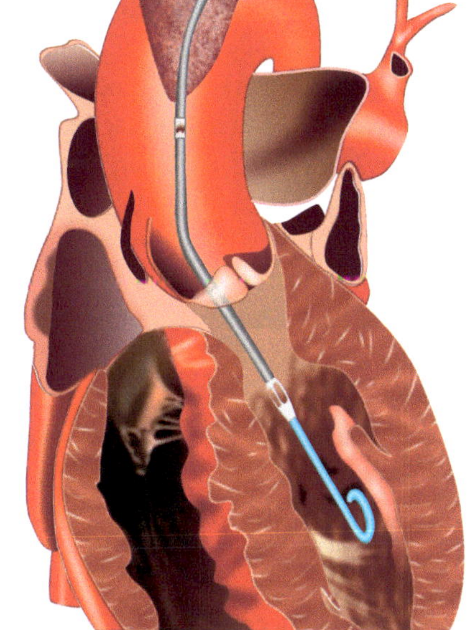

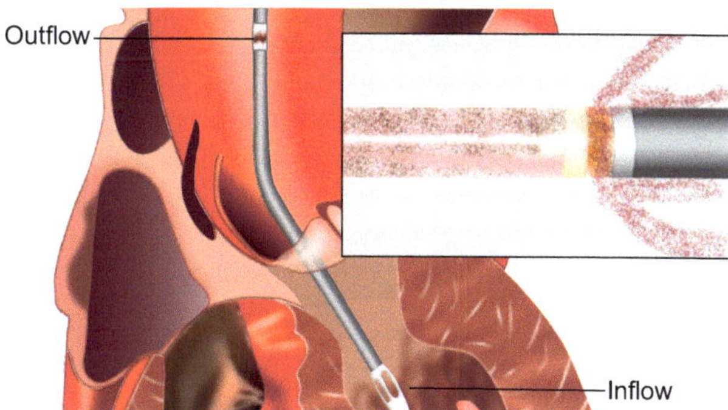

Figure 2: Impella device for temporarily increasing cardiac output

Percutaneous coronary artery intervention (PTCA)

PTCA has become a common procedure for coronary stenosis. It is a significant advancement in the treatment of coronary stenosis.[20] PTCA is the treatment of choice for patients with STEMI, where time is of the essence. The culprit vessel causing an MI can be stented emergently to achieve reperfusion.[21,22] Angioplasty almost always involves implantation of a stent made of nitinol (Figure 3). The incidence of restenosis is 30% to 40% with bare metal stents. Recent advances using drug-eluting stents have reduced restenosis significantly. The drug-eluting stents are coated with drugs such as sirolimus which inhibits interleukin-2 or the rapamycin pathway, or paclitaxel that works by an antimitotic mechanism. The antiproliferative effects of these drugs reduce restenosis by preventing scarring and neo-endothelial coverage of the stents. All patients are therefore put on dual antiplatelet therapy for one year. Late thrombosis is an unresolved issue, and both the short- and long-term effect of GpIIb/IIIa platelet inhibitors is variable. It is a minimally invasive procedure. PTCA is also used as an initial procedure in NSTEMI when a high-risk culprit vessel can be identified in the absence of complex multivessel disease.[23] Use of stenting in multivessel disease, left main stem disease, and unstable angina is questionable, and the decision should be made on an individual basis. Restenosis rates and the need for repeat procedures are higher with the use of multiple stents, long stents, and in complex lesions. Due to the overall costs, benefits, and recent results, there is an increasing trend to have a multi-disciplinary cardiac care team approach towards decision making in coronary revascularization. The choice of the procedure is directed towards reducing major adverse cardiovascular events (MACE) and the patient is fully informed of the risks and benefits whenever time permits.

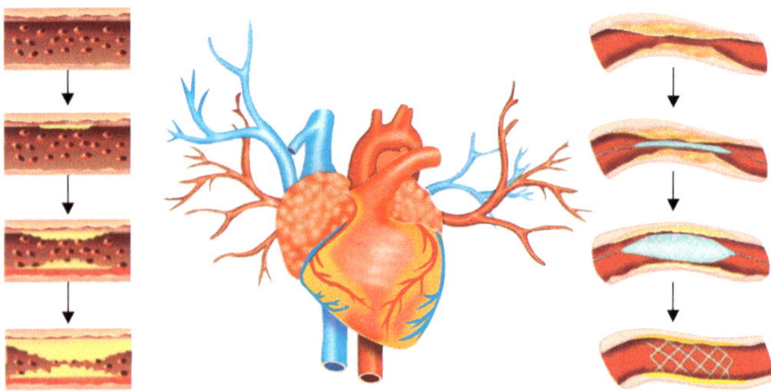

Figure 3: Angioplasty for Coronary Artery Disease

Coronary artery surgery

Coronary artery bypass grafting (CABG) is the most definitive and logical treatment for CAD. It is also the most analyzed. The superiority of CABG over medical management and PTCA has been clearly shown in many subsets of patients.[24,25]

The standard CABG procedure involves cardiopulmonary bypass. The heart is stopped and protected by infusing a high potassium solution called cardioplegia into the coronary circulation.[26] The procedure is done in a static bloodless field. The conduits used are the internal thoracic arteries, radial arteries, and the greater saphenous veins. The distal anastomosis is done end-to-side to the coronary artery distal to the stenosis, and the proximal anastomosis is done end-to-side to the aorta if free conduits are used. The internal thoracic arteries are left attached to their subclavian origin as pedicled grafts and anastomosed end-to-side to the coronary artery. The internal thoracic artery conduits have significantly longer patency rates (Figure 4). Complete revascularization is possible, as it is important for long-term results.[27]

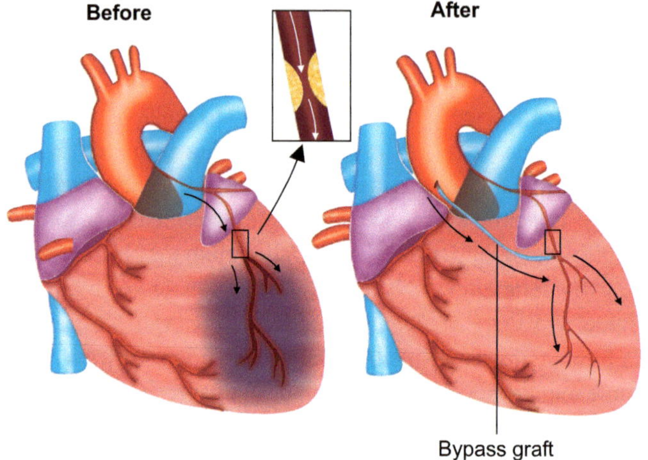

Figure 4: Coronary artery bypass graft

Recently off-pump CABG was introduced to reduce the incidence of stroke and neuro-psychiatric complications caused by cardiopulmonary bypass. The heart is stabilized using suction-based devices and the coronary bypass surgery can be safely accomplished with only brief regional ischemia. The procedure can be converted to on-pump in case of hemodynamic instability, though the mortality of conversion is higher. Several randomized studies showed no difference in the outcomes between the two techniques, with only a trend towards reduced patency rates of grafts to the posterior wall of the heart.[28] It can be done in all high-risk groups of patients with a low mortality rate and possible reduction of stroke.[29,30] Patients with severe ischemic LV dysfunction should be carefully assessed and selected for surgery.[31] The off-pump procedure is widely popular in the developing world because of lower costs due to the possibility of reusing the heart stabilizing devices in many patients. Other minimally invasive robotically assisted CABG procedures are available, and a hybrid approach combining angioplasty and minimally invasive surgery is feasible.

There is a small group of patients with diffuse CAD not amenable to bypass surgery or angioplasty. They can be treated with trans-myocardial laser revascularization (TMLR), which punches small holes with carbon dioxide or a Holmium laser in areas that cannot be grafted during CABG or as a stand-alone procedure. The mechanism of angina relief is related denervation and stimulation of endothelial growth factors.[32]

The serious complications of ischemic heart disease are ventricular aneurysm, mitral regurgitation, and post-infarction ventricular septal defect. The patients may present with cardiogenic shock or severe chronic heart failure. The patients are stabilized using an intra-aortic balloon pump support before and after surgery in acute cases, and then the lesions are corrected. The ventricular septal defect is closed with a patch through left ventriculostomy by incising the infarcted area.[33] Ventricular aneurysms and large akinetic ventricles with heart failure are treated by aneurysm resection and the Dor procedure, where an intraventricular patch is used to reduce the LV volume.[34] Mitral valve damage due to papillary muscle rupture can be repaired or replaced.

Post-operative care

After cardiac surgery, the majority of patients develop a significant systemic inflammatory response and vasodilation, as well as some myocardial stunning due to cardio-pulmonary bypass and cardioplegic arrest during surgery. Patients need vasopressors and inotropes to initially maintain normal hemodynamics. Severe complications such as heart and respiratory failure, stroke, bleeding, and wound infection are exceedingly rare in spite of patients having multiple comorbid factors. The results of cardiac surgery have significantly improved over the years. There is a trend towards extubating these patients early. Patients rarely require mechanical support using, most commonly, an intra-aortic balloon pump (IABP) both before and after revascularization. IABP provides diastolic augmentation of blood pressure and helps reduce the afterload effect on the LV. In the western world, temporary and permanent implantable ventricular assist devices are available if the patient's own heart is unable to sustain life.

The mortality of CABG is less than 2%. Outcomes have improved due to continuous quality improvement (CQI) using multiple national databases and mandatory reporting. Predictors of death and complications are clearly stated, and the risks and benefits can be clearly explained.

Future of coronary revascularization

Percutaneous and surgical coronary revascularization is one of the remarkable advances in improving the quality of life of patients. The most important decision in coronary artery revascularization is the choice of the procedure for the individual patient. The benefits of CABG over medical and PTCA management are clearly demonstrated in patients with left main disease, multivessel disease with proximal LAD stenosis, patients with LV dysfunction, diabetes, renal dysfunction, and diffuse disease.[35,36] PTCA is an excellent treatment for patients with STEMI due to the speed of revascularization in an acutely ill patient.[37] Patients with single or two-vessel disease can also have PTCA in specific situations if they have medical refractory angina. A few groups of patients who have high-risk for complications after CABG surgery due to severe comorbid factors can benefit from angioplasty and stenting. A multidisciplinary team approach is needed to tailor the treatment for individual patients and diseases. This approach is important to produce long-term benefit in the form of survival, freedom from symptoms, and need for repeat procedures. It has also become imperative to take a team approach in the treatment of CAD due to increased healthcare costs and long-term results.[38-40]

The results of the following studies are frequently used in deciding the method of revascularization in patients with angina.

1. BARI trial (Bypass Angioplasty Revascularization Investigation)
   - No difference in mortality and 5-year survival.
   - Rate of repeat vascularization was 54% in the angioplasty group compared to 8% in the CABG group.
   - 31% of patients in the angioplasty group subsequently underwent surgery.
   - The major difference was due to diabetic patients and ones with complex coronary lesions. The findings have been confirmed by other trials.
2. SoS trial (Surgery or Stent)
   - Repeat revascularization was 20.7% in the PTCA group compared to 6% in the surgery group.
   - In a 2-year follow up, mortality was 4.5% in the angioplasty group and 1.6% in the surgery group.
   - Diabetics do significantly better with surgery.
3. SYNTAX trial (SYNergy between PTCA with TAXus and cardiac surgery trial)[41]
   - This is the most important trial, and it reflects real clinical practice rather than the select groups included in the other trials.[42] Almost 79% of patients with three-vessel CAD and 66% of patients with left main disease had survival benefits and marked reduction in repeated revascularizations with CABG in 3 years.
   - For less severe CAD, the survival is similar, but the repeat revascularization is still a problem.[43] CABG benefits most of the patients. Significant repeat vascularization and increased adverse cardiovascular events occurred in the angioplasty group, the adverse events were mainly related to disease complexity. This resulted in the creation of a specific scoring system known as the "syntax" score. This score is used to grade the complexity of the coronary lesions and to help with the decision of choosing the better procedure for the individual patient.
4. ASCERT study (Clinical registry data and longitudinal claims data)[44]
   - Ability to predict long-term survival following PTCA or CABG based on available data.

Surgical revascularization will continue to be the dominant strategy to treat coronary ischemic heart disease as it is based on a simple, logical approach and it has stood the test of time. It is important to educate and involve patients in making the right choice.[45]

REFERENCES

1. van der Horst A, Boogaard FL, Van't Veer M, et al. Towards patient-specific modeling of coronary hemodynamics in healthy and diseased state. Comput Math Methods Med. 2013;2013:393792, Epub 2013 Mar 4.
2. Lee J, Smith NP. The multi-scale modeling of coronary blood flow. Ann Biomed Eng. 2012 Nov;40(11):2399-413.
3. Messer JV, Wagman RJ, Levine HJ, et al. Patterns of myocardial oxygen extraction during rest and exercise. J Clin Invest 1962;41:725.
4. Pijls NH. Fractional flow reserve to guide coronary revascularization. Cic J. 2013 Feb 25;77(3):561-9.
5. Park SJ, Ahn JM. Should we be using fractional flow reserve more routinely to select stable coronary patients for percutaneous coronary intervention? Curr Opin Cardiol. 2012 Nov;27(6):675-81.
6. Takahashi K, Oharaseki T, Yokouchi Y, et al. Kawasaki disease: basic and pathological findings. Clin Exp Nephrol. 2012 Nov 28.
7. Daniels LB, Tjajadi MS, Walford HH, et al. Prevalence of Kawasaki disease in young adults with suspected myocardial ischemia. Circulation. 2012 May 22;125(20):2447-53.
8. Wood FO, Trivax JE, Safian RD. Coronary artery aneurysms: Case report and review of transcatheter strategies. Catheter Cardiovasc Interv. 2013 Feb 15.
9. Layland J, Wilson AM, Lim I, Whitbourn RJ. Virtual histology: a window to the heart of atherosclerosis. Heart Lung Circ. 2011 Oct;20(10):615-21.
10. Eshtehardi P, MaDaniel MC, Suo J, et al. Association of coronary wall shear stress with atheroscelerotic plaque burden, composition, and distribution in patients with coronary artery disease. J Am Heart Assoc. 2012 Aug;1(4):e002543.
11. Crea F, Liuzzo G. Pathogenesis of acute coronary syndromes. J Am Coll Cardiol. 2013 Jan 8;61(1):1-11.
12. Shah PK. Pathophysiology of coronary thrombosis: role of plaque rupture and plaque erosion. Prog Cardiovasc Dis. 2002 Mar-Apr;44(5):357-68.
13. Fihn SD, Gardin JM, Abrams J, et al. 2012 ACCF/AHA/ACP/AATS/PCNA/SCAI/STS Guideline for the diagnosis and management of patients with stable ischemic heart disease. J Am Coll Cardiol. 2012 Dec 18;60(24):e44-e164.
14. Kones R. Recent advances in the management of chronic stable angina II. Anti-ischemic therapy, options for refractory angina, risk factor reduction and revascularization. Vasc Health Risk Manag. 2010 Sep 7;6:749-74.
15. Tarkin JM, Kaski JC. Pharmacological treatment of chronic angina pectoris. Clin Med. 2013 Feb;13(1):63-70.
16. Behnke LM, Solis A, Shulman SA, Skoufalos A. A targeted approach to reducing overutilization: Use of percutaneous coronary intervention in stable coronary artery disease. Popul Health Manag. 2012 Oct 31. (Epub).
17. Thomas S, Gokhale R, Boden WE, Devereaux PJ. A meta-analysis of randomized controlled trials comparing percutaneous coronary intervention with medical therapy in stable angina pectoris. Can J Cardiol. 2013 Apr;29(4):472-82.
18. Nauta ST, Gaspersz M, Deckers JW. The new European society of cardiology guideline on myocardial revascularization: an appraisal. Heart. 2012 Jan;98(1):11-4.
19. Osnabrugge RL, Head SJ, Bogers AJ, Kappetein AP. Appropriate coronary artery bypass grafting use in the percutaneoius coronary intervention era: are we finally making progress? Semin Thorac Cardiovasc Surg. 2012 winter;24(4):241-3.
20. Iqbal J, Gunn J, Serruys PW. Coronary stents: historical development, current status and future directions. Br Med Bull. 2013 Mar 26 (Epub ahead of print).
21. Jneid H, Anderson JL, Wright RS, et al. 2012 ACCF/AHA focused update of the guideline for the management of patients with unstable angina/non-ST-elevation myocardial infarction. J Am Coll Cardiol. 2012 Aug 14;60(7):645-81.
22. Yiadom MY. Emergency department treatment of acute coronary syndromes. Emer Med Clin North Am. 2011 Nov;29(4):699-710.
23. Bawamia B, Mehran R, Qiu W, Kunadian V. Risk score in acute coronary syndrome and percutaneous coronary intervention: A review. Am Heart J. 2013 Apr;165(4):441-50.
24. Hlatky MA, Boothroyd DB, Baker L, et al. Comparative effectiveness of multivessel coronary bypass surgery and multi-vessel percutaneous coronary intervention: A cohort study. Ann Inter Med. 2013 Apr 23 (Epub).
25. Farkouh ME, Domanski M, Sleeper LA et al. Strategies for multivessel revascularization in patients with diabetes. N Engl J Med. 2012 Dec 20;367(25): 2375-84.

26. Algarni KD, Weisel RD, Caldarone CA, et al. Microplegia during coronary artery bypass grafting was associated with less low cardiac output syndrome: a propensity-matched comparison. Ann Thorac Surg. 2013 May;95(5):1532-8.
27. Farooq V, Serruys PW, Garcia-Garcia HM, et al. The negative impact of incomplete angiographic revascularization on clinical outcomes and its association with total occlusions: the SYNTAX trial. J Am Coll Cardiol. 2013 Jan 22;61(3):282-94.
28. Shroyer AL, Grover FL, Hattler B, et al. On-pump versus off-pump coronary-artery bypass surgery. N engl J Med. 2009 Nov 5;361(19):1827-37.
29. Polomsky M, He X, O'Brien SM, Puskas JD. Outcomes of off-pump versus on-pump coronary artery bypass grafting: Impact of preoperative risk. J Thorac Cardiovasc Surg. 2013 MAY;145(5):1193-8.
30. Sa MP, Ferraz PE, Escobar RR, et al. Off-pump versus on-pump coronary artery bypass surgery: meta-analysis and meta-regression of 13,524 patients from randomized trials. Rev Bras Cir Cardiovasc. 2012 Dec;27(4):631-41.
31. Kwon DH, Hachamovitch R, Popovic ZB, et al. Survival in patients with severe ischemic cardiomyopathy undergoing revascularization versus medical therapy: association with end-systolic volume and viability. Circulation. 2012 Sep 11;126(11 suppl 1):S3-8.
32. Manchanda A, Aggarwal A, Aggarwal N, Soran O. Management of refractory angina pectoris. Cardiol J. 2011;18(4):343-51.
33. Management and mid-term outcomes of post-infarction ventricular septa defect.
34. Chen X, Qiu ZB, Xu M, Liu LL, Jiang YS, Wang LM. Surgery for left ventricular aneurysm after myocardial infarction: techniques selection and results assessment. Chin Med J (Engl). 2012 Dec;125(24):4373-9.
35. Farooq V, van Klaveren D, Steyerberg ew, et al. Anatomical and clinical characteristics to guide decision making between coronary artery bypass surgery and percutaneous coronary intervention for individual patients: development and validation of SYNTAX score II. Lancet.2013 Feb 23;381(9867):639-50.
36. Hee L, Mussap CJ, Yang L, et al. Outcomes of coronary revascularization (percutaneous or bypass) in patients with diabetes and multivessel coronary disease. Am J Cardiol. 2012 Sep 1;110(5):643-8.
37. Comparison of clinical and angiographic prognostic risk scores in patients with acute coronary syndromes: Analysis from the Acute Catheterization and Urgent Intervention Triage StrategY (ACUITY) trial.
38. Mohr FW, Morice MC, Kappetein AP, et al. Coronary artery bypass graft surgery versus percutaneous coronary intervention in patients with three-vessel disease and left main coronary disease: 5-year follow-up of the randomised, clinical SYNTAX trial. Lancet. 2013 Feb 23;381(9867):629-38.
39. Tong BC, Huber JC, Ascheim DD, et al. Weighting composite endpoints in clinical trials: essential evidence for the heart team. Ann Thorac Surg. 2012 Dec;94(6):1908-13.
40. Holmes DR, Rich JB, Zoghbi WA, Mack MJ. The heart team of cardiovascular care. J Amer Coll Cardiol. 2013;61:903-7.
41. Taggart DP. Lessons learned from the SYNTAX trial for multivessel and left main stem coronary artery disease. Curr Opin Cardiol. 2011 Nov;26(6):502-7.
42. Yan TD, Padang R, Cao C, et al. Drug-eluting a-stents versus coronary artery bypass grafting for the treatment of coronary artery disease: A meta-analysis of randomized and non-randomized studies. J Thorac cardiovasc Surg 2011;141:1134-44.
43. Shiomi H, Morimoto T, Hayano M, et al. Comparison of long-term outcome after percutaneous coronary intervention versus coronary artery bypass grafting in patients with unprotected left main coronary artery disease (from the CREDO-Kyoto PCI/CABG Registry Cohort-2) Am J Cardiol. 2012 Oct 1;110(7):924-32.
44. Shahian DM, O'Brien SM, Sheng S, et al. Predictors of long-term survival after coronary artery bypass grafting surgery: results from the Society of Thoracic Surgeons Adult Cardiac Surgery Database (the ASCERT study). Circulation. 2012 Mar 27;125(12):1491-500.
45. Kawasuji M. Clinical evidence versus patients' perception of coronary revascularization. Surg Today. 2013 Jan 3.
46. Palmerini T, Caixeta A, Genereux P, et al. Am Heart J. 2012 Mar;163(3):383-91.

❑❑❑

64

CHAPTER

Pericardial Disease, Myocardia Disease, and Cardiac Tumors

Wickii T. Vigneswaran, MD, FACS, FCCP

Pericardial diseases result in severe diastolic heart failure and ultimately a low-output state due to constriction and restriction. A myocardial disease of surgical importance is hypertrophic cardiomyopathy, which is both restrictive and obstructive. Cardiac tumors can be either infiltrative or may present as obstructive lesions.

Pericardial Disease

The causes of pericarditis are idiopathic, infective (e.g., viral, bacterial, tuberculous), immune diseases (e.g., rheumatoid, SLE, renal failure), mediastinal irradiation, post-cardiac surgery, end-stage renal disease, and metastatic malignancy.[1]

Many of these conditions resolve after initial inflammation and effusion (Figure 1). However, some patients continue to develop scarring, leading to constrictive pericarditis. The pericardium in these cases is thick, fibrosed, and often calcified. This results in significant diastolic restriction and ultimately a low-output state and heart failure. It is difficult to distinguish between pericardial constriction from restrictive myocardial diseases in late cases because the physiological basis is quite similar and visceral pericardium is indistinguishable from epicardium.[2,3]

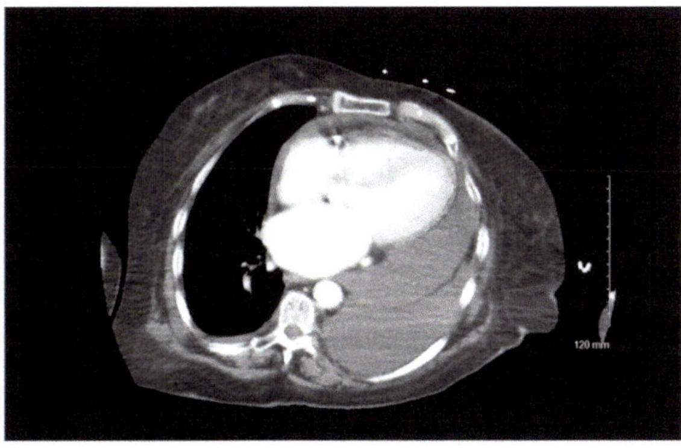

Figure 1: Pericardial effusion

Clinical features

Patients develop biventricular failure, but signs and symptoms of right heart failure such as peripheral edema, ascites, and liver congestion predominate the clinical picture. Left ventricular (LV) diastolic failure and the resulting pulmonary hypertension further aggravate the right heart failure. Patients are tired, weak, malnourished, and dyspneic. Frequently, they present in late-stage heart failure, as it is difficult to recognize the subtle signs as it develops.[4] It takes a longer time to recognize pericardial constriction after cardiac surgery.[5]

The clinical exam includes muffled heart sounds and elevated jugular venous pressure (JVP) even during inspiration, a phenomenon known as Kussmal's sign. It is possible to detect the rapid 'y' descent on inspection of JVP during diastole after the second heart sound. Electrocardiogram (ECG) shows low voltage QRS complexes and chest X-ray may show pericardial calcifications. Computed tomography (CT), magnetic resonance imaging (MRI), or echocardiogram can be done to obtain confirmation. Cardiac catheterization is needed only in cases where the diagnosis is equivocal. The classic signs include the square-root sign, where one sees a dip-plateau pattern of the ventricular pressure during diastole, a prominent 'y' descent on right atrial tracing, and equalization of the right and LV end-diastolic pressures. Equalization of pressures and right ventricular diastolic restriction are also diagnosed by echocardiogram.

The treatment for pericardial constriction is total pericardiectomy, taking care to preserve the phrenic nerves. This can b e accomplished by both sternotomy and left thoracotomy approaches. It is possible to remove both the anterior and posterior pericardium without cardiopulmonary bypass through a left thoracotomy. If problems arise, requiring cardio-pulmonary bypass, the incision will have to be extended across the sternum to get to the atrium. Sternotomy is preferred to remove all the pericardium over the right atrium, vena cava, right ventricle, and anterolateral LV. This can be accomplished without bypass. Bypass can be initiated to remove the fibrocalcific posterior pericardium. Care must be taken to preserve both phrenic nerves.[6,7] The results are excellent if the surgery is performed before the onset of liver failure and significant ascites.[8] Some patients require prolonged pharmacological support of their heart failure after surgery before feeling its benefits.

Hypertrophic Cardiomyopathy

Hypertrophic cardiomyopathy is a genetic cardiac disease affecting myocardial fibers.[9] Many patients who have hypertrophic cardiomyopathy are asymptomatic. Mild to moderate symptoms can easily be managed medically. In the presence of LV outflow tract obstruction, the patient develops classic symptoms of dyspnea on exertion, angina, and palpitations if they have atrial arrhythmias.

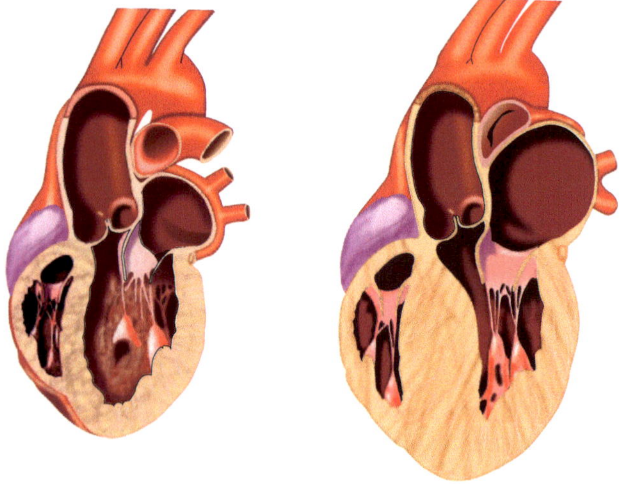

Figure 2: Hypertrophic cardiomyopathy

The major components of surgical disease are severe LV myocardial hypertrophy (LVH) where the septum bulges into the outflow tract and there is systolic anterior motion of the mitral valve (MV). It is important to understand the structural abnormalities of the MV. The MV has large leaflets and anterior displacement of the papillary muscle and chordae. The final result is dynamic obstruction of the outflow tract. The other complications of this disease include atrial and ventricular arrhythmias, and sudden death. LVH can also be seen in atypical forms such as severe concentric hypertrophy (e.g., papillary muscles) or asymmetric apical hypertrophy. This is a complex disease where patients require life-long treatment and follow-up.[10]

Hypertrophic cardiomyopathy is diagnosed by typical echocardiographic findings of hypertrophy and systolic anterior motion of the MV leaflet. For diagnostic and treatment purposes, cardiac catheterization is necessary for measuring gradients and coronary angiography. Some patients have a high gradient seen at rest whereas others must be provoked by amyl nitrate inhalation or postextrasystolic potentiation. These maneuvers needed to increase the myocardial contractility, increase obstruction. Another important symptom in this group of patients is ventricular arrhythmias and sudden death. These symptoms correlate with the severity of the disease and family history. Additional treatment with implantable defibrillators may be necessary in such cases.

The initial treatment of obstructive symptoms is beta-blockers and/or calcium channel blockers.[11] Some patients can also be treated with disopyramide. The goal is to produce myocardial depression that leads to relaxation of the outflow tract. Patients who can tolerate high doses of these drugs can be medically managed in the long-term.

Complete relief of obstruction can be achieved with excellent short- and long-term success and low mortality by surgery using cardiopulmonary bypass.[12] It is important to clearly delineate the extent and thickness of the myocardium that needs to be removed by using transesophageal echocardiogram during surgery.

Surgery involves resection of the hypertrophic septum; in some cases, it involves resection all the way down to the papillary muscle. This can be done by a transaortic approach alone or in combination with a trans-mitral approach. The large anterior leaflet of the MV may require plication procedures in some cases.[13,14] Occasionally, the surgeon can suture the anterior and posterior leaflets to produce a double opening (Alfieri stitch) and an annuloplasty to prevent systolic anterior motion (SAM) of the MV. In centers with limited experience, and in cases of extensive hypertrophy, outflow obstruction relief can be achieved by MV replacement. In this case, surgeons use a low-profile valve with or without septal myomectomy. Patients will have to face the long-term complications of prosthetic MV. Severe organic disease of the MV may also necessitate MV replacement. Significant survival benefit is achieved in spite of the multiple surgical procedures needed to treat this condition.[15]

Similar symptomatic relief of obstruction can be achieved by destroying the septal bulge in appropriate cases. This is done by injecting alcohol into the first septal artery.[16] It is a less invasive procedure, but there is concern about the long-term arrhythmogenic potential of producing a myocardial infarction and scar.[17] The long-term results and complications are more predictable with surgery than alcohol ablation since surgical expertise is available to produce consistent results. Further studies are warranted. Similar to the trend that is occurring in complex coronary artery disease and valve diseases, a multidisciplinary approach and decision making is important to provide the right care for this group of patients.[18]

Cardiac Tumors

Cardiac tumors are primary or metastatic, benign, or malignant, and can be myocardial or endocardial.[19] The type of tumor varies based on the age at presentation.[20] They are in general very rare. The symptoms vary depending on the location. Endocardial tumors such as fibroelastomas and myxomas cause obstructive or embolic symptoms mimicking valve lesions.[21] Myocardial tumors that are usually metastatic cause restrictive cardiomyopathy and dysrhythmias leading to death. Intracardiac thrombus can occasionally mimic tumors.

Benign tumors

Cardiac myxomas are the most common and dramatic intracardiac tumors. Myxomas are usually sporadic and about 7% occur as part of an autosomal dominant syndrome. They are discrete masses attached to the atrial septum on the left side in 75% of cases. In 15% to 20% of patients, they occur in the right atrium and bilaterally.[22,23] They rarely occur in the ventricles.[24] The myxomas associated with genetic syndromes tend to be indiscrete and can be attached to various areas of the atria and atrioventricular valves. They also have a higher recurrence rate after surgery.[25]

Clinical features and diagnosis

Asymptomatic myxomas are frequently diagnosed when screening for other problems. Sometimes large atrial myxomas cause MV and tricuspid valve obstructive signs and symptoms. They are also responsible for a syndrome causing peripheral emboli and immune reactions with fever, rash, and myalgia. Only a transthoracic echocardiography is needed for investigation.

Treatment

Surgical removal is achieved through cardiopulmonary bypass. To prevent recurrence, it is important to remove the myocardium or the septum where the pedicle is attached in the case of an atrial myxoma.[26] Then the defect is closed with a patch.[26]

Other benign tumors are rhabdomyomas, lipomas, and papillary fibroelastomas. The tumors need surgical resection only when they cause symptoms of obstruction, arrhythmias, or recurrent systemic emboli.[27,28]

Malignant tumors, both primary sarcomas and metastatic tumors, are rarely removed by surgery as the prognosis is poor. Frequently, metastasis affects both the parietal and visceral pericardium with effusion. Palliative treatment is achieved by performing a pericardial window to relieve symptoms of compression.

REFERENCES

1. Khandaker MH, Espinosa RE, Nishimura RA, et al. Pericardial disease: diagnosis and management. Mayo Clin Proc. 2010 Jun;85(6):572-93.
2. Kusunose K, Dahiva A, Motoki H, et al. Biventricular mechanics in constrictive pericarditis comparison with restrictive cardiomyopathy and impact of pericardiectomy. Cic Cardiovasc Imaging. 2013, Mar 26.
3. Zwas DR, Gotsman I, Admon D, Keren A. Advances in the differentiation of constrictive pericarditis and restrictive cardiomyopathy. Herz. 2012 Sep;37(6):664-73.
4. Schdoeder JR, Osorno H, Chait R, Fischer A. Hiding in plain sight; constrictive pericarditis. BMJ Case Rep.
5. Gaudino M, Anselmi A, Pavone M, Massetti M. Constrictive pericarditis after cardiac surgery. Ann Thorac Surg. 2013 Feb;95(2):731-6.
6. Chowdhury UK, Subramaniam GK, Kumar AS, et al. Pericardiectomy for constrictive pericarditis: a clinical, echocardiographic and hemodynamic evaluation of two surgical techniques. Ann Thorac Surg 2006;81:522-9.
7. Ariyoshi, Hashizume K, Taniguchi S, et al. Surgical experience with chronic constrictive pericarditis. Gen Thorac Cardiovasc Surg. 2012 Dec;60(12):796-802.
8. Kang SH, Song JM, Kim M, et al. Prognostic factors in pericardiectomy for constrictive pericarditis. J Thorac Cardiovasc Surg. 2013 Feb 1.
9. Ivens E. Hypertrophic cardiomyopathy. Heart Lung Circ. 2004;13 Sppl 3:S48-55.
10. Gersh BJ, Maron BJ, Bonow RO, Dearani JA, et al. 2011 ACCF/AHA guideline for the diagnosis and treatment of hypertrophic cardiomyopathy. J Thorac Cardiovasc Surg. 2011 Dec;142(6):e153-203.
11. Elmariah S, Fifer MA. Medical, surgical and interventional management of hypertrophic cardiomyopathy with obstruction. Curr Treat Options Cardiovasc Med. 2012 Dec;14(6):665-78.
12. Swistel DG, Balaram SK. Surgical myomectomy for hypertrophic cardiomyopathy in the 21st century, the evolution of the "RPR" repair: resection, plication, and release. Prog Cardiovasc Dis. 2012 May-Jun;54(6):498-502.
13. Anagnostopoulos PV, Johnson NC, Robertson L, Sapru A, Azakie A. Surgical management of left ventricular outflow tract obstruction. J Card Surg. 2012 Jan;27(1):103-11.
14. Altarabsheh SE, Dearani JA, Burkhart HM, et al. Outcome of septal myomectomy for obstructive

hypertrophic cardiomyopathy in children and young adults. Ann Thorac Surg. 2013 Feb;95920663-9.

15. Woo A, Rakowski H. Does myectomy convey survival benefit in hypertrophic cardiomyopathy? Heart Fail Clin. 2007 Jul;3(3):275-88.
16. Firoozi S, Elliott PM, Sharma S, et al. Septal myotomy-myectomy and trancoronary septal alcohol ablation in hypertrophic obstructive cardiomyopathy. A comparison of clinical, haemodynamic and exercise outcomes. Eur Heart J. 2002 Oct;23(20):1617-24.
17. Sorajja P. Binder J, Nishimura RA, et al. Predictors of an optimal clinical outcome with alcohol septal ablation for obstructive hypertrophic cardiomyopathy. Catheter Cardiovasc Interv. 2013 Jan 1;18(1):E58-67.
18. Lacovoni A, Spirito P, Simon C, et al. A contemporary European experience with surgical septal myomectomy in hypertrophic cardiomyopathy. Eur Heart J. 2012 Aug;33(16):2080-7.
19. Amano J, Nakayama J, Yoshimura Y, Ikeda U. Clinical classification of cardiovascular tumors and tumor-like lesions, and its incidences. Gen Thorac Cardiovasc Surg. 2013 Mar 5 (Epub ahead of print).
20. Penha JG, Zorzanelli L, Barbosa-Lopes AA, et al. Heart neoplasms in children: retrospective analysis. Arg Bras Cardiol. 2013 Feb;100(2) 120-126.
21. Val-Barnal JF, Mayorga M, Garijo MF, et al. Cardiac papillary fibroelastoma: retrospective clinicopathologic study of 17 tumors with resection at a single institution and literature review. Pathol Res Pract. 2013 Apr;209(4):208-14.
22. Smith M, Chaudhry MA, Lozano P, Humphrey MB. Cardiac myxoma induced paraneoplastic syndrome: a review of the literature. Eur J Inter Med. 2012 Dec;23(8):669-73.
23. Yuan SM, Sternik L. Mitral valve myxoma: a large scale collective review. J BUON. 2012 Jul-sep; 17(3):543-53.
24. Simsek E, Durdu S, Hodo B, Yazicioglu L, Uysalel A. Left ventricular myxoma producing cardiac failure. Heart Surg Forum. 2013 Feb 1;16(1):E57-9.
25. Sheng WB, Luo BE, Liu Y, et al. Risk factors for post-operative recurrence of cardiac myxoma and the clinical managements: a report of 5 cases in one center and review of literature. Chin Med J (Engl). 2012 Aug;125(16):2914-8.
26. Garatti A, Nano G, Canziani A, et al. Surgical excision of cardiac myxomas: twenty years experience at a single institution. Ann Thorac Surg. 2012 Mar;93(3):825-31.
27. Restrepo CS, Betacourt SL, Martinez-Jimenez S, Gutierrez FR. Tumors of the pulmonary artery and veins. Semin Ultrasound CT MR. 2012 Dec;33(6):580-90.
28. Kumar N, Agarwal S, Ahuja A, et al. Spectrum of cardiac tumors excluding myxoma: Experience of a tertiary center with review of literature. Pathol Res Pract. 2011 dec 15;207(12):769-74.

❑❑❑

65

CHAPTER

Transplant Surgery: Kidney Liver, Pancreas

Dinesh Ranjan, MD, FACS
Gazi Zabari, MD, FACS
Wickii T. Vigneswaran, MD, FACS
Reza F. Saidi, MD
Vijay K. Mittal, MD, MS, FICS, FACS

INTRODUCTION

Organ transplantation is now accepted therapy for end-stage organ failure. Significant advances have taken place over the previous half century resulting in further refinement of surgical technique, anesthesia and critical care, organ preservation, and immunosuppression. This has resulted in significant improvements in allograft and patient's survival. This chapter provides a very brief review of the current status of kidney, liver and pancreas transplantation.

KIDNEY TRANSPLANTATION

The first successful kidney transplantation was done in 1954. This was performed between 2 identical twins thus obviating the need for immunosuppression. With improvements in immunosuppression, now it is possible to achieve a high degree of allograft function and longevity even in poorly matched kidneys. However, most centers believe (and it is supported by UNOS) that even from a random (as compared to a blood relative) donor, a zero mismatch between the live donor and the recipient imparts significant immunological advantages. It is routine for all kidney transplant programs to do an HLA type matching between donors and recipients and it is required to perform a crossmatch prior to transplantation to virtually eliminate the probability of antibody based hyperacute rejection. Presence of alloreactive preformed antibodies can be known by the mandatorily used PRA (Panel Reactive Antibody) test as most human beings are supposed to have a PRA of 0%. Common causes of high PRA include previous transplantation, blood transfusions, pregnancy, and idiopathic.

Technique of Kidney Transplantation

Kidney transplantation is performed in the heterotopic location into iliac fossa in the retroperitoneal location. A curvilinear incision is made medial to the anterior superior iliac spine extending medially and inferiorly towards the suprapubic region. The fascia is divided, and the muscles are either reflected medially (preferred) or divided as need be. The retroperitoneal space is identified deeper to the fascia transversalis by identifying the inferior epigastric vessels and spermatic cord/round ligament of the uterus entering the deep inguinal ring. Inferior epigastric vessels are routinely ligated and divided; however, some surgeons preserve the inferior epigastric artery as an inflow of smaller lower polar artery if present in the donor kidney. Subsequently the external iliac artery and vein are isolated and dissected to free up enough length to allow proximal and distal control. The artery typically has lymphatic channels along its surface and many surgeons believe that these need to be carefully ligated to prevent postoperative lymphocele. Once sufficient mobilization has occurred, the donor kidney, usually sitting preserved in an ice-bath at 4°C, is brought in. Both venous and arterial anastomoses are done with end-to-side technique, in that order. Most transplant programs prefer to start induction immunosuppression according to their center specific protocols prior to completion of vascular anastomosis, often dictated by the quality of HLA matching and other immunologic variables. The organ is then allowed to be perfused with warm blood from the recipient. A well-prepared donor organ usually does not require too much hemostasis. Subsequently the ureteric anastomosis is performed. This is the proverbial Achilles' heel of the kidney transplant operation because of the tenuous blood supply of the ureter. The blood supply of the donor ureter comes from an arterial network along the lower pole of the kidney with the network descending down around the ureter in the surrounding tissue. Therefore, the length of the ureter should be kept shortest feasible, and the cut edge of the ureter should demonstrate adequate vascularity. Multiple techniques of ureteral neo-cystostomy have been described in transplantation. Most surgeons believe in creation of a short submucosal tunnel with the belief that this should reduce retrograde reflux. Additionally, there continues to be discussion regarding the use of a ureteric stent for this anastomosis, typically for 1-3 months. Again, this is determined by the surgeons' preference and/or center specific protocols. Just before this anastomosis has been started, the Foley catheter that was placed prior to the incision and used to fill and irrigate the bladder with antibacterial solutions, is unclamped and a record of urine output is maintained from this moment on. A drain may be left in the transplant fossa depending on the surgeons' preference. A kidney transplant is demonstrated in Figure 1.

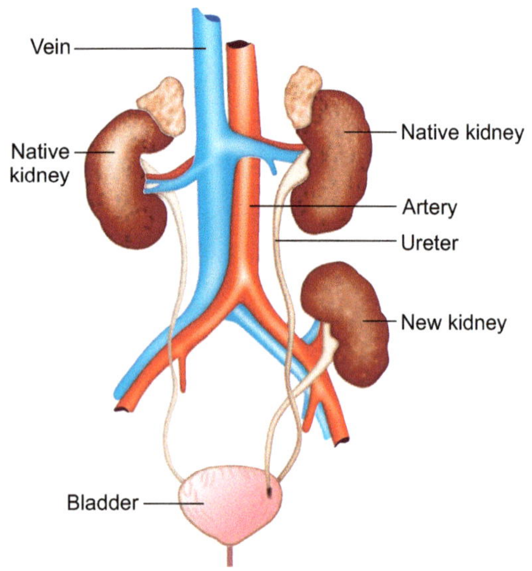

Figure 1: Kidney transplant

Postoperative Management

Most patients can be managed without placing them in the ICU. During the first 24-48 hours, the urine output is replaced cc/cc with a sugarless electrolyte solution as the kidney has lost its concentrating ability and therefore the patient runs the risk of dehydration. However, as the renal function improves, evidenced with rapidly falling serum creatinine, this can be tapered off by the 2nd or 3rd postoperative day. Since the patient undergoes this operation via a retroperitoneal approach, they are allowed to have liquids the day of surgery that can be gradually advanced.

Immunosuppression Management

This is highly center specific; however, most centers prefer to use an induction bolus of steroid (IV Methylprednisolone 500-1000mg) before unclamping the kidney and then a rapid or slow taper protocol of steroids. A calcineurin inhibitor of choice (Cyclosporine or Tacrolimus) and an antimetabolite (Mycophenolate Mofetil) is added in the immediate perioperative phase. The dose of calcineurin inhibitors is tightly managed based on its trough serum levels during the postoperative period due to its nephrotoxic effects.

Acute Rejection

Often, a diagnosis is made based on presumptive clinical findings, most prominently due to a rise in serum creatinine. Most centers, however, prefer to substantiate this clinical impression with a percutaneous core biopsy, either done blindly since the allograft is palpable, or under ultrasound guidance. Treatment is given with either escalation of steroid dosing, with or without a bolus dose, or for more severe or recurrent rejections; a course of antilymphocyte antibody therapy. Each episode of rejection requires the team to re-examine the immunosuppression strategy, as a lost nephron never regenerates back.

Chronic Allograft Nephropathy

This much discussed problem is usually multifactorial: immunologic (chronic rejection which is usually humoral mediated); other physiologic factors (hypertension, diabetes, myocardial disease); drug related (calcineurin inhibitor toxicity, contrast exposure); anatomic problems (renal artery stenosis) or other structural issues such as reflux nephropathy, chronic UTI etc. Unfortunately, unless a clear-cut correctable cause, most commonly anatomic, is found, this problem results in a gradual loss of the allograft and the need for re-transplantation.

Surgical Management of the Renal Transplant Recipient

During the early postoperative period, the care is directed towards monitoring for bleeding and allograft function.

Allograft Function: hourly measurement of urine output during the first 24-48 hours is routine for most transplant programs. In addition, a daily measurement of serum creatinine is routinely done. In patients with significant polyuria (>250cc/h of urine) daily, sometimes twice daily monitoring of serum electrolytes is necessary.

Management of Allograft Dysfunction: Allograft dysfunction work-up typically involves a set algorithm using three tests that rule out various commonly encountered etiologies of renal allograft dysfunction.

1. An ultrasound with Doppler (duplex) examination is extremely valuable because it provides a noninvasive bed-side image-based differentiation of commonly encountered problems:
   a. Large collection of fluid in the allograft fossa: urine leak, lymphocele, hematoma, abscess

b. Resistive index of renal artery: a high RI (>0.75) indicates a swollen allograft as would be seen in a rejection, infection, or venous outflow problem. Very low RI can be seen with renal artery stenosis

c. No flow in renal artery or renal infarction: this is ominous. Even if there is documented flow in the renal artery, it is often needed to interrogate both poles of the kidney as loss of blood flow to a segment could result in renal dysfunction and hypertension. In addition, loss of blood flow to the lower pole is associated with ureteric necrosis.

d. Hydroureter or hydronephrosis: this in itself does not necessarily imply a problem as a denervated ureter can sometimes dilate. However, in a patient with allograft dysfunction, it is necessary to take further steps to rule out a true structural problem.

2. Renal Scan: A nuclear medicine-based test that allows the clinicians to gauge the function of allograft based on efficiency of radio-isotope uptake and excretion in the allograft and subsequent transit to the urinary bladder.

   a. By measuring the intensity of uptake between the iliac artery and the allograft the radiologist can comment on the appropriateness of arterial inflow.

   b. The image of the allograft provides a pictorial representation of uniformity of renal blood flow or segmental infarction

   c. The loss of radioisotope from the allograft in the ureter and then to the bladder and their respective transit time and intensity allows a calculation that can effectively differentiate between intrinsic allograft dysfunction vs obstruction.

   d. Radio-isotope leak in the renal fossa would indicate ureteric necrosis and/or anastomotic leak.

3. Histology (Renal Biopsy): This is the definitive examination to rule in or rule out rejection and other inflammatory processes (i.e., CMV infection or BK-Polyomavirus infection). This test is also valuable in kidneys that are suffering from ATN in the immediate post-transplant phase (approximately 10-20% of cadaveric allografts) thus precluding the use of serum creatinine as a test to monitor allograft and suspect rejection. The biopsy can often be done at the bedside with or without ultrasound visualization as the allograft is mostly palpable. Despite being invasive, it is a fairly safe test. Significant complications are rare (1-2%) and may include bleeding resulting in hematuria (usually self-limited), an arteriovenous fistula or pseudoaneurysm, and uretero-pelvic injury.

Common causes of allograft dysfunction (rising or high serum creatinine), their diagnostic criteria and very abbreviated treatment strategy:

1. ATN: Good flow in renal scan but poor or no function. Histology is diagnostic. No treatment is necessary, only supportive treatment is needed.
2. Acute rejection: High RI on duplex, somewhat diminished flow on renal scan. Histology is diagnostic. Treated with Steroid bolus with pulse and/or antilymphocyte therapy.
3. Obstruction: dilated ureteral-calyceal system. Renal scan shows good function (uptake and elimination from renal parenchyma) but slow transit to the bladder. A cystoscopic retrograde urethrogram with stenting or antegrade nephro-urethrogram is often needed as the first step. Surgical revision of ureteroneocystostomy or surgical correction of the offending cause may be needed.
4. Lymphocele: fluid collection in the allograft fossa with or without obstructive features as above. An incidentally discovered lymphocele does not need treatment. If obstruction is seen, then percutaneous ultrasound guided actuator placement is done. This may require alcohol sclerosis as well vs laparoscopic or open marsupialization of the lymphocele to drain it into the peritoneal cavity.
5. Urine leak: fluid collection in the allograft fossa and radioisotope leak in the allograft fossa. Sometimes seen with loss of arterial flow to lower pole of the kidney and lower polar infarction on the renal scan. The first step is to decompress the urinary bladder. An early urine leak (within 2-3 weeks of transplantation) will require surgical revision by resecting the distal ureter and performing ureteroneocystostomy. A later leak can often be managed with bladder decompression and stenting (retrograde or antegrade).
6. Calcineurin inhibitor toxicity: high drug levels coupled with lack of anatomical findings as above. Histology may show vacuolization. This is treated by adjusting the offending medications' dose and patience.
7. Viral infection: similar to acute rejection as above, histology is definitive. Other signs of viral infection such as fever, malaise, peripheral viral markers etc. help. CMV is treated with antiviral therapy and temporary reduction in immunosuppression. BKPV infection is treated with reduction in immunosuppression. More recently, Leflunomide has been utilized in Rx patients with BKPV.

LIVER TRANSPLANTATION

The first human liver transplantation was done by Thomas Starzl in Colorado in 1966. It took more than a decade for the technique, immunosuppression, and organ preservation to reach a point where the results are now predictably good. Once thought of as the "mother of all operations" – due to the skills required to perform hepatectomy in a coagulopathic patient with portal hypertension and adhesions and then do meticulous implantation and limited to a very few centers and with huge, reported requirements for blood products – liver transplantation now is performed in 140+ centers in the USA, with survivals matching other organ transplant survivals. Whereas the western world benefits from a well-developed system in cadaveric organ donation, many of the underdeveloped countries have to rely on living donation solely or primarily. This has resulted in further refinement in the techniques of both liver implantation and partial donor hepatectomy for transplantation purposes.

Immunologic Considerations

The liver is an immunologically privileged organ. It has a tremendous mass of non-reactive hepatocytes that do not express class II antigen and therefore are not targeted by alloreactive immune processes. Indeed, the presence of alloreactive donor specific antibodies does not present as a contraindication to liver transplantation. Therefore, for liver transplantation the only matching that is necessary is the blood type matching, and just as in blood transfusions – a blood type O donor is a universal donor while a blood type AB recipient is a universal recipient. Despite attempts at flushing the donor organ off the passenger blood cells from the donor, passenger leukocytes invariably accompany the donor liver and must be considered for infectious and immunologic purposes.

Operative Technique

The most difficult part of liver transplantation is the hepatectomy. This is due to the fact that there is portal hypertension resulting in high pressure, thin-walled collaterals around the liver in an already coagulopathic patient. Many of these patients also have had upper abdominal surgery resulting in highly vascular adhesions. Typically, hepatectomy is done in stages, most often starting with mobilization of the triangular (phreno-hepatic) ligaments. The lesser omentum is divided carefully, ligating the venous and arterial (accessory left hepatic artery in around 10% arises from left gastric artery) channels. The hilum is then dissected carefully, ligating and dividing the bile duct and hepatic artery with enough length to be used in implantation. The portal vein is then skeletonized to the bifurcation and then clamped and divided. The liver can then be mobilized quickly by encircling infrahepatic and suprahepatic cava and then placing clamps and dividing at these sites with care to leave enough length on the body side to perform the anastomosis. Many surgeons use a "piggy-back" technique where instead of dividing the supra and infrahepatic cava, the liver is dissected off the cava by individually ligating and dividing short hepatic veins and then securing the right hepatic vein and the confluence of the middle and left hepatic veins. A common conduit can then be created at the confluence of all three hepatic veins to which the donor liver's suprahepatic cava is anastomosed, thus the name "piggy-back". In this case, the infrahepatic cava of the donor liver is simply ligated. However, more traditional technique is to perform a suprahepatic and infrahepatic caval anastomoses between the respective donor and recipient vessels, thus restoring the caval continuity by the donor cava conduit.

A veno-venous bypass cannula can be placed in the portal vein at this time and carefully secured in place. This cannula will connect to a cannula in the femoral vein and jugular vein to complete the bypass of venous blood from portal and femoral veins to the jugular vein. A flow of 1.5L/min is needed to prevent clots from developing in the system and resulting in a pulmonary embolism. In earlier times, the femoral and jugular cannulas were placed by surgically cutting down on femoral and axillary veins, but now it is customary to have these placed percutaneously either by the surgeon or the anesthesiologist. Indeed, veno-venous bypass, once used quite commonly in most transplant programs, is now used much less frequently since the anesthesia team is often able to compensate for the loss of blood flow from the lower part of the body by volume infusions.

Most teams flush the donor liver with an electrolyte or colloid solution of choice, as the preservative fluid of choice (UW/Belzer's solution) carries a very high concentration of potassium. This is usually done via donor portal vein while the caval anastomosis is being done. Failure to flush the liver will result in refractory cardiac standstill once blood is circulated through the liver. There are other alternate preservative solutions that are not as toxic and have become popular with some transplant teams. Once the caval anastomosis is done, the portal venous anastomosis is made, making sure to not leave any redundancy in length. The anastomosis itself however is completed with a "growth factor", an air-knot that allows the portal vein to grow and expand once flow is restored. This is considered important to prevent recurrence of portal hypertension. Up until this time, the liver is kept cooled and preserved; however now warm blood can be circulated through the liver as portal venous blood has enough oxygen. It is imperative that the anesthesiology team is alerted prior to this, since there is almost invariably a short period of hemodynamic instability following liver reperfusion, often referred to as "reperfusion syndrome". If proper precautions have been taken (including hemodynamic support and electrolyte management), then this is a short period. However, this is the time that many teams experience hemodynamic, cardiac, or bleeding problems that can have serious consequences. Patients that were on veno-venous bypass can now be taken-off. The next anastomosis is hepatic arterial, and this is usually done at a bifurcation patch of hepatic artery to the aortic patch of the donor celiac trunk. The last anastomosis is the biliary anastomosis and in most cases is done between the donor and recipient common bile duct. Some surgeons stent this with a t-tube introduced via the side of the recipient duct away from anastomosis, while other surgeons place an ERCP type of internal biliary stent. If needed, this can be used postoperatively to study the bile duct radiographically and is usually removed after 6-8 weeks. A cholecystectomy is usually done just prior to placing drains (subdiaphragmatic and subhepatic) and closing the fascia in layers. In many cases, instead of a direct choledochocholedochostomy, an anastomosis between the donor duct and Roux-en-Y bowel loop has to be made if the recipient duct is unsuitable (as in patients with primary or secondary sclerosing cholangitis). The different liver techniques are demonstrated in Figure 2.

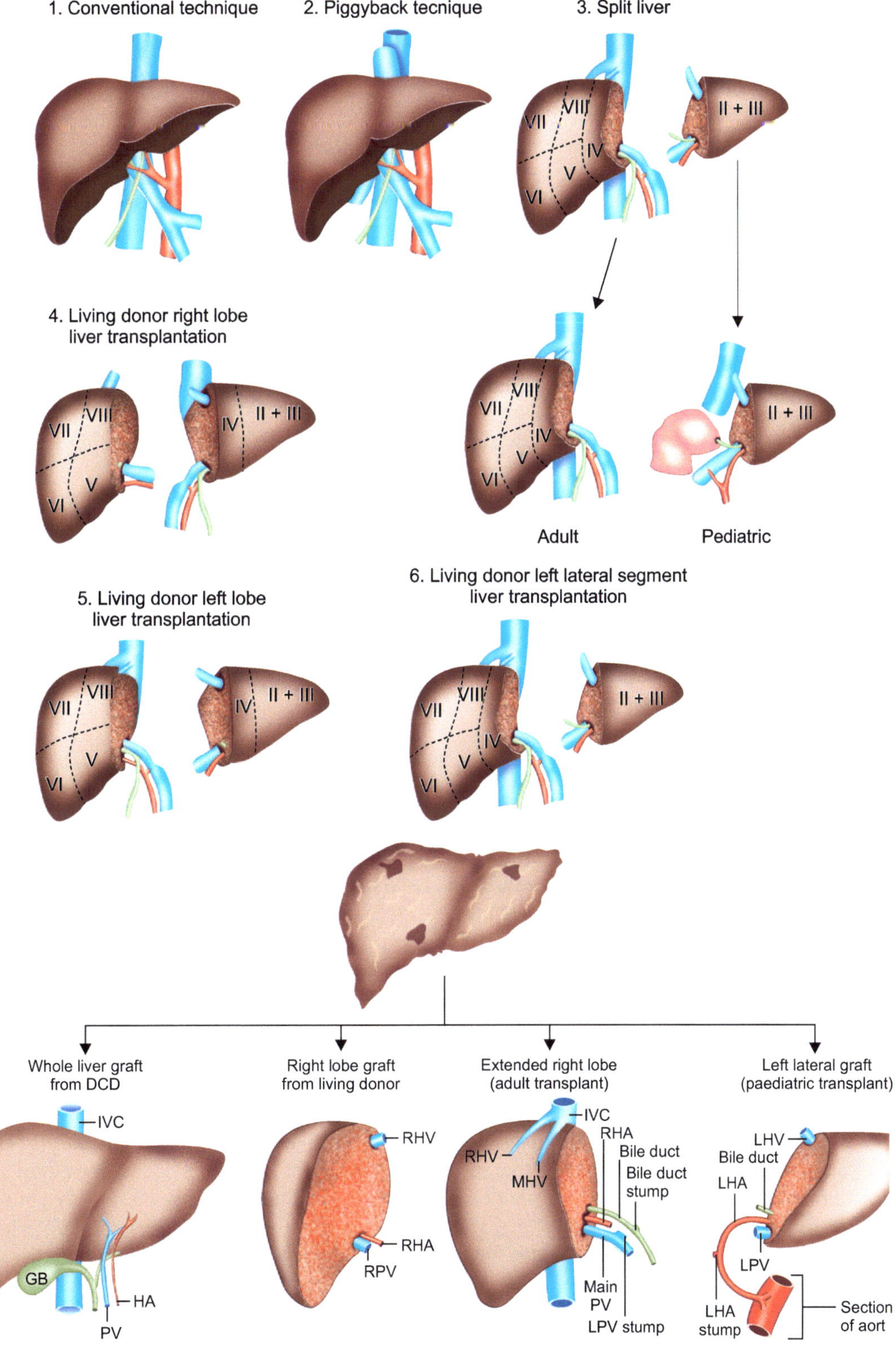

Figure 2: Different liver transplant techniques.

Immunosuppression

Almost all programs use an induction dose of corticosteroid similar to kidney transplantation. However, subsequently the liver patients can be tapered rapidly, and many (if not most) liver transplant patients are on very low doses of immunosuppression by the end of 12 months; namely a calcineurin inhibitor or mycophenolate mofetil with or without a low dose oral steroid.

Postoperative Care

In an uneventful case, the patient is typically given low volume crystalloids postoperatively as they are expected to have a total body surplus of salt and water due to precedent cirrhosis pathophysiology. The following specific facts have to be kept in consideration: (1) recovery of brain function from anesthesia is considered an important demonstration of liver function, therefore sedatives and narcotics are kept at a minimum. The following serves as a guide to monitoring the function of a liver on the recovery path: (1) neurologic recovery, (2) correction of acidosis, (3) absence of hypoglycemia, (4) correction of coagulopathy, (5) golden-brown (as compared to colorless or green) bile if a t-tube was placed, and (6) hemodynamic stabilization. It is important to not incorrectly characterize the hyperdynamic circulation seen in liver disease patients with sepsis. Postoperative antibiotics are typically stopped after 24-72 hours. Drains, if only draining serous or serosanguinous fluid, can be removed in 2-3 days.

Postoperative Problems

Allograft dysfunction after liver transplantation is typically investigated with triple-testing: Doppler ultrasound, biliary study (t-tube cholangiogram or ERCP), and a liver biopsy. Between these three modalities, the clinical team can often discern the differential between the most common postoperative problems in >90% of cases.

1. Primary Non-function (PNF): This is the most feared postoperative problem and is a true emergency as the patient is running on a very short time and needs to be urgently re-listed for re-transplantation. Common causes are donor factors including advanced age and steatosis, excessive ischemic times, poor blood supply to the donor organ, intraoperative factors, hemodynamic instability, immunologic phenomena, etc. Recognition of PNF is through awareness of the above-mentioned signs. These patients manifest immediate signs of severe liver injury with transaminases in the five digits, climbing bilirubin, and INR.
2. Initial Poor Function (IPF): This is more common, especially since with improving overall outcomes, transplant teams have ventured into previously unchartered territories, most prominently including using marginal donors. These patients eventually recover their liver function due to the tremendous regeneration capacity of the liver. However, the recipient needs to be supported during recovery with judicious nutrition (i.e., substitution for fat-soluble vitamins), watching for immunologic events, and viral infections (i.e., CMV).
3. Bleeding: Many patients require some blood transfusion postoperatively. However, enough bleeding to cause hemodynamic instability and rapid filling of drain reservoirs is cause for re-exploration. Common bleeding sites include the sites of caval anastomoses and the phrenic veins.
4. Hepatic Artery Thrombosis (HAT): Another feared complication since surgeons often take this complication as a comment on their surgical technique. This may be the reason for the routine practice of postoperative Doppler ultrasound on the 1st postoperative day. While the hepatic parenchyma can live off the oxygen supply from the portal venous blood, the bile ducts are dependent on the oxygen from the hepatic artery. Early hepatic artery thrombosis within 14 days almost always requires re-exploration, thrombectomy, and/or revision of the anastomosis. Late thromboses are often managed expectantly as it is believed that enough collateralization from the diaphragm, lesser omentum, and along the hepatic hilum is available to support the arterial blood supply to the bile ducts. However, in most instances, these patients end up with biliary strictures. Isolated strictures can often be managed with stenting (ERCP or percutaneous). In some patients, however, with extensive intrahepatic biliary strictures; the only true option is re-transplantation. For this reason, the treatment paradigm has shifted to an aggressive approach to treat HAT even when it is discovered late.
5. Biliary leak: A bile leak after liver transplantation should prompt a search for hepatic artery thrombosis or stenosis. If occurring within a month, then an operative intervention and refashioning of anastomosis is required, ideally a Roux-en-Y conversion in case of an earlier duct-to-duct anastomosis. A minor leak can be temporary, even in the early phase, with an ERCP stent; however, the endoscopist must exercise caution in handling a recently anastomosed bile duct. A late bile leak is usually seen after removal of a biliary stent, such as a t-tube after the center preferred period which is typically >6 weeks considering the inability of steroid treated transplant patients to form well-formed tracts. Despite a peritoneal reaction that is not uncommonly

seen after removal of the t-tube, most patients can avoid direct surgical intervention. Sometimes an ERCP and stent placement is required.

6. Biliary strictures: This was discussed above.
7. Recurrent disease: This often manifests weeks or months later. Hepatitis C recurrence in the transplanted liver is almost universal and no true proven treatment exists for this problem. HCV recurrence can be severe and result in allograft loss, especially if virulent viral genomes are involved. There is also the risk of HBV recurrence, but it has been reduced to an insignificant problem due to the prevalent use of antiviral therapy starting with Lamivudine, while this problem was highly prevalent and rapidly destructive when HBIg was the only option. Even now, many centers prefer to add HBIg therapy to their antiviral treatment for Hepatitis B. Autoimmune diseases can also recur, especially autoimmune hepatitis. For this reason, caution is used when reducing immunosuppression in these patients. Other recurrences to watch for include recidivism in patients with a history of alcoholism and recurrence of hepatocellular carcinoma.

Living Liver Transplant

Living related liver transplantation has helped to increase the number of available organs for transplantation. This has been of tremendous help especially in pediatric patients where the donor operation is much less risky than living donor hepatectomy for adult patients. In countries where brain dead criteria for cadaveric organ donation have not been accepted, living related liver transplantation is the only way patients with ELSD can receive their liver transplant; though in countries that have cadaveric organ donation, living related liver transplant is practiced in less than 10% of patients. The amount of liver tissue taken from the donor is the most important factor in the safety of the donor. Adult donor hepatectomy, most commonly a right hepatectomy, is the most difficult and complicated surgery. Due to the complexity of donor hepatectomy, strict rules and regulations are governing the practice of living related liver transplant. In spite of these strict rules, there have been donor mortalities which negatively affected the practice of living liver transplantation. Donor selection is very strict and only around 10 to 40% of potential donors end up donating part of their liver to the recipients.

Donors go through psychological evaluations before a thorough medical evaluation to ascertain their willingness and suitability for donation. Medical Evaluations include age, size (i.e., height, weight, BMI), blood type, liver function, and renal function. Additionally, CT/MRI/MRCP of the liver with volumetry is completed to access the anatomy and adequacy of both donated part and remaining part of liver so as not to jeopardize the life of both the donor and recipient. There have been a lot of technical advancements in both assessing the vascular and biliary anatomy of the liver. Also, different technologically advanced instruments are being used, especially for parenchymal transection which has made the donor surgery safer.

Some centers are considering using two donors (two left lobes) if the right lobe of the donor is not adequate for the recipient, this brings an ethical issue which is difficult to address since it is increasing the potential risk for two donors. This is currently practiced in certain Asian countries with apparently good results. Some centers in the Western hemisphere also have returned to using left lobe transplant with apparent equal results and less risk to the donor.

Usually, a multi-disciplinary team consisting of hepatologist, transplant surgeons, independent donor advocates, social workers, coordinates, financial advisors, and psychologists are involved in selecting the donor.

Strategically, a living related liver transplant is very demanding, requiring two to three experienced transplant surgeons who have previously performed HPB surgery, in addition to having two operating rooms with experienced staff available. Hepatectomy in the recipient is similar to cadaveric liver transplant using the piggyback technique. Implantation starts with upper venous outflow anastomosis which is between the stump of right hepatic vein of the graft and either the right hepatic vein of recipient, the confluence of the left and middle hepatic veins, or directly to the anterior aspect of the vena cava. The right portal vein of the graft is anastomosed to the recipient's portal vein and usually the right hepatic artery of the recipient is anastomosed to the right hepatic artery of the graft. The bile duct, which has been cut sharply at the level of parenchymal transection, can be anastomosed either to the recipient's common bile duct or to a Roux-en-Y loop constructed in the recipient. Placement of the T-tube for biliary stenting has become optional based on the surgeon's preference and the complexity of the biliary anatomy in the graft. Some types of extra vascular reconstruction may become necessary in up to 25% of cases for venous outflow or portal vein reconstruction. A right lobe liver transplant is demonstrated in Figure 3.

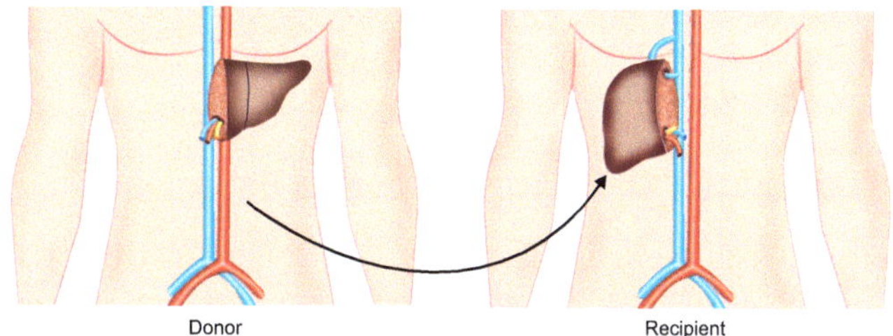

Figure 3: Right lobe liver transplant

The major morbidity in LRLT is from small for size syndrome (inadequate liver tissue to sustain life in the recipient) and biliary complications, since smaller bile ducts and more than one bile duct must be anastomosed directly to the recipient bile duct or use Roux-en-Y for biliary drainage. There should always be a cadaveric re-transplant option available in case the transplanted organ fails due to primary non-function or vascular catastrophe. In countries without this option this usually ends in the recipient's demise if they cannot get another living donor urgently.

Immunosuppression for LR liver transplant is no different than cadaveric liver transplant and the outcome is as good as a liver transplant from a cadaveric donor.

Pancreas and Islet Cell Transplantation

Diabetes mellitus affects around 6% of the general population. In the United States, it is the third most common disease and the fourth leading cause of death by disease. There are an estimated 21 million diabetic individuals in the United States and 1 to 2 million have insulin-dependent diabetes mellitus (IDDM). Every year, there are almost 300,000 new IDDM cases diagnosed, and this incidence continues to increase.[1] Due to its prevalence, pancreas transplantation has become increasingly important in IDDM treatment. Currently, pancreas transplantation is the only available treatment that can reliably result in an insulin-independent state, where patients can become euglycemia and obtain a normal glycosylated hemoglobin level; reestablishing normal feedback controls that can produce endogenous insulin secretion.[2]

Pancreas transplantation was initially described in 1967,[3] however, the results of the first pancreas grafts and patient survival rates were poor. Since then, there have been significant improvements in graft and patient survival due to several factors such as advances in surgical techniques, graft preservation techniques, immunosuppression, diagnostic methods of transplant rejection and its treatment, and the management of common post-transplant complications. Therefore, more pancreas transplants are being reported to United Network of Organ Sharing (UNOS) and the International Pancreas Transplant Registry (IPTR) and this number continues to increase, with 26,571 cases between December 1966 and October 2006, 20,014 of which were performed in the United States.[4]

Indications for and Types of Pancreas Transplantation

Patients with type 1 diabetes and end stage renal disease (ESRD) three transplant procedure options: (1) a kidney transplant only, (2) a simultaneous pancreas-kidney transplant, or (3) a kidney transplant with a subsequent pancreas transplant (pancreas-after-kidney transplant), where the kidney graft can be obtained from either a living or deceased donor.

1. **Simultaneous pancreas-kidney transplantation:** In simultaneous pancreas-kidney transplant (SPK), the pancreas and kidney are usually obtained from the same deceased donor; therefore, changes in kidney function can be used to determine whether rejection is occurring in either organ.[5,6] In case of SPK, the kidney is usually transplanted first, as a functioning kidney transplant offers the advantage of protecting the transplant pancreas from edema.
2. **Pancreas-after-kidney (PAK) transplantation:** This is the second most common pancreas transplant procedure. The indication for this procedure is a patient with type 1 diabetes who has identified a living donor for kidney transplant and wants to plan a later pancreas-after-kidney transplant, or the type 1 diabetes patient who already has a kidney transplant that has stable graft function, desires the potential benefits of normoglycemia, and has the cardiac reserve to undergo the procedure.[5,6]
3. **Pancreas transplant alone (PTA):** Pancreas transplant alone is the least common pancreas transplant procedure performed. Frequent, severe, hypoglycemic events are the most common indication for this procedure. The American Diabetes Association position statement suggests that indications for pancreas transplant (in the absence of kidney failure) are "frequent, acute and severe metabolic complications (hypoglycemia, hyperglycemia, and ketoacidosis) requiring medical attention" as well as "clinical and emotional problems with exogenous insulin therapy that are so severe as to be incapacitating; and consistent failure of insulin-based management to prevent acute complications".[8]

Patient Selection

Prior to transplantation, a multidisciplinary team must complete a comprehensive medical evaluation of the patient to confirm an IDDM diagnosis, determine if the patient can tolerate the operative procedure, and document end-organ complications to be used in the future for tracking after transplantation. SPK is considered in patients with IDDM with advanced nephropathy. These are patients who were dependent or would have been imminently dependent on dialysis and have a creatinine clearance <30 mL/min. PTA selection criteria include the patient having early diabetic complications associated with either hypoglycemia unawareness or exogenous insulin failure with hyper-labile diabetes. Additionally, they must have marked impairment in their quality of life. PTA generally requires a creatinine clearance >60 mL/min prior to transplantation since immunosuppression can accelerate renal function deterioration if the patient has a lower creatinine clearance. Another potential candidate for PAK includes diabetic patients with a previously renal allograft, from a living or cadaver donor if they had a creatinine clearance >40 mL/min on immunosuppression.[9-17]

Donor Selection

There is a gap between the organ supply and the number of patients awaiting donations for all transplantations. Since the donor criteria has extended ('marginal' donors) for kidney, cardiac, and liver transplantation, the donor pool has expanded significantly. For pancreas transplants, only 35% of pancreases are recovered from deceased donors, resulting in an underutilization of these grafts. Many surgeons continue to be reluctant to use the pancreata of 'marginal' or non-heart beating donors, even though recent literature suggests this can expand the donor pool safely and effectively. The outcome of the pancreas transplant is highly dependent on donor factors. However, if approached judiciously, using 'extreme' donors can greatly increase the availability of organs, shorten the waiting list burden, and minimize additional risks.

Pancreas Preservation

Oftentimes, pancreas organ donors are multi-organ donors. Liver surgeons, not pancreas surgeons, choose a solution to use for preservation. Currently, the two major solutions include (1) University of Wisconsin solution (UW, Viaspan; Bristol-Myers Squibb, Brussels, Belgium) and (2) histidine–tryptophan–ketoglutarate solution (HTK, Custodiol; Essential Pharmaceuticals, Newtown, Pennsylvania, USA).[17-21] These solutions can then be divided into either intracellular or extracellular solutions, depending on their high sodium and low potassium content, or vice versa, respectively. The UW solution is considered an intracellular solution. The HTK is considered an extracellular solution with a low sodium and potassium content, however it uses histidine to maintain osmotic pressure.

Results of studies analyzing whole pancreas preservation solutions have been controversial. There have been four recent studies[17-20] that compared the HTK with UW solutions in clinical pancreas transplantation. In a multi-institutional study, Englesbe[17] et al. showed no difference of graft and patient survival in early outcomes. However, Malek[19] et al. reported higher rates of edema in HTK preserved pancreases, but similar complication rates in both groups. Becker[20] et al. had similar clinical results, however, this study concluded there are many factors (i.e., donor and recipient factors) that must be considered for a successful pancreas transplantation. In this setting, the organ preservation solutions used will contribute to the transplant outcomes, but it is a limited impact.

Gonzalez[21] et al. studied the costs of organ retrieval and preservation. They adjusted the flushing procedure with UW solution; first to flush the pancreas with 1 liter of Euro-Collins solution, then to flush with 1 liter of UW solution. In the study, they observed that the patients who were transplanted with pancreases treated with this sequential technique had comparable outcomes as patients who received grafts flushed with 2 liters of UW solution. The results showed no significant differences in postsurgical complications, graft survival and functionality, or in patient survival and hospitalization time. Thus, this flushing technique can reduce the cost of harvesting the pancreas with similar clinical results. Additionally, it is important to mention that intra-abdominal organs treated with HTK require a larger volume of UW solution due to its lower viscosity, and thus faster perfusion speed. This therefore offsets the higher cost of the UW solution per volume.

Operative Technique in Pancreas Transplantation

Surgical Issues in Pancreas Transplantation

Currently, with more than 26,000 PTX reported to the international registry, and some 1900 new cases added annually,[4] the surgical debate continues regarding venous drainage (i.e., systemic vs. portal) and duct management (i.e., bladder vs. enteric).[22-27] The first PT involved a duct-ligated segmental graft implanted extra-peritoneally to the left iliac fossa. It functioned for 6 days but was eventually lost due to pancreatic fistula.[3] The next case was a pancreatic-duodenal graft, placed in the same location, with the first jejunal loop exteriorized to allow exocrine drainage. The graft functioned but was rejected early.

During recovery of the pancreas, en-bloc removal of pancreas, duodenum and spleen is part of a multi-organ retrieval. The pancreas graft is prepared on the back table in cold UW or HTK solution. Arterial reconstruction is completed with the donor iliac artery Y graft by anastomosing the superior mesenteric artery with the external iliac artery and the splenic artery with the internal iliac artery, or vice versa.

Pancreas transplantation can be carried out through J-shaped iliac incisions, transverse abdominal incisions, or midline abdominal incisions. The pancreas can either be placed extra-peritoneally or intraperitoneally. Extraperitoneal pancreas placement through J-shaped iliac or transverse abdominal incisions allows good pelvic exposure but it is usually associated with increased incidence of peri-graft and wound infections. Creation of a peritoneal window can facilitate absorption of potential leaks. When the pancreas is placed in the pelvis, it is usually transplanted on the right iliac vessels because of their favorable anatomic disposition. Simultaneous kidney transplantation is preferentially done on the contralateral side, either intraperitoneally or extra-peritoneally. When drained via the portal system, the pancreas is placed in a mid-abdominal position or behind the right colon.

In enteric drainage method, the stumps of the graft duodenum can be closed with a linear stapler, reinforced with absorbable sutures, and inverted. Duodenal anastomosis can be stapled, or hand sewn. Duodenocystostomy complication rate is not different between the two methods. Stapled duodenocystostomy can be inspected through an anterior cystotomy and reinforced with running absorbable sutures. Hand-sewn bladder or enteric anastomosis are usually constructed with an external layer of interrupted nonabsorbable sutures and an internal layer of continuous absorbable material. Stapled enteric anastomosis can employ either a circular or a linear device.

Enteric anastomosis involves either the distal ileum or the proximal jejunum. It can be constructed end-to-end, end-to-side, and side-to-side. Some groups prefer to use a Roux-en-Y loop, while other surgeons choose direct anastomosis.

Bladder versus Enteric Duct Management

With bladder drainage (BD), graft function can be determined using urine amylase as a marker. Pancreas graft biopsies can be obtained by going across the bladder wall using cystoscopy (Figure 4). However, there are a few potential complications with this procedure. Metabolic acidosis and extracellular volume depletion are both very common and can occasionally be severe enough to necessitate hospitalization. These complications result from the urine losing sodium bicarbonate-rich pancreatic secretions. Other BD complications include bladder leak, chemical cystitis/urethritis, reflux pancreatitis (especially with neurogenic bladder), duodenitis in the connecting segment, frequent bladder infections, bladder calculi, bladder tumors, urethral stricture and erosion, prostatitis, epididymitis, and prostatic abscess. There is a high frequency of urological complications (50–77%), however, graft or patient losses are rare.

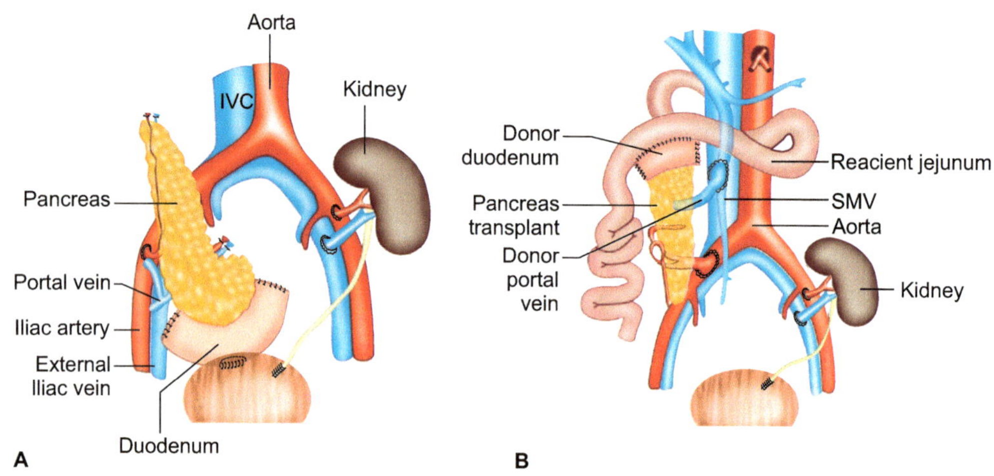

Figure 4. Old (left) and new (right) technique for kidney-pancreas transplantation

Enteric drainage (ED) of the exocrine duct is an alternative to BD. During ED, the pancreatic duct is inserted into the small bowel using a small duodenum "button" or using a Roux-en-Y limb. Overall, since immunosuppression has improved and there is a lower frequency of rejection episodes, pancreas transplants of all types require less monitoring of the pancreas graft. Enteric conversion surgery (20-25%) is indicated when there are frequent episodes of severe extracellular volume depletion, severe metabolic acidosis, problems with the duodenal segment, or urological complications.

There are equal rates of graft survival for simultaneous pancreas-kidney transplants performed with either BD or ED.

Portal versus Systemic Venous Drainage

Systemic venous drainage (SVD) is when insulin is secreted in the systemic circulation, or the pancreatic venous effluent. Thus, the insulin is not immediately extracted by the liver, as would be the case if it were emptied into the portal circulation. This results in elevated systemic concentrations of insulin, both fasting and postprandial. Subsequently, another procedure was developed which consisted of the graft being placed in the portal circulation and the pancreatic duct drained into the small intestine. The portal venous drainage (PVD) combined with the ED procedure resulted in significantly decreased peripheral insulin concentrations compared to pancreas transplant recipients with SVD, these results are comparable to nondiabetic kidney transplants receiving similar immunosuppression.

Complications

Pancreas transplantation is a very complex procedure. In addition to the complexity of the procedure, many patients have a high likelihood of having pre-existing disease secondary to their diabetes, thus, there are significant operative and postoperative risks to the recipient. These risks likely limited the acceptance of pancreas transplantation early in its development. Serious postoperative surgical complications consist of intra-abdominal hemorrhage, thrombosis of graft vessels, graft pancreatitis, anastomotic leak (enteric or bladder), intra-abdominal sepsis, and pancreatic fistula formation. All of these complications can result in the need for relaparotomy and have the potential of graft loss. More recently, due to improvements in donor and recipient selection criteria, immunosuppression protocols (decreased incidence of early, acute rejection) surgical technique, and prophylaxis regimens (i.e., antibacterial, antiviral, and anti-thrombosis), the overall incidence of serious complications and the rate of relaparotomy have significantly decreased.[28-36]

Most of the problems are due to the exocrine pancreas, namely pancreatitis, enzyme leak, and the most feared complication of venous thrombosis. Additionally, in patients with a bladder drained pancreas, there is the added complication of dehydration, acidosis, and reflux pancreatitis from an over-distended bladder.

1. Allograft Pancreatitis: Some degree of allograft pancreatitis is universal and is managed with patience and bowel rest. A well-procured pancreas usually has self-limited brief pancreatitis that resolves itself.
2. Acidosis and dehydration: A careful monitoring of serum electrolytes, acid-base status, and hydration is mandatory.
3. Anastomotic leak: In a patient with a bladder drained pancreas, the leak from duodenocystostomy can be managed with a Foley catheter placed in the bladder for the long-term. However, in a patient with an enteric drained pancreas, an anastomotic leak will always require re-exploration, drainage of bowel leak or sepsis, and re-doing the anastomosis.
4. Allograft venous thrombosis: This complication results in allograft loss, although there are sporadic reports of successful thrombectomy of the allograft portosplenic vein. It is believed that venous thrombosis is secondary to increased pressure in the transplanted organ, as would be seen in pancreatitis or venous outflow obstruction. Additionally, the incidence of this severe complication is higher in donor organs with excessive fat content, which is the reason most transplant programs stay away from pancreata procured from obese (BMI >35) and/or elderly donors (age >50 years). This complication is also reported to be higher in small petite female recipients; this may be a factor of small vessel size and use of oral contraception.
5. Infectious complications: These are more common with the pancreas transplantation as compared with the kidney or liver transplantation. Pancreatitis results in inflammation and necrosis in the peri-graft area, predisposing to bacterial and fungal infections.
6. Hematuria secondary to hemorrhage cystitis.

Postoperative Management

Patients are volume resuscitated, more than what would be needed for kidney transplantation alone, as these patients also develop ileus postoperatively. It is critical that the patients are kept well hydrated and often clinical guidance is taken from central venous pressure or pulmonary artery catheter monitoring. Blood glucose is closely monitored as there is a risk of hypoglycemia for 1 to 2 days, in a well-functioning pancreas transplantation. Patients are also monitored for bleeding and significant pancreatitis (serum and drain fluid amylase) as any inflammation increases the risk of graft edema and reduced flow to the organ. Most patients can take oral feeds by the 3rd or 4th postoperative day and can be discharged by the 7th to 10th day. Immunosuppressive protocols for these patients are very similar to kidney transplantation, including induction therapy using antilymphocyte antibodies and prolonged use of triple immunosuppression (calcineurin inhibitor, antimetabolite, and steroid).

Immunosuppression

In 2000, the most common pancreas transplant regimen consisted of tacrolimus/mycophenolate mofetil (MMF; nearly 80%) and the distant second most commonly used regiment was cyclosporine/MMF (5%–20%).[37] Tacrolimus/MMF largely replaced cyclosporine/MMF due to evidence of lower rejection rates, and better lipids and blood pressure. Other immunosuppression combinations include tacrolimus-sirolimus-MMF, tacrolimus-sirolimus cyclosporine-sirolimus, MMF-sirolimus, and sirolimus only.

Many centers continue to include corticosteroids in their immunosuppression protocol, allowing for a reduced calcineurin inhibitor dose, but others are attempting to use a "steroid-free" protocol to hopefully decrease the risk of weight gain, dyslipidemia, glucose intolerance, and bone loss.

Pancreas transplantation results continue to improve with increasingly targeted immunosuppressive strategies. Withdrawal from or avoidance of corticosteroids is becoming a clinical reality, particularly in SPK and PAK recipients, however, minimizing or eliminating CNI is still a work in progress. For whole pancreas transplantation, induction immunosuppression is routinely used, with >75% of recipients receiving either: (1) a T-cell depleting polyclonal antibody (Thymoglobulin, ATGAM) or monoclonal antibody (OKT3, Campath), (2) a non-depleting monoclonal anti-CD25 antibody (Zenapax, Simulect), or (3) both.

Alemtuzumab induction's initial results appear to be quite promising; however, it seems to be more effective when used as a conventional induction agent instead of a tolerance inducing or maintenance immunosuppressant. SPK recipients use both T-cell depleting and non-depleting antibody agents for induction, whereas solitary PTX more often uses T-cell depleting antibodies. Some patients can use monotherapy, but which regimen is most safe and effective remains unclear. Clinical studies in the future will continue focusing on the long-term outcomes, immunologic monitoring, immunosuppressive reduction, appropriate donor and recipient selection, and outcomes-based research.

Long-term use of immunosuppression has many significant side effects and complications. Such side effects associated with standard maintenance immunosuppression include hypertension, microvascular disease, nephrotoxicity, hyperlipidemia, glucose intolerance, weight gain, gastrointestinal problems, skin changes, alopecia, and hirsutism. Immunosuppression-related side effects include malignancy (skin, lymphoproliferative genitourinary) and infections (viral, bacterial, fungal, parasitic). Infection risk is dependent on the degree of immune system compromise from the immunosuppressive regimen and the pathogen exposure, either through re-activation of preexisting infection (e.g., viral, tuberculosis) or introduction during the transplant process (e.g., transfer from donor, surgical technique). The risk of skin cancer for a renal transplantation patient on immunosuppression is cumulative, ranging from 10% at 10 years to 40% at 20 years, with a 2:1 ratio of squamous cell to basal cell carcinoma. The prevalence of post-transplant lymphoproliferative disease and leukemia varies from 1% to 2%.

Results and Outcome

Simultaneous pancreas-kidney transplant patient survival is consistently better than survival observed during cadaveric-donor kidney transplant, possibly except for recipients >50 years old. Part of this advantage may be attributed to improved glucose levels after pancreas-kidney transplant when compared with kidney transplant alone. Additionally, other survival factors include the differences of the recipients and the donor grafts used for these two procedures. Simultaneous pancreas-kidney transplant mortality is equal to living-donor kidney transplant alone after 10 years. Both pancreas-after-kidney and pancreas transplant alone can potentially increase 4-year mortality compared to remaining on the waiting list. Before considering these procedures for these patients, it is important to account for specific quality of life (QOL) concerns and the impact of pancreas transplant on specific diabetic complications in addition to the potential early increase in mortality

In the United States, whole pancreas transplantation has proven to be a safe procedure, with a 1-year survival rate of 95%- and 5-year survival rate of 89% for all forms of pancreas transplant (SPK, PAK, PTA) since 1998 (unadjusted patient survival rates, 2005 OPTN/SRTR Annual Report).[37]

Immediately after the pancreas transplant, the patient's glucose normalizes. If SVD is used, there is an additional expense of hyperinsulinemia. Despite denervation, insulin secretion demonstrates oscillations with normal first- and second-phase secretion responses, unless graft function decreases or insulin resistance increases. There is often a slight elevation of C-peptide concentrations, both basally and after mixed meal stimulus, however, these elevations are similar to nondiabetic kidney transplant recipients. Although fasting proinsulin does increase, it is not necessarily representative of failing graft function. Glucagon response to hypoglycemia improves with time, eventually returning to normal or near normal. Epinephrine and growth hormone responses improve but never reach normal after pancreas transplant. Documented hypoglycemic symptoms and events are uncommon and generally diminish with time, but this can be attributed to a variety of factors. It should be cautioned that glucagon response to hypoglycemia does not improve with allo- or auto-transplantation of islets into the liver, in animal and human studies, as described with pancreas transplant. This may be due to being located in the liver.[16]

After more than 5-years of normal pancreas function, a functioning pancreas graft can prevent diabetic nephropathy and reverse pathological changes of diabetes.[7, 10] Initially, diabetic retinopathy can worsen following pancreas transplantation with sudden glucose level improvement; thus it is important to evaluate and treat any preexisting retinopathy when considering pancreas transplant surgery.[9] However, after 3 years of pancreas graft function, fewer retinal surgeries are required after simultaneous pancreas-kidney transplant compared with kidney transplant alone as long as the patient does not have end-stage eye disease. Lifelong eye surveillance exams are necessary for patients who undergo pancreas transplant, and laser surgery may still be required, particularly early after the procedure. Also, eye screenings are important to evaluate for new or progressing cataracts, especially in patients treated with corticosteroids. Sensory and motor neuropathy improvements are seen after both simultaneous pancreas-kidney and kidney transplant alone, with simultaneous pancreas-kidney transplants showing greater improvements and ongoing improvements up to 10-year post-transplant. Autonomic neuropathies may require >10 years to show improvement and may only show partial reversal or no reverse at all. Some autonomic neuropathy parameters have shown improvement in some studies, particularly autonomic response to hypoglycemia, hypoglycemia awareness, and cardiac autonomic neuropathies.[12]

Vascular disease is the most common cause of death in patients with diabetes and who undergo transplantation. Simultaneous pancreas-kidney transplant can improve glucose control, which can then improve vascular reactivity and microvascular integrity and responses. However, there are other post-transplant factors that may prevent or minimize these improvements in some cases.[11] Risk over time is impacted by (1) changes in renal function, (2) genetic predisposition to hypertension, dyslipidemia, or insulin resistance, (3) the type and dose of immunosuppressants, (4) patient behavior including weight gain or smoking cessation, and (5) donor and graft variables that contribute to delayed or decreased renal function, or frequency of rejection that increases the need for immunosuppression. However, current results suggest that simultaneous pancreas-kidney transplant improves macrovascular disease in most patients, but there is not adequate data available to draw conclusions for pancreas transplant alone or pancreas-after-kidney transplant.

Advantages of Pancreas Transplantation

Other than the significant life-style advantages from not being tethered to a glucometer and insulin injections, it is well accepted that a successful pancreas transplantation provides numerous physiologic advantages that include stabilization or improvement of diabetic neuropathy, retinopathy, and vasculopathy. Indeed, there is documented histological evidence of improved early diabetic nephropathy (KW lesions) in diabetic patients who received pancreas transplantation alone (PTA). There are also studies showing improvement in myocardial function. All in all, it appears that a successful pancreas transplant halts, or partially reverses the ravages of long-standing diabetes on various organ systems. Therefore, while earlier it was argued that the pancreas transplantation was merely exchanging insulin injections for a major surgical procedure, most now agree to the tremendous physiological advantages presented by this organ transplantation.

Islet Cell Transplantation

An alternative therapy to insulin treatment or pancreas transplant for type 1 diabetic patients is islet cell transplantation. Islet cells are isolated from a donor pancreata and embolized into the liver of the recipient via the portal vein. Islet cell transplantation is a much similar procedure compared to pancreas transplantation with lower morbidity and the ability to store the islet graft in tissue culture or cryopreservation for banking.[38-43]

Recent advances in islet cell isolation methods and the introduction of more potent and less diabetogenic immunosuppressive therapies, have enabled islet cell transplantation to progress from research to clinical reality. To date, several international institutions have demonstrated that islet cell transplantations can have successful clinical outcomes with high rates of insulin independence.[41] There continue to be refinements in donor pancreas procurement and processing, developments in islet isolation and purification technology. These advances in novel immunological conditioning and induction therapies have resulted in the acceptance of islet transplantation as a safe and effective therapy for patients with type 1 diabetes.

Tremendous progress has been made in clinical islet cell transplantation over the past few years, such progress includes refinement of the Edmonton Protocol and novel strategies for improved islet isolation, implantation, and recipient immunosuppression. The islet cell isolation procedure continues to be one of the most critical areas of research, being highly labor intensive, expensive, and relatively inconsistent. The highest-grade preparations are only able to recover about 20 to 50% of the potential islet mass. Additionally, rates for successful islet cell isolation at leading centers vary from 25 to 75% and are highly dependent on the quality of the pancreas, the amount of cold storage and the heterogeneity of collagenase preparations.[42,43]

Moving forward, one of the more focused challenges is to achieve reliable insulin independence with single-donor grafts. Prior experience with islet cells auto-transplantation after total pancreatectomy has shown the need for a minimum of 300,000 islets to achieve insulin independence in 70% of patients.[42] This can be compared to the 850,000 islets needed for the Edmonton series of patients. These results suggest that the presence of autoimmunity, diabetogenic immunosuppression, and brain death of the donor may have detrimental effects on islet cell engraftment and function. These effects may be due to the fact that cadaveric brain-dead organ donors are often hemodynamically unstable, need high doses of inotropic support, and circulating brain-derived inflammatory peptides can be directly toxic to the pancreas prior to retrieval. As there continue to be advances in cadaveric donor procurement techniques and improvements with less toxic and more potent immunosuppression, fewer islet cells will be required to achieve normoglycemia.

The development of novel immunosuppressive protocols which consist of using more specific and less toxic drugs, and moving towards inducing tolerance, is important to applying islet cell transplantation earlier in the course of the disease, including transplantation in the pediatric population. Moreover, further advancements in identifying other sources of islet cells and better understanding the biology of diabetes, will aid in increasing the limited supply of islets through gene therapy, stem-cell biology techniques, or xenotransplantation. Continued international collaboration is anticipated to further stimulate excitement in the field, as novel solutions are generated to address the remarkable challenges that lie ahead.

REFERENCES

1. National Diabetes Information Clearing House. Diabetes Statistics. Bethesda, MD: The National Institutes of Health, National Institute of Diabetes and Digestive and Kidney Diseases, 2006.
2. American Diabetes Association Pancreas Transplantation for patients with Type 1 diabetes. *Diabetes Care* 2004; 27 (Suppl. 1): S105.
3. W.D. Kelly, R.C. Lillehei and F.K. Merkel *et al.*, Allotransplantation of the pancreas and duodenum along with the kidney in diabetic nephropathy, *Surgery* 1967; 61:827-31
4. International Pancreas Transplant Registry. Newsletter 2004; Vol. 16, No. 1.
5. Sutherland DER, Gruessner RW, Dunn DL *et al.* Lessons learned from more than 1,000 pancreas transplants at a single institution. *Ann Surg* 2001; 233: 463–501.
6. Reddy KS, Stablein D, Taranto S *et al.* Long-term survival following simultaneous kidney-pancreas transplantation versus kidney transplantation alone in patients with type 1 diabetes mellitus and renal failure. *Am J Kidney Dis* 2003; 41: 464–470.
7. Venstrom JM, McBride MA, Rother KI, Hirshberg B, Orchard TJ, Harlan DM. Survival after pancreas transplantation in patients with diabetes and preserved kidney function. *JAMA* 2003; 290: 2817–2823.
8. Humar A, Kandaswamy R, Granger D, Gruessner RW, Gruessner AC, Sutherland DER. Decreased surgical risks of pancreas transplantation in the modern era. *Ann Surg* 2000; 231: 269–275.
9. Königsrainer A, Miller K, Steurer W *et al.* Does pancreas transplantation influence the course of diabetic retinopathy? *Diabetologia* 1991; 34 (Suppl. 1): S86–S88.
10. Fioretto P, Steffes MW, Sutherland DER, Goetz FC, Mauer M. Reversal of lesions of diabetic nephropathy after pancreas transplantation. *N Engl J Med* 1998; 339: 69–75.
11. Jukema JW, Smets YFC, van der Pijl JW *et al.* Impact of simultaneous pancreas and kidney transplantation on progression of coronary atherosclerosis in patients with end-stage renal failure due to Type 1 diabetes. *Diabetes Care* 2002; 25: 906–911.
12. Navarro X, Sutherland DER, Kennedy WR. Long-term effects of pancreatic transplantation on diabetic neuropathy. *Ann Neurol* 2003; 42: 727–736.
13. Paty BW, Lanz K, Kendall DM, Sutherland DE, Robertson RP. Restored hypoglycemic counterregulation is stable in successful pancreas transplant recipients for up to 19 years after transplantation. *Transplantation* 2001; 72: 1103–1107.
14. Robertson RP, Davis C, Larsen J, Stratta R, Sutherland DER. Pancreas, and islet transplantation for patients with diabetes. *Diabetes Care* 2000; 23: 112–116.
15. Ryan EA, Lakey JRT, Paty BW *et al.* Successful islet transplantation. Continued insulin reserve provides long-term glycemic control. *Diabetes* 2002; 51: 2148–2157.
16. Ryan EA, Shandro T, Green K *et al.* Assessment of the severity of hypoglycemia and glycemic lability in Type 1 diabetic subjects undergoing islet transplantation. *Diabetes* 2004; 53: 955–962.
17. Englesbe MJ, Moyer A, Kim DY, et al. Early pancreas transplant outcomes with histidine–tryptophan–ketoglutarate preservation: a multicenter study. Transplantation 2006; 82:136–139.
18. Agarwal A, Murdock P, Pescovitz MD, et al. Follow-up experience using histidine–tryptophan–ketoglutarate solution in clinical pancreas transplantation. Transplant Proc 2005; 37:3523–3526.
19. Malek PS, Eghtesad B, Shapiro R, et al. Initial experience using histidine–tryptophan–ketoglutarate solution in clinical pancreas transplantation. Clin Transplant 2004; 18:661–665.
20. Becker T, Ringe B, Nyibata M, et al. Pancreas transplantation with histidine–tryptophan–ketoglutarate (HTK) solution and University of Wisconsin (UW) solution: is there a difference? JOP 2007; 8:304–311.
21. Gonzalez AM, Filho GJ, Pestana JO, et al. Effects of Eurocollins solution as aortic flush for the procurement of human pancreas. Transplantation 2005; 80:1269–1274.
22. Stratta RJ, Gaber AO, Shokouh-Amiri MH, et al. Evolution in pancreas transplantation techniques: simultaneous kidney-pancreas transplantation using portal-enteric drainage without antilymphocyte induction. Ann Surg 1999; 229:701-712.
23. Sollinger HW, Knechtle SJ, Reed A, et al. Experience with 100 consecutive simultaneous kidney-pancreas transplants with bladder drainage. Ann Surg 1991; 214:703-711.
24. Mittal VK, Toledo-Pereyra LH. Long-term function and rehabilitation in combined kidney and pancreatic transplants. Transplant Proc. 1991 Oct;23(5):2469.

25. Kaufman DB, Leventhal JR, Gallon LG, et al. Technical and immunologic progress in simultaneous pancreas-kidney transplantation. Surgery 2002; 132:545-553.
26. Farney AC, Cho E, Schweitzer EJ, et al. Simultaneous cadaver pancreas living-donor kidney transplantation: a new approach for the type 1 diabetic uremic patient. Ann Surg 2000; 232:696-703.
27. Tyden G, Lundgren G, Ostman J, et al. Grafted pancreas with portal venous drainage. Lancet 1984; ii: 964-965.
28. Toledo–Pereyra LH, Mittal VK: Complications of pancreas transplantation—effect of technique. Transplant Proc 1987, 19:2319–2322.
29. Mühlbacher F, Gnant MF, Auinger M, et al. Pancreatic venous drainage to the portal vein: a new method in pancreas transplantation. Transplant Proc 1990; 22:636-637.
30. Mittal VK, Toledo-Pereyra LH. Management of delayed complications of the duodenal loop in whole organ pancreatic duodenal transplantation. *Transplant Proc.* 1990 Apr; 22(2):580-1.
31. Shokouh-Amiri MH, Gaber AO, Gaber LW, et al. Pancreas transplantation with portal venous drainage and enteric exocrine diversion: a new technique. Transplant Proc 1992; 24:776-777.
32. Zibari GB, Aultman DF, Abreo KD, et al. Roux-en-Y venting jejunostomy in pancreatic transplantation: a novel approach to monitor rejection and prevent anastomotic leak. Clin Transplant 2000; 14:380-385.
33. Toledo–Pereyra LH, Mittal VK. Effect of duodenal culture and postoperative infection on the long-term function of pancreaticoduodenal grafts.
34. Di Carlo V, Castoldi R, Cristallo M, et al. Techniques of pancreas transplantation through the world: an IPITA center survey. Transplant Proc 1998; 30:231-241.
35. Toledo–Pereyra LH, Mittal VK. Complications of pancreas transplantation-effect of technique. *Transplant Proc.* 1987 Feb;19(1 Pt 3):2319-22.
36. Hakim NS, Zarka ZA, El-Tayar A, et al. A new technique for kidney-pancreas transplantation. Transplant Proc 2003; 35:2803-2804.
37. OPTN/SRTR, HHS/HRSA/HSB/DOT. 2005 OPTN/SRTR Annual Report 1995-2004. www.ustransplant.org/annual_reports, 2005.
38. Villiger P, Ryan EA, Owen R, O'Kelly K, Oberholzer J, Al Saif F, Kin T, Wang H, Larsen I, Blitz SL, Menon V, Senior P, Bigam DL, Paty B, Kneteman NM, Lakey JR, Shapiro AM. Prevention of bleeding after islet transplantation: lessons learned from a multivariate analysis of 132 cases at a single institution. *Am J Transplant* 2005; 5: 2992-2998.
39. Sutherland DE, Gruessner R, Kandswamy R, Humar A, Hering B, Gruessner A. Beta-cell replacement therapy (pancreas and islet transplantation) for treatment of diabetes mellitus: an integrated approach. *Transplant Proc* 2004; 36: 1697-1699.
40. Hering BJ. Achieving and maintaining insulin independence in human islet transplant recipients. *Transplantation* 2005; 79: 1296-1297.
41. Merani S, Shapiro AM. Current status of pancreatic islet transplantation. *Clin Sci* (Lond) 2006; 110: 611-625.
42. Ryan EA, Bigam D, Shapiro AM. Current indications for pancreas or islet transplant. *Diabetes Obes Metab* 2006; 8: 1-7.
43. Ryan EA, Paty BW, Senior PA, Bigam D, Alfadhli E, Kneteman NM, Lakey JR, Shapiro AM. Five-year follow-up after clinical islet transplantation. *Diabetes* 2005; 54: 2060-2069.

SECTION 8: MISCELLANEOUS

66. Basic Urology
67. Bladder Dysfunction
68. Prostate
69. Urogenital Malignancies
70. Gynecology
71. Orthopedics
72. Pediatric Surgery
73. Neurosurgery
74. Updates of TNM Classification from 7th to 8th Edition

66

CHAPTER

Basic Urology

Pankaj Dangle, MD
Pasala Ravichandran, MD

INTRODUCTION

This chapter is an overview of the common urologic disorders with an emphasis on urolithiasis, bladder cancer, penile cancer, and renal masses. With the advent of advanced and frequent imaging, the incidence of renal mass diagnosis appears to be on the rise. Here, we give simplified algorithms for the diagnosis and management of these urologic disorders.

Urolithiasis

Since 1991, the American Urological Association (AUA) has led the formulation of urolithiasis guidelines. Many editions of these guidelines have come out since then, with the most recent being the 2005 guidelines on staghorn calculi.[1] Additionally since 2000, similar guidelines have been published by the European association of urology (EAU), with the most recent being published in 2010.[2]

This chapter covers the indications and techniques of general and special circumstances for percutaneous nephrolithotomy (PCNL).[3]

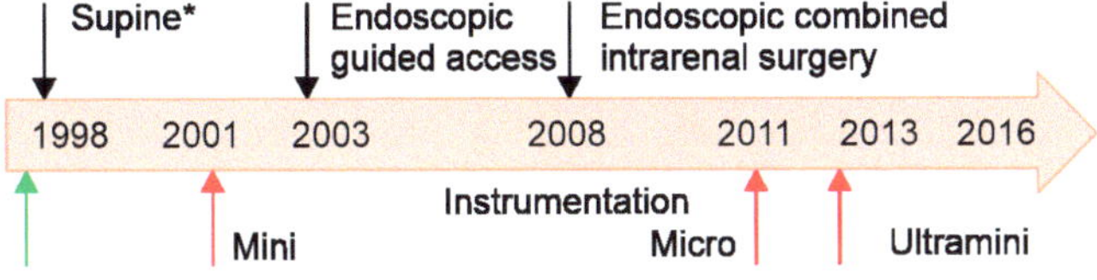

Figure 1: Innovations of PCNL

Preoperative Work Up

The gold standard for the work up of urolithiasis is non-contrast computerized tomography (NCCT) scans. In acute flank pain, randomized studies showed that NCCT has equivalent or superior results to excretory urography.[4] Furthermore, when creatinine is elevated or in pregnant or lactating patients, contrast media should be avoided.[5,6] Computerized tomographic urography (CTU) can provide more information; however, at the moment, level 1 evidence is not present to support that CTU is superior to IVU when working up urolithiasis.[7] Besides identifying stones, computerized tomography (CT) helps provide information such as presence, size, number, attenuation number, and degree of hydronephrosis, which is the skin to stone distance (Figure 2). This information is useful for selecting the appropriate treatment modality. Some clinicians use ultrasound and X-ray KUB as preoperative investigations. These methods are not considered standard but help when planning access and predicting the potential success rates. If the access method is ultrasound guided, then ultrasound could be useful as a tool in the preoperative workup.

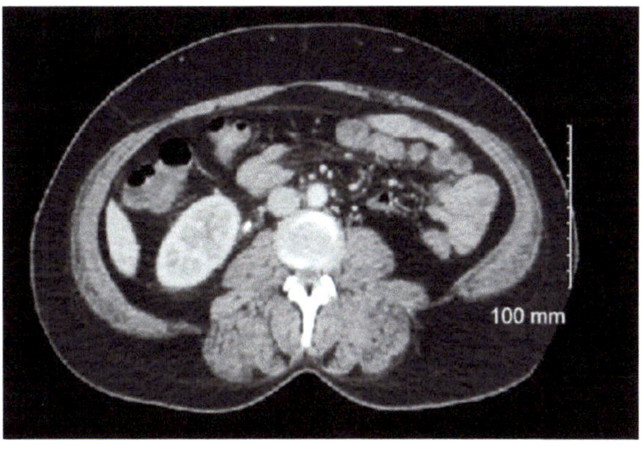

Figure 2: Proximal ureter stone

The applicability of three-dimensional reconstruction is described for planning percutaneous access. Staghorn stone distribution (also known as 'staghorn morphometry') and volume predicts the necessity of tract and stage for percutaneous nephrolithotomy (PCNL) monotherapy. The authors who described this application theorized that CT urography-based staghorn morphometry can predict tracts and stages for PCNL monotherapy, and that it can also help classify staghorn calculi accordingly. Staghorn morphometry differentiates staghorns into type 1 (single tract and single stage), type 2 (multiple tracts and single stage; single tract and single/multiple stages), and type 3 (multiple tracts and multiple stages).[8]

The EAU guidelines state that a patient should be administered antibiotics prior to removing the stone and at least 4 days after the procedure if they have an infection associated with their stone, for example bacteriuria and a recent urinary tract infection. Septic patients who have obstructing stones require urgent collecting system decompression with either percutaneous drainage or ureteral stenting. Sepsis should be resolved before definitive stone treatment is started.[2]

Indications for PCNL

PCNL is indicated based on stone factors (i.e., the composition of the stone, the size of the stone, and the location of the stone), patient factors (i.e., renal anomalies and habitus), and failure of other treatments (i.e., flexible ureteroscopy, ESWL). PCNL is generally indicated in patients with stones that are >20 mm,[2] have partial or complete staghorn calculi, and if the patient has stones in addition to chronic kidney disease. PCNL is contraindicated in pregnant patients, patients with bleeding disorders, and patients with uncontrolled urinary tract infections.[2]

Stone Factors

Stone Size

The treatment for large stones (> 2cm) is PCNL monotherapy. The stone free rate of PCNL is up to 95% since it directly removes stone fragments through the nephrostomy tract. Smaller stones (<2 cm) (Figure 3) have a more complicated treatment algorithm because there are multiple variables involved. PCNL is recommended for staghorn calculi according to the AUA guidelines. This is because in one retrospective study of 200 patients with staghorn calculi, 28% who were treated conservatively had renal deterioration. This indicates that aggressive surgical management of staghorn stones is very important.[10] PCNL results in >3 times the clearance rate compared to ESWL.[11] Treatment options for staghorn calculi are as follows:[1]

1. The treatment of choice is percutaneous nephrolithotomy for most patients. This treatment shows level 2 evidence.
2. For staghorn stones, ESWL is not the preferred treatment modality.
3. If the stone is not expected to be removed over the course of a reasonable number of stages, open surgery is recommended.
4. In non-functioning kidneys, nephrectomy should be considered.[1]

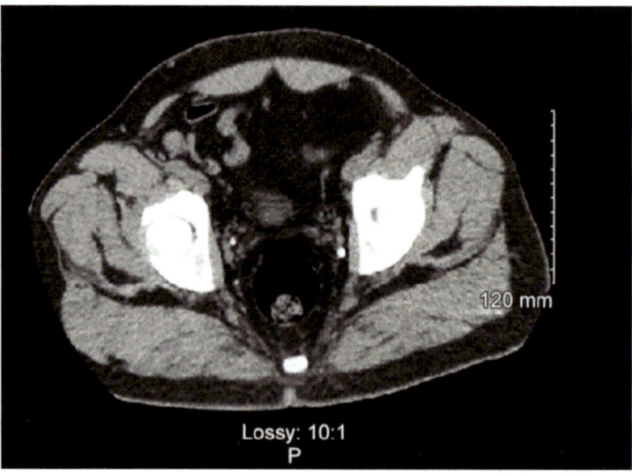

Figure 3: Less than 1 cm ureter stone in pelvic ureter junction

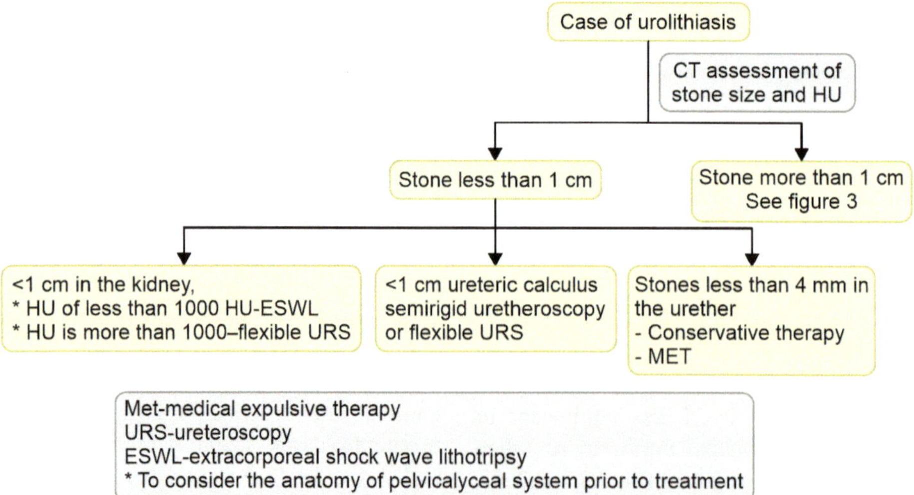

Figure 4: Algorithm for management of kidney stones less than one centimeter in size

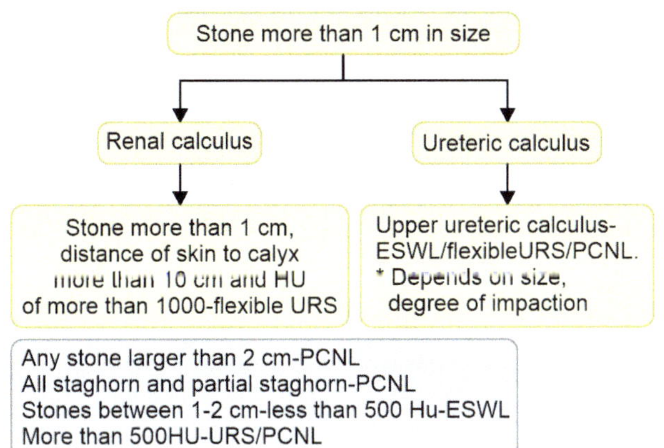

Figure 5: Algorithm for management of kidney stones more than one centimeter in size

Location of Stones

If the stone is large and located in the lower pole, PCNL is recommended as a first-line treatment option, irrespective of the anatomy of the lower pole.[3] The stone diameter should guide treatment of lower pole stones. Meta-analysis data suggests that larger, lower pole stones have higher retreatment rates and lower clearance rates (level 1 evidence).[11] A large multicenter prospective randomized trial which compared both ESWL and PCNL demonstrated that PCNL had significantly higher stone free rates (91%) than ESWL (21%). Additionally, ESWL required both more ancillary procedures and more frequent retreatment when compared to PCNL (level 1 evidence).[12,13] While considering the stone location, the number one factor in predicting the clearance of a stone is the calyceal stone burden.

A calyceal diverticulum is the non-secretory urothelium that lines the compartments in communication with the renal collecting system. If a stone in the diverticulum is asymptomatic, they can be left alone. However, treatment is required if a patient is symptomatic and the stone causes pain, hematuria, or infection. PCNL results in higher stone free rates; however, no randomized trials have compared laparoscopy with PCNL and ureteroscopy. PCNL is also the gold standard treatment for calyceal diverticular stones. PCNL has higher stone free rates (between 85 and 93%) compared to ESWL and has similar recurrence and complication rates.[14] PCNL is additionally advantageous because it provides excellent access for diverticular sac obliteration.[15]

Composition and Hardness of Stone

Another important factor in determining treatment modality is the stone composition and fragility. Different stone compositions result in different rates of clearance due to the different stone fragilities. For example, it is difficult to fragment cystine stones, therefore if the stone is >15 mm, PCNL is recommended over ESWL.[2] Stone density measurements using NCCT enables predicting the success rates of ESWL and, if the predicted success rate is low, then PCNL is indicated. If a stone has >1,000 Hounsfield units (HU), this indicates poor ESWL results.[16,17] PCNL is also the best treatment for struvite stones. EAU guidelines state that if a stone is large and ESWL-resistant, then PCNL is recommended for the efficient removal of the stone, thereby avoiding the renal tissue from receiving excess shock-wave energy.[2]

PCNL Technique Recommendations[3]

Traditionally, PCNL is performed with the patient in the prone position, but it can be performed in the lateral decubitus or supine positions as well. Guided ultrasound or fluoroscopy enables collecting system access, depending on instrument availability and operator expertise. When possible, the access site should be the posterior calyx because it is the shortest tract between the skin and the calyx transversing the papilla. Additionally, the stone configuration should be studied when selecting the calyx (supracostal, infracostal, or subcostal) to enable the maximum stone bulk to clear the minimum number of tracts. Dilation of the renal tract can be done by either the balloon amplatz or metallic dilators. However, balloon dilators are considered the gold standard. A nephrostomy tube is placed during complicated cases or if a secondary intervention is needed because it can function as a tamponade and a conduit for a second look. If a case is uncomplicated, a tubeless PCNL either with or without the application of tissue sealants is a safe alternative.

PCNL in Special Situations

Anomalous Kidneys

Anomalous kidneys include horseshoe kidneys, stones in ectopic, or kidneys with fusion anomalies. The management of anomalous kidneys should be individualized and should take into account the stone bulk, stone location, the vascular anatomy, and the pelvicalyceal anatomy of the pelvicalyceal system. Diagnosis and accessing ectopic kidney are complete through ultrasound. CT is crucial in deciding which management and treatment method to use in an anomalous kidney.

CT will also provide attenuation values and help determine if one should use ESWL or a flexible ureteroscopy. For the treatment of small burden stones, flexible ureteroscopy is helpful due to the availability of smaller flexible ureteroscopes and access sheaths. However, surgeons should also consider a complete "on table" clearance because these patients often have impaired drainage. A surgeon should be well versed in the USG guided approach before utilizing it to treat ectopic kidneys. Laparoscopic assisted PCNL has shown good clearance rates, decreased need for ancillary procedures, and minimal morbidity. Even though ESWL can obtain adequate fragmentation, there may be impaired drainage of the fragments due to anatomical abnormalities. Choosing to treat with ESWL versus flexible ureteroscopy should be done prudently

Pediatric urolithiasis

Pediatric treatment modalities are the same as those used in adults. ESWL is indicated in conditions similarly to adults. Ideally, a stone in a child will have a diameter <20 mm. There is a decrease in success rate as stone burden increases. PCNL is indicated for larger stones.[2] Children require knowledge of a few important points which are as follows:

1. Children tend to pass larger stone fragments
2. Ultrasound should be used to localize stones when ESWL is the chosen modality for treatment
3. Endourologic manipulations require smaller instruments[2]

Percutaneous Antegrade Ureteroscopy

The removal of ureteral stones may be done with percutaneous antegrade in certain cases including when ESWL is not indicated or failed to treat adequately and when the upper urinary tract cannot tolerate retrograde URS. It may be indicated when treating large (>15 mm diameter) impacted stones located in the proximal ureter between the lover 4th lumbar vertebra boarder and the ureteropelvic junction. In these cases, percutaneous antegrade ureteroscopy has demonstrated stone-free rates between 85% and 100%.[2]

Urolithiasis in pregnancy

Urolithiasis in pregnant women has been and remains to be a diagnostic and therapeutic challenge. Ultrasound is safe and practical and has therefore been used to evaluate pregnant women who have urolithiasis. The time of stone presentation and the degree of obstruction are important in determining the management of these patients. A temporary diversion is warranted if conservative methods failed. ESWL and PCNL are contraindicated during pregnancy because they risk the growing fetus being exposed to radiation.[2]

Evaluation of a Case of Hematuria (Figure 6)

Hematuria is one of the commonest presenting symptoms in the urology clinic. The urologist should evaluate a case of hematuria after considering the age, type, comorbidity, and drug history of patients. The evaluation should involve pertinent laboratory tests and clinical evaluations to ascertain the cause of hematuria.

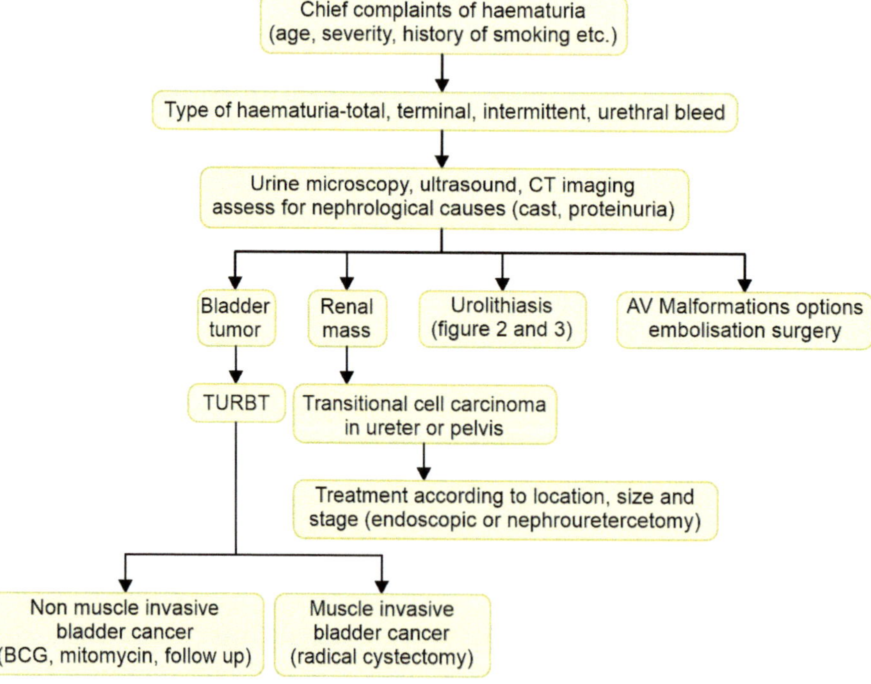

Figure 6: Algorithm for the evaluation of hematuria

Clinical Examination

Smoking and a history of contact with hair dyes and paints constitutes risk factors for bladder cancer. If the hematuria is total, a suspicion of bladder mass should be entertained; a terminal hematuria suggests pathology at the bladder neck; hematuria with amorphous clots suggest a pathology in the bladder, while long serpentine clots suggest an upper tract pathology. An advanced malignancy with lymphadenopathy will present with pedal edema. The urologist should also look for a palpable bladder lump or renal lump in the flank.

Urine Examination

A urine microscopy examination provides a wealth of information. Significant hematuria is defined as more than 3 RBC in a high-power field. A freshly voided sample is useful for detecting urinary acid-fast bacilli. Similarly, a urine cytology examination should be collected in the morning. Atypical cells or cell atypia is typically defined as irregular cells with large nucleoli. The examination requires a skilled cytopathologist. Urinary protein levels >300 mg is considered significant, and if seen along with casts, should raise suspicion for a nephrological cause of hematuria. However, the presence of crystals in the urine suggests urolithiasis.

Imaging

Ultrasound examination of the kidney, ureter, and the bladder is the key in deciding further line of evaluation. Ultrasound will show the presence of tumors in the renal medulla or cortex (renal cell carcinoma) (Figure 7), and renal pelvis (transitional cell carcinoma). Ultrasound will give information regarding the presence of a bladder tumor (i.e., size, number, broad based, sessile), and the status of the upper tract. In addition, urolithiasis can be diagnosed on ultrasound.

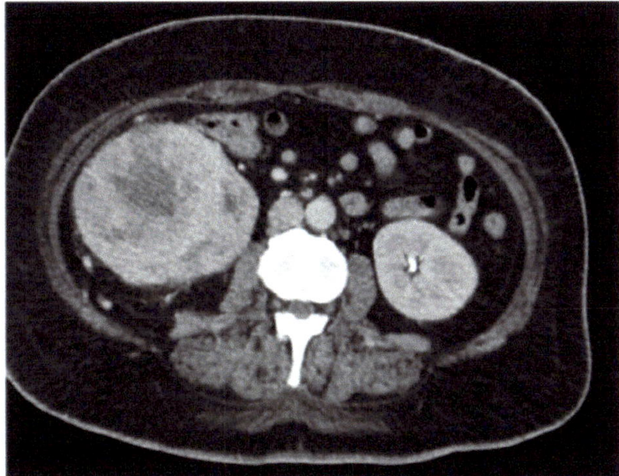

Figure 7: Renal cell carcinoma

Ultrasound is advantageous because it is radiation free and easily available. The downside is that it is operator dependent, and the results may not be reproducible.

Triple phase CT is helpful in the diagnosis of common urological conditions such as urolithiasis, bladder tumor, and upper tract malignancy, and other rare causes of hematuria including arteriovenous fistulas, and pseudoaneurysms etc. The indications for performing a CT scan in bladder tumors include a broad-based tumor, upper tract changes, and the presence of multiple tumors. Once the diagnosis of hematuria is confirmed, further management depends on the diagnosis

Bladder Cancer

It is crucial to establish the clinical stage of the disease to determine the treatment of choice for bladder cancer. A transurethral bladder tumor (TURBT) biopsy establishes the clinical stage. Prior to transurethral resection, a cystourethroscopy should be performed to assess the urethra and the bladder. The presence of a bladder tumor, number of lesions, and size of the lesions should be ascertained. The bladder capacity should be noted. The TURBT biopsy should be obtained with a thin loop. The specimen should be sent in two containers: one container should be for superficial chips, while the other should be for deeper chips.

Non-invasive bladder cancer

The management of non-invasive bladder cancer involves regular surveillance with cystoscopies, and intravesical chemotherapy (BCG 6 +3 protocol). Studies have shown that immediate intravesical mitomycin helps decrease the chance of recurrence in these patients.

Invasive bladder cancer

The indications for radical cystectomy are recurrent T1G3 non-invasive cancer, BCG refractory bladder cancer, and muscle invasive bladder cancer. Radical cystectomy specimens include the tumor bearing bladder with prostate in men, and lymph nodes which include the internal and external iliac group, the obturator nodes, and nodes along the bifurcation of the aorta. The choice of diversion after radical cystectomy depends on the histopathology of the urethral margin. If the urethral margin is positive for malignancy, an iliac conduit diversion is preferable. If the urethral margin is negative, either a continent stoma (Indian pouch or Kochs pouch), or an orthotopic neobladder is preferred. The role of neoadjuvant and adjuvant therapy, although limited, is seen in T3 lesions. Radical cystectomy with diversion can be performed either with robotic, laparoscopic, or open procedures. The approach to radical cystectomy is a matter of surgeon preference and expertise.

Renal Masses

The frequent use of CT and MRI has led to the increasingly frequent diagnosis of smaller renal masses. Small renal masses are defined as small (<4 cm), solid, sporadic, and apparently organ-confined tumors that are suspicious for RCC, based on imaging characteristics.[18] This has led to the ongoing debate regarding the applicability of radical nephrectomy in this subgroup of patients. There are issues including a lack of improvement in cancer rates, and a potential overkill by offering RNs in SRM.

The treatment options available for SRM are active surveillance, radiofrequency ablation, cryotherapy, and partial nephrectomy. Several studies have shown that radical nephrectomy can be overkill in patients with T1a disease. In a study by Lau et. al., there was no significant difference with respect to overall survival (P = 0.88) or cancer-specific survival (P = 0.71). There was a significant increase in risk for proteinuria (protein/osmolality radio of ≥0.12) in patients undergoing RN and after 10 years, the cumulative incidence of chronic renal insufficiency (creatinine >2.0 mg/dL at least 30 days post-surgery) was 22.4% and 11.6%, respectively.[19] Radical nephrectomy involves removal of the tumor bearing kidney; adrenalectomy is indicated in upper polar tumors, and in cases wherein imaging is suggestive of gross invasion in the adrenal area. Lymphadenectomy is indicated if the tumor is >10 cm and shows areas of necrosis, or if there is radiologic suggestion of lymphadenopathy. The lymphadenectomy is performed from the renal ostium to the bifurcation of the aorta. Partial nephrectomy involves enucleation or excision of the tumor with adequate margins. The approach may be open, laparoscopic, or robotic.

Penile Cancers (Figure 8)

Squamous cell carcinomas account for 95% of the malignancies. The premalignant conditions for penile cancer include balanitis xerotica obliterans, cutaneous horn, and Bowenoid carcinoid.

Biopsy of the lesion is indicated if there is doubt regarding the nature of the lesion and if, in the opinion of the physician, this will dictate the therapy for lymph nodes. On physical exam, details of a lesion suspicious of penile cancer include lesion diameter, suspicious lesion areas on the penis, number of lesions, and morphology of the lesions. The physical examination should include the examination of both groins. Ultrasound guided FNAC or sentinel node biopsy is indicated. If nodes are negative, a PET scan or CT scan can be useful for diagnosis and staging.

The treatment options for Tis, Ta, T1a (G1, G2) CO2 or Nd: YAG lesions are glands resurfacing, laser surgery-wide local excision, Mohs' micrographic surgery, glans resection, or photodynamic therapy. The treatment for T1b(G3) and T2 (glans only) is Glansectomy, and may or may not include tips amputation or reconstruction is recommended.

The management for T2 lesions is partial amputation with perineal urethrostomy. In T3 lesions the treatment of choice is total amputation. In T4 lesions the treatment of choice is followed by adjuvant chemotherapy.

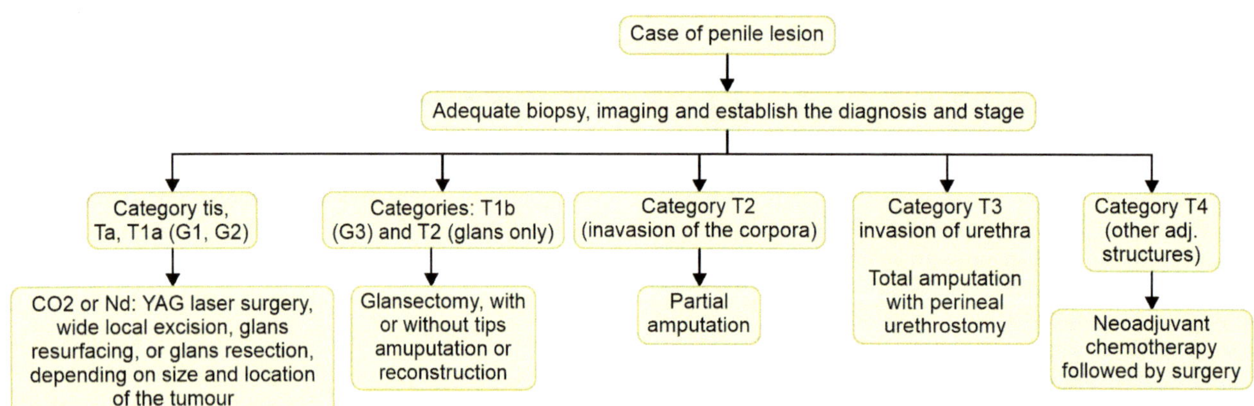

Figure 8: Management of penile lesions

REFERENCE

1. Preminger GM, Assimos DG, Lingeman JE, et al. Nephrolithiasis guideline panel Chapter 1 AUA guideline on management of staghorn calculi: Diagnosis and treatment recommendation J Urol 2005; 173:1991-2000.
2. Turk I, Knoll T, Petrik A, Sarica K, Seitz C, Straub M, Traxer O. EAU guidelines on Urolithiasis, 2010.
3. Stone disease Ed J Denstedt S Khoary edition 2008, 2nd international consultation on Stone disease.
4. Worster A, Preyra I, Weaver B, Haines T. The accuracy of non-contrast helical computed tomography versus intravenous pyelography in the diagnosis of suspected acute urolithiasis A metaanalysis Ann emerg Med 2002 ;40(3):280-6.
5. Morcos SK, Thomsen HS, Webb JA. Contrast media safety committee of the European society of urogenital radiology prevention of generalized reactions to contrast media: A consensus report and guidelines Eur Radiol 2001; 11(9):1720-8.
6. Thomsen HS, Morcos SK. Contrast media and the kidney: European society of urogenital radiology (ESUR) guidelines Br J Radiol 2003; 76(908):513-8.
7. Aga P, Bansal R. Is intravenous urogram no longer an imaging of choice for percutaneous nephrolithotomy Indian J Urol 2010;26:303-4.
8. Mishra S, Bhattu AS, Sabnis RB, Desai MR. Staghorn classification: Platform for morphometry assessment. Indian J Urol. 2014 Jan;30(1):80-3. doi: 10.4103/0970-1591.124212. PMID: 24497688; PMCID: PMC3897060.
9. Tiselius HG, Ackermann D, Alken P, Buck C, Conort P, Gallucci M. Working party on Lithiasis, European association of urology. Eur Urol 2001; 40(4):362-371.
10. Tiechman JM, Long RD, Hulbert JC. Long term renal fate and prognosis after staghorn calculus management Jurol 1995.153:1403.
11. Mertyk S, Gofrit ON, Gafni O, Pode D, Shapiro A, Verstandig A, et al. Complete staghorn calculi;Randomized prospective comparison between extracorporeal shock wave lithotripsy monotherapy and combined with percutaneous nephrolithotomy J Urol, 1997.157:780.
12. Lingeman JE, Siegel YI, Steele B. Management of lower pole nephrolithiasis J Urol 2005; 173:469-473.
13. Albala DM, Assimos DG, Clayman RV, et al. A prospective randomized trial of extracorporeal shock wave lithotripsy and percutaneous nephrostlithotomy for lower pole nephrolithiasis: initial results J Urol 2001:166:2072-2080.
14. Turna B, Raza A, Moussa S, Smith G, Tolley DA. Management of calyceal Diverticular stones with extracorporeal shock wave lithotripsy and percutaneous nephrolithotomy;long term outcome.BJU Int 2007;100:151-156.
15. CC Wen, SY Nakada. Treatment selection outcomes: renal calculi Urol Clin N Am 34(3), 409-419.
16. Shah K, Kurien A, Mishra S, GanpuleA, Muthu V, Sabnis RB, Desai M. predicting effectiveness of extracorporeal shockwave lithotripsy by stone attenuation value J Endourol 2010;24(7);1169-73.
17. El Nahas AR, El Assmy AM, Manour O, Sheir KZ. A prospective multivariate analysis of factors predicting stone disintegration by extracorporeal shock wave lithotripsy: The value of high resolution non contrast computed tomography Eur Urol 2007; 51(6):1688-93.
18. Lane BR, Campbell SC. AUA Update series Lesson 34, volume 28,2009.
19. Lau WK, et al. Matched comparison of radical nephrectomy vs nephron-sparing surgery in patients with unilateral renal cell carcinoma and a normal contralateral kidney. Mayo Clin Proc. 2000 Dec; 75(12):1236-42.

❑❑❑

67

CHAPTER

Bladder Dysfunction

Nirmish Singla, MD
Ajay Singla, MD

INTRODUCTION

The main functions of the urinary bladder are storage and emptying. Problems of storage are more common and cover the majority of this chapter.

We will discuss two types of urinary storage problems: bladder overactivity and stress urinary incontinence.

Overactive Bladder (OAB)

Overactive bladder is a clinical diagnosis that usually presents with irritative urinary symptoms mainly urinary frequency, urgency, nocturia with or without urge incontinence, in the absence of urinary tract infection (UTI) or other obvious pathology.[1] Urgency is defined by the ICS as the "complaint of a sudden, compelling desire to pass urine which is difficult to defer.[1]

Urinary frequency is the complaint of frequent urination. Urinary frequency up to 6-7 micturition episodes during waking hours is considered normal,[2] but this number may vary depending upon fluid intake, underlying comorbid medical conditions, and other factors.

Nocturia is defined as getting up from sleep at night to void.[1] Like daytime frequency, nocturia often may be due to factors related to excessive nighttime urine production, sleep apnea, and/or the amount of fluid intake or consumption of bladder stimulants. For practical purposes, getting up twice or more to urinate at night constitutes abnormal.

Urgency urinary incontinence is defined as the involuntary loss of urine, associated with a sudden strong desire to void. Some patients may complain of both urge and stress incontinence known as mixed urinary incontinence.

Epidemiology

OAB is more common in women than men. The prevalence rates range from 9 to 43% in women and 7 to 27% in men.[3] The prevalence and severity tend to increase with age.[4]

Etiology

The exact etiology of OAB is not known. In the majority of women, no underlying cause is found (idiopathic), while there may be an underlying bladder outlet obstruction causing OAB in men. In some patients, any bladder irritation such as a UTI, bladder calculi, or bladder cancer can cause symptoms of OAB while prostatic obstruction may be the leading cause of OAB symptoms in men.

Clinical Presentation

OAB is a symptom-based diagnosis, where patients complain of urinary frequency (both day and night) and urgency, with or without urgency incontinence. These symptoms may present only at night as nocturia associated with urgency incontinence. This should be differentiated from nocturnal polyuria (the production of greater than 20 to 33% of total 24-hour urine output during sleep) and polydipsia. These can easily be distinguished with a bladder diary. A similar clinical presentation is seen in patients with interstitial cystitis or bladder pain syndrome. Even though bladder/pelvic pain or dyspareunia are usually not present in OAB patients. Interstitial cystitis is less common than OAB and should be ruled out with proper evaluation in refractory OAB patients.

Evaluation

The American Urological Association (AUA) has recently published clinical practice guidelines on overactive bladder.[5]

A careful history, physical examination and urinalysis are necessary to document typical OAB symptoms and to rule out other urinary disorders which may cause similar symptoms. History should assess both storage symptoms (e.g., frequency, urgency, nocturia, urinary incontinence) and bladder emptying symptoms (e.g., hesitancy, weak stream, intermittency of stream). The amount and type of fluids consumed by the patient should be inquired. Patients should be asked to fill out a 3-day bladder diary to document the amount of fluid intake and voids per day. Bowel habits should also be inquired. Comorbid conditions including diabetes and underlying neurologic diseases (i.e., stroke, multiple sclerosis, spinal cord injury etc.) which can affect bladder function should also be inquired.

Physical examination: A directed physical examination of the abdomen and genitalia, and a pelvic examination should be carried out. A focused neurological examination of the perineal and perianal area to assess perineal sensations and anal sphincter tone should be carried out.

Urinalysis: All patients should be asked to provide a clean catch midstream urine specimen to rule out a UTI and hematuria.

Post-void residual (PVR): Initial PVR is recommended in patients with complex symptoms, both obstructive and irritative. This helps to rule out overflow incontinence as well as bladder outlet obstruction, especially in men.

Further work-up: Per AUA guidelines, urodynamics, cystoscopy, and renal ultrasound are not recommended in the initial workup of uncomplicated patient unless they have failed conservative management with medical therapy.[5]

Management

OAB is a symptom complex that generally impacts patient quality of life. Patients should be offered treatment if the symptoms are bothersome and affecting daily life routine.

Behavioral Therapies

These are usually the first-line treatment and best suited for patients with bothersome sensory urgency. This involves changing individual lifestyles. Patients are asked to maintain a 3-day bladder diary. This will provide information on patient fluid intake and voiding habit. Components of behavioral therapy include modifying fluid intake and restricting the consumption of bladder stimulants such as caffeine, carbonated, alcohol, and acidic beverages. In addition, changing bladder behavior by changing voiding habits with bladder retraining exercises may help to improve urinary frequency and urgency. Patients are instructed in various techniques of urge suppression and thus increasing the voiding interval. These may include a pelvic floor muscle training program by pelvic floor contraction, normal voiding techniques by proper pelvic floor relaxation, use of biofeedback techniques, and electric stimulation. The literature supports the effectiveness of bladder training and pelvic floor muscle training programs with a 50 to 80% improvement in reducing incontinence episodes.[6] Even weight loss programs in obese women may improve incontinence episodes by 47%.[7]

Pharmacotherapy

Two muscarinic receptors subtypes, M2 and M3, are present in the bladder muscle. Although M2 is most abundant in the detrusor muscle (70 to 80%), the M3 subtype is the major receptor mediating detrusor contraction. Antimuscarinic agents block these receptors. Behavioral and drug therapies are often used in combination in clinical practice to control patients' symptoms and improve quality of life. Anti-muscarinic agents are used as second-line treatment. A number of these agents have been introduced over the years and are used extensively for the treatment of OAB. These include older agents which may have to be administered more than once a day or newer agents which are long-acting and can be used as once a day.

Antimuscarinic agents have been effective in reducing symptoms in a number of clinical trials but also can cause side effects which can be bothersome to patients, and even rarely may be life-threatening. The most common side effects reported are dry mouth, constipation, dry eyes, blurred vision, dyspepsia, urinary retention, and impaired cognitive function. Rarely, cardiac arrhythmias have been reported. This is in part due to the effects on muscarinic receptors on other organs in the body. A number of randomized trials with placebos and/or trials comparing different medications, revealed no difference in efficacy across medications.[8,9] Because of these side effects, patient compliance with these medications has been a problem. Extended-release preparation has improved the compliance in patients with OAB.[10] Other preparations with different modes of drug delivery may be used (e.g., transdermal oxybutynin patch or gel) to improve compliance and to minimize the side effects. Antimuscarinics are contraindicated in patients with untreated narrow-angle glaucoma and in patients with impaired gastric or bladder emptying. These medications should also be used with extreme caution in elderly patients as some of these agents cross the blood-brain barrier and may affect cognitive function.

Beta-3-adrenoceptor agonists (mirabegron) have also been approved for use in patients with OAB. Mirabegron is a selective B3-adrenoceptor agonist and by virtue of its action on beta adrenergic receptors in the detrusor muscle, it decreases the frequency of detrusor muscle contraction. It enhances urine storage function by significantly decreasing the mean number of micturition, urgency and urge incontinence episodes. The main side effects reported are headache, blurred vision, and vascular disorders.[11]

More recently, another Beta-3 agonist, vibegron (gemtesa) has been approved by the FDA.

Neuromodulation Therapies

Patients who have failed behavioral and antimuscarinic therapy may be offered neuromodulation. These therapies are approved by the FDA for the treatment of idiopathic OAB.

Sacral neuromodulation (SNS) was introduced in 1997 as the open placement of an electrode in the third sacral foramen (S3) but was modified to percutaneous placement of an electrode in 2002. This is connected to a battery-operated energy generator which is implanted in the buttock area. This provides continuous stimulation of the S3 nerve root and in turn results in a decrease in detrusor contraction. The exact mechanism of action is not clearly understood. Multiple studies in patients with refractory OAB have reported an improvement of 68% in urge incontinence at 5 years.[12] Frequent adverse events reported are pain at the stimulator site, infection/irritation, electric shock, and the need for surgical revision. AUA guidelines panel recommended that, in carefully selected patients, SNS is an appropriate therapy with durable effects but may require additional surgical revisions or re-programming.[5] The main limitation that patients should be counseled on is the inability to undergo MRI scanning after implantation.

Posterior tibial nerve stimulation (PTNS) is FDA approved for symptoms of OAB. This is less invasive than SNS and is performed in an office setting. Stimulation is applied to the post tibial nerve for 30 minutes once a week for 12 weeks. Multiple studies have reported efficacy of PTNS in treating refractory OAB symptoms.[13] The AUA guideline panel recommends PTNS in selected patients with refractory symptoms and who are willing to comply with PTNS protocol.[5]

Other Treatment (OnabotulinumtoxinA)

OnabotulinumtoxinA is injected into the detrusor muscle during cystoscopy. A total dose of 100-200 units may be injected at multiple sites excluding the trigone. The procedure may be performed in the office under local anesthesia. This is currently approved by the FDA for both idiopathic and neurogenic OAB. Multiple randomized trials with placebo control groups evaluated the efficacy of onabotulinumtoxinA in patients with non-neurogenic OAB who were refractory to anti-muscarinic medications.[14] All studies reported a significant reduction in urgency and incontinence episodes. The main reported risks of injection are urinary retention as high as 30% and UTI. All patients undergoing onabotulinumtoxinA treatment should be counseled regarding the possible need for self-catheterization and should be willing to accept this risk. Further, the effects diminish overtime and patients may require repeat injections every 9 to 12 months.[14]

Additional Treatments

In rare cases of severe, refractory OAB, surgery such as augmentation cystoplasty or urinary diversion may be considered. These major procedures are associated with significant morbidity and the need for repeat surgery for possible complications.

Stress Urinary Incontinence

Prevalence: The exact prevalence of urinary incontinence is not clear, but it is estimated that 30% of women between the ages of 30 to 60 years suffer with urinary incontinence, and approximately half of these are attributed to stress urinary incontinence (SUI).[15]

Definition: It is defined as the leakage of urine with any increase in abdominal pressure such as coughing, sneezing, laughing, exercise, lifting, etc. without an increase in detrusor pressure. It should be differentiated from urge urinary incontinence which is involuntary leakage accompanied by urgency. It may present in conjunction with urge incontinence which is referred to as mixed incontinence.

Evaluation: The American Urological Association has published guidelines in the evaluation and management of female stress urinary incontinence in 1997, which was later updated in 2010.[16] The diagnosis of SUI is fairly straightforward with a focused history and physical examination. Patients should be asked about the duration of incontinence, severity of leakage, precipitating factors, and degree of bothersome. Any associated voiding problems should also be discussed, in particular bladder emptying to rule out overflow incontinence. Any history suggestive of concurrent urge incontinence should also be inquired. In patients with total incontinence or urinary leakage per vagina would raise suspicion for a urinary fistula.

A detailed pelvic examination with an objective demonstration of urinary leakage from the urethral meatus with valsalva or cough (positive stress test) would confirm the diagnosis. Assessment to determine the presence of pelvic organ prolapse should be performed along with the assessment of general hormonal status. A urine analysis should be carried out in all patients with urinary incontinence. Postvoid residual urine volume estimation should be done to rule out overflow incontinence.

Additional diagnostic tests can be performed to assess the lower urinary tract function which includes urodynamic testing with the measurement of valsalva leak point pressure, imaging, and cystoscopy. The role of additional testing continues to be controversial in the management of uncomplicated stress urinary incontinence. The AUA guideline panel recommends additional tests in the following cases:[16] mixed incontinence, inability to make a definitive diagnosis based on history and examination, prior failed anti-incontinence procedures, known or suspected neurogenic bladder, negative stress test, abnormal postvoid residual urine volume, history of voiding dysfunction, and the presence of a high degree of pelvic organ prolapse.

Management

Nonsurgical Treatment: Conservative management of SUI includes behavioral and pharmacological treatment.

Behavioral treatment involves bladder retraining and a pelvic floor muscle rehabilitation program. The main goal for a bladder retraining program is to control frequency and urgency. This increases the time interval between each void.

Pelvic floor muscle training consists of repetitive episodic contractions of the pelvic floor muscles, performed overtime. Patients are instructed in these exercises or preferably given a printed handout. This training program is based on "Kegel" exercises and is commonly referred to by that name. These can be performed under the direct supervision of a trained nurse or physiotherapist and incorporate biofeedback technology in the form of a perineometer. These exercises strengthen the levator muscles (sphincter muscles) thereby decreasing lower urinary tract symptoms of incontinence, urgency, and frenquency.[17] In the biofeedback technology, both audio and visual signals are used to identify the appropriate muscles. To obtain the signals either vaginal (in women) or rectal (in men) probes are used. In women with SUI simple vaginal cones can also be used to aid in the contraction of pelvic floor muscles. Low grade electrical stimulation to the pelvic floor muscles can be applied to aid in pelvic floor muscle contraction and to inhibit unwanted detrusor contractions by reflex inhibition of the detrusor muscle.

Pharmacotherapy: There are no currently approved drugs for SUI in the United States. There are two main groups of drugs used for SUI:

- Alpha-adrenergic agonists like phenylpropanolamine, ephedrine, and pseudoephedrine have been used for patients with SUI in the past but the efficacy is poor. These agents would act by increasing urethral smooth muscle tone mediated by alpha-adrenergic receptors. Their use is discouraged due to a lack of efficacy and high risk of adverse effects.
- Duloxetine is a serotonin-norepinephrine reuptake inhibitor that has been approved in other countries at a dose of 40 mg twice a day for the treatment of SUI. This drug is not approved by the FDA for SUIs but approved for depression. A North American, double blind, placebo-controlled study showed a decrease in incontinence episodes in 51% of subjects in the treatment group.[18]

Estrogen replacement therapy orally or transvaginally, has been controversial and is being used routinely by some clinicians in postmenopausal women with urogenital atrophy.

Surgical Treatments

There has been an evolution in the surgical procedures for SUI due to a lack of an ideal procedure. There are four main categories of surgical procedures for SUI: retropubic suspensions, slings, injectable agents, and artificial urinary sphincters (AUS).

Retropubic suspensions: The retropubic suspensions can be performed either with open procedure or by laparoscopic method. The retropubic suspension involves the elevation of the bladder neck and proximal urethra, and anchoring it to either Cooper's ligament (Burch colposuspension) or the pubic symphysis (Marshall-Marchetti-Krantz). These procedures have proven to be effective in curing stress urinary incontinence both in the short- and long-term. The reported cured/dry rates at 12 to 23 months for open Burch suspension are 82% while the cured/dry rates for laparoscopic Burch suspension are lower around 69%. The long-term overall cured/dry rates for all open procedures range from 74 to 76%.[16]

Post-operative complications specific to retropubic suspensions include voiding dysfunction, de novo urge incontinence, and vaginal prolapse.

Sling procedures: The slings are designed to support the bladder neck and urethra. The commonly known bladder neck sling is the pubovaginal sling, which is a type of compressive sling that helps in urethral coaptation. A number of sling materials (e.g., allograft, xenograft or autologous) have been used to construct the sling. Autologous fascial slings are still considered the "gold standard" sling used for female stress urinary incontinence. The cured/dry rates reported in the literature range between 90% at 12 to 23 months and 82% at 48 months or longer.[16] The main complications are similar to retropubic suspensions such as voiding dysfunction, de novo urge incontinence, and bladder injury.

Midurethral slings: More recently, minimally invasive tension free vaginal tapes have become very popular. These use a synthetic mesh which is placed in the mid urethra (TVT, suprapubic arc sling, TOT). Their cured/dry rates are comparable to suspensions and bladder neck slings in the range of 81 to 84%.[16] The main complications reported are bladder injuries, vascular injuries, and mesh complications.

Injectable agents: Patients who are elderly, do not wish to

undergo invasive surgery, or have failed prior surgeries may elect to have agents like collagen, coaptite, or durasphere injected at the bladder neck and proximal urethra. But the efficacy is much inferior to surgery.

Artificial Urinary Sphincter (AUS): The implantation of this device around the urethra helps to close the urethral lumen in cases with severe SUI due to intrinsic sphincter deficiency following prior failed anti-incontinence surgeries. This can be a salvage therapy with high rates of dryness. Complications include urethral erosions, malfunction, and infection.

REFERENCES

1. Haylen BT, de Ridder D, Freeman RM, et al. An International Urogynecological Association (IUGA)/ International Continence Society (ICS) joint report on the terminology for female pelvic floor dysfunction. Neurourol Urodyn 2010; 29:4.
2. Fitzgerald MP, Brubaker L. Variability of 24-hour voiding diary variables among asymptomatic women. J Urol 2003; 169:207.
3. Coyne KS, Sexton CC, Vats V, et al. National community prevalence of overactive bladder in the United States stratified by sex and age. Urology 2011; 77: 1081.
4. Donaldson MM, Thompson JR, Mathews RJ, et al The natural history of overactive bladder and stress urinary incontinence in older women in the community: a 3-year prospective cohort study. Neurourol Urodyn 2006; 25: 709.
5. Gormley EA, Lightner DJ, Burgio KL, Chai TC, et al. Diagnosis and Treatment of Overactive Bladder (Non-Neurogenic) in Adults: AUA/SUFU Guideline. J Urol 2012; 188(6): 2455-2463.
6. Fantl JA, Wyman JF, McClish DK, et al. Efficacy of bladder training in older women with urinary incontinence. JAMA 1991; 265: 609.
7. Subak LL, Wing R, West DS, et al. Weight loss to treat urinary incontinence in overweight and obese women. NEJM 2009; 360: 481.
8. Anderson RU, Mobley D, Blank B, et al. Once daily controlled versus immediate release oxybutynin chloride for urge urinary incontinence. OROS Oxybutynin Study Group. J Urol 199; 161: 1809.
9. Chappel CR, Martinez-Garcia R, Selvaggi L, et al. A comparison of the efficacy and tolerability of solifenacin succinate and extended release tolterodine at treating overactive bladder syndrome: Results of the STAR trial. European Urol 2005; 48: 464.
10. D'Souza AO, Smith MJ, Miller LA, et al. Persistence, adherence, and switch rates among extended-release and immediate-release overactive bladder medications in a regional managed care plan. J Manag Care Pharm 2008; 14: 291.
11. Nitti V, Herschorn S, Ayers M, Lee M, Martin N. The Selective (beta) 3-adrenoreceptor agonist mirabegron is effective and well tolerated in patients with overactive bladder syndrome. J Urol 2011; 185(4): 783-784.
12. van Kerrebroeck PE, van Voskuilen AC, Heesakkers JP, et al. Results of sacral modulation therapy for urinary voiding dysfunction: outcomes of a prospective, worldwide clinical study. J Urol 2007; 178: 2029.
13. MacDiarmid SA, Peters KM, Shobeiri SA, et al. Long-term durability of percutaneous tibial nerve stimulation for the treatment of overactive bladder. J Urol 2010; 183: 1438.
14. Dmochowski R, Chapple C, Nitti V, et al. Efficacy and safety of onabotulinumtoxinA for idiopathic overactive bladder: A double-blind, placebo controlled, randomized, dose ranging trial. J Urol 2010; 184: 2416.
15. Hampel C, Weinhold D, Benken N, et al. Definition of overactive bladder and epidemiology of urinary incontinence. Urology 1997; 50:4.
16. Dmochowski RR, Blaivas JM, Gormley EA, et al. Update of AUA guideline on the surgical management of female stress urinary incontinence. J Urol 2010; 183(5): 1906-14.
17. Fantl J, Newman D, Colling J, et al. Urinary incontinence in adults: Acute and chronic management. Clinical practice guideline No. 2: Update (AHCPR Publication No. 96-0692). Rockville, MD: Agency for Healthcare and Policy Research.
18. Dmochowski RR, Miklos JR, Norton PA, et al. Duloxetine versus placebo for the treatment of North American women with stress urinary incontinence. J Urol 2003; 170(4 pt 1): 1259-1263.

❑❑❑

68

CHAPTER

Prostate

Nirmish Singla, MD
Ajay Singla, MD

Benign Enlargement of Prostate

Benign enlargement of prostate (BEP) is the most common urological disease affecting older men after the age of 50 years.[1] Benign prostatic hyperplasia (BPH) is a histological diagnosis which refers to hyperplasia of smooth muscle cell and epithelial cell causing an enlargement of the prostate gland. The prevalence of histologic BPH is age dependent, usually starting after 40 years of age. At 40 years, only 8% of men have BPH.[2] It increases to 50% at or after age 60 years, and as high as 90% at or after 85 years.[2] BPH may be asymptomatic or sometimes associated with lower urinary tract symptoms (LUTS). These symptoms may or may not be bothersome to patients and sometimes may affect quality of life. There is, however, no strong relationship between prostate size and symptoms. While about 50% of men eventually develop histologic BPH, only a subset of those will develop bothersome LUTS or bladder outlet obstruction (BOO).[3]

The exact etiology is not known, but various extrinsic and intrinsic factors are thought to a play role as proposed by Lee et al.[4] There is strong evidence that a family history of BPH predisposes to the disease. Sanda et al found a strong relationship for first degree relatives of BPH treated patients to have the disease, indicating a mendelian autosomal-dominant inheritance pattern.[5] The enlarged prostate gland may contribute to LUTS by two different mechanisms. One by obstructing the bladder outlet by its enlarged size, the static component. The second by increasing bladder outlet resistance by increasing the smooth muscle tone, the dynamic component. It is important to understand that the bladder plays a role in the development of these complex symptoms. Some of these symptoms are a direct result of outlet obstruction while others are from urinary storage problems.

The American Urological Association (AUA) first published BPH guidelines in 2003 and later revised them in 2010. It provides the most detailed reference document for physicians.[6,7]

Urinary symptoms negatively impact quality of life depending upon the degree of bother and interference with daily activities. To assess the severity of these symptoms the AUA introduced a 7-questions, self-administered questionnaire which has been validated and is used worldwide. It is known as AUA Symptom Index/International Prostate Symptom Score-IPSS. The total score is 35 points. Patients with scores between 1 to 7 are classified as mild, 8 to 18 as moderate, and 19 to 35 as severely symptomatic. This questionnaire comprises a combination of both irritative and obstructive symptoms.[8] Irritative symptoms include urinary frequency, nocturia, and urgency with or without urge incontinence. Obstructive Symptoms include weak stream, hesitancy, and incomplete bladder emptying.

BPH is not a life-threatening disease but, if untreated over a long period, it can lead to complications. The most common complications are acute or chronic retention, hematuria, urinary incontinence, urinary tract infections (UTI), bladder stones, and obstructive uropathy leading to renal failure.

Evaluation

Evaluation and treatment of BPH depend upon the impact on quality of life. Some men are found to have enlarged prostate on routine physical examination and are asymptomatic. These men do not need any further evaluation. The scientific committee of the 6th International Consultation on Incontinence (ICI) formulated recommendations for the evaluation which were divided into basic, advanced, and optional tests.[9] The AUA established similar guidelines for BPH in 2003. An algorithm is being suggested for diagnosis and treatment.[6,7]

Basic evaluation:

- Medical history to identify other causes of voiding dysfunction.
- Physical examination, including a genitourinary exam, a digital rectal exam, and a focused neurologic examination.
- AUA symptom index (IPSS) questionnaire in the assessment of symptoms and degree of bother.
- Urinalysis.
- Prostate specific antigen (PSA) blood test.

Recommended before non-invasive therapy:

- Uroflow measurement and post-void residual estimation (PVR)

Recommended before invasive therapy

- Pressure/flow study by urodynamics

Optional tests:

- Urine cytology
- Upper tract imaging studies
- Prostate ultrasound
- Cystoscopy
- Serum creatinine routine screening is not recommended.

Management

The treatment of BPH depends on the seriousness of symptoms and degree of bother.

AUA guidelines recommend that patients with mild symptoms (AUA/IPSS score of 7 or less) or patients with moderate symptoms (score of 8-17) but who are not bothered by their symptoms should ideally be managed with watchful waiting.

Patients with bothersome moderate to severe symptoms should be counseled regarding various treatment options including watchful waiting, medical therapy, minimally invasive, or surgical therapies. They should also be counseled regarding the benefits and risks of each therapy.

Watchful Waiting

Watchful waiting is the most conservative treatment for LUTS. It is considered as the first line in the management for patients with mild symptoms (AUA score of 7 or less) or may be appropriate for patients with moderate symptoms (AUA score of 8-17) who are not bothered with their symptoms. Patients are monitored very closely by the physician, but do not receive active intervention for BPH. Patients may be advised with behavioral modifications such as decreasing coffee, alcohol, and fluid intake at bedtime. This may help improve some of their symptoms. Patients on watchful waiting are reexamined yearly, repeating the initial evaluation.

Medical Therapy

Medical therapy is aimed to relieve symptoms, reduce prostate enlargement, and prevent long term disease outcomes and/or complications. This is generally preferred as first-line treatment for men with bothersome symptoms. Medical therapy includes α-adrenergic receptor antagonists (α-blockers), 5 α-reductase inhibitors (5ARI), and combination therapy.

Alpha Blockers

The α-blocker inhibits α-1 adrenergic mediated activation of prostatic smooth muscle, leading to a decrease in smooth muscle tone and decreasing bladder outlet resistance and hence relieving bladder outlet obstruction.[10]

There are five α-blockers commonly used in the treatment of LUTS: tamsulosin, alfuzosin, doxazosin, terazosin, and silodosin. These drugs are comparable in their effectiveness in treating LUTS. Some of them differ in their selectivity for receptors and, in turn, the side effects associated with them. The most commonly reported adverse side effects include dizziness in 2% to 14% of patients, headache, postural hypotension, nasal congestion, and ejaculatory dysfunction in about 5% to 9%.[7] The side effects appear slightly different between older versus newer α-blockers, for example, tamsulosin seems to have a lower incidence of orthostatic hypotension but a higher likelihood of ejaculatory dysfunction than the other α-blockers. Tamsulosin has also been linked with the development of intraoperative floppy iris syndrome.[11] The risk of this complication seems to be much lower with older α-blockers. Patients should be warned in case of planned cataract surgery. The older α-1 blockers like doxazosin and terazosin were initially used for treating hypertension and binding selectively to α-1 receptors, but they do not exhibit α-1 subtype selectivity. The dose may be titrated to achieve the maximum response. These may also be associated with orthostatic hypotension and may require blood pressure monitoring. Patients are advised to take these medications at bedtime to avoid dizzy spells. Unlike other treatments, tamsulosin selectively binds to α-1a and α-1d subtypes. This reduces the incidence of dizziness in elderly men and can safely be taken during the daytime without requiring dose titration.

5-Alpha Reductase Inhibitors

The male hormone testosterone is converted to dihydrotestosterone (DHT) by 5-α-reductase enzyme. DHT is a more potent anabolic steroid, responsible for cellular growth and causing prostatic hyperplasia. There are two types of enzymes type 1 and type 2. Two 5-α reductase inhibitors (5-ARIs) have been approved by the FDA, finasteride and dutasteride. Finasteride inhibits the 5-AR type 2 isoenzyme while dutasteride inhibits both type 1 and type 2 isoenzymes.[12] 5-ARIs lower both serum and intraprostatic dihydrotestosterone levels. These drugs have been shown to decrease overall prostate size, improve urinary flow, and help to reduce BPH symptoms. The clinical efficacy of the two 5-ARIs is very similar except finasteride takes longer than dutasteride to start shrinking the prostate size (6 months versus 3 months). Even the side effects profile for both 5-ARIs is comparable, mainly erectile dysfunction, decreased libido, and ejaculatory dysfunction. AUA guidelines have suggested that the use of these drugs is an appropriate and effective treatment for patients with LUTS secondary to BPH and who have demonstrable prostate enlargement. These drugs have been shown to reduce the risk of urinary retention and likelihood of undergoing future prostate related surgery. It was recommended that 5-ARIs should not be used in men with LUTS secondary to BPH without prostatic enlargement.[6,7]

Combination Therapy

AUA guidelines suggest that the combination therapy with α-adrenergic blocker and a 5α-reductase inhibitor is efficacious treatment for patients with LUTS due to prostatic enlargement. In multiple studies, combination therapy is shown to be better at relieving and preventing the progression of symptoms than singular α-blocker therapy including the long-term risk of acute urinary retention and the future need for BPH-related surgery.

Minimally Invasive Therapies

Recently, many minimally invasive procedures which can be performed in the physician office have been approved by the FDA. These include Rezum which is a water vapor therapy using thermal energy, Aquablation which uses high pressure waterjet to ablate prostatic tissue. Another minimally invasive therapy called UroLift which uses small implants to retract the obstructing prostatic lobes away from each other in an attempt to remove the obstruction. Men who have failed medical therapy as first line treatment, could not tolerate the medication, do not wish to remain on medication, or who are not suitable for invasive surgery may be considered for any of these office-based procedures.

Thermal-based therapies take advantage of high temperatures to cause coagulation necrosis of prostatic tissues at temperatures over 45°C. This causes shrinkage of the prostate and partial relief in symptoms. Similar to TUMT, TUNA also causes prostatic tissue necrosis by using radiofrequency waves which heat the prostatic tissue from 90°C to 100°C. The clinical effect is thought to be secondary to denervation of intraprostatic nerve fibers leading to smooth muscle relaxation.[13] The ideal candidate for TUNA is a patient with an obstructive prostate of less than 60 grams with predominantly lateral lobe enlargement. Both of these therapies were recently discontinued for the treatment of LUTS secondary to BPH.

These minimally invasive procedures have the advantage of not involving any cutting or blood loss and seems to be more effective than medical therapy in the average patient, but it is less effective than surgery in relieving symptoms.

Surgical Treatments

Surgery remains the most definitive treatment for BPH. It is indicated for moderate-to-severe LUTS or patients who are unresponsive to medical therapy and in patients with acute urinary retention or other BPH-related complications. Ideally, patients should try and fail medical therapy before pursuing surgery. Surgery offers the greatest improvement in symptom and flow rate improvement but is also associated with a greater likelihood of complications. The choice of surgical approach is based on the patient's prostate size, associated comorbidities, and surgeon's preference. Surgical options include laser treatment or conventional prostatectomy.

Laser Treatment

Laser treatment was first used for the treatment of BPH in 1990.[14] Compared with conventional TURP, it is less morbid and has quicker recovery with comparable improvements in LUTS. There are two main techniques in which lasers can be used to destroy prostate tissue. These include (1) tissue vaporization with contact versus non-contact laser and (2) enucleation or resection of tissue based on type of laser wavelength. The main advantage of laser prostatectomy over conventional prostatectomy is decreased morbidity, catheterization time, and length of stay. There is also a decreased risk of perioperative TUR syndrome complications, bleeding, and need for blood transfusion. Because of minimal or no bleeding, laser treatment remains a suitable option for men taking anticoagulant medication.

Conventional Prostatectomy

The choice of surgical approach, open versus transurethral, is based on the prostate size, comorbidities, and individual surgeon's preference.

Transurethral resection of prostate (TURP) remains the "gold standard" treatment for BPH, despite the advent of new technologies. Randomized clinical trials with long term follow-up demonstrates that TURP improves symptoms and flow rates better than other available treatments. It is associated with a higher incidence of bleeding, urethral stricture, and

TUR syndrome. Additional complications may include UTI, incontinence, erectile dysfunction, and retrograde ejaculation. TUR syndrome is a unique complication characterized by hypotension, bradycardia, nausea, vomiting, and mental confusion. This is caused by dilutional hyponatremia that occurs with the absorption of irrigate fluid into the bloodstream.[15] Bipolar TURP utilizes normal saline instead of glycine as in conventional TURP for irrigation. The risk of TUR syndrome is eliminated by using bipolar technology (gyrus).

Open prostatectomy is reserved for patients with prostate glands too large to be removed safely endoscopically (volumes >80 to 100 grams). Additional indications for open enucleation include concomitant bladder diverticula and bladder calculi.

On the other hand, transurethral incision of the prostate (TUIP) is an appropriate surgical option for men with moderate to severe symptoms with smaller prostates (i.e., <30 grams). The incision opens the bladder neck and prostatic urethra, and results in subjective and objective improvements in symptoms equivalent to those experienced after TURP. Advantages of TUIP over TURP include outpatient procedure, less bleeding, less risk of retrograde ejaculation, and shorter operative time.

Prostate Cancer

Prostate cancer remains one of the most common cancers diagnosed in men and is the second leading cause of death in American men, after lung cancer. Since 1995, about 2.6 million men in the United States have received a diagnosis of prostate cancer, and almost 375,000 men have died from the disease.[16] According to the American Cancer Society, a total of 248,530 new cases of prostate cancer is predicted to be diagnosed and about 34,130 will die of the disease in 2021.[17] Higher risk men include African American men, men older than 65 years of age, and men with a family history of prostate cancer. About 1 man in 8 will be diagnosed with prostate cancer during his lifetime and 1 man in 41 will die of their disease (cancer.org).

Screening

The debate continues regarding prostate cancer screening. The American Urological Association continues to advocate for annual screening while the United States task force against annual screening. Patients with localized prostate cancer in early stages are usually asymptomatic. Slowing of the stream and/or nocturia, are common symptoms in old men secondary to BPH and may be unrelated to the presence of prostate cancer. These patients may only be diagnosed with prostate cancer screening modalities. The two most commonly used methods are blood test (serum prostate specific antigen (PSA) levels and a digital rectal examination (DRE). Transrectal ultrasound, when used in combination with PSA and DRE, may be utilized and may improve the diagnostic yield of prostate cancer; these screening methods, however, are linked to high false-positive rates and may also identify some tumors that are insignificant and not life-threatening.[18,19]

More recently, MRI technology has been used as an additional tool for screening in patients with abnormal PSA or DRE to identify prostate cancer.

Prostate Specific Antigen

PSA is a glycoprotein secreted by prostatic epithelial cells and can be measured in the blood. Normal Serum PSA levels are within range from 0-4 ng/dL. While a high PSA level is often seen in men with prostate cancer, PSA elevation is not specific for prostate cancer. Currently, PSA elevation continues to be used as the most common test used to detect prostate cancer in the United States.

Digital Rectal Examination

A DRE enables a physician to palpate the prostate gland to detect any abnormality. DRE may detect asymmetry of prostate gland or a hard nodule which may be suspicious of cancer.

Prostate Biopsy

Prostate cancer diagnosis is confirmed with a prostate biopsy. Traditional prostate biopsy is carried out under local anesthesia using a needle passed through a rectal probe under trans-rectal ultrasound guidance and multiple cores of tissue taken from different parts of the prostate gland are removed. These are then sent for pathology. More recently, MRI technology is being used to target suspicious areas precisely rather than taken randomly during traditional ultrasound biopsy.

Tumor Characteristics

Tumors are classified based on grade, using the Gleason grading system. [20] This system assigns a grade based on the degree of architectural differentiation of the tumor, from 1 being the least aggressive to 5 being the most aggressive. The Gleason score is obtained by adding a primary grade which is the most prevalent in the biopsy, with a secondary grade or second most prevalent grade in the tissue. Generally, a Gleason score of 7 or above refers to a high-grade tumor.

Tumor Staging

Prostate cancer clinical staging depends upon if the cancer is localized in the prostate gland either in one lobe or in both lobes of the prostate, or if it has spread into the surrounding tissue called extraprostatic extension involving seminal vesicles etc. The American Joint Committee on Cancer (AJCC) has established prostate cancer staging.[21]

Using the AJCC nomenclature, stage T1 is localized to prostate with a normal DRE or stage T2 will be palpable disease on DRE but no evidence of disease beyond the confines of the prostate, N0 to NX (LN status) and M0 (no evidence of metastatic spread) (Figure 1). An advanced cancer stage will be stage T3 to T4 (locally advanced tumors with cancer spread outside prostate gland) with N1 or M1 (nodal or distant metastasis). Imaging modalities like computed tomography (CT) scan, magnetic resonance imaging (MRI), radionuclide bone scans are currently the most widely used imaging tools for detecting cancer spread outside the prostate gland either in the pelvic lymph nodes or distant spread in the bones. Pelvic lymph node dissection (PLND) remains the most accurate method to assess metastases to pelvic nodes and is usually performed during radical prostatectomy either open or robot assisted laparoscopic dissection. Computed tomography (CT) scan can detect grossly enlarged nodes but is not as reliable as surgical staging at staging pelvic node disease.[22,23] Similarly MRI is a poor tool for evaluating nodal disease. MRI prostate imaging, has shown to be highest sensitivity and specificity for identifying organ confined and extraprostatic disease.[24]

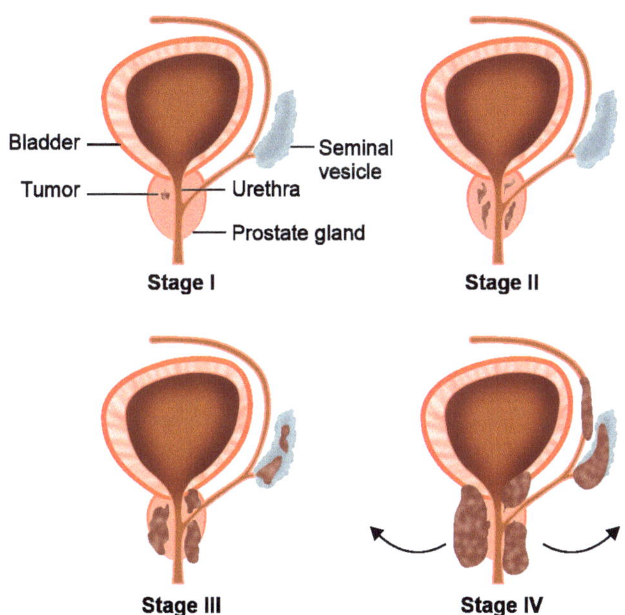

Figure 1: Staging of Prostate Cancer

Treatment Options

Clinical guidelines for the management of clinically localized prostate cancer were published by the national urological society (American Urological Association) in 2007.[16] Based on the review of data and panel consensus, the AUA recommends that the patient's life expectancy, overall health status, and cancer grade and stage should be examined before any treatment decisions are finalized. Life expectancy should also be considered in the assessment. The panel did not specify a chronological age cut off. Because many older patients with localized tumors, may die of other medical illnesses like heart attack or stroke rather from prostate cancer. Since the complications from prostate cancer treatment could be disabling and significantly affect quality of life, these should also be taken in consideration in selecting the appropriate management for individual patients. Patient's overall health status, life expectancy and any associated coexisting medical diseases should also be considered before a definitive treatment is planned.

There are number of treatment options which may be offered to the patient with clinically localized prostate cancer:

- Watchful waiting and active surveillance
- Interstitial brachytherapy
- External beam radiotherapy
- Surgery
- Cryotherapy
- Hormonal therapy

Watchful Waiting and Active Surveillance

Men who are older, with low grade disease and localized low volume disease with insignificant tumors may be offered a watchful waiting program or active surveillance. Watchful waiting is offered to patients who are unlikely to benefit from definitive treatment of prostate cancer or risks of the treatment outweighs the benefits achieved from invasive treatment. Active surveillance includes periodic physical examinations and PSA testing, or periodic repeated prostate biopsies. Patients with lower risk tumors (low Gleason score, PSA level, and clinical stage) are considered suitable candidates for this treatment option. During surveillance period, if the tumor shows evidence of progression (e.g., increased grade, volume, or stage) based upon repeat imaging (MRI) or biopsy, surveillance is discontinued, and patient is offered curative treatment.[25]

Interstitial Brachytherapy

Interstitial prostate brachytherapy with placement of radioactive Iodine 125 seeds as a treatment for prostate cancer has been performed since the 1960s.[26] It was started as open placement of 125 seeds. But in the late 1980s, a trans-perineal approach under transrectal ultrasound guidance was developed for replacement of radioactive iodine 125 seeds.[27] Two most commonly used radioactive seeds in this treatment regimen employ 120 Gy (palladium) or 140 Gy (I^{125}) (Figure

2). Patients with clinically localized prostate cancer and low risk disease (i.e., low PSA and low Gleason score) are considered suitable candidates for interstitial prostate brachytherapy. Complications may include urethritis causing irritative urinary symptoms and, in more severe cases, fistula formation from urethral necrosis.

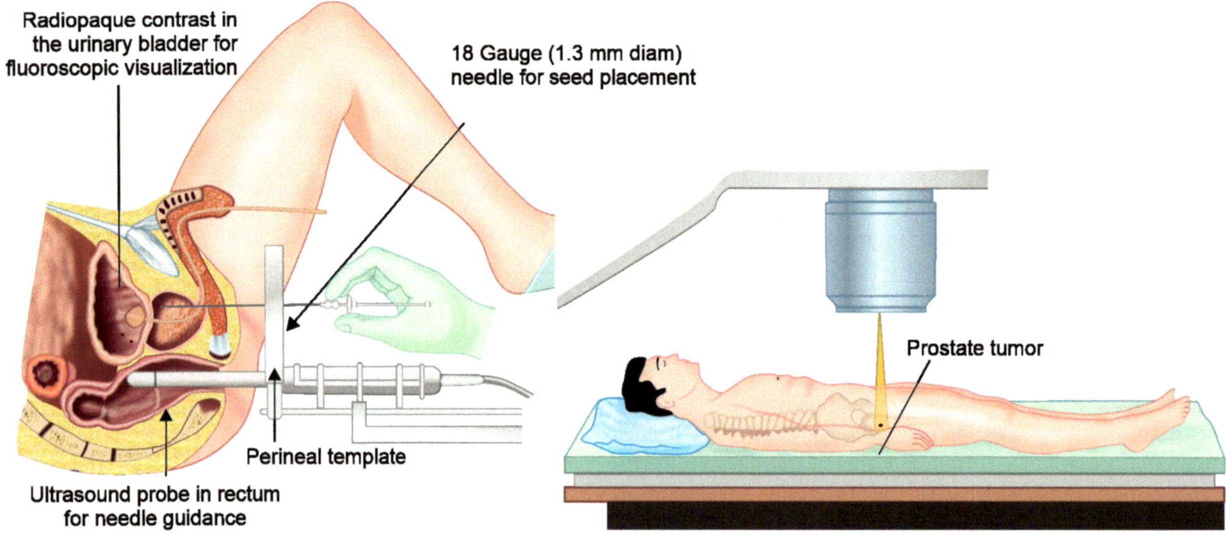

Figure 2: Brachytherapy for prostate cancer. Seeds are inserted through the skin of the perineum. Each seed is placed in a predetermined location. Beams of high-energy radiation are focused on the target area. The radiation attempts to kill cancer cells in the affected areas.

External Beam Radiotherapy

External beam radiotherapy has been utilized for the treatment of localized prostate cancer since the 1930s, with orthovoltage equipment.[16] However, in the 1960s, megavoltage irradiation was used to deliver high radiation doses.[16] In the 1980s, CT scan planning was incorporated to target the prostate more precisely which limited the toxicity to surrounding structures in the radiation field such as the bladder, rectum and small bowel. As a result, radiation doses were increased safely from 65 Gy to 75 Gy. This technique resulted in fewer radiation-related complications.

Radiation therapy is only suitable for localized prostate cancer. Patients should have negative workup for metastatic disease by CT scan and/or bone scan. Patients considered poor medical candidates for surgery or who refused surgery may be treated with radiotherapy which has acceptably low complication rates.[28]. A retrospective review that included 999 patients treated with megavoltage radiation therapy showed cause-specific survival rates to be significantly different at 10 years when looking at T-stage: T1 (79%), T2 (66%), T3 (55%), and T4 (22%).[29] For patients with high risk disease (high PSA and Gleason score), a short course of hormonal therapy (3-6 months) in conjunction with standard dose external beam radiotherapy (approximately 70 Gy) is often utilized.[16] The main complications after radiation therapy include radiation cystitis presenting as hematuria and radiation proctitis. These problems may become chronic and recurring, but rarely require surgical intervention.

Surgery

Surgery is usually offered to patients in good health and reasonably good life expectancy. These patients should have disease confined to the prostate gland (stage T1 to T2). Surgery of choice is radical prostatectomy which involves removal of the entire prostate gland with the attached seminal vesicles and the ampulla of the vas deferens. Radical prostatectomy can be conducted using an open retropubic or perineal approach, or through a laparoscopic or robotic-assisted technique. Depending on Gleason grade and patient's sexual function, nerve-sparing to preserve erectile function can be performed. Otherwise, non-nerve-sparing radical prostatectomy is preferred.[30]

Pelvic lymphadenectomy is sometimes performed concurrently with radical prostatectomy and is generally reserved for patients with higher risk of nodal involvement (large tumor volume, high PSA, and high Gleason grade).[31] Radical prostatectomy is usually not performed if the pre-op evaluation reveals grossly enlarged lymph nodes or on frozen section of the pelvic nodes reveals metastatic disease.

All patients undergoing surgery should be warned of the possible risk of complications such as urinary incontinence, impotence and urethral stricture, and the need for blood transfusion.

Cryotherapy

This technique involves the intermittent freezing and thawing of the prostate tissue with cryoprobes.[32] Cryotherapy is less established than standard prostatectomy, meaning long-term outcomes are not as well studied as with prostatectomy or radiation therapy. Patients with low risk, clinically localized prostate cancer (low PSA level, low Gleason score, and stage T1 to T2) are considered suitable candidates for cryotherapy. Complications include impotence, urinary incontinence, urethral sloughing, and rectal injury.

Hormonal Therapy

Primary androgen deprivation therapy (ADT) may be utilized for patients in whom definitive treatment with surgery or radiation is not possible because of presence of locally advanced disease or distant metastatic disease. Primary ADT is not considered a "standard" treatment option for localized disease.[16] Several different hormonal approaches may be used in the management of advanced prostate cancer. These include bilateral orchiectomy, LHRH agonists, antiandrogens, estrogen therapy, and more. The benefits of bilateral orchiectomy include immediate lowering of testosterone, compliance, and low cost. The disadvantages include psychological effects, loss of libido, impotence, hot flashes, and osteoporosis. With hormonal therapy, there is also an increased risk of cardiovascular disease such as coronary heart disease, myocardial infarction, and stroke. While castration with bilateral orchiectomy is permanent, it is reversible with LHRH agonist. Tumor flare reactions may occur transiently but can be prevented by the concurrent use of antiandrogens.

REFERENCES

1. Girman CJ, Guess HA. Epidemiology of benign prostatic hyperplasia. In: Lepor H, Lawson RK: Prostatic Diseases, Milwaukee, WI, WB Saunders Co, 1993, pp 116-126.
2. Barry MJ. Epidemiology and natural history of benign prostatic hyperplasia. Urol Clin North Am 1990; 17: 495-507.
3. Janetschek G. Future trends in benign prostatic hyperplasia. In: Narayan Perichery, ed: Benign Prostatic Hyperplasia. Gainsville, FL, Churchill Livingstone, 2000, pp 385-395.
4. Lee C, Kozlowski JM, Grayhack JT. Intrinsic and extrinsic factors controlling benign prostatic growth. Prostate 1997; 31: 131-138.
5. Sanda MG, Doehring CB, Binkowitz B, et al. Clinical and biological characteristics of familial benign prostatic hyperplasia. J Urol 1997; 157: 876-879.
6. AUA Practice Guidelines Committee (2003): AUA Guideline on the management of benign prostatic hyperplasia. (2003) Chapter 1: Diagnosis and treatment recommendations. J Urol 2003; 170 (2): 530-547.
7. McVary KT, Roehrborn CG, Avins AL, et al. Update on AUA Guideline on the Management of Benign Prostatic Hyperplasia. J Urol 2011; 185: 1793-1803.
8. Barry MJ, Fowler FJ Jr, O' Leary MP, et al. The American Urological Association symptom index for benign prostatic hyperplasia. The measurement committee of the American Urological Association. J Urol 1992; 148: 1549-1557.
9. Roehrborn CG. Contemporary Diagnosis and Management of Benign Prostatic Hyperplasia. In: Benign Prostatic Hyperplasia, Handbooks in Health Care Co., Newton, Pennsylvania, USA, 2007.
10. Narayan P, Tewari A. Alpha blockers in clinical management. In: Narayan P, ed: Benign Prostatic Hyperplasia. Gainsville, FL, Churchill Livingston, 2000, pp 155-169.
11. Chang D, Campbell J. Intraoperative floppy iris syndrome associated with tamsulosin. J Cataract Refrac Surg 2005; 31:664.
12. Roehrborn C, Andriole G, et al. Effect of the dual 5 alpha reductase inhibitor dutasteride on endocrine parameters and prostate volume. Eur Urol 2002; 1(suppl 1): 107.
13. Zlotta AR, Giannakopoulos X, Maehlum O, et al. Long term evaluation of transurethral needle ablation of the prostate (TUNA) for treatment of symptomatic benign prostatic hyperplasia: clinical outcome upto five years from three centers. Eur Urol 2003; 44: 89-93.
14. Costello AJ, Bowsher WG, Bolton DM, et al. Laser ablation of the prostate in patients with benign prostatic hypertrophy. Br J Urol 1992; 69: 603-608.
15. Hahn RG. Fluid absorption in endoscopic surgery. Br J Anaesth 2006; 96: 8-20.
16. Thompson, I, Thrasher JB, Aus G, Burnett AL, et al. Guideline for the Management of Clinically Localized Prostate Cancer: 2007 Update. J Urol 2007; 177(6): 2106-2131.
17. American cancer Society: Cancer Facts and Figures 2012. Atlanta, Ga: American Cancer Society, 2012. Available online. Last accessed November 23, 2012.
18. Hinman F Jr. Screening for prostatic carcinoma. J Urol 1991; 145(1): 126-129.
19. Gerber GS, Chodak GW. Routine screening for cancer of the prostate. J Natl Cancer Inst 1991; 83(5): 329-335.
20. Gleason, DF. Histologic grading and clinical staging of prostatic carcinoma. In: Urology Pathology; The

Prostate. Edited by M. Tannenbaum. Philadelphia: Lea & Febiger, chapter 9, 1977.

21. American Joint Committee on Cancer (AJCC).
22. Gerber GS, Goldberg R, Chodak GW. Local staging of prostate cancer by tumor volume, prostatic-specific antigen, and transrectal ultrasound. Urology 1992; 40(4): 311-316.
23. Hanks GE, Krall JM, Pilepich MV, et al. Comparison of pathologic and clinical evaluation of lymph nodes in prostate cancer: implications of RTOG data for patient management and trial design and stratification. Int J Radiat Oncol Biol Phys 1992; 23(2): 293-298.
24. Schiebler ML, Schall MD, Pollack HM, et al. Current role of MR imaging in the staging of adenocarcinoma of the prostate. Radiology 1993; 189(2): 339-352.
25. Warlick C, Trock BJ, Landis P, et al. Delayed versus immediate surgical intervention and prostate cancer outcome. J Natl Cancer Inst 2006; 98: 355.
26. Sogani PC, Whitmore WF Jr, Hilaris BS, Batata MA. Experience with interstitial implantation of iodine 125 in the treatment of prostatic carcinoma. Scand J Urol Nephrol Suppl 1980; 55: 205.
27. Balasko JC, Ragde H, Grimm PD. Transperineal ultrasound-guided implantation of the prostate: morbidity and complications. Scan J Urol Nephrol Suppl 1991; 137: 113.
28. Forman JD, Order SE, Zinreich ES, et al. Carcinoma of the prostate in the elderly: the therapeutic ratio of definitive radiotherapy. J Urol 1986; 136(6): 1238-1241.
29. Duncan W, Warde P, Catton CN, et al. Carcinoma of the prostate: results of radical radiotherapy (1970-1985) Int J Radiat Oncol Biol Phys 1993; 26(2): 203-210.
30. Walsh PC. Patient-reported impotence and incontinence after nerve-sparing radical prostatectomy. J Urol 1988; 159: 308.
31. Carroll P, Coley C, McLeod D, Schelhammer P, Sweat G, Wasson J, et al. Prostate-specific antigen best practice policy-part II: prostate cancer staging and post-treatment follow-up. Urology 2002; 57: 225.
32. Robinson JW, Saliken JC, Donnelly BJ, et al. Quality-of-life outcomes for men treated with cryosurgery for localized prostate carcinoma. Cancer 1999; 86(9): 1793-1801.

❑❑❑

69

CHAPTER

Urogenital Malignancies

Claire de la Calle, MD
Nirmish Singla, MD

INTRODUCTION

Urologic cancers comprise a large proportion of malignancies worldwide and include prostate, urothelial, kidney, testicular, penile, and adrenal cancers. In many countries prostate cancer is the number one cancer diagnosis in men, and globally it is the second most common cancer in men with 1.4 million new cases a year. Bladder and kidney cancer also comprise a significant portion of urology practices. Worldwide bladder and kidney cancers are the 6th and 9th most common malignancies in men, with around 570,000 and 430,000 diagnoses yearly respectively. Testis cancer is much less prevalent, with 74,000 newly diagnosed men yearly worldwide. Other rare urologic cancers include penile cancer, with around 36,000 diagnoses yearly worldwide, and even less common cancers such as primary cancers of the urethra and adrenal gland.[1]

In this chapter, we will provide an overview of the diagnosis and management of the most commonly encountered non-prostate urologic malignancies: bladder cancer, kidney cancer and testis cancer. Prostate cancer was discussed in a previous chapter.

Urothelial Carcinoma of the Bladder

Histopathology

The bladder is comprised of 4 layers: the urothelium, the lamina propria, the muscularis propria and the serosa. The urothelium is a specialized stratified epithelium comprised of 5 to 6 layers of cells when the bladder is empty. It is also called 'transitional epithelium' as it restructures to accommodate the urine, becoming 2 to 3 layers.[2]

The vast majority of bladder cancers are epithelial malignancies, and around 96% of those are urothelial carcinomas, also called transitional cell carcinomas. These are further subdivided into low-grade or high-grade urothelial carcinomas. The remaining 4% are called 'variant histology' bladder cancers and include primary adenocarcinomas and squamous cell carcinomas of the bladder, micropapillary, sarcomatoid, small cell, and other histologies.[3] Many tumors with variant histology are primarily composed of urothelial carcinoma histology, with a fraction of variant histology. Bladder cancers with any amount of variant histology tend to have more aggressive courses with worse prognosis and are usually treated more aggressively than the pure urothelial carcinoma tumors.[4]

Most bladder cancers are papillary tumors that protrude into the bladder lumen. Low-grade noninvasive tumors tend to be papillary, and they are often attached to the bladder wall via a thin stalk, whereas high-grade and more invasive tumors can be sessile or ulcerated. Carcinoma in situ (CIS) lesions are the exception as they are flat high-grade tumors that can easily be missed or confused with simple inflammation of the bladder wall on cystoscopy. CIS is also often considered to be a misnomer as these lesions can progress to become invasive.[5]

Risk Factors

Tobacco smoking is the number one bladder cancer risk factor, likely attributable for at least 50-60% of bladder cancers. Current and past smokers have a 2- to 4-fold higher risk of developing bladder cancer but are also at higher risk of harboring a higher stage and grade and a worse mortality risk.[6,7] Several occupational exposures have been associated with increased bladder cancer risk. Chemical industry workers exposed to different aromatic hydrocarbons, painters and hairdressers exposed to aromatic amines in dyes, and rubber and latex manufacturing workers exposed to N-nitrosamines are some of the occupational exposures that have been associated with increased bladder cancer risk.[8] Other risk factors include chronic urinary tract infections, bladder trauma, schistosomiasis, phenacetin, cyclophosphamide, and radiation therapy. The role of genetics and inherited bladder cancer risk is poorly understood.

Presentation and Diagnosis

Bladder cancer is diagnosed at an average age of 70 years.[9] It is more common in men with a 3:1 male-to-female ratio,[3] and in the United States, it is more common in Caucasians than in African Americans, but women and African Americans tend to be diagnosed at later stages and have a worse prognosis.[10,11] For most patients, hematuria (gross or microscopic) is the only presenting symptom.[12] A small fraction will present with irritative voiding symptoms such as urgency and frequency, particularly those with CIS.

The differential diagnosis of hematuria is broad including stones, urinary tract infection, strictures, urothelial cancers, kidney cancer, urinary fistulas, trauma, and instrumentation of the urinary tract. The American Urological Association (AUA) has put forth a guideline for the workup of patients with hematuria.[13] Per the AUA, all patients with microscopic hematuria and over 60 years of age or over 30 pack-year smoking history should be evaluated with a cystoscopy and a 4-phase CT Urogram of the abdomen and pelvis. All patients with over 25 red blood cells per high-power field or any history of gross hematuria should also be evaluated with the same diagnostic modalities. For the patients not meeting these criteria, considered to be at lower risk, cystoscopy with renal bladder ultrasound or repeat urinalysis in 6 months followed by cystoscopy and renal bladder ultrasound if the hematuria persists can be considered.

In patients with a known bladder tumor identified on imaging, a pre-operative cystoscopy can be omitted as this can be performed in the operating room at the time of tumor biopsy. Patients with bladder masses identified on cystoscopy still require a CT urogram however for local, nodal, and distant staging purposes but also because up to 2% of patients with bladder cancer will also have an upper urinary tract tumor.[14] A urine cytology can be considered in patients at high risk for developing bladder cancer and otherwise negative hematuria workup. In those cases, if the urine cytology is positive for high-grade urothelial carcinoma, random bladder biopsies (including a biopsy of the prostatic urethra) to look for CIS, upper urinary tract cytologies and endoscopic evaluation of the upper urinary tract might be necessary to identify the source of the positive cytology.[15] Blue light cystoscopy and narrow band imaging are two forms of enhanced cystoscopy that improve the visualization and detection of small papillary tumors and CIS. Either modality can be considered in cases of suspected CIS or known CIS, as in addition to being associated with increased detection, their use also reduces recurrences.[16-18]

Staging and Risk Categories

For management purposes, bladder cancers are grouped into non-muscle invasive bladder cancers (NMIBC; Ta, Tis, T1) and muscle invasive bladder cancers (MIBC; T2, T3, T4) (Figure 1, Table 1).[19] Most patients present with NMIBC (around 75%).[20] Clinical T stage is determined by endoscopic transurethral resection of the bladder tumor. For tumors that are suspected to be at least muscle invasive, a bimanual examination after visually complete endoscopic resection of the tumor is important to identify extravesical extension (i.e., cT3 or higher). MRI of the pelvis can also aid to evaluate for tumor invasion beyond the bladder. Chest imaging is indicated in all patients with cT2, or higher tumors and a bone scan should be obtained if there is clinical suspicion for bone metastases or if alkaline phosphatase is elevated.

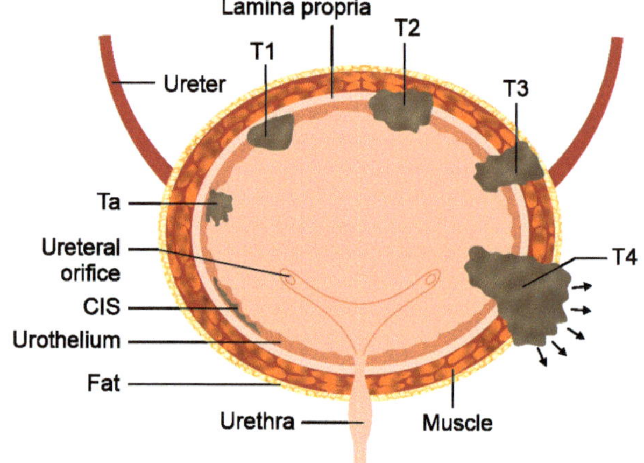

Figure 1: Diagram of bladder cancer staging. CIS: carcinoma in situ.

Table 1: Bladder cancer staging. Adapted from the American Joint Committee on Cancer (AJCC) TNM Staging System for Bladder Cancer 8th ed. 2017.[19]

T stage	Primary Tumor
Tx	Cannot assess the primary tumor
T0	There is no evidence of a primary tumor
Ta	The papillary carcinoma is noninvasive
Tis	Urothelial carcinoma in situ also known as a "flat tumor"
T1	The tumor invades the lamina propria
T2	Tumor invades muscularis propria
T2a	The tumor invades the inner portion of the muscularis propria
T2b	Tumor invades the outer half of the muscularis propria
T3	Tumor invades perivesical tissue
T3a	Tumor invades perivesical tissue microscopically

T3b	Tumor invades perivesical tissue macroscopically
T4	The extravesical tumor directly invades an adjacent structure (i.e., seminal vesicles, prostatic stroma, vagina, uterus, abdominal wall, pelvic wall
T4a	The extravesical tumor directly invades the seminal vesicles, prostatic stroma, vagina, uterus
T4b	The extravesical tumor directly invades the abdominal and/or pelvic wall
N	**Regional Lymph Nodes**
Nx	Cannot assess the lymph nodes
N0	There is no metastasis to the lymph nodes
N1	Metastasis to a single regional lymph node located in the true pelvis (i.e., obturator, perivesical, sacral, or internal and external iliac lymph node)
N2	Metastasis to multiple regional lymph nodes in the true pelvis
N3	Metastasis to the common iliac lymph nodes
M	**Distant Metastasis**
M0	There is no distant metastasis
M1	There is distant metastasis
M1a	The distant metastasis is limited to lymph nodes past the common iliacs
M1b	The distant metastasis is non-lymph-node

Treatment

Treatment of NMIBC is based on the AUA risk stratification (Table 2).[21] For all NMIBCs, transurethral resection of the bladder tumor (TURBT) is the gold standard. TURBTs must be visually complete, and the resection must include the muscularis propria for appropriate staging. Low-risk and most intermediate-risk tumors can be treated with a single transurethral resection, provided the resection is visually complete. In high-grade or high-risk tumors, a second transurethral resection should be considered as many will be under-staged during the first resection. For high-grade T1 tumors, re-resection is strongly recommended as at least 30% will be upstaged to MIBC at re-resection.[22]

Table 2: AUA Risk Stratification for Non-Muscle Invasive Bladder Cancer.[21]

Low Risk	Intermediate Risk	High Risk
Low-grade solitary Ta 3 cm	Recurrence within 1 year, LGTa	High-grade T1
Papillary urothelial neoplasm of low malignant potential	Solitary low-grade Ta >3 cm	Any recurrent high-grade Ta
	Low-grade Ta, multifocal	High-grade Ta >3 cm (or multifocal)
	High-grade Ta 3 cm	Any carcinoma in situ
	Low-grade T1	Any BCG failure in High-Grade patient
		Any variant histology
		Any lymphovascular invasion
		Any high-grade prostatic urethral involvement

Up to 50% of NMIBC will recur at least once and around 11% will progress to MIBC so adjuvant intravesical therapies are recommended to reduce the risk of recurrence and progression.[5] A single post-operative dose of intravesical chemotherapy (e.g., gemcitabine, mitomycin or epirubicin) given within 24 hours of surgery, is recommended in cases of suspected or known low- to intermediate-risk bladder cancers as these agents can reduce recurrence by 10 to 15%.[23,24] Gemcitabine is usually favored due to its low side effect profile. In high-risk patients and 'higher risk' intermediate risk patients, a 6-week induction course of weekly intravesical BCG (Bacillus Calmette-Guérin) instillations is considered to be the gold standard.[25] BCG is an attenuated strain of *Mycobacterium bovis* that produces immune mediated antitumor activity but its exact mechanism of action is unclear.[26] The patients who respond to a BCG induction course will then benefit from maintenance BCG (1 year for intermediate-risk patients, 3 years for high-risk patients) consisting of 3-week courses of weekly instillations at months 3, 6, 12, 18, 24, and 36.[27,28] BCG will reduce around 50% of recurrences,[29] but another 50% will benefit from a second induction course if they do recur once.[30]

Patients that are found to have high-grade T1 disease after an induction course, or those that do not respond to a second induction course or one induction course plus a maintenance course, are considered BCG unresponsive. In these patients and those with adverse features such as variant histology, lymphovascular invasion, or persistent high-grade T1 after second TURBT, early radical cystectomy is recommended as NMIBC patients that progress to MIBC tend to have a worse prognosis than those who initially present with MIBC,[31,32] particularly those with high-grade T1 disease.[33]

For patients that are not medically fit for radical cystectomy or those who are unwilling to undergo radical cystectomy, alternative intravesical treatments exist such as valrubicin,[34] gemcitabine,[35] docetaxel,[36] or combination gemcitabine/docetaxel.[37] Systemic pembrolizumab is another alternative option for patients with BCG unresponsive NMIBC and CIS.[38] It is important to recognize however that these alternative treatments provide only a modest reduction in recurrence-free survival and therefore radical cystectomy should be strongly considered in these BCG-unresponsive patients. This is an active area of research however, and it is expected that more treatment alternatives will be incorporated in the guidelines in the near future.[39] It is also important to recognize that while most patients will suffer from treatable BCG side effects, mostly lower urinary tract symptoms, 8% will have symptoms severe enough to warrant treatment discontinuation.[40] For these patients, the same alternative treatments given for BCG unresponsive disease can be considered.

If left untreated MIBC progresses rapidly to metastasis and death (around 24 months).[41] The gold standard treatment for MIBC is neoadjuvant cisplatin-based chemotherapy followed by radical cystectomy. Neoadjuvant chemotherapy (NAC) (usually gemcitabine with cisplatin or MVAC which consists of methotrexate, vinblastine, adriamycin, and cisplatin) should be strongly recommended to all patients who are candidates for receiving cisplatin, as NAC can increase 5-year survival by around 5 to 7%.[42,43] Patients who are ineligible to receive cisplatin should proceed with upfront cystectomy, and those that underwent cystectomy without receiving NAC and have pT3+ disease or nodal disease should be considered for adjuvant cisplatin-based chemotherapy at this appears to at least prolong progression-free survival.[44] Adjuvant nivolumab can also be considered in patients that did not receive NAC or those that have persistent invasive or nodal disease after NAC and cystectomy.[45] For patients who are not medically fit to undergo surgery or unwilling to undergo cystectomy, trimodal therapy is an alternative. Trimodal therapy consists of maximal TURBT, external beam radiation therapy, and concurrent radiosensitizing chemotherapy. A complete resection of all visible disease is key in trimodal therapy as it will increase the rates of local control by 20%.[46,47] Therefore, ideal candidates for trimodal therapy have small tumors, do not have multifocal tumors or high-volume CIS, and do not have hydronephrosis (as this can be a sign of locally advanced disease).[48] Other bladder preserving options include partial cystectomy, TURBT alone or radiation alone; however, only trimodal therapy seems to provide comparable survival rates to cystectomy provided a prompt salvage cystectomy is performed for non-responders.[49] Close follow-up is important for all patients after bladder preserving therapies, as locoregional recurrences tend to be higher.[50] MIBC recurrences require salvage cystectomy, and patients desiring a bladder preserving approach must understand that salvage cystectomies have higher complication rates, especially after radiation.[51]

In men, radical cystectomy involves removal of the bladder, prostate, and seminal vesicles. In women, in addition to the bladder the gynecologic organs might need to be resected if there is concern for direct invasion on preoperative workup, but often they can safely be spared.[52,53] A bilateral pelvic lymph node dissection should be performed at the time of surgery as this provides staging information, can improve survival, and decrease recurrences.[54] The appropriate extent of the lymph node dissection is debated but most agree that it should include the bilateral common iliac, external iliac, internal iliac, and obturator lymph nodes for adequate staging.[55,56] Radical cystectomy can be performed robotically or via an open incision. Several trials have compared the two techniques and have failed to demonstrate non-equivalence.[57-60]

The ileal conduit is made from a small segment of distal ileum and is the most commonly performed urinary diversion. It is an incontinent diversion that requires the use of an ostomy bag, it is the easiest diversion to perform and is associated with less complications than the other diversions.[61,62] The orthotopic neobladder and various cutaneous pouches are continent alternatives to the ileal conduit, however these cannot be considered if the patient has significant renal or liver dysfunction, if the patient has limited bowel length, if the patient is physically unable or unwilling to catheterize, or if cancer is identified at the urethral margin during surgery (the latter applies to orthotopic diversions only).[48] Each type of diversion affects quality of life differently and is associated with different possible complications, often related to the bowel segment used and the degree of urinary continence provided by the diversion (ranging from incontinence to hyper-continence). Radical cystectomy is a major surgery associated with a high complication rate of around 65% at 90 days post-surgery,[60] which is further complicated by the fact that MIBC patients tend to be older with multiple comorbid conditions. At least a quarter of patients are readmitted[63] and most peri-operative complications are related to the urinary diversion.[64] Most centers that perform cystectomies follow an ERAS (enhanced recovery after surgery) pathway, similar to the protocols used in patients undergoing colorectal surgery, and these have been shown to decrease some of the bowel related complications.[65] The vast majority of patients will also experience long term complications including, but not limited to, ureteral strictures, stoma related complications such as parastomal hernia, continence issues in those with 'continent' diversions, recurrent urinary tract infections, pouch stones, impaired sexual and bowel function, decline in renal function and metabolic/electrolyte abnormalities, body image issues, and skeletal fractures.

Metastatic bladder cancer is not considered to be a surgical disease, unless required for palliative reasons, and the systemic therapies for metastatic bladder cancer are outside the scope of this chapter. However, it is important to recognize that the treatment of metastatic bladder cancer is rapidly evolving, especially with the advent of immune checkpoint inhibitors and other targeted therapies. As these treatments improve, the role of consolidative surgery in advanced stage bladder cancer might evolve as well.

Prognosis and Surveillance

The 5-year survival for NMIBC is around 96%.[66] However, given the high recurrence rate, these patients need to be regularly monitored with cystoscopies, as well as a cytology for the high-risk patients. In fact, it has been shown that up to 45% of patients will have a tumor noted on their first surveillance cystoscopy.[67] Intermediate and high-risk patients also require upper tract imaging every 1-2 years, as up to 10% of these patients will have recurrence in the upper tracts.[21] The 5-year survival of MIBC is considerably lower at 69%. Similar surveillance protocols combining cystoscopy and upper tract imaging are utilized after the bladder preserving treatment of MIBC, and those treated with cystectomy are followed with imaging and cytology.[48]

Upper Tract Urothelial Carcinoma (UTUC)

The renal pelvis and ureters are lined by a similar urothelium as the bladder. Only 5 to 10% of all urothelial carcinomas involve the upper urinary tract.[68] Because of its low incidence, much of the treatment principles of UTUC have been extrapolated from what is known about bladder cancer.

The risk factors associated with UTUC are largely similar to the ones for bladder cancer. Interestingly, germline carriers of the Lynch Syndrome DNA mismatch repair genes (*MLH1*, *MSH2*, *MSH6*, *PMS2*, *EPCAM*) are at an increased risk of developing a UTUC. Patients with an *MSH2* pathogenic mutation seem to be at the highest risk.[69,70] Surveillance protocols have been suggested for these patients, but none have been established to change outcomes. Exposure to aristolochic acid, which is endemic to the Balkan regions and a common ingredient in Chinese herbs, is another unique risk factor for the development of UTUC.[71] Also similar to bladder cancer, most patients with UTUCs present with hematuria, however some patients can present with flank pain from hydronephrosis caused by malignant obstruction. The initial hematuria workup of these patients is the same with cystoscopy and CT urogram. Once an upper urinary tract tumor is suspected however, either due to a positive urine cytology without evidence of tumor in the lower urinary tract, or due to a tumor or a filling defect in the upper urinary tract noted on CT urogram, further endoscopic evaluation with ureteroscopy and biopsy and/or upper tract selective cytologies is warranted. The grading system for UTUC is the same as for lower urinary tract urothelial carcinomas. T staging is also similar with Ta tumors representing superficial noninvasive tumors, Tis is carcinoma in situ, T1 tumors invade the lamina propria, T2 tumors invade the muscularis, T3 tumors invade the periureteral or renal sinus fat or renal parenchyma, and T4 tumors invade adjacent organs.[19] Clinical staging however is notoriously inaccurate in UTUC, as the tissue samples obtained from ureteroscopic biopsies tend to be too small to properly assess staging.

The gold standard treatment for UTUC is radical nephroureterectomy, which involves the removal of the kidney and entire ureter with a small cuff of bladder around the ureteral orifice, performed via an open incision, laparoscopically, robotically, or in a combined approach.[72] Nephroureterectomy is often recommended if the patient has high-risk features such as high-grade pathology, large tumor size (>2 cm), multifocal disease or variant histology.[73-75] Regional lymph node dissection is also recommended in patients with high-grade disease.[76,77] Distal ureteral masses however can be managed by distal ureterectomy and ureteral reimplantation when renal sparing is desired.[78] At the time of surgery or shortly thereafter, many surgeons will administer one intravesical dose of chemotherapy (mitomycin, gemcitabine or pirarubicin) as this has been shown to reduce bladder recurrences.[79]

Low-grade tumors are preferentially treated with organ sparing approaches, especially if the tumor is unifocal and the disease burden is low (<2 cm).[74,80] This is most commonly done endoscopically via laser or cautery ablation; however, percutaneous resection and/or ablation is a possible alternative for renal pelvis tumors. Complete tumor eradication is often accomplished only after several endoscopic interventions which is why these patients and all patients that are managed with organ sparing approaches require close surveillance of their upper urinary tracts with regular imaging, cystoscopy, cytology, and/or ureteroscopy. Patients that experience recurrence after organ sparing approaches should be considered for nephroureterectomy. For patients with recurrent low-grade tumors or with high-grade tumors who are not medically fit for nephroureterectomy, or those with a solitary kidney or significant kidney disease, topical BCG, mitomycin or gemcitabine instillations can be considered via a percutaneous nephrostomy tube or retrograde via a ureteral stent. The efficacy of these instillations is limited due to limited dwell time and contact with the upper tract urothelium.[81-83] A mitomycin containing reverse thermal hydrogel that is liquid at cold temperatures but solidifies into a gelatinous fluid at body temperature, was developed allowing for easy instillation in the liquid form but longer dwell time in the upper urinary tract due to its increased viscosity in the body. This is a novel, FDA-approved mode of drug delivery that can be used for low-grade UTUC tumors that are difficult to control endoscopically.[84]

The benefit of NAC prior to nephroureterectomy in UTUC is not as well established as it is for MIBC, but a growing body of literature is now suggesting oncologic benefit in administering cisplatin-based NAC.[85,86] In the adjuvant setting, the POUT randomized controlled trial demonstrated a disease-free survival benefit for patients with pT2-4 or pN1-3 disease receiving adjuvant gemcitabine with cisplatin or carboplatin.[87] However, as renal function can be decreased after surgery, NAC might be increasingly favored as more prospective data becomes available in the neoadjuvant space. Just like for urothelial carcinoma of the bladder, surgery plays a limited role in metastatic UTUC for which systemic therapy is the mainstay.

Renal Cell Carcinoma (RCC)

Histopathology

The functional unit of the kidney is the nephron. Over 90% of renal cortical malignant tumors are renal cell carcinomas (RCC), most of which are clear cell RCCs that arise from the proximal convoluted tubule of the nephron (Figure 2B). Other RCC sub-classifications include papillary RCC also arising from the proximal convoluted tubule, chromophobe and collecting duct RCCs both arising from the collecting duct, unclassified RCC, and renal medullary carcinoma.[88] With the exception of chromophobe RCC, RCCs are further sub-classified by nucleolar grade, ranging from 1 to 4, with higher grades associated with larger and more aggressive tumors.[89,90]

Risk Factors and Inherited Cancers

Similar to urothelial cancers, male gender, age and smoking are risk factors for developing RCC.[91] Obesity, hypertension, and dialysis dependence for end stage renal disease are also well established RCC risk factors.[92-95] RCC may also manifest as a hereditary disease, and therefore a positive family history can be a risk factor. Several autosomal dominant familial RCC syndromes have been described, such as von Hippel Lindau (VHL), hereditary papillary RCC (HPRC), Birt-Hogg-Dubé (BHD), and hereditary leiomyoma RCC (HLRCC) among others. Around 2 to 6% of RCC cases are thought to be related to these hereditary syndromes.[96,97]

Clinical Presentation and Diagnosis

In contemporary practice, over 50% of renal cortical tumors are incidentally diagnosed on imaging obtained for unrelated reasons. Prior to such high usage of cross-sectional imaging, RCCs were often diagnosed at advanced stages, once symptoms of locally advanced or metastatic disease developed or when associated with paraneoplastic syndromes such as Stauffer's syndrome. In fact, the classic triad of flank pain, hematuria, and a palpable mass occur in less than 10% of patients. As renal cancers tend to be silent until advanced stages, 30% of patients already have distant disease at diagnosis.[68] Patients that do present with hematuria should be evaluated per the AUA hematuria guidelines as described earlier.[13] Otherwise, patients known to have a renal mass are best evaluated with multi-phase contrast-enhanced cross-sectional imaging of the abdomen in order to best characterize the mass and its stage. As diagnostic modalities for renal masses, CT and MRI are considered equivalent, however for the evaluation of renal vein or IVC tumor thrombus, invasion MRI is often considered superior.[98,99]

Solid, rounded, enhancing renal masses without evidence of fat are suspicious for RCC (Figure 2A). Complex cystic renal masses also raise concern for cystic RCC.[100] It is thought that 15 to 20% of renal parenchymal masses that are less than 4 cm are benign masses such as oncocytomas or angiomyolipomas (AML).[101,102] With the exception of fat-containing AMLs, benign tumors can be hard to distinguish from malignant tumors on imaging, so when the diagnosis is in doubt, a renal mass biopsy can be considered.[98,99] Renal mass biopsies are considered safe and are highly accurate in histologic determination when malignant cells are sampled. However, the non-diagnostic rate is around 14% and renal tumors can be heterogeneous, so a benign biopsy does not rule out the presence of cancer.[103,104] This is a regularly encountered issue when oncocytic histology is noted on biopsy as oncocytic tumors can co-exist with chromophobe RCCs.[105] In this setting, a sestamibi PET scan may be informative to differentiate between benign and malignant lesions.[106]

Owing to the fact that 2 to 6% of RCCs are related to a familial syndrome, the AUA also recommends genetic consultation for young patients diagnosed with RCC (<46 years), those with bilateral or multifocal tumors, positive family history, or any other clinical signs of one of the familial RCC syndromes.[98,99]

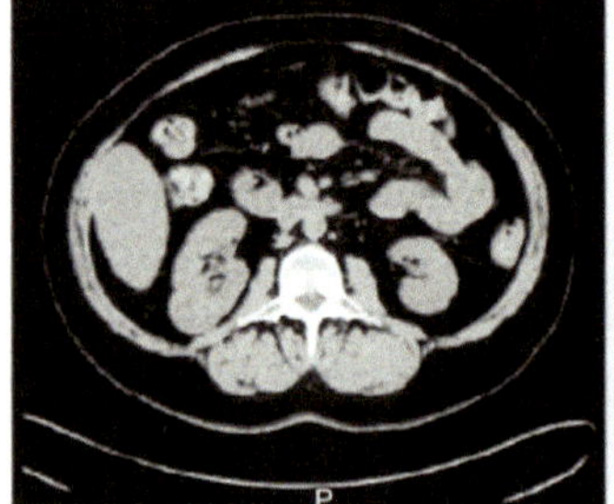
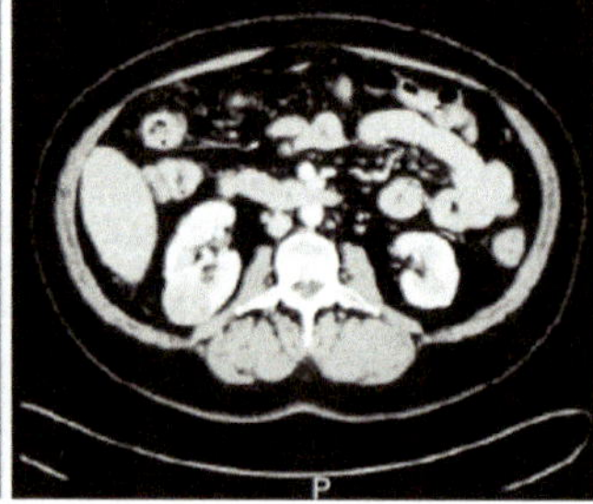

Figure 2A: Axial cut of an abdominal CT with and without intravenous contrast demonstrating a single enhancing 4 cm mass in the posterior mid-right kidney, concerning for clear cell RCC.

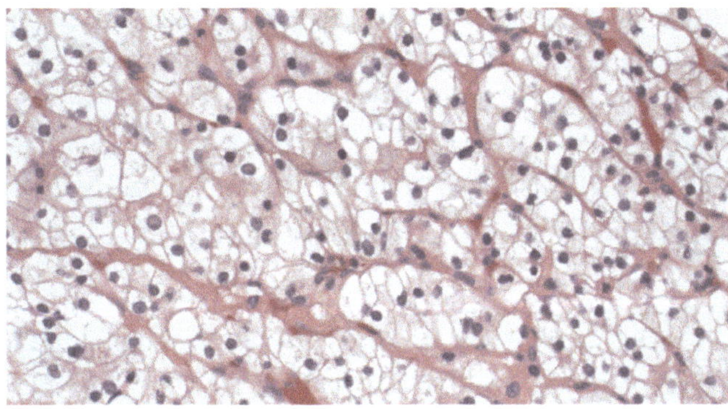

Figure 2B: Representative image of the tumor's histology (obtained after partial nephrectomy), demonstrating RCC cells rich in intracellular lipids giving them their clear appearance. Magnification 40X.

Figure 2: Localized clear cell RCC of the kidney.

Staging

Clinical stage T1 and T2 tumors are limited to the kidney, while T3 tumors exhibit varying degrees of renal sinus or venous invasion and/or perirenal fat invasion, and T4 tumors extend beyond Gerota's fascia and can invade into adjacent organs such as the adrenal gland (Table 3).[19] Clinical staging is based on cross sectional imaging findings. Chest imaging is also indicated in all patients with known or suspected RCC for staging purposes. Bone scan and brain imaging are warranted only if there is clinical suspicion for bone or brain metastases. Sixty-five to seventy percent of RCCs present with localized disease, and 30-35% present with regional or distant spread.[68]

Table 3: Kidney cancer staging. Adapted from the American Joint Committee on Cancer (AJCC) TNM Staging System for Testis Cancer 8th ed. 2017.[19]

T stage	Primary Tumor
Tx	Cannot assess the primary tumor
T0	There is no evidence of a primary tumor
T1	Tumor <7 cm, limited to the kidney
T1a	Tumor >4 cm, limited to the kidney
T1b	Tumor >4 cm but , limited to the kidney
T2	Tumor >7 cm, limited to the kidney
T2a	Tumor >7 cm but , and is limited to the kidney
T2b	Tumor >10 cm, limited to the kidney
T3	Tumor invades the perinephric tissues or major veins, but does not invade the ipsilateral adrenal gland and does not move past Gerota's fascia
T3a	Tumor invades ethers the renal vein or a its branches, the pelvicalyceal system, or the perirenal and/or renal sinus fat. Gerota's fascia
T3b	Tumor invades into the vena cava under the diaphragm
T3c	Tumor invades into the vena cava above the diaphragm or the vena cava wall
T4	Tumor invades past Gerota's fascia (including direct extension into the ipsilateral adrenal gland)
N	**Regional Lymph Nodes**
Nx	Cannot assess the lymph nodes
N0	There is no metastasis to the lymph nodes
N1	There is metastasis to the regional lymph node(s)
M	**Distant Metastasis**
M0	There is no distant metastasis
M1	There is distant metastasis

Treatment

Historically, radical nephrectomy was considered the gold standard for the treatment of localized RCCs. This involves removal of the kidney and its enveloping Gerota's fascia, proximal ureter, and adrenal gland if there is concern for local extension, and regional lymph nodes in cases of resectable lymphadenopathy.[107,108] Depending on tumor size and its invasion into adjacent structures, radical nephrectomy can be performed laparoscopically, robotically, or via an open incision.[109] Tumors that invade the IVC often require a multidisciplinary surgical approach at high volume centers. Depending on the cephalad level of IVC and tributary vein invasions and occasional IVC wall invasion, assistance of vascular surgeons might be needed for IVC reconstruction, hepatobiliary surgeons for liver mobilization, and cardiothoracic surgeons for resection of tumor thrombus in the right atrium, typically with cardiopulmonary bypass.

Partial nephrectomy is now a widely favored alternative to radical nephrectomy for most cT1a and many cT1b/cT2 tumors, provided they can be safely resected without affecting oncologic outcomes.[110,111] Nowadays most partial nephrectomies are performed robotically unless the surgical complexity is very high favoring an open approach. Partial nephrectomy allows for nephron-sparing and results in less postoperative CKD than radical nephrectomy.[112] However, partial nephrectomies tend to be associated with a higher risk of postoperative complications than radical nephrectomies, including an increased need for blood transfusions, urine leaks potentially requiring ureteral stent and/or abdominal drain placement, and pseudoaneurysms requiring embolization.[113,114] Partial nephrectomy is particularly encouraged for patients with RCC familial syndromes as these patients are at high risk for having multiple tumors throughout their lifetime. In fact, enucleation is often favored for these patients, leaving minimal to no renal parenchymal margin around the tumor, in order to spare as much parenchyma as possible.[115,116]

Furthermore, these masses are often observed until the largest tumor reaches 3 cm to limit repeated surgical interventions.[117] Two exceptions are patients with HLRCC and succinate dehydrogenase deficiency RCC as these tumors tend to be more aggressive, and therefore radical nephrectomy is often the favored approach.[118]

Thermal ablation, usually performed percutaneously, is a minimally invasive approach that is often considered for patients that are not surgical candidates and have small renal masses (usually <3 cm) in a favorable location (usually peripheral).[98,99] The most widely used thermal ablation techniques include radiofrequency ablation (RFA) and cryoablation, both of which provide similar oncologic outcomes.[119] Compared to surgical excision, local recurrences tend to be higher for thermal ablative techniques and may require a salvage ablation or surgical resection, but metastasis-free and cancer specific-free survival are similar, particularly for renal masses less than 3 cm.[120,121]

Small renal masses, defined as those less than 4 cm in size (cT1a), can also be safely monitored on active surveillance as only 1 to 2% of these patients will progress to metastatic disease.[122-124] Predominantly cystic masses also tend to have indolent courses clinically and can therefore be good candidates for surveillance.[125,126] For active surveillance patients, guidelines recommend regular imaging (usually every 3-6 months) and treatment is recommended if the growth rate exceeds 5 mm per year, if clinical stage migration is noted, if aggressive pathology is uncovered by a biopsy, or if the patient elects to pursue active treatment.[127]

The role of adjuvant therapy after nephrectomy performed in patients with localized disease continues to evolve. The S-TRAC trial evaluated the role of the adjuvant tyrosine kinase inhibitor sunitinib for patients at high risk of recurrence. This trial demonstrated improvement in disease-free survival, but this did not translate into improved overall survival.[128,129] Although this led to the approval of sunitinib in an adjuvant setting, the lack of proven survival benefit and side effect profile have largely limited its widespread use. More recently, adjuvant pembrolizumab was approved based on the improvement in disease-free survival seen in the KEYNOTE-564 trial, but further follow-up is needed to elucidate whether these benefits will ultimately translate to improvements in overall survival.[130,131]

The role and timing of cytoreductive nephrectomy, metastasectomy, and metastasis-directed radiation therapy is evolving in the era of immune checkpoint inhibitors. Patient selection is paramount when offering cytoreductive nephrectomy for metastatic RCC and must be counterbalanced by the use of systemic therapies.[132, 133] Surgical candidates with otherwise oligometastatic disease likely benefit from multimodal approaches, including systemic therapy, nephrectomy, and locoregional control of metastatic sites either surgically or via stereotactic radiation. Nephrectomy may also be pursued for palliative indications, most commonly refractory hematuria or intractable pain.[134]

Prognosis

Overall, the 5-year survival of localized kidney cancers is 93%. This decreases to 70% for regional disease, 50% for patients with IVC tumor thrombus, and 13% for distant disease.[68] These numbers are likely to improve as treatment paradigms for metastatic disease continue to evolve.

Testis Cancer

Histopathology

Ninety-five percent of testicular cancers are germ cell tumors (GCT), while the remainder are sex cord stromal tumors (Leydig cell and Sertoli cell tumors).[135] Germ cell neoplasia in situ (GCNIS), the precursor lesion of GCTs, first arises from transformed primordial germ cells and eventually most will become GCTs.[136] GCTs are further divided into seminoma and non-seminoma germ cell tumors (NSGCT). The NSGCT subtypes include embryonal carcinoma, yolk sac, choriocarcinoma, and teratoma. Most NSCGTs are mixed, containing at least two histologic subtypes, including seminoma.[137] The presence of any NSGCT histologic subtype will characterize the tumor as an NSGCT. Pure seminomas tend to present at earlier stages, in older men, and tend to grow at a slower rate than NSGCTs.[135]

Risk Factors

One of the most well-established risk factors for developing testicular cancer is a history of cryptorchidism, undescended testis. Cryptorchidism increases the testicular cancer risk by 4- to 6-fold, but this risk decreases to a 2- to 3-fold risk if an orchiopexy is performed before puberty.[138-140] Studies have even suggested an increased risk for testicular cancer in the contralateral testis as well.[141] Other risk factors include a personal history of testicular cancer. In fact, 2% of patients will ultimately have a tumor in the contralateral testicle, and the median time to developing the second tumor is 6 years, so these patients need to be surveilled long term.[142,143] A positive family history and disorders of sex differentiation are other risk factors.[144]

Clinical Presentation and Diagnosis

Testicular cancer is overall a rare cancer, but in men aged 20 to 40 years it is the most common solid malignancy.[145] In young men presenting with a retroperitoneal mass or metastatic disease of unknown origin, testicular cancer must be considered on the differential. Most patients with testis cancer present with a painless testicular mass and the first diagnostic test ordered is the scrotal ultrasound. Scrotal ultrasound is highly sensitive for the detection of solid testicular masses.[146] Heterogeneous lesions are more likely to be NSGCTs while seminomas tend to appear more homogeneous on ultrasound.[147] If a testicular mass is identified on ultrasound, the tumor markers alpha-fetoprotein (AFP), human chorionic gonadotropin (HCG, specifically the beta subunit), and lactate dehydrogenase (LDH) should be obtained as these can inform histology, staging, treatment selection, prognostication, surveillance, and response to therapy. Notably, pure seminomas never secrete AFP, but 15% can exhibit elevated HCG.[148] Yolk sac tumors and choriocarcinomas have a propensity to secrete AFP and HCG, respectively. It is important to note, however, that these tumor markers suffer from limited sensitivity and may even be elevated in other malignancies or medical conditions. After the diagnosis of testicular cancer is confirmed, staging evaluation with abdominopelvic and chest imaging is recommended.[149] Brain MRI should be considered if tumors markers are very elevated (AFP >10,000 ng/mL and HCG >5000 IU/L), if the primary tumor has choriocarcinoma, or if there is a high volume of metastatic disease.[150]

Staging

Testicular cancers follow predictable patterns of spread to regional lymph nodes in the retroperitoneum based on the lymphatic drainage of the testicle. Right sided tumors first spread to the inter-aortocaval nodes followed by the paracaval and para-aortic nodes. Left sided tumors first spread to the para-aortic lymph nodes but, because lymphatic drainage in the retroperitoneum is from right to left, it is uncommon for left sided tumors to spread to the right side of the retroperitoneum. Staging is based on the degree of invasiveness of the testicular tumor (pT stage), retroperitoneal disease burden (N stage), and distant disease (M stage) (Table 4). Unique to testis cancer staging, an additional 'S' stage is assigned based on post-orchiectomy nadir serum tumor markers.[19] Elevated nadir tumor markers post-orchiectomy are assigned to stages S1 through S3 based on the degree of elevation and reflect the presence of remaining metastatic GCT. Aside from the AJCC TNMS staging classification, GCT patients are also assigned to an AJCC prognostic stage group (Table 5). Patients with advanced disease (stage IIC or III) are also assigned an International Germ Cell Cancer Collaborative Group (IGCCCG) risk classification based on tumor markers and sites of metastasis (Table 6).[151]

Table 4: Testis cancer staging. Adapted from the American Joint Committee on Cancer (AJCC) TNM- Staging System for Testis Cancer 8th ed. 2017.[19]

T stage	Primary Tumor (pathologic staging)
Tx	Cannot assess the primary tumor
T0	There is no evidence of a primary tumor
Tis	Germ cell neoplasia in situ
T1	The tumor invades into the lamina propria
T2	The tumor is limited to the testis (rete testis invasion included) there is no lymphovascular invasion
T1a	Tumor <3 cm
T1b	Tumor ≥3 cm
T2	The tumor is limited to the testis (rete testis invasion included) and there is lymphovascular invasion OR the tumor invades the hilar soft tissue, epididymis, or the penetrating visceral mesothelial layer that covers the external surface of the tunica albuginea +/- lymphovascular invasion
T3	The tumor directly invades the spermatic cord soft tissue +/- lymphovascular invasion
T4	Tumor invades scrotum +/- lymphovascular invasion
N	**Regional Lymph Nodes (pathologic staging)**
Nx	Cannot assess the lymph nodes
N0	There is no metastasis to the regional lymph node
N1	Metastasis and a lymph node mass of ≤2 cm in greatest dimension and ≤5 positive nodes none of which are >2 cm in greatest dimension
N2	Metastasis with lymph node mass of >2 cm but <5 cm in greatest dimension; or >5 positive nodes none of which are >5 cm; or there is evidence of the tumor with extranodal extension
N3	Metastasis and a lymph node mass >5 cm in greatest dimension
M	**Distant Metastasis**
M0	There is no distant metastasis
M1	There is distant metastasis
M1a	Metastasis is non-retroperitoneal nodal or pulmonary
M1b	Metastasis is non-pulmonary visceral
S	**Serum Markers**
Sx	Not available or did not perform a marker study
S0	The marker study results were within normal limits
S1	LDH <1.5 times the upper limit of normal and HCG <5,000 mIU/mL and AFP <1,000 ng/mL
S2	LDH 1.5-10 times the upper limit of normal or HCG 5,000-50,000 mIU/mL and AFP 1,000-10,000 ng/mL
S3	LDH >10 times the upper limit of normal or HCG >50,000 mIU/mL and AFP >10,000 ng/mL

Legend: LDH: lactate dehydrogenase; AFP: alpha-fetoprotein; HCG: human chorionic gonadotropin

Table 5: AJCC Prognostic Stage Groups. Adapted from the American Joint Committee on Cancer (AJCC) TNMS Staging System for Testis Cancer 8th ed. 2017.[19]

Tumor	Node	Metastasis	Stage	
Stage 0	pTis	Node 0	Metastasis 0	Stage 0
Stage I	pT1-T4	Node 0	Metastasis 0	Stage x
Stage IA	pT1	Node 0	Metastasis 0	Stage 0
Stage IB	pT2	Node 0	Metastasis 0	Stage 0
	pT3	Node 0	Metastasis 0	Stage 0
	pT4	Node 0	Metastasis 0	Stage 0
Stage IS	Any pT/Tx	Node 0	Metastasis 0	Stage 1-3
Stage II	Any pT/Tx	Node 1-3	Metastasis 0	Stage x
Stage IIA	Any pT/Tx	Node 1	Metastasis 0	Stage 0
	Any pT/Tx	Node 1	Metastasis 0	Stage 1
Stage IIB	Any pT/Tx	Node 2	Metastasis 0	Stage 0
	Any pT/Tx	Node 2	Metastasis 0	Stage 1
Stage IIC	Any pT/Tx	Node 3	Metastasis 0	Stage 0
	Any pT/Tx	Node 3	Metastasis 0	Stage 1
Stage III	Any pT/Tx	Any Node	Metastasis 1	Stage x
Stage IIIA	Any pT/Tx	Any Node	Metastasis 1a	Stage 0
	Any pT/Tx	Any N Node	Metastasis 1a	Stage 1
Stage IIIB	Any pT/Tx	Node 1-3	Metastasis 0	Stage 2
	Any pT/Tx	Any Node	Metastasis 1a	Stage 2
Stage IIIC	Any pT/Tx	Node 1-3	Metastasis 0	Stage 3
	Any pT/Tx	Any Node	Metastasis 1a	Stage 3
	Any pT/Tx	Any Node 0	Metastasis 1b	Any Stage

Table 6: International Germ Cell Cancer Collaborative Group (IGCCCG) risk classification. Adapted from the International Germ Cell Cancer Collaborative Group consensus classification.[151]

Risk Status	Non-seminoma	Seminoma
Good Risk	There is a testicular or retroperitoneal primary tumor, metastasis is not non-pulmonary visceral, and markers post-orchiectomy are as follows: AFP <1,000 ng/mL HCG <5,000 IU/L LDH <1.5 times the upper limit of normal	The tumor is at any primary site, metastasis is not non-pulmonary visceral, and markers are as follows: AFP is normal HCG is any value LDH is any value
Intermediate Risk	There is a testicular or retroperitoneal primary tumor, metastasis is not non-pulmonary visceral, and markers post-orchiectomy are as follows: AFP 1,000 – 10,000 ng/mL HCG 5,000 – 50,000 IU/L LDH 1.5 – 10 times the upper limit of normal	The tumor is at any primary site, metastasis is non-pulmonary visceral, and markers are as follows: AFP is normal HCG is any value LDH is any value
Poor Risk	There is a mediastinal primary tumor, a metastasis is non-pulmonary visceral, or markers post-orchiectomy are as follows: AFP >10,000 ng/mL HCG >50,000 IU/L LDH >10 x upper limit of normal	No patients classified as poor risk
Legend: LDH: lactate dehydrogenase; AFP: alpha-fetoprotein; HCG: human chorionic gonadotropin		

Treatment

The vast majority of patients newly diagnosed with testicular cancer first undergo a radical orchiectomy. Most men with localized testis cancer (clinical stage I) are cured by orchiectomy alone.[152] A small fraction presenting with widely metastatic disease may benefit from starting chemotherapy urgently, even prior to orchiectomy. Radical orchiectomy is performed via an inguinal approach to avoid altering lymphatic drainage patterns via scrotal skin disruption. High ligation of the spermatic cord at the internal inguinal ring is performed for easy removal of the spermatic cord stump at the time of retroperitoneal lymph node dissection if indicated. Partial orchiectomy with intraoperative frozen sections may be considered in selected patients with solitary testicles, bilateral masses or small (<2 cm) benign appearing masses on imaging.[153-155] Subsequent management is then based on the TNM-S stage.

For patients with stage I pure seminoma, surveillance with regular cross-sectional imaging of the abdomen and pelvis is favored, as more than 80% of these patients are cured with orchiectomy alone.[156,157] Adjuvant options for patients who do not wish to proceed with surveillance include 1 cycle of carboplatin or radiotherapy to the retroperitoneum, both reducing relapse rates to <5%.[158-160] Similarly, surveillance is favored for most patients with stage IA NSGCT,[161-163] as the relapse rate following orchiectomy is around 10 to 20%.[164,165] However, patients with stage IB NSGCT, particularly those with lymphovascular invasion or embryonal carcinoma histologic predominance, tend to have higher relapse rates and often benefit from adjuvant treatment.[166] Adjuvant options for patients with stage I NSGCT include retroperitoneal lymph node dissection (RPLND) or 1-2 cycles of bleomycin, etoposide and cisplatin (BEPx1-2), both reducing relapse rates.[164,167-171] Chemotherapy following RPLND may be pursued depending on the pathologic nodal (pN) stage, usually with 2-3 cycles of BEP.[172-174] It is important to note that relapses on surveillance are still highly treatable for both pure seminomas and NSGCTs. Ultimately, the management of stage I GCTs is based on shared decision making between the patient and clinician.[149]

For patients with stage II pure seminoma, induction chemotherapy (BEPx3 versus EPx4) is often favored; however, if the retroperitoneal adenopathy is not bulky (<3 cm) and the patient wishes to avoid chemotherapy, radiation is also an accepted alternative, though less often pursued.[175-179] For patients with stage IIA NSGCT, options include RPLND or induction chemotherapy.[180,181] RPLND is an attractive option in this setting, especially in the presence of a single retroperitoneal mass, as many patients will be cured with surgery alone and avoid the need for chemotherapy.[167,182] Those who are found to harbor pN2 or pN3 disease at RPLND, however, should be recommended to receive chemotherapy.[172-174,180] Induction chemotherapy is generally recommended for all stage IIC-III pure seminoma, stage IIB-III NSGCT, and all patients with elevated and rising post-orchiectomy markers.[150]

The goal of a bilateral full-template RPLND is to remove all lymph nodes bounded by the renal hilum and crus of the diaphragm superiorly, ureters laterally, and common iliac arteries inferiorly at the level where they are traversed by the ureters. Bilateral template RPLND is recommended in patients with any evidence of nodal disease on imaging and in the post-chemotherapy setting; however, for clinical stage I patients, various modified templates have been proposed. Historically, the bilateral template has been associated with the lowest recurrence rates.[183,184] The most common long-term complication after RPLND is retrograde ejaculation due to injury to the postganglionic fibers exiting the sympathetic trunks; however, nerve sparing techniques may preserve antegrade ejaculation in 90% of cases even with a full bilateral template dissection, and should always be performed when feasible, as long as it does not affect oncologic outcomes.[185-187] The ipsilateral gonadal vessels and vas deferens should also be removed, down to the level of the internal inguinal ring. Traditionally, RPLNDs are performed via an open midline laparotomy incision (Figure 3). The role of minimally invasive RPLND has been explored but remains controversial at this time. Early studies suggest that it could be a safe alternative when performed by experienced surgeons, but long-term oncologic data are currently lacking.[188,189]

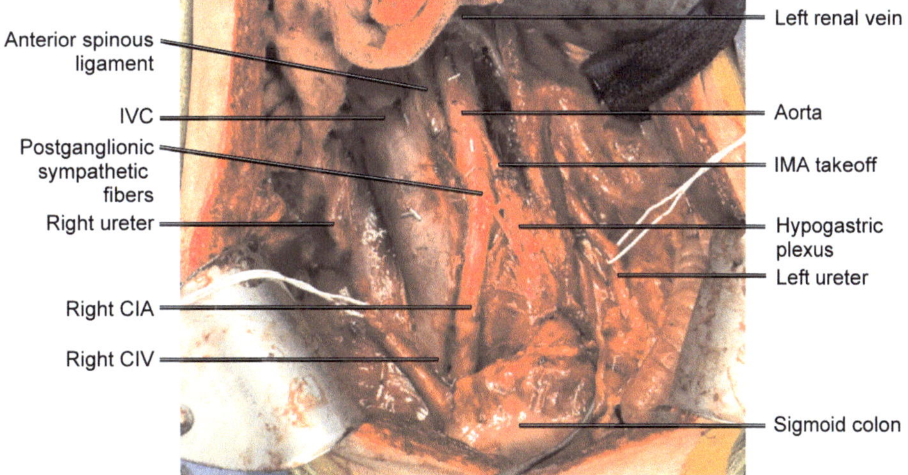

Figure 3: Nerve sparing retroperitoneal lymph node dissection. IVC: inferior vena cava; IMA: inferior mesenteric artery; CIA: common iliac artery; CIV: common iliac vein.

Following induction chemotherapy for advanced seminoma, up to 80% of patients may have persistent tumors on imaging, of which 10% will have viable tumor.[190] FDG PET imaging can help identify viable tumor in post-chemotherapy masses greater than 3 cm for patients with seminoma.[190,191] If PET positive, surgical resection of the mass should be considered. Masses less than 3 cm can be monitored with imaging. Conversely for NSGCT, surgical resection should be attempted for all post-chemotherapy masses greater than 1 cm. Around 10% will have a viable tumor and 30% a teratoma.[192] In NSGCT, the presence of a teratoma in the primary tumor or within metastases has important management implications. Teratoma can grow slowly and in some cases be indolent, but it can also become locally invasive and grow into adjacent structures, and/or transform into somatic malignancies such as sarcoma or adenocarcinoma.[193] Teratomas are also notoriously resistant to chemotherapy and patients can have negative tumor markers yet growing masses on imaging ('growing teratoma syndrome') requiring surgical resection.[194]

Prognosis

Overall, the 5-year survival rate for men with testicular cancer is excellent, at 95% across all stages. For stage I disease, the survival rate approaches 100% and for stage III disease, the 5-year survival rate is 73%.[145] Close surveillance is necessary as relapses are not uncommon, but they are almost always curable. The risk of relapse follows a conditional probability, with the highest risk within the first 2 years; thereafter, the risk drops considerably. Given that most men are cured and live many years after their treatments, GCT survivors should be monitored for long term survivorship issues such as the development of secondary cancers, cardiovascular toxicities, and mental health issues.[195,196]

REFERENCES

1. Sung H, Ferlay J, Siegel RL, et al. Global Cancer Statistics 2020: GLOBOCAN Estimates of Incidence and Mortality Worldwide for 36 Cancers in 185 Countries. *CA Cancer J Clin.* 2021;71:209-249.
2. Bolla SR, Odeluga N, Jetti R. *Histology, Bladder*: StatPearls Publishing; 2022.
3. de la Calle CM, Washington SL 3rd, Lonergan PE, Meng MV, Porten SP. Bladder cancer in patients younger than 40 years: outcomes from the National Cancer Database. *World J Urol.* 2021;39:1911-1916.
4. Porten SP, Willis D, Kamat AM. Variant histology: role in management and prognosis of nonmuscle invasive bladder cancer. *Curr Opin Urol.* 2014;24:517-523.
5. Sylvester RJ, van der Meijden AP, Oosterlinck W, et al. Predicting recurrence and progression in individual patients with stage Ta T1 bladder cancer using EORTC risk tables: a combined analysis of 2596 patients from seven EORTC trials. *Eur Urol.* 2006;49:466-465; discussion 475-467.
6. Freedman ND, Silverman DT, Hollenbeck AR, Schatzkin A, Abnet CC. Association between smoking and risk of bladder cancer among men and women. *JAMA.* 2011;306:737-745.
7. Cumberbatch MG, Rota M, Catto JW, La Vecchia C. The Role of Tobacco Smoke in Bladder and Kidney Carcinogenesis: A Comparison of Exposures and Meta-analysis of Incidence and Mortality Risks. *Eur Urol.* 2016;70:458-466.
8. Cumberbatch MGK, Jubber I, Black PC, et al. Epidemiology of Bladder Cancer: A Systematic Review and Contemporary Update of Risk Factors in 2018. *Eur Urol.* 2018;74:784-795.
9. Howlader N NA, Krapcho M, Miller D, Bishop K, Kosary CL, Yu M, Ruhl J, Tatalovich Z, Mariotto A, Lewis DR, Chen HS, Feuer EJ, Cronin KA (eds). SEER Cancer Statistics Review, 1975-2014, National Cancer Institute. Bethesda, MD.
10. Williams SB, Huo J, Dafashy TJ, et al. Survival differences among patients with bladder cancer according to sex: Critical evaluation of radical cystectomy use and delay to treatment. *Urol Oncol.* 2017;35:602 e601-602 e609.
11. Weiner AB, Keeter MK, Manjunath A, Meeks JJ. Discrepancies in staging, treatment, and delays to treatment may explain disparities in bladder cancer outcomes: An update from the National Cancer Data Base (2004-2013). *Urol Oncol.* 2018;36:237 e239-237 e217.
12. Lenis AT, Lec PM, Chamie K, Mshs MD. Bladder Cancer: A Review. *JAMA.* 2020;324:1980-1991.
13. Barocas DA, Boorjian SA, Alvarez RD, et al. Microhematuria: AUA/SUFU Guideline. *J Urol.* 2020;204:778-786.
14. Palou J, Rodriguez-Rubio F, Huguet J, et al. Multivariate analysis of clinical parameters of synchronous primary superficial bladder cancer and upper urinary tract tumor. *J Urol.* 2005;174:859-861; discussion 861.
15. Hara T, Takahashi M, Gondo T, et al. Risk of concomitant carcinoma in situ determining biopsy candidates among primary non-muscle-invasive bladder cancer patients: retrospective analysis of 173 Japanese cases. *Int J Urol.* 2009;16:293-298.
16. Daneshmand S, Schuckman AK, Bochner BH, et al. Hexaminolevulinate blue-light cystoscopy in non-muscle-invasive bladder cancer: review of the clinical

evidence and consensus statement on appropriate use in the USA. *Nat Rev Urol.* 2014;11:589-596.

17. Yuan H, Qiu J, Liu L, et al. Therapeutic outcome of fluorescence cystoscopy guided transurethral resection in patients with non-muscle invasive bladder cancer: a meta-analysis of randomized controlled trials. *PLoS One.* 2013;8:e74142.
18. Xiong Y, Li J, Ma S, et al. A meta-analysis of narrow band imaging for the diagnosis and therapeutic outcome of non-muscle invasive bladder cancer. *PLoS One.* 2017;12:e0170819.
19. Amin MB, Greene FL, Edge SB, et al. The Eighth Edition AJCC Cancer Staging Manual: Continuing to build a bridge from a population-based to a more "personalized" approach to cancer staging. *CA Cancer J Clin.* 2017;67:93-99.
20. Pasin E, Josephson DY, Mitra AP, Cote RJ, Stein JP. Superficial bladder cancer: an update on etiology, molecular development, classification, and natural history. *Rev Urol.* 2008;10:31-43.
21. Chang SS, Boorjian SA, Chou R, et al. Diagnosis and Treatment of Non-Muscle Invasive Bladder Cancer: AUA/SUO Guideline. *J Urol.* 2016;196:1021-1029.
22. Herr HW. Role of Repeat Resection in Non-Muscle-Invasive Bladder Cancer. *J Natl Compr Canc Netw.* 2015;13:1041-1046.
23. Abern MR, Owusu RA, Anderson MR, Rampersaud EN, Inman BA. Perioperative intravesical chemotherapy in non-muscle-invasive bladder cancer: a systematic review and meta-analysis. *J Natl Compr Canc Netw.* 2013;11:477-484.
24. Messing EM, Tangen CM, Lerner SP, et al. Effect of Intravesical Instillation of Gemcitabine vs Saline Immediately Following Resection of Suspected Low-Grade Non-Muscle-Invasive Bladder Cancer on Tumor Recurrence: SWOG S0337 Randomized Clinical Trial. *JAMA.* 2018;319:1880-1888.
25. Han RF, Pan JG. Can intravesical bacillus Calmette-Guerin reduce recurrence in patients with superficial bladder cancer? A meta-analysis of randomized trials. *Urology.* 2006;67:1216-1223.
26. Pettenati C, Ingersoll MA. Mechanisms of BCG immunotherapy and its outlook for bladder cancer. *Nat Rev Urol.* 2018;15:615-625.
27. Oddens J, Brausi M, Sylvester R, et al. Final results of an EORTC-GU cancers group randomized study of maintenance bacillus Calmette-Guerin in intermediate- and high-risk Ta, T1 papillary carcinoma of the urinary bladder: one-third dose versus full dose and 1 year versus 3 years of maintenance. *Eur Urol.* 2013;63:462-472.
28. Lamm DL, Blumenstein BA, Crissman JD, et al. Maintenance bacillus Calmette-Guerin immunotherapy for recurrent TA, T1 and carcinoma in situ transitional cell carcinoma of the bladder: a randomized Southwest Oncology Group Study. *J Urol.* 2000;163:1124-1129.
29. Chou R, Buckley D, Fu R, et al. *Emerging Approaches to Diagnosis and Treatment of Non-Muscle-Invasive Bladder Cancer.* Rockville (MD)2015.
30. Bui TT, Schellhammer PF. Additional bacillus Calmette-Guerin therapy for recurrent transitional cell carcinoma after an initial complete response. *Urology.* 1997;49:687-690; discussion 690-681.
31. Schrier BP, Hollander MP, van Rhijn BW, Kiemeney LA, Witjes JA. Prognosis of muscle-invasive bladder cancer: difference between primary and progressive tumours and implications for therapy. *Eur Urol.* 2004;45:292-296.
32. van den Bosch S, Alfred Witjes J. Long-term cancer-specific survival in patients with high-risk, non-muscle-invasive bladder cancer and tumour progression: a systematic review. *Eur Urol.* 2011;60:493-500.
33. Raj GV, Herr H, Serio AM, et al. Treatment paradigm shift may improve survival of patients with high risk superficial bladder cancer. *J Urol.* 2007;177:1283-1286; discussion 1286.
34. Dinney CP, Greenberg RE, Steinberg GD. Intravesical valrubicin in patients with bladder carcinoma in situ and contraindication to or failure after bacillus Calmette-Guerin. *Urol Oncol.* 2013;31:1635-1642.
35. Addeo R, Caraglia M, Bellini S, et al. Randomized phase III trial on gemcitabine versus mytomicin in recurrent superficial bladder cancer: evaluation of efficacy and tolerance. *J Clin Oncol.* 2010;28:543-548.
36. McKiernan JM, Masson P, Murphy AM, et al. Phase I trial of intravesical docetaxel in the management of superficial bladder cancer refractory to standard intravesical therapy. *J Clin Oncol.* 2006;24:3075-3080.
37. Steinberg RL, Thomas LJ, Brooks N, et al. Multi-Institution Evaluation of Sequential Gemcitabine and Docetaxel as Rescue Therapy for Nonmuscle Invasive Bladder Cancer. *J Urol.* 2020;203:902-909.
38. Balar AV, Kamat AM, Kulkarni GS, et al. Pembrolizumab monotherapy for the treatment of high-risk non-muscle-invasive bladder cancer unresponsive to BCG (KEYNOTE-057): an open-label, single-arm, multicentre, phase 2 study. *Lancet Oncol.* 2021;22:919-930.
39. Kamat AM, Colombel M, Sundi D, et al. BCG-unresponsive non-muscle-invasive bladder cancer: recommendations from the IBCG. *Nat Rev Urol.* 2017;14:244-255.

40. Brausi M, Oddens J, Sylvester R, et al. Side effects of Bacillus Calmette-Guerin (BCG) in the treatment of intermediate- and high-risk Ta, T1 papillary carcinoma of the bladder: results of the EORTC genito-urinary cancers group randomised phase 3 study comparing one-third dose with full dose and 1 year with 3 years of maintenance BCG. *Eur Urol.* 2014;65:69-76.
41. Prout GR, Marshall VF. The prognosis with untreated bladder tumors. *Cancer.* 1956;9:551-558.
42. Grossman HB, Natale RB, Tangen CM, et al. Neoadjuvant chemotherapy plus cystectomy compared with cystectomy alone for locally advanced bladder cancer. *N Engl J Med.* 2003;349:859-866.
43. Advanced Bladder Cancer Meta-analysis C. Neoadjuvant chemotherapy in invasive bladder cancer: update of a systematic review and meta-analysis of individual patient data advanced bladder cancer (ABC) meta-analysis collaboration. *Eur Urol.* 2005;48:202-205; discussion 205-206.
44. Sternberg CN, Skoneczna I, Kerst JM, et al. Immediate versus deferred chemotherapy after radical cystectomy in patients with pT3-pT4 or N+ M0 urothelial carcinoma of the bladder (EORTC 30994): an intergroup, open-label, randomised phase 3 trial. *Lancet Oncol.* 2015;16:76-86.
45. Bajorin DF, Witjes JA, Gschwend JE, et al. Adjuvant Nivolumab versus Placebo in Muscle-Invasive Urothelial Carcinoma. *N Engl J Med.* 2021;384:2102-2114.
46. Kaufman DS, Winter KA, Shipley WU, et al. The initial results in muscle-invading bladder cancer of RTOG 95-06: phase I/II trial of transurethral surgery plus radiation therapy with concurrent cisplatin and 5-fluorouracil followed by selective bladder preservation or cystectomy depending on the initial response. *Oncologist.* 2000;5:471-476.
47. Kaufman DS, Winter KA, Shipley WU, et al. Phase I-II RTOG study (99-06) of patients with muscle-invasive bladder cancer undergoing transurethral surgery, paclitaxel, cisplatin, and twice-daily radiotherapy followed by selective bladder preservation or radical cystectomy and adjuvant chemotherapy. *Urology.* 2009;73:833-837.
48. Chang SS, Bochner BH, Chou R, et al. Treatment of Non-Metastatic Muscle-Invasive Bladder Cancer: AUA/ASCO/ASTRO/SUO Guideline. *J Urol.* 2017;198:552-559.
49. Ploussard G, Daneshmand S, Efstathiou JA, et al. Critical analysis of bladder sparing with trimodal therapy in muscle-invasive bladder cancer: a systematic review. *Eur Urol.* 2014;66:120-137.
50. Mak RH, Hunt D, Shipley WU, et al. Long-term outcomes in patients with muscle-invasive bladder cancer after selective bladder-preserving combined-modality therapy: a pooled analysis of Radiation Therapy Oncology Group protocols 8802, 8903, 9506, 9706, 9906, and 0233. *J Clin Oncol.* 2014;32:3801-3809.
51. Pieretti A, Krasnow R, Drumm M, et al. Complications and Outcomes of Salvage Cystectomy after Trimodality Therapy. *J Urol.* 2021;206:29-36.
52. Bree KK, Hensley PJ, Westerman ME, et al. Contemporary Rates of Gynecologic Organ Involvement in Females with Muscle Invasive Bladder Cancer: A Retrospective Review of Women Undergoing Radical Cystectomy following Neoadjuvant Chemotherapy. *J Urol.* 2021;206:577-585.
53. Patel SH, Wang S, Metcalf MR, et al. Safety and Efficacy of Reproductive Organ-Sparing Radical Cystectomy in Women With Variant Histology and Advanced Stage. *Clin Genitourin Cancer.* 2022;20:60-68.
54. Tilki D, Brausi M, Colombo R, et al. Lymphadenectomy for bladder cancer at the time of radical cystectomy. *Eur Urol.* 2013;64:266-276.
55. Hwang EC, Sathianathen NJ, Imamura M, Kuntz GM, Risk MC, Dahm P. Extended versus standard lymph node dissection for urothelial carcinoma of the bladder in patients undergoing radical cystectomy. *Cochrane Database Syst Rev.* 2019;5:CD013336.
56. Bi L, Huang H, Fan X, et al. Extended vs non-extended pelvic lymph node dissection and their influence on recurrence-free survival in patients undergoing radical cystectomy for bladder cancer: a systematic review and meta-analysis of comparative studies. *BJU Int.* 2014;113:E39-48.
57. Parekh DJ, Reis IM, Castle EP, et al. Robot-assisted radical cystectomy versus open radical cystectomy in patients with bladder cancer (RAZOR): an open-label, randomised, phase 3, non-inferiority trial. *Lancet.* 2018;391:2525-2536.
58. Yuh B, Wilson T, Bochner B, et al. Systematic review and cumulative analysis of oncologic and functional outcomes after robot-assisted radical cystectomy. *Eur Urol.* 2015;67:402-422.
59. Venkatramani V, Reis IM, Gonzalgo ML, et al. Comparison of Robot-Assisted and Open Radical Cystectomy in Recovery of Patient-Reported and Performance-Related Measures of Independence: A Secondary Analysis of a Randomized Clinical Trial. *JAMA Netw Open.* 2022;5:e2148329.
60. Bochner BH, Dalbagni G, Sjoberg DD, et al. Comparing Open Radical Cystectomy and Robot-assisted

Laparoscopic Radical Cystectomy: A Randomized Clinical Trial. *Eur Urol.* 2015;67:1042-1050.

61. Lee RK, Abol-Enein H, Artibani W, et al. Urinary diversion after radical cystectomy for bladder cancer: options, patient selection, and outcomes. *BJU Int.* 2014;113:11-23.
62. Nieuwenhuijzen JA, de Vries RR, Bex A, et al. Urinary diversions after cystectomy: the association of clinical factors, complications and functional results of four different diversions. *Eur Urol.* 2008;53:834-842; discussion 842-834.
63. Stimson CJ, Chang SS, Barocas DA, et al. Early and late perioperative outcomes following radical cystectomy: 90-day readmissions, morbidity and mortality in a contemporary series. *J Urol.* 2010;184:1296-1300.
64. Froehner M, Brausi MA, Herr HW, Muto G, Studer UE. Complications following radical cystectomy for bladder cancer in the elderly. *Eur Urol.* 2009;56:443-454.
65. Cerantola Y, Valerio M, Persson B, et al. Guidelines for perioperative care after radical cystectomy for bladder cancer: Enhanced Recovery After Surgery (ERAS((R))) society recommendations. *Clin Nutr.* 2013;32:879-887.
66. Society AC. Cancer Facts & Figures 2021. www.cancer.org: Atlanta, Ga: American Cancer Society; 2021.; 2021.
67. Brausi M, Collette L, Kurth K, et al. Variability in the recurrence rate at first follow-up cystoscopy after TUR in stage Ta T1 transitional cell carcinoma of the bladder: a combined analysis of seven EORTC studies. *Eur Urol.* 2002;41:523-531.
68. Siegel RL, Miller KD, Fuchs HE, Jemal A. Cancer Statistics, 2021. *CA Cancer J Clin.* 2021;71:7-33.
69. Lonati C, Necchi A, Gomez Rivas J, et al. Upper Tract Urothelial Carcinoma in the Lynch Syndrome Tumour Spectrum: A Comprehensive Overview from the European Association of Urology - Young Academic Urologists and the Global Society of Rare Genitourinary Tumors. *Eur Urol Oncol.* 2021.
70. Carlo MI, Ravichandran V, Srinavasan P, et al. Cancer Susceptibility Mutations in Patients With Urothelial Malignancies. *J Clin Oncol.* 2020;38:406-414.
71. Wu F, Wang T. Risk assessment of upper tract urothelial carcinoma related to aristolochic acid. *Cancer Epidemiol Biomarkers Prev.* 2013;22:812-820.
72. Veccia A, Antonelli A, Francavilla S, et al. Robotic versus other nephroureterectomy techniques: a systematic review and meta-analysis of over 87,000 cases. *World J Urol.* 2020;38:845-852.
73. Margulis V, Shariat SF, Matin SF, et al. Outcomes of radical nephroureterectomy: a series from the Upper Tract Urothelial Carcinoma Collaboration. *Cancer.* 2009;115:1224-1233.
74. Flaig TW. NCCN Clinical Practice Guidelines in Oncology - Bladder Cancer. Version 1.2022 - February 11, 2022 ed2022.
75. Cutress ML, Stewart GD, Zakikhani P, Phipps S, Thomas BG, Tolley DA. Ureteroscopic and percutaneous management of upper tract urothelial carcinoma (UTUC): systematic review. *BJU Int.* 2012;110:614-628.
76. Zareba P, Rosenzweig B, Winer AG, Coleman JA. Association between lymph node yield and survival among patients undergoing radical nephroureterectomy for urothelial carcinoma of the upper tract. *Cancer.* 2017;123:1741-1750.
77. Roscigno M, Shariat SF, Margulis V, et al. The extent of lymphadenectomy seems to be associated with better survival in patients with nonmetastatic upper-tract urothelial carcinoma: how many lymph nodes should be removed? *Eur Urol.* 2009;56:512-518.
78. Bagrodia A, Kuehhas FE, Gayed BA, et al. Comparative analysis of oncologic outcomes of partial ureterectomy vs radical nephroureterectomy in upper tract urothelial carcinoma. *Urology.* 2013;81:972-977.
79. Yoo SH, Jeong CW, Kwak C, Kim HH, Choo MS, Ku JH. Intravesical Chemotherapy after Radical Nephroureterectomy for Primary Upper Tract Urothelial Carcinoma: A Systematic Review and Network Meta-Analysis. *J Clin Med.* 2019;8.
80. Gadzinski AJ, Roberts WW, Faerber GJ, Wolf JS Jr. Long-term outcomes of immediate versus delayed nephroureterectomy for upper tract urothelial carcinoma. *J Endourol.* 2012;26:566-573.
81. Bachir BG, Kassouf W. Efficacy of instillations with chemotherapy or immunotherapy following endoscopic resection for upper tract urothelial carcinoma. *Expert Rev Anticancer Ther.* 2012;12:63-75.
82. Giannarini G, Kessler TM, Birkhauser FD, Thalmann GN, Studer UE. Antegrade perfusion with bacillus Calmette-Guerin in patients with non-muscle-invasive urothelial carcinoma of the upper urinary tract: who may benefit? *Eur Urol.* 2011;60:955-960.
83. Metcalfe M, Wagenheim G, Xiao L, et al. Induction and Maintenance Adjuvant Mitomycin C Topical Therapy for Upper Tract Urothelial Carcinoma: Tolerability and Intermediate Term Outcomes. *J Endourol.* 2017;31:946-953.

84. Kleinmann N, Matin SF, Pierorazio PM, et al. Primary chemoablation of low-grade upper tract urothelial carcinoma using UGN-101, a mitomycin-containing reverse thermal gel (OLYMPUS): an open-label, single-arm, phase 3 trial. *Lancet Oncol.* 2020;21:776-785.
85. Leow JJ, Chong YL, Chang SL, Valderrama BP, Powles T, Bellmunt J. Neoadjuvant and Adjuvant Chemotherapy for Upper Tract Urothelial Carcinoma: A 2020 Systematic Review and Meta-analysis, and Future Perspectives on Systemic Therapy. *Eur Urol.* 2021;79:635-654.
86. Margulis V, Puligandla M, Trabulsi EJ, et al. Phase II Trial of Neoadjuvant Systemic Chemotherapy Followed by Extirpative Surgery in Patients with High Grade Upper Tract Urothelial Carcinoma. *J Urol.* 2020;203:690-698.
87. Birtle A, Johnson M, Chester J, et al. Adjuvant chemotherapy in upper tract urothelial carcinoma (the POUT trial): a phase 3, open-label, randomised controlled trial. *Lancet.* 2020;395:1268-1277.
88. Srigley JR, Delahunt B, Eble JN, et al. The International Society of Urological Pathology (ISUP) Vancouver Classification of Renal Neoplasia. *Am J Surg Pathol.* 2013;37:1469-1489.
89. Delahunt B, Cheville JC, Martignoni G, et al. The International Society of Urological Pathology (ISUP) grading system for renal cell carcinoma and other prognostic parameters. *Am J Surg Pathol.* 2013;37:1490-1504.
90. Keegan KA, Schupp CW, Chamie K, Hellenthal NJ, Evans CP, Koppie TM. Histopathology of surgically treated renal cell carcinoma: survival differences by subtype and stage. *J Urol.* 2012;188:391-397.
91. Hunt JD, van der Hel OL, McMillan GP, Boffetta P, Brennan P. Renal cell carcinoma in relation to cigarette smoking: meta-analysis of 24 studies. *Int J Cancer.* 2005;114:101-108.
92. Bjorge T, Tretli S, Engeland A. Relation of height and body mass index to renal cell carcinoma in two million Norwegian men and women. *Am J Epidemiol.* 2004;160:1168-1176.
93. Renehan AG, Tyson M, Egger M, Heller RF, Zwahlen M. Body-mass index and incidence of cancer: a systematic review and meta-analysis of prospective observational studies. *Lancet.* 2008;371:569-578.
94. Weikert S, Boeing H, Pischon T, et al. Blood pressure and risk of renal cell carcinoma in the European prospective investigation into cancer and nutrition. *Am J Epidemiol.* 2008;167:438-446.
95. Stewart JH, Buccianti G, Agodoa L, et al. Cancers of the kidney and urinary tract in patients on dialysis for end-stage renal disease: analysis of data from the United States, Europe, and Australia and New Zealand. *J Am Soc Nephrol.* 2003;14:197-207.
96. Menko FH, Maher ER. Diagnosis and Management of Hereditary Renal Cell Cancer. *Recent Results Cancer Res.* 2016;205:85-104.
97. Carlo MI, Mukherjee S, Mandelker D, et al. Prevalence of Germline Mutations in Cancer Susceptibility Genes in Patients With Advanced Renal Cell Carcinoma. *JAMA Oncol.* 2018;4:1228-1235.
98. Campbell SC, Clark PE, Chang SS, Karam JA, Souter L, Uzzo RG. Renal Mass and Localized Renal Cancer: Evaluation, Management, and Follow-Up: AUA Guideline: Part I. *J Urol.* 2021;206:199-208.
99. Campbell SC, Uzzo RG, Karam JA, Chang SS, Clark PE, Souter L. Renal Mass and Localized Renal Cancer: Evaluation, Management, and Follow-up: AUA Guideline: Part II. *J Urol.* 2021;206:209-218.
100. Schoots IG, Zaccai K, Hunink MG, Verhagen P. Bosniak Classification for Complex Renal Cysts Reevaluated: A Systematic Review. *J Urol.* 2017;198:12-21.
101. Kutikov A, Fossett LK, Ramchandani P, et al. Incidence of benign pathologic findings at partial nephrectomy for solitary renal mass presumed to be renal cell carcinoma on preoperative imaging. *Urology.* 2006;68:737-740.
102. Johnson DC, Vukina J, Smith AB, et al. Preoperatively misclassified, surgically removed benign renal masses: a systematic review of surgical series and United States population level burden estimate. *J Urol.* 2015;193:30-35.
103. Patel HD, Johnson MH, Pierorazio PM, et al. Diagnostic Accuracy and Risks of Biopsy in the Diagnosis of a Renal Mass Suspicious for Localized Renal Cell Carcinoma: Systematic Review of the Literature. *J Urol.* 2016;195:1340-1347.
104. Richard PO, Jewett MA, Bhatt JR, et al. Renal Tumor Biopsy for Small Renal Masses: A Single-center 13-year Experience. *Eur Urol.* 2015;68:1007-1013.
105. Ginzburg S, Uzzo R, Al-Saleem T, et al. Coexisting hybrid malignancy in a solitary sporadic solid benign renal mass: implications for treating patients following renal biopsy. *J Urol.* 2014;191:296-300.
106. Gorin MA, Rowe SP, Baras AS, et al. Prospective Evaluation of (99m)Tc-sestamibi SPECT/CT for the Diagnosis of Renal Oncocytomas and Hybrid Oncocytic/Chromophobe Tumors. *Eur Urol.* 2016;69:413-416.
107. Bekema HJ, MacLennan S, Imamura M, et al. Systematic review of adrenalectomy and lymph node

dissection in locally advanced renal cell carcinoma. *Eur Urol.* 2013;64:799-810.

108. John NT, Blum KA, Hakimi AA. Role of lymph node dissection in renal cell cancer. *Urol Oncol.* 2019;37:187-192.

109. Asimakopoulos AD, Miano R, Annino F, et al. Robotic radical nephrectomy for renal cell carcinoma: a systematic review. *BMC Urol.* 2014;14:75.

110. Kim SP, Thompson RH, Boorjian SA, et al. Comparative effectiveness for survival and renal function of partial and radical nephrectomy for localized renal tumors: a systematic review and meta-analysis. *J Urol.* 2012;188:51-57.

111. Jang HA, Kim JW, Byun SS, et al. Oncologic and Functional Outcomes after Partial Nephrectomy Versus Radical Nephrectomy in T1b Renal Cell Carcinoma: A Multicenter, Matched Case-Control Study in Korean Patients. *Cancer Res Treat.* 2016;48:612-620.

112. Gershman B, Thompson RH, Boorjian SA, et al. Radical Versus Partial Nephrectomy for cT1 Renal Cell Carcinoma. *Eur Urol.* 2018;74:825-832.

113. Lowrance WT, Yee DS, Savage C, et al. Complications after radical and partial nephrectomy as a function of age. *J Urol.* 2010;183:1725-1730.

114. Spana G, Haber GP, Dulabon LM, et al. Complications after robotic partial nephrectomy at centers of excellence: multi-institutional analysis of 450 cases. *J Urol.* 2011;186:417-421.

115. Minervini A, Campi R, Sessa F, et al. Positive surgical margins and local recurrence after simple enucleation and standard partial nephrectomy for malignant renal tumors: systematic review of the literature and meta-analysis of prevalence. *Minerva Urol Nefrol.* 2017;69:523-538.

116. Capitanio U, Rosiello G, Erdem S, et al. Clinical, surgical, pathological and follow-up features of kidney cancer patients with Von Hippel-Lindau syndrome: novel insights from a large consortium. *World J Urol.* 2021;39:2969-2975.

117. Duffey BG, Choyke PL, Glenn G, et al. The relationship between renal tumor size and metastases in patients with von Hippel-Lindau disease. *J Urol.* 2004;172:63-65.

118. Menko FH, Maher ER, Schmidt LS, et al. Hereditary leiomyomatosis and renal cell cancer (HLRCC): renal cancer risk, surveillance and treatment. *Fam Cancer.* 2014;13:637-644.

119. El Dib R, Touma NJ, Kapoor A. Cryoablation vs radiofrequency ablation for the treatment of renal cell carcinoma: a meta-analysis of case series studies. *BJU Int.* 2012;110:510-516.

120. Pierorazio PM, Johnson MH, Patel HD, et al. Management of Renal Masses and Localized Renal Cancer: Systematic Review and Meta-Analysis. *J Urol.* 2016;196:989-999.

121. Salagierski M, Wojciechowska A, Zajac K, et al. The Role of Ablation and Minimally Invasive Techniques in the Management of Small Renal Masses. *Eur Urol Oncol.* 2018;1:395-402.

122. Pierorazio PM, Johnson MH, Ball MW, et al. Five-year analysis of a multi-institutional prospective clinical trial of delayed intervention and surveillance for small renal masses: the DISSRM registry. *Eur Urol.* 2015;68:408-415.

123. Jewett MA, Mattar K, Basiuk J, et al. Active surveillance of small renal masses: progression patterns of early stage kidney cancer. *Eur Urol.* 2011;60:39-44.

124. Mason RJ, Abdolell M, Trottier G, et al. Growth kinetics of renal masses: analysis of a prospective cohort of patients undergoing active surveillance. *Eur Urol.* 2011;59:863-867.

125. Westerman ME, Cheville JC, Lohse CM, et al. Long-Term Outcomes of Patients With Low Grade Cystic Renal Epithelial Neoplasms. *Urology.* 2019;133:145-150.

126. Chandrasekar T, Ahmad AE, Fadaak K, et al. Natural History of Complex Renal Cysts: Clinical Evidence Supporting Active Surveillance. *J Urol.* 2018;199:633-640.

127. Crispen PL, Viterbo R, Boorjian SA, Greenberg RE, Chen DY, Uzzo RG. Natural history, growth kinetics, and outcomes of untreated clinically localized renal tumors under active surveillance. *Cancer.* 2009;115:2844-2852.

128. Ravaud A, Motzer RJ, Pandha HS, et al. Adjuvant Sunitinib in High-Risk Renal-Cell Carcinoma after Nephrectomy. *N Engl J Med.* 2016;375:2246-2254.

129. Motzer RJ, Ravaud A, Patard JJ, et al. Adjuvant Sunitinib for High-risk Renal Cell Carcinoma After Nephrectomy: Subgroup Analyses and Updated Overall Survival Results. *Eur Urol.* 2018;73:62-68.

130. Choueiri TK, Powles T. Adjuvant Pembrolizumab after Nephrectomy in Renal-Cell Carcinoma. Reply. *N Engl J Med.* 2021;385:1920.

131. Laukhtina E, Quhal F, Mori K, et al. Pembrolizumab outperforms tyrosine kinase inhibitors as adjuvant treatment in patients with high-risk renal cell carcinoma after nephrectomy. *Eur Urol Oncol.* 2022.

132. Mejean A, Ravaud A, Thezenas S, et al. Sunitinib Alone or after Nephrectomy in Metastatic Renal-Cell Carcinoma. *N Engl J Med.* 2018;379:417-427.

133. Mejean A, Ravaud A, Thezenas S, et al. Sunitinib Alone or After Nephrectomy for Patients with Metastatic Renal Cell Carcinoma: Is There Still a Role for Cytoreductive Nephrectomy? *Eur Urol.* 2021;80:417-424.
134. Motzer RJ. NCCN Clinical practice guidelines in oncology - Kidney Cancer. Version 4.2022 - December 21, 2021 ed2022.
135. Cheville JC. Classification and pathology of testicular germ cell and sex cord-stromal tumors. *Urol Clin North Am.* 1999;26:595-609.
136. Montironi R. Intratubular germ cell neoplasia of the testis: testicular intraepithelial neoplasia. *Eur Urol.* 2002;41:651-654.
137. Vasdev N, Moon A, Thorpe AC. Classification, epidemiology and therapies for testicular germ cell tumours. *Int J Dev Biol.* 2013;57:133-139.
138. Wood HM, Elder JS. Cryptorchidism and testicular cancer: separating fact from fiction. *J Urol.* 2009;181:452-461.
139. Lip SZ, Murchison LE, Cullis PS, Govan L, Carachi R. A meta-analysis of the risk of boys with isolated cryptorchidism developing testicular cancer in later life. *Arch Dis Child.* 2013;98:20-26.
140. Pettersson A, Richiardi L, Nordenskjold A, Kaijser M, Akre O. Age at surgery for undescended testis and risk of testicular cancer. *N Engl J Med.* 2007;356:1835-1841.
141. Akre O, Pettersson A, Richiardi L. Risk of contralateral testicular cancer among men with unilaterally undescended testis: a meta analysis. *Int J Cancer.* 2009;124:687-689.
142. Fossa SD, Chen J, Schonfeld SJ, et al. Risk of contralateral testicular cancer: a population-based study of 29,515 U.S. men. *J Natl Cancer Inst.* 2005;97:1056-1066.
143. Che M, Tamboli P, Ro JY, et al. Bilateral testicular germ cell tumors: twenty-year experience at M. D. Anderson Cancer Center. *Cancer.* 2002;95:1228-1233.
144. Mai PL, Chen BE, Tucker K, et al. Younger age-at-diagnosis for familial malignant testicular germ cell tumor. *Fam Cancer.* 2009;8:451-456.
145. Bethesda, MD. SEER Cancer Stat Facts: Testicular cancer . National Cancer Institute.
146. Rifkin MD, Kurtz AB, Pasto ME, Goldberg BB. Diagnostic capabilities of high-resolution scrotal ultrasonography: prospective evaluation. *J Ultrasound Med.* 1985;4:13-19.
147. McDonald MW, Reed AB, Tran PT, Evans LA. Testicular tumor ultrasound characteristics and association with histopathology. *Urol Int.* 2012;89:196-202.
148. Gilligan TD, Seidenfeld J, Basch EM, et al. American Society of Clinical Oncology Clinical Practice Guideline on uses of serum tumor markers in adult males with germ cell tumors. *J Clin Oncol.* 2010;28:3388-3404.
149. Stephenson A, Eggener SE, Bass EB, et al. Diagnosis and Treatment of Early Stage Testicular Cancer: AUA Guideline. *J Urol.* 2019;202:272-281.
150. Gilligan T. NCCN Clinical practice guidelines in oncology - Testicular cancer. Version 2.2022 - January 4, 2022 ed2022.
151. International Germ Cell Consensus Classification: a prognostic factor-based staging system for metastatic germ cell cancers. International Germ Cell Cancer Collaborative Group. *J Clin Oncol.* 1997;15:594-603.
152. Pierorazio PM, Cheaib JG, Patel HD, et al. Comparative Effectiveness of Surveillance, Primary Chemotherapy, Radiotherapy and Retroperitoneal Lymph Node Dissection for the Management of Early Stage Testicular Germ Cell Tumors: A Systematic Review. *J Urol.* 2021;205:370-382.
153. Bojanic N, Bumbasirevic U, Bojanic G, Vukovic I, Milojevic B, Pekmezovic T. Testis sparing surgery for treatment of small testicular lesions: Is it feasible even in germ cell tumors? *J Surg Oncol.* 2017;115:287-290.
154. Xiao F, Shi JZ, Liu Y, et al. Radical and testis-sparing surgery for primary testicular tumors: A single-center experience. *Mol Clin Oncol.* 2019;10:343-351.
155. Ory J, Blankstein U, Gonzalez DC, et al. Outcomes of organ-sparing surgery for adult testicular tumors: A systematic review of the literature. *BJUI Compass.* 2021;2:306-321.
156. Groll RJ, Warde P, Jewett MA. A comprehensive systematic review of testicular germ cell tumor surveillance. *Crit Rev Oncol Hematol.* 2007;64:182-197.
157. Tandstad T, Stahl O, Dahl O, et al. Treatment of stage I seminoma, with one course of adjuvant carboplatin or surveillance, risk-adapted recommendations implementing patient autonomy: a report from the Swedish and Norwegian Testicular Cancer Group (SWENOTECA). *Ann Oncol.* 2016;27:1299-1304.
158. Mead GM, Fossa SD, Oliver RT, et al. Randomized trials in 2466 patients with stage I seminoma: patterns of relapse and follow-up. *J Natl Cancer Inst.* 2011;103:241-249.
159. Soper MS, Hastings JR, Cosmatos HA, Slezak JM, Wang R, Lodin K. Observation versus adjuvant radiation or chemotherapy in the management of stage

I seminoma: clinical outcomes and prognostic factors for relapse in a large US cohort. *Am J Clin Oncol.* 2014;37:356-359.

160. Dieckmann KP, Dralle-Filiz I, Matthies C, et al. Testicular seminoma clinical stage 1: treatment outcome on a routine care level. *J Cancer Res Clin Oncol.* 2016;142:1599-1607.

161. Sturgeon JF, Moore MJ, Kakiashvili DM, et al. Non-risk-adapted surveillance in clinical stage I nonseminomatous germ cell tumors: the Princess Margaret Hospital's experience. *Eur Urol.* 2011;59:556-562.

162. Daugaard G, Gundgaard MG, Mortensen MS, et al. Surveillance for stage I nonseminoma testicular cancer: outcomes and long-term follow-up in a population-based cohort. *J Clin Oncol.* 2014;32:3817-3823.

163. Weiner AB, Pearce SM, Eggener SE. Management trends for men with early-stage nonseminomatous germ cell tumors of the testicle: An analysis of the National Cancer Database. *Cancer.* 2017;123:245-252.

164. Tandstad T, Dahl O, Cohn-Cedermark G, et al. Risk-adapted treatment in clinical stage I nonseminomatous germ cell testicular cancer: the SWENOTECA management program. *J Clin Oncol.* 2009;27:2122-2128.

165. Kollmannsberger C, Moore C, Chi KN, et al. Non-risk-adapted surveillance for patients with stage I nonseminomatous testicular germ-cell tumors: diminishing treatment-related morbidity while maintaining efficacy. *Ann Oncol.* 2010;21:1296-1301.

166. Blok JM, Pluim I, Daugaard G, et al. Lymphovascular invasion and presence of embryonal carcinoma as risk factors for occult metastatic disease in clinical stage I nonseminomatous germ cell tumour: a systematic review and meta-analysis. *BJU Int.* 2020;125:355-368.

167. Stephenson AJ, Bosl GJ, Motzer RJ, et al. Retroperitoneal lymph node dissection for nonseminomatous germ cell testicular cancer: impact of patient selection factors on outcome. *J Clin Oncol.* 2005;23:2781-2788.

168. Albers P, Siener R, Krege S, et al. Randomized phase III trial comparing retroperitoneal lymph node dissection with one course of bleomycin and etoposide plus cisplatin chemotherapy in the adjuvant treatment of clinical stage I Nonseminomatous testicular germ cell tumors: AUO trial AH 01/94 by the German Testicular Cancer Study Group. *J Clin Oncol.* 2008;26:2966-2972.

169. Stephenson AJ, Sheinfeld J. Management of patients with low-stage nonseminomatous germ cell testicular cancer. *Curr Treat Options Oncol.* 2005;6:367-377.

170. Al-Tourah AJ, Murray N, Coppin C, Kollmannsberger C, Man A, Chi KN. Minimizing treatment without compromising cure with primary surveillance for clinical stage I embryonal predominant nonseminomatous testicular cancer: a population based analysis from British Columbia. *J Urol.* 2005;174:2209-2213, discussion 2213.

171. Stephenson AJ, Bosl GJ, Bajorin DF, Stasi J, Motzer RJ, Sheinfeld J. Retroperitoneal lymph node dissection in patients with low stage testicular cancer with embryonal carcinoma predominance and/or lymphovascular invasion. *J Urol.* 2005;174:557-560; discussion 560.

172. Behnia M, Foster R, Einhorn LH, Donohue J, Nichols CR. Adjuvant bleomycin, etoposide and cisplatin in pathological stage II non-seminomatous testicular cancer. the Indiana University experience. *Eur J Cancer.* 2000;36:472-475.

173. Kondagunta GV, Sheinfeld J, Mazumdar M, et al. Relapse-free and overall survival in patients with pathologic stage II nonseminomatous germ cell cancer treated with etoposide and cisplatin adjuvant chemotherapy. *J Clin Oncol.* 2004;22:464-467.

174. McHugh DJ, Funt SA, Silber D, et al. Adjuvant Chemotherapy With Etoposide Plus Cisplatin for Patients With Pathologic Stage II Nonseminomatous Germ Cell Tumors. *J Clin Oncol.* 2020;38:1332-1337.

175. von Amsberg G, Hamilton R, Papachristofilou A. Clinical Stage IIA-IIC Seminoma: Radiation Therapy versus Systemic Chemotherapy versus Retroperitoneal Lymph Node Dissection. *Oncol Res Treat.* 2018;41:360-363.

176. Garcia-del-Muro X, Maroto P, Guma J, et al. Chemotherapy as an alternative to radiotherapy in the treatment of stage IIA and IIB testicular seminoma: a Spanish Germ Cell Cancer Group Study. *J Clin Oncol.* 2008;26:5416-5421.

177. Tandstad T, Smaaland R, Solberg A, et al. Management of seminomatous testicular cancer: a binational prospective population-based study from the Swedish norwegian testicular cancer study group. *J Clin Oncol.* 2011;29:719-725.

178. Classen J, Schmidberger H, Meisner C, et al. Radiotherapy for stages IIA/B testicular seminoma: final report of a prospective multicenter clinical trial. *J Clin Oncol.* 2003;21:1101-1106.

179. Detti B, Livi L, Scoccianti S, et al. Management of Stage II testicular seminoma over a period of 40 years. *Urol Oncol.* 2009;27:534-538.

180. Weissbach L, Bussar-Maatz R, Flechtner H, Pichlmeier U, Hartmann M, Keller L. RPLND or primary

chemotherapy in clinical stage IIA/B nonseminomatous germ cell tumors? Results of a prospective multicenter trial including quality of life assessment. *Eur Urol.* 2000;37:582-594.

181. Stephenson AJ, Bosl GJ, Motzer RJ, Bajorin DF, Stasi JP, Sheinfeld J. Nonrandomized comparison of primary chemotherapy and retroperitoneal lymph node dissection for clinical stage IIA and IIB nonseminomatous germ cell testicular cancer. *J Clin Oncol.* 2007;25:5597-5602.
182. Donohue JP, Thornhill JA, Foster RS, Bihrle R, Rowland RG, Einhorn LH. The role of retroperitoneal lymphadenectomy in clinical stage B testis cancer: the Indiana University experience (1965 to 1989). *J Urol.* 1995;153:85-89.
183. Eggener SE, Carver BS, Sharp DS, Motzer RJ, Bosl GJ, Sheinfeld J. Incidence of disease outside modified retroperitoneal lymph node dissection templates in clinical stage I or IIA nonseminomatous germ cell testicular cancer. *J Urol.* 2007;177:937-942; discussion 942-933.
184. Large MC, Sheinfeld J, Eggener SE. Retroperitoneal lymph node dissection: reassessment of modified templates. *BJU Int.* 2009;104:1369-1375.
185. Pettus JA, Carver BS, Masterson T, Stasi J, Sheinfeld J. Preservation of ejaculation in patients undergoing nerve-sparing postchemotherapy retroperitoneal lymph node dissection for metastatic testicular cancer. *Urology.* 2009;73:328-331; discussion 331-322.
186. Nonomura N, Nishimura K, Takaha N, et al. Nerve-sparing retroperitoneal lymph node dissection for advanced testicular cancer after chemotherapy. *Int J Urol.* 2002;9:539-544.
187. Klein EA. Open technique for nerve-sparing retroperitoneal lymphadenectomy. *Urology.* 2000;55:132-135.
188. Abdul-Muhsin H, Rocco N, Navaratnam A, et al. Outcomes of post-chemotherapy robot-assisted retroperitoneal lymph node dissection in testicular cancer: multi-institutional study. *World J Urol.* 2021;39:3833-3838.
189. Taylor J, Becher E, Wysock JS, et al. Primary Robot-assisted Retroperitoneal Lymph Node Dissection for Men with Nonseminomatous Germ Cell Tumor: Experience from a Multi-institutional Cohort. *Eur Urol Focus.* 2021;7:1403-1408.
190. De Santis M, Becherer A, Bokemeyer C, et al. 2-18fluoro-deoxy-D-glucose positron emission tomography is a reliable predictor for viable tumor in postchemotherapy seminoma: an update of the prospective multicentric SEMPET trial. *J Clin Oncol.* 2004;22:1034-1039.
191. Treglia G, Sadeghi R, Annunziata S, Caldarella C, Bertagna F, Giovanella L. Diagnostic performance of fluorine-18-fluorodeoxyglucose positron emission tomography in the postchemotherapy management of patients with seminoma: systematic review and meta-analysis. *Biomed Res Int.* 2014;2014:852681.
192. Stephenson AJ, Sheinfeld J. The role of retroperitoneal lymph node dissection in the management of testicular cancer. *Urol Oncol.* 2004;22:225-233; discussion 234-225.
193. Motzer RJ, Amsterdam A, Prieto V, et al. Teratoma with malignant transformation: diverse malignant histologies arising in men with germ cell tumors. *J Urol.* 1998;159:133-138.
194. Hiester A, Nettersheim D, Nini A, Lusch A, Albers P. Management, Treatment, and Molecular Background of the Growing Teratoma Syndrome. *Urol Clin North Am.* 2019;46:419-427.
195. Travis LB, Fossa SD, Schonfeld SJ, et al. Second cancers among 40,576 testicular cancer patients: focus on long-term survivors. *J Natl Cancer Inst.* 2005;97:1354-1365.
196. Lavi A, Clark R, Ly TL, et al. Long-term Testis Cancer Survivors in Canada-Mortality Risks in a Large Population-based Cohort. *Eur Urol Open Sci.* 2020;22:54-60.

□□□

70

CHAPTER

Gynecology

Amanpreet Kaur Bhullar, MD, DGO
Sreeja Biswas-Roy, MD, MS
Jasneet Singh Bhullar, MD
Kayla K. Umemoto, BA
Pooja Mittal, MD, FACS

INTRODUCTION TO FEMALE PELVIC ANATOMY

Genital Tract Viscera

The female internal genitalia, also known as the upper genital tract, consists of the cervix, uterine corpus (uterus), fallopian tubes, and ovaries. A sagittal view of the female pelvis is shown in Figure 1.

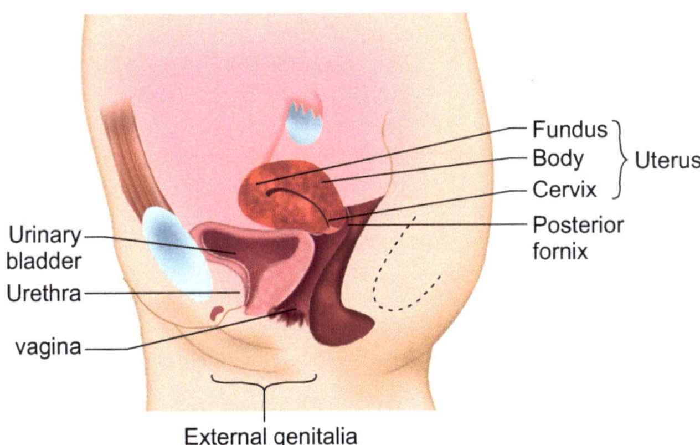

Figure 1: Sagittal view of the female pelvis

Uterus

The uterus (womb) is the pelvic organ where an embryo is implanted and develops into a fetus. The uterus is a pear shaped, thick, muscular organ located in the middle of the pelvis. The uterus is mainly divided into two parts: the uterine corpus (main body) and the uterine cervix. Histologically, the three tissue layers of the uterus are:

- Endometrium: The endometrium is the innermost and superficial layer of the uterine cavity which consists of glandular epithelium and stroma. The endometrium is made up of 2 layers: the deep stratum basalis and superficial stratum functionalis. The thickness of the endometrium varies during different stages of the menstrual cycle in response to hormonal stimulation.
- Myometrium: The myometrium is a thick muscular layer present between the endometrium and the outer serosal layer. It is the thickest layer of the uterus and is made up of smooth muscle fibers. The smooth muscle fibers of the myometrium undergo hypertrophy and hyperplasia during pregnancy.
- Serosa/Perimetrium: The serosa is the outer layer of the uterus, investing the body of the uterus. It is a thin layer and consists of visceral peritoneum.

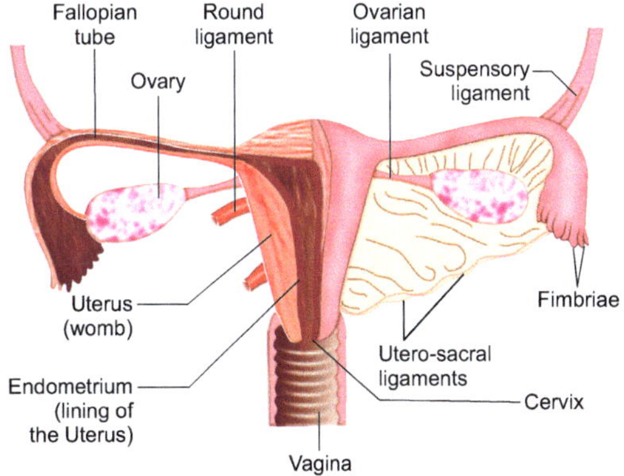

Figure 2: The structures of the uterus, fallopian tubes, and ovaries.

Adnexa

The ovaries and fallopian tubes are two structures making the uterine adnexa. The ovaries present as a pair of round, grape size, ovum (egg) producing organs. The ovaries, also known as the female gonads, and are the primary reproductive organs in women, similar to the testes in men. Beside producing eggs, the ovaries also produce hormones, mainly estrogen and progesterone, which are essential for female reproductive development and fertility. The ovaries are suspended lateral and/or posterior to the uterus by the utero-ovarian ligament. The infundibulo-pelvic ligament (also known as the suspensory ligament of the ovary) is another important supporting structure of the ovaries. The ovarian vessels travel through the infundibulo-pelvic ligament. Another important structure supporting the ovaries is the broad ligament, which condenses to form the mesovarium.

The fallopian tubes also known as the oviducts are a pair of long narrow tubes that arise from the uterine corpus, posterior and superior to the round ligaments. The fallopian tubes are supported by the broad ligaments through the mesosalpinx. They are about 10-13 cm long and extend from the uterus towards the ovaries bilaterally. Each tube is divided into four portions: the interstitial portion where the oviducts pass through the uterine cornu; the isthmus, a narrow portion of the fallopian tube connecting the ampulla to the uterine cavity; the ampulla which is the widest portion of the tubes with a larger lumen and mucosal folds; and the fimbria which are frond like projections located at the end of the tube. These projections increase the surface area at the end of the tubes, and help facilitate contact with the ovulated ova. The fallopian tube lumen communicates with the uterine cavity and the intra-abdominal cavity. Anatomically, the fallopian tubes are made up of an outer muscularis layer consisting of longitudinal smooth muscle fibers and an inner layer consisting of circular fibers. The mucosa of the fallopian tubes is composed of a number of delicate papillary folds (plica) which consist of three different types of cells: (1) ciliated columnar epithelial cells, (2) non ciliated, columnar secretory cells (Peg cells), and (3) intercalated cells, which are simply inactive secretory cells.[1]

Uterine Support

There are mainly three ligaments that support the uterus:

1. Uterosacral and cardinal ligament complex: The uterosacral/cardinal ligament complex suspends the uterus and upper vagina into its normal orientation.[2] The uterosacral ligament is composed of connective tissue bands, fused with the cardinal ligaments where they intersect in the cervix. The uterosacral ligaments pass posteriorly and inferiorly where they attach to the ischial spine and sacrum. Their function is to maintain the length of the vagina and the near horizontal axis of the vagina in a standing woman so that the levator plate can support it. If this support is lost, the uterus and/or vaginal apex can prolapse. The uterine vessels remain mostly in the cardinal ligaments.
2. Round ligaments: The round ligaments are extensions of the uterine musculature. They begin at the uterine fundus anterior and inferior to the fallopian tubes, cross retroperitoneally through the layers of the broad ligament, and enter the inguinal canal where they then terminate in the labia majora. The male homolog of the round ligaments is the gubernaculum testis.
3. Broad ligament: The broad ligament is a peritoneum sheet covering the lateral uterine corpus and upper cervix and is made of both visceral and parietal peritoneum containing smooth muscle and connective tissue. The boundaries of the broad ligament are the round ligaments superiorly, the infundibulopelvic ligaments posteriorly, and the cardinal and uterosacral ligaments inferiorly. Structures contained in the broad ligament are considered retroperitoneal.

Diseases of Female Genital Tract

This chapter is a brief focused overview of common diseases affecting the vulva, vagina, cervix, corpus uteri, and adnexa (fallopian tube, and ovary).

According to the International Society for the Study of Vulvar Disease (ISSVD) 1989, benign diseases of vulva can be categorized into several categories:

- Inflammatory
- Blistering
- Pigmentary changes.
- Benign tumors, hamartomas, and cysts
- Congenital malformations.

Table 1: Inflammatory Diseases of the Female Genital Tract

1. Lichen sclerosus	11. Seborrheic dermatitis
2. Squamous cell hyperplasia (+/- atypia)	12. Psoriasis
3. Lichen simplex chronicus (localized neurodermatitis)	13. Reiter disease
4. Primary irritant dermatitis	14. Lichen planus
5. Intertrigo	15. Lupus erythematosus
6. Allergic contact dermatitis	16. Darier disease
7. Fixed drug eruption	17. Aphthosis and Behcet disease

8. Erythema multiforme	18. Pyoderma gangrenosum
9. Toxic epidermal necrolysis	19. Crohn disease
10. Atopic dermatitis	20. Hidradenitis suppurativa
	21. Fox-Fordyce disease
	22. Plasma cell vulvitis
	23. Vulvar vestibulitis syndrome

Table 2: Blistering Diseases of the Female Genital Tract

1. Familial benign chronic pemphigus (Hailey-Hailey disease)
2. Bullous pemphigoid
3. Cicatricial pemphigoid
4. Pemphigus vulgaris
5. Erythema multiforme
6. Epidermolysis bullosa

Table 3: Pigmentary Changes of the Female Genital Tract

1. Acanthosis nigricans
2. Lentigo
3. Melanocytic nevus
4. Post inflammatory hyperpigmentation
5. Post inflammatory hypopigmentation
6. Vitiligo

Table 4: Benign Tumors, Hamartomas, and Cysts

1. Bartholin cysts	9. Hidradenoma
2. Epidermal inclusion cyst (Dermoid cyst)	10. Lipoma
3. Endometriosis	11. Chronic Inflammatory swellings
4. Hydrocele of the canal of Nuck	12. Hemangioma
5. Skene duct cyst	13. Lymphangioma
6. Seborrheic keratosis	14. Angiokeratoma
7. Acrochordon (fibroepithelial polyp)	15. Pyogenic granuloma
8. Fibroma, fibromyoma, and dermatofibroma	16. Sebaceous gland hyperplasia
	17. Papillomatosis

Vulvar Lichen Sclerosus et Atrophicus

Lichen sclerosus (LS) is a chronic, benign and progressive dermatologic condition. It shows marked inflammation, epithelial thinning, and distinctive dermal changes along with symptoms of pain and pruritus.[3] Vulvar LS shows a bimodal age distribution with peaks of onset being in prepubertal girls and perimenopausal or postmenopausal women.[4] Vulvar LS is one of the most commonly seen conditions treated in vulvar clinics.

Etiology: The etiology of lichen sclerosus (LS) is unknown. A number of mechanisms proposed based upon epidemiologic data are as follows:

Table 5: Etiologies of lichen sclerosus

Etiology
• Genetic factors
• Local factors
• Immunologic abnormality: alopecia areata, vitiligo, thyroid disorders, pernicious anemia, and diabetes mellitus
• Hormonal factors: low estrogen
• Infection: Borrelia burgdorferi, human papillomavirus (HPV)

Clinical Features: LS can be asymptomatic however the most common symptoms of vulvar LS are pruritus and soreness or irritation. In some patients, nonspecific, dull, vulvar discomfort is a prodrome of the gross lesions. Classic vulvar LS presents as white, atrophic, glistening papules that may later coalesce to form large plaques; in early lesions, follicular plugging may also be observed. LS can also present as hemorrhagic, purpuric, hyperkeratotic, bullous, eroded, or ulcerated lesions.[5] Vulvar LS lesions most frequently affect the labia minora and/or labia majora, however the whitening may extend over the perineum and around the anus in a keyhole fashion. Lesions can also extend onto the genitocrural folds or buttocks.[6] Fissuring can also be frequently seen in the perianal region in the interlabial folds, or around the clitoris.

- Vulvar pruritus: Vulvar pruritus, which is the hallmark of the disease, is often so intense that it interferes with sleep.
- Dyspareunia: Dyspareunia is often times a late symptom associated with introital stenosis, fissures, or posterior deflection of fused labial tissues at the time of intromission. Marked dyspareunia may occur in perimenopausal or postmenopausal women with a deficiency in estrogen in addition to vulvar LS.
- Anal discomfort: Patients with vulvar LS may also have involvement of perianal skin. Pruritus ani, painful defecation, anal fissures, and rectal bleeding are common symptoms.
- Dysuria: Dysuria and difficulty voiding may occur, particularly when the labia minora shows fusion over the urethra with advanced disease.

Diagnosis: Vulvar LS is diagnosed by the characteristic clinical manifestations and ideally should be confirmed histologically.[5] In children, the diagnosis of vulvar LS is often made based upon the clinical examination. Biopsy may be reserved for children with atypical clinical features or treatment-refractory disease.[7,8]

The routine biopsy of adult-onset vulvar LS is recommended rather than biopsy only after failure of empiric therapy because of the broad differential diagnosis of vulvar whitening, the possibility of underlying atypia or malignancy, and because biopsy should not be performed in women who have used corticosteroids within the previous two weeks. A 3 mm vulvar punch biopsy typically provides sufficient tissue to confirm the diagnosis and evaluate for atypical histologic features.

Additional diagnostic studies should be based upon any suspected autoimmune disease (e.g., thyroid disease, diabetes, pernicious anemia).

Histopathology: On histologic examination, the epidermis is typically thinned, although areas of hyperkeratosis may be observed and early lesions may demonstrate mild, irregular epidermal acanthosis.[9] The upper dermis is hyalinized with a band of lymphocytes below.

Table 6: Differential diagnosis of lichen sclerosus

Differential Diagnosis
• Lichen planus
• Lichen simplex chronicus
• Vitiligo
• Mucous membrane pemphigoid
• IAnal fissures and hemorrhoids
• Candidiasis
• Psoriasis
• Estrogen deficiency

Associated Malignancy: Women who are diagnosed with vulvar LS are at an increased risk of developing squamous cell cancer (SCC) of the vulva.[10-12] There have been case reports of verrucous carcinoma and basal cell carcinoma with LS. Differentiated vulvar intraepithelial neoplasia (VIN) is a precursor to SCC and is often associated with LS.

Management: Early treatment of vulvar LS is preferred whenever feasible. Treatment is strongly recommended for all women with vulvar LS, even if a woman is asymptomatic. This is done to prevent disease progression. Vulvar LS can result in physical dysfunction, disfigurement, and an impaired quality of life. Successful treatment is determined by relief of pruritus and pain, and resolution of fissuring, hyperkeratosis, and ecchymoses.[6] Treatment sometimes improves atrophy and depigmentation; however, any scarring present will remain.

First-line Therapy: The initial management of LS involves patient education and medical therapy. Patient education includes discussion of good vulvar hygiene and the importance of scratching cessation to minimize exposure to factors that may exacerbate symptoms.

Medical Therapy: Topical corticosteroids are the mainstay of therapy. Intralesional corticosteroid therapy is another option that is useful mainly for the treatment of thick hypertrophic plaques in which the topical corticosteroids may not penetrate adequately.

Treatment with a super high potency topical corticosteroid (group 1) (e.g., clobetasol propionate, halobetasol, fluocinonide) is considered the standard of care for vulvar LS. Some evidence suggests mometasone furoate, a less potent (group 3) topical corticosteroid may be an effective alternative. The daily use of topical emollients may help maintain symptom relief after topical corticosteroid treatment.[14]

Intralesional Corticosteroids: Intralesional corticosteroids are recommended in patients with thickened hypertrophic plaques who generally respond poorly to topical corticosteroids. In these cases, a monthly injection of triamcinolone hexacetonide or triamcinolone acetonide directly into the area of involvement for three months is suggested.[13]

Second-line Therapy: When topical corticosteroid therapy is ineffective or poorly tolerated, the preferred second-line treatment is a topical calcineurin inhibitor.

- Topical calcineurin inhibitors: Topical calcineurin inhibitors like tacrolimus and pimecrolimus appear to have efficacy for the treatment of vulvar LS, but may be less potent therapies than clobetasol propionate.
- Oral Acitretin: Retinoids appear to reduce the connective tissue degeneration seen in LS.[15] However, the use of acitretin is limited by significant and potentially harmful side effects.
- UVA1 phototherapy and Photodynamic therapy: UVA1 phototherapy may be an additional treatment option for vulvar LS. The long-term safety of UVA1 phototherapy for vulvar LS is unknown.
- Topical progesterone and topical testosterone: Historically, topical progesterone and topical testosterone creams were considered treatments for vulvar LS, but trials suggested less efficacy when compared to clobetasol.

Because of the often-chronic course of vulvar LS, long-term follow-up is recommended. Patients with well-controlled disease and a stable treatment plan should be examined at least once yearly after the initial treatment period. Closer follow-up with a specialist is indicated for patients with atypical features, previous vulvar cancer or vulvar intraepithelial neoplasia, or persistent symptoms.[6]

Bartholin's Gland Abscess

Bartholin Cyst

The Bartholin glands (or greater vestibular glands) are the homologues of the bulbourethral glands (Cowper's glands) in the male. These glands are the size of a pea (approximately 0.5 cm in size) and are located bilaterally at the base of the labia minora (Figure 3). The Bartholin glands drains tiny drops of mucus through 2 to 2.5 cm long ducts emptying into the vestibule at about the 4 o'clock and 8 o'clock positions. Obstruction of the orifice of the Bartholin gland duct results in the accumulation of mucus produced by the gland and leads to cystic dilatation of the duct proximal to the obstruction, forming a Bartholin duct cyst. Obstruction is often caused by local or diffuse vulvar edema. Bartholin duct cysts are usually sterile but can become infected resulting in the formation of a Bartholin gland abscess.

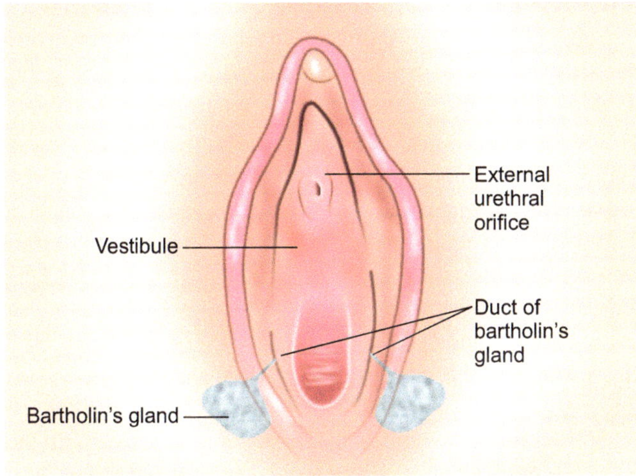

Figure 3: Anatomy of the external female genitalia

Clinical Manifestations and Diagnosis: Bartholin duct cysts are usually unilateral, an average size of 1 to 3 cm, and can be nonpalpable and asymptomatic. When cysts grow larger in size, they present as a protruding mass in the posterior introitus where the duct opens into the vestibule. Large cysts get indurated and may cause discomfort and pain, typically during sexual intercourse, sitting, or ambulating.

The diagnosis is clinical and based upon findings of a soft, painless mass in the area of the Bartholin gland (i.e., medial labia majora or lower vestibular area). Most cysts are detected during a routine pelvic examination or by the woman herself. For a patient presenting with a Bartholin cyst, endocervical specimen should be obtained to identify the presence of Chlamydia trachomatis and Neisseria gonorrhoeae.

Table 7: Clinical characteristics to differentiate between a Bartholin abscess and cyst

Character	Bartholin Abscess	Bartholin Cyst
Size	Enlarged Bartholin gland	Enlarged gland
Erythema	Skin overlying the gland feels warm to touch	No erythema
Temperature	Fever and tachycardia	No temperature increase No fever
Associated symptoms	An advancing cellulitis may be present	No cellulitis
Complications Labs	Leukocytosis and the pus from the Bartholin gland contain bacteria and WBCs	Normal WBC count and no bacteria and WBCs present in the fluid. Usually, serous fluid is contained within the cyst.

Management: No intervention is necessary for an asymptomatic Bartholin cyst. A possible exception is for women over the age of 40, for whom some experts suggest drainage and biopsy to exclude carcinoma. A biopsy is required for women of any age if there are findings suggestive of malignancy of the Bartholin gland or other vulvar site.

The treatment of a Bartholin abscess is done by different surgical procedures like, the marsupialization of the abscess, incision and drainage of the abscess, or by placement of a Word catheter. Incision and drainage of the abscess is a relatively quick procedure and can provide immediate relief of symptoms; however, it is usually discouraged because the recurrence rate of another Bartholin duct cysts/abscess is high after incision and drainage (Figure 4). Also, if the placement of a Word catheter is needed later on, it becomes difficult after an incision and drainage procedure. Marsupialization and Word catheter placement results in more definitive drainage of a Bartholin gland abscess. The catheter is left in place to facilitate the epithelization of the tract which usually occurs after 3 to 6 weeks. The catheter is left in place until it falls out spontaneously. The patients are usually given antibiotics to cover against C. trachomatis, N. gonorrhoeae, and other gram-positive and negative facultative and obligate anaerobes. The usual regimen is 500 mg of metronidazole every 8 hours with 500 mg of oral levofloxacin every 24 hours for 7 to 10 days. The patient should be reevaluated within 3 weeks and then at 6 weeks to rule out any signs of septicemia.

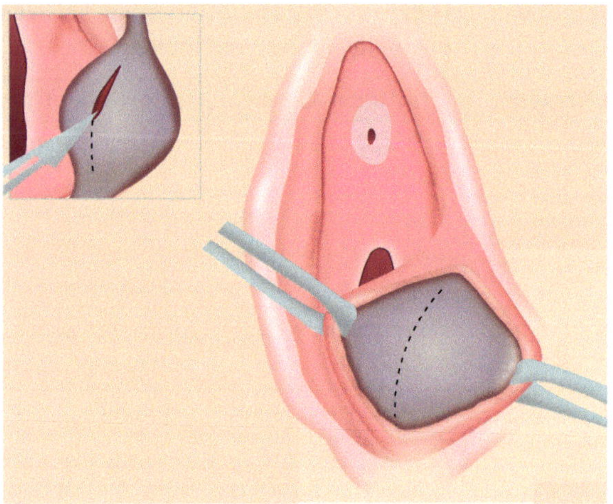

Figure 4: Incision and drainage of Bartholin's cyst and abscess

Marsupialization is another procedure done to treat Bartholin's cyst. This procedure should be avoided if there is an abscess. Marsupialization is an easy and quick procedure and can be performed in the office or in an outpatient surgical suite if the cyst is deeply seated.

Endometriosis

Introduction

Endometriosis is a common clinical and pathological condition which was initially described by Von Rokitansky in 1860. It affects approximately 2-10% of females who are of childbearing age. Endometriosis is characterized by the presence of endometrial tissue outside the uterine cavity. This ectopic tissue can be found implanted throughout the pelvic cavity, including the ovaries, uterine ligaments, rectovaginal septum, parietal peritoneum, intestinal serosa, and appendix. Less commonly the ectopic tissue can be found on hernia sacs, the umbilicus, laparotomy and episiotomy scars, and the pleural and pericardial cavities.

Histogenesis: The exact mechanism of endometriosis development is unknown, although there has been much discussion as to its origin. Four major theories have been proposed; however, the most widely accepted and earliest theory is the 'Refluxed Menstruation' theory in which it is hypothesized that menstrual blood is refluxed into the pelvic cavity and embeds into different intra-abdominal sites. The fact that the most commonly affected sites with endometriosis are near the fallopian tube, in some way supports the theory of reflux menstruation as an etiology of endometriosis.

Risk Factors: Many risk factors have been cited, the most common among them include early menarche and late menopause resulting in increased duration of menstruation exposure. Other risk factors include-low BMI, nulliparity, heavy and prolonged menstruation (bleeding >5 days), shorter length of menstrual cycle (<28 days), and presence of Mullerian abnormalities

Clinical Characteristics: The clinical features of endometriosis vary, ranging from no symptoms to debilitating pelvic pain and infertility. The clinical presentation depends mainly on the site of endometriosis and the severity of disease. The characteristic of the disease is described by the classical triad of dysmenorrhea, dyspareunia, and infertility. Other less common symptoms include dyschezia, non-menstrual pelvic pain, lateral pelvic pain, lower back pain, bladder pain, frequency and dysuria, partial bowel obstruction, irritable bowel syndrome, and abdominal wall pain.

Diagnosis: Endometriosis is diagnosed clinically, and a good history and pelvic examination findings are mandatory to reach the diagnosis. As endometriosis is the most common cause of pelvic pain in childbearing age groups, it should always be first on the list of differential diagnoses. In most of the patients, a presumptive diagnosis of endometriosis can be made on the basis of characteristic findings on pelvic examination. Laparoscopy is usually confirmatory.

Pelvic Examination: Speculum examination can reveal hemorrhagic spots on the cervix. Endometriosis of the uterosacral ligaments or cul-de-sac invading the posterior fornix of the vagina can be seen as nodules on the surface of vagina if the speculum is directed posteriorly, enabling examination of the posterior vaginal fornix. Bimanual pelvic examination should focus on the uterus, bilateral uterosacral ligaments, and the cul-de-sac. The size, shape, position, and consistency of the uterus and degree of tenderness on bimanual palpation should be noted. The normal ovaries are usually not palpable on the pelvic exam but enlarged ovaries are easier to detect. In advanced cases of endometriosis where there are severe adhesions, the uterus and enlarged ovaries may form an indistinct mass.

Diagnostic Tests

The cancer antigen-125 (CA-125) assay has been researched extensively but the overall value in establishing the diagnosis of endometriosis is limited. Elevated levels of CA-125 and placental protein-14 (PP14) have been associated specifically with the presence of endometriosis cysts and severe deep endometriosis.

Another diagnostic tool available includes the transvaginal ultrasound which can detect the endometrial cysts reliably with a sensitivity of 89% and specificity of 91%, making it the imaging modality of choice. The ultrasound however cannot reliably detect the smaller endometrial implants. Magnetic resonance imaging (MRI) may be of help in assessing deep pelvic and extra-pelvic endometriosis.

Treatment

General Approach: The goal of therapy is to relieve the clinical manifestations of endometriosis which fall into three general categories: pelvic pain, infertility, and pelvic mass. Various types of medical management modalities are available to treat the symptoms of endometriosis; however, NSAIDs remain the first-line treatment modality to treat the pelvic pain. There is no evidence supporting the benefits and superiority of one type of medical therapy over another for the treatment of endometriosis symptoms or their effects on future fertility. Therefore, treatment is mostly individualized, based on the severity of symptoms, the extent and location of disease, the age of the patient, whether there is a desire for pregnancy, medication tolerance and adverse effects, cost of treatment, and candidacy of surgical treatment.

Different treatment approaches include:

- Expectant management
- Pain control
- Hormonal medical therapy which includes estrogen-progestin oral contraceptives (cyclic or continuous), gonadotropin-releasing hormone (GnRH) agonists, and progestins (oral, parenteral, or intrauterine). Danazol (an androgen) is also used effectively to treat the pelvic pain.
- Aromatase inhibitors (i.e., letrozole, anastrozole, mifepristone, and exemestane or Aromasin) are several other medications that are under evaluation for the treatment of endometriosis.
- Surgical options include a conservative approach (retain the uterus and ovarian tissue) or a definitive treatment with hysterectomy and possible bilateral oophorectomy.
- Combination therapy in which medical therapy is given either initially and/or post-surgery.

Surgical Management

Indications: Surgery allows for both the diagnosis and management of women with known or suspected endometriosis. Indications for surgery include:

- Failure of medical therapy to ameliorate symptoms.
- Women who decline or have contraindications to medical therapy.
- When there is a need for a definitive diagnosis of endometriosis: Making a definitive diagnosis requires surgery to visualize and/or biopsy lesions. Women with mild symptoms suggestive of endometriosis are often treated empirically with first-line therapies (e.g., NSAIDs, estrogen-progestin contraceptives). If such therapy is unsuccessful, a definitive diagnosis may be preferred prior to treating with therapies that are difficult to tolerate and/or have potential adverse effects (e.g., GnRH agonists).
- Exclude malignancy in an adnexal mass: Endometriotic implants may develop into an ovarian cyst (endometrioma). Endometriosis may also result in pelvic adhesions that form a peritoneal inclusion cyst. Such cysts may have features suggestive of malignancy, and surgery may be required for diagnosis and treatment.
- Treatment of infertility in selected women: Historically, a diagnostic laparoscopy to evaluate for endometriosis was a standard part of the evaluation of infertility. However, current practice varies. Some experts advise that women with infertility and symptoms suggestive of endometriosis undergo laparoscopy prior to other treatments, while others do not perform laparoscopy and treat these patients in the same stepwise manner as other women (ovulation induction with intrauterine insemination followed by in vitro fertilization or IVF). In some cases, women are not able to undergo ovulation induction or IVF, and laparoscopy should be performed.
- Obstruction of the urinary tract or gastrointestinal tract.

Contraindications: Relative contraindications to the surgical management of endometriosis include:

- Incomplete evaluation of the patient's pain: Etiologies that do not require surgical evaluation or treatment should be excluded prior to surgery (primary dysmenorrhea, interstitial cystitis/bladder pain syndrome, irritable bowel syndrome).
- Repeated surgeries for endometriosis without sustained relief.
- Women who are approaching menopause: Endometriosis symptoms typically resolve with menopause. Menopause can be anticipated in a patient who is close to the average age (51 years) or has symptoms of the menopausal transition. These patients may choose to tolerate symptoms that are not completely controlled with medical therapy in order to avoid surgery. This decision depends upon patient preferences regarding the symptoms impact on their quality of life and the value placed on avoiding potential surgical morbidity.

Conservative versus Definitive Surgery: Conservative surgery is typically used as the initial surgical treatment for endometriosis. This is usually effective in the short term, but many women eventually develop recurrent symptoms. Women with recurrent symptoms may be treated with either repeat conservative surgery or definitive surgery.

These two approaches to surgical treatment are:

- Conservative surgery involves the excision or ablation of endometriotic lesions with the intent of preserving the uterus and as much of the ovarian tissue as possible.[3] Laparoscopic removal of an endometrioma, and excision and/or ablation of lesions are the most common conservative treatment procedures.
- Definitive surgery consists of hysterectomy combined with bilateral salpingo-oophorectomy.

Adnexal Mass

Introduction

An adnexal mass or adnexal tumor is a common gynecologic condition and is usually described as a growth near the uterus (mass of the ovary, fallopian tube, or surrounding connective tissues). Adnexal masses can have gynecological or non-gynecological causes. Adnexal masses are found in women of all ages, from fetuses to the elderly, and they consist of a wide variety of types (Table 8). The principal goals of the evaluation of the adnexal mass are to (1) address the acute conditions (e.g., ectopic pregnancy) and (2) to determine whether a mass is malignant or benign

Table 8: Differential diagnosis of adnexal masses in women

Differential diagnosis of adnexal masses in women
Benign masses:
• Extraovarian mass
• Ectopic pregnancy
• Hydrosalpinx or tubo ovarian abscess
• Peritoneal inclusion cyst
• Paraovarian cyst
• Pedunculated fibroid
• Diverticular abscess
• Appendiceal abscess or tumor
• Pelvic kidney
• Inflammatory or malignant bowel disease
Ovarian mass
• Theca lutein cysts
• Simple or hemorrhagic physiologic cysts (e.g., follicular, corpus luteum)
• Endometrioma
Malignant masses
• Fallopian tube cancer
• Ovarian cancer (e.g., epithelial, germ cell, sex-cord)
• Metastatic carcinoma (e.g., breast, colon, endometrium)

Prevalence

The reported prevalence of adnexal masses varies widely and mainly depends upon the population studied and the criteria employed. In a study with 335 asymptomatic women aged 25 to 40 years old, the point prevalence of an adnexal lesion on ultrasound examination was 7.8% (prevalence of ovarian cysts 6.6%).[16] In another random study, transvaginal ultrasonography was performed on 8,794 asymptomatic postmenopausal women as part of their routine gynecological check-up and 2.5% had a simple unilocular adnexal cyst.[17]

Clinical Approach

The main goal of the clinical approach toward the patient with an adnexal mass is to determine the gynecological or non-gynecological etiology of the mass.

The evaluation of the adnexal mass is guided mainly by the age of the patient, reproductive status of the patient, anatomic location of the mass, and clinical presentation. As an example, findings of a solid ovarian mass in a postmenopausal female raises a high suspicion of ovarian cancer. Alternatively, in a woman of reproductive age, a mass of the fallopian tube accompanied by pain and bleeding requires the exclusion of an ectopic pregnancy through an immediate pregnancy test.

Risk of Malignancy

The most serious concern when an adnexal mass is found is the possibility of malignancy. clinical factors that increase the likelihood of malignancy include:

- Prepubescent (girls <15 years of age) or postmenopausal females
- A complex or solid appearing mass on imaging
- A known genetic predisposition
- An adnexal mass in a woman known to have a non-gynecological cancer (e.g., breast or gastric cancer)
- Presence of Ascites

In girls younger than 15 years of age, there is a high percent of malignant ovarian tumors.[18] The overall risk of malignancy of an adnexal mass increase with age and is 29 to 35% in postmenopausal women as compared to 6 to 11% in premenopausal women.[19]

Imaging characteristics suggestive of a malignant mass: Sonographic characteristics that have been typically associated with malignancy are shown in Table 9.

Table 9: Imaging characteristics suggestive of a malignant mass

1. Solid component that is often nodular or papillary and is not hyperechoic
2. Septations, if present, which are >2 to 3 mm thick
3. Color Doppler demonstrates flow in the solid component
4. Presence of ascites (usually postmenopausal women with any peritoneal fluid and premenopausal women with more than a small amount of peritoneal fluid is abnormal)
5. Peritoneal masses, enlarged lymph nodes, or findings of matted bowel

Additional Techniques to Diagnose Adnexal Mass

Combined Grayscale and Doppler Evaluation: When a mass does not have a typical benign appearance, using color Doppler to look for the presence or absence of flow in solid areas or septations can be useful. Doppler evaluation of adnexal masses decreases the false positive rate of sonography findings of ovarian carcinoma.[20]

CA-125: The use of cancer antigen-125 (CA-125) as a biomarker for epithelial ovarian cancer (EOC) was first described in 1983[21] and is currently the most widely used biomarker for EOC. CA-125 combined with sonographic features of the adnexal mass appears to have a higher specificity for ovarian malignancy than CA-125 alone.

Treatment

The management of an adnexal mass depends upon different factors which includes mainly the location of the mass, the etiology of the mass, and the clinical presentation. In general, the three options for adnexal mass management are as follows:

- Surgery: The main indications for surgery include a high suspicion of malignancy, complications and risks associated with the mass (e.g., infection or torsion), or when symptoms arise due to the mass. Surgical exploration can be done laparoscopically (conventional or robotic) or through a laparotomy. Using a surgical approach depends on the degree of suspicion of a malignancy, and the preference of both the surgeon and patient. Staging a patient with ovarian cancer is completed through either an open or laparoscopic approach, however, most currently practicing surgeons continue to prefer laparotomy if they are suspicious of malignancy. In patients with a low to moderate suspicion of malignancy, laparoscopy is generally preferred over laparotomy because it is minimally invasive, associated with fewer complication, has a much shorter recovery period, and has a decreased perioperative morbidity. Oophorectomy or ovarian cystectomy is performed for ovarian masses. biopsy and resection can be performed for other adnexal masses.
- Continued surveillance: If there is low suspicion of malignancy, continued surveillance is indicated, the differential is just not completely excluded. Continued surveillance is usually done with serial pelvic ultrasounds and/or serum tumor marker measurements.
- Expectant management: Patients with an apparent mass of benign etiology have no indication for surgery or surveillance and no further follow-up is recommended

Uterine Leiomyomas

Introduction

Uterine leiomyomas, also known as uterine fibroids or myomas, represent the most common gynecological problem in women of reproductive age and are the most common pelvic tumor in females (Figure 5).[22-24] They are benign neoplasms arising from the smooth muscle cells of the myometrium. While most of the leiomyomas are asymptomatic, they can typically present with symptoms of heavy or prolonged menstrual bleeding, pelvic pain/pressure, and can have reproductive effects.

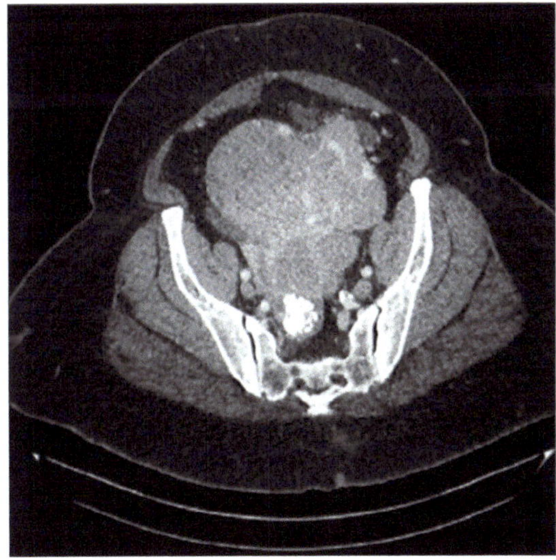

Figure 5: Uterine mass

Classification

Fibroids are often classified according to their location in the uterus, although many fibroids have more than one location designation. The International Federation of Gynecology and Obstetrics (FIGO) staging scheme for fibroids is shown below.[25]

- Intramural myomas (FIGO type 3, 4, and 5): These develop in the uterine wall and can grow large enough to cause distortion of the uterine cavity, extend out from the serosal surface, or can be transmural and extend from the serosa to the mucosal surface.
- Submucosal myomas (FIGO type 0, 1, and 2): These originate from myometrial cells located just below the endometrium and protrude into the uterine cavity. The FIGO/European Society of Hysteroscopy classification system describes the extent of protrusion of submucosal fibroids into the cavity, and it is important to know for predicting the outcome of a hysteroscopic myomectomy. Type 0 fibroids are completely intracavitary, type I fibroids have <50% of their volume in the uterine wall, and type II fibroids have ≥50% of their volume in the uterine wall. Only types 0 and I fibroids can be resected hysteroscopically, although type I fibroid resection requires significant hysteroscopic expertise.
- Subserosal myomas (FIGO type 6 and 7): These originate in the myometrium at the uterus' serosal surface and have a broad or pedunculated base that sometimes extends between the folds of the broad ligament (i.e., intraligamentary).
- Cervical myomas (FIGO type 8): These are located in the cervix and can cause significant hindrance while performing hysterectomy or C-section.

Prevalence

The exact prevalence of uterine fibroid in women who are at reproductive age is hard to determine due to several reasons. Most fibroids are asymptomatic, and therefore have low rates of clinical detection. One hysterectomy study found that myomas were in 77% of uterine specimens.[26]

The epidemiology of uterine leiomyomas parallels the ontogeny and life cycle changes of the reproductive hormones. Their growth is dependent on estrogen and progesterone. Studies have shown significant growth reduction in the fibroids with the use of gonadotropin-releasing hormones (GnRH) analogs.

Uterine leiomyomas are rare before puberty, an increase in prevalence is noted during the reproductive years, and these tumors usually decrease in size after menopause.

Risk Factors

Race: Epidemiologically, the most significant risk factors for fibroid development are increasing age (until menopause) and race (African descent as compared to white). Fibroid incidence rates are around 2-3-fold higher in African women than in white women.[22,28,29]

Age: Usually found in women 30-40 years old. Rare before 30 or after 40 years old.

Menstrual History: There is an increased risk of fibroid development with early menarche in girls (<10 years old).

Parity: Common in nulliparas or patients with low parity. It is rare in multiparas women.

Hyperestrogenemia: Estrogen receptors (ER) more than the surrounding myometrium but less than those in the endometrium:

- Common in low parity.
- Atrophies and shrinks after menopause.
- Common association with other hyperestrenic conditions such as endometriosis, endometrial hyperplasia, and endometrial carcinoma.

Hormonal Contraception: Low dose oral contraceptives (OCs) use does not result in an increased growth of the fibroids and therefore administration of these drugs is not contraindicated in women with fibroids.[30-34]

Obesity: A strong relationship between fibroids and an increased body mass index has been shown in most studies.

Smoking: Smoking decreases the risk of fibroids although the mechanism is unknown.

Heredity: Familial predisposition to leiomyomas in some women is implied in studies.

Other Factors: Hypertension increase the risks of leiomyoma development.

Clinical Presentation

Symptoms attributable to uterine fibroids can generally be classified into three distinct categories:

- Abnormal uterine bleeding
- Pelvic pressure and pain
- Reproductive dysfunction

Abnormal Uterine Bleeding: Heavy and/or prolonged menses is the typical bleeding pattern with myomas and the most common fibroid symptom.[35] Intermenstrual bleeding and postmenopausal bleeding are not characteristic of myomas and should be investigated to exclude an endometrial pathology. Heavy uterine bleeding may be responsible for associated problems such as iron deficiency anemia.

The severity of abnormal uterine bleeding usually depends upon the size and location of the fibroid. Significant menorrhagia[23,37,38] is most frequently related to submucosal fibroids that protrude into the uterine cavity (e.g., types 0 and I). However, women who have intramural myomas may also have symptoms of heavy or prolonged menstrual bleeding. The clear mechanism(s) of heavy bleeding is unclear but some believe it may be due to impaired endometrial hemostasis, molecular dysregulation of angiogenic factors, or abnormalities of both microscopic and macroscopic uterine vasculature caused by the fibroids.[39]

Pelvic Pressure and Pain: Pelvic pressure and pain are the second most common symptoms reported with the diagnosis of fibroids. The uterus with leiomyomas is irregularly shaped, thus causing specific symptoms related to pressure caused by the myoma at different locations. Such symptoms include increased urinary frequency, incomplete or difficulty emptying the bladder, and rarely urinary obstruction and retention; constipation is seen in patients with fibroids putting pressure on the rectum. An enlarged uterus may compress the vena cava and can lead to an increase in thromboembolic risk.[40-42] Infrequently, fibroids can cause acute pain from degeneration (e.g., carneous or red degeneration) or torsion of a pedunculated tumor.

Reproductive Dysfunction: In clinical practice, leiomyomas are often used to explain infertility. Leiomyomas may cause infertility by distorting the uterine cavity, especially with submucosal or intramural leiomyomas. Additionally, leiomyomas are associated with adverse pregnancy outcomes including fetal growth restriction, placental abruption, malpresentation, and preterm labor and birth.

Other: Rarely a leiomyoma can present with transcervical prolapse, which can result in infection or ulceration of the tumor.

Other rare symptoms of fibroid associated with ectopic hormone production include:

- Autonomous production of erythropoietin resulting in polycythemia[43]
- Autonomous production of PTHrP resulting in hypercalcemia[44]
- Hyperprolactinemia[45]

Diagnosis

A careful detailed history and pelvic examination is crucial for the diagnosis of uterine fibroids. Findings on bimanual pelvic exam of an enlarged, mobile uterus with irregular contours is suggestive of uterine leiomyoma. Ultrasound is typically used to confirm the diagnosis.

Pelvic Examination: On bimanual pelvic exam, a uterus with leiomyomas can be felt as a bulky, enlarged, mobile uterus with an irregular contour. Other findings (e.g., adnexal mass, cervical mass) along with the size, contour, and mobility of the uterus help with following progressive uterine changes over time and also help with surgical planning (e.g., plan transverse or vertical incision). The speculum exam has low yield, however occasionally a prolapsed submucosal fibroid can be seen at the external cervical os.

Imaging: When a myoma is suspected, imaging or hysteroscopy is used to exclude other types of uterine or adnexal mass. Transvaginal ultrasounds are the most commonly used, and computed tomography has little use in determining fibroid position.

Ultrasound: Transvaginal ultrasound is the most widely used modality with a high sensitivity (95 to 100%) for detecting myomas in uterus <10 weeks size. Ultrasounds are easily available and cost effective. Localization of fibroids in an enlarged uterus >10 weeks size is limited.[46]

Diagnostic Hysteroscopy: The gold standard for evaluating the intrauterine extension of fibroids is hysteroscopy. This is an outpatient clinic procedure, performed with a flexible or rigid hysteroscope. The lesions are hysteroscopically classified as intracavitary when the whole fibroid can be seen arising from a pedicle or if it has a broad base. However, the depth of penetration cannot be determined with a hysteroscope if the fibroid abuts the endometrium or extends into the myometrium. Additionally, hysteroscopy has very low accuracy in accurately predicting the fibroid size compared to ultrasound and sonohysterography.

Magnetic Resonance Imaging: The accurate visualization of uterine fibroid size and location is best done with magnetic resonance imaging (MRI). MRI also helps distinguish leiomyomas, adenomyosis, and adenomyomas, and to differentiate leiomyosarcoma from the leiomyomas. Since it is expensive, MRI is generally reserved for the surgical planning of complicated procedures, or prior to uterine artery embolization because imaging patterns can predict the outcome of this procedure.

Hysterosalpingography: Hysterosalpingography (HSG) is a common diagnostic test to assess tubal pregnancy. A hysterosalpingogram (HSG) is helpful in defining endometrial cavity contour. However, is offers poor visualization of the remainder of the myometrium and can result in the false identification of an intramural fibroid impinging on the uterine cavity as a submucosal fibroid. It is most often specifically used for visualization of myomas only when an HSG is required for tubal patency evaluation of women coming in with infertility.

Management

A vast majority of uterine myomas are asymptomatic and often require no treatment. In patients who present with symptoms of myoma (e.g., abnormal uterine bleeding, pain, pressure), the major goal of treatment is to provide relief of symptoms.[24] Patients are offered several options for management ranging from expectant management to medical treatment, surgical treatment, and embolization. The type and timing of intervention is determined by the type and severity of the following symptoms:[27]

- Myoma(s) size
- Myoma(s) location
- Age of patient
- Reproductive plans and obstetrical history

Expectant Management: Expectant management is usually indicated for very small asymptomatic fibroids or fibroids in pregnancy. There is no strong data available with guidelines regarding follow-up of fibroids in patients with no symptoms or patients who refuse any medical or surgical treatment. However, given data that fibroids can shrink substantially and that there is substantial regression during the postpartum period, expectant management appears to be a reasonable option for some women.[28,29]

Medical Therapy: Anecdotal data suggest that medical therapy can achieve adequate symptom relief in some women, primarily in patients where the main or only symptom is excessive menstrual bleeding. In general, 75% of women were observed to have some improvement in their symptoms over the period of one year of medical therapy, but there are high rates of failure in the long-term.[47] Many different modalities have been used to date to treat leiomyomas, but the six primary modalities used are: OCP for endometrial suppression, GnRH agonist therapy, anti-steroidal therapy, androgen therapy, leiomyoma receptor growth factor antagonists, and uterine blood flow (altering drugs).

Hormonal Therapies: Oral combined hormonal contraceptives and progestational agents have long been prescribed to regulate abnormal uterine bleeding but appear to have limited efficacy in the treatment of uterine leiomyomas.[48-49]

Levonorgestrel-Releasing Intrauterine System: In contrast to oral combined use, levonorgestrel intrauterine contraceptive systems (LN-IUS) can reduce uterine volume and fibroid related menorrhagia. This therapy is advantageous because it is a form of contraception for women desiring not to become pregnant. A strong relative contraindication of LN-IUS is the presence of intracavitary leiomyomas that can be treated with hysteroscopic resection.

Progestin Implants, Injections, and Pills: The progestin-only contraceptives provide relief of abnormal uterine bleeding by causing endometrial atrophy. In contrast to gonadotropin-releasing agonists and antagonists, most of these «contraceptives» provide continuous exposure to low doses of hormones, which should minimize deleterious effects.

Gonadotropin-Releasing Hormone Agonists: Gonadotropin-releasing hormone (GnRH) agonists are the most effective and most commonly used medical therapy for leiomyoma-related symptom treatment. These drugs work by initially increasing the release of gonadotropins, followed by desensitization and downregulation to a hypogonadotropic, hypogonadal state that clinically resembles menopause. Most women will develop amenorrhea, improvement in anemia (if present), and significantly reduced (35 to 60%) uterine size within three months of initiating this therapy, thus achieving improvements in both categories of myoma symptomatology.[50-52]

Antiprogestins and Progesterone Receptor Modulators: Antiprogestins (i.e., mifepristone or RU 486) are sometimes used to treat leiomyomas. Selective progesterone receptor modulators (SPMs) are a fairly new drug class that act as both agonist and antagonists at progesterone, glucocorticoid, and androgen receptors.

Raloxifene: Raloxifene has antiestrogenic activity which aids in reducing the volume of fibroids (also clomiphene citrate and tamoxifen). The efficacy of selective estrogen receptor modulators (SERM) for the treatment of leiomyomas is unclear and they have the additional concern of potentially increasing the risk of venous thrombosis when used at high doses.

Aromatase Inhibitors: A few small series and a randomized clinical trial that studied aromatase inhibitors have observed the decrease in size of symptomatic leiomyomas and reduction in the symptoms of leiomyomas in perimenopausal women.[53,54]

Antifibrinolytic Agents: Antifibrinolytic agents, mostly used in the treatment of idiopathic menorrhagia, have not been well studied in the treatment of menorrhagia related to leiomyomas. Tranexamic acid is now FDA approved for the treatment of heavy menstrual bleeding and is available in the United States.[55]

Nonsteroidal Anti-Inflammatory Drugs: Nonsteroidal anti-inflammatory drugs (NSAIDs) have not been extensively studied as an effective treatment in leiomyoma-related menorrhagia,[56,57] NSAIDs reduce pain during menses and can be useful in this population.

Androgens: Danazol and gestrinone are androgenic steroids used in the treatment of fibroids by the inhibition of pituitary gonadotropin secretion, by the direct inhibition of endometriotic implant growth, and by the inhibition of ovarian enzymes responsible for estrogen production.

Surgery: Uterine leiomyomas are generally treated with surgery. The definitive treatment is hysterectomy, but other procedures include myomectomy, endometrial ablation, uterine artery embolization (UAE), magnetic resonance-guided focused-ultrasound surgery (MRgFUS), and myolysis.

Indications: Surgical therapy indications are as follows:

- Abnormal uterine bleeding
- Bulk-related symptoms
- Uterus larger than 12 weeks size

- Infertility or recurrent pregnancy loss
- Suspected malignancy (rapidly enlarging or post-menopausal growth)

Multiple huge fibroids liable to complications

Hysterectomy: Hysterectomy is the definitive therapy for:

1. Women who have acute hemorrhage and who failed to respond to other therapies.
2. Women who do not desire more pregnancies and have a higher risk of diseases (e.g., endometriosis, cervical intraepithelial neoplasia, endometrial hyperplasia, adenomyosis, or uterine or ovarian cancer) that can be treated or decrease the risk with hysterectomy.
3. Women where other minimally invasive therapies attempting to treat leiomyomas have failed.
4. Women with significant symptoms, multiple leiomyomas, and who want a definitive end to their symptoms.

Myomectomy: Myomectomy aims at the removal of all myomas, with conservation of a functioning uterus to preserve a woman's reproductive function, thus it is used for women who wish to have more children or wish to keep their uterus. This procedure can be performed through different techniques. The removal of subserosal or intramural myomas has classically been done by a laparotomy incision, although it is now also common to see laparoscopic and robotic-assisted procedures. Hysteroscopic myomectomy is the most common procedure used to remove intracavitary myomas (submucosal and intramural myomas that protrude into the uterine cavity). A vaginal myomectomy can be done if a fibroid prolapses through the cervix.

Endometrial Ablation: Endometrial ablation is used to treat bleeding abnormalities in women who do not desire future pregnancy. Endometrial ablation can be performed alone or with a hysteroscopic myomectomy.

Myolysis: Laparoscopic myolysis is a procedure used for patients with fibroids, but who cannot undergo a myomectomy. Myolysis refers to the procedure in which there is laparoscopic thermal coagulation or cryoablation (cryomyolysis) of the leiomyoma.[58,59]

Uterine Artery Occlusion: Occlusion of uterine vessels either via laparoscopy or a vaginally placed clamp has also been proposed as an alternative to uterine artery embolization (UAE), but experience is limited.[60,61] Currently, it appears that UAE is preferable to laparoscopic uterine artery occlusion.

Uterine Artery Embolization: This procedure was developed because it is known that decreasing uterine blood flow can significantly decrease fibroid size and uterine volume. Uterine artery embolization (UAE), or uterine fibroid embolization (UFE), are minimally invasive treatments of leiomyoma-related symptoms. For women not interested in fertility, but would like to keep their uterus, UAE is an effective treatment option.

Magnetic Resonance Guided Focused Ultrasound: In premenopausal women who have completed childbearing, magnetic resonance guided focused ultrasound surgery (MRgFUS) (e.g., ExAblate 2000) has more recently been used to treat uterine leiomyomas. This noninvasive thermal ablative technique converges multiple waves of ultrasound energy on a small volume of tissue. This leads to the thermal destruction of the tissue. MRgFUS is often an outpatient procedure.[62,63]

Pelvic Inflammatory Disease

Introduction

Pelvic inflammatory disease (PID) has been and continues to be a debilitating condition that primarily affects younger women of reproductive age. PID is an acute infection of the female internal genital organs that involves the uterus, the oviducts, and/or the ovaries; and often involves other neighboring organs in the pelvis. PID is caused by a sexually transmitted agent which ascends the external genitalia and infects the upper genital tract.

Prevalence

Over the last decade, there has been a decrease in PID prevalence in the United States and in developing countries.[65,65] In the United States, over the course of a year, there are roughly 106,000 outpatient visits and 60,000 hospitalizations for PID. Additionally, PID is often seen in the emergency department.[66]

Microbiology

The two most common sexually transmitted bacteria that cause PID among sexually active pre-menopausal females are Neisseria gonorrhoeae and Chlamydia trachomatis. Mycoplasma genitalium is also likely to be a cause in the pre-menopausal group. E. coli and colonic anaerobes may be responsible for the rare cases of PID seen in post-menopausal women. Very rare pathogens identified include Mycobacterium tuberculosis and the agents of actinomycosis. Regardless of the pathogen initiating the disease, PID is clinically considered a mixed infection.

Risk Factors

Table 10: Pelvic Inflammatory Disease Risk Factors

Risk Factors for Pelvic Inflammatory Disease Acquisition	
• Sex is the primary risk factor for pelvic inflammatory disease (PID).	• Age: most commonly affects patients 15 to 25 years of age.
• Young age at first sex	• Contraceptive method: barrier contraception protects against PID
• Multiple sexual partners	• Illicit drug use
• STI in the partner	• Delayed and decreased access to care
• Previous PID or history of STD	• Cervical ectopy

Clinical Signs and Symptoms

Lower abdominal or Pelvic pain is the cardinal presenting symptom in women with PID. The acute onset of pain that worsens during intercourse or with jarring movement may sometimes be the only presenting symptom of PID; the onset of pain during or shortly after menses is particularly suggestive as well.[67] Abdominal pain is usually bilateral and rarely of more than two weeks' duration.[68]

Other associated signs include unusual vaginal discharge, urethritis, proctitis, fever, chills, and abnormal uterine bleeding.

On Exam, only about one-half of PID patients were found to have fever during the physical exam. Diffuse tenderness greatest in the lower quadrants is evident on abdomen exam. Roughly 10% of patients will have perihepatitis (Fitz-Hugh Curtis syndrome) and exhibit marked tenderness in the right upper quadrant

Pelvic examination findings include the presence of endocervical discharge that is purulent, and acute cervical motion tenderness and adnexal tenderness on the bimanual examination.

Perihepatitis (Fitz-Hugh Curtis Syndrome) is an infection of the liver capsule and peritoneum of the anterior right upper quadrant. It was first associated with gonococcal salpingitis[69] and subsequently with C. trachomatis.[70,71] Acute phase manifestations include a patchy purulent and fibrinous exudate ("violin string" adhesions), and generally affects the liver's anterior surfaces, not the liver parenchyma.

Diagnostic Criteria and Guidelines: Clinical diagnosis should raise high suspicion for PID, particularly if the patient is an adolescent woman, and even in women denying sexual activity.

The CDC has recommended a minimal set of clinical criteria for the empirical treatment of PID which includes cervical motion tenderness or uterine/adnexal tenderness on bimanual exam in the presence of lower abdominal or pelvic pain.

Table 11: Clinical criteria for the empirical treatment of PID

CDC recommendation for the clinical criteria required for the empirical treatment of PID
• Oral temperature >101° F (>38.3°C)
• Abnormal cervical or vaginal mucopurulent discharge
• Presence of abundant numbers of white blood cells (WBCs) on saline microscopy of vaginal secretions
• Elevated erythrocyte sedimentation rate
• Elevated C-reactive protein

Table 12: Additional criteria used to support a clinical diagnosis in patients with pelvic pain

Additional criteria used to support a clinical diagnosis in patients with pelvic pain and tenderness include one or more of the following:
• Histologic results from biopsy demonstrate acute or chronic (plasma cell) endometritis or acute salpingitis
• C. trachomatis or N. gonorrhoeae is shown to be in the genital tract
• Laparotomy or laparoscopy demonstrate gross salpingitis
• Ability to isolate a pathogenic bacterium from an upper genital tract specimen
• Inflammatory/purulent pelvic peritoneal fluid showing no evidence of another cause

The CDC also has issued guidelines for the "definitive" diagnosis of PID in patients who are symptomatic.[72] One or more of the following three findings should be present to establish the diagnosis:

- Biopsy of the endometrium histologically shows evidence of endometritis
- Imaging displays thickened fluid-filled tubes/oviducts with or without tuboovarian complex or free pelvic fluid
- Laparoscopic examination abnormalities are consistent with PID (e.g., edema, tubal erythema, adhesions, abnormal fimbriae, purulent exudate or cul-de-sac fluid)

Guidelines for subclinical PID diagnosis remain to be established.

Differential Diagnosis

Table 13: Differential diagnosis of Pelvic Inflammatory Disease

• Endometriosis
• Appendicitis & other gastro conditions
• Appendicitis is unilateral and right sided
• PID is bilateral
• Ectopic pregnancy
• Always do a pregnancy test
• Urinary tract infection or stone
• "Ovarian cysts," ovarian torsion, ovarian tumor

Diagnostic Testing

There is no single test or combination of tests that are both sensitive and specific for the diagnosis of PID. The diagnostic tests for PID include laboratory studies beginning with a pregnancy test, urine and culture testing, looking for signs of inflammation, imaging studies, and microscopic evaluation of cervical or vaginal secretions. If the patient is diagnosed with acute PID, they should also receive an HIV test.[73]

Gram stain and microscopic examination of vaginal secretions may provide useful information. If a cervical Gram stain is positive for Gram negative intracellular diplococci the probability of PID greatly increases; if negative, it is of little use.[74]

Table 14: Recommended laboratory tests for diagnosing pelvic inflammatory disease

Recommended laboratory tests
• Pregnancy test
• Complete blood counts
• Urinalysis
• C-reactive protein (optional)
• Microscopic exam of vaginal discharge in saline
• Nucleic acid amplification tests for C. trachomatis and N. gonorrhoeae
• Hepatitis B surface antigen and surface antibody
• HIV testing
• Testing for syphilis

Imaging Techniques: A transvaginal ultrasound is better for the diagnosis of PID. The findings of thickened, fluid-filled oviducts support a PID diagnosis.

Laparoscopy: Laparoscopy is valuable in confirming a PID diagnosis. However, laparoscopy is not considered the gold standard for diagnosis because it is not sensitive enough. Laparoscopy is recommended for:

- A patient who is sick and there is a high suspicion other diagnosis (normally appendicitis)
- A patient who is acutely ill and failed outpatient PID treatment
- A patient who is not clearly improving after roughly 72 hours of inpatient PID treatment

Management

Pelvic inflammatory disease can be treated on an outpatient bases and necessity of hospitalization should be determined based on the severity of the disease. In patients with mild or moderate PID, the clinical trial data support an outpatient treatment approach. Early diagnosis and initiation of treatment are the key elements in preventing long-term sequelae, such as infertility and ectopic pregnancy. Recommended indications for hospitalization and parenteral antibiotics include:[75]

- Pregnancy
- Tolerance or no response to oral medications
- Therapy nonadherence
- Nausea and vomiting causing an inability to take oral medications
- Severe clinical illness (nausea, vomiting, high fever, severe abdominal pain)
- Complicated PID with pelvic abscess (including tubo-ovarian abscess)
- Potential need for surgery or diagnostic exploration for another etiology (e.g., appendicitis)

Recommended Regimens: The choice of antimicrobial therapy is determined mainly by the patient's need to be treated as an inpatient or outpatient. Patients who are candidates for outpatient treatment should be started on antibiotics with good activity against Neisseria gonorrhoeae and Chlamydia trachomatis. Anaerobic bacteria are frequently found in the patient with acute PID however there is no consensus whether anaerobic coverage is needed at all.[76,77]

First-Line Therapies for Inpatient Treatment of PID: In severe cases of PID requiring hospitalization, CDC recommendations include:

- Parenteral antibiotics: 2 g intravenous cefoxitin every 6 hours; 2 g intravenous cefotetan every 12 hours and 100 mg oral doxycycline every 12 hours.
- 900 mg intravenous clindamycin every 8 hours and gentamicin loading dose (2 mg/kg of body weight) then a maintenance dose (1.5 mg/kg) every 8 hours.
- 100 mg doxycycline twice daily for 14 days is given to complete the antibiotics.

Alternative Regimens: Alternative regimen offered by the CDC

- 3g intravenous ampicillin-sulbactam every 6 hours and 100 mg doxycycline twice daily; or 2 g cefoxitin every 6 hours and 100 mg doxycycline twice daily
- Monotherapy of azithromycin, azithromycin and metronidazole, or a combination regimen including a beta-lactam[78]

Outpatient Therapy: Patients who have mild or moderate PID can receive oral therapy as an outpatient. The clinical outcomes are equivalent with parenteral or oral therapy.

First-Line Regimens for Outpatient Treatment: The CDC recommendation for the outpatient treatment of PID, with or without metronidazole (500 mg twice a day for 14 days), includes:

- A single dose of 250 mg intramuscular ceftriaxone and 100 mg oral doxycycline twice a day for 14 days
- A single dose of 2 g intramuscular cefoxitin and a single dose of 1 g oral probenecid and 100 mg oral doxycycline twice a day for 14 days
- Another parenteral third-generation cephalosporins, such as a single dose of 1 g intramuscular cefotaxime or a single dose of 1 g intramuscular ceftizoxime with 100 mg oral doxycycline twice a day for 14 days
- Metronidazole is indicated in cases of Trichomonas vaginalis or if the woman has a recent history of uterine instrumentation.

Pregnant Patient: PID during pregnancy is quite a rare entity, however there is risk of infection during the first 12 weeks of gestation because the mucus plug and decidua have not yet sealed off the uterus from ascending bacteria. Pregnant patients with PID should be hospitalized for administration of parenteral antibiotics. The first-line treatment of PID in pregnant patients includes a second generation cephalosporin such as intravenous cefoxitin or cefotetan and 1 gram oral azithromycin (azithromycin is used instead of doxycycline).

Sex Partners: Along with the treatment of patient, it is important to also evaluate and treat the sex partner to reduce reinfection risk. If a male sex partner had sexual contact with a woman with PID within 60 days prior to the woman's symptoms, he should also have an examination and be treated, regardless of the woman's test results of a sexually transmitted infection. Treatment consists of antibiotics that are effective against Chlamydia trachomatis and Neisseria gonorrhoeae including intramuscular ceftriaxone (250 mg) and either a single dose of oral azithromycin (1 gram) or oral doxycycline (100 mg) twice daily for seven days.

Ectopic Pregnancy

Introduction

An ectopic pregnancy is an extrauterine pregnancy where the blastocyst does not implant into the uterine endometrium; the most common site of implantation being the fallopian tube (Figure 6).

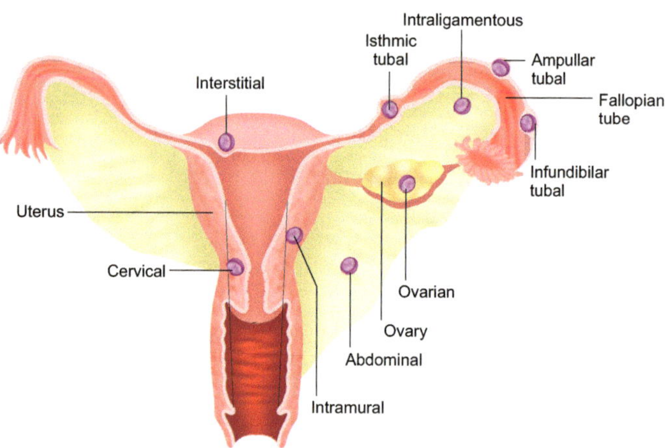

Figure 6: Locations of ectopic pregnancies

Epidemiology

The prevalence of ectopic pregnancy among women who present in the emergency department with first trimester bleeding, pain, or both, ranges from 6 to 16%.[79] In the United States between 1980 and 2007, 876 deaths were attributed to ectopic pregnancies.

Risk Factors

Risk factors for ectopic pregnancy can be separated into high, moderate, or low risk (Table 15).

Table 15: Risk factors for ectopic pregnancy

High Risk Factors	Previous ectopic pregnancy
	Previous tubal surgery
	Tubal pathology
	Tubal ligation
	In-utero DES exposure
	Current IUD use
Moderate Risk Factors	Infertility
	Previous cervicitis/genital infections (gonorrhea, Chlamydia)
	Multiple sexual partners
	In vitro fertilization
	History of pelvic inflammatory disease
	smoking
Low Risk Factors	Previous pelvic or abdominal surgery
	Vaginal douching
	Early age of intercourse (<18 years)

Pathology

The most common location of an ectopic pregnancy is in the fallopian tube (98%) especially in the ampulla (70%). The rest of ectopic pregnancies are approximately equally divided between the isthmus and fimbriae ends. Several factors may be involved in the pathogenesis of tubal pregnancies, and they are generally believed to be due to (1) conditions that prevent or delay fertilized oocyte passage into the uterine cavity (e.g., salpingitis isthmica nodosa or chronic salpingitis) or (2) inherent factors of the embryo resulting in premature implantation.

Clinical Presentation

A first trimester ectopic pregnancy will often present with vaginal bleeding and/or abdominal pain six to eight weeks after the woman's last normal menstrual period. However, symptoms may present later, or some patients may even be asymptomatic, especially in an extrauterine, non-fallopian tube ectopic pregnancy.

Tubal rupture (or rupture of the affected structures) can lead to life-threatening hemorrhage. Therefore, it is important to note any symptoms that suggest rupture (e.g., abdominal pain that is severe or persistent) or symptoms that suggest ongoing bleeding (e.g., loss of consciousness or feeling faint).

Evaluation of Women with Suspected Ectopic Pregnancy

History: A complete history including menstrual history and a calculated estimate of the gestational age should be taken. The history should focus on the presence and characteristics of vaginal bleeding and abdominal pain.

Physical Examination: The patient's hemodynamic status should be assessed immediately by measuring the complete set of vital signs. An abdominal exam is generally either unremarkable or shows tenderness of the lower abdomen. In cases of rupture with significant bleeding, the patient may have a distended abdomen, or localized and/or rebound tenderness to palpation.

It is mandatory to perform a complete pelvic exam. The speculum exam confirms a uterine source of bleeding, instead of a vaginal or cervical source, and assesses the volume of blood by the amount in the vagina and seeing if there is active bleeding from the cervix.

It is common for the bimanual pelvic exam to be unremarkable if the woman has a small, unruptured pregnancy. Findings on examination may include cervical motion, adnexal, and/or abdominal tenderness. An adnexal mass is noted in some women.

Transvaginal Ultrasound: TVS is the most useful imaging test and is the principal approach used for sonographic evaluation of pregnancy of unknown location. TVS should be performed as part of the initial evaluation and may need to be repeated, depending upon the hCG level or a suspicion of rupture. An adnexal mass is present on ultrasound in 89% or more of ectopic pregnancies.[80,81]

Human Chorionic Gonadotropin: hCG measurements are obtained for pregnancy diagnosis and then used to test for an ectopic pregnancy. During diagnosis of a suspected ectopic pregnancy, a serial serum hCG is obtained (typically every two days) to see if there are increased levels which is consistent with an abnormal pregnancy

Laparoscopy: If hCG levels and ultrasound are inconclusive, laparoscopy can confirm a diagnosis of ectopic pregnancy. In the case where an ectopic pregnancy is discovered laparoscopy, it should be treated immediately with surgery because additional risk comes with a medical approach, and it has not been proven to be beneficial.

Culdocentesis: Culdocentesis used to be used to detect blood in the posterior cul-de-sac. Now transvaginal ultrasound is also used. Bleeding due to an unruptured or ruptured tubal pregnancy can result in blood in the posterior cul-de-sac. However, the blood can also be from a ruptured ovarian cyst, thus a culdocentesis with blood is nondiagnostic of an ectopic pregnancy.

Uncommon Sites of Ectopic Pregnancy: Though uncommon, it is possible for an ectopic pregnancy to occur in other locations, or even bilaterally, and thus must be considered by the physician. Such locations include a hysterotomy scar, cervical, interstitial, abdominal, rudimentary uterine horn, and ovarian.

Management

Ectopic pregnancy is a potentially life-threatening condition. Surgery has been the mainstay treatment; however, in the 1980s, medical therapy (i.e., methotrexate or MTX) was introduced with advances in early diagnosis.[82] Early diagnosis due to routine ultrasounds in infertile patients who conceive has enabled the use of medical treatment for ectopic pregnancy. Ectopic pregnancy can be managed with surgery (salpingostomy or salpingectomy), medical therapy (MTX), or expectant management. About one-third of women can use MTX as management.[83] Everyone else requires surgery due to various reasons including a large ectopic pregnancy, suspicion of a ruptured tube, inability of patients to comply with follow-up during MTX therapy, or a preference for surgery. Few patients will be eligible for expectant management.

Expectant Management: When an ectopic pregnancy is suspected, expectant management is employed only for patients who meet the following criteria:

- Transvaginal ultrasound (TVUS) does not show a gestational sac or demonstrate an extrauterine mass suspicious for an ectopic pregnancy

- The beta-human chorionic gonadotropin (hCG) concentration is low (≤200 mIU/mL) and declining.[101]

Patients treated with expectant management should be monitored closely. Tubal rupture has been reported in women with low and declining hCG levels. Following the hCG level every 48 hours for three measurements is suggested to confirm continual declining of hCG, and then weekly until it is undetectable, at which point tubal rupture is highly unlikely.

Medical Treatment: MTX therapy provides a noninvasive, safe treatment with comparable efficacy and fertility outcomes when compared to laparoscopic salpingostomy. Additionally, it avoids surgical complications.[84,85] The optimal candidates for MTX treatment of ectopic pregnancy are:

- Hemodynamically stable patient
- hCG ≤5000 mIU/mL
- Absent cardiac activity of the fetus
- Ectopic mass <3 to 4 cm in size
- Patient can and will comply with post-treatment follow-up

Surgical Management: Surgical treatment of an ectopic pregnancy is advantageous because it requires less time to treat and avoids the need for prolonged monitoring. Surgery is indicated for emergency or urgent cases, if MTX is contraindicated or will probably be unsuccessful, or if the patient is already undergoing another surgical procedure. If a woman is hemodynamically stable, surgery is only performed if transvaginal ultrasound clearly shows an adnexal mass suggestive of ectopic pregnancy or shows a tubal ectopic pregnancy.

Table 16: Indications for surgery in patients with ectopic pregnancy

Surgical Indications	
1. Emergency surgery is required	• Hemodynamically unstable
	• If the patient is showing signs and symptoms of approaching or ongoing ectopic mass rupture (e.g., abdominal or pelvic pain or intraperitoneal bleeding suggesting rupture)
2. Indications for concurrent surgical procedure	• Patient desires sterilization
	• There is a plan for futurein vitro fertilization (IVF) with known hydrosalpinx (removing the hydrosalpinges increase the chances of a successful IVF)
3. Contraindications to MTX therapy	
4. Failed medical therapy	

Salpingostomy versus Salpingectomy: The two options for treating tubal pregnancy include salpingostomy (fallopian tube removal) and salpingectomy (tube incision to remove the gestation, leaving the rest of the tube intact). The standard procedure has traditionally been performing a salpingectomy; however, salpingostomy is a more conservative option for women and is also performed often.[100] The choice of salpingostomy or salpingectomy relies upon many factors and includes shared decision-making between the surgeon and patient. Both procedures have shown similar fertility outcomes in future pregnancies.

Salpingectomy: Salpingectomy is the standard procedure if the condition of the tube is compromised (ruptured or disrupted), the gestation seems too large for removal with salpingostomy, or there is uncontrolled bleeding. Salpingectomy is advantageous for other cases because the future need for treatment can be avoided. For women who have completed childbearing, bilateral salpingectomy may be performed as permanent sterilization. Salpingectomy is required for women with:

- Ruptured tube
- Uncontrolled tubal bleeding
- Moderately or severely damaged tube
- A large tubal pregnancy. In our practice, we use 3 cm as the threshold

Salpingostomy: Salpingostomy consists of making an incision in the fallopian tube and removing the ectopic gestation. The advantage of salpingostomy is preservation of the tube for potential future fertility. Persistent ectopic pregnancy after salpingostomy occurs in 4 to 15% of cases.

Laparoscopy versus Laparotomy: The standard treatment of ectopic pregnancies is a laparoscopic surgery, including ectopic pregnancies with complications such as hemoperitoneum. However, if there is acute bleeding, laparotomy is sometimes preferred. The choice of which surgical approach to use is made by the surgeon with an anesthesiologist consult and consideration of the patient's clinical status.

Gynecologic Oncology

The general surgeon may often encounter common gynecologic malignancies in his or her practice. These include, and are not exclusive to, endometrial and ovarian cancer. Cervical cancer, though common in the reproductive-age group of women, is less commonly encountered in general surgical practice.

Endometrial Cancer

Introduction

Endometrial cancer is the fourth most common cancer in women, after breast, lung, and colorectal cancer. It remains the most common gynecologic malignancy in the United States.[85] About 70% of patients present with disease confined to the uterus at diagnosis, leading to a better overall prognosis.

Epidemiology and Risk Factors

Patients with endometrial cancers are usually older with multiple medical comorbidities. The peak age at diagnosis of ovarian cancer is between 65 and 69 years old.

There are two pathogenetic types of endometrial cancers:[86] Type I cancers (90%) are associated with unopposed estrogen exposure and have endometrioid pathology, are low grade, are diagnosed at an early stage, and have an excellent prognosis.

Type II cancers are high grade, they often have a papillary serous or clear cell pathology, are diagnosed at a later stage, and have a poorer prognosis overall.

Factors which increase the risk for endometrial cancer include increasing age, nulliparity, infertility, menstrual irregularities, early menarche and late menopause, estrogen use, tamoxifen use, polycystic ovarian syndrome, obesity, high fat diet, and hereditary nonpolyposis colon cancer (HNPCC) syndrome.[87,88]

Factors which decrease the risk for endometrial cancer include the use of oral contraceptives, the use of non-medicated IUDs, phytoestrogens in diet, and physical activity.

Screening: Patients with HNPCC may consider chemoprevention with OCPs, and surveillance with serial endometrial biopsies and TVS, or risk-reducing surgery with hysterectomy and bilateral salpingo-oophorectomy.

Diagnosis

The most common presenting symptom of uterine cancer is post-menopausal bleeding. In pre-menopausal women, irregular or heavy vaginal bleeding is the most common presentation. All patients with post-menopausal bleeding, and any woman older than 35 years old with abnormal bleeding, should have endometrial sampling for possible endometrial cancer. Young women with risk factors such as PCOS, obesity, and early menarche should also undergo endometrial sampling.

A thorough history and physical is important to assess for symptoms of metastatic disease, such as abdominal/pelvic pain, bowel or bladder symptoms, lower extremity pain or swelling, early satiety, shortness of breath, or cough. The medical history gives information of cardiovascular risk and comorbid conditions.

A physical examination is helpful to look for signs of metastatic disease such as supraclavicular lymphadenopathy, ascites, palpable abdominal masses, and bipedal edema. A pelvic examination is mandatory as part of the initial physical examination to assess for uterine size and mobility, and evidence of extrauterine extension such as nodularity in the cul-de-sac or adnexal mass.

Transvaginal pelvic ultrasound to evaluate for endometrial thickness should be used as a first step in evaluation of post-menopausal bleeding.[89] An endometrial stripe thickness >4 mm is further evaluated with an office endometrial biopsy.[90,91] D&C is reserved for those in whom endometrial sampling is unsuccessful or inadequate (Figure 7).

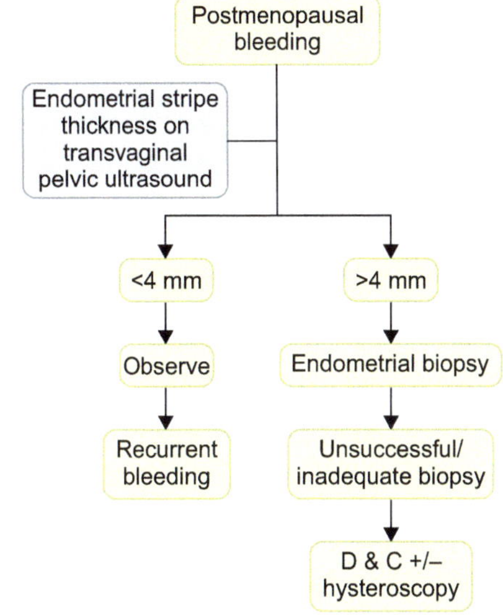

Figure 7: Management of postmenopausal bleeding

Treatment

Treatment of endometrial cancers is primarily surgical and based on the staging of the tumor.

Table 17: The current FIGO staging of endometrial cancer

Stage I	Tumor confined to body of uterus
IA	Limited to endometrium or invades <½ of myometrium
IB	Invades ≥½ of myometrium
Stage II	Invades cervix but does not extend beyond uterus
Stage III	Extension beyond the uterus
IIIA	Involves serosa and/or adnexa
IIIB	Vaginal or parametrial involvement
IIIC	Pelvic/paraaortic node involvement
Stage IV	Invades bladder, or bowel mucosa, or distant metastases

Risk Stratification

A full set of pre-operative labs should be ordered. This includes a complete blood count, electrolytes, hepatic, and renal function tests. An EKG helps with cardiac risk stratification. A chest X-ray should be obtained for pulmonary evaluation as well as to look for metastatic disease. A preoperative anesthesia consultation should be obtained for surgery clearance. The patient should be medically optimized before surgery is planned.

Surgery

In patients who are at acceptable surgical risk, surgery is the primary mode of treatment. In patients with Stage III or IV endometrial cancer, cytoreductive surgery has a survival benefit.[91,92] Patients with Stage I or II uterine cancers who are not surgical candidates, can be treated with primary pelvic radiotherapy, although the median survival is poorer in this group than operable patients.[93] Vaginal hysterectomy is another option for selected patients who are poor candidates due to comorbid conditions.

Steps of surgery include the following:

- Incision: Lower midline incision
- Peritoneal washings: Pelvic organs are washed with 50-100 cc of saline, and the fluid is sent for malignant cells
- Systematic exploration of the peritoneal cavity: This is done to look for pelvic/peritoneal metastasis. This includes inspecting the omentum, stomach, liver, peritoneal surfaces, paracolic gutters, kidneys, undersurface of the diaphragm, anterior surface of the colon and small bowel, and nodal palpation from the lower border of the pancreas down to the pelvic nodes. The three most common lymphatic basins of spread for uterine cancer include pelvic (paracervical and parametrial lymphatics), paraaortic (ovarian lymphatics), and inguinal (round ligament lymphatics).
- Grasp the cornua: After Trendelenburg positioning, packing of the bowel, and application of retractors, the uterine cornua are grasped with Kelly clamps to prevent spillage of cancer cells through the fallopian tubes.
- Ligation and transection of the round ligament
- Incision of the pelvic peritoneum 1 cm lateral and parallel to the infundibulopelvic ligament
- Identification and preservation of the ureters: The ureter is most easy to identify as it crosses the common iliac bifurcation at the pelvic brim. Visible peristalsis and palpation are used to confirm the ureter.
- Division of the infundibulopelvic ligament
- Skeletonization of the utero-ovarian ligament
- Incision of the vesicoureteral ligament and dissection of the bladder
- Clamping and division of the uterine arteries
- Clamping and division of the cardinal ligament: It is important to apply the clamp with the tip perpendicular to the cervix, with 1-1.5 centimeters of tissue in each bite, with subsequent clamps being applied medial to the previous clamps to avoid ureteric injury.
- Transection of the cervicovaginal junction, and closure of the vaginal stump
- Pelvic lymphadenectomy: Remove all tissue anterior and medial to the common and external iliac arteries, medial to the external iliac vein, and anterior to the hypogastric artery, extending distally to crossing of the circumflex iliac vein over the common iliac artery.
- Paraaortic lymphadenectomy: From the level of the inferior mesenteric artery to the level of the common iliac bifurcation on the anterior surface of the aorta and inferior vena cava.

Adjuvant Treatment

For Stage IA or IB, grade 1 or 2 uterine cancers, no further treatment is required postoperatively.[94] Patients with Stage IB, grade 2 or 3, and stage IC, grade 1 or 2 cancers have shown reduced rates of pelvic recurrence after adjuvant pelvic radiation.[95] Stage IC, grade 3 patients do better with adjuvant radiation in terms of 5-year survival, but the survival benefit should be balanced against the risk of pelvic complications. Positive lymph nodes warrant postoperative external beam radiotherapy to the involved nodal basins.[94]

Systemic chemotherapy with doxorubicin and platinum is reserved for recurrent or advanced endometrial cancer. Hormonal therapy with progestins and tamoxifen is another option for advanced endometrial cancers.

Follow-Up

Surveillance includes a physical exam every 3 months for 2 years, then every 6 to 12 months. A CT scan should be done every 3 to 6 months for 2 to 3 years, then every 6 months for the next 2 years, or as clinically indicated.[96]

Ovarian Cancer

Introduction

The incidence of epithelial ovarian cancer is relatively low when compared with that of breast, colon, and lung cancer. Ninety percent of primary ovarian tumors are derived from epithelial cells. When an ovarian mass is detected, biopsy is not routinely recommended as this can disseminate tumor cells in the peritoneal cavity. Surgery is typically required for definitive diagnosis.

Epidemiology and Risk Factors

Ovarian cancer is predominantly a disease of postmenopausal women. The peak age of ovarian cancer diagnosis is 65 to 75 years old. It is rare in premenopausal women under 40 years old, unless they have a genetic predisposition for the disease like BRCA1/BRCA2 gene mutations, and MSH2 and MLH1 mutations in hereditary nonpolyposis colorectal cancer syndrome.

Factors which increase the risk for ovarian cancer include nulliparity,[97] estrogen use, talc use,[98] and a positive family history. Factors which decrease the risk for ovarian cancer include multiparity, breastfeeding and tubal ligation, and use of oral contraceptives (OCPs).[99] OCPs decrease the risk of ovarian cancer by as much as 50%, with the protective effect lasting up to 20 years after OCP cessation.

Screening: A trans-vaginal ultrasound and a serum CA-125 assay are most effective for the screening of ovarian cancer. In a postmenopausal patient, a CA-125 value greater than 65 units/mL is almost diagnostic of malignancy, with 98% specificity. In premenopausal patients, elevations between 35 and 65 units/mL are associated with a 50% to 60% risk of cancer.

Diagnosis

The symptoms of early-stage ovarian cancer are vague and nonspecific, including abdominal bloating or pain, indigestion, urinary frequency, and constipation. Most patients tend to ignore their symptoms, or a wrong diagnosis is made because of the non-specific nature of their symptoms. Symptoms of advanced ovarian cancer include abdominal distention, fatigue, and weight loss. Metastatic disease may present as vaginal bleeding (uterine involvement or excess estrogen production by ovarian stromal tumor), shortness of breath (pleural effusion), or palpable inguinal nodes.

Abdominal examination often shows signs of ascites with distention and a fluid wave. The presence of a pelvic or adnexal mass in a postmenopausal woman is suspicious for ovarian cancer. A similar mass in a premenopausal woman has a much lower predictive value for the presence of cancer.

Elevated serum CA-125 values (normal <35 units/mL) are found in more than 80% of patients with advanced ovarian cancer. CA-125 is elevated only in 25-50% of early ovarian cancer women.

Findings on ultrasonography suggestive of ovarian cancer include a solid mass, a cyst with thick septations, and ascites. Transvaginal ultrasound (TVS) is most accurate in assessing tumor size and morphology. An abdominal ultrasound may also be necessary in some patents to determine the full extent of their tumor. TVS also gives information about intrauterine tumors and ascites. A CT scan of the abdomen and pelvis is recommended to define the extent of disease. However, results of these imaging techniques are not sensitive enough to outweigh findings based on the history and physical examination when establishing the diagnosis. PET scanning and MRI are not usually recommended. If the imaging is strongly suggestive of ovarian cancer, the diagnosis may be made at the time of a surgical debulking procedure.

Table 18: Staging for ovarian cancer

Stage I	Limited to ovaries
IA	Limited to one ovary
IB	Limited to both ovaries
IC	IA or IB with tumor on the surface, capsule rupture, malignant ascites, or positive peritoneal washings
Stage II	Involving one or both ovaries with pelvic extension
IIA	Involvement of uterus or fallopian tubes
IIB	Extension to other pelvic tissues
IIC	IIA or IIB with tumor on the surface, capsule rupture, malignant ascites, or positive peritoneal washings
Stage III	Involving one or both ovaries with extension or metastases outside the true pelvis
IIIA	No gross extra-pelvic tumor, + microscopic seeding on histology
IIIB	Histologically confirmed peritoneal implants <2 cm, negative nodes
IIIC	>2 cm implants, and/or + retroperitoneal/inguinal nodes
Stage IV	Distant metastasis

Risk Stratification

Every patient with an ovarian tumor should undergo medical risk stratification for surgery. This includes routine hematologic and biochemical testing, chest X-ray, EKG (if >40 years old), and evaluation of their cardiac and functional status.

Surgery

Surgery is needed for tumor diagnosis, staging, and treatment. The extent of cancer found at surgery defines the stage and guides further treatment decisions. Surgery involves the evaluation of the primary tumor and the potential sites of intra-abdominal spread.

Optimal surgical staging includes the following steps (Figure 8):

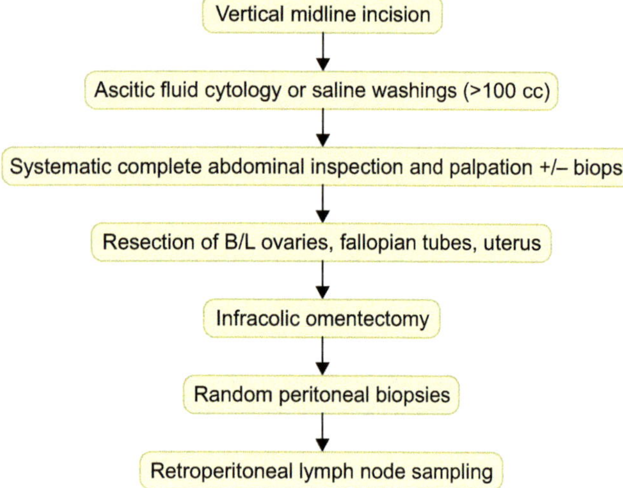

Figure 8: Optimal surgical staging

Adjuvant Treatment

For patients with malignant ovarian germ cell tumors, post operative chemotherapy with BEP (Bleomycin, Etoposide, Cisplatin) is the standard treatment.[101] For high-risk early-stage sex-cord stromal tumors, either the BEP regime or paclitaxel-carboplatin combination chemotherapy may be used.

Follow-Up

After completion of treatment, follow-ups are scheduled every 3 to 6 months for 5 years, then annually. A follow-up visit includes a history and physical exam including a pelvic exam and obtaining CA-125 level, a complete blood count, and a chemistry panel. An ultrasound performed as indicated. Clinical relapse is treated with surgical debulking if appropriate with or without adjuvant chemotherapy or hypecthesmic intrapecitoreal chemotherapy (HIPIEC).

REFERENCES

1. Kumar V, Abbas AK, Fausto N, et al. Robbins and Cotran Pathologic Basis of Disease, Professional Edition, 8th ed, Saunders, Philadelphia 2009.
2. Ramanah R, Berger MB, Parratte BM, DeLancey JO, Int Urogynecol J. Anatomy and histology of apical support: a literature review concerning cardinal and uterosacral ligaments. 2012 Nov;23(11):1483-94. Epub 2012 May 23.
3. Black MM, McKay M, Braude PR. Color atlas and text of obstetric and gynecologic dermatology, Mosby Wolfe, London 1995. p.119.
4. McPherson T, Cooper S. Vulval lichen sclerosus and lichen planus. Dermatol Ther. 2010 Sep-Oct;23(5):523-32. doi: 10.1111/j.1529-8019.2010.01355.x. PMID: 20868406.
5. Funaro D. Lichen sclerosus: a review and practical approach. Dermatol Ther. 2004;17(1):28.
6. Neill SM, Lewis FM, Tatnall FM, Cox NH. British Association of Dermatologists ' guidelines for the management of lichen sclerosus 2010. British Association of Dermatologists. Br J Dermatol. 2010;163(4):672.
7. Bercaw-Pratt JL, Boardman LA, Simms-Cendan JS. Clinical recommendation: pediatric lichen sclerosus. North American Society for Pediatric and Adolescent Gynecology. J Pediatr Adolesc Gynecol. 2014 Apr;27(2):111-6.
8. Dendrinos ML, Quint EH. Lichen sclerosus in children and adolescents. Curr Opin Obstet Gynecol. 2013 Oct;25(5):370-4.
9. Regauer S, Liegl B, Reich O. Early vulvar lichen sclerosus: a histopathological challenge. Histopathology. 2005 Oct;47(4):340-7.
10. Carli P, Cattaneo A, De Magnis A, Biggeri A, Taddei G, Giannotti B. Squamous cell carcinoma arising in vulval lichen sclerosus: a longitudinal cohort study. Eur J Cancer Prev. 1995;4(6):491.
11. Leibowitch M, Neill S, Pelisse M, Moyal-Baracco M. The epithelial changes associated with squamous cell carcinoma of the vulva: a review of the clinical, histological, and viral findings in 78 women. Br J Obstet Gynaecol. 1990;97(12):1135.
12. Zaki I, Dalziel KL, Solomonsz FA, Stevens A. The under-reporting of skin disease in association with squamous cell carcinoma of the vulva. Clin Exp Dermatol. 1996;21(5):334.
13. Mazdisnian F, Degregorio F, Mazdisnian F, Palmieri A. Intralesional injection of triamcinolone in the treatment of lichen sclerosus. J Reprod Med. 1999;44(4):332.
14. Simonart T, Lahaye M, Simonart JM. Vulvar lichen sclerosus: effect of maintenance treatment with a moisturizer on the course of the disease. Menopause. 2008 Jan;15(1):74-7.
15. Niinimäki A, Kallioinen M, Oikarinen A. Etretinate reduces connective tissue degeneration in lichen sclerosus et atrophicus. Acta Derm Venereol. 1989;69(5):439.
16. Borgfeldt C, Andolf E. Transvaginal sonographic ovarian findings in a random sample of women 25-40 years old. Ultrasound Obstet Gynecol. 1999;13(5):345.

17. Castillo G, Alcázar JL, Jurado M. Natural history of sonographically detected simple unilocular adnexal cysts in asymptomatic postmenopausal women. Gynecol Oncol. 2004;92(3):965.

18. Norris HJ, Jensen RD. Relative frequency of ovarian neoplasms in children and adolescents. Cancer 1972;30(3):713.

19. Kinkel K, Lu Y, Mehdizade A, Pelte MF, Hricak H. Indeterminate ovarian mass at US: incremental value of second imaging test for characterization--meta-analysis and Bayesian analysis. Radiology. 2005;236(1):85.

20. Bourne T, Campbell S, Steer C, Whitehead MI, Collins WP. Transvaginal colour flow imaging: a possible new screening technique for ovarian cancer. BMJ. 1989;299(6712):1367.

21. Bast RC Jr, Klug TL, St John E, et al. A radioimmunoassay using a monoclonal antibody to monitor the course of epithelial ovarian cancer. N Engl J Med.1983;309(15):883.

22. Baird DD, Dunson DB, Hill MC, Cousins D, Schectman JM. High cumulative incidence of uterine leiomyoma in black and white women: ultrasound evidence. Am J Obstet Gynecol. 2003;188(1):100.

23. Buttram VC Jr, Reiter RC. Uterine leiomyomata: etiology, symptomatology, and management. Fertil Steril. 1981;36(4):433.

24. Serden SP, Brooks PG. Treatment of abnormal uterine bleeding with the gynecologic resectoscope. J Reprod Med. 1991;36(10):697.

25. Munro MG, Critchley HO, Fraser IS. The FIGO classification of causes of abnormal uterine bleeding in the reproductive years. FIGO Menstrual Disorders Working Group. Fertil Steril. 2011 Jun;95(7):2204-8, 2208.

26. Cramer SF, Patel A. The frequency of uterine leiomyomas. Am J Clin Pathol. 1990;94(4):435.

27. Downes E, Sikirica V, Gilabert- Estelles J, Bolge SC, Dodd SL, Maroulis C, Subramanian D. The burden of uterine fibroids in five European countries. Eur J Obstet Gynecol Reprod Biol. 2010;152(1):96.

28. Templeman C, Marshall SF, Clarke CA, et al. Risk factors for surgically removed fibroids in a large cohort of teachers. Fertil Steril. 2009;92(4):1436.

29. Marshall LM, Spiegelman D, Barbieri RL, Goldman MB, Manson JE, Colditz GA, Willett WC, Hunter DJ. Variation in the incidence of uterine leiomyoma among premenopausal women by age and race. Obstet Gynecol. 1997;90(6):967.

30. Wise LA, Palmer JR, Harlow BL, Spiegelman D, Stewart EA, Adams-Campbell LL, Rosenberg L. Reproductive factors, hormonal contraception, and risk of uterine leiomyomata in African-American women: a prospective study. Am J Epidemiol. 2004;159(2):113.

31. Ross RK, Pike MC, Vessey MP, Bull D, Yeates D, Casagrande JT. Risk factors for uterine fibroids: reduced risk associated with oral contraceptives. Br Med J (Clin Res Ed). 1986;293(6543):359.

32. Chiaffarino F, Parazzini F, La Vecchia C, Marsico S, Surace M, Ricci E. Use of oral contraceptives and uterine fibroids: results from a case-control study. Br J Obstet Gynaecol. 1999;106(8):857.

33. Parazzini F, Negri E, La Vecchia C, Fedele L, Rabaiotti M, Luchini L. Oral contraceptive use and risk of uterine fibroids. Obstet Gynecol. 1992;79(3):430.

34. Lumbiganon P, Rugpao S, Phandhu-fung S, Laopaiboon M, Vudhikamraksa N, Werawatakul Y. Protective effect of depot-medroxyprogesterone acetate on surgically treated uterine leiomyomas: a multicentre case--control study. Br J Obstet Gynaecol. 1996;103(9):909.

35. Fraser IS, Critchley HO, Munro MG, Broder M. A process designed to lead to international agreement on terminologies and definitions used to describe abnormalities of menstrual bleeding. Writing Group for this Menstrual Agreement Process. Fertil Steril. 2007;87(3):466.

36. Wamsteker K, Emanuel MH, de Kruif JH. Transcervical hysteroscopic resection of submucous fibroids for abnormal uterine bleeding: results regarding the degree of intramural extension. Obstet Gynecol. 1993;82(5):736.

37. Wegienka G, Baird DD, Hertz-Picciotto I, et al. Self-reported heavy bleeding associated with uterine leiomyomata. Obstet Gynecol. 2003;101(3):431.

38. Puri K, Famuyide AO, Erwin PJ, Stewart EA, Laughlin-Tommaso SK. Submucosal fibroids and the relation to heavy menstrual bleeding and anemia. Am J Obstet Gynecol. 2014 Jan;210(1):38.e1-7.

39. Stewart EA, Nowak RA. Leiomyoma-related bleeding: a classic hypothesis updated for the molecular era. Hum Reprod Update. 1996;2(4):295.

40. Fletcher H, Wharfe G, Williams NP, Gordon-Strachan G, Pedican M, Brooks A. Venous thromboembolism as a complication of uterine fibroids: a retrospective descriptive study. J Obstet Gynaecol. 2009 Nov;29(8):732-6.

41. Shiota M, Kotani Y, Umemoto M, Tobiume T, Tsuritani M, Shimaoka M, Hoshiai H. Deep-vein thrombosis is associated with large uterine fibroids. Tohoku J Exp Med. 2011;224(2):87-9.

42. Rosenfeld H, Byard RW. Lower extremity deep venous thrombosis with fatal pulmonary thromboembolism caused by benign pelvic space-occupying lesions--an overview. J Forensic Sci. 2012;57(3):665.
43. Yoshida M, Koshiyama M, Fujii H, Konishi M. Erythrocytosis and a fibroid. Lancet. 1999;354(9174):216.
44. Ravakhah K, Gover A, Mukunda BN. Humoral hypercalcemia associated with a uterine fibroid. Ann Intern Med. 1999;130(8):702. 10215576.
45. Bradley LD, Falcone T, Magen AB. Complete remission of hyperprolactinemia and erythrocytosis after hysterectomy for a uterine fibroid in a woman with a previous diagnosis of prolactin-secreting pituitary microadenoma. Cordiano V.Ann Hematol. 2005;84(3):200.61.
46. Dueholm M, Lundorf E, Hansen ES, Ledertoug S, Olesen F. Accuracy of magnetic resonance imaging and transvaginal ultrasonography in the diagnosis, mapping, and measurement of uterine myomas. Am J Obstet Gynecol. 2002;186(3):409.
47. Carlson KJ, Miller BA, Fowler FJ Jr. The Maine Women and Health Study: II. Outcomes of nonsurgical management of leiomyomas, abnormal bleeding, and chronic pelvic pain. Obstet Gynecol. 1994;83(4):566.
48. Friedman AJ, Barbieri RL, Doubilet PM, Fine C, Schiff I. A randomized, double-blind trial of a gonadotropin releasing-hormone agonist (leuprolide) with or without medroxyprogesterone acetate in the treatment of leiomyomata uteri. Fertil Steril.1988;49(3):404.
49. Carr BR, Marshburn PB, Weatherall PT, et al. An evaluation of the effect of gonadotropin-releasing hormone analogs and medroxyprogesterone acetate on uterine leiomyomata volume by magnetic resonance imaging: a prospective, randomized, double blind, placebo-controlled, crossover trial. J ClinEndocrinol Metab. 1993;76(5):1217.
50. Friedman AJ, Barbieri RL, Doubilet PM, Fine C, Schiff I. A randomized, double-blind trial of a gonadotropin releasing-hormone agonist (leuprolide) with or without medroxyprogesterone acetate in the treatment of leiomyomata uteri. Fertil Steril. 1988;49(3):404.
51. Carr BR, Marshburn PB, Weatherall PT, Bradshaw KD, Breslau NA, Byrd W, Roark M, Steinkampf MP. An evaluation of the effect of gonadotropin-releasing hormone analogs and medroxyprogesterone acetate on uterine leiomyomata volume by magnetic resonance imaging: a prospective, randomized, double blind, placebo-controlled, crossover trial. J Clin Endocrinol Metab. 1993;76(5):1217.
52. Minaguchi H, Wong JM, Snabes MC. Clinical use of nafarelin in the treatment of leiomyomas. A review of the literature. J Reprod Med. 2000;45(6):481.
53. Shozu M, Murakami K, Segawa T, Kasai T, Inoue M. Successful treatment of a symptomatic uterine leiomyoma in a perimenopausal woman with a nonsteroidal aromatase inhibitor. Fertil Steril. 2003;79(3):628.
54. Parsanezhad ME, Azmoon M, Alborzi S, Rajaeefard A, Zarei A, Kazerooni T, Frank V, Schmidt EH. A randomized, controlled clinical trial comparing the effects of aromatase inhibitor (letrozole) and gonadotropin-releasing hormone agonist (triptorelin) on uterine leiomyoma volume and hormonal status. Fertil Steril. 2010 Jan;93(1):192-8. Epub 2009 Jan9.
55. Lethaby A, Farquhar C, Cooke I. Antifibrinolytics for heavy menstrual bleeding. Cochrane Database Syst Rev 2000:CD000249.
56. Mäkäräinen L, Ylikorkala O. Primary and myoma-associated menorrhagia: role of prostaglandins and effects of ibuprofen. Br J Obstet Gynaecol. 1986;93(9):974.
57. Ylikorkala O, Pekonen F. Naproxen reduces idiopathic but not fibromyoma-induced menorrhagia. Obstet Gynecol. 1986;68(1):10.
58. Goldfarb HA. Laparoscopic coagulation of myoma (myolysis). Obstet Gynecol Clin North Am. 1995;22(4):807.
59. Zupi E, Piredda A, Marconi D, Townsend D, Exacoustos C, Arduini D, Szabolcs B. Directed laparoscopic cryomyolysis: a possible alternative to myomectomy and/or hysterectomy for symptomatic leiomyomas. Am J Obstet Gynecol. 2004;190(3):639.
60. Hald K, Langebrekke A, Kløw NE, Noreng HJ, Berge AB, Istre O. Laparoscopic occlusion of uterine vessels for the treatment of symptomatic fibroids: Initial experience and comparison to uterine artery embolization. Am J Obstet Gynecol. 2004;190(1):37.
61. Lichtinger M, Hallson L, Calvo P, Adeboyejo G. Laparoscopic uterine artery occlusion for symptomatic leiomyomas. J Am Assoc Gynecol Laparosc. 2002;9(2):191.
62. Hesley GK, Felmlee JP, Gebhart JB, Dunagan KT, Gorny KR, Kesler JB, Brandt KR, Glantz JN, Gostout BS. Noninvasive treatment of uterine fibroids: early Mayo Clinic experience with magnetic resonance imaging-guided focused ultrasound. Mayo Clin Proc. 2006;81(7):936.
63. Smart OC, Hindley JT, Regan L, Gedroyc WG. Gonadotrophin-releasing hormone and magnetic-

resonance-guided ultrasound surgery for uterine leiomyomata. Obstet Gynecol. 2006;108(1):49.

64. French CE, Hughes G, Nicholson A, Yung M, Ross JD, Williams T, Soldan K. Estimation of the rate of pelvic inflammatory disease diagnoses: trends in England, 2000-2008. Sex Transm Dis. 2011 Mar;38(3):158-62.
65. Galask RP, Larsen B, Ohm MJ, Vaginal flora and its role in disease entities. Clin Obstet Gynecol. 1976;19(1):61.
66. Centers for Disease Control and Prevention (CDC). Pelvic Inflammatory Disease (PID). http://www.cdc.gov/std/pid/stats.htm (Accessed on January 05, 2015).
67. Korn AP, Hessol NA, Padian NS, Bolan GA, Donegan E, Landers DV, Schachter J. Risk factors for plasma cell endometritis among women with cervical Neisseria gonorrhoeae, cervical Chlamydia trachomatis, or bacterial vaginosis. Am J Obstet Gynecol. 1998;178(5):987.
68. Westrom L, Mardh PA. Epidemiology, etiology, and prognosis of acute salpingitis: A study of 1,457 laparoscopically verified cases. In: Nongonococcal Urethritis and Related Diseases, Hobson D, Holmes KK (Eds), Am Soc Microbiol, Washington, DC 1977. p.84.
69. Stajano C. La reaccio and frenich en ginecologia. Semana Méd. 1920;27:243.
70. Müller-Schoop JW, Wang SP, Munzinger J, Schläpfer HU, Knoblauch M, Tammann RW. Chlamydia trachomatis as possible cause of peritonitis and perihepatitis in young women. Br Med J. 1978;1(6119):1022.
71. Wang SP, Eschenbach DA, Holmes KK, Wager G, Grayston JT. Chlamydia trachomatis infection in Fitz-Hugh-Curtis syndrome. Am J Obstet Gynecol. 1980;138(7 Pt 2):1034.
72. "CDC - STD Treatment." Centers for Disease Control and Prevention, Centers for Disease Control and Prevention, 24 Jan. 2022, https://www.cdc.gov/std/treatment/default.htm.
73. Eschenbach DA, Buchanan TM, Pollock HM, Forsyth PS, Alexander ER, Lin JS, Wang SP, Wentworth BB, MacCormack WM, Holmes KK. Polymicrobial etiology of acute pelvic inflammatory disease. N Engl J Med. 1975;293(4):166.
74. Sellors J, Mahony J, Goldsmith C, Rath D, Mander R, Hunter B, Taylor C, Groves D, Richardson H, Chernesky M. The accuracy of clinical findings and laparoscopy in pelvic inflammatory disease. Am J Obstet Gynecol. 1991;164(1 Pt 1):113.
75. Irwin KL, Moorman AC, Sullivan MJ, Sperling R, Koestler ME, Soto I, Rice R, Brodman M, Yasin S, Droese A, Zhang D, Schwartz DA, Byers RH. Influence of human immunodeficiency virus infection on pelvic inflammatory disease. Obstet Gynecol.2000;95(4):525.
76. McGregor JA, Crombleholme WR, Newton E, Sweet RL, Tuomala R, Gibbs RS. Randomized comparison of ampicillin-sulbactam to cefoxitin and doxycycline or clindamycin and gentamicin in the treatment of pelvic inflammatory disease or endometritis. Obstet Gynecol. 1994;83(6):998.
77. Comparative evaluation of clindamycin/gentamicin and cefoxitin/doxycycline for treatment of pelvic inflammatory disease: a multi-center trial. The European Study Group. Acta Obstet Gynecol Scand. 1992;71(2):129.
78. Murray H, Baakdah H, Bardell T, Tulandi T. Diagnosis and treatment of ectopic pregnancy. CMAJ. 2005;173(8):905.
79. Bouyer J, Coste J, Fernandez H, Pouly JL, Job-Spira N. Sites of ectopic pregnancy: a 10 year population-based study of 1800 cases. Hum Reprod. 2002;17(12):3224.
80. Condous G, Kirk E, Lu C, Van Huffel S, Gevaert O, De Moor B, De Smet F, Timmerman D, Bourne T. Diagnostic accuracy of varying discriminatory zones for the prediction of ectopic pregnancy in women with a pregnancy of unknown location. Ultrasound Obstet Gynecol. 2005;26(7):770.
81. Cepni I, Ocal P, Erkan S, Erzik B. Conservative treatment of cervical ectopic pregnancy with transvaginal ultrasound-guided aspiration and single-dose methotrexate. Fertil Steril. 2004;81(4):1130.
82. Stovall TG, Ling FW, Buster JE. Outpatient chemotherapy of unruptured ectopic pregnancy. Fertil Steril. 1989;51(3):435.
83. Hajenius PJ, Mol F, Mol BW, Bossuyt PM, Ankum WM, van der Veen F. Interventions for tubal ectopic pregnancy. Cochrane Database Syst Rev. 2007.
84. Korhonen J, Stenman UH, Ylöstalo P. Low-dose oral methotrexate with expectant management of ectopic pregnancy. Obstet Gynecol. 1996;88(5):775.
85. American Cancer Society. Cancer Facts and Figures 2015. Atlanta, GA: American Cancer Society; 2015.
86. Bockhman JV. Two pathogenetic types of endometrial carcinoma. Gynecol Oncol 1983;15:10.
87. Beral V, Bull D, Reeves G. Million Women Study Collaborators. Endometrial cancer and hormone-replacement therapy in the Million Women Study. Lancet 2005; 365:1543.
88. Brinton LA, Berman ML, Mortel R, et al. reproductive, menstrual and medical risk factors for endometrial

cancer: results of a case control study. Am J Obstet Gynecol 1992; 167:1317.

89. Clark TJ, Barton PM, Coomarsamy A, et al. Investigating postmenopausal bleeding for endometrial cancer: cost-effectiveness of initial diagnostic strategies. BJOG 2006;113:502.
90. Moodley M, Roberts C. Clinical pathway for the evaluation of postmenopausal bleeding with an emphasis on endometrial cancer detection. J Obstet Gynecol. 2004;24:736.
91. Gupta JK, Chien PF, Voit D, et al. Ultrasonographic endome trial thickness for diagnosing endometrial pathology in women with postmenopausal bleeding: a meta-analysis. Acta Obstet Gynecol Scand 2002;81:799.
92. Goff BA, Goodman A, Muntz HG. Surgical Stage IV endometrial carcinoma: a study of 47 cases. Gynecol Oncol 1994;52:237.
93. Fishman D, Roberts K, Chambers J, Kohorn E, Schwartz P, et al. Radiation therapy as exclusive treatment for medically inoperable patients with Stage I and II endometrioid carcinoma of the endometrium.
94. Creutzberg CL, Nout RA, Lybeert ML, Wárlám-Rodenhuis CC, Jobsen JJ, Mens JW, Lutgens LC, Pras E, van de Poll-Franse LV, van Putten WL. PORTEC Study Group. Fifteen-year radiotherapy outcomes of the randomized PORTEC-1 trial for endometrial carcinoma. Int J Radiat Oncol Biol Phys. 2011 Nov 15;81(4).
95. Straughn JM Jr, Huh WK, Kelly FJ, et al. Stage IC adenocarcinoma of the endometrium: survival comparisions of surgically staged patients with and without adjuvant therapy. Gynecol Oncol 2001;89:295.
96. Version 2. 2015. National Comprehensive Cancer Network Guidelines.
97. Whittemore AS, Harris R, Itnyre J. Corroborative Ovarian Cancer Group: characteristics relating to ovarian cancer risk, collaborative analysis of 12 U.S. case control studies. II. Invasive epithelial ovarian cancers in white women. Am J Epidemiol 1992; 136:1184.
98. Cook LS, Kamb ML, Weiss NS, et al. perineal powder exposure and risk of ovarian cancer. Am J Epidemiol 1997; 145:459.
99. Riman T, Dickman PW, Nilsson S, et al. Hormonal replacement therapy and risk of invasive epithelial ovarian cancer in Swedish women. J Natl Cancer Inst 2002;94:497.
100. Leblan E, Querleu D, Narducci F, et al. Lapaoscopic staging of early-stage invasive adnexal tumors: a 10-year experience. Gynecol Oncol 2004;94-624.
101. Homesley HD, Bundy BN, Huteau JA, et al. Bleomycin, etoposide, and cisplatinum combination therapy of ovarian granulose cell tumors and other stromal malignancies: a Gynecologic Oncology Group study. Gynecol Oncol 1999;72:131.

❑❑❑

71

CHAPTER

Orthopedics

Jonathan Egle, MD
Vijay K. Mittal, MD, FACS

INTRODUCTION

Orthopedics is "the medical specialty concerned with the preservation, restoration, and development of form and function of the musculoskeletal system, extremities, spine, and associated structures by medical, surgical, and physical methods."[1] The bulk of the specialty encompasses dealing with fractures to the axial and appendicular skeletons.

Prior to discussing specific pathologies, it is prudent to review some terminology specific to orthopedics, in order to facilitate comprehensive understanding:[1]

- Comminuted: broken into several pieces
- Diaphysis: the shaft of a long bone
- Displacement: the change in the form or position of tissues as a result of pressure
- Epiphysis: part of a long bone developed from a separate center of ossification than the diaphysis and separated from the diaphysis by a layer of cartilage
- External fixation: firmly attaching or setting by pins or screws drilled into the bony part through the overlying skin and connected by a metal bar
- Internal fixation: stabilization of fractured bony parts by direct attachment to one another with surgical wires, screws, pins, or plates
- Lamellar: a thin sheet or layer, such as compact bone
- Medulla: the soft center portion of bones
- Metaphysis: growth zone between the epiphysis and diaphysis during the development of a bone
- Reduction: restoration by manipulative procedures, of a part to its normal anatomical relation

Fracture Healing

Knowledge of the fundamentals of bony growth and healing patterns is critical to the understanding of proper management of orthopedic pathology. Bone has the ability to heal without forming a fibrous scar.[2] The remarkable regenerative capacity of bone, however, sometimes fails as bones heal in dysfunctional positions, do not heal in a timely fashion, or sometimes do not heal together at all. Fracture healing can be classified into one of two patterns: indirect or secondary healing, and direct or primary healing.

Indirect Healing

The most common form of bone healing is indirect.[2] This is the natural history of fracture healing, and it also occurs with casting, traction, external fixation, or intramedullary nailing. Micro-motion and weight bearing stimulate indirect fracture healing, though too much movement can be detrimental.

The mechanism of indirect healing is as follows: a hematoma forms around the fracture site following the initial trauma.[2] The ensuing inflammatory response causes coagulation of the hematoma, forming a template for callus formation. A brief period of pro-inflammatory state, marked by tumor necrosis factor-α (TNF-α), interleukin-1 (IL-1), IL-6, IL-11, and IL-18. Mesenchymal stem cells are recruited to the fracture site, proliferate, and form osteogenic cells. These osteogenic cells form a collagenous soft callus in the hematoma. Simultaneously, intramembranous ossification occurs subperiosteally at the proximal and distal ends of the fracture, bridging the gap between bones with a hard callus. To facilitate this process, angiopoietin and vascular endothelial growth factors act to promote angiogenesis, providing a blood supply for the newly forming bone.

Fracture chondrocytes, which produce the soft cartilaginous callus, proliferate, become hypertrophic, and the extracellular matrix becomes calcified. Osteoclasts and bone cells reabsorb this mineralized cartilage and form woven bone. As this occurs, the callus becomes more rigid. Finally, the remodeling phase begins with the high expression of IL-1 and TNF-α. Remodeling is a balance of callus resorption by osteoclasts and lamellar bone formation by osteoblasts which may take years to be fully complete. Axial loading causes temporary polarity of the long bone, which stimulates osteoblasts and osteoclasts to actively remodel the outer callus into lamellar bone and the inner callus into a medullary cavity.

Direct Healing

Direct healing, or primary healing, only occurs when fractures are adequately reduced and have no movement, as is the case after open reduction and internal fixation. Depending on the precision of reduction, primary healing occurs via either contact healing or gap healing.[2] When the gap between bone ends is less than 0.01 mm and there is less than 2% strain from one fragment to the next, contact healing occurs as osteoclasts cross the fracture line. These osteoclasts form longitudinal cavities which are filled in later by osteoblasts, thus bridging the fracture line and reconstructing the bone in the axial direction. The bony union is later remodeled, and lamellar bone is laid down. Thus, the bone heals without forming a periosteal callus.

Gap healing occurs when the fragments are within 0.8-1.0 mm. The fracture site is initially filled in by lamellar bone. This is subsequently replaced by osteoblasts, which produce lamellar bone perpendicular to the long axis. A secondary remodeling phase is necessary to restore the normal axis of the lamellar bone, and therefore the anatomical and biomechanical properties of the bone.

Factors Influencing Healing

The process of fracture healing is complex, and many factors can impede its progress. Disturbing the blood flow to the fracture will disrupt the supply of oxygen, inflammatory mediators, and osteoprogenitor cells.[3] Insufficient mechanical stability may cause too much motion for even indirect healing to take place. A poor nutritional state and age may serve as comorbidities that prevent the patient's reserve status from being able to accommodate an increased anabolic state. Smoking can decrease the microvascular supply to a healing fracture site. Also, medications such as steroids, chemotherapeutic agents, antibiotics, and NSAIDS have been shown to delay or impede fracture healing. However, a recent review has questioned the impact of NSAIDS, citing discrepancies within the published studies.[3]

Upper Extremity

Humerus

The humerus is the long bone of the proximal arm. The radial nerve travels in close proximity to the bone, traveling in the spiral groove posteriorly, placing it in significant risk of injury in association with a humeral shaft fracture.

Fractures of the humerus are a common orthopedic injury, accounting for 3% of all fractures (Figure 1). The management of humeral shaft fractures is largely non-operative. Alignment with a brace or sling can provide a sufficient degree of stabilization to allow for healing via callus formation.[4] Most patients can tolerate some degree of malalignment without untoward effects, including up to 20° in the sagittal plane and 30° degrees in the coronal plane. Success of union in non-surgical cases is typically reported to be greater than 90%.

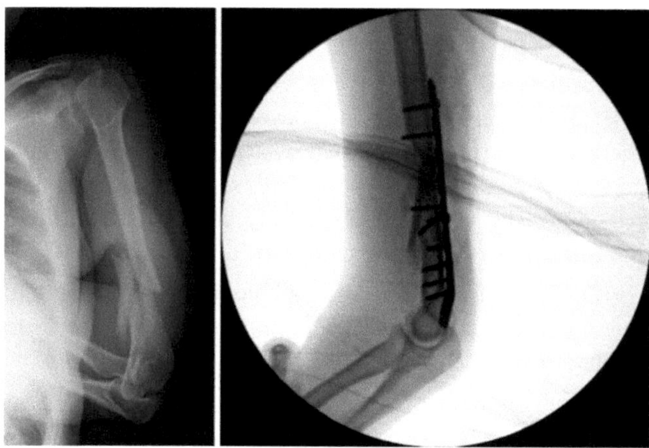

Figure 1: Fracture of humeral diaphysis with subsequent fixation

Stabilization of humeral shaft fractures can be attained via coaptation splinting. In order to prevent varus angulation, one must ensure that the axillary portion of the U-shaped splint terminates proximal to the fracture site. Coaptation splinting, however, is often poorly tolerated. Alternatively, posterior splints may be used for distal fractures, and slings can be considered for proximal fractures.

A circumferential brace, referred to as a Sarmiento brace, provides pressure and allows continued function with the injured limb, and has become the standard of care for most humeral shaft fractures.[4] The brace is left in place for 5-7 days before continuing with more traditional coaptation splinting. The Sarmiento brace allows for immediate initiation of range of elbow motion exercises, though shoulder immobility must be maintained.

Not all patients are candidates for non-operative management. Patients with open fractures, articular extension of the fractures, neurovascular injuries, floating elbow, or failure of closed management must be considered for surgical repair. Open fractures of the humerus, like other open fractures, are managed with debridement and antibiotics. Fixation is mandatory to prevent further tissue trauma, but may be accomplished in a staged fashion, with external fixation preceding internal fixation. Humeral fractures with joint involvement should also receive early fixation so that therapy may be initiated, preventing joint stiffness

Operative fixation of the humerus is via external fixation, open reduction and internal fixation (ORIF), intramedullary nailing, or minimally invasive percutaneous osteosynthesis. External fixation is rarely used as definitive treatment, but rather can be used in the setting of soft tissue injuries, burns, vascular compromise, or open fractures as a bridge to internal fixation. Internal fixation allows for direct visualization of the fracture site, and thus permits anatomic reduction while preserving adjacent anatomic structures. Fixation is usually via a plate-and-screw technique. Care must be taken to avoid excessive dissection of soft tissues. Traditionally three to four screws were placed both proximally and distally to the fracture, but recent trends emphasize the length of the plate on each side of the fracture rather than the number of screws.

Intramedullary (IM) nailing provides an alternative to ORIF, minimizing disruption to the surrounding tissues and preserving periosteal blood supply. This technique allows for lower infection rates and similar rates of iatrogenic radial nerve injury. However, IM nailing generally results in decreased elbow and shoulder range of motion compared to plating, and typically has a higher need for reoperation.

Minimally invasive percutaneous osteosynthesis is a technique which has grown in popularity due to its ability to provide adequate stability to allow for early motion yet minimize the amount of soft tissue dissection at the time of operative fixation.[5] This method includes reduction of the fracture segments, often through a closed technique. A plate is slid through an incision over the deltoid along the humerus, passing between the bursa and the greater tuberosity. The axillary and radial nerves are palpated and protected during this process. Finally, small incisions are made over the screw holes to facilitate fixation of the plate to the humerus.

Forearm

Two million emergency room visits per year are attributable to forearm fractures.[6] Of these, 18% are humeral fractures, 31% are radial or ulnar fractures, and 51% are for carpal, metacarpal, or phalangeal fractures. A thorough history, physical exam, and radiologic exam are necessary to correctly classify the type of fracture, which will then guide the management.

Colles fractures are fractures of the distal radius, representing up to one-sixth of all fractures treated.[6] Elderly patients may sustain these injuries with a low-energy fall, whereas younger patients typically sustain high-energy trauma in order to cause a Colles fracture. There is no consensus on whether operative fixation is necessary or closed reduction and casting is sufficient. Minimally displaced fractures, those with preservation of volar tilt, preserved radial inclination, and minimal radial shortening are most likely to be successful with non-operative management.

Non-surgical immobilization begins with a volar or sugar-tong splint for four-to-eight weeks. When additional concern lingers, a short arm case can be added to protect fractures within osteoporotic bones. Surveillance with weekly x-rays will detect any displacement which forms within the first several weeks of treatment.

Isolated fractures of the shaft of the ulna, or nightstick fractures, typically result from direct impact to the forearm.[6] They can be seen on AP and lateral x-rays of the forearm. Special attention must be paid to the elbow and wrist to rule out concomitant injuries. Ulnar shaft fractures are managed successfully with non-operative means via short arm case or forearm brace for four-to-eight weeks. When accompanied with a dislocation of the radial head, they are termed Monteggia fractures and frequently require operative intervention due to the associated angulation and shortening of the ulna.

Galeazzi fractures are fractures of the distal radius with associated disruption of the distal radioulnar joint (DRUJ).[7] The radius fracture is commonly in the middle to distal third of the bone, and this is often the result of a fall on the outstretched hand with the wrist in extension and arm in marked pronation or supination. In children, the preferred treatment is closed reduction and an above-elbow cast of the arm in supination for 4-6 weeks. If reduction is not possible or this strategy does not maintain reduction, ORIF is indicated with Kirschner wires, IM nailing, or dorsal plate fixation. In adults, all Galeazzi fractures require ORIF of the radius with a dynamic compression plate with intraoperative assessment of the DRUJ. Depending on the stability of the DRUJ, it may require fixation of the ulna to radius and further casting in a fashion similar to that described for pediatric patients.

Combined fractures of both the radius and ulna shaft are often treated with closed reduction and cast immobilization.[8] However, when fractures are open, segments are angulated, completely displaced, or have significant malrotation, operative fixation may be necessary (Figure 2). Single-bone fixation is possible but results in an increased likelihood of loss of reduction post-operatively. Plates or IM fixation are possible with both the radius and ulna. IM fixation has a higher rate of nonunion when open reduction is necessary. However, overall, plating has higher operating times, duration of hospitalization, and cosmesis. Duration and methods of post-operative immobilization are controversial.

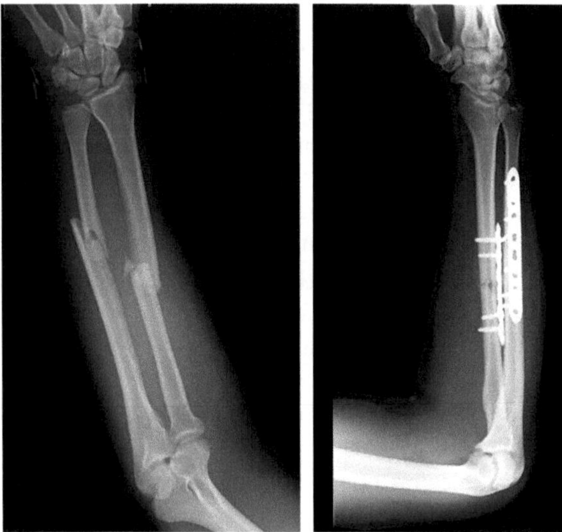

Figure 2: Fracture of radius and ulna with subsequent internal fixation

Radial head fractures are caused by forceful axial loads with the arm in a pronated position, direct blow to the lateral elbow, or falls with the elbow slightly flexed.[6] These are seen with AP and lateral radiographs, though oblique supplemental views are occasionally helpful. They are graded according to the Mason classification system. Grade I fractures are non-displaced, grade II have displacement >2 mm or angulation >30°, grade III are comminuted, and grade IV have associated elbow dislocation. Grade I injuries are managed with a posterior splint for five-to-seven days, and then a sling for comfort. Grades II-VI injuries require surgical fixation.

Olecranon fractures are usually intra-articular, and they are often the result of direct impact to the flexed elbow. These are best visualized with lateral radiographs of the elbow. Occasionally a triceps avulsion injury causes an extra-articular olecranon fracture, but this is less common. Extra-articular olecranon fractures require only non-surgical therapy, whereas intra-articular fractures often require operative fixation, particularly in active patients with significant displacement, unstable elbows, comminution, or interrupted extensor mechanisms.

Coronoid process fractures are unusual injuries that are often encountered in conjunction with elbow dislocation. These are best visualized with lateral radiographs of the elbow. The primary objective of treatment of these injuries is to reduce the elbow and preserve neurovascular function of the extremity. Isolated injuries are managed with long-arm splinting of the elbow in 90° flexion for one-to-three weeks.

Lower Extremity

Femur

The lower extremity articulates with the axial skeleton at the hip joint, with the head of the femur joining with the acetabulum of the pelvis. The neck of the femur connects the head to the shaft and is vulnerable to injury. Fractures of the neck of the femur can be broadly categorized based on mechanism of injury, with high-energy injuries more common in younger patients, and low-energy mechanisms more common in the elderly.[9] Elderly patients require more urgent intervention because of the associated poor functional outcomes and high mortality rate, though early surgery has not proven to reduce long-term outcomes.[9]

Approximately one-third of younger patients who sustain a femoral neck fracture will develop avascular necrosis.[9] These rates are reduced with early fixation, but long-term functional improvement has not been shown to be improved.

Femoral shaft fractures can result in septic complications and pulmonary failure, and thus, immediate stabilization is the standard of care.[10] Fat emboli is a serious, potentially fatal, complication of femur fractures, and the incidence is decreased by a 20 to 63% reduction with early stabilization, and delay of fixation for even as short a time as 48 hours can have significantly inferior results.[10]

The traditional method of treating femoral shaft fractures is traction and bedrest for 4-6 weeks.[11] This method has a high degree of success, and inadequate bone alignment or shortening only occurs in approximately 2% of cases. However, the obvious downsides of prolonged immobility have led operative intervention to supplant traction as the mainstay of treatment. Surgical fixation is most commonly via IM nailing, though plate fixation is an alternative option (Figure 3).[12] The transition in standard of care has been so dramatic that there has even been the development of low-cost methods of IM nailing that are being utilized in third-world countries.[13]

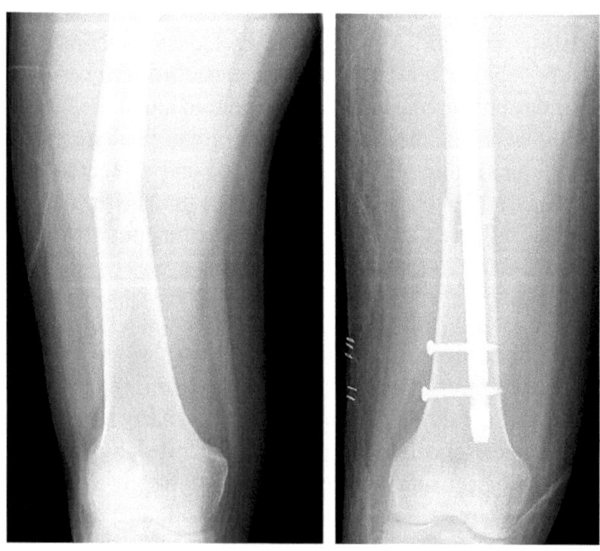

Figure 3: Femoral shaft fracture with subsequent IM nail

Lower Leg

Tibial shaft fractures have traditionally been treated with closed reduction and casting (Figure 4).[14] Fractures in which reduction was not possible or could not be maintained were treated by ORIF beginning in the 1950s, but this presented the potential drawbacks of extensive tissue dissection and devitalization. The development of IM nailing has presented a way of providing early stabilization, allowing for early mobility without the higher likelihood of nonunion or infection that may result from iatrogenic trauma inherent to ORIF. IM nailing has become the standard of care for tibial shaft fractures.[12]

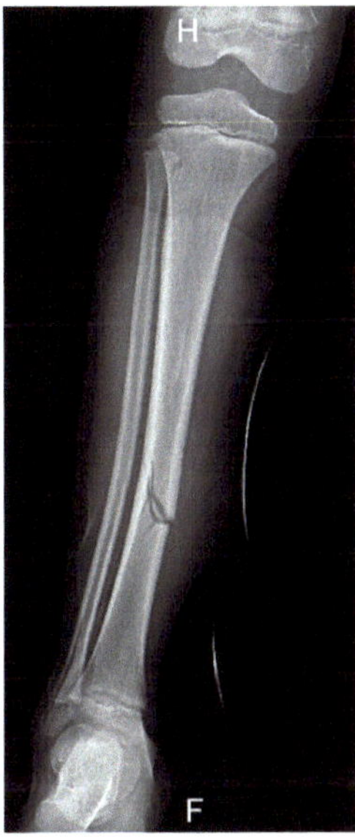

Figure 4: Isolated tibial diaphysis fracture

Proximal tibial fractures initially had a poor rate of union (16%) with nailing, but this has improved with more involved techniques. Unfortunately, the placement of an IM nail for a proximal tibial fracture is a time-intensive process, not suitable for the polytrauma patient. Distal tibial fractures can be successfully managed with IM nailing so long as the ankle joint involvement can be managed with a percutaneous screw. Union rates have been reported from 96 to 100%.[12] Patients whose tibial fractures are managed with IM nailing are permitted to do range of motion within 1-2 days and are non-weight-bearing for 6-8 weeks.

Fibula fractures are clinically relevant when they involve the ankle joint. Pilon fractures are often accompanied by distal fibula fractures. These fibula fractures should be stabilized in order to optimize functional outcomes.[15] Stabilization of the fibula with a plate, or slightly less effectively with a pin, results in better ankle stability and less post-traumatic ankle arthrosis.[15]

Torso

Ribs

Rib fractures are historically a non-operative injury (Figure 5). The morbidity and mortality associated with chest wall injury is oftentimes more directly attributable to the underlying injury to the lungs and subsequent impaired ventilation and oxygenation. In recent years, the indication for surgical stabilization of rib fractures has grown to include pain reduction, chronic malunion, overriding ribs, and flail chest.[16] Specific indications for rib fixation are still controversial, though some authors propose scoring systems that include such characteristics as patient age, number of fractured ribs, presence of a pulmonary contusion, and contralateral rib fractures.[17]

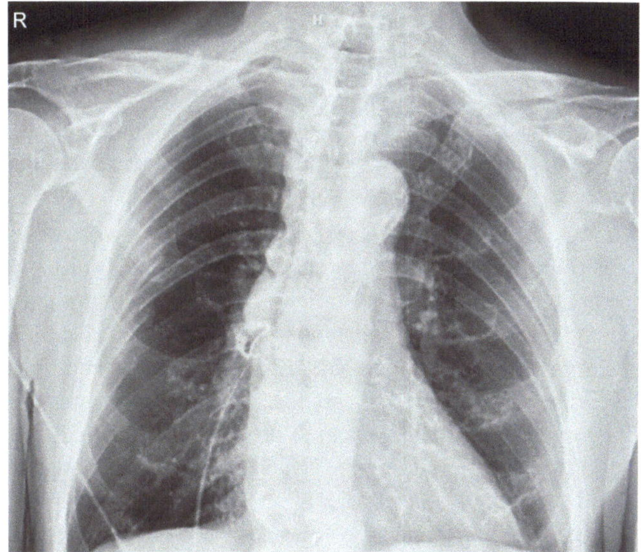

Figure 5: Fractures of right sixth through tenth ribs

The surgical fixation of ribs was accomplished with Kirshner wires or other orthopedic devices used for lack of a better alternative for years.[18] Attempts at external splinting for flail segments failed to improve outcomes in the early 1900s. In the 1950s, the concept of "internal splinting" via positive pressure ventilation grew in popularity, but beginning in the 1960s, reports began to surface of operative fixation improving outcomes.

Recently, implants specifically for rib fixation have been introduced.[18] Options for rib fixation now include anatomically contoured plates or intramedullary rib splints. These have both been shown to simplify the operative fixation of ribs and to improve respiratory function and pain control in certain rib fracture patients.

Scapula

Scapula fractures only account for 1% of all fractures.[19] Scapula body fractures are traditionally treated non-operatively.[20] However, indications for operative fixation do exist. If the lateral fragments are completely displaced there is greater than 30° angulation of the lateral border and glenoid fossa, or if a fragment has penetrated the thoracic wall, ORIF is indicated.[20]

Furthermore, fractures of the acromion and coracoid processes have historically been managed nonoperatively.[19] Acromion process fractures occur due to direct trauma, dislocation of the humeral head causing indirect trauma, avulsion by the deltoid muscle, and stress fractures in athletes. Coracoid process fractures result from direct trauma, dislocation of the humeral head, axial loading of an ipsilateral clavicle fracture, or avulsion during acromioclavicular joint separation. Complications resulting from non-operative management can include symptomatic non-union, compression of the brachial plexus, pain, reduced motion, rotator cuff tears, AC joint separation, humeral head subluxation, and shoulder weakness.

There are no widely accepted criteria for an operative intervention for either an acromion or coracoid process fracture, though proposed criteria include symptomatic nonunion, concomitant ipsilateral scapula fracture, ≥1 cm of displacement upon radiographic evaluation, and/or multiple disruption of the superior shoulder suspensory complex.[19] Fixation options for the acromion process include ORIF via plates, tension band wiring for distal fractures, interfragment screw fixation, or Kirshner wires. Options for coracoid process fractures are interfragment screw fixation with cortical lag screws for larger fragments and non-absorbable sutures for smaller fragments, with or without supplementation of a plate.

Clavicle

Fractures of the clavicle are a frequent occurrence in adults, representing 5 to 10% of all fractures.[21] About 80% of these fractures occur in the mid-shaft portion of the clavicle, and the mainstay of treatment has been non-operative management with a sling (Figure 6). More recent reports favor operative fixation. Complication rates are reported to be as high as 15% with non-operative approaches, whereas operative interventions typically report non-union and infection rates less than 10%.[22] However, irritation or failure of the plate ranges from 9 to 65%, depending on the series, necessitating additional operations in at least 10% of patients.

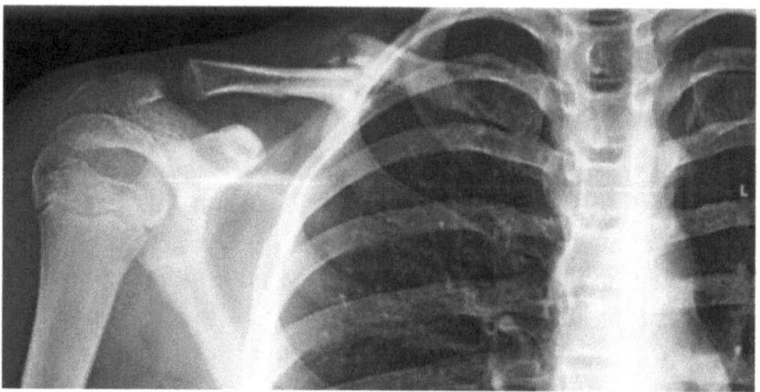

Figure 6: Mid-clavicle fracture

Currently accepted indications for surgical fixation of clavicle fractures include significant displacement, fracture comminution, threatened skin integrity, and unstable lateral fractures.[21] Options for stabilization include Kirshner wire fixation, coracoclavicular screw fixation, tension band wiring, and clavicular plate fixation.

Life-Threatening Injuries

Open Fractures

Approximately 3% of all fractures are open.[23] Open fractures have a high risk of deep tissue infection, prompting emergent intervention by the trauma or orthopedic surgeon. Sepsis and death were such formidable complications that up until 150 years ago, the treatment for an open fracture was amputation.[24] These complications are much less frequent with advances in antibiotics, wound management, and orthopedic techniques, but the historical "six-hour rule," mandating operative intervention in the immediate post-injury period, has remained.

The traditional management of open long-bone fractures includes initial debridement, often with placement of an external fixator. This is followed by serial washouts, as necessary, until the wound bed is clean and healthy, with no signs of infection, at which point internal fixation may be considered.

Some trace the "six hour rule" back to an 1898 study by Friedrich, but it was perpetuated by a 1973 Robson et al. study that quantified the density of bacteria in an open fracture wound and determined that they reached a clinically significant concentration of 10^5 organisms per gram of tissue in 5.17 hours.[24] However, recent retrospective studies in multiple countries have questioned the correlation between time-to-operation and rates of infection.[24,25] Prospective studies are still lacking to definitively invalidate the "six hour rule."

Regardless of the timing of operative intervention, antibiotics are a critical component of management of open fractures. Open fractures can be classified according to the soft tissue damage and associated injuries, based on the Gustilo classification system

(Table 1).[26] This classification system can be used to help guide antibiotic regimen. Gustilo types 1 and 2 fractures mandate a cephalosporin, whereas Gustilo type 3 fractures should be treated with a first-generation cephalosporin plus an aminoglycoside or a third-generation cephalosporin.

Table 1: Gustilo classification

Gustilo Type	Definition
I	Open fracture, clean wound, wound length <1 cm
II	Open fracture, wound >1 cm in length, no extensive soft-tissue damage, avulsions, flaps
III	Open fracture, extensive soft-tissue damage, loss, or laceration; or an open segmental fracture. Open fractures due to farm injuries, fractures needing vascular repair, or fractures open >8 hrs prior to treatment
IIIA	Fracture with extensive soft-tissue damage or laceration, but has adequate periosteal coverage of the fracture bone
IIIB	Fracture with extensive soft-tissue loss, bone damage, and periosteal stripping. Massive contamination is often associated with the fracture. Often requires further soft-tissue coverage procedure (i.e., rotational or free flap)
IIIC	Fracture with an arterial injury requiring repair, irrespective of the amount of soft-tissue injury.

Sternoclavicular Dislocations

An uncommon injury is a sternoclavicular joint dislocation which represents 3% of shoulder injuries, and less than 1% of all joint dislocations.[27] Most of these injuries involve the anterior displacement of the medial head of the clavicle. However, posterior displacement is of greater concern, as the superior mediastinum is vulnerable to injury. These injuries can present with pain and swelling at the medial clavicular head, but also dyspnea, dysphagia, and dysphonia, depending on the involved structures. Diagnosis is usually via CT scan, as plain chest radiograph findings are subtle and nonspecific. Treatment is reduction, either closed or open. Closed reduction is generally accomplished by positioning the patient supine with a shoulder roll between the scapulae and manipulation of the ipsilateral arm.[28]

Mangled Extremities

Limb injuries typically result from direct force, bone fragment mobilization, or from burns.[29] When severe, these can present a difficult decision for the surgeon: attempt at salvaging the extremity and increase the risk of mortality or primary amputation of the injured extremity to increase likelihood of patient survival.[30] Preserving a limb may avoid the emotionally-charged idea of amputation, but it can subject a patient to an increased risk of numerous surgical reconstructive procedures, sepsis, and potentially death. Furthermore, it remains difficult to predict at the time of injury which limbs are not only salvageable, but also have the potential for long-term functional recovery.[30]

A number of different clinical predictors have been developed to help clinicians decide whether to preserve a limb or amputate: Mangled Extremity Severity Score (MESS), Predictive Salvage Index (PSI), Limb Salvage Index (LSI), Mangled Extremity Syndrome Index (MESI), Nerve Injury, Ischemia, Soft Tissue, Skeletal Injury, Shock, Age of Patient Score (NISSSA), and Hannover Fracture Scale.[29] The most widely utilized of these is the MESS system, which was designed specifically for lower extremities but has been extrapolated to upper extremities by some (Table 2).

Table 2: Mangled Extremity Severity Score

	Score
Skeletal/Soft Tissue Injury	1 Point: Low energy injury 2 Points: Medium energy injury 3 Points: High energy injury 4 Points: Very high energy injury
Limb Ischemia	1 Point: Normal perfusion with reduced or absent pulse 2 Points: Absent pulse, paresthesia, diminished capillary refill 3 Points: Cool, paralyzed, insensate limb
Shock	0 Points: Systolic blood pressure >90 mmHg 1 Point: Hypotensive transiently 2 Points: Hypotensive persistently
Age	0 Points: <30 years old 1 Point: 30-50 years old 2 Points: >50 years old
*Overall score is doubled for ischemia >6 hours MESS >7 is predictive of need for amputation.	

Multiple reports, however, have indicated shortcomings of each of these scoring systems, reporting that they are not predictive of the need for amputation.[29,30] Moreover, many authors argue that the scoring systems are even weaker at determining long-term functional outcomes of salvaged extremities.[31] There is a predominance of data on combat injuries where "life before limb" is a frequent attitude.[29] There is a relative paucity of civilian literature, particularly with pediatric patients, limiting the surgeon's ability to generalize the data available.

Fat Emboli

Fractures, particularly of long bones, can cause the release of fat particles into the circulatory system, occluding vessels and causing ischemia, most commonly of the lung.[32] Trauma is the cause in 90% of fat emboli cases. Other causes include syndromes that increase hydrolysis of fat to fatty acids.[33] Factors that increase the risk of fat emboli include young age, closed fractures, multiple fractures, and conservative management of long-bone fractures.[32] Virtually all patients with long-bone fractures develop subclinical fat emboli, but in a small subset of patients, the emboli become symptomatic.[33]

Symptoms usually present 12-36 hours after a trauma. Many symptoms of fat emboli are similar to those of other pulmonary emboli (e.g., hypoxemia, tachypnea, dyspnea, and tachycardia).[32] Other symptoms include agitation, delirium, seizures or coma in 86% of patients. Petechial rash, especially within the torso and conjunctiva, presents in 60% of cases. Mortality is 5 to 15% overall, and 36% in patients with ventilator-dependent respiratory failure.

Diagnosis is clinical, based on the constellation of symptoms.[33] Many advocate using Gurd's criteria (Table 3). Treatment is supportive, consisting of fluid resuscitation to maintain hemodynamic stability, and ventilatory support as needed.[33] Some recommend albumin to restore intravascular volume and bind fatty acids to reduce further pulmonary injury. The use of steroids is controversial for treatment or prophylaxis.

Table 3: Gurd's Criteria for Fat Embolism Syndrome

	Criteria
Major Criteria	Petechial Rash Respiratory Insufficiency Cerebral Involvement
Minor Criteria	Fever Retinal Changes Jaundice Renal signs Thrombocytopenia Anemia Elevated ESR Fat Macroglobulinemia
Diagnosis requires at least two major criteria or one major and four minor criteria	

Special circumstances

Compartment Syndrome

Long-bone fractures occurring within the confines of the fascial compartments of the extremities can lead to a build-up of pressure from the subsequent bleeding or edema. This pressure reduces capillary flow and causes local tissue hypoxia and necrosis. Increased pressure in a limited space that compromises the perfusion and function of the contents of that space is designated as acute compartment syndrome.[34] When sustained, the muscles within such a space will necrose, fibrose, and become contracted. Both muscles and nerves can tolerate ischemia for four hours and begin to experience irreversible damage beyond eight hours. Other causes of compartment syndrome include arterial obstruction, lithotomy position.

Compartment syndrome is largely a clinical diagnosis. Pain is the predominant symptom, but may also be accompanied by paresthesia, paresis, pulselessness, and tense compartments.[35] However, these signs and symptoms have a high sensitivity but low specificity, making them appropriate for ruling out a diagnosis of compartment syndrome but not confirming a diagnosis. When the diagnosis is in doubt, confirmation can be obtained by directly measuring compartment pressure. Normal compartment pressure is 0-8 mmHg and signs of ischemia develop at pressures of >20 mmHg.[35] Pressures in excess of 30 mmHg exceed the fascia's compliance, and compartment syndrome ensues.

Compartment syndrome from fractures is more common in the lower extremities than the upper extremities, but it can happen in either. It can also occur within the hands or feet.[34,35] Following tibial fractures, the incidence of compartment syndrome ranges from 2.7 to 11%, more often from open fractures than closed.[35] Conversely, 36% of lower leg compartment syndrome occurrences are due to tibial fractures.

Management of compartment syndrome focuses on restoring perfusion to the affected limb. Initially, these measures can focus on easily identifiable sources of perfusion compromise. This includes removing external dressings and casts, particularly ones which are circumferential, maintaining normotension, and administering supplemental oxygen.[34] Definitive treatment is fasciotomy. Discrete indications are controversial, but most argue for mandatory fasciotomy when the compartment pressure is greater than 30 mmHg or within 15-20 mmHg of diastolic blood pressure, when there has been six hours of limb ischemia prior to reperfusion, or when clinical findings are equivocal.

Multiply-Injured Patients

Patients presenting with fractures often have concomitant injuries and consideration must be given to the sequence of treatment. Initial management decisions vary based on whether the patient is hemodynamically stable or unstable.[9] Delayed, or limited orthopedic intervention may play a role in poly-trauma patients. Definitive fixation of long bones within the first 24 hours of injury, previously the standard of care, often requires long surgical procedures which can cause injury to the lungs and other end organs, rather than minimizing hemorrhage and fat embolization as previously hypothesized.

Hemodynamically unstable multiply-injured blunt trauma patients with pelvic fractures present clinical dilemmas. If pelvic fractures appear unstable, they are likely to be the primary source of bleeding, and mortality can be reduced by 35% if angiography precedes laparotomy.[9] If ongoing thoracic or abdominal bleeding is suspected to be the patient's primary problem, orthopedic fixation beyond placement of a pelvic binder is delayed.

When index of suspicion is high for pelvic fractures as the primary source of bleeding, usually based on extravasation on CT scan, the sequence of external fixation and angiography with embolization is controversial.[9] Some studies have demonstrated that a high percentage of pelvic fractures are amenable to embolization, and therefore angiography should be given priority. Other studies, though, have shown that embolization is successful only in rare cases, and fixation is more likely to be beneficial.

When fractures are associated with major vascular injuries, there is debate about the order of repair. Some advocate bony stabilization to protect the subsequent vascular repair, while others argue that prolonged ischemia is more detrimental than the theoretical risk of disruption to a vascular repair. A retrospective analysis by McHenry et al. found that patients undergoing fixation prior to revascularization had higher rates of fasciotomies and longer hospital stays.[36] No disruptions of vascular repair were noted when revascularization was undertaken prior to bony stabilization. The authors suggested initial placement of a temporary intravascular shunt, followed by bony fixation via either internal or external fixation, and then definitive vascular repair. This could be followed by definitive fracture stabilization, if not performed initially, in the same setting or in a delayed fashion.

Pediatrics

Children frequently sustain orthopedic injuries. The average boy has a 42 to 64% risk of fracturing a bone during childhood, and the average girl has a 27 to 40% risk.[37] Most fractures in children affect the upper extremity (84.1%), while lower extremity fractures account for nearly all others.

Some aspects of fractures within the pediatric population differ significantly from adults. Due to the increased compliance of the pediatric skeleton, more force is necessary to actually cause a bone to fracture.[38] Therefore, when fractures are seen within the axial skeleton, particularly rib fractures, the surgeon must consider the force transmitted to the underlying organs. For example, a significant lung injury may be associated with no rib fractures or only a single rib fracture, whereas adults who sustain pulmonary contusions typically have multiple rib fractures.

Another consideration in pediatric patients with fractures is child abuse. Skin lesions and bruises are the most common finding in child abuse, but fractures are the second most common finding.[39] Furthermore, in a majority of cases, fractures are not accompanied by any external signs of abuse such as hematomas. Because fractures are not only a common finding in accidental injuries in children but are also one of the most common findings in non-accidental trauma, the differentiation is both difficult and important.

Stigmata that suggest that fractures are caused by non-accidental trauma include the following:[39]

- Rib fractures
- Classic metaphyseal fractures (corner fractures of the distal femur, distal or proximal tibia/fibula, or proximal humerus)
- Scapula fractures
- Spinous process fractures
- Sternal fractures
- Multiple fractures in different stages of healing

Rib fractures are the most common fracture in child abuse.[39] The positive predictive value of rib fractures for abuse is 95% in children less than 3 years old. Posterior fractures, in particular, are indicative of abuse, as anterior-posterior compression of the thoracic cage causes ribs to bend over the transverse processes to the point of fracturing.

Part of the work-up for suspected child abuse should include a systematic radiologic survey of the entire skeleton to identify all fractures. This includes more than twenty plane x-rays of the entire skeleton. This is more sensitive for classic metaphyseal lesions than either a CT scan or bone scintigraphy.

REFERENCES

1. Stedman's Medical Dictionary. 25th ed. 1990. Williams and Wilkins. Baltimore, MD.
2. Marsell R, Einhorn TA. "The biology of fracture healing." Injury. 2011 Jun;42(9):551-5.
3. Pountos I, Georgouli T, Calori GM, Giannoudis PV. "Do nonsteroidal anti-inflammatory drugs affect bone healing? A critical analysis." ScientificWorldJournal. 2012;2012:606404.

4. Carroll EA, Schweppe M, Langfitt M, Miller AN, Halvorson JJ. "Management of humeral shaft fractures." J Am Acad Orthop Surg. 2012 Jul;20(10):423-33.
5. Altman GT, Gallo RA, Molinero KG, Muffly MT, Mascarenhas L. "Minimally invasive plate osteosynthesis for proximal humerus fractures: functional results of treatment." Am J Orthop (Belle Mead NJ). 2011 Mar;40(6):E40-7.
6. Black WS, Becker JA. "Common forearm fractures in adults." Am Fam Physician. 2009 Nov 15;80(14):1096-102.
7. Atesok KI, Jupiter JB, Weiss AP. "Galeazzi fracture." J Am Acad Orthop Surg. 2011 Oct;19(14):623-33.
8. Weiss JM, Mencio GA. "Forearm shaft fractures: does fixation improve outcomes?" J Pediatr Orthop. 2012 Jun;32 Suppl 1:S22-4.
9. Fulkerson EW, Egol KA. "Timing issues in fracture management: a review of current concepts." Bull NYU Hosp Jt Dis. 2009;67(4):58-67.
10. Bone LB, Johnson KD, Weigelt J, Scheinberg R. "Early versus delayed stabilization of femoral fractures. A prospective randomized study." J Bone Joint Surg Am. 1989 Mar;71(6):336-40.
11. Akinyoola AL, Orekha OO, Taiwo FO, Odunsi AO. "Outcome of non-operative management of femoral shaft fractures in children." Afr J Paediatr Surg. 2011 Jan-Apr;8(4):34-9.
12. Wood GW 2nd. "Intramedullary nailing of femoral and tibial shaft fractures." J Orthop Sci. 2006 Nov;11(9):657-69.
13. Zirkle LG Jr. "Injuries in developing countries--how can we help? The role of orthopaedic surgeons." Clin Orthop Relat Res. 2008 Oct;466(14):2443-50.
14. Janssen KW, Biert J, van Kampen A. Treatment of distal tibial fractures: plate versus nail: a retrospective outcome analysis of matched pairs of patients. Int Orthop. 2007 Oct;31(8):709-14.
15. Lee YS, Chen SW, Chen SH, Chen WC, Lau MJ, Hsu TL. "Stabilisation of the fractured fibula plays an important role in the treatment of pilon fractures: a retrospective comparison of fibular fixation methods." Int Orthop. 2009 Jun;33(6):695-9.
16. Bottlang M, Walleser S, Noll M, Honold S, Madey SM, Fitzpatrick D, Long WB. "Biomechanical rationale and evaluation of an implant system for rib fracture fixation." Eur J Trauma Emerg Surg. 2010 Oct;36(8):417-426.
17. Pressley CM, Fry WR, Philp AS, Berry SD, Smith RS. "Predicting outcome of patients with chest wall injury." Am J Surg. 2012 Dec;204(9):910-4.
18. Fitzpatrick DC, Denard PJ, Phelan D, Long WB, Madey SM, Bottlang M. "Operative stabilization of flail chest injuries: review of literature and fixation options." Eur J Trauma Emerg Surg. 2010 Oct;36(8):427-433.
19. Anavian J, Wijdicks CA, Schroder LK, Vang S, Cole PA. "Surgery for scapula process fractures: good outcome in 26 patients." Acta Orthop. 2009 Jun;80(6):344-50.
20. Bartoníček J, Frič V. "Scapular body fractures: results of operative treatment." Int Orthop. 2011 May;35(8):747-53.
21. Bajuri MY, Maidin S, Rauf A, Baharuddin M, Harjeet S. "Functional outcomes of conservatively treated clavicle fractures." Clinics (Sao Paulo). 2011;66(7):635-9.
22. Wijdicks FJ, Van der Meijden OA, Millett PJ, Verleisdonk EJ, Houwert RM. "Systematic review of the complications of plate fixation of clavicle fractures." Arch Orthop Trauma Surg. 2012 May;132(8):617-25.
23. Cross WW 3rd, Swiontkowski MF. "Treatment principles in the management of open fractures." Indian J Orthop. 2008 Oct;42(7):377-86.
24. Schenker ML, Yannascoli S, Baldwin KD, Ahn J, Mehta S. "Does timing to operative debridement affect infectious complications in open long-bone fractures? A systematic review." J Bone Joint Surg Am. 2012 Jun 20;94(15):1057-64.
25. Kamat AS."Infection rates in open fractures of the tibia: is the 6-hour rule fact or fiction?" Adv Orthop. 2011;2011:943495.
26. Gustilo RB, Mendoza RM, Williams DN. Problems in the management of type III (severe) open fractures: A new classification of type III open fractures. J Trauma. 1984;24:742–6.
27. Ciftdemir M, Copuroglu C, Ozcan M. "Posterior dislocation of the sternoclavicular joint." Hippokratia. 2011 Jul;15(6):284.
28. Hoekzema N, Torchia M, Adkins M, Cassivi SD. "Posterior sternoclavicular joint dislocation." Can J Surg. 2008 Feb;51(4):E19-20.
29. Fodor L, Sobec R, Sita-Alb L, Fodor M, Ciuce C. Mangled lower extremity: can we trust the amputation scores?" Int J Burns Trauma. 2012;2(4):51-8.
30. Korompilias AV, Beris AE, Lykissas MG, Vekris MD, Kontogeorgakos VA, Soucacos PN. "The mangled extremity and attempt for limb salvage." J Orthop Surg Res. 2009 Feb 13;4:4.

31. Ly TV, Travison TG, Castillo RC, Bosse MJ, MacKenzie EJ. LEAP Study Group. "Ability of lower-extremity injury severity scores to predict functional outcome after limb salvage." J Bone Joint Surg Am. 2008 Aug;90(11):1738-43.
32. Porpodis K, Karanikas M, Zarogoulidis P, Konoglou M, Domvri K, Mitrakas A, Boglou P, Bakali S, Iordanidis A, Zervas V, Courcoutsakis N, Katsikogiannis N, Zarogoulidis K. "Fat embolism due to bilateral femoral fracture: a case report." Int J Gen Med. 2012;5:59-63.
33. Shaikh N, Parchani A, Bhat V, Kattren MA. "Fat embolism syndrome: clinical and imaging considerations: case report and review of literature." Indian J Crit Care Med. 2008 Jan;12(4):32-6.
34. Chandraprakasam T, Kumar RA. "Acute compartment syndrome of forearm and hand." Indian J Plast Surg. 2011 May;44(5):212-8.
35. Shadgan B, Menon M, Sanders D, Berry G, Martin C Jr, Duffy P, Stephen D, O'Brien PJ. "Current thinking about acute compartment syndrome of the lower extremity." Can J Surg. 2010 Oct;53(8):329-34.
36. McHenry TP, Holcomb JB, Aoki N, Lindsey RW. "Fractures with major vascular injuries from gunshot wounds: implications of surgical sequence." J Trauma. 2002 Oct;53(7):717-21.
37. Valerio G, Gallè F, Mancusi C, Di Onofrio V, Colapietro M, Guida P, Liguori G. "Pattern of fractures across pediatric age groups: analysis of individual and lifestyle factors." BMC Public Health. 2010 Oct 30;10:656.
38. Karadayi S, Nadir A, Sahin E, Celik B, Arslan S, Kaptanoglu M. "An analysis of 214 cases of rib fractures." Clinics (Sao Paulo). 2011;66(6):449-51.
39. van Rijn RR, Sieswerda-Hoogendoorn T. "Educational paper: imaging child abuse: the bare bones." Eur J Pediatr. 2012 Feb;171(5):215-24.

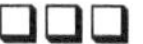

72

CHAPTER

Pediatric Surgery

Tarun Kumar, MD
Kayla K. Umemoto, BA
Pankaj Dangle, MD

PHYSIOLOGY

Pediatric patients necessitate a unique surgical intervention due to the distinctive physiologic and anatomic causes for a variety of illness. Additionally, the management of prepubertal patients is immensely different than in adults.

PHYSIOLOGICAL ASPECT OF CHILDREN

Metabolism/Nutrition

During the growth phase, the metabolic requirements in children are geared towards different goals compared to adults. Both the neonatal and juvenile age group necessitates substantially higher energy requirements as compared to adults due to a higher basal metabolic rate, and a majority of energy being utilized for growth. In the pediatric population the pattern on the "Growth Curve" is unique and substantially well defined. Thus, any deviation in the normal growth is preliminary evidence of a pathological process.

In the neonatal age group, the birth weight is two times greater by 5 months, three times by 1 year, and 4 times by 3 years with a subsequent decline until puberty. Energy consumption at a baseline resting energy expenditure in neonates is twofold (45-50 kcal/kg/day) as compared to adolescents and adults (20-25 kcal/kg/day) (Table 1). Due to the higher energy requirements, children are at a higher risk of switching to a catabolic state during periods of stress.

Table 1: Calorie requirements of children separated by age groups.[1]

Age in Years	Kcal/kg/day
0 to 1	90 to 120
1 to 7	75 to 90
7 to 12	60 to 75
12 to 18	30 to 60

In many instances, starvation and/or the stress response is the primary initiators of catabolic metabolism. During starvation metabolism, the energy source for most vital organs is via ketogenesis. While with any stress response in reaction to, for example, surgery and/or acute illness, the pathway of ketogenesis is inhibited, making tissue glucose requirements critically important.

Glucose is the major source of energy in the neonatal age group. At birth, after the separation of the placenta, glycogenolysis is the vital source of glucose until feeding is commenced. Since, the major source of glycogen stores is produced 36-40 weeks of gestation, preterm infants are at an increased risk for starvation metabolism.

In premature infants, the skeletal muscle and fat represent only 1% of body weight compared to term infants (15%) making both lipolysis and gluconeogenesis a trivial reserve for providing an alternative source of energy supply. When enteral feeding cannot be initiated or tolerated, alternative forms of energy in the form of total parenteral nutrition should be commenced. During fasting, neonates and young children can tolerate 1 week without nutritional support, whereas older children and adolescents are comparable to adults who can go up to 1-3 weeks without nutrition.

During the first year of life, newborns require at least 100-120 kcal/kg/day to meet baseline resting energy and growth requirements. Both breast milk and formula contain 0.67 kcal/ml (20 kcal/oz). To calculate, 3-hour oral requirements based on gastric emptying equals the child's weight in kg times 22.5, where 22.5 is a coefficient derived from the energy requirements and the kcal density of standard formula; for continuous feedings via feeding tubes, the coefficient is 7.3 (i.e., 22 / 3).

Renal Physiology and Fluids/Electrolytes

A deficient homeostatic mechanism and even a trivial derangement in chemistry can lead to significant changes and responses in both neonates and small children. In neonates, the majority (75-80%) of their total body weight is due to water. Immediately post-delivery, the decreased vascular resistance leads to an increase in renal blood flow, thereby giving 3 distinct phases of fluid management. There is a slow decline to the adult level of renal blood flow and glomerular filtration rate. Thus, it is important to be aware that weight loss in the first week of life is a normal phenomenon related to the diuretic phase event in preterm infants.

Renal concentrating capacity (RCC): The serum osmolality in children, especially in infants, is lower at roughly 600-700 mOsm/L compared to adults which is about 1,200-1,400 mOsm/L. Despite a lower GFR, the lower concentrating capacity of the kidneys makes handling a large water load uncomplicated. As compared to adults (70-100 mOsm/L), infants can make diluted urine up to 50 mOsm/L.

Urine output is the most reliable indicator of fluid balance in all age groups. Renal solute excretion is maintained at a rate of 0.5 ml/kg/hr. Pediatric patients require an elevated fluid turnover secondary to the augmented metabolic demand from growth. This is different depending on the age of the patient which is as follows:

- Premature infants: 4 ml/kg/hr
- Infants: 2 ml/kg/hr
- Toddlers: 1 ml/kg/hr

In pediatric patients, maintenance fluid requirements per hour can be roughly calculated as shown in Table 2.

Table 2: Maintenance fluid requirements per hour

Weight	Maintenance fluid per hour
First 10 kg	4 ml/kg/hr
Next 10 kg	2 ml/kg/hr
Additional kg	1 ml/kg/hr

Physiological handling of sodium: Term infants and young children require approximately 2-3 mEq/kg/day of sodium. Whereas premature infants are "salt-wasters" and require relatively higher levels of sodium replacement. In healthy young children D10 ¼ NS is used, whereas in preterm infants D10 ½ NS will meet the required sodium requirements.[2] Both the third space losses and electrolyte shifts requiring a change in fluid administration are of paramount importance in post-surgical patients. The preferred fluids for managing these patients are shown in Table 3.

Table 3: Preferred fluids for managing sodium replacement in children

Age	Type of Solution	Rate for Initial 12 hours
<6 months	D10 ½ NS	1.5 times maintenance
>6 months	D10 Lactated Ringer's	1.5 times maintenance

Pulmonary Physiology

There are 5 phases of pulmonary development:

- Embryonic (gestation week 3)
- Pseudo glandular (week 7-16)
- Canalicular (week 17-24)
- Terminal saccular (week 24-40)
- Alveolar (birth to 8 years)

The type II pneumocytes responsible for surfactant production develop in the canalicular phase (i.e., phase 3). The canalicular phase is critical in preterm babies as this is the earliest time at which functional gas exchange occurs and is thus the earliest survivable gestational age of birth (currently 22-24 weeks gestation). The term infants are born with roughly 20 million alveolar units during the alveolar phase as compared to the adults with 300 million alveolar units.

When understanding the lung, it is important to know the following equation: total lung capacity (TLC) = inspiratory reserve volume (IRV) + tidal volume (TV) + expiratory reserve volume (ERV) + and residual volume (RV). The 2 critical measures within the combined spectrum of the ERV and RV are the Functional Residual Capacity (FRC) and Closing capacity (CC). FRC is the volume of air at the end of a tidal breath. CC is the volume at which alveolar units begin to collapse.

Role of Surfactant

Surfactant is produced by type II pneumocytes during the terminal saccular phase and reduces the surface tension in the alveoli. This reduction in surface tension results in a reduction in the CC based on the Laplace relationship of $P = 2T / R$ (P = pressure, T = wall tension, R = radius). Due to the direct relationship, reducing T reduces the pressure at which low radii alveoli must be maintained to resist elastic recoil and collapse. Thus, the CC is reduced.

Respiratory distress syndrome (RDS) of the newborn with resultant alveolar collapse secondary to insufficient surfactant is seen in neonates born during the late canalicular to early terminal saccular phases of development.

Cardiac Physiology

The transition from placental to postnatal circulation is the critical difference between pediatric and adult cardiac physiology. In the intrauterine phase, two physiologic shunts allow the oxygenated blood from the placenta to pass directly into the systemic circulation. The right and left flow shunts run in parallel rather than series. The two shunts include the:

- Foramen ovale: Window between the right and left atria.
- Ductus arteriosus: Vascular connection between the pulmonary artery and the aorta letting diversion of right heart blood away from the unexpanded fetal lungs.

Changes in Circulation After Birth

As the baby is compressed going through the birth canal, amniotic fluid is expelled from the lungs. Then, with the first breath, the lungs expand, and the pulmonary vascular resistance drops. Having a low vascular resistance leads to increased blood flow into the lungs with increased preload to the left atrium. The flap over the foramen ovale closes secondary to higher pressures in the left atrium, thus closing the first of the two shunts. A patent foramen of ovale occurs when the flap over the foramen ovale does not close. This condition generally remains asymptomatic but can occasionally be symptomatic.

Another change after birth is closure of the ductus arteriosus. The ductus arteriosus mostly closes within 24 hours of birth due to decreased levels of circulating placental prostaglandins and increased levels of oxygen. One condition related to the ductus arteriosus that may arise is a patent ductus arteriosus (PDA). This is common in preterm babies and is based on the pressure difference between the pulmonary artery and aorta. It can lead to (1) a right to left shunt leading to pulmonary hypertension and congestive heart failure or (2) a left to right shunt causing hypoxia. Additionally, the ductus venosus/umbilical vein and flow through the umbilical arteries close shut. In extreme circumstances, the umbilical vein may be kept open via catheterization and used as venous access.

Differences in Pediatric and Adult Cardiac Physiology

Cardiac output is determined by preload/heart rate and contractility/afterload:

- Preload: The main determining factor is venous return, which increases myocardial stretch with the increased blood volume at end-diastole. The neonatal heart is less compliant than the adult heart. The neonatal myocardium characteristically fills maximally at diastole with consequential maximal stretch at baseline.
- Contractility: The neonatal myocardium has decreased contractility secondary to lesser contractile fibers when compared to adults. The neonate myocardium is more sensitive to negative ionotropic stimuli secondary to an immature sympathetic system which results in a dominant parasympathetic system. The neonatal myocardium is more resistant to the negative effects of hypoxia and acidosis as compared to adults.
- Afterload: Following the first breath, a resultant lowering of the vascular resistance decreases right heart afterload, whereas the shunt closure on the left simultaneously increases the left afterload. Increased systemic afterload during the initial 2-3 years of life leads to left heart hypertrophy. The neonatal myocardium in early life is exquisitely sensitive to a high afterload such as seen with aortic stenosis or coarctation of the aorta.

Neonates have a lower cardiac reserve and is rate-dependent for cardiac output; secondary to immature myocardium it is unable to adjust preload, contractility, and afterload effectively as compared to adults.

TORTICOLLIS

Congenital

Torticollis is derived from the Latin word "toquere" for twisted and "collum" for neck.[3] This condition is a congenital shortening of the sternocleidomastoid muscle, and it may be secondary to two possible causes:

1. Being in a fixed position in the uterus leads to shortening and tightening of one sternocleidomastoid muscle.
2. Trauma during passage through the birth canal due to a large baby or abnormal presentation.

Acquired

The acquired type of torticollis is due to a variety of causes: (1) atlanto-axial subluxation, (2) brainstem tumors, (3) infectious causes like tonsillitis, retropharyngeal abscess, and cervical lymphadenopathy. On physical examination, the newborn's head will be tilted toward the involved side with the chin slightly rotated away from the involved muscle.

Management

The management of torticollis is physiotherapy which involves gentle stretching of the neck muscle. If the condition does not improve with physiotherapy, then surgical intervention may be required. Surgery consists of dividing the involved sternocleidomastoid muscle.

CYSTIC HYGROMA

Embryologically, the lymphatics begin to develop from the mesenchymal clefts during the 6th gestational week. A cystic hygroma is a benign multiloculated lymphatic malformation due to failure of the lymphatics and the venous system to fuse. This results in a malformed collection of blind-ending lymphatics, causing a hygroma. Sixty to seventy percent of cystic hygromas present at birth, the remainder present within the first two years of life, occurring mostly in the neck or axilla, but they may appear anywhere in the body.

Presentation

Most cystic hygromas are asymptomatic. If they are symptomatic, they may have various presentations including (1) respiratory distress due to airways obstruction or due to the huge size of the hygroma, this may be life-threatening, (2) infections that present with erythema, fever, and pain and may lead to septicemia if it is not treated with antibiotics during the infective stage, and (3) hemorrhage in 10 to 15% of cases which presents with a rapidly enlarging, painful mass.

Management

Imaging studies such as CT or MRI scans may be obtained depending on their availability; however, an MRI is preferred because it can delineate the lesion and its relation to adjacent vital structures.

Treatment

Medical treatment consists of injecting sclerosing agents for example bleomycin, ethanol, and OK-432 a derivative of penicillin and heat inactivated Streptococcus pyogenes. OK-432 is a trial drug that has been effective in large, cystic lesions and less effective in multicystic lesions. Though it may be treated medically, surgical resection is the treatment of choice. However, if the mass is asymptomatic and increasing in size, surgery may be delayed for 6 to 12 months. Immediate surgery is indicated if there is airway obstruction. Complications include persistent leak of lymph, fistula formation, chylothorax, or hemorrhage.

BRANCHIAL CLEFT REMNANTS

A branchial cleft remnant is a congenital anomaly of the neck due to the persistence of the fetal branchial clefts.

Embryology

The branchial clefts form in the 4th to 8th week of gestation and four pairs of branchial arches form in the cervicofacial region of the embryo, with clefts expressed externally and pouches expressed internally. The clefts and their adult equivalents are as follows:[4]

- Cleft I becomes the Eustachian tube and a portion of the external auditory canal.
- Cleft II is obliterated without a distinct adult counterpart.
- Cleft III migrates inferiorly to form the inferior parathyroid glands and the thymus.
- Cleft IV migrates inferiorly but stops above the final level of cleft III, forming the superior parathyroid glands and thyroid C-cells.

Pathophysiology

Branchial cleft remnants are due to the incomplete obliteration of the clefts as the fetal neck develops. It may form cysts, sinuses, fistulas, cartilaginous remnants, and cleft remnants.

- Cleft I remnants occur along the angle of the mandible and sinuses/fistulas may extend to the external auditory canal.
- Cleft II remnants occur along the anterior border of the sternocleidomastoid muscle and may communicate with the tonsillar fossa (the most common form).
- Cleft III and IV remnants are rare and communicate between the piriform sinus and the glands that they form or the neck lower than the 2nd cleft remnant.

Management

Diagnosis is made by the clinical presentation which includes a discharging sinus or cystic mass at the location mentioned above.

- Cleft I remnants may present as sinuses or fistulas draining along the angle of the mandible and the patient will have a history of recurrent watery discharge with or without infection.
- Cleft II remnants are by far the most common and present as fistulas or sinuses along the anterior border of the sternocleidomastoid (fistulous tracts cross the bifurcation of the carotid artery between the internal and external carotid arteries, and they may end in the tonsillar fossa).
- Cleft III and IV remnants typically present as thyroid lobe abscesses at a later age in childhood. A CT scan may be helpful in diagnosis.

The treatment of choice consists of complete surgical excision after treating the infection.

THYROGLOSSAL DUCT CYSTS

Thyroglossal duct cysts are cyst formed from the thyroglossal duct remnant (Figure 1), which is the path of downward migration of the thyroid gland from the base of the tongue to its adult location. It is found in the midline and may contain thyroid tissue. Sometimes, it is the only thyroid tissue in the body.

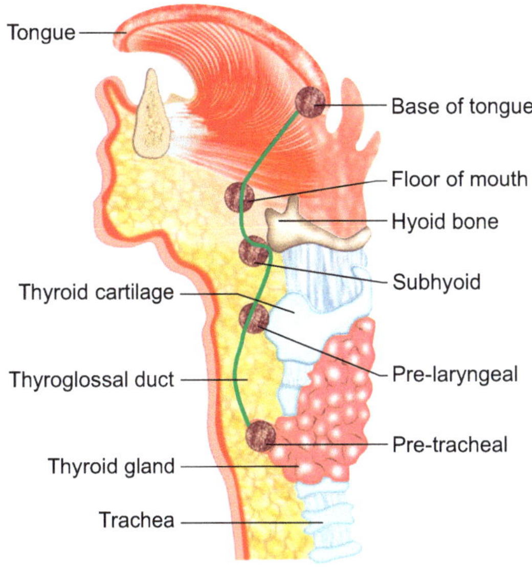

Figure 1: Thyroglossal duct remnant

Pathophysiology

Thyroglossal duct cysts develop when the thyroglossal duct fails to obliterate following migration of the thyroid gland from the foramen cecum at the base of the tongue to the neck, also passing through the central portion of the hyoid bone during its descent. It may occur anywhere along the path of the thyroglossal duct. The ectopic thyroid tissue may be the patient's only functioning thyroid tissue in rare cases, and papillary adenocarcinoma may develop along the duct.

Management

Diagnosis is made through the clinical presentation which often displays a mass in the midline between the submental region and the superior aspect of the trachea. It can potentially present as a midline abscess in the neck if there is communication with the base of the tongue and can result in contamination. Non-infected cysts are soft, smooth, and non-tender and may move with swallowing or protrusion of the tongue.

The treatment of choice is surgical excision. It should include excision of the cyst, tract, and the entire central portion of the hyoid bone, carried up the foramen cecum at the base of the tongue. If there is thyroid tissue present in the resected specimen, thyroid function tests should be performed to rule out iatrogenic hypothyroidism. If it is left untreated or inadequately treated, there is a possibility of recurrence or thyroid carcinoma development.

THORAX

Chest wall anomalies represent deformities in the development of the chest's supportive architecture and their functional impairment.

The ribs are formed by segmental somites that advance ventrally toward the sternum. They develop from two mesoderm bands that eventually fuse in the center. The costal cartilages link the developing ribs to the sternum.

There are three types of chest wall anomalies which include, (1) pectus excavatum, (2) pectus carinatum, and (3) sternal cleft.

Pectus Excavatum

The most common chest wall deformity, present in 1 of 300 to 1 of 400 live births. It can be unilateral or bilateral, but typically involves 3 or more ribs on the affected side. The degree of deformity can vary due to abnormal growth regulation of the costal cartilages. It rarely affects cardiopulmonary function, and it may lead to psychosocial impairment due to the cosmetic look. Mostly it is asymptomatic but may be symptomatic depending on the severity of the deformity which can compromise cardiopulmonary functions. Pectus excavatum is diagnosed by chest X-ray, and a CT scan may be helpful.

Treatment involves surgical correction during late childhood or adolescence. It is performed later in life because earlier correction can lead to thoracic dystrophy. The surgical techniques, as described by Ravitch, involve resection of the costal cartilages, elevation of the sternum off of mediastinal and muscular structures, osteotomy of the sternum, and reinforcement of the sternum with a strut.

The Nuss procedure is a minimally invasive technique in which a metal bar is advanced under the sternum. The bar is then left in place to push the defect back into a normal position. The bar is usually removed after 2 years.

Pectus Carinatum

Pectus carinatum has a protrusive appearance due to the outward displacement of the sternum. It becomes more pronounced and disfiguring in adolescence.

Management can be either nonoperative or operative. Nonoperative treatment involves a brass application. Operative treatment involves surgical correction. This is purely cosmetic as no physiologic deficits occur with pectus carinatum. The procedure includes osteotomies that flatten the sternum.

Sternal Cleft

A sternal cleft occurs when the sternal bars of the mesoderm fail to completely fuse during development. It usually occurs as a part of the pentalogy of Cantrell: sternal cleft, omphalocele, diaphragmatic defect, pericardial defect, and intracardiac defect.

Sternal clefts may be surgically corrected by reapproximating the cleft in the midline which is curative. If it is incomplete, the cleft must be divided completely for adequate healing.

PULMONARY SEQUESTRATION

Pulmonary sequestration is abnormal lung tissue that develops without normal communication between the trachea or a bronchus with an aberrant blood supply. Arterial supply from the aorta and venous drainage is either from the pulmonary or systemic circulation. It is more common in males at a 4:1 male to female ratio. There are two types of pulmonary sequestration, intralobar and extralobar (Table 2).

Table 2: Intralobar vs. extralobar pulmonary sequestration

	Intralobar	Extralobar
Location	Within chest/medial aspect of lower lobes	Chest/diaphragm or retroperitoneum
Covering	Visceral pleura	No pleura
Blood Supply	Mostly vessel from infradiaphragmatic aorta	Mostly vessel from infradiaphragmatic aorta

Intralobar sequestrations are essentially within the chest, are invested by visceral pleura, and are located in the medial posterior segments of the lower lobes. A majority are fed by vessels arising from the infra-diaphragmatic aorta running through the inferior pulmonary ligament.

Extralobar sequestrations are not invested by pulmonary pleura and may occur within the chest, diaphragm, or the retroperitoneum. Most often, it is incidentally detected and is frequently associated with other congenital anomalies. The left side is more commonly affected and there is rare communication with the foregut.

The pathogenesis of pulmonary sequestration is not completely understood. There is a possible origin from either the accessory lung bud or primitive foregut with angiogenesis occurring from the aorta. In the intralobar variant, there is no distinctive bronchus present, but usually there are micro communications with the airways leading to infection of the lung sequestration. The most common presentation is recurrent lung infections in early childhood.

Pulmonary sequestration is diagnosed with chest X-ray which reveals an inferiorly located consolidation with aeration. Recently, contrast CT scans and MRI have replaced the need for angiography. The extra lobar variety is diagnosed during an evaluation for a different congenital anomaly. It is rarely associated with aeration unless there is communication with the foregut.

Management

In symptomatic cases of intralobar sequestration, surgical resection is the standard of care. Due to an inability to distinguish between sequestration segments and the surrounding pulmonary lobe, a completion lobectomy is frequently required.

Cases of extralobar sequestration are typically observed unless there is communication between the foregut with the resultant infection or an extrinsic compression on the gastrointestinal tract.

ESOPHAGEAL ATREASIA AND TRACHEOESOPHAGEAL FISTUAL

Esophageal atresia is defined as a congenital disruption of esophageal development that results in a blind ending esophagus with obstruction.

A tracheoesophageal (TE) fistula is defined as an abnormal fistulous communication between the trachea and esophagus that often occurs in conjunction with esophageal atresia.

Anatomical variants of esophageal atresias and TE fistulas are as follows (Figure 2):

Type A: Blind ending proximal pouch, distal pouch, and no TE fistula (6%)

Type B: Proximal TE fistula and distal blind pouch (2%)

Type C: Proximal blind pouch and distal TE fistula (85%)

Type D: Proximal pouch, distal pouch, and TE fistula (1%)

Type E: Pure TE fistula and no esophageal atresia (2%)

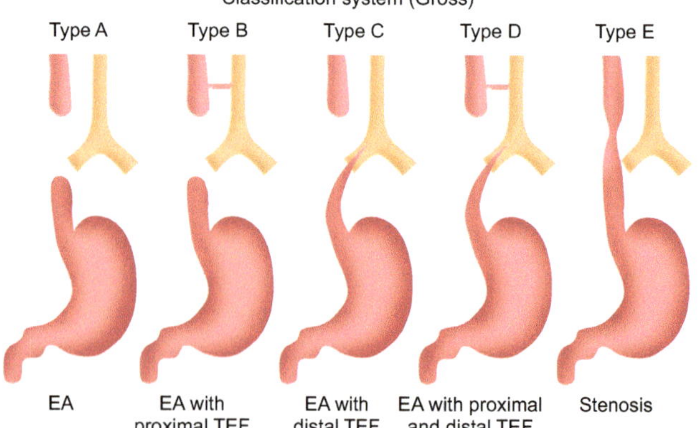

Figure 2

Both esophageal atresias and TE fistulas are frequently seen with a constellation of several other anomalies known as the VACTERL syndrome (V = Vertebral Anomalies, A = Anorectal Malformation, C = Cardiac Abnormalities, TE = Tracheoesophageal Fistula, R = Renal Anomalies, L = Limb Deformity). In a patient, either one, multiple, or all anomalies may be present together.

Pathogenesis

During the 4th week of gestation, the laryngotracheal tube, the common embryologic source for both the trachea and esophagus, forms. A tracheoesophageal septum formed by lateral invagination divides the tube into the trachea and esophagus. A defect in the formation of the septum or the division results in an esophageal atresia and TE fistula.

Management

Diagnosis is established at birth due to excessive secretion and an inability to pass the nasogastric tube. Once the primary diagnosis is established, imaging to rule out associated VACTERL anomalies should be performed. Workup includes imaging of the chest and spine, an echocardiogram, a renal ultrasonography, examination of the anus and limbs, and a genetic workup.

Treatment is surgical, consisting of dividing the TE fistula and anastomosis of the esophageal ends. The procedure depends on if the atresia has a short or long gap. A short gap atresia (<2½ vertebral body height) requires a single stage repair. A long gap atresia requires a staged procedure based on the length and type of defect. It also requires a feeding gastrostomy prior to anastomosis. The procedure consists of stretching both pouches by serial dilation, surgical fistulization and suture placement at both ends, a circular esophagomyotomy with primary anastomosis, and a cervical spit fistula of the proximal end with sequential lengthening down the neck.

CONGENITAL DIAPHRAGMATIC HERNIA (CDH)

CDH is defined as a congenital defect in the development of the diaphragm that allows the migration of peritoneal contents into the chest cavity leading to pulmonary hypoplasia. There are two distinct types of CDH (Figure 3):

- Bochdalek: The most common type, with a defect in the posterolateral location
- Morgagni: A rare anteromedial defect located behind the sternum.

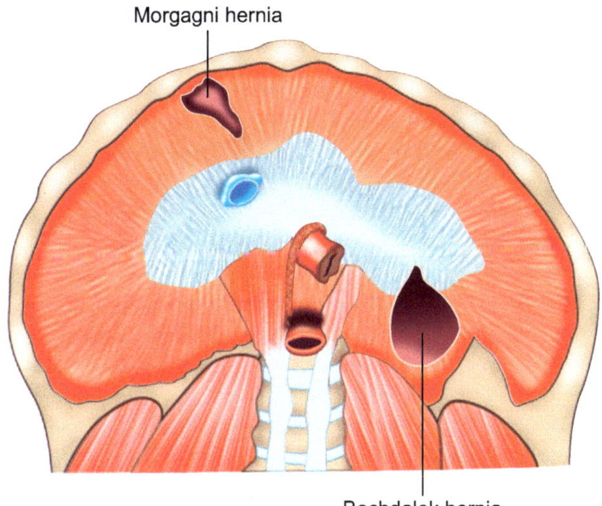

Figure 3: Locations of Bochdalek and Morgagni congenital diaphragmatic hernias

Pathophysiology

The muscular diaphragm is formed by a combination of inward growth of the lateral body musculature and the primordial diaphragm formed by the pleuroperitoneal membranes. Closure failure of the pleuroperitoneal membranes lead to CDH. Right sided defects are less common due to earlier closure of the right pleuroperitoneal membrane and the protective mass effect of the liver. The overall mortality rate is about 30 to 40%.

Management

Occasionally, CDH is difficult to differentiate from eventration of the diaphragm, either congenital or acquired, due to paralysis of the phrenic nerve. It is classically diagnosed on prenatal ultrasound showing polyhydramnios (80%), and at birth, neonates present with cyanosis and respiratory distress. Mild cases may remain asymptomatic or present with chronic respiratory infections, pneumonia, feeding difficulty, or bowel obstruction. Most cases are usually confirmed with a chest X-ray.

Treatment involves in utero fetal surgery at select centers using the EXIT procedure. Postnatally, management includes treatment in the neonatal intensive care unit with pulmonary support, extracorporeal membrane oxygenation (ECMO), high oscillation ventilation, partial liquid ventilation, and inhaled nitric oxide and exogenous surfactant. The mainstay of treatment is surgical repair, which reduces the abdominal contents.

In spite of improved diagnosis, surgical care and postnatal care survival is significantly dependent on the degree of pulmonary hypoplasia.

ABNORMALITIES OF THE ABDOMINAL WALL GASTROSCHISIS

Gastroschisis or "split stomach" is a misnomer. The condition is actually secondary to a defect of the anterior abdominal wall musculature. Patients always present with protrusion of the intestines through the abdominal wall defect into the amniotic cavity (Figure 4). This condition is more common in males, with the defect being exclusively on the right side, the umbilicus is always spared. This subgroup of patients has a low risk of having other congenital or genetic anomalies.

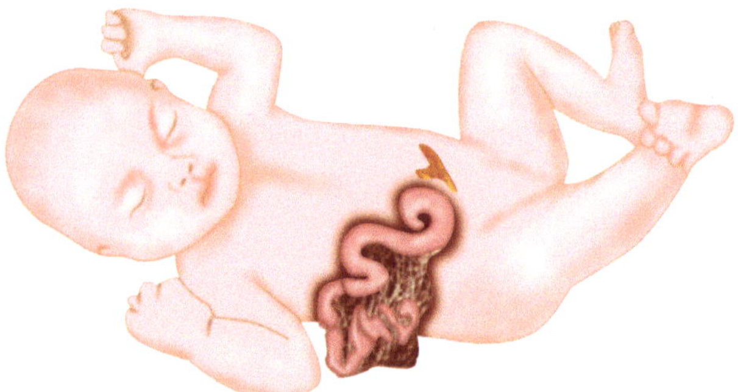

Figure 4: Gastroschisis, a defect of the anterior abdominal wall musculature resulting in intestine protrusion

Pathogenesis

There are no well-defined etiological causes known, but the proposed etiological agents are as follows: (1) maternal age <20 years old, (2) increased use of cigarettes, alcohol, and recreational drugs, and (3) increased use of aspirin, ibuprofen, and pseudoephedrine. The intestine is typically shortened, thickened, and matted or adherent together. Occasionally, 15% of cases present with intestinal atresia.

Management

Gastroschisis is routinely detected on prenatal ultrasound. Once diagnosed, patients should be managed at a facility with neonatal intensive care, pediatric surgery, and high-risk obstetrics coverage.

The immediate post-delivery care includes covering the intestine in a moist and sterile dressing, nasogastric tube decompression, and intravenous access with hydration and broad antibiotic coverage.

For definitive treatment, if the abdominal contents are easily reducible the gastroschisis requires primary closure. If unable to reduce the defect, a silo bag is applied with sequential tightening until the intestines are reduce back and the abdominal wall closes without much tension.

The postoperative course is prolonged with an inevitable postoperative ileus. Patients are managed with parenteral nutrition and frequent monitoring of liver function tests.

OMPHALOCELE

An omphalocele is an abdominal wall defect in which the viscera extrude through the umbilicus and is covered by a peritoneal and amniotic sac (Figure 5). This condition is highly associated with genetic and congenital abnormalities including (1) trisomy 13, 18, and 21, (2) cardiac, musculoskeletal, and gastrointestinal anomalies, (3) Beckwith-Wiedemann syndrome which includes exomphalos (omphalocele) macroglossia, gigantism, hyperinsulinemia, and hypoglycemia. Regarding prevalence, 1 of 5,000 live births have an omphalocele with herniation of the intestines, and 1 of 10,000 live births have an omphalocele with herniation of both the intestines and solid organs.

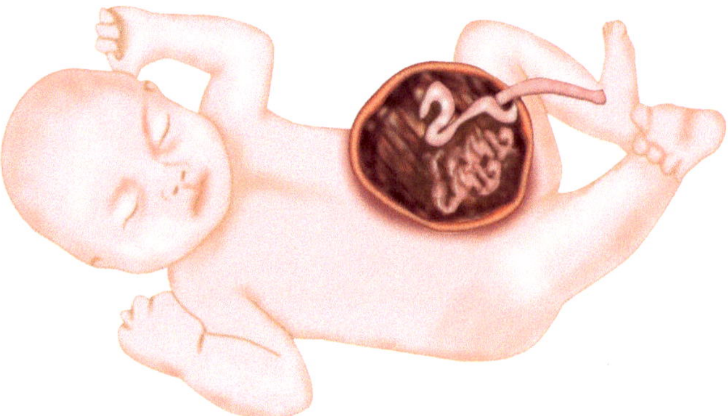

Figure 5: Omphalocele, a defect where the viscera extrude through the umbilicus. It is covered by a peritoneal and amniotic sac.

Pathogenesis

Between the 6th and 10th weeks of normal gestation, the abdominal contents herniate into the umbilicus and undergo a series of coordinated rotations before returning to the peritoneal cavity after which the abdominal wall closes. An omphalocele occurs when the intestines fail to return to the abdominal cavity. The inner lining of the omphalocele sac is peritoneum and the outer covering is umbilical cord epithelium derived from the amniotic sac.

Management

Omphaloceles are typically diagnosed by prenatal ultrasound. Pre- and postnatal care are essentially the same for both an omphalocele and gastroschisis. Additionally, a workup for associated anomalies should be undertaken.

The inital managment is conservative, followed by surgical closure of the defect.

EXSTROPHY OF THE BLADDER

Exstrophy of the bladder is a defect in the infraumbilical abdominal wall where there is failure of the median inferior portion to close, resulting in exposure and protrusion of the posterior wall of the urinary bladder through the defect. This is almost uniformly associated with male patients who have epispadias, and female patients with a bifid clitoris. Exstrophy of the bladder occurs in 1 in 10,000 to 1 in 40,000 live births.

Pathophysiology

During the 4th week of gestation, mesenchymal cells migrate into the space between the cloaca and ectoderm of the primitive abdomen. A failure to migrate leads to no development of the abdominal musculature in this position. Eventually, there is rupture of the thin epidermis and anterior wall of the bladder, allowing wide exposure of the bladder mucous membrane.

Management

Exstrophy of the bladder is diagnosed by clinical inspection. Treatment consists of surgical correction which closes the bladder plate and concurrently repairs epispadias in boys. Surgical repair should proceed within 72 hours of birth.

UMBILICAL HERNIA

An umbilical hernia is a defect in the connective tissue around the umbilicus present at birth. It is the most common abdominal wall defect in the newborn and tends to occur more commonly in African American infants than in Caucasian infants.

Pathophysiology

An umbilical hernia is due to lack of complete closure of the linea alba at the umbilicus. The umbilicus is reinforced by the paired umbilical ligaments (umbilical artery remnants), the round ligament (umbilical vein remnant), the urachus (primitive allantois remnant), and the transversalis fascia. Weakness or failure of any of these reinforcing structures can predispose one to an umbilical hernia.

Management

The diagnosis of an umbilical hernia is by clinical inspection and palpation. In most cases of congenital umbilical hernia, the defect will close spontaneously during the first three years of life. If the hernia persists at five years of age, surgical closure is indicated.

CONGENITAL INGUINAL HERNIA/HYDROCELE

An inguinal hernia is due to failure of the processus vaginalis to close, allowing abdominal contents to herniate through the inguinal ring and possibly the scrotum. A hydrocele is a collection of fluid around the testicle within the tunica vaginalis. Predisposing factors include prematurity. Congenital inguinal hernias and hydroceles are the most common indication for surgery in the infant population.

Pathophysiology

The testes develop intra-abdominally and migrate along a path created by the gubernaculum. The testes descend into the scrotum through the processus vaginalis, a canal which protrudes through the abdominal wall into the inguinal canal. After the descent of the testes, the processus vaginalis closes and obliterates. Failure of the processus vaginalis to close allows herniation of intra-abdominal contents resulting in a congenital inguinal hernia.

Partial closure of the processus vaginalis with a resultant collection of fluid results in a hydrocele. A hydrocele may be communicating, which is when a small opening in the proximal processus vaginalis remains open, allowing fluid passage but not herniation. A non-communicating hydrocele is when there is proximal closure of the processus vaginalis and resultant distal fluid collection.

Management

The diagnosis of a congenital inguinal hernia/hydrocele is clinical. The typical history of a hernia is a groin bulge that enlarges with crying or straining. The typical history of a hydrocele is a stable scrotal or groin swelling and on clinical exam, it will transilluminate. Most reduce spontaneously or with gentle applied pressure.

Surgical treatment is indicated at the time of diagnosis of an inguinal hernia and a communicating hydrocele which has a tendency to develop into a true hernia. A non-communicating hydrocele may be observed since they tend to resolve spontaneously during the first two years of life.

COMMON CYSTIC LESIONS IN THE ABDOMINAL CAVITY

Mesenteric Cyst: A mesenteric cyst is a cystic intra-abdominal mass with associated pain and emesis. It is mostly located at the mesenteric side of the intestine.

Duplication Cyst: A duplication cyst occurs anywhere along the gastrointestinal tract. In this type of cyst, all three layers of intestine are present in the cyst. There are two types, the tubular (communicating) type and the cystic (non-communicating) type. Diagnosis is made by physical findings, an abdominal X-ray, ultrasonography, and abdominal CT.

Treatment involves surgery where the cyst is excised with or without bowel resection depending on the extent of the lesion.

Omental Cyst: An omental cyst is a cyst filled with lymphatic fluid. It is a tender, palpable mass. Treatment involves a laparoscopic or an open exploratory laparotomy.

Hepatic Cyst (single or multiple): A hepatic cyst can be congenital or acquired. Clinical features include abdominal pain and jaundice if the cyst is big enough to cause pressure over the biliary tree. Imaging studies used for the diagnosis of a complicated cyst include an abdominal ultrasound, abdominal CT scan, and an MRCP or abdominal MRI. Also, a HIDA scan can be used to rule out biliary connectors. Treatment involves surgery. For a non-communicating cyst, a laparoscopic or open marsupialization can be used. For a communicating cyst, Roux-en-Y drainage is performed.

Choledochal Cyst: A choledochal cyst is a cystic malformation of the biliary tree. This cyst may involve saccular or diffuse dilatation of the extra hepatic bile duct, a diverticulum of the extrahepatic bile duct, a choledochocele, multiple cysts of the extra- or intrahepatic bile duct, or single or multiple intrahepatic bile ducts. Clinical features include a palpable mass and abdominal pain (cholangitis), cholestatic jaundice (obstructive), and clay-colored stools (alcoholic). Diagnosis involves obtaining lab values of conjugated hyperbilirubinemia, an abdominal ultrasound, an abdominal CT, an MRCP (superior to an abdominal CT), and a HIDA scan. Additionally, an ERCP may be useful in late presentation, as kids are grown up. Treatment includes a cystectomy with Roux-en-Y end-to-side hepaticojejunostomy.

Lymphangioma: A lymphangioma is an abnormal cystic collection of lymph, mostly in the retroperitoneum. It presents as a painful, palpable mass. Treatment involves a laparoscopic or open operation. The procedures include marsupialization of the cystic area with drainage and total excision if possible.

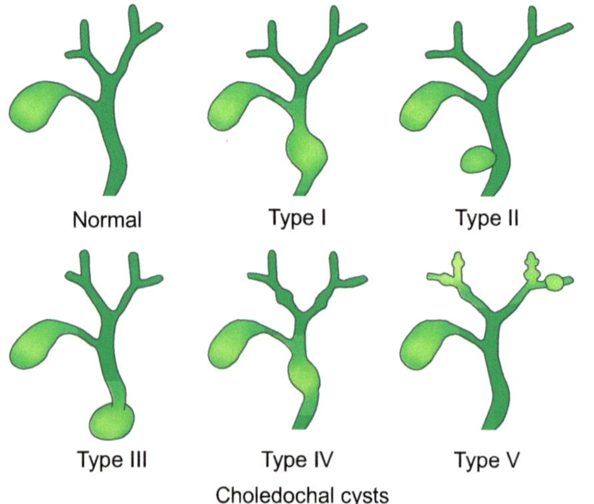

Figure 6

Urachal Remnant: A urachal remnant is a lower abdominal mass, mostly in the midline running along the course of the urachus. It presents with a discharging umbilicus. Diagnosis is made through abdominal and pelvic ultrasound and cystourethrogram. Treatment involves excision of the urachal remnant with repair of the urinary bladder if it is involved.

GASTROINTESTINAL TRACT HYPERTROPHIC PYLORIC STENOSIS

Hypertrophic pyloric stenosis is caused by gastric outlet obstruction secondary to hypertrophy of the pyloric muscle, resulting in narrowing of the pyloric lumen. It is more commonly seen in males than females.

Pathophysiology

The pathophysiology is not clear. A few theories have been proposed, the most commonly accepted one is a deficiency of nitric oxide synthase in the pylorus resulting in an inability of the pyloric muscle to relax and muscular hypertrophy. The maximum thickness occurs between the 4th and 8th week of age.

Management

Hypertrophic pyloric stenosis is diagnosed by clinical presentation. Symptoms include projectile, non-bilious emesis beginning in the 2nd to 4th weeks of life, a palpable abdominal mass or "olive" in the epigastrium, and hypokalemic-hypochloremic alkalosis on blood workup. The diagnostic procedure of choice is a pyloric ultrasonography that shows a thickened pyloric muscle (≥4 mm) and pyloric channel length (≥17 mm). A contrast upper GI series is required when physical examination and abdominal ultrasonography are not conclusive.

Treatment involves preoperative fluid resuscitation, IV hydration and serum electrolyte correction. A surgical pyloromyotomy (laparoscopic or open Ramstedt) is performed. This procedure involves dividing all layers, except for the mucosa, along the entire hypertrophied segment.

DUODENAL ATRESIA/STENOSIS/WEB

Duodenal atresia is due to the obliteration of a segment of the duodenum during development that results in a stricture or blind-ending obstruction (atresia). It may also be due to (1) a narrowing of the duodenal lumen secondary to an annular pancreas (stenosis) or (2) a diaphragm with or without a hole blocking the duodenal lumen (web). The incidence of a duodenal atresia is 1 in 6,000 to 1 in 10,000. There are three types of duodenal atresia as follows:

- Type 1 (92%): An intraluminal web or diaphragm with an intact mesentery and intact seromuscular layers in the involved intestinal segment.

- Type 2 (1%): The fibromuscular cord replaces the intestinal segment on an intact mesentery.
- Type 3 (7%): A complete atretic segment with a mesenteric gap, and proximal/distal blind-ending intestinal pouches.

Pathophysiology

This condition is due to either (1) failure of duodenal recanalization, (2) vascular disruptions during development, or (3) an annular pancreas.

Management

Diagnosis is made through maternal history-polyhydramnios, birth history of prematurity, epigastric fullness, bilious emesis, and a double-bubble sign on abdominal X-ray.

Treatment includes IV fluids, antibiotics, and a nasogastric or orogastric tube. Surgical options include a duodenoduodenostomy or duodenojejunostomy.

INTESTINAL ATRESIA/STENOSIS

An intestinal atresia/stenosis is due to the obliteration of a segment of the intestine during development that results in a stricture or blind-ending obstruction of the intestine. The incidence is 1 in 500 to 1 in 1,500 live births, and it occurs in about 15% of gastroschisis cases.

There are four types which include:

- Type I: Intraluminal web or diaphragm with intact mesentery and seromuscular layers in the involved intestinal segment.
- Type II: Fibromuscular cord replaces the intestinal segment on an intact mesentery.
- Type III: There are two subtypes (1) 3a which is when there is a complete atretic segment with a mesenteric gap, and proximal/distal blind-ending intestinal pouches and (2) 3b which is when there is a complete atretic segment with a mesenteric gap, and with a distal pouch corkscrewed around a single mesenteric vessel (Apple Peel or Christmas Tree).
- Type IV: Multiple atretic segments are in succession with the mesenteric gaps. This is also known as a string of sausages.

Pathophysiology

The fetal intestine develops from the midgut and undergoes a sequence of elongation, herniation from the coelomic cavity, rotation, return to the coelomic cavity, and fixation to the posterior abdominal wall. The blood supply is derived from the superior mesenteric artery which arises off of the dorsal aorta during development. Atresia occurs when there are vascular disruptions during development. The greater the vascular insult, the more severe the atresia type.

Management

Diagnosis is made with a maternal history of polyhydramnios, a birth history of prematurity, bilious emesis, abdominal distension, and failure to pass meconium. Then plain abdominal films are obtained which show a dilated proximal intestine and a decompressed distal intestine/colon. Additionally, a barium enema will show a microcolon.

Treatment includes initiating nasogastric suction upon diagnosis and correcting any fluid or electrolyte imbalances prior to surgery. Surgery may be performed semi-electively after stabilization and involves a tapering jejunoplasty and end-to-back anastomosis.

NECROTIZING ENTEROCOLITIS (NEC)

Necrotizing enterocolitis occurs when there is intestinal ischemic injury that begins in the mucosa. However, it may progress to full-thickness necrosis of small bowel or colon segments. This condition occurs most commonly in premature infants and is associated with the initiation of enteral feeding. The incidence is increasing because neonatal intensive care advances allow younger gestational age infants to survive past delivery.

Pathophysiology

The etiology of necrotizing enterocolitis is multifactorial. It is due to decreased perfusion leading to hypoxia in the intestine. It is associated with cardiac defects with shunting, respiratory failure, and hypotension. It also has an infectious etiology evident by the clustering of the condition. Infectious agents include Clostridium, Pseudomonas, Klebsiella, Enterobacter, and Staphylococcus species. Finally, there are immunologic factors. The host inflammatory response and free radical damage play a role and may help to propagate and worsen an existing case of NEC.

Management

Clinical features include abdominal distention, bloody stools, bilious emesis, and feeding intolerance. Physical examination shows abdominal distention with tenderness, decreased bowel sounds, blood per rectum, and abdominal wall erythema. Lab values may show thrombocytopenia, neutropenia, elevated PT/PTT, metabolic acidosis, and/or hyponatremia. Imaging may reveal diffuse bowel distention or ileus, pneumatosis intestinalis, fixed loops on serial X-rays, and portal venous air or free air.

Treatment includes both medical and surgical management. Medical management is the mainstay treatment and includes nasogastric decompression, total parenteral nutrition, broad-spectrum intravenous antibiotics, close monitoring and correction of fluid and electrolyte abnormalities, and proper ventilation to avoid hypoxemia. Surgical intervention is indicated in any case of bowel perforation or necrosis with pneumoperitoneum, abdominal compartment syndrome, and failure of medical management. The goal of surgery is to resect necrotic segments while maintaining as much viable bowel as possible to avoid short bowel syndrome. The standard surgical approach is to create an ostomy rather than primary anastomosis as the disease process may still progress. Overal survival of NEC at a tertiary or quaternary case center is close to 80%.

MECONIUM ILEUS

Meconium ileus occurs when the distal ileum is obstructed in a newborn infant with cystic fibrosis due to an inspissated meconium. In 10 to 20% of patients with the disease, it is the presenting symptom of cystic fibrosis.

Pathophysiology

Cystic fibrosis is a disorder of chloride channels caused by a single base deletion in the cystic fibrosis transmembrane conductance regulator (CFTR) gene. These patients have abnormally thickened gastrointestinal and pulmonary secretions due to a diminished volume of secretions and increased reabsorption of sodium chloride via the normal functioning of the sodium-potassium pump, thus leading to further dehydration of the secretions. Additionally, since the pancreatic and gastrointestinal secretions are abnormally thick, these patients will usually require pancreatic enzyme replacement. Death typically occurs by age 30 due to progressive pulmonary disease; however, with improved treatments and therapies, this age is gradually increasing.

Management

Clinical features include failure to pass meconium, abdominal distention, and bilious emesis. Abdominal X-ray shows dilated loops of small bowel and the soap bubble sign (ground-glass appearance due to meconium mixed with air). An enema study shows a microcolon. Additionally, there will be a family history of cystic fibrosis.

Treatment is conservative (effective in up to 70% of cases) and includes saline enemas or irrigation, gastrograffin enemas, and dilute N-Acetylcysteine enemas. If medical management fails, surgery is indicated. Surgery involves an exploratory laparotomy with enterotomy and manual removal of the meconium and a simple enterotomy with primary closure. If there is doubtful bowel viability, an intestinal resection ostomy (proximal and mucus fistula) is indicated. T-tube placement into the terminal ileum for continued irrigation may also be used. Postoperatively, the continued irrigation of the bowel with dilute N-Acetylcysteine via nasogastric tube or enema may be helpful for the passage of meconium.

MALROTATION

Malrotation occurs when there is an abnormal anatomic position of the bowel due to aberrant or absent embryologic rotation of the gut occurring in the 5th to 10th weeks of gestation. This results in a shortened intestine with abnormal attachments to the peritoneal wall. Ladd bands are the dense attachments between the body wall and cecum in incomplete rotation. They pass anterior to the small intestine and may serve as a point of obstruction. There are three variations which are as follows:

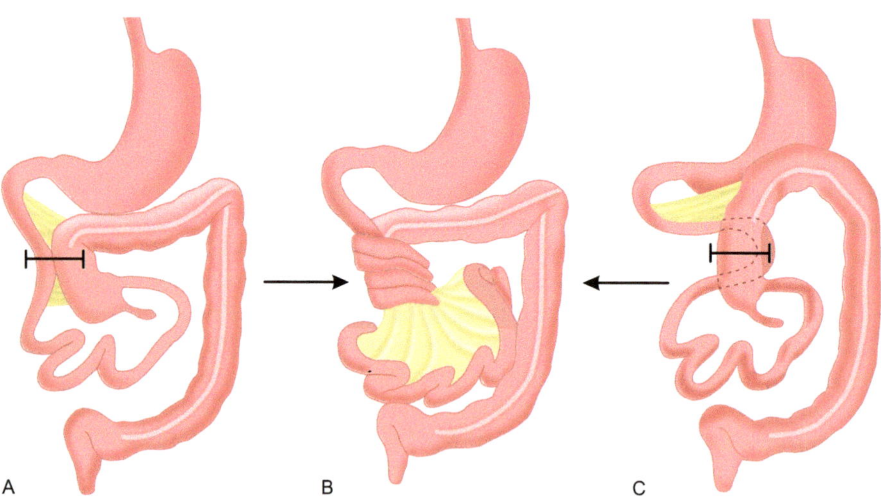

Figure 7. Malrotation of intestine

- Nonrotation: Very shortened small intestine on the right, the duodenum does not cross the midline, the cecum is at the midline, and the colon is on the left.
- Incomplete rotation: The small intestine is mostly on the right and the colon is on the left with the cecum in the left upper quadrant densely affixed to the right posterior body wall.
- Mesocolic hernia: There is incomplete rotation resulting in an essentially normal length of bowel, but with non-fixation of the right or left colon creating potential space for internal herniation of the bowel to occur.

Pathophysiology

Normal midgut rotation occurs along the axis of the superior mesenteric artery (SMA) with a 270° counterclockwise rotation resulting in an anteriorly located colon and posteriorly located small intestine. Rotation occurs during the physiologic herniation that occurs outside of the coelomic cavity between the 5th and 10th weeks of normal gestation. There is a significant lengthening of the jejunoileal segment during this time. The failure or cessation of rotation and fixation due to unknown causes is the source of malrotation.

Management

Diagnosis is made when there is evidence of bilious emesis and a volvulus due to non-fixation and a narrow base of mesentery. Many patients will remain asymptomatic and the malrotation may be discovered incidentally due to studies performed for other reasons. The diagnostic study of choice is an upper GI series with small bowel follow-through. The duodenum does not cross the midline and most of the small bowel loops are on the right side.

Treatment involves exploratory laparotomy and repair even in asymptomatic patients, or the Ladd's procedure. The Ladd's procedure involves detorsion of the midgut, division of Ladd bands, placement of the cecum in the left upper quadrant, and placement of the duodenum in the right upper quadrant. Then there is passage of a catheter through the duodenum to rule out associated duodenal obstruction, widening of the base of the mesentery, and appendectomy to prevent future misdiagnosis.

HIRSCHSPRUNG'S DISEASE

Hirschsprung's disease is a functional, rather than mechanical obstruction of the colon due to failure of ganglion development in a segment of the colon. This leads to failure of colonic peristalsis and obstruction.

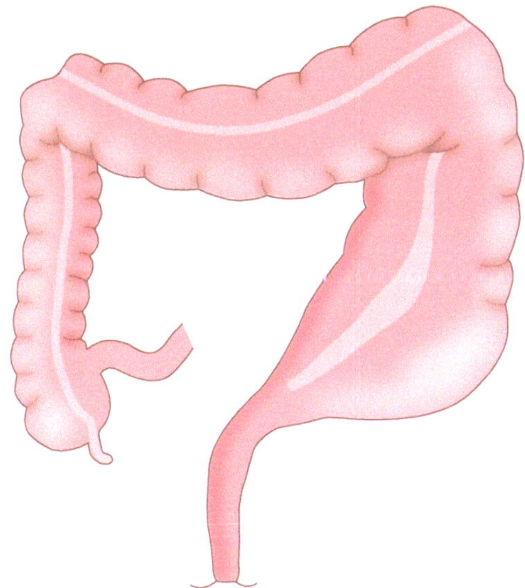

Figure 8. Hirschprung

Pathophysiology

From the 5th to 7th gestational weeks, neural crest cells migrate (craniocaudal migration) into the wall of the colon forming Auerbach's myenteric plexus and Meissner's submucosal plexus. Hirschsprung's disease occurs when there is failure of neural crest cell migration into the colon wall or subsequent failure of micro-environmental support. Genetic theory believes that there are several genes involved including the RET proto-oncogene, endothelin 3 gene, and endothelin B receptor gene. Aganglionosis occurs in a distal to proximal manner.

Management

The clinical presentation includes bilious emesis, abdominal distention, infrequent bowel movements or constipation, and failure to thrive. In neonates, a delayed passage of meconium (>24 hours) is noted. Additionally, one must perform an anorectal exam to rule out an anorectal anomaly, an abdominal X-ray to rule out other sources of obstruction and the absence of gas in the pelvis, a barium enema to identify the transition zone, anorectal manometery, and a biopsy. Rectal suction biopsy should show an absence of ganglion cells to confirm the diagnosis and a hypertrophic nerve bundle is a supportive finding. A full thickness rectal biopsy (FTRB) is required if suction biopsy is inconclusive, and the biopsy should have AChE staining.

Treatment includes staged repair surgical correction which is curative. One procedure involves primary pull through with or without ostomy. A temporary colostomy proximal to the transition zone is required, then there is pull through (Duhamel/Soave/Swenson). Figure 9 and closure of the ostomy (either colostomy or ileostomy depending on the length of diseased segment). The definitive procedure is performed at age 6 to 12 months and can be one of the following:

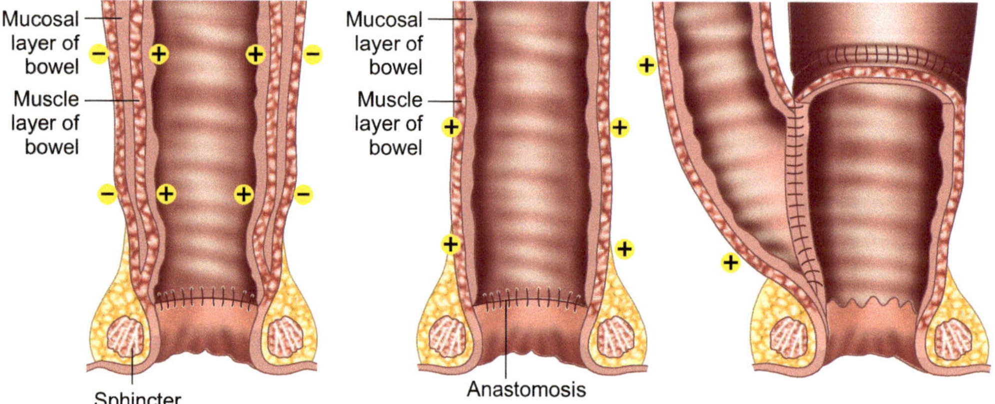

Figure 9. Swenson and Duhamel's procedure

- Duhamel-Martin procedure: This involves resection of the aganglionic segment with colorectal anastomosis of the normal colon posteriorly to the aganglionic remnant of the rectum anteriorly (retrorectal colonic pull trough).
- Soave procedure: This involves division of the colon at the transition point with transanal mucosal proctectomy and transrectal pull-through (endorectal pull through) excision of aganglionic segment, and colorectal anastomosis.
- Laparoscopic assisted pull through.

INTUSSUSCEPTION

Intussusception is the invagination or "telescoping" of a segment of bowel into itself causing mechanical obstruction (Figure 10). It may occur in any segment of the intestine, but ileocolic intussusception is the most common type. Intussusception is more common in infants and young children, but it can happen in adults.

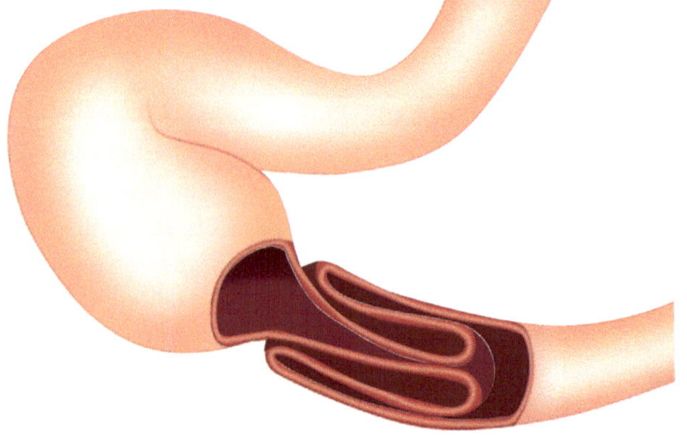

Figure 10: Sketch of intussusception

Pathophysiology

Intussusception mostly occurs due to a "lead point" at which the intussusception initiates and peristalsis propagates. The lead point may be lymphoid hyperplasia due to viral infections, Meckel's diverticulum, polyps, lymphoma, or another space occupying lesion in the gastrointestinal tract.

Management

Intussusception will present as a young child with colicky abdominal pain (severe alternating pain with pain free intervals). They may also have bilious vomiting and abdominal distention with a sausage-shaped right lower quadrant mass. Rectal exam shows "currant jelly stools" (stool mixed with blood and mucus). Guaiac positive stools occur in 90 to 95% of cases. The diagnostic procedure of choice is a contrast enema, which is also therapeutic in roughly 80 to 90% of cases, depending on the experience of the radiologist.

The initial therapeutic procedure involves hydrostatic reduction with contrast enema. Then one may try, pneumatic reduction with air-contrast enema. Pressures are 80 mmHg for infants and 120 mmHg for young children. Success is seen in up to 80 to 90% of patients depending on the duration of disease. Surgery is indicated for peritonitis, shock, or with failure of nonoperative means. Manual reduction on exploratory laparotomy (open or laparoscopic) is usually sufficient in uncomplicated cases. Resection may be required if there is bowel necrosis or if the lead point is suspected to be a malignancy. Most surgeons will perform an appendectomy to prevent future misdiagnoses. Patients should be kept in the hospital post-reduction as approximately 10% of intussusceptions may recur, most often recurring within 24 hours. Six months after the first episode, the incidence of recurrence is equal to the rest of the population. Recurrent intussusceptions in older children warrant exploratory surgery to rule out tumors as a causative lead point.

IMPERFORATED ANUS

An imperforated anus is when the anorectal orifice fails to develop. It is associated with the VACTERL syndrome. There are several types of this condition which include the following (Figure 11):

- Low: Located distal to the puborectalis muscle. This frequently presents with a perineal meconium fistula and does not require a colostomy.
- High: Located above the puborectalis muscle. This mostly occurs with fistualization with the urethra, bladder, or vagina and does require a colostomy.

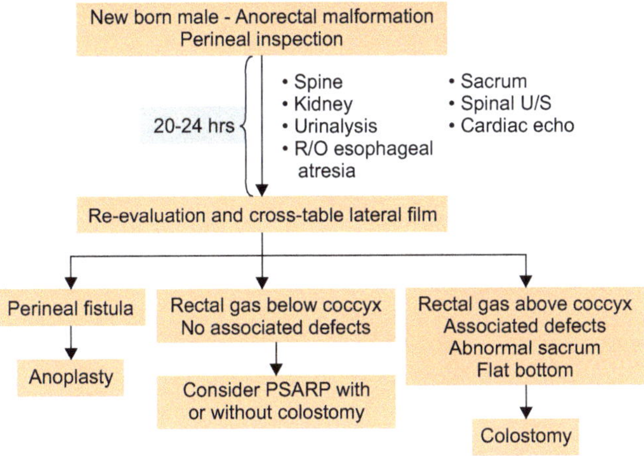

Figure 11. Algorithm of anorectal malformation management

Pathophysiology

An imperforated anus occurs due to the abnormal development of the urorectal septum, which results in the incomplete division of the fetal cloaca into its urogenital and anorectal portions. The abnormal connection between the rectum and urogenital systems may occur anywhere in the pelvis.

Management

Diagnosis is made through clinical examination, followed by a plain X-ray of the pelvis (pronogram) 24 hours after birth to allow for the distal passage of swallowed air, with the infant held upside down or placed in the prone position to helps assess the level of involvement.

Treatment depends on the type of imperforated anus. For the low type, primary repair is done with the perineal approach (cut back anoplasty) or limited PSARP. For the high type, colostomy is performed in infancy followed by a posterior sagittal anorectoplasty (PSARP) at age 4-8 months. Laparoscopic-assisted anorectoplasty (LARP) can be used.

BILIARY ATRESIA

Biliary atresia is the obliteration of the biliary tract in infants resulting in neonatal cholestatic jaundice. It can be classified as either (1) intrahepatic which is biliary hypoplasia, a rare condition that has a patent but underdeveloped biliary system and (2) extrahepatic which is the more common form and has atrophied extrahepatic bile ducts and an atrophied gallbladder. These can be classified into several types as follows:[5] (Figure 12)

- Type I: Obliteration of the common bile duct.
- Type IIa: Obliteration of the proper hepatic duct with cystic dilation of the porta hepatis.
- Type IIb: Atresia of the left and right hepatic ducts extending up to the level of the porta hepatic.
- Type III: Complete extrahepatic biliary atresia, the most common type.

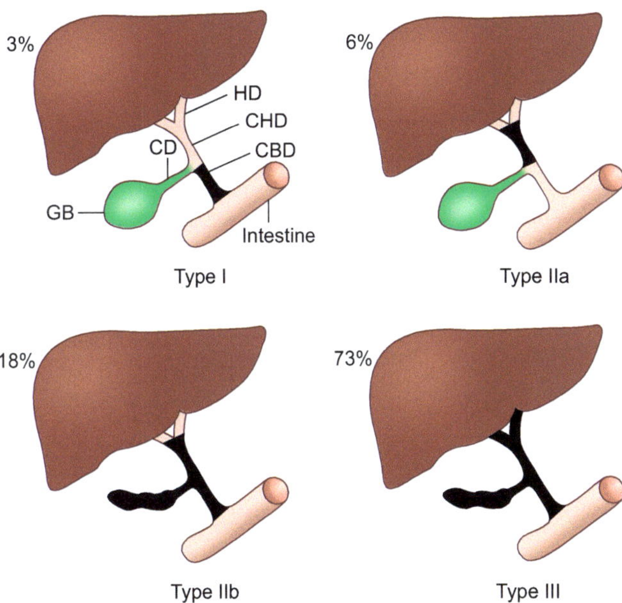

Figure 12. Biliary atresia

Pathophysiology

Biliary atresia is mostly of idiopathic etiology. Possible causes include an inflammatory process of the biliary ductal system after birth and viral infection (e.g., CMV) or toxin exposure in the ductal system. It is rare in premature infants. If left untreated, it will progress to cirrhosis and hepatic failure.

Management

Biliary atresia is suspected when there is neonatal jaundice lasting more than 2 to 4 weeks, dark colored urine, and alcoholic, clay-colored stools. Laboratory values will show elevated direct bilirubin. Additionally, an α1-antitrypsin with Pi typing should be completed to rule out enzyme deficiency, and a sweat chloride test should be done to rule out cystic fibrosis.

Imaging studies include a HIDA scan which will show rapid liver uptake with no excretion of radiotracer into the bowel. Also, a liver ultrasound which will show increased liver echogenicity and biliary dilation with a small, shrunken, or atrophied gallbladder. Liver biopsy is the most important diagnostic and prognostic test and has a high sensitivity in a suggestive clinical picture. Intraoperative cholangiogram via gallbladder cannulation should be done at the time of surgery.

Treatment is different from intrahepatic versus extrahepatic biliary atresia. For the intrahepatic form, an orthotropic liver transplant is required. For the extrahepatic form, portoenterostomy is the procedure of choice.

The Kasai procedure (Figure 13) involves resection of the atretic biliary ductal system and anastomosis of a Roux-en-Y limb to the porta hepatic. The level of resection is determined by frozen section to assess duct diameter.

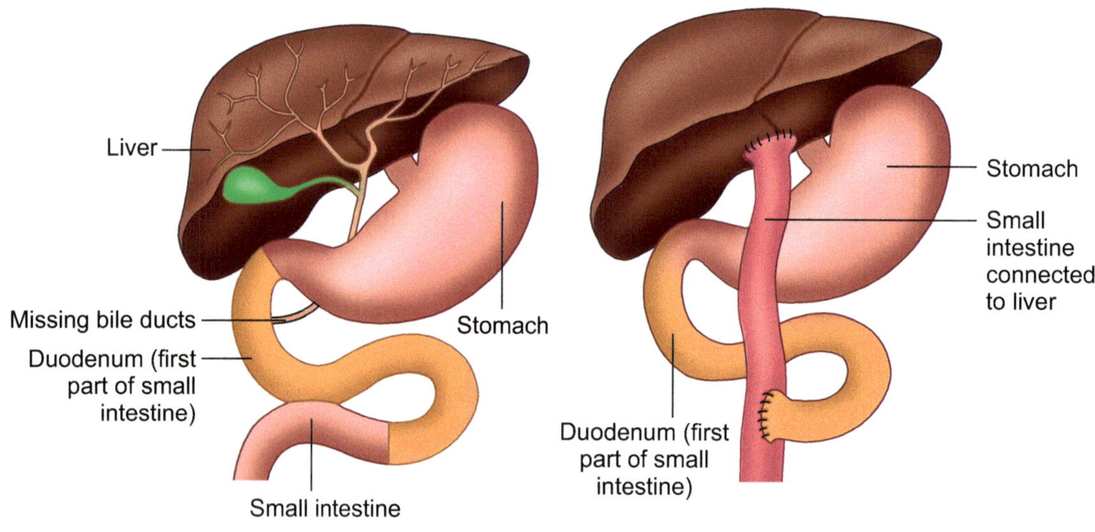

Figure 13. Kasai procedure for biliary atersia

Complications of these procedures include cholangitis. Twenty-five to thirty-five percent of patients have a 10-year survival without liver transplant, the remaining two-thirds of patients will eventually need liver transplant.

ONCOLOGY

Leukemia and lymphoma represent the most common cancer diagnoses in children and the most common solid tumors of infancy and childhood. General pediatric surgical therapy is the mainstay of treatment.

NEUROBLASTOMA

Neuroblastomas occur in 1 in 8,000 to 1 in 10,000. It represents 10% of childhood tumors with more than 50% presenting within the first 2 years of life. These tumors occur in various locations including the adrenal gland (50%), paraspinal (25%), mediastinum (20%), cervical (5%), and pelvis (<5%) pelvic organ of Zuckerkandl.

A neuroblastoma is a solid tumor arising from primitive neural crest cells and these tumors tend to be located in the distribution of neural crest cell derivatives. They represent the most common extracranial solid tumor in children.

Pathophysiology

Neuroblastomas are associated with the N-myc oncogene. Additionally, deletions on chromosome p11 and gain of DNA on chromosome 17q both confer a worse prognosis. They are high cellularity, uniform tumors with varying degrees of stroma within the tumor.

They are graded on the Shimada scale which is as follows:

- Favorable factors are tumors rich in stroma, young age of patient, and a low mitosis/karyorrhexis index (MKI).
- Unfavorable factors are tumors of nodular pattern, greater age at diagnosis, poor differentiation, and high MKI.

MKI assesses the number of mitoses and karyorrhexis per 5,000 cells in the tumor

The typical presentation is a cervical, abdominal, or pelvic solid mass. Cervical masses occasionally present as an airway obstruction depending on the tumor size. Its origin is from the cervical sympathetic chain and therefore can cause Horner's syndrome on the involved side. It rarely metastasizes and involves the lymph nodes. Abdominal masses mostly present as a hard mass in the abdomen arising from the adrenal medulla or midline sympathetic chain, and it involves the lymph node along the aorta. Pelvic masses present with intestinal or ureteral obstruction. There is sacral nerve involvement affecting the motor function of the lower extremities and anal sphincter tone. Other signs and symptoms of neuroblastomas include periorbital ecchymosis due to venous congestion or rupture with metastasis to the eyes, myoclonus due to anti-tumor antibody cross-reaction with purine fibers in the cerebellum, and secretory diarrhea syndrome due to secretion of vasoactive intestinal peptide (VIPOMA)

Management

When working up a neuroblastoma, contrast CT or MRI are used to show tumor extent. Additionally, one can use a MIBG scan. Serum and urinary markers are obtained to look for increased levels of serum and urinary catecholamines and by products. Biopsy is the mainstay of diagnosis and staging.

Staging is as follows:

- I: Tumor localized to site of origin with no nodal or distant metastasis.
- 2A: Unilateral tumor with incomplete gross excision without metastasis.
- 2B: Unilateral tumor with ipsilateral positive nodes, no contralateral nodal or distant metastasis.
- 3: Unilateral tumor with bilateral nodal involvement or tumor that crosses the midline.
- 4: Distant metastasis to nodes, bone marrow, bone, or liver.
- Stage 4S: Localized primary tumor as in stage 1 and 2, with dissemination limited to the liver or skin (limited to infants <1 year of age).

Treatment for low-risk tumors involve resection alone. Treatment for high-risk tumors involve resection and central venous access device placement for chemotherapy and radiation.

NEPHROBLASTOMA (WILMS TUMOR)

Wilms tumor is a tumor of primitive metanephric blastema cells. This is the most common pediatric renal tumor and the 5th most common pediatric cancer (Figure 14).

Pathophysiology

Wilms tumors are seen in several forms. These include the following:

- Sporadic form: Results from two allele loss in a specific tumor suppressor gene. The WT1 gene, an oncogene located on chromosome 11 is involved in the development of Wilms tumor.
- Denys-Drash syndrome: Wilms tumor, pseudohermaphroditism, and glomerulonephropathy.
- WAGR syndrome: Wilms tumor, Aniridia, Genitourinary malformation, mental Retardation.
- Beckwith-Wiedemann syndrome: Hemihypertrophy

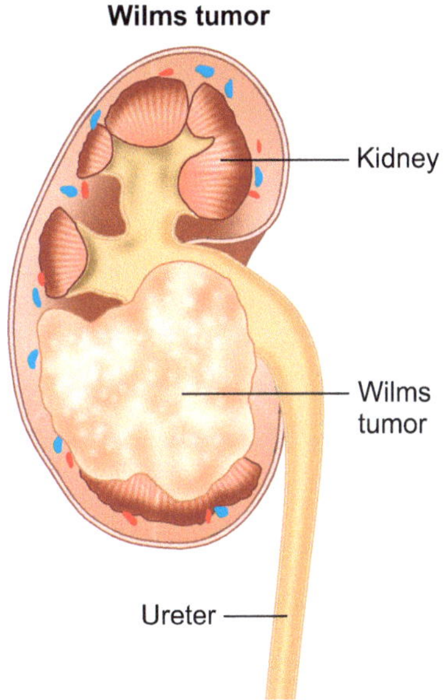

Figure 14. Wilms tumor

Management

Wilms tumor is seen as a palpable abdominal or flank mass, with or without abdominal pain. Additionally, the patient may have hematuria, hypertension, and fever. Renal ultrasound is obtained to assess the renal mass and renal vascular involvement. CT of the chest, abdomen, and pelvis allows for assessment of the tumor, differentiation from a neuroblastoma of the adrenal, assessment of the opposite kidney, and nodal or distant metastasis.

Staging is as follows:

- I: Tumor is confined to the kidney and can be completely resected.
- II: Tumor is completely excised, but with extension beyond the renal capsule, or biopsy of the confined tumor with local spillage.
- III: Tumor is incompletely excised, there are positive lymph nodes, or peritoneal seeding, or there is intra-abdominal tumor spillage.
- IV: There is hematogenous or lymph node metastasis beyond the abdominal cavity.
- V: Simultaneous bilateral involvement.

Surgical resection is required for treatment and staging. Additionally, chemotherapy is required for all Wilms tumor diagnoses and consists typically of doxorubicin, dactinomycin, and vincristine. Radiation therapy is used for stage 3-5 disease. If CT scan determines the tumor to be inoperable, then neoadjuvant cytoreductive chemotherapy should be given.

HEPATOBLASTOMA

A hepatoblastoma is the most common liver cancer in the pediatric age group. Its occurrence is 1 in 1 million children. It typically presents 6 months to 3 years of age. It may be epithelial or mixed epithelial and mesenchymal. Epithelial tumors are fetal (31%), embryonic (19%), macrotrabecular (3%), and anaplastic (3%). The remaining 44% is mixed epithelial and mesenchymal. These tumors are associated with Beckwith-Wiedemann syndrome and familial adenomatous polyposis (FAP).

Management

Hepatoblastomas present as a palpable abdominal mass with or without abdominal swelling, pain, irritability, gastrointestinal disturbances, fever, pallor, and/or failure to thrive. Alpha-fetoprotein (AFP) levels are significantly elevated with hepatoblastoma (>90%). Abdominal X-ray may show hepatomegaly. CT reveals a heterogeneous mass and is the imaging procedure of choice to assess for metastasis but is less sensitive than MRI for the primary diagnosis. MRI is the imaging of choice for diagnosis.

Staging is as follows:

- I: Complete surgical resection.
- II: Microscopic positive margins without regional spread, confined to one lobe of the liver.
- III: Partially resected tumor, spillage of the tumor at the time of surgery, involving two lobes of the liver and with positive lymph nodes.
- IV: Distant metastasis

Treatment includes neoadjuvant chemotherapy with doxorubicin and cisplatin prior to surgical resection. After reducing the tumor load, surgical resection with hepatic lobectomy is the procedure of choice, though in rare instances, a wedge resection may be used for small, peripherally located tumors. Liver transplantation will be required in up to 5 to 7% of patients.

TESTICULAR TUMORS

Testicular tumors are most commonly seen in children 2 to 4 years old. Diagnosis involves the presence of a nontender, solid scrotal mass and imaging. Imaging includes an ultrasonography of the scrotum and a CT scan of the abdomen and pelvis. Additionally, levels of the tumor markers alfa fetoprotein (yolk sac tumors) and beta-hCG (seminoma and choriocarcinoma) will be increased. Treatment involves radical orchiectomy and retroperitoneal lymph node dissection (RPLND) if needed.

PEDIATRIC UROLOGY. POSTERIOR URETHRAL VALVE (PUV)

A PUV has thin mucosal folds that look like a membrane causing varying degrees of obstruction during the act of urination (Figure 6). This is only seen in males and can lead to urethral obstruction in infants or newborns. The incidence is 1 in 8,000 to 1 in 15,000 live births. One third of PUVs progress to end stage renal disease and children will require renal transplant. Ten to fifteen percent of children who undergo renal transplant have PUV. There are three types of PUV defined by Young's classification. They include

- I: Abnormally high insertion and fusion (95%).
- II: Hypertrophy of the plicae colliculi.
- III: Septum at the junction of the anterior and posterior urethra.

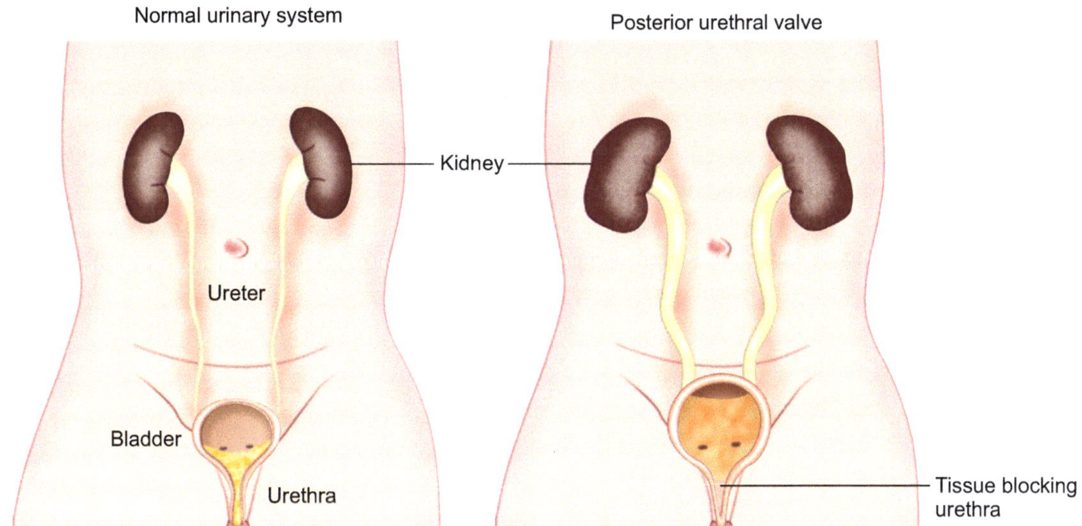

Figure 15: Posterior urethral valve

Management

Patients will present with various degrees of obstruction (mild/moderate/severe). They will have a poor, intermittent, dribbling stream of urine. Additionally, they may have frequent urinary infections, sepsis, symptoms related to severe obstruction (e.g., abdominal mass, distended midline bladder), and failure to thrive.

Laboratory findings include azotemia and a poor concentrating ability of the kidneys and chronic anemia. Diagnostic tests include (1) a voiding cystourethrogram (VCUG) showing the most common type (type I), associated reflux, elongation, and dilation of the posterior urethra with a prominent bladder neck, (2) an excretory urogram which will show a hydroureter and hydronephrosis in severe cases, (3) a ultrasonogram which can detect PUV prenatally as early as 28 weeks of gestation, and (4) cystoscopy which will confirm the diagnosis, when there is the presence of vesical trabeculation, diverticuli, bladder neck, and trigone hypertrophy.

Treatment depends on the degree of obstruction and the health of the child. Mild to moderate obstruction is treated with minimal azotemia-transurethral fulguration of the valve. Severe obstruction requires an individualized approach. If there is associated sepsis the child will require bladder drainage. Additionally, any fluid and electrolyte imbalances must be corrected. A vesicostomy or percutaneous urostomy may be indicated. The prognosis of a child with PUV depends on the presence of azotemia, the degree of sepsis, and the age of presentation.

HYPOSPADIAS

Hypospadias is a condition in which the urethral opening is seen on the ventral aspect of the penis. It occurs in about 1 in 250 male births, is more common in white children, and has a 7% familial rate.

Pathophysiology

Sexual and urethral development begins on the 8th week of gestation and completes at the 15th week. Failure of canalization of the ectodermal cord that has grown through the urethral folds results in hypospadias. There is a genetic association, where there is an 8-fold increase, polygenic inheritance with 8 to 14% history in brothers and fathers. It may be due to a decrease in available androgen or inability to use available androgen. Additionally, there may be endocrine disruption by environmental factors. Combination theory believes that there are two or more causes that work together that result in hypospadias. The type of hypospadias depends on the location of the urethral meatus. They include the following:

- Glandular: Opening is proximal to the glans penis (most common)
- Coronal: At the coronal sulcus (most common)
- Penile shaft: Can be either proximal, mid, or distal
- Penoscrotal
- Perineal

Management

Patients will present with an abnormal urethral opening at different sites, and it is associated with curvature (Chordee) of the penis, generally ventral bending. Additionally, it is associated with undescended testis. In more proximal (penoscrotal, scrotal) hypospadias it is essential to rule out ambiguous genitalia by buccal smear and karyotyping.

Treatment involves surgery. The aim of surgical repair includes orthoplasty (straight penis), urethroplasty (meatus at tip of penis), and glansplasty (conical glans). It is essential to repair the hypospadias before the child reaches school age for psychological reason, this is generally between 1 to 2 years of age.

Multiple techniques are described; especially since the repair depends on the type of hypospadias.

- Tabularized incised plate (TIP) urethroplasty: This is the most common technique where the urethral plate is incised in the midline to increase the width of the urethra for the tubularization.

Single stage repair:

- Duckett's procedure: Preputial flap.
- Koyanagi and modified Koyanagi repair: Using the preputial flap with variation in division of the flap by either dividing at 12 o'clock or through a buttonhole procedure.
- Denise-Brown technique: With burial of the skin strip with spontaneous re-epithelialization.

URETEROCELE

A ureterocele is a terminal dilatation, sacculation of the terminal portion of the ureter. The type is based on the number of renal units and the location of the opening. The types include the single system ureterocele, the duplex system ureterocele, the orthotopic (within the bladder), and ectopic. The other classification is based on features of the affected ureter. These include stenotic, sphincteric, sphincterostenotic, and cecoureterocele. The incidence of ureteroceles is 1 in 4,000 live births and it is more common in white females than in males.

The precise etiology is unknown; however, there are a few theories. The most accepted theory is a ureteral orifice obstruction with incomplete dissolution of the Chwalla membrane. The Chwalla membrane is a primitive thin membrane separating the ureteral bud from the urogenital sinus.

Management

Patients will present with urinary tract infections, urosepsis, obstructive voiding symptoms, urinary retention, failure to thrive, ureteral calculi, and hematuria.

Diagnosis is made by ultrasound which will show evidence of a cyst in a cyst sign fluid filled cystic cavity in the bladder. There will also be associated hydronephrosis and duplication of the renal units. Voiding cystourethrography (VCUG) is performed to rule out lower urinary tract anomalies. A nuclear renal scan is obtained to assess the split renal function. Other studies obtained include an intravenous urogram (IVU), a CT scan in equivocal cases, and the dropping lily sign to determine if there is a hydronephrotic upper pole displacing a lower moiety and a Cobra head extension in the bladder.

Surgery is the mainstay of treatment. The aims of surgery are to control the infection, preserve renal function, protect ipsilateral and contralateral renal units, and maintain urinary continence. The surgical approach depends on the site of the ureterocele, the clinical situation, and renal anomalies and size. Techniques used include endoscopic incision, transurethral unroofing, upper pole heminephrectomy and partial ureterectomy, ureteropyelostomy, excision of the ureterocele and ureteral reimplantation, and nephrectomy.

CONGENITAL URETEROPELVIC JUNCTION (UPJ) OBSTRUCTION

UPJ obstruction is the most common cause of an upper urinary tract obstruction in children and is secondary to a functional impairment of urine transport from the pelvis to the ureter. The incidence of urinary tract obstruction in children is 1 in 500 to 1 in 700 pregnancies, of which 40 to 50% are secondary to a UPJ obstruction.

Pathophysiology

A UPJ obstruction is due to either an intrinsic narrowing of the lumen at the UPJ secondary to an aperistaltic segment, an abnormal recanalization of the ureter, or an extrinsic-aberrant or supernumerary vessel.

Patients are generally asymptomatic, and the obstruction is often detected prenatally or incidentally. If a patient is symptomatic, they will have symptoms of episodic flank pain, a flank mass, urinary tract infections, nausea, vomiting, failure to thrive, and hematuria secondary to blunt abdominal trauma.

Management

Diagnosis is normally made through prenatal ultrasound by measuring the AP diameter of the renal pelvis. Dimensions will include 4 mm in fetuses less than 33 weeks gestation, and greater than 7 mm in fetuses greater than 33 weeks gestation. Additionally, patients often incidentally discover a UPJ obstruction on intravenous urograms, CT scans, or MRIs performed for other reasons. A nuclear renal scan is done to assess renal function.

Surgery is the mainstay treatment, and the procedure is based on the etiology. Pyeloplasty is an open, minimally invasive (endoscopic/laparoscopic/robotic) procedure. The principles of surgery are to form a tunnel at the ureteropelvic anastomosis. It includes dependent drainage, watertight anastomosis, and tension free anastomosis. In failed primary surgery, one must perform either a ureterocalostomy or place an interventional radiology assisted drain or nephrostomy.

VESICOURETERAL REFLUX (VUR)

VUR is an abnormal movement of urine from the bladder to the ureter or kidneys. The incidence is unknown as most children are asymptomatic. It is more commonly seen in children with urinary tract infection (15 to 70%), siblings of children with VURs (25 to 33%), and in white children.

Management

There are two groups of VUR based on the time of diagnosis. Children are prenatally detected. If symptomatic, children will present with urinary tract infections, failure to thrive, abdominal pain, pyelonephritis, sterile reflux with episodic abdominal pain, and reflux nephropathy. The etiology for primary reflux is unknown, but a few theories exist such as having a genetic predisposition, previous urinary tract infections, congenital bladder obstruction, and dysfunctional voiding.

Diagnostic tests include ultrasound and voiding cystourethrogram (VCUG). Children will receive these diagnostic tests during the evaluation of a urinary tract infection if <5 years, they have a febrile urinary tract infection, or if they are a boy with a urinary tract infection.

The VUR is classified into the following based on the VCUG:

- Grade I: Reflux into a nondilated ureter.
- Grade II: Reflux into the renal pelvis and calyces without dilation.
- Grade III: Reflux with mild-to-moderate dilation and minimal blunting of the fornices.
- Grade IV: Reflux with moderate ureteral tortuosity and dilation of the renal pelvis and calyces.
- Grade V: Reflux with gross dilation of the ureter, pelvis, and calyces, loss of papillary impressions, and ureteral tortuosity.

Treatment of VUR aims to prevent renal infection, damage, and complications of renal damage. Newly diagnosed urinary tract infections require antibiotic therapy with prophylaxis until imaging reveals reflux. All newly diagnosed grades I-IV and some grade V refluxes are treated with antibiotics.

Surgery is indicated when there are breakthrough urinary tract infections despite antibiotics, severe (grade V or bilateral IV reflux), mild to moderate reflux in pubertal females, poor compliance with medications, and poor renal growth. The surgical approach is an endoscopic reflux procedure, open intravesical/extravesical.

UNDESCENDED TESTIS

Undescended testis is the absence of one or both testicles from the scrotum at birth. The incidence is in 3% of full-term and 30% of premature infants. It is more commonly seen in infants who are premature or low birth weight, who encountered an environmental chemical endocrine disruptor, who have a family history of cryptorchidism (4% in fathers and 6 to 10% in brothers), and who have a congenital malformation syndrome (e.g., Prader-Willi syndrome, Noonan syndrome, Cloacal extrophy).

Management

This is a clinical diagnosis with findings of an empty scrotum or testes palpable in the inguinal canal. Imaging has limited value, but a diagnostic laparoscopy can be used in cases where the testis is not palpable on imaging.

Treatment is surgery. The aim of surgery is to increase the likelihood of fertility, self-examination, to correct the psychological effects of an empty scrotum, to correct an associated hernia, and to prevent torsion. The surgical approach is based on whether the testis is palpable or non-palpable with inguinal, extended inguinal/abdominal approach, or laparoscopy.

RENAL ECTOPIA

Renal ectopia is due to failure of kidney ascent during embryogenesis. The types of renal ectopia include simple, crossed without fusion/fusion. These patients have an associated abnormal vasculature from local tissue and have a predilection for infection and obstruction.

Diagnosis is made with a clinically palpable mass, confirmed with imaging. Additionally, renal ectopia may be incidentally detected during the workup for other issues. Treatment is not required, but it is provided for any associated complications of obstruction and infection.

RENAL AGENESIS

Renal agenesis is the absence of one or both renal units. It is an extremely rare condition, with less than 400 cases reported. This condition is not compatible with life. The incidence of renal agenesis is 1 in 500 to 1 in 1,000 live births.

Workup is done in prenatally suspected patients. They may have oligohydramnios, associated pulmonary hypoplasia, and facial deformities (Potters syndrome).

AUTOSOMAL RECESSIVE POLYCYSTIC RENAL DISEASE

Autosomal recessive polycystic renal disease is seen in 1 in 10,000 live births. In this condition, cysts are on both renal units and on the liver. They will have varying presentations based on the degree of renal and/or liver failure. Many patients present with a palpable masses, renal failure, and portal hypertension secondary to fibrosis. Many neonates will die in the first few weeks of life, secondary to pulmonary hypoplasia and insufficiency. If they survive, most will present with renal and hepatic failure. Treatment is based on presentation, either with replacement therapy or renal and/or liver transplantation.

HORSESHOE KIDNEY

Horseshoe kidney is the most common fusion anomaly. It is due to the fusion of both kidneys, most commonly occurring at the lower pole. Other sites of fusion include the isthmus and the upper pole. The horseshoe kidney is commonly located at vertebral level L4 since the inferior epigastric artery impedes the ascent of the kidney.

Patients will present with a lump in the abdomen, infections, renal stones, and ureteropelvic obstruction. Diagnosis is made through ultrasound, CT scan, or intravenous urogram. Functional imaging is done by nuclear imaging studies. Treatment is based on the mode of presentation, either by an open or laparoscopic route.

OTHER TYPES OF FUSION

Other types of fusion include crossed fused renal ectopia and fused pelvic kidney (pancake kidney).

REFERENCES

1. Pediatric Surgery General Principles and Newborn Surgery. 2020. Springer Science and Business Media LLC.
2. Greenbaum LA, Kliegman RM, Stanton BF, St. Geme JW. Pathophysiology of body fluids and fluid therapy. Nelson Textbook of Pediatrics. 2011. pp. 212-49.
3. Atlas of Pediatric Surgery Principles and Treatment. 2020. Springer Science and Business Media LLC.
4. Adams A, Mankad K, Offiah C, Childs L. Branchial cleft anomalies: a pictorial review of embryological development and spectrum of imaging findings. Insights Imaging. 2016 Feb;7(1):69-76. doi: 10.1007/s13244-015-0454-5. Epub 2015 Dec 10. PMID: 26661849; PMCID: PMC4729717.
5. Hartley JL, Davenport M, Kelly DA. Biliary atresia. The Lancet. 2009. doi: https://doi.org/10.1016/S0140-6736(09)60946-6.

73

CHAPTER

Neurosurgery

Y.S. Mohan MD
Chandramani N. Rao MD
Binit Katuwal MD
Vijay Mittal MD

INTRODUCTION

An understanding of basic neurosurgical concepts and management strategies is vital in the care of all patients among all fields of medicine and surgery. The following subchapters describe some of the important concepts within the field of neurosurgery, which might aid a general surgeon in caring for the patients.

COMA

Coma is a clinical state of cognitive dysfunction with impairment of the arousal mechanism.[1] Coma evaluation is designated based on the Glasgow Coma Scale (GCS). The scale evaluates for communication between all the sensory response centers and is administered based on eye opening (scored from 1-4, with 4 being highest), verbal response (scored from 1-5, with 5 being highest), and motor response (scored from 1-6, with 6 being highest), with a normal total score of 15/15.[2–4]

Table 1: Glasgow Coma Scale.[5]

Feature	Response	Score
Eye Opening	Spontaneous	4
	To Speech	3
	To Pain	2
	None	1
Verbal Response	Oriented	5
	Confused conversation	4
	Words inappropriate	3
	Incomprehensible	2
	None	1
Motor Response	Obeys Commands	6
	Localizes to pain	5
	Normal Flexion	4
	Abnormal Flexion	3
	Extension	2
	None	1
Total GCS Score		Between 3-15

If the patient's verbal access cannot be assessed due to intubation, a 'T' may be recorded next to the total score.[6,7]

Patients with a total GCS less than 8 signifies greater degree of impairment and increased mortality. Coma results from bilateral hemispheric injury, cortical or subcortical white matter injury, dysfunction of the diencephalic system, or dysfunction of central pons or midbrain.

Various types of body posturing may be observed in comatose patients. "Decorticate" posturing occurs because of removal of the corticospinal pathways above the midbrain which results in abnormal flexion of the upper extremities and the extension of the lower extremities. "Decerebrate" posturing is attributed to inhibition of the vestibulospinal tract and removal of the inhibition of the medullary reticular formation, resulting in abnormal extension of the upper and lower extremities.[8,9] These have also been incorporated in the GCS scoring system.

ETIOLOGY OF THE COMATOSE PATIENT

Table 2: Etiology of coma[10]

	Diffuse Neuronal Dysfunction		
Structural Etiologies	**Toxic Etiologies**	**Metabolic Etiologies**	**Etiologies that Mimic Coma**
• Hydrocephalus • Neoplasia • Vascular occlusion • Intracranial hemorrhage	• Sedative-hypnotics agents • Dissociative agents • Opioids • Carbon monoxide • Antidepressants • Toxic alcohols • Antiepileptics • Simple asphyxiants • Agents of histotoxic hypoxia • Serotonin syndrome • Neuroleptic malignant syndrome • Clonidine	• Respiratory insufficiency • Dysglycemia • Dysthermia • Electrolyte disorders • Hypothyroidism • Infection • Nonconvulsive status epilepticus • Thiamine deficiency	• Neuromuscular paralysis • Locked-in syndrome • Psychogenic unresponsiveness • Akinetic mutism

Approaching the comatose patient

A structured approach is necessary in evaluation and the treatment of a comatose patient. The initial stabilization is the same as all the patients who present to the emergency. The ABCs of acute care management which includes securing an airway, breathing and circulation needs to be done keeping in mind to give close attention to the spine. It is generally recommended that GCS less than 8 necessitates intubation to secure the airway, especially in traumatic patients.[11,12]

History and Physical examination

History is usually very limited in a comatose patient. Information from the EMT, family members, any bracelets or medical records might aid in evaluating the probable cause and the progression of the symptoms.

Vitals signs should be clearly recorded and evaluated which might provide strong clues in diagnosis especially in comatose patients with intoxication. It can also provide clues in the severity of the brain injury.

Breathing patterns

Various breathing patterns can be seen in comatose patients, and identification of the specific breathing pattern can aid in finding the cause of coma.[13]

- Cheyne-Stokes breathing gradually crescendos in amplitude followed by an expiratory pause and then the pattern repeats. This pattern of breathing is usually seen in diencephalic lesions or bilateral cerebral hemispheric lesions.
- Hyperventilation (i.e., rapid breathing) usually occurs in response to hypoxemia, metabolic acidosis, aspirations, and pulmonary edema. True central neurogenic hyperventilation is rare and usually results from dysfunction in the pons.
- Cluster breathing involves periods of rapid irregular breathing separated from an apneic spell. This is usually seen in high medullary or lower pons lesions.
- Apneustic breathing which is signified by a pause at full inspiration, is quite rare. It may occur in cases of pontine lesions with basilar artery occlusion.
- Ataxic breathing involves breathing with no pattern either in the rate or depth of breaths. These can be seen in medullary lesions.

Pupillary Response

A proper eye examination is another important tool to identify the severity of a coma and even provide information as to the cause of a coma. Both pupils should be examined in ambient light and reaction to direct and consensual light should be observed for both pupils. The pupillary response is the most useful sign to distinguish metabolic from structural comas.[14]

The metabolic causes of fixed and dilated pupils are glutethimide toxicity, anoxic encephalopathy and topically applied atropine.

- Fixed dilated pupils are usually due to oculomotor palsy or possibly herniation. If the larger pupil is associated with an ipsilateral third nerve lesion, the eye will focus downward and/or outward.
- Bilateral fixed and dilated pupils that are between 7 mm to 10 mm occur during subtotal damage to the medulla, post-anoxic brain damage, and hypothermia (with core temperature below 32.2 degrees Centigrade or below 90 degrees Fahrenheit).
- Midposition of the pupils between 4 mm to 6 mm with no light reactivity indicates a more extensive midbrain lesion due to interruption of the sympathetic and parasympathetic at the same time.
- Pinpoint pupil with limited light reactivity that can only be detected with a magnifying glass is usually seen in pontine lesions involving the Edinger-Westphal nucleus. Bilateral meiosis is often seen in narcotics usage.

Extraocular Muscle Movements

In addition to pupillary response, extraocular muscle movements can provide significant clues as well.[15]

- Bilateral conjugate deviation is often seen in frontal lobe lesions. In such lesions, eyes gaze towards the side of the destructive lesion and away from the hemiparesis. In pontine lesions and medial thalamic hemorrhage, the eyes gaze away from the lesion and towards the hemiparesis. During seizures, eyes typically gaze away from the seizure focus.
- Parinaud syndrome includes downward deviation of the eye and difficulty in moving the eyeballs upwards. This may be caused by thalamic or midbrain pretectal lesions or even due to metabolic coma following a seizure.
- Unilateral outward gaze deviation on the side of the larger pupil is seen during uncal herniation.
- Unilateral inward gaze deviation is seen during sixth nerve palsy.
- Internuclear ophthalmoplegia may occur due to a lesion in the medial longitudinal fasciculus (MLF). In this case, the eye ipsilateral to the MLF lesion does not adduct during spontaneous eye movements or in response to reflex maneuvers.

Other physical findings might include bilateral orbital ecchymosis (Raccoon Eyes), postauricular bruising (Battle's sign) and hemotympanum in case of base of skull fractures, skin rashes in case of infection.

Management of comatose patients

Blood should be obtained for stat electrolytes, sodium, glucose, blood urea nitrogen (BUN), ammonia and complete blood count (CBC) with differential and ABG.

Emergency supportive medications should be administered, thiamine 50 mg to 100 mg IV push, followed by glucose at least 25 mL of D50 intravenous (IV) push especially if there is indication of hypoglycemia.

Naloxone should be given in a suspected case of narcotic overdose with a 0.4 mg IV push.

Flumazenil should be given in a suspected case of benzodiazepine overdose, starting with 0.2 mg IV over 30 seconds, wait for 30 seconds and then give 0.3 mg over 30 seconds at 1-minute intervals up to a total of 3 mg until the patient becomes arousable.

Imaging should be obtained when a structural cause is suspected, particularly in the setting of trauma. In these cases, usually the culprit is identified. CT is the commonly used modality for the evaluation of comatose patients. MRI might be of benefit in providing greater definition of cortical and subcortical structures which might not be apparent in a CT scan. Magnetic Resonance Angiography (MRA) or CT angiography (CTA) can be utilized to evaluate the arterial system.

If herniation syndromes or signs of expanding posterior fossa lesion with compression of the brainstem are detected, initiate measures to lower the intracranial pressure (ICP). LP should never be performed in cases of suspected herniation. Herniation syndromes include unilateral sensory or motor deficit, progressive obtundation to coma, unilateral third nerve palsy, and decorticate or decerebrate posturing. If there are no signs of herniation or posterior fossa mass or no focal deficits and if there is no papilledema, perform LP and start antibiotics immediately. Treat generalized seizures if present and try to get an emergency EEG. Treat metabolic, electrolyte, acid-base, and body temperature abnormalities.

Brain Death

Brain death is defined by the irreversible loss of all functions of the brain including the absence of brainstem reflexes.[16] Pupils are fixed with no response to light, corneal reflexes are absent, oculovestibular reflexes diagnosed with a caloric testing are absent, oculocephalogyric reflexes tested by doll's eye movement are absent, and gag or cough reflex is absent. Apnea is seen with arterial PCO2 more than 60 mmHg and there is no response to deep central pain. It is important to check all brainstem reflexes as a positive reflex excludes brain death. Oculovestibular reflex is measured/quantified/ using the cold-water caloric test. Instill 50 ml of cold water into one ear with the head elevated at 30 degrees. (Do NOT perform this test if the tympanic membrane is perforated). Wait at least 1 minute for a response and more than 5 minutes before testing the opposite side.[16,17] All the other reversible causes of altered consciousness like intoxication, medications, hypothermia and shock should be excluded.

The Apnea Test

Apnea is confirmed when no breathing effort is observed at a PaCO2 of 60 mm Hg or with a 20 mmHg increment from baseline, which implies that the apnea test is positive. During the test, to prevent hypoxemia and reduce the risk of cardiac arrhythmia or myocardial infarction, 100% FiO2 ventilation is administered for 15 minutes prior to the apnea test. The ventilator should be adjusted to bring the $PaCO_2$ to 40 mmHg to shorten the test time and thus reduce the risk of hypoxemia. During the test, a passive O2 flow should be administered at 6 liters per minute either via a pediatric oxygen cannula or a #14 French tracheal suction catheter. The test is aborted prematurely if the patient's breathing is incompatible with brain death, significant hypotension occurs, the O2 saturation level drops below 80%, or a significant cardiac arrhythmia occurs.[18]

Clinical confirmatory tests include cerebral angiography and no of intracranial flow at the circle of Willis or at the level of the carotid bifurcation. Cerebral radionuclide angiogram can be performed at the bedside with a general purpose scintillation camera with a low-energy collimator. Brain death is confirmed if there is no uptake in the brain parenchyma, which is known as the hollow skull phenomenon. Alternative tests include transcranial Doppler and somatosensory evoked potentials.

INTRACRANIAL PRESSURE (ICP)

In adults and older children, the normal range of ICP is between 10 and 15 mmHg, younger children will be between 3 and 7 mmHg and at term infants will be between 1.5 to 6 mmHg.[19] Intracranial hypertension due to trauma may occur due to cerebral edema, hyperemia, traumatically induced masses like a subdural or epidural hematoma, intraparenchymal hemorrhage, foreign bodies, and depressed skull fracture. Increased ICP may also be seen in hydrocephalus, hypoventilation, systemic hypertension, venous thrombosis, increased muscle tone, and sustained posttraumatic seizures.

A secondary increase in the intracranial pressure is occasionally seen 3 to 10 days after trauma and may indicate a worse prognosis. This may be due to delayed epidural hematoma, delayed acute subdural hematoma, delayed traumatic intracerebral hemorrhage, cerebrovascular spasm, and severe adult respiratory distress syndrome. Edema formation, which is more common in pediatric patients and in cases of hyponatremia, may also cause a delayed secondary increase in ICP.

Indications for ICP Monitoring

ICP monitoring is indicated for patients who cannot follow commands with a GCS below 9.[20] ICP monitoring is also indicated during multiple system injuries with altered level of consciousness especially when treating other injuries can potentially have adverse effects on ICP including high levels of positive end-expiratory pressure (PEEP), large volume IV fluid resuscitation, and heavy sedation. In cases of epidural hematomas, subdural hematomas, or depressed skull fractures, a physician may choose to monitor ICP during the postoperative period after evacuation of the material.

Monitoring ICP in patients who have acute fulminant liver with an INR more than 1.5 and a grade 3 or grade 4 coma occurs in some centers.[21,22] Patients may be administered factor VII (40 mcg/kg IV over 1 to 2 minutes) and then a subarachnoid Bolt catheter. The Bolt should be inserted within 15 minutes and no more than 2 hours after administration to reduce hemorrhage risk.

An ICP monitor should not be placed on a patient that is awake or a patient with coagulopathy such as DIC (which is frequently seen in severe head injury). If ICP monitoring is essential, steps must be taken to correct the coagulation by giving fresh frozen plasma and platelets. A subarachnoid Bolt or epidural monitor should be considered. Intraventricular or trans parenchymal monitors are contraindicated in such patients.

Treatment

The cerebral perfusion pressure (CPP) which directly relates to the ability of blood to perfuse within the brain, is calculated as the difference between mean arterial pressure (MAP) and ICP.

CPP = MAP- ICP

The usual CPP is above 50 mmHg. An ICP more than 20 to 25 thus significantly reduces CPP and is associated with a high mortality and worse outcome. So ICP should be kept below 20. The primary goal is to control the ICP which simultaneously controls the CPP. The CPP threshold for ischemia is in the range of 50 to 60 mmHg. It is therefore better to maintain pressure above 70 mmHg.

Measures which can be used to prophylactically control intracranial hypertension include:[23]

1. Elevate the head of the bed by 30 to 45 degrees
2. Keep the neck straight and avoid tight tracheostomy or endotracheal tube tape
3. Avoid hypotension, keeping systolic blood pressure above 90 mmHg, control hypertension if present
4. Avoid hypoxia {PaO2 less than 60 mmHg or O2 saturation less than 93%.}, maintain airway adequate oxygenation, ventilate to normocarbia $PaCO_2$ 35 to 40 mmHg
5. Add sedation such as codeine 30 to 60 mg every 4 hours as needed

Sequence of steps to medically control intracranial hypertension includes:*

1. Heavy sedation such as fentanyl 1 to 2 mL or magnesium sulfate 2 to 4 mg IV every hour and/or paralytic agents like vecuronium 8 mg IV
2. If an intraventricular catheter is present, drain 3 to 5 mL of CSF.
3. Hyperventilate $PaCO_2$ 30 to 35 mmHg.
4. Administer mannitol 0.25 to 1g/Kg then 0.25 g/Kg every 6 hours; dose can be increased if high ICP persists and serum osmolarity is less than 320. If there is an osmotic room (serum osmolarity less than 320), a mannitol bolus can be administered with 10 to 20 mL of 23.4% hypertonic saline.
5. Hyperventilate $PaCO_2$ 25 to 30 mmHg.
6. Prevent hyperglycemia, which can aggravate cerebral edema and is usually present in head injury. It may be exacerbated by steroids.
7. Intubate the patient if GCS is less than or equal to 8.

*Avoid prolonged hyperventilation and keep $PaCO_2$ to eucapnia level of 35 mmHg.

CSF drainage can be utilized to manage ICP. 3 to 5 mL of CSF can be drained with a drip chamber at below or equal to 10 cm above the external auditory meatus. Osmotic therapy is recommended when there is evidence of raised intracranial pressure. A 0.25 g to 1g/kg bolus of mannitol can be given in less than 20 minutes followed by 0.25g/kg intravenous push over 20 minutes every 6 hours as needed. Keeping the patient euvolemic or slightly hypervolemic is considered acceptable in the management of increased ICP. If the increased intracranial pressure persists, serum osmolarity can be brought lower than 320 mOsm/L by increasing mannitol up to 1g/kg and then shortening the dosing interval. If ICP remains refractory to Mannitol, hypertonic saline can be added either as continuous 3% saline infusion or as a bolus 23.4% at 10 to 20 mL. Hypertonic saline therapy should be discontinued after 72 hours to avoid rebound edema. Serum osmotic therapy should be paused if serum osmolarity is more than 320 mOsm/L. Pediatric dosage is mannitol 1 mg/kg IV up to a maximum of 6 mg every six hours as needed. Hyperventilation (keeping the $PaCO_2$ to 30 to 35 mmHg) can also be used to temporarily reduce ICP. This should be used only for short periods of acute neurological deterioration, documented ICP unresponsive to sedation, paralyzing agents, CSF drainage and osmotic therapy. Hyperventilation should not be used prophylactically, and aggressive hyperventilation should be avoided, as this increases risk of ischemia especially within 24 hours of injury.

Heavy sedation may be required in patients who are agitated.

1. Morphine sulfate: 2 mg to 4 mg per hour IV drip can be established.
2. Fentanyl: 1 mg to 2 mg IV every hour, or 2 μg – 5 μg / kg/hr IV drip.
3. Sufentanil 10 μg: 30 μg test dose and then 0.05 μg - 2 μg /kg/hr IV drip.
4. Midazolam: 2 mg test dose, and then 2 mg - 4 mg/hr IV drip.
5. Propofol drip: 0.5 mg/kg test dose and 20 μg to 75 μg/kg/min IV drip. Avoid high-dose Propofol; dosage should not exceed more than 83/kg per minute.
6. Phenobarbital: adult dose is 100 mg IV every 4 hours, pediatric dose is 2 to 5 mg/kg IV every 4 hours

In case of failure to control ICP with the above measures, decompressive craniectomy may be considered. Craniectomy decreases the intracranial pressure to less than 20 mmHg, regardless of the pupillary response to light, timing of craniectomy, brain shift, and age.

Patients who will undergo emergency surgery for extradural or subdural hematomas may consider having early decompressive craniectomy. The flap should have a diameter of at least 12 cm, and duraplasty is a must.[23] Temporal tip lobectomy up to 5 cm on the dominant side and 7 cm on the non-dominant side are acceptable options.

HYDROCEPHALUS

Hydrocephalus, literally meaning "water in the brain," occurs due to excessive accumulation of cerebrospinal fluid (CSF) in the brain.[24] In normal circumstances, the majority of CSF is created via the choroid plexus within the ventricular system. It then travels through the lateral ventricles, to the foramen of Monro, into the third ventricle, through the cerebral aqueduct (aqueduct of Sylvius), into the fourth ventricle, through the foramen of Magendie (medially) and foramen of Luschka (laterally), to finally empty into the subarachnoid space of the brain and spinal cord. CSF is then reabsorbed at arachnoid granulations into the dural venous sinuses. When the normal flow of CSF is altered, hydrocephalus ensues.

The two main types of hydrocephalus include obstructive hydrocephalus and communicating hydrocephalus. In obstructive (noncommunicating) hydrocephalus, a blockage occurs proximal to the arachnoid granulations within the path of CSF flow. Computed tomography (CT) or magnetic resonance imaging (MRI) demonstrates enlarged ventricles proximal to the block. In communicating (nonobstructive) hydrocephalus, CSF circulation is blocked at the level of arachnoid granulation. CT or MRI demonstrates diffuse enlargement of the ventricular system.

Table 3: Causes of hydrocephalus

Common Etiologies for hydrocephalus:
Congenital
Chiari type II malformation with myelomeningocele
Chiari type I malformation ~ fourth ventricle outlet obstruction
Primary aqueductal stenosis
Secondary aqueductal gliosis due to intrauterine infection or germinal matrix hemorrhage
Dandy-Walker malformations
Acquired
Infections - post-meningitic, post cysticercosis
Posthemorrhagic - post-subarachnoid bleed, post intraventricular hemorrhage.

Signs and Symptoms

In neonates and young infants, hydrocephalus is commonly identified by a cranium that enlarges at a faster rate than the child's height and weight. In addition, these children present with bulging fontanels, splaying of cranial sutures, enlarged scalp veins, poor head control, and irregular respiration with apneic spells. Macewen sign is specific to children with hydrocephalus in which percussion of the dilated ventricles produces a unique sound like the sound of striking a cracked pot. Both children and adults may also present with the sunset sign (as part of Parinaud syndrome) in which eyes gaze downward with eyelid retraction. Other common symptoms in children and adults include headache, papilledema, nausea, vomiting, cranial nerve deficits, spasticity, hyperactive reflexes, change in gait, personality changes, and irritability.

CT/MRI Criteria for Identification of Hydrocephalus

1. Temporal horn width more than 2 mm (temporal horn is barely seen under normal circumstances)
2. Ballooning of the frontal horns of the lateral ventricle.
3. Enlarged third ventricle (typically a slit in most normal MRIs)
4. Thinning or upper bowing of the corpus callosum on sagittal MRI
5. Periventricular low density on CT or periventricular high intensity signal on T2-weighted MR showing trans ependymal absorption of CSF
6. Evan's ratio: A ratio of the maximal frontal horn ventricular width to the maximal transverse inner diameter of the skull measured from the same CT slice; a value more than 0.3 suggests hydrocephalus.

Treatment

Treatment should start with diuretic therapy consisting of acetazolamide 25 mg/kg per day until a dosage of 100 mg/kg per day is reached. In addition, the patient should be given furosemide 1 mg/kg per day orally three times daily. Electrolyte levels should be carefully monitored for signs of imbalance and CSF pressure should be monitored via spinal taps. Hydrocephalus occurring as a result of intraventricular hemorrhage may be transient. Thus, in this situation, frequent monitoring of CSF pressure with serial spinal taps or lumbar punctures may suffice. When hydrocephalus persists, treatment is surgical with the insertion of a ventricular shunt. Ventriculoperitoneal shunt, ventriculopleural or ventriculoarterial shunt can be placed to divert the CSF into the peritoneal, pleural or atrium respectively.[25] Endoscopic third ventriculostomy is an alternative to shunt procedures.

Normal Pressure Hydrocephalus

Some forms of hydrocephalus may occur as a syndrome such as occurs in Normal Pressure Hydrocephalus (NPH). NPH is manifested by a triad of dementia, gait disturbance, and urinary incontinence. It is identified as a communicating hydrocephalus on CT and MRI with normal pressure on random lumbar puncture. Symptoms are often resolved with CSF shunting. Gait disturbance is usually seen as a wide-based stance with short shuffling steps and unsteadiness on turning. NPH is usually seen in patients older than 60 years of age with a male predominance. Speech is often disturbed by impaired motivation or executive dysfunction. Aphasia is atypical in NPH.

As normal pressure hydrocephalus progresses, the patient may experience more generalized cognitive impairment and a decreased responsive to treatment. Symptoms may occur that are like those of idiopathic Parkinson's (which occurs in about 11% of the patients). After the onset of symptoms, brain imaging on CT or MRI must show ventricular enlargement which is not due to congenital enlargement or cerebral atrophy. Imaging must also demonstrate an Evan's index of more than 0.3 with no apparent microscopic obstruction of the CSF flow. In addition, more than one of the following supporting features must be seen: enlarged temporal horns, a callosal angle of over 40 degrees, evidence of brain water content changes, periventricular change not due to micro-vascular or ischemic changes or demyelination, and aqueductal or fourth ventricle flow void.

Pseudo-Hydrocephalus

Describes situations that mimic hydrocephalus but lack the excessive accumulation of CSF. Hydrocephalus ex vacuo is such a condition and occurs as a result of enlargement of the ventricles due to loss of cerebral tissue. This can occur as a function of normal aging but can be accelerated by traumatic brain injury and certain diseases such as Alzheimer's and Creutzfeldt–Jakob. External hydrocephalus is another condition which may be seen in neonates presenting with enlarged subarachnoid space, increasing head circumference, and normal or mildly dilated ventricles. This condition is benign and self-limited and is thus rarely treated. Hydranencephaly describes total or near total absence of cerebrum and is most commonly due to bilateral internal cerebral artery infarcts. Treatment for this condition is only supportive and prognosis is poor with death usually occurring in the first year of life.

INFECTIONS OF THE NERVOUS SYSTEM

Cerebral Abscess

Cerebral abscess may arise from blood spread, contiguous spread, or direct trauma. Risk factors include pre existing pulmonary abscess, AV fistula, congenital cyanotic heart disease, immune compromise, chronic sinusitis, chronic otitis, and dental procedures. Peripheral white blood cell (WBC) counts may be normal or slightly increased. CRP is usually increased. Streptococcus is the most implicated bacteria in cerebral abscesses, while up to 60% are polymicrobial.

Abscess maturation occurs in four stages: early cerebritis, late cerebritis, early capsule formation, and late capsule formation.[26] Early cerebritis describes early infection and inflammation that occurs in days 1 to 3 and presents with lesions that are poorly demarcated from the surrounding brain, perivascular infiltrates, and toxic changes in involved neurons. Late cerebritis occurs in days 4 to 9 and presents with the development of a necrotic center. Early capsule formation occurs between days 10 to 13, with further development of the necrotic center and neovascularization. Late capsule formation is seen over 14 days and presents with a collagen capsule, a well-developed necrotic center, and gliosis around the capsule.

Symptoms

No symptoms are specific for brain abscesses. Symptoms are typically due to edema surrounding the lesion and increased ICP, which often results in headache, nausea, vomiting, and lethargy. Hemiparesis and seizures develop in 30-50% of the patients. Papilledema may also be seen but is rare before two years of age.[27]

Diagnostic Tests

Peripheral WBC may be normal or only mildly elevated in 70% of cases. Blood cultures should be obtained when an abscess is suspected, but results are usually negative. Erythrocyte sedimentation rate and C-reactive protein levels may be elevated but are non-specific for abscesses. There is no characteristic diagnostic finding on LP in a case of cerebral abscess. Opening pressure will be increased and WBC count and protein may be elevated. Technetium tagged WBC scan with a labeled molecule and is near 100% sensitive and specific for abscesses.

Imaging

CT typically demonstrates ring-enhancing lesions with sensitivity close to 100% (Figure 1). MRI shows high intensity T1W1 thin-walled ring-enhancing lesions with a low intensity central region. Fluid filled levels may also be seen within the lesions. Diffusion weighted imaging (DWI) typically shows bright signal suggesting viscous fluid in contrast to the dark signal seen in tumors.[28] MR spectroscopy may show increased peaks of amino acid acetate and lactate which are also diagnostic of an abscess.

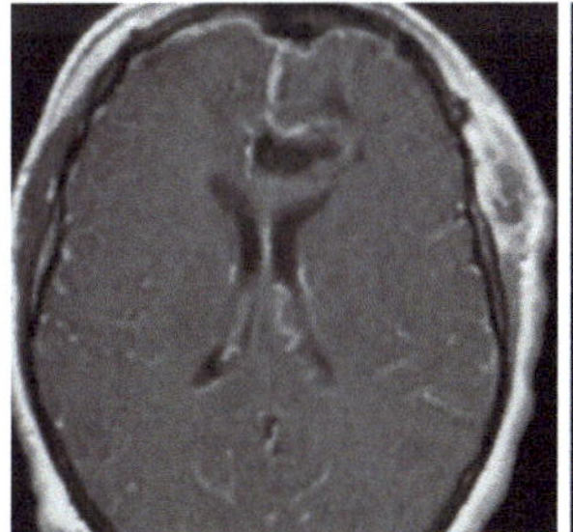
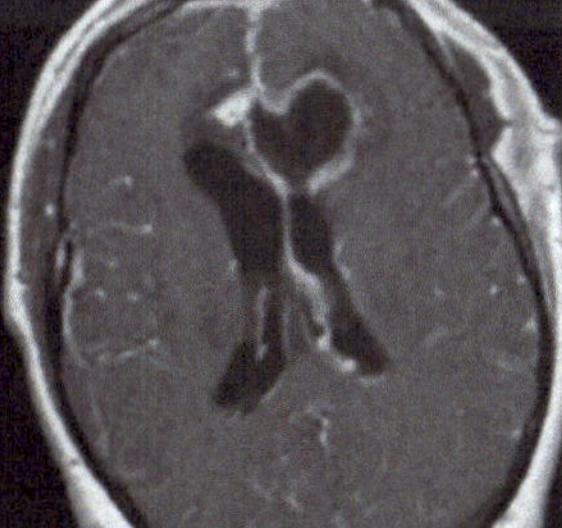

Figure 1: Cerebral abscess

During the cerebritis stages, T1W1 MRI will demonstrate low intensity regions and T2W1 MRI will demonstrate high intensity regions. During the capsular stage, T1W1 MRI will demonstrate a low signal central region, a mildly high signal capsule, and low signal perilesional edema. T2W1 MRI will show an iso/hyper intense central region, a low intensity capsule, and high signal perilesional edema.[29]

Treatment

Surgical management of cerebral abscesses is indicated if:

1. The abscess causes significant mass effect as seen on CT and MRI

2. There is evidence of significantly increased intracranial pressure
3. The abscess is in close proximity to a ventricle, thereby increasing risk of intraventricular rupture (associated with poor outcome)
4. The abscess contains foreign material (as seen in traumatic cases), contains fungi, is drug-resistant, or is multiloculated
5. Adequate diagnosis is difficult to achieve (especially in adults)
6. Follow-up CT/MRI scan cannot be obtained every one to two weeks

Management typically consists of IV antibiotics; however, some patients may require drainage (via syringe). Steroids are reserved for patients showing evidence of deterioration from marked mass effect on clinical imaging. Treatment of cerebral abscess with steroids reduces the edema and decreases the likelihood of fibrous encapsulation. The duration of steroid therapy should be minimized. 95% of the lesion will resolve with antibiotics alone within one month. Follow-up imaging should show a decrease in the degrees of ring enhancement, edema, mass effect, and size of the lesion in 1 to 4 weeks.

Spine Infections

Spine infections and spinal epidural abscesses should be considered in patients with low back pain, fever, and spine tenderness. Major risk factors for the development of spinal infections include diabetes, IV drug abuse, chronic renal failure, previous spine surgery and alcoholism. Primary infection of the nucleus pulposus may start in the cartilaginous endplate and spread to the disc and vertebral body. This can occur following several procedures or may occur spontaneously as a self-limited disease. The usual organisms encountered are *Staphylococcus aureus, Escherichia coli, Pseudomonas aeruginosa, Streptococcus pneumoniae,* Enterobacter species, and *Mycobacterium tuberculosis*. Multiple organisms are found in less than 10% of patients and anaerobes are cultured in less than 8%.[30]

Symptoms

Fevers, chills, sweats, and rigors are common, but a normal WBC and temperature is not uncommon. Progressive myelopathy may occur as the abscess compresses on neural structures. Typical symptoms include moderate to severe pain which is exacerbated by any motion of the spine. This pain is usually well localized to the level of involvement, radiating to the abdomen, hip, legs, scrotum, groin, and perineum. Patients will have point tenderness, paravertebral muscle spasms, and limitation of movement.

Diagnostic Tests

Blood tests will typically show increases in WBC, ESR, and CRP levels. An echocardiogram should be conducted to rule out endocarditis or valvular vegetations. Percutaneous needle biopsies are often required to identify the organisms. Blood cultures may also be helpful in identifying the organism in some cases. While WBC, ESR, and CRP may be elevated in acute abscesses, these values are usually normal in chronic abscesses.

Imaging

Plain radiographs will show destruction of the disc space, which is highly suggestive of infection. Tumors do not typically cross into the disc space. Plain x-rays will show interspace narrowing with some demineralization of the vertebral body. This is not usually apparent after four weeks. Between four and twelve weeks following the onset of clinical symptoms, the adjacent cortical margins appear sclerotic and adjacent areas of the vertebral body demonstrate increased density, representing new bone formation. The adjacent vertebral endplates also appear irregular with sparing of the pedicle, except in cases of tuberculosis which may involve the pedicles. In 50% of cases, the infection remains confined to the disc space; however, in the other 50%, the infection may spread to the adjacent vertebral body. A late finding is widening of the disc space with erosion of the vertebral body. Circumferential bone formation may lead to exuberant spur formation between the vertebral bodies, which may occur 6 to 8 months after the onset of infection. Spontaneous fusion of the vertebral body may also occur. Plain films also help to identify the presence of osteomyelitis, heralded by the presence of lytic lesions, demineralization, and scalloping of the endplates. Osteomyelitis takes about four to six weeks to present.

MRI has a high sensitivity and specificity in diagnosing spinal infections and as such it is the most reliable imaging in evaluating spinal infections (Figure 2).[31] Its utility is not only limited to evaluate spinal infections, but it is useful in evaluating extra or paraspinal spread of infections. In epidural spread, T1W1 MRI will demonstrate a hypo- or isointense epidural mass and T2 MRI will demonstrate a high intensity epidural mass. Vertebral osteomyelitis will appear as a reduced signal in bone. With gadolinium enhancement, lesions may appear as a dense homogeneous enhancement, an inhomogeneous region without areas of uptake, or as a lesion with a thin peripheral enhancement. MRI is also useful in ruling out paravertebral or epidural spinal abscesses versus recurrent residual disc herniation. Characteristic findings include decreased signal from the disc and adjacent portion of the vertebral body on T1W1 and increased signal from the structures on T2W1 (Figure 2). These findings may occur after three to five days of symptoms.

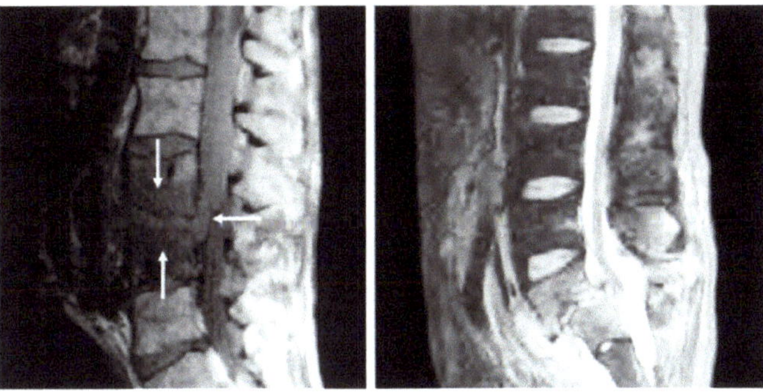

Figure 2: Spinal infections as seen in the MRI imaging

Additional studies include myelogram, which shows findings of extradural compression, and post-myelographic CT (typically more sensitive than myelogram).

Treatment

Treatment of spinal infections is controversial. Often times, patients will improve with only antibiotics, and other deteriorate rapidly despite medical treatment, thus requiring immediate surgical intervention. The first line treatment is medical management with antibiotics, especially for patients with contraindications/risk factors for surgery, involvement of a large segment of the spinal canal, and three or more days of complete paralysis. Treatment consists of three to four weeks of IV antibiotics, then four weeks of oral antibiotics. Longer duration of IV antibiotics (6-12 weeks) is recommended if there is documented concomitant vertebral osteomyelitis or discitis. Antibiotics are often given alongside immobilization and strict bed rest. Patients are fitted with a plastic-type body jacket where they can move around but must remain inside for about six to eight weeks. Other immobilization forms include a spica cast and a corset type brace. Treatment outcome is generally good.

Surgery is indicated in cases of unclear diagnosis or if culture of the causative organism is required. Surgery is also indicated if neoplasm cannot be ruled out. Surgery may be required for decompression of neural structures and drainage of associated spinal epidural abscess. This is especially the case for septated abscesses or compressive granulation tissue that is difficult to remove via CT-guided percutaneous needle. Surgery is especially indicated in case of acute or progressive neurological deficit, intraspinal lesion, instability or ineffective conservative therapy (Figure 3).

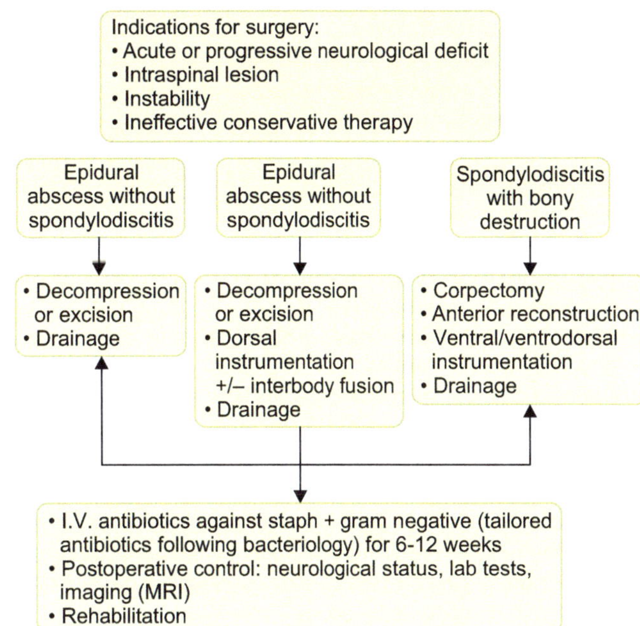

Figure 3: Operative treatment algorithm of Spinal infections[32]

BRAIN TUMORS

Primary brain tumors refer to a wide group of tumors arising from cells within the CNS. The most common presentation of a brain tumor is progressive neurological deficit which occurs in about 68% of affected individuals. Other presenting symptoms include headaches which occur in 30% of patients, motor weakness which occurs in 45% of patients, and seizures which occur in about 50% of patients.[33] The headache associated with brain tumors is caused by an increase in intracranial pressure and can be secondary to hydrocephalus, tumor mass effect, associated cerebral edema, hemorrhage, or from the invasion or compression of pain-sensitive structures on the dura, blood vessels, and periosteum. Tumors may have different manifestations depending on location of presentation.

Supratentorial Tumors

Supratentorial tumors represent about 50% of the intracranial neoplasms. In adults, the incidence may reach as high as 75%. Gliomas are the most common subtypes.[34] These tumors typically manifest with increased ICP due to mass effect of the tumor and/or cerebral edema. These tumors may block CSF drainage, resulting in an obstructive hydrocephalus which could manifest as a headache. Progressive focal deficits may occur due to destruction of the brain parenchyma by tumor invasion, by compression of the brain parenchyma by mass or peritumoral edema, or by compression of the cranial nerves.

Mental status changes may occur including depression, lethargy, apathy, and confusion. Symptoms suggestive of transient ischemic attack or stroke may be due to occlusion of the blood vessel by the tumor cells or hemorrhage into the tumor. In special cases of pituitary tumors, patients may present with endocrine disturbances, pituitary apoplexy, or a spontaneous CSF leak.

Infratentorial Tumors

Infratentorial tumors comprises about 50-55 % of all tumors, more common in children. Metastasis, hemangioblastoma, medulloblastoma, glioma and lymphoma are the common subtypes of infratentorial CNS tumors.[35] Most posterior fossa tumors present with signs and symptoms of increased intracranial pressure which consist of headache, nausea, vomiting, papilledema, gait disturbance, ataxia, and vertigo. If diplopia is present, it may be due to sixth nerve palsy. Lesions of the cerebellar hemisphere may cause ataxia of the extremities, dysmetria (or intentional tremor) and nystagmus. Cerebellar vermis lesions may result in a broad-based gait and truncal ataxia. Brain stem involvement usually results in the deficit of multiple cranial nerves and long tract abnormalities.

Focal Neurological Deficits Associated with Brain Tumors

If the tumors are found in the frontal lobe, patients may exhibit non-lateralizing symptoms such as abulia, dementia, and personality changes, or lateralizing symptoms such as hemiparesis, apraxia, and dysphasia with dominant (left) hemispheric involvement. Temporal lobe tumors manifest with hallucinations (i.e., auditory or olfactory), memory impairment, déjà vu, and contralateral superior quadrantanopia found on visual field testing. Tumors of the parietal lobe manifest with contralateral motor or sensory impairment, apraxias, homonymous hemianopsia, and agnosia with dominant hemisphere involvement. Occipital lobe tumors manifest with contralateral visual field deficits and alexia (especially with corpus callosum involvement). Posterior fossa tumors usually manifest with cranial nerve deficits and truncal/appendicular ataxia.[36]

Steroid Use in Brain Tumors

For patients not previously on steroids, patients can be given a dexamethasone 10 mg intravenous (IV) push as a loading dose and then 6 mg orally or dexamethasone 10mg IV push every six hours. Patients with severe vasogenic edema may be given dexamethasone 10 mg every 4 hours.[37] In pediatric cases dexamethasone should be given as a 0.5 to 1mg /kg IV push as a loading dose followed by 0.25 to 0.5mg/kg/day orally or as dexamethasone 0.5 to 1mg /kg IV push every six hours. Prolonged steroid use should be avoided because of the growth suppression effect. For patients who are already on steroids in the setting of acute deterioration, one should try approximately doubling the usual dose.

CRANIAL TRAUMA

Cranial trauma may result in a variety of penetrating or non-penetrating injuries to the brain and it is important to have a good understanding of the fundamentals of cranial trauma.

Head injuries are graded based on the Glasgow Coma Scale (GCS), loss of consciousness, and presentation of neurological deficits.

- Mild head injury: presents with a GCS equal to 13-15 plus either brief loss of consciousness less than 30 minutes, or impaired alertness or memory
- Moderate head injury: presents with a GCS between 9 and 12, loss of consciousness more than 30 minutes to 6 hours, or persistent focal neurological deficits
- Severe head injury: presents with a GCS less than 8

Various types of non-penetrating cranial trauma can present including concussion, contusion, and diffuse axonal injury.

Concussion

A concussion is defined as an injury as a result of a non-penetrating brain injury resulting in alteration of consciousness or brain functioning without structural damage.[38] Possible findings in a concussion include a vacant stare or confused expression, delayed verbal or motor response, increased inattentiveness, inability to perform normal activities, and disorientation. Patients may be seen walking in the wrong directions, unaware of the date, time, or place. Speech alterations can manifest with slurred or in-coherent statements. Patients may lack coordination presenting with stumbling and inability to tandem walk. Exaggerated emotionality may be seen such as inappropriate crying. Memory deficits may manifest with the inability to recall three objects after five minutes and the patient repeatedly asking the same question which has already been answered.

Severity of a concussion used to be graded according to standards set by the American Association of Neurologic Surgeons in 1997 and Colorado Medical Society Guidelines:[39]

Grade 1 concussions: are mild concussions that present with transient confusion, no loss of consciousness, and resolution of symptoms in less than 15 minutes. These patients should be removed from their activity and examined every five minutes for amnesia or post concussion symptoms. Patients may return to their activity if symptoms are clear within 15 minutes.

Grade 2 concussions: are moderate concussions that present with transient confusion, no loss of consciousness, but with symptoms that persist more than 15 minutes. These patients should be removed from their activity and not be allowed to return to the activity on the same day. Patients should be examined onsite often to search for signs of evolving intracranial pathology and reexamined the following day by trained health professionals. CT or MRI may be necessary if headache or other symptoms worsen or last more than one week. Patients may return to their activity after one full week without symptoms.

Grade 3 concussions: are severe concussions that present with any loss of consciousness. Patients should be taken to the ER if they remain unconscious or if concerning neurological signs are present. Patients should have a full neurological exam, with the appropriate neurological imaging as necessary. The patient may go home with head injury instructions if they present with normal findings at the time of initial neurologic exam. Otherwise, they should be admitted to the hospital if they show any signs of pathology or continued abnormal mental status. Daily neural status assessments should be done until there has been stabilization or resolution of all symptoms. After a brief (i.e., less than one minute), grade 3 concussion, patients must not return to their activity until they are asymptomatic for one full week. After a prolonged (i.e., more than one minute), grade 3 concussion, patients must not return to their activity until they are asymptomatic for two full weeks.

These guidelines has been changed as per 2013 AAN guidelines and now the guidance focuses on more detailed neurocognitive assessment prior to return of play.[40]

Contusion

A contusion is a head injury with CT findings that may include areas of low attenuation (representing associated edema) and high attenuation (representing hemorrhagic lesions). The hemorrhagic lesions generally have less mass effect relative to their apparent (edema) size. Contusions most commonly occur at locations where sudden head deceleration causes the brain to be impacted on bony prominences. These can show as coup injuries (brain injured directly under the point of impact) or contrecoup injuries (brain injured opposite to the point of impact). The common locations for contusions are at the temporal, frontal and the occipital lobes. Contusions can progress or blossom at the impacted areas. Surgical decompression may be necessary if the contusion progresses to cause a herniation.

Diffuse Axonal Injury

A diffuse axonal injury (DAI) is a primary lesion caused by a rotational acceleration/deceleration head injury. In its severe form, hemorrhagic foci can be seen in the corpus callosum and the dorsolateral rostral brainstem with microscopic evidence of diffuse injury to the axons. DAI may be diagnosed clinically when loss of consciousness lasts more than 6 hours in the absence of an intracranial mass or ischemia.

- Mild DAI: is diagnosed if the coma persists more than 6 to 24 hours followed by mild-to-moderate memory impairment, and mild-to-moderate disabilities.
- Moderate DAI: is diagnosed if the coma persists for more than 24 hrs followed by confusion, long lasting amnesia, and mild-to-severe memory, behavioral and cognitive deficits.
- Severe DAI: is diagnosed if the coma lasts months or longer with flexor-extensor posturing and deficits in cognition, memory, speech, sensation, motor control, or personality. Dysautonomia may also occur in severe DAI.

Management of Head Injury

Adequate acute management in the Emergency Room consists of a thorough neurosurgical exam including identification of the following:

1. Signs of basal skull fracture: 'Raccoon eyes' (periorbital ecchymosis) or Battle's sign (postauricular ecchymosis around the mastoid), CSF rhinorrhea, otorrhea, hemotympanum, or laceration of the external auditory canal
2. Signs of facial fractures including Le Fort fractures (palpable instability of facial bones) and Orbital rim fracture (palpable step off)
3. Craniocervical auscultation: bruit over the carotid artery may be associated with carotid dissection, bruit over eye may indicate traumatic carotid cavernous fistula.
4. Physical signs of trauma to spine: bruising over the spine and visible deformity.
5. Identification and management of seizures: single, multiple, or continuing status epilepticus.

Neurological examination should include a thorough cranial nerve exam and a fundoscopic exam. Pupillary size in ambient light and its reaction to both direct and consensual light should be noted. The seventh cranial nerve should be checked for peripheral facial nerve palsy. The sixth cranial nerve should be checked for signs of raised intracranial pressure. The level of consciousness should be documented as per the Glasgow Coma Scale. Orientation status should be assessed if the patient is able to communicate. If the patient is cooperative, motor strength should be assessed in all four extremities. If the patient is uncooperative, movement of all four extremities should be assessed via noxious stimuli. Integrity of the spinal cord can be checked by observation of the resting tone of the anal sphincter on rectal exam. If the patient can cooperate, voluntary sphincter contractions should be evaluated. Pin prick sensation should be assessed on the trunk and all four extremities (major dermatomes C4 to S1). If the patient is uncooperative, pain sensation can be identified via central response to noxious stimuli by either grimace or vocalization. Flexion withdrawal response can be a false positive reaction to pain, as it is a spinal cord mediated reflex. Reflexes should be assessed. If a flaccid limb has preserved reflexes, it indicates a CNS injury over a nerve root injury. Check plantar reflexes for up going toes (Babinksi reflex). For suspected spinal cord injury, anal wink and bulbo-cavernosus reflexes can be assessed via rectal exam. Patients at moderate risk for intracranial injury include patients with a history of change or loss of consciousness during or after the injury, progressive headache, intoxication with alcohol or drugs, posttraumatic seizures, unreliable or inadequate history, age less than 2 years, vomiting, postraumatic amnesia, signs of basilar skull fracture, multiple traumas, serious facial injury, possible skull penetration or depressed fractures, suspected child abuse, and significant subgaleal swelling.

Imaging

An initial CT scan is indicated in the presence of any moderate or high-risk criteria including a GCS less than 14, unresponsiveness, focal deficits, amnesia for injury, altered mental status, deteriorating neural status, and signs of basal or calvarial skull fractures. CT scan is also indicated prior to initiation of general anesthesia for patients that are unable to be assessed via neurological exam for detection of deterioration. Emergent CT is indicated to rule out suspected extra-axial blood collections as seen in epidural hematomas, subdural hematomas or subarachnoid bleeds, intracerebral hemorrhages, hemorrhagic contusions, intraventricular hemorrhages, hydrocephalus, cerebral swelling, suspected cerebral anoxia, skull fractures, ischemic infarctions, pneumocephalus, and shift of midline structures due to extra or intra-axial hematomas. In addition, the cervical spine must be cleared radiographically from craniocervical junction to C7-T1 junction after a cranial injury. Thoracic or lumbosacral spine film may also be necessary based on the mechanism of injury and physical findings.

Follow-up CT scans should be done for stable patients and should be repeated in 3 to 5 days. Some centers recommend a follow-up CT scan at 24 hours and some centers only repeat CT scan prior to discharge. Prior to discharge, at least one repeat CT scan should be taken for patients with mild-to-moderate head injuries who had an abnormal initial CT. Such a repeat CT is not required for stable patients who had a mild head injury and normal initial CT.

Treatment

Patients with minor cranial injuries may be observed at home if they meet the following criteria: a normal cranial CT, initial GCS more than 14 or equal to 14, no high-risk criteria, and no moderate risk criteria except loss of consciousness. The patient should be neurologically intact, and a responsible sober adult should be available that can observe the patient. The patient should have reasonable access to return to the hospital or ER if needed. There should be no suspicion of domestic violence or child abuse as a cause of the injury. The patient should be instructed to seek medical attention if they experience a change in level of consciousness, decreased arousal, abnormal behavior, increased headache, slurred speech, weakness or numbness in the extremities, persistent vomiting, dilation of one or both pupils, increased cranial swelling, or development of seizures. Patients should be instructed not to take any sedatives or pain medications except for acetaminophen for headaches and muscle aches. Aspirin and non-steroidal anti-inflammatory drugs should be avoided.

For patients to be admitted with a minor head injury (GCS more than or equal to 14), patient care should include bed rest with the head of the bed elevated to 35 to 40 degree. Neurological checks should be conducted at least every two hours, with a shorter duration if symptoms are concerning. Intensive Care Unit (ICU) admission should be considered for at risk patients. Physicians should be contacted immediately for signs of neurological deterioration. The patient should receive nil per os (npo) until they are alert, after which they can receive clear liquids and advance in diet as tolerated. Isotonic IV fluids should be given with normal saline at 20 mEq of KCL/liter administered at 11 cc/hr (i.e., maintenance level for an average size adult). In pediatric patients saline should be administered IV at 2L/m2/d. Mild analgesics such as acetaminophen (with codeine if necessary) may be given orally or rectally as needed. Antiemetics should be given sparingly to avoid excessive sedation. Phenothiazines should be avoided. To treat nausea in the adult patient 200 mg Tigan may be given intramuscularly every 8 hours as needed.

For patients with moderate head injury (GCS between 9 and 13), patients should be admitted to the ICU. Patients that fail to reach a GCS between 14 and 15 within 12 hours should have a repeat CT. Patients should be intubated if they demonstrate a depressed level of consciousness, cannot protect their airway (usually seen in GCS less than 7), or have severe maxillofacial trauma with poor airway patency.

If a basal skull fracture through the cribriform plate is possible, nasotracheal intubation should be avoided to prevent intracranial entry of the tube. Oro-tracheal intubation should be utilized instead. It is important to understand that intubation prevents the assessment of the patient's ability to verbalize thus reducing the Glasgow Coma Scale score. In addition, there is increased risk of pneumonia with intubation.

Cranial injury may progress leading to increased intracranial pressure (ICP) and increased risk of herniation. Clinical signs of intracranial hypertension include pupillary dilatation, (unilateral or bilateral), asymmetric pupillary reaction to light, and decerebrate or decorticate posturing (usually contralateral to blown pupil). Hyperventilation may be used as a temporary measure for patients with signs of transtentorial herniation or progressive neurological deterioration until an ICP monitoring system is introduced. Hyperventilation should be avoided during the first 24 hours after traumatic brain injury as cerebral blood flow is typically decreased, and hyperventilation may exacerbate cerebral ischemia. Hyperventilation should not be used prophylactically. With appropriate indications, hyperventilation to a $PaCO_2$ equal to 30 to 35 mmHg is advisable. A $PaCO_2$ of less than 30 mmHg further reduces the cerebral blood flow, without significant effect in reducing the ICP.

Mannitol may be given before ICP monitoring in patients who are adequately volume resuscitated with signs of transtentorial herniation or progressive neurological deterioration. Such patients should have evidence of mass effect and focal deficits, or present with sudden deterioration prior to CT including pupillary dilatation. Mannitol may be given after CT if a lesion is identified that is associated with increased ICP. Mannitol may also be given while going to the operating room to assess salvageability in patients with no evidence of brain stem function (assessed via return of brain stem reflexes). Prophylactic administration of mannitol is not recommended due to its volume depletion of effect. The dose of mannitol should be 0.25 to 1g/kg over 20 minutes. An average adult will require about 350 mL of 20% solution. The peak effect of mannitol administration occurs in 20 minutes.

Conditions associated with an increased risk of posttraumatic seizures include acute subdural, epidural, intracerebral hematomas, open depressed skull fractures with parenchymal injury, penetrating brain injury, history of significant alcohol abuse, cortical contusions on CT, and a GCS less than 10. Seizures may occur within the first 24 hours of injury. In such patients, antiepileptic drug prophylaxis may be administered. For suspected traumatic subarachnoid hemorrhage, nimodipine 60 mg orally every 4 hours may be given to improve patient outcome. Nimodipine should not be given in the presence of hypotension.

Exploratory Burr Holes

In patients with a rapidly deteriorating neurological exam that does not improve or stabilize with mannitol or hyperventilation, patients may require placement of exploratory burr holes to avoid rapid transtentorial herniation or brain stem compression. In such a situation, the patient may experience a sudden drop in the GCS, one pupil fixed and dilated, and paralysis or decerebration is seen contralateral to the blown pupil.

The first burr hole may be placed in the middle cranial fossa just superior to the zygomatic arch. This location provides access to the middle fossa and is the most common site of epidural hematoma formation. This site also allows access to the most convexity, ease of access to subdural hematomas, as well as access proximally to the midline meningeal artery and the region of the pterion.

If no epidural hematoma is seen, the dura may be opened if it has a bluish discoloration suggesting a subdural hematoma. If there is strong suspicion of a mass lesion on the opposite side, a second temporal burr hole can be placed on the contralateral side. If the second burr hole is negative, further burr holes may be placed beginning with an ipsilateral frontal burr hole. Subsequent burr holes may be placed in the parietal region and lastly in the posterior fossa.

Skull Fractures

Skull fractures may occur due to a variety of injuries and may be symptomatic or asymptomatic. CT imaging aids in identification of skull fractures. Linear skull fractures are dark black in color, very thin, and usually straight with no branching. Vessel grooves appear gray in density and are usually seen curving and branching. They are thicker in width compared to fracture lines. Suture lines are also gray in density and follow the course of known suture lines while joining other suture lines. They are jagged in appearance.

No surgery is indicated if there is no:

1. Dural penetration (intra-dural pneumocephalus, CSF leak) clinical or CT evidence
2. Significant intracranial hematoma
3. Depression <1 cm
4. Involvement of the frontal sinus
5. Gross contamination or wound infection
6. Gross cosmetic deformity

Surgical management of a depressed skull fracture is indicated in open (i.e., compound) fractures. Surgical methods involve elevation and debridement of the depressed fragment. Consider primary bone replacement if there is no infection of the wound. All compound depressed fractures should be treated with antibiotics. Depressed skull fracture elevation has shown no evidence of reducing post-traumatic seizures development.

Epidural Hematoma

Epidural hematomas occur with an incidence about 2% of all head traumas, with a male to female predominance of 4:1.[41] These are usually seen in young adults and is rarely seen in infants before 2 years old or elderly patients after 60 years old since the dura is more strongly adherent to the inner table in these populations.[42] The source of the bleeding is arterial in 85% of cases with bleeding from the middle meningeal artery as the most common cause. The remainder of cases may be due to bleeding from the middle meningeal vein or dural sinuses. Less than 10% of patients have the classic presentation of brief post traumatic loss of consciousness followed by a lucid interval, followed by obtundation, contralateral hemiparesis, and ipsilateral pupillary dilatation. The biconvex shaped CT finding is classical for epidural hematomas (Figure 4). Prompt surgical evacuation is strongly recommended in cases of epidural hematoma with a GCS less than 9 and isocoria or an extradural hematoma volume more than 30cc regardless of the GCS.

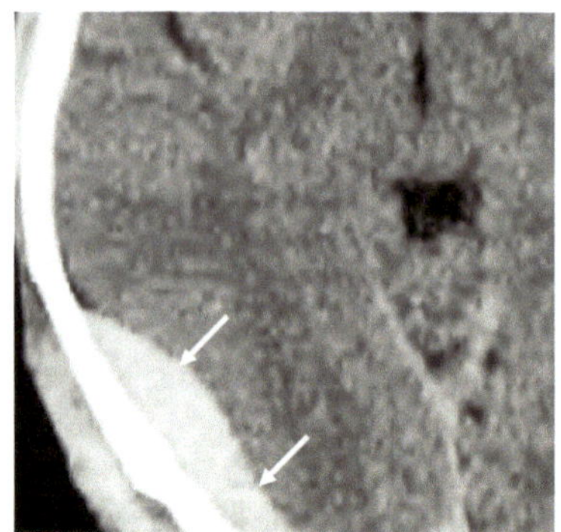

Figure 4: CT finding in epidural hematoma as a lanceolate(biconvex) hemorrhagic collection in the epidural space

Epidural hematoma may be managed nonsurgically if the hemorrhage volume is less than 30 cc, the thickness is less than 1.5 cm, the midline shift is less than 5 mm, the GCS is more than 8, and there is no focal neurological deficit. Patients are taken to a neurosurgical center and managed with serial CT scans followed by close neurological observation.

Acute Subdural Hematoma

Acute subdural hematomas are often caused by impacts that are more severe than those seen in epidural hematoma, thus causing underlying brain contusions that are more lethal than the epidural hematoma.[43] Shearing of surface or bridging vessels from cerebral acceleration-deceleration during the injury is the causative factor. Accumulation of blood may be seen around the parenchymal laceration. CT scans are diagnostic, displaying a crescentic mass of increased attenuation adjacent to the inner table. Edema is often present over convexities but may also be interhemispheric along the tentorium or in the posterior fossa (Figure 5). Membrane formation usually occurs after 4 days, and blood becomes isodense after two weeks. Surgical evacuation is indicated if the hematoma has a thickness more than 10 mm or midline shift more than 5mm regardless of the Glasgow Coma Scale. Surgical evacuation is also indicated if the hematoma has a thickness less than 10 mm, midline shift less than 5mm, but there is a drop in GCS of 2 points, asymmetric, fixed and dilated pupils, or if the ICP is above 20 mmHg. All patients with an acute subdural hematoma with a GCS less than 9 should have ICP monitoring.

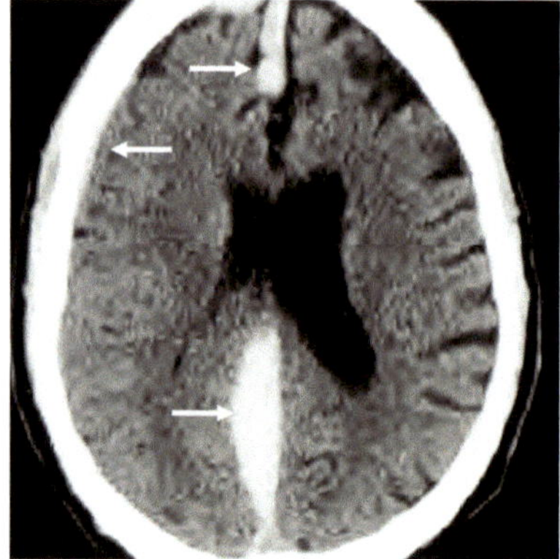

Figure 5: Computed scan in subdural hematoma showing a accumulation of blood in the subdural space

CSF FISTULAS

Cerebrospinal fluid (CSF) fistulas may develop for a variety of reasons. The common causes of CSF fistula development are iatrogenic causes, which typically present post-procedural after pituitary surgery, skull-base surgery, and after post-traumatic surgeries. CSF fistulas can also present after trauma (acutely or delayed) or as a result of high-pressure hydrocephalus. Tumors, infections, focal olfactory/sellar region atrophy, and necrosis may erode bone of the skull also causing fistulas. Fistulas may also develop as a result of congenital defects. After development of a CSF fistula, CSF may leak via mastoid air cells, sphenoid air cells, frontal air cells, at the cribriform plate of the ethmoid bone, along the sheath of the internal carotid artery, along Rosenmuller's fossa, or percutaneously through a surgical or traumatic wound. CSF leaks along the internal auditory canal, middle ear, or Eustachian tube may manifest with rhinorrhea in the nasopharynx. CSF leaks along the external auditory canal or through a perforated tympanic membrane may manifest as otorrhea.

Diagnostic Tests

A variety of techniques can be used to evaluate suspected cases of CSF leak. Suspect CSF fluid is as clear as water. The fluid does not cause excoriation within or outside the nose, and the taste is described as salty. Patients may also complain of anosmia. Confirmatory laboratory tests include the beta-2 transferrin test which is very sensitive and specific for CSF. For this test, 0.5 mL of the fluid must be placed in a sterile container with dry ice and shipped to a lab that can perform the study. CSF can also be identified via quantitative glucose estimation. Normal CSF glucose is typically more than 30 mg% (may be lower in meningitis) whereas lacrimal secretions and mucus are usually less than 5 mg%. If the fluid is blood tinged, the Ring sign can be seen by allowing the fluid to drip onto a piece of linen. A ring of blood with a larger concentric ring of clear fluid is known as a double ring or halo sign and is suggestive of CSF leak (Figure 6).

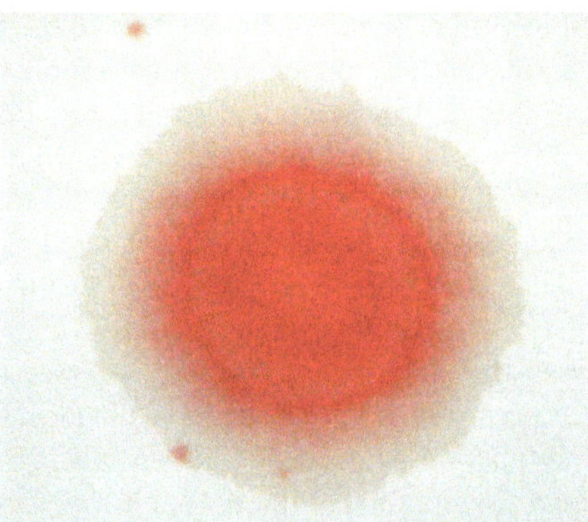

Figure 6: Ring sign to identify CSF leak, see the characteristic halo formed around the blood in cases of CSF leak

A Reservoir sign may also be seen where a gush of fluid occurs with certain head positions. Radiographic signs of CSF leak include pneumocephalus (air in the brain) on a CT image or a skull x-ray image. Pneumocephalus occurs in about 20% of patients with CSF leak. Other radiography tests include a cisternogram (intrathecal injection of radionuclide traces followed by scintigram) or CT scan with contrast.

Localization of the CSF Fistula

After confirming the presence of a CSF leak, it is important to identify the location of the fistula. CT can be a good first test to detect the pneumocephalus, fracture of the skull-base, hydrocephalus, and destructive neoplasms. CT should be gathered via thin coronal cuts and reconstruction from the anterior fossa all the way back to the Sella turcica. CT with IV contrast can help determine the leak site by identifying abnormal enhancement of the adjacent brain parenchyma due to inflammation. MRI may also provide additional information. When no site of leakage is identified on brain CT, water-soluble contrast cisternography is the procedure of choice to help identify the leakage site.

Treatment

Observation is justified in most cases as leaks may spontaneously close. Usage of prophylactic antibiotics is controversial for patients with posttraumatic or postoperative leaks. Nonsurgical treatment may include ICP control, bed rest, avoidance of straining, acetazolamide 250 mg orally four times daily (to reduce CSF production), and fluid restriction to 1.5 liters per day in adults or 75% of the maintenance per day in pediatric patients. If the leak persists, obstructive hydrocephalus should be ruled out via CT or MRI. Surgery may be indicated for traumatic CSF leak persisting more than 2 weeks despite nonsurgical measures, leaks complicated by meningitis, and spontaneous leaks or delayed-onset post-trauma/post-surgery leaks due to a high incidence of recurrence. Smaller CSF leaks especially in the spinal cord can be managed by dural blood patch. Larger cranial CSF leaks needs surgical correction which might use direct suturing or using pedicled pericranial flaps, fascia lata grafts or muscle flaps.[44]

GUNSHOT WOUND TO THE HEAD

The initial steps of management for gunshot wounds to the head include control of bleeding from the scalp associated with the wound. The scalp must be shaved to properly identify the entrance wound, the exit wound, and to decrease the time required in the operating room. AP and lateral skull radiographic evaluation should be conducted to localize bone and metal fragments and to help identify entrance and exit sites. Brain non-contrast CT scans help to identify the blood track, intracranial hematomas, and intraparenchymal location of metal and bone fragments. The ICP is assumed to be elevated in all cases of gunshot wounds.

Other initial steps for management of gunshot wounds to the head should include:

1. Elevation of the head end to 35 to 40 degrees with the head midline
2. Mannitol 1g/kg/bolus as tolerated by blood pressure
3. Hyperventilate with $PaCO_2$ of 30 to 35
4. Prophylaxis against GI ulcer via an H2 antagonist
5. Acute seizures control via phenytoin
6. Antibiotics
7. Tetanus toxoid

Surgical treatment for gunshot wounds to the head is controversial. Operation should not be performed in patients that are not in shock with good oxygenation and poor cognitive and neurological status including fixed/dilated pupils and decorticate/decerebrate posturing due to the possibility of no meaningful recovery. Urgent operation should be considered in patients with less severe injuries. Goals of surgery include evacuation of the subdural or intraparenchymal hematoma, accessible bone fragment removal, accessible bullet fragment retrieval for forensics, and return of hemostasis with watertight dural closure (usually requires dural graft).

Poor Prognostic Factors

The most important prognostic factor is the patient's level of consciousness. Ninety-four percent of comatose patients with absent or inappropriate responses to noxious stimuli at the time of admission will be permanently severely disabled. Other poor prognostic factors include bullets crossing the midline, passing geographic centers of the brain, and transversing the ventricles. Suicide attempts are more likely to be fatal.

SPINAL INJURIES

Spinal injuries may present with incomplete lesions or complete lesions.

Incomplete lesions describe any persistence of residual motor or sensory function more than 3 segments below the level of the injury.

Incomplete lesions may present with sensation (including position sense), voluntary movement in the lower extremities, sacral sparing, preserved sensation around the anus, voluntary rectal sphincter contractions, and voluntary toe flexion. The types of incomplete lesions include central cord syndrome, Brown Sequard syndrome, anterior cord syndrome, and posterior cord syndromes.

In contrast, of patients with complete lesions present without any motor preservation or sensory function greater than 3 segments below the injury level, 3% have some recovery within 24 hours. However, if the injury is complete and not treated for more than 72 hours, recovery is essentially zero.

A variety of conditions may present along with acute cases of spinal injury. Spinal shock defines a hypotensive state that follows spinal cord injury in which systolic blood pressure may be equal to or less than 80 mmHg. The cause is interruption of sympathetic pathways, thus implying spinal cord injury above T1. Patients may present with bradycardia due to loss of vasculature tone (vasoconstrictors) below the level of injury, thus leaving parasympathetic pathways relatively unopposed. Loss of muscle tone due to skeletal muscle paralysis below the level of the injury may result in venous pooling, which can lead to relative hypovolemia.

Acute Spinal Injury

Every patient with significant trauma and with (1) loss of consciousness, (2) referred spine, neck, or back complaints, and (3) new onset tingling, numbness, abnormal breathing, extremity weakness, or priapism should be managed as if they have an acute spinal cord injury until further proof is ascertained. Patients that are awake, alert, oriented, with no mental status changes (including no alcohol or drug intoxication) and patients with no neck pain, back pain or neurological deficits can be reasonably considered to have cervical spine stability.

Initial Management

When first approaching a patient with a spinal cord injury, the patient must be log-rolled (keeping spine stable) supine onto a backboard. Sandbags should be placed on both sides of the head to keep the head straight. 3" adhesive tape may also be used to further secure head position to the backboard across the forehead. The upper and lower spine should be immobilized, and a rigid cervical collar (or Philadelphia collar) should be placed to keep the cervical spine stable. Blood pressure should be maintained above 90 mmHg with IV fluids, vasopressors (such as dopamine), and in some cases military (pneumatic) anti-shock trousers. A mean arterial pressure (MAP) of 85 to 90 mmHg should be maintained for the first 7 days after spinal cord injury to improve spinal cord perfusion. Oxygen should be administered via face mask, nasal cannula, or intubation as needed. Caution must be exercised with intubation in situations with an uncleared C-spine. The chin-lift maneuver should be used without neck extension. Nasotracheal intubation may also be used to avoid movement of the C-spine. Tracheostomy or cricothyroidotomy should be avoided, if possible, as they may compromise later anterior cervical spine surgical approaches. Patients should be in the ICU and cardiac, respiratory, and hemodynamic status must be monitored to identify any rapidly progressive decline in neural status.

Assessment of the spinal cord injury

Once the patient is stabilized, a full neurological and functional assessment is crucial to evaluate the extent of spinal cord injury. The history or mechanism of injury should be elicited to determine hyperflexion vs. extension, axial loading, history suggestive of loss of consciousness, history of weakness of the arms and legs below the level of the injury following trauma, and the occurrence of numbness or tingling at any time following the injury.

Neurological/functional Physical Exam should include:

1. Palpation of the spine for point of tenderness, step-offs, or widened interspinous spaces
2. Motor level assessments including rectal exam for voluntary anal sphincter contraction

3. Sensory level assessments including sensation to pinprick on extremities, body, and face (spinal trigeminal tract), light touch (anterior spinothalamic tract), and proprioception (the posterior columns)
4. Reflexes assessment (deep tendon reflexes may be absent initially in the cord injury; abdominal cutaneous, cremasteric, bulbocavernosus and anal cutaneous reflexes may also be absent)
5. Examination for autonomic dysfunction including altered patterns of perspiration, bowel-bladder incontinence, and priapism

Motor level classification in the extremities is graded from 0 to 5 with 5 being normal muscle strength, 0 being no muscle strength, and 3 being antigravity muscle strength. Key muscles include:

- C4: Deltoid, abduct the shoulder
- C5: Biceps, flex the elbow
- C6: Wrist extensor, cockup the wrist
- C7: Triceps, extend the elbow
- C8: Flexor digitorum profundus, flex middle distal phalanx
- T1: Hand intrinsic, abduct little finger
- L2: Iliopsoas, ask the patient to flex the hip
- L3: Quadriceps, straighten the knee
- L4: Tibialis anterior, dorsiflex the foot
- L5: Extensor hallucis Longus (EHL), dorsiflex the big toe
- S1: Gastrocnemius, plantar flex the foot

The ASIA Internal Standard for neurological and functional assessment of spinal cord injuries can be used to classify the severity of the spinal cord injury as follows (Figure 7):[45]

- ASIA A is considered a complete spinal cord injury: no motor/no sensory function preserved below the neurological level
- ASIA B is considered an incomplete spinal cord injury: sensory findings are preserved but no motor function preserved below the neurological level
- ASIA C is considered an incomplete spinal cord injury: motor function is preserved below the neurological level, but the muscle strength is below grade 3
- ASIA D is considered an incomplete spinal cord injury: motor function is preserved below the neurological level and the muscle strength is above grade 3
- ASIA E is considered normal sensorimotor function

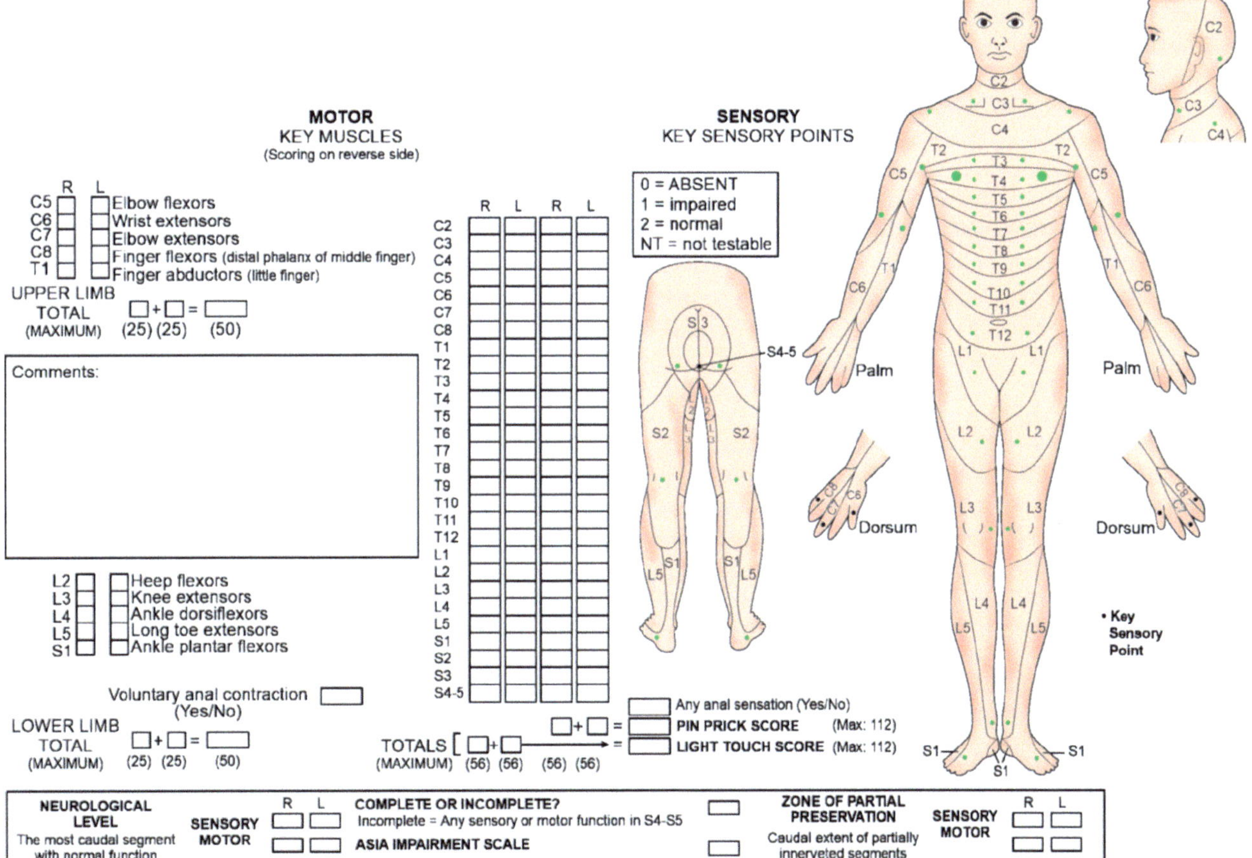

Figure 7: The ASIA scale for assessment of spinal cord injuries

Imaging

In assessing plain films of the spine, it is important to identify the normal alignment of the anterior longitudinal ligament, the posterior longitudinal ligament, and the spino-laminar line (Figure 8). The laminar distance should then be identified as equal and aligned. Unequal or misaligned laminar distances may indicate vertebral subluxation.

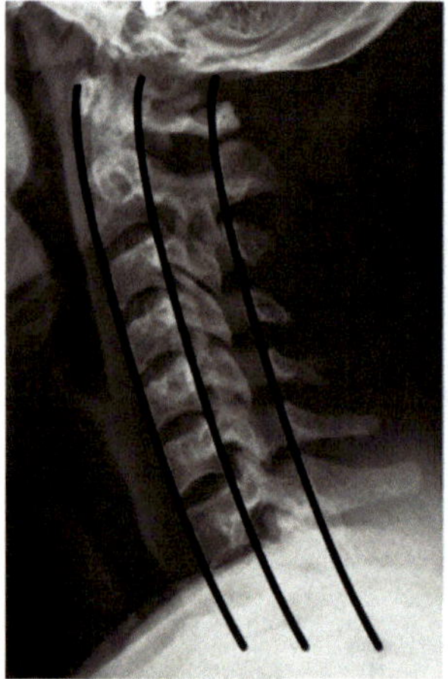

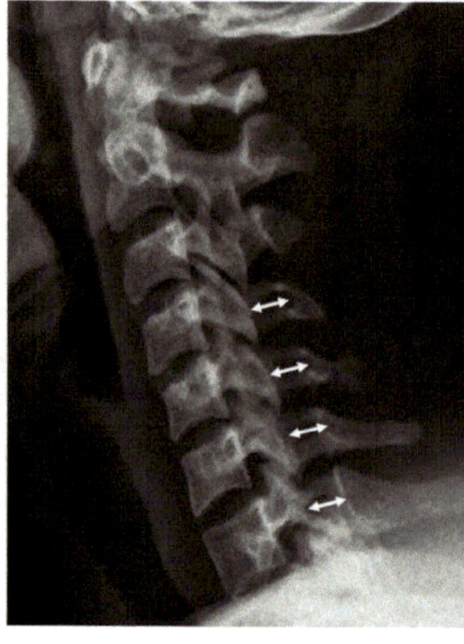

Figure 8: C-spine x-rays demonstrating (A) alignment of the anterior longitudinal ligament, the posterior longitudinal ligament, and the spino-laminar line and (B) equal and aligned laminar distances (arrows)

Cervical spine (C-spine) trauma may be identified radiographically by the following signs: a retropharyngeal space more than 7 mm, a retrotracheal space more than 14 mm or 22 mm in pediatric patients, a displaced prevertebral fat stripe, tracheal deviation, or laryngeal dislocation. Vertebral segment components may display loss of lordosis, acute kyphotic angulation, torticollis, widened interspinous spaces, axial rotation of the vertebra, and discontinuity of contour lines. Abnormal joint findings may include an atlantodental interspace more than 3 mm in adults and more than 4 mm in pediatric patients, narrowed or widened disc spaces, and widening of the apophyseal joints.

Flexion-extension plain films of the cervical spine may be necessary to disclose occult instability. Not all ligamentous injuries that involve the posterior ligamentous complex have bony fractures. A lateral flexion-extension film is helpful in detecting such injuries. Acquiring a flexion-extension films requires a cooperative patient without mental impairment. There must be no evidence of head injury, or any subluxation more than 3.5 mm at any level via cross table C-spine X-ray, and the patient should be neurologically intact. If there is any degree of spinal cord injury, MRI should be performed rather than other studies. Flexion-extension X-rays are no longer recommended in an obtunded patient due to a low yield of positive results. A normal flexion-extension view shows slight anterior subluxation at all cervical levels and there will be preserved normal contour lines. Spinous process flaring is an abnormal finding (exaggerated widening).

Urgent MRI of the spine may be necessary in cases of incomplete spinal cord injury, neurological deterioration, and worsening deficit not explained by radiographic findings. Such neurological deficits may include a fracture level different from the level of the deficit and lack of identifiable bony injuries. MRI can also rule out soft tissue compressions such as disc herniation and hematomas in situations that might require surgery.

Treatment

Management of acute spinal injuries may include use of analgesics, reduction with traction, or surgery.

Treatment with methylprednisolone for 24 to 48 hours after a spinal cord injury used to be commonly utilized in the past. This has largely been disregarded as the treatment of acute spinal trauma as it was seen to be associated with more deleterious effects including increased risk of death.[46]

In some cases, a closed reduction of the C-spine may be used to restore anatomic alignment in an awake patient. Patients should have an MRI prior to an attempted reduction if they cannot be examined during a closed reduction or before an open posterior reduction. A significant herniated disc is a relative indication for anterior decompressive surgery before the reduction. Cervical MRI should be recommended to patients who fail an attempted closed reduction.

Closed reduction should not be used in cases of atlanto-occipital dislocation, type 2A or 3 Hangman's fracture, skull defect/ fracture at anticipated pin site, patients younger than 3 years, elderly patients, patients with demineralized skull (seen in patients with osteogenesis imperfecta and some elderly patients), patients who also have rostral injury, and patients with movement disorders (a pin erosion through the skull can be due to constant motion).

During the reduction, pins are placed at various positions depending on the etiology of the injury. For neutral position injuries, pins are placed in the temporal ridge above the temporalis muscle which is about the breadth of three fingers directly over the external acoustic meatus. For flexion injuries (as occurs in locked facets), pins should be placed three fingers above and 3 cm posterior to the external acoustic meatus. For extension injuries, pins may be placed 3 cm above and 3 cm anterior to the external acoustic meatus. After placement of the pins, a Halo ring or tongs are attached to the pins, which connect to varying weights for constant application of neck traction. Traction is usually applied for 3 days.

In some cases, early laminectomy in acute spinal cord injury has been associated with increased risk of neurological deterioration. Generally, surgery is reserved for some instances of incomplete lesions such as compound fractures or penetrating trauma to the spine, acute anterior spinal cord syndrome, and cases of non-reducible fracture dislocation. Myelogram, CT, and MRI may show bone fragments or soft tissue elements (such as hematoma) in the spinal canal causing spinal cord compression. Emergency decompressive surgery should not be done in patients that present with complete spinal cord injury over 24 hours post injury, patients with central cord syndrome, medically unstable patients, and those with no motor/sensory function below the level of the lesion.

Incomplete Spinal Cord Injuries

Incomplete spinal cord injuries may present in a variety of different syndromes including central cord syndrome, Brown-Sequard syndrome, and Posterior cord syndrome. Central cord syndrome presents with motor deficit that is worse in the upper extremities than the lower extremities. Patients may also present with varying sensory deficits below the lesion, myelopathic findings, sphincter disturbances, and hyperpathia to either noxious and non-noxious stimuli. The most commonly seen incomplete spinal cord injury is central cord syndrome and usually presents after an acute hyperextension injury in an older patient. Patients typically have preexisting congenital or acquired spinal stenosis as a result of bony hypertrophy (osteophytic spur) or in folding of redundant ligamentum flavum.

Patients with central cord syndrome often experience an initial phase of improvement. Lower extremities recover first, bladder function recovers next, and upper extremities recover last after which patients experience a plateau phase followed by later deterioration. 90% of the patients are usually able to walk with assistance within five days. Diagnostic MRI shows compromise of the anterior spinal canal by discs or osteophytes. The addition of plain C-spine x-rays helps to differentiate osteophytic spurs from traumatic disc herniation. MRI is useful for evaluation of redundant ligamentum flavum. T2W MRI demonstrates spinal cord edema acutely and detects development of hematomyelia. Patients should be kept in the ICU with MAP maintenance between 85 and 90 mmHg. Early reduction of fractures, dislocations, and other injuries is recommended to avoid neurological sequelae.

Anterior cord syndrome may occur due to spinal cord infarction in the territory supplied by the anterior spinal artery or as a result of anterior cord compression by a dislocated bone fragment or herniated disc.

Patients will typically present with paraplegia. If the lesion is higher than C7, patients will present with quadriplegia. Patients experience dissociated sensory loss below the lesion, loss of pain and temperature sensation and preserved two-point discrimination, joint position sense, and deep pressure sensation (posterior column sensation). Only 10% to 20% of patients recover functional motor control. Sensation may return enough to help prevent injuries. Surgical decompression, particularly for compressive lesions, can be considered with an anterior surgical approach.

Brown-Sequard syndrome presents as a spinal cord hemisection injury. Neurological findings consist of ipsilateral motor paralysis below the lesion, loss of posterior column function (proprioception and vibratory sensation), and contralateral loss of pain and temperature sensation two segments inferior to the lesion. Light touch is usually preserved. Brown-Sequard syndrome is usually due to a penetrating trauma but can also happen as a result of spinal cord tumor, spinal AVM, cervical spondylosis, and spinal cord herniation. 90% of patients with this condition will regain anal and sphincter continence as well as the ability to ambulate independently.

Posterior cord syndrome is a rare syndrome that produces pain and paresthesias often of burning quality in the neck, upper arm, and torso. Mild paresis of the upper extremities may also be seen.

INDICATIONS FOR SURGERY

Surgery may be indicated for incomplete spinal cord injuries with continued compression of the spinal cord that correlates with the level of the deficit. Patients present with persistent significant motor deficit following a varying period of recovery, deterioration of function, and continued significant dysesthesia. Patients with progressive deterioration should be decompressed as soon as possible to preserve neurological function. Surgery may also be indicated for patients with gross spinal instability and patients with hematomyelia. Patients with hematomyelia may recover some lower extremity strength after surgery.

Atlanto-Occipital Dislocation

Atlanto-occipital dislocation (AOD) is a rare injury in which the atlas becomes misaligned in reference to the occiput.

- Type 1 AOD: describes anterior dislocation of the occiput relative to the atlas.
- Type-2 AOD: describes longitudinal dislocation between the occiput and the atlas.
- Type-3 AOD: describes posterior dislocation of the occiput relative to the atlas.

Evaluation of suspected AOD with lateral C-spine x-ray and calculation of BAI (Basion-axial interval) and BDI (Basion Dental Interval) are recommended for confirmation of diagnosis.

BAI is the measurement of the distance between the basion (the inferior tip of the clivus) and the axial interval (rostral extension of the posterior axial line).

The Power ratio (BC/AO) is calculated by dividing the distance between the basion and the posterior arch of the atlas (BC) by the distance between the anterior arch of the atlas and the opisthion (AO). A power ratio more than 1 is diagnostic of an AOD.

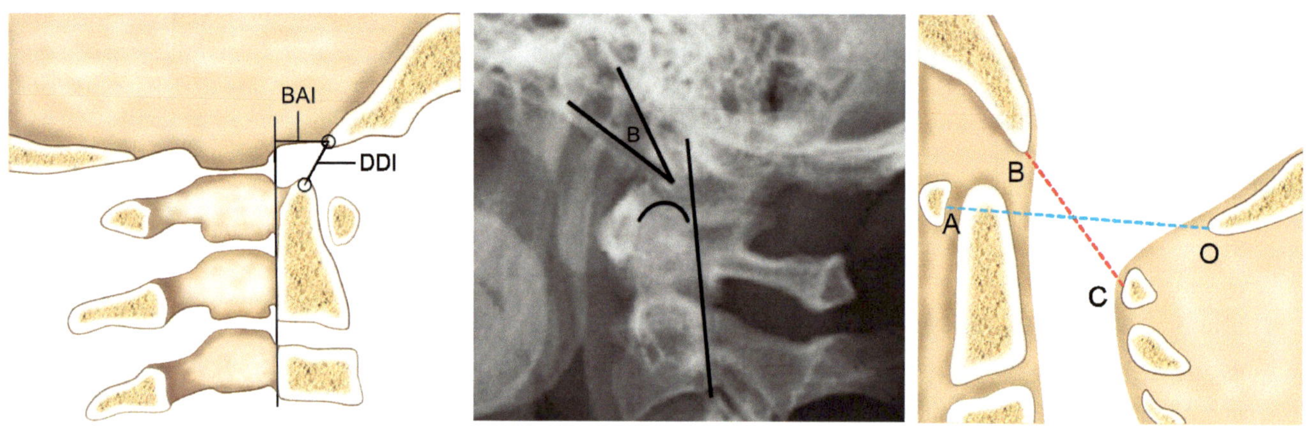

Figure 9: Radiographic evaluation of Atlanto-Occipital dislocations.

Upper cervical prevertebral soft tissue swelling on an otherwise non-diagnostic plain lateral x-ray should prompt additional imaging. Abnormal T2W1 MRI findings typically include abnormal high signal in the atlanto-occipital joints or in the posterior occipital atlantal ligaments. Management of AOD involves immobilization of the neck with a halo orthosis or with sandbags. Cervical traction should not be attempted to reduce AOD because of the risk of neurological deterioration.

Atlanto-Axial Subluxation

Atlanto-axial subluxation (AAS) involves partial dislocation between C1 and C2 that may occur in association with trauma, rheumatoid arthritis, and respiratory tract infections (as seen in Grisel syndrome). Rotary AAS is usually seen in children. Anterior AAS is more common in adults and has the worst prognosis. Posterior AAS is rare and usually due to erosion of the odontoid process, thus necessitating fusion to ensure stability of the joint. In anterior AAS, assessment of the integrity of the transverse ligament is essential to determine management. Spence's rule states that on open mouth odontoid x-ray, a total overhang distance between the lateral mass of C1 and C2 more than 7 mm indicates a ruptured transverse ligament (Figure 10).

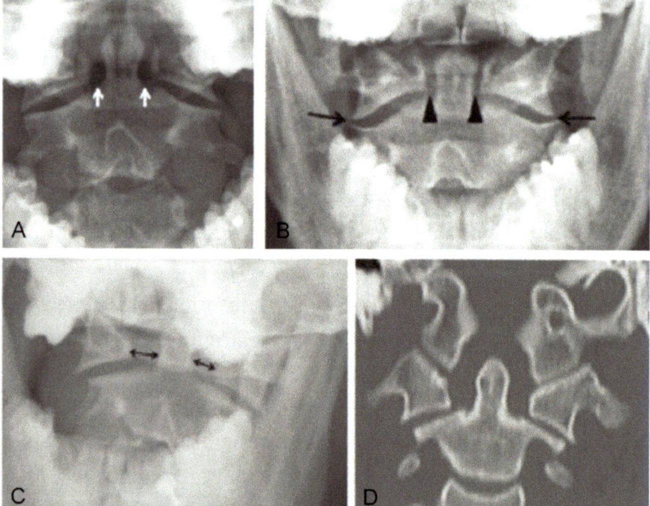

Figure 10: Open mouth odontoid x-rays demonstrating increasing overhang distance between C1 and C2; (A) normal; (B) slightly increased overhang distance; (C) moderately increased overhang distance, and (D) severely increased overhang distance.

MRI may show transverse atlantal ligament injury. Early traction is often successful in the treatment of AAS. Predisposing infections (as in Grisel syndrome) should be treated. Subluxations that are irreducible by traction may need trans-oral subluxation release.

Occipital Condyle Fracture

- Type 1 occipital condyle (OC) fractures are comminuted and may occur after impact with axial loading.
- Type 2 OC fractures involve extension of a linear basilar skull fracture.
- Type 3 OC fractures occur with avulsion of the condylar fragment which may result from rotation of the head.

In all cases of OC fracture, MRI is recommended to assess the integrity of the craniocervical ligaments. Type 1 and 2 fractures are considered as stable and can be treated with or without external immobilization, cervical collar, or halo. Type 3 fractures are unstable and have higher risk of delayed deficits. External immobilization is recommended for six to eight weeks. Indications for occipitocervical fusion or halo immobilization include craniocervical misalignment and an occipital-C1 interval more than 2 mm.

C1 Fracture:

- Type 1 C1 fractures involve fracture of a single arch of C1.
- Type 2 C1 fractures are known as Burst fractures or classic Jefferson's fractures and may include fracture of multiple arches of C1 (Figure 11)
- Type 3 C1 fractures involve fracture of the lateral mass of C1.

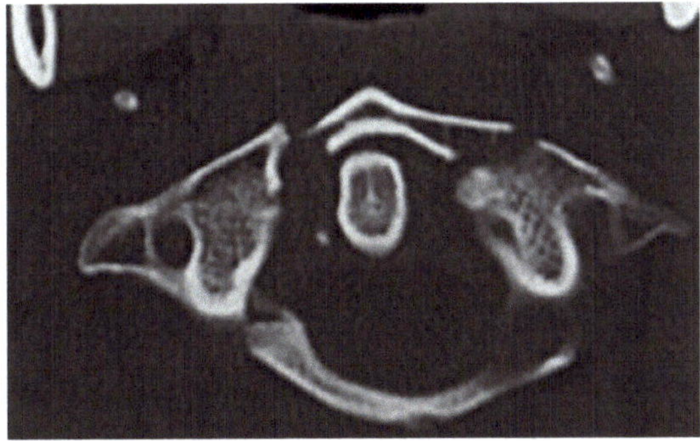

Figure 11: CT image of C1 fracture

If the transverse atlantal ligament is intact, type 2 fractures are considered as stable. Patients may be treated with placement of a collar, sternal-occipital-mandibular immobilizer (SOMI), or halo immobilization. A disrupted ligament with a burst fracture necessitates stabilization and fusion of the C1-C2 joint. For lateral mass fractures and transverse process fractures, collar placement is sufficient for treatment.

C2 Fracture

1. Odontoid fracture. (The most common is injury to the axis)
2. Hangman's fracture
3. Miscellaneous C2 fractures

Hangman's Fractures

Hangman's fractures are bilateral fractures through the pars interarticularis of C2 with traumatic subluxation of C2 on C3. These injuries are most often due to hyperextension of the neck. Most fractures are stable with no neurological deficits and do well with non-halo external immobilization for 14 weeks. Radiological studies should include cervical CT with sagittal and coronal reconstruction, cervical MRI to assess the C2-3 disruption, and CT angiography to screen for dissection of the vertebral artery. Surgical stabilization should be considered in cases of severe angulation of C2 on C3, disruption of the C2-3 disc space, or inability to establish or maintain alignment with external immobilization.

Odontoid Fractures

- Type 1 odontoid fractures occur just through the tip of the odontoid above the transverse ligament.
- Type 2 fractures occur through the base of the neck, most commonly as a dens fracture.
- Type 2A fractures are similar to type 2 but with a large bone chip at the fracture site.
- Type 3 fractures occur throughout the body, usually involving marrow space, and may involve the superior articular surface.

Only Type 3 fractures are considered stable. Type 1, 2, and 3 fractures may be managed initially with external cervical immobilization. Children younger than 7 years almost always heal with immobilization alone.

Surgery is recommended for odontoid type 2 fractures in patients with displacement more than 5 mm, instability at the fracture site in the halo vest, and older than 50 years. A degree of displacement more than 4-6 mm increases the risk of nonunion. Nonunion, including from fibrous union, is associated with delayed instability. This is especially true if accompanied by myelopathy and disruption of the transverse ligament.

Instability of Mid and Lower C-spine

Mid and lower C-spine instability can be diagnosed if the following radiographic criteria are met (Figure 12):

1. Sagittal plane displacement more than 3.5 mm on neutral position x-ray

2. Relative sagittal plane angulation more than 11 degrees
3. Sagittal plane translation by 3.5 mm on flexion/ extension views
4. Rotation more than 20 degrees

Figure 12: Evaluation of instability of C spine injuries

Element	Point Value
Destroyed or non-functioning anterior element	2
Destroyed or non-functioning posterior element	2
Positive stretch test	2
X-Ray criteria A. Flexion-extension a. Sagittal plane translation 20% or >3.5 mm b. Sagittal plane rotation >20 degrees or B. Resting a. Sagittal plane displacement 20% or >3.5 mm b. Relative sagittal plane angulation >11 degrees	2
Spinal canal narrowed developmentally (Pavlov radio <0.8 or sagittal diameter <13 mm)	1
Abnormal disk narrowing	1
Damage to spinal cord	2
Damage to nerve root	1
Anticipated dangerous loading	1
Patient is unstable if ≥5	

Distinguishing Between the Teardrop Fracture and Avulsion Fracture

A small bone chip from the inferior anterior portion of the vertebral body is known as a teardrop fracture. This may need to be distinguished from an avulsion fracture if it meets the following criteria:

1. The bone fragment is too small to be properly assessed
2. The vertebral bodies are aligned
3. No vertebral fracture is seen on AP, C-spine x-rays or CT\MRI of the sagittal plane
4. No posterior element fracture on X-ray or CT scan
5. No prevertebral soft tissue swelling at the level of the fragment
6. No loss of vertebral body height or disc space height.

If the above criteria are met, flexion and extension C-spine x-rays should be obtained. If there is no abnormal movement, the patient may be discharged in a rigid collar with follow-up scans to be performed in 4 to 7 days. If the pain has subsided and the second set of films is normal, the collar may be removed. If the fracture does not meet the above criteria, the fracture must be treated as an unstable fracture.

Locked Facets

Locked facets are also known as 'jumped' facets due to a reversed normal shingled relationship between the facets; mainly the inferior facet of the above level is located posteriorly to the superior facet of the below level. This involves disruption of the facet capsule. Perched facets are incompletely locked facets but with significant ligamentous disruption after distraction (just short of locking).

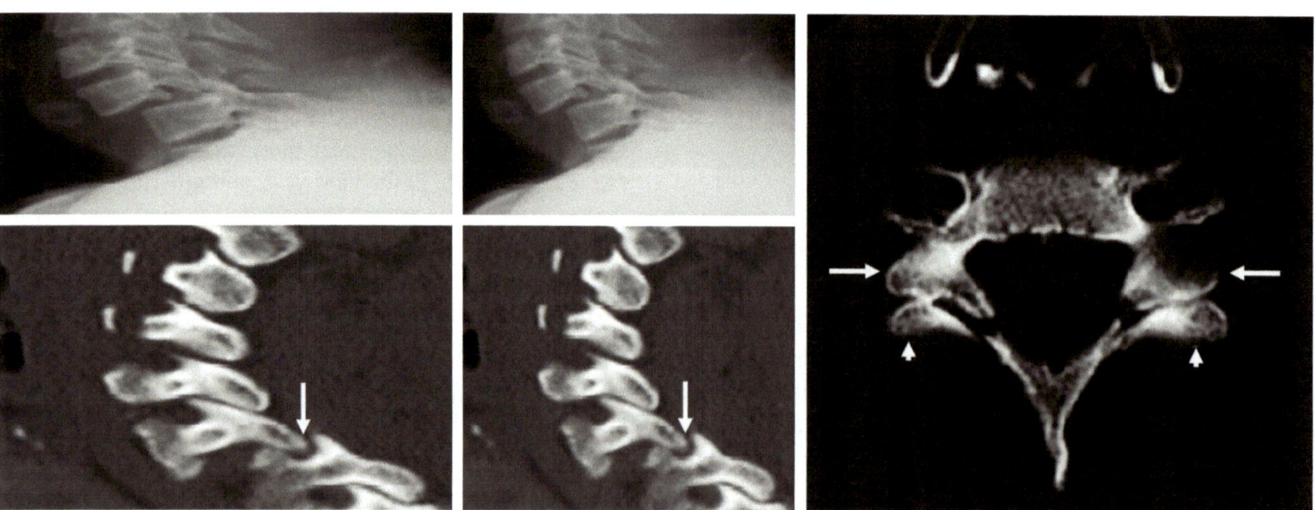

Figure 12: Locked facets: see the characteristic locking of facets as pointed by the arrows

Unilateral locked facets may present as neurologically intact in 25% of patients, as incomplete spinal cord injuries in 22% of patients, or as complete spinal cord injuries and quadriplegic in 15% of patients.

Bilateral locked facets are very common at C5-6 and C6-7 levels, with most presenting with complete quadriplegia. Both unilateral and bilateral locked facets will produce subluxation as seen on C-spine x-ray. The spinous process above the subluxation can be seen rotating to the same side as the locked facet. Oblique x-rays may demonstrate the locked facets, which can be seen blocking the neural foramen. A 60-degree left anterior oblique image can be used for the left locked facet and 60-degree right anterior oblique image can be used for the right facet. Treatment involves traction, with an initial weight equal to three times the cervical vertebral level. Weights should be increased in 5 to 10 lb increments with 10 to 15 minutes intervals with regular neurological assessment, SSEP, and MEP monitoring. Traction should be stopped if occipitocervical instability develops, if disk space height exceeds 10 mm (considered as over distraction) or if there are somatosensary evoked potential (SSEP) and motor evoked potential (MEP).

Clay-shoveler's fracture is an avulsion of the spinal process usually at the C7 level (Figure 14). This fracture is stable and itself poses little risk. Rigid collar may be used on an as-needed basis for pain.

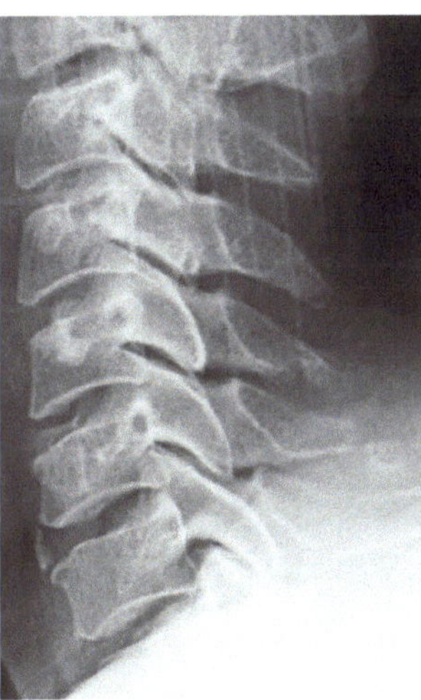

Figure 14: Clay Shoveler fracture: Avulsion of spinal process of C7

Thoracic and Lumbar Spine Fractures

Characterization of thoracic and lumbar spine fractures is based on a three-column model (Figure 15). The anterior column consists of the anterior half of the vertebral body, annulus fibrosus, anterior longitudinal ligament, and nucleus pulposus (disc). The middle column consists of the posterior half of the disc and vertebral body, posterior longitudinal ligament, and the pedicles. The posterior column consists of the posterior bony complex, posterior arch with interposed posterior ligamentous complex, supraspinous and interspinous ligament, facet joints, capsule, and ligamentum flavum. Injury to the posterior column alone does not cause instability.

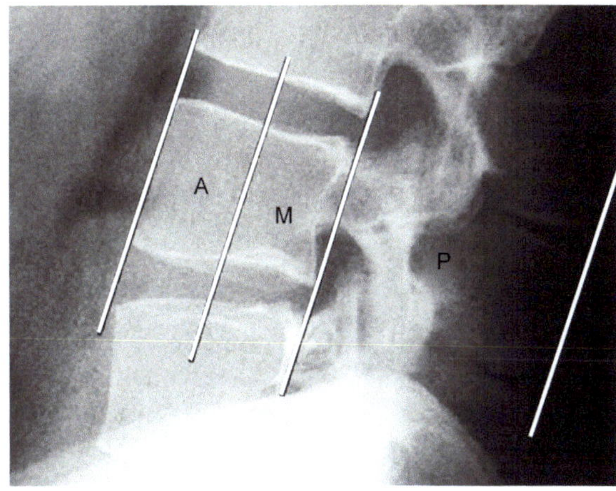

Figure 15: The 3-column model used to assess the alignment of spine

Fracture of the transverse process usually presents with no neurological deficits. Exceptions to this include fractures at L4-L5 (associated with lumbosacral plexus injuries) and T1-T2 (associated with brachial plexus injuries). Compression fractures most commonly occur in the anterior column between T6-8 and T12-L3. Lateral x-rays show anterior wedging of the vertebral body with no posterior loss of height and no associated subluxation. On CT, the spinal canal is intact. Disruption of the anterior endplate is often seen. Neurologically, the patient is intact.

Burst fractures occur mainly at the thoracolumbar (TL) junction between T10 and L2 (Figure 16). L5 burst fractures are rare. Fracture of both end plates is seen in the lower lumbar region. Fracture of the superior endplate is the most common burst fracture seen at the TL junction. Fracture of the inferior endplate is rare.

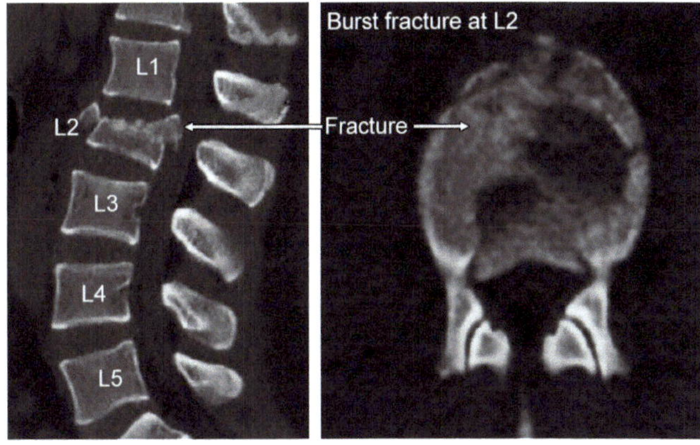

Figure 16: Burst fracture at the level of L2

Lateral x-rays demonstrate cortical fracture of the posterior vertebral body wall, loss of the posterior vertebral height, retropulsion of the bone fragment from the endplate into the canal, an increase in interpedicular distance, and vertical fracture of the lamina displaying the facet joints. CT demonstrates a break in the posterior wall of the vertebral body with a retropulsed bone fragment into the spinal canal. Fifty percent of the canal area can become obstructed. Myelogram may show a large central defect.

Seat Belt Injury

Seat belt injuries occur with flexion across the fulcrum anterior to the anterior column. Plain x-ray shows increase in the interspinous distance, pars interarticularis fracture, and horizontal split of the pedicles and transverse process. There is usually no subluxation. Treatment of stable anterior and middle column thoracolumbar spine injuries includes treatment with analgesics, recumbency, bed rest, and comfort care for one to three weeks. Thordco Lumbo Sacral Orthosis (TLSO) brace is recommended for 12 weeks. Vertebroplasty may be an option for some cases. Serial x-ray may be necessary to rule out progressive deformity. Unstable compression fractures occur in single compression fractures with loss of more than 50% of the height with kyphotic angulation more than 30 degrees, and in cases of three or more contiguous compression fractures. Neurological deficit generally does not occur with pure compression fracture. Middle column fractures are generally always unstable except in cases where fracture is above T8 with intact ribs and sternum, or below L4 with intact posterior elements. Typical features of middle column fractures include an anterior vertebral body height less than 50% of the posterior vertebral body height, a residual canal diameter less than 50%, kyphotic angulation more than 20 degrees, neurological deficits, and progressive kyphosis.

Osteoporotic Compression Fractures

Patients may present initially with severe pain necessitating hospital or subacute care facility admission for adequate pain control. Bedrest is recommended for approximately 7 to 10 days with prophylactic prevention of deep vein thrombosis. Physical therapy should be initiated after 7 to 10 days. Kyphoplasty may be indicated for painful osteoporotic compression fractures, severe pain that interferes with patient activity, and pain refractory to oral pain medications. Fractures producing less than 5% to 10% loss of height are not typically treated. Kyphoplasty does not give as rapid pain relief as the compression fractures secondary to metastatic disease. Kyphoplasty should not be used in patients with coagulopathy, a completely healed fracture, no edema on MRI, active infections (i.e., sepsis), osteomyelitis, discitis, epidural abscess, or spinal instability. Complications include cement leakage, radiculopathy, pedicle fracture, rib fracture, transverse process fracture, anterior penetration with needle, puncture of the great vessels, pneumothorax, and possible vertebral body compression fracture at adjacent levels.

Gunshot Wounds to the Spine

Gunshot wounds to the spine should be managed according to normal trauma protocol. Once the patient is stabilized and assessed, management can be determined based on location of wound and radiographic imaging. Emergent surgical management is required with injury to the cauda equina, neurological deterioration with epidural hematoma, compression of a nerve root, and CSF leak.

Low Back Pain and Radiculopathy

Low back pain is an over whelming public health problem and prevalence rates may be as high as 85%. Mechanical low back pain, which comprises most of the low back pain cases, describes musculoskeletal (from paraspinal muscles) ligament injury and irritation of the facet joints. Initial assessment of the patient with back pain is based on history and physical examination. History should include age of onset, history of trauma, history of persistent numbness and weakness of the extremities, response to previous therapy, and pain that is worse at rest. Cancer or osteomyelitis should be suspected in patients older than 50 years or younger than 20 years of age with a history of malignancies that are prone to skeletal metastatic disease, unexplained weight loss, immunosuppression, urinary tract infections, IV drug abuse, fever and chills, back pain not improved with rest, and pain radiating below the knee. Spinal fracture should be considered in patients with any history of significant trauma, prolonged use of steroids, and age over 70 years. Cauda equina syndrome should be considered if there is a history of acute onset urinary retention or overflow incontinence, fecal incontinence, saddle anesthesia, and global progressive weakness in one or both lower extremities. While taking the history, it is also important to determine psychological and socioeconomic factors that may influence the pain such as work status, typical job tasks, educational level, pending litigations, workers compensations, previous treatment failures, substance abuse, and depression.

A targeted physical exam is crucial in assessing lower back pain and vital for determining the etiology of the pain. Findings suggestive of nerve root impingement include pain radiating down the lower extremity, motor weakness, dermatomal sensory changes, reflex abnormalities, tenderness over the sciatic notch, and a positive nerve root tension sign such as Lasegue sign (Straight leg raise test). More than 90% of cases of radiculopathy are due to a herniated nucleus pulposus and involve L4-L5 or L5-S1 nerve roots. Such patients present with dorsiflexion weakness at the ankle and great toe, suggesting L5 and some L4 dysfunction. Sensory loss over the medial malleolus and medial foot suggests L4 radiculopathy, sensory loss over the dorsum of the foot suggests L5 radiculopathy, and sensory loss over the lateral malleolus and lateral foot suggest S1 radiculopathy. Proper examination of reflexes is also important. In the presence of a hyperactive knee jerk, contralateral thigh adductor contraction may indicate an upper motor neuron lesion. A diminished Achilles reflex may suggest an S1 root dysfunction.

The straight leg raise (SLR) test helps to differentiate sciatica from pain due to hip pathology. In this test, with the patient supine, the affected limb is raised by the ankle until pain is elicited. Pain should occur at an angle less than 60 degrees as tension in the nerve increases little above this angle. A positive test consists of leg pain or paresthesia in the distribution of pain (back pain alone does not qualify). In addition, the patient will try to extend their hip by lifting off the table to reduce the angle. Ankle dorsiflexion along with the SLR test usually augments the pain in suspected cases of nerve root compression. The SLR test primarily increases tension in L5 and S1, less often in L4 and very little to none in the more proximal root. In the crossed straight leg raise test, testing of the painless leg causes contralateral limb pain. Although a larger angle of elevation is usually required than the painful side, this test is more specific but less sensitive than the SLR test.

In the Patrick's test (FABER – flexion, abduction, and external rotation), the hip and knee are flexed, and the lateral malleolus is placed on the contralateral knee. The ipsilateral knee is then gently displaced downwards towards the exam table. This maneuver stresses the hip joint, thus exaggerating pathological pain in the hip joint, which rules out the nerve stretch phenomenon caused by physical stretching of the nerve causing localized pain symptoms.

Diagnostic Tests

Initial investigations may include CBC differential, ESR, CRP, blood cultures, urine cultures, plain x-ray, bone scan, CT scan, and MRI with contrast. MRI is the diagnostic modality of choice for evaluation of lumbar radiculopathy. MRI in the sagittal plane provides information regarding tissue outside the spinal canal, is noninvasive, and does not involve ionizing radiation. It also helps to evaluate suspected cauda equina lesions. CT with Myelography with soluble contrast is about 60% to 100% sensitive and 83% to 94% specific for suspected cases of radiculopathy. It also provides functional information about varying degrees of stenosis. Myelography can be used to identify a herniated nucleus pulposus which produces extradural filling defects at the level of the intervertebral disc herniation. Massive disc herniation or severe lumbar stenosis can be seen as total or near total block on myelography.

Treatment

Conservative treatment consists of activity modification and bed rest for two to three days. The objective is to reduce symptoms by reducing pressure on the nerve roots. Patients should avoid heavy lifting, prolonged sitting, and bending or twisting of the back. During the first two weeks of recovery, walking, bicycling, and swimming are allowed and encouraged. Analgesics may be used for a short period of time for acute symptomatic relief. Opioids may be required for severe pain, especially in cases of severe radicular pain. If desired, muscle relaxants can be used for less than two to three weeks. An epidural steroid injection is an alternative option for short-term relief of radicular pain.

Usually about 85% to 90% of the patients with acute disc herniation will improve without surgical intervention on an average of 6 weeks. Surgical indications include development of cauda equina syndrome, progressive symptoms, or persistence of neurological deficit despite conservative treatment of severe radicular pain for more than six weeks. Emergent surgeries are required in the presence of cauda equina syndrome, progressive motor deficits, and intolerable pain despite adequate narcotic pain medications. Surgery may also be indicated if nonsurgical management fails to control the pain after 5 to 8 weeks.

Treatments that are still offered but not recommended for acute low back pain consist of oral steroids, colchicine, antidepressant medications, transcutaneous electrical nerve stimulation (TENS), traction, heat therapy and lumbar corsets, biofeedback, acupuncture, trigger point and ligamentous injection, facet steroid injection in absence of facet arthritis, and epidural steroid injection in absence of radiculopathy.

REFERENCES

1. Eelco FM.The Comatose Patient - Wijdicks - Google Books. Accessed November 30, 2021. https://books.google.com/books?hl=en&lr=&id=HpCtAwAAQBAJ&oi=fnd&pg=PT14&ots=TY-Ym5C_8_&sig=Zjk-2bGA-34dCGfcdm3mYlM65qA#v=onepage&q&f=false.
2. Teasdale G, Jennett B. ASSESSMENT OF COMA AND IMPAIRED CONSCIOUSNESS: A Practical Scale. *Lancet*. 1974;304(7872):81-84. doi:10.1016/S0140-6736(74)91639-0.
3. Teasdale G, Knill-Jones R, Van Der Sande J. Observer variability in assessing impaired consciousness and coma. *J Neurol Neurosurg Psychiatry*. 1978;41(7):603-610. doi:10.1136/JNNP.41.7.603.

4. Bouzarth WF. Neurosurgical watch sheet for craniocerebral trauma. *J Trauma Acute Care Surg.* 1968;8(1):29-31.
5. Teasdale G, Jennett B. Assessment and prognosis of coma after head injury. *Acta Neurochir 1976 341.* 1976;34(1):45-55. doi:10.1007/BF01405862.
6. Rutledge R, Lentz CW, Fakhry S, Hunt J. Appropriate use of the Glasgow Coma Scale in intubated patients: a linear regression prediction of the Glasgow verbal score from the Glasgow eye and motor scores. *J Trauma Acute Care Surg.* 1996;41(3):514-522.
7. Stocchetti N, Pagan F, Calappi E, et al. Inaccurate Early Assessment of Neurological Severity in Head Injury. *https://home.liebertpub.com/neu.* 2004;21(9):1131-1140. doi:10.1089/NEU.2004.21.1131.
8. Davis RA, Davis L. Decerebrate Rigidity in Humans. *Neurosurgery.* 1982;10(5):635-642. doi:10.1227/00006123-198205000-00017.
9. Plum F, Posner JB. The diagnosis of stupor and coma. *Contemp Neurol Ser.* 1972;10:1-286.
10. Traub SJ, Wijdicks EF. Initial Diagnosis and Management of Coma. *Emerg Med Clin North Am.* 2016;34(4):777-793. doi:10.1016/J.EMC.2016.06.017.
11. Student Course Manual ATLS ® Advanced Trauma Life Support ®. Published online 2018.
12. Mayglothling J, Duane TM, Gibbs M, et al. Emergency tracheal intubation immediately following traumatic injury: An eastern association for the surgery of trauma practice management guideline. *J Trauma Acute Care Surg.* 2012;73(5 SUPPL.4). doi:10.1097/TA.0B013E31827018A5.
13. Whited L, Graham DD. Abnormal Respirations. *StatPearls.* Published online December 22, 2017. Accessed November 30, 2021. http://europepmc.org/books/NBK470309.
14. James B. The Pupils. *Ophthalmol Investig Exam Tech.* Published online 1990:123-127. doi:10.1016/B978-0-7506-7586-4.50015-5.
15. Wiwatwongwana A, Lyons CJ. Eye movement control and its disorders. *Handb Clin Neurol.* 2013;113:1505-1513. doi:10.1016/B978-0-444-59565-2.00021-6.
16. Goila A, Pawar M. The diagnosis of brain death. *Indian J Crit Care Med.* 2009;13(1):7. doi:10.4103/0972-5229.53108.
17. Zakaria Z, Abdullah MM, Halim SA, Izaini Ghani AR, Idris Z, Abdullah JM. The Neurological Exam of a Comatose Patient: An Essential Practical Guide. *Malays J Med Sci.* 2020;27(5):108. doi:10.21315/MJMS2020.27.5.11.
18. MacHado C, Perez J, Scherle C, Areu A, Pando A. Brain death diagnosis and apnea test safety. *Ann Indian Acad Neurol.* 2009;12(3):197. doi:10.4103/0972-2327.56326.
19. Smith M. Monitoring intracranial pressure in traumatic brain injury. *Anesth Analg.* 2008;106(1):240-248. doi:10.1213/01.ANE.0000297296.52006.8E.
20. Bratton SL, Chestnut RM, Ghajar J, et al. VI. Indications for Intracranial Pressure Monitoring. *https://home.liebertpub.com/neu.* 2007;24(SUPPL. 1). doi:10.1089/NEU.2007.9990.
21. Raghavan M, Marik PE. Therapy of intracranial hypertension in patients with fulminant hepatic failure. *Neurocritical Care 2006 42.* 2006;4(2):179-189. doi:10.1385/NCC:4:2:179.
22. Stravitz RT, Kramer AH, Davern T, et al. Intensive care of patients with acute liver failure: Recommendations of the U.S. Acute Liver Failure Study Group. Crit Care Med. 2007;35(10). doi:10.1097/01.CCM.0000287592.94554.5F.
23. Carney N, Totten AM, O'Reilly C, et al. Guidelines for the Management of Severe Traumatic Brain Injury, Fourth Edition. Neurosurgery. 2017;80(1):6-15. doi:10.1227/NEU.0000000000001432.
24. Rekate HL. A Contemporary Definition and Classification of Hydrocephalus. Semin Pediatr Neurol. 2009;16(1):9-15. doi:10.1016/J.SPEN.2009.01.002.
25. Hamilton MG. Treatment of Hydrocephalus in Adults. Semin Pediatr Neurol. 2009;16(1):34-41. doi:10.1016/J.SPEN.2009.02.001.
26. Erdo an E, Cansever T. Pyogenic brain abscess. Neurosurg Focus. 2008;24(6):E2. doi:10.3171/FOC/2008/24/6/E2.
27. Smail], Tekk6k H, Erbengi A. m NS Management of brain abscess in children: review of 130 cases over a period of 21 years. Child's Nerv Syst. 1992;8:411-416.
28. Desprechins B, Stadnik T, Koerts G, Shabana W, Breucq C, Osteaux M. Use of Diffusion-Weighted MR Imaging in Differential Diagnosis Between Intracerebral Necrotic Tumors and Cerebral Abscesses. Am J Neuroradiol. 1999;20(7).
29. Haimes AB, Zimmerman RD, Morgello S, et al. MR Imaging of Brain Abscesses. Am J Neuroradiol. 1989;10(2).
30. Sapico FL. Microbiology and Antimicrobial Therapy of Spinal Infections. Orthop Clin North Am. 1996;27(1):9-13. doi:10.1016/S0030-5898(20)32045-9.
31. Leone A, Dell'Atti C, Magarelli N, et al. Imaging of spondylodiscitis. Eur Rev Med Pharmacol Sci. 2012;16(Suppl 2):8-19.

32. Lener S, Hartmann S, Barbagallo GM V, Certo F, Thomé C, Tschugg A. Management of spinal infection: a review of the literature. Acta Neurochir (Wien). 2018;160(3):487-496. doi:10.1007/s00701-018-3467-2.
33. Lapointe S, Perry A, Butowski NA. Primary brain tumours in adults. Lancet. 2018;392(10145):432-446. doi:10.1016/S0140-6736(18)30990-5.
34. Di Rocco C, Lannelli A. Intracranial supratentorial tumors: classification, clinical findings, surgical management. Rays. 1996;21(1):9-25. Accessed December 31, 2021. https://europepmc.org/article/med/8677342.
35. Bilaniuk LT. Adult infratentorial tumors. Semin Roentgenol. 1990;25(2):155-173. doi:10.1016/0037-198X(90)90047-8.
36. Amidei C, Kushner DS. Clinical implications of motor deficits related to brain tumors. Neuro-Oncology Pract. 2015;2(4):179-184. doi:10.1093/NOP/NPV017.
37. Ryken TC, Kuo JS, Prabhu RS, Sherman JH, Kalkanis SN, Olson JJ. Congress of Neurological Surgeons Systematic Review and Evidence-Based Guidelines on the Role of Steroids in the Treatment of Adults with Metastatic Brain Tumors. Clin Neurosurg. 2019;84(3):E189-E191. doi:10.1093/NEUROS/NYY546.
38. McCrory P, Meeuwisse WH, Aubry M, et al. Consensus statement on concussion in sport: the 4th International Conference on Concussion in Sport held in Zurich, November 2012. Br J Sports Med. 2013;47(5):250-258. doi:10.1136/BJSPORTS-2013-092313.
39. Practice parameter: the management of concussion in sports (summary statement). Report of the Quality Standards Subcommittee. Neurology. 1997;48(3):581-585. doi:10.1212/WNL.48.3.581.
40. Giza CC, Kutcher JS, Ashwal S, et al. Summary of evidence-based guideline update: Evaluation and management of concussion in sports: Report of the Guideline Development Subcommittee of the American Academy of Neurology. Neurology. 2013;80(24):2250. doi:10.1212/WNL.0B013E31828D57DD.
41. Khairat A, Waseem M. Epidural Hematoma. StatPearls. Published online August 2, 2021. Accessed January 1, 2022. https://www.ncbi.nlm.nih.gov/books/NBK518982/.
42. Chicote Álvarez E, González Castro A, Ortiz Lasa M, et al. Epidemiology of traumatic brain injury in the elderly over a 25 year period. Rev Española Anestesiol y Reanim (English Ed. 2018;65(10):546-551. doi:10.1016/J.REDARE.2018.11.005.
43. Aromatario M, Torsello A, D'errico S, et al. Traumatic Epidural and Subdural Hematoma: Epidemiology, Outcome, and Dating. Medicina (Kaunas). 2021;57(2):1-16. doi:10.3390/MEDICINA57020125.
44. Oakley GM, Orlandi RR, Woodworth BA, Batra PS, Alt JA. Management of cerebrospinal fluid rhinorrhea: an evidence-based review with recommendations. Int Forum Allergy Rhinol. 2016;6(1):17-24. doi:10.1002/ALR.21627.
45. Maynard FM, Bracken MB, Creasey G, et al. International Standards for Neurological and Functional Classification of Spinal Cord Injury. American Spinal Injury Association. Spinal Cord. 1997;35(5):266-274. doi:10.1038/SJ.SC.3100432.
46. Walters BC, Hadley MN, Hurlbert RJ, et al. Guidelines for the Management of Acute Cervical Spine and Spinal Cord Injuries2013 Update. Neurosurgery. 2013;60(CN_suppl_1):82-91. doi:10.1227/01.NEU.0000430319.32247.7F.

74

CHAPTER

Updates of TNM Classification from 7th to 8th Edition

Yavar Abgin
Ethan Tabaie
Lawrence Chen
Austin Lee
Kayla Umemoto
Dinesh Vyas

INTRODUCTION

The TNM classification of malignant tumors developed by Pierre Denoix between 1943 and 1952, have since been used to quantify and categorize clinical stages and extensions of malignancies to easily communicate the amount of spreading and prognosis of tumors. As some classifications within the TNM grading system were once binary, particularly the N and M categories, over many years the Union for International Cancer Control (UICC) has developed a more precise tumor, lymph node, and metastasis classification system. In 1995, a project titled *Prognostic Factors in Cancer* introduced a compilation of prognostic factors, both anatomical and non-anatomical, at each body site.[1] TNM-8 - the newest edition of classifications - took effect at the start of 2017. This paper focuses on the changes made between the previous and current classification systems.[1]

To begin, new classifications in TNM-8 include abdominal viscera cancers, head and neck cancers, thoracic cavity cancers, retroperitoneal sarcomas, pelvic and spine osteosarcomas, oropharynx p16-positive malignant tumors, thymus tumors, unknown primary cervical lymph nodes, neuroendocrine tumors, and head and neck skin cancers.

Moreover, there have been modifications to:

- Lung Tumors*
- Nasopharyngeal Tumors
- Head and Neck Nodes
- Prostate Tumors
- Ovary Tumors
- Anal Tumors
- Liver Tumors
- Stomach Tumors
- Thyroid Tumors
- Esophagus Tumors

* Though TNM-8 allows physicians to classify lung tumors with better precision, a few interpretation pitfalls exist, and physicians are still met with cases that are not yet classified with respect to staging using imaging.

Issues include lymphangitis carcinomatosis, lung cancers with multiple pulmonary involvements, and imagining of pleural invasion.[7] Overall, radiologists work to better understand the major changes brought about within TNM-8.

Of note, other areas of the body have also seen either slight or no modifications. These include other carcinomas of the head and neck, bone and soft tissue sarcomas, skin carcinomas, malignant lymphomas and melanomas, ophthalmic tumors, pleura tumors, small intestine tumors, colon tumors, rectum tumors, kidneys tumors, ovary tumors, penis tumors, urethra tumors, and hepatobiliary tumors.[3] Some new structures have also been added into TNM-8 including prognostic grids, a clarification of isolated tumor cells (ITC), and pediatric malignancies.[3] C factor has been removed from the introduction.[3]

Table 1. Summary of changes from TNM 7th to 8th Edition

	New to TNM-8	Significant Modifications in TNM-8	Minor/No Modifications in TNM-8
Head and Neck Tumors	• Unknown Primary Cervical Lymph Nodes	• Nasopharynx • Oropharynx: p16 positive malignant tumors • Thyroid	• Lip • Oral Cavity • Pharynx • Larynx • Paranasal Sinuses • Major Salivary Glands • Malignant Melanoma of Upper Respiratory Tract
Digestive System Tumors	• Well Differentiated Neuroendocrine Tumors of the GI Tract • Abdominal Viscera Cancers	• Esophagus • Stomach • Anal Canal and Perianal Skin • Liver	• Small Intestine • Appendix • Colon and Rectum • Intrahepatic Bile Ducts • Gallbladder • Perihilar Bile Ducts • Distal Extrahepatic Bile Duct • Ampulla of Vater • Pancreas
Lung and Pleural Tumors	• Thymic Tumors	• Lung Tumors	• Pleural Tumors
Bone and Soft Tissue Tumors	• Retroperitoneal Sarcomas • Spine Osteosarcomas		• Bone • Soft Tissues • Gastrointestinal Stromal Tumors
Skin Tumors	• Skin Carcinoma of the Head and Neck	• Isolated Tumor Cells (ITCs) in lymph nodes/distant sites suggest N0 or M0 classification, except in malignant skin melanomas and Merkel cell carcinomas it is classified as N1a or N2a	• Carcinoma of Skin • Carcinoma of Skin of the Eyelid • Malignant Melanoma of Skin • Merkel Cell Carcinoma of Skin
Breast Tumors		• Breast: tumor grade, estrogen and progesterone receptor expression, HER2 expression	
Gynecological Tumors	• Primary Peritoneal Carcinoma • Pelvic Osteosarcomas		• Gestational Trophoblastic Neoplasms • Vulva • Vagina • Cervix Uteri • Endometrium • Uterine Sarcomas • Fallopian Tube • Ovaries

	New to TNM-8	Significant Modifications in TNM-8	Minor/No Modifications in TNM-8
Urological Tumors		- Prostate	• Urethra • Penis • Urinary Bladder • Testis • Ureter • Kidney • Renal Pelvis
Adrenal Cortex Tumors	No Changes		
Ophthalmic Tumors			• Carcinoma and Malignant Melanoma of Conjunctiva • Malignant Melanoma of Uvea • Sarcoma of Orbit • Carcinoma of Lacrimal Gland • Retinoblastoma
Hodgkin Lymphoma	No Changes		
Non-Hodgkin Lymphomas	No Changes		
Others	• Pediatric Malignancies: stage by population, still under development • Prognostic Factors for Cancers		

Isolated Tumor Cells (ITC) Propositions: Important for Malignant Melanomas of the Skin and for Merkel Cell Carcinomas

There is much discussion on the standardization of pathology. Although there are trends toward standardizing histopathology via the development of guidelines, morphology remains foiled by subjectivity. Further, it is noted that guidelines and databases of classifications and grading will help pathologists in working with more precision in order to assist with difficult cases and promote consistency.[8] Additionally, there are definitions of ITC's that vary by size, with propositions arguing for clusters of <200 cells on histology in breast cancers versus <20 cells.[1] These discussions may potentially yield additional criteria to the accepted size of ITC's which would be visualized under immunohistochemistry.

It is important to clarify the difference between ITCs from micrometastasis. ITCs are currently defined in TNM-8 as single cells or clusters of cells that do not have any metastatic activity or penetration into the vessels or lymphatics.[1] Previously in a 1999 paper, ITCs were defined as circulating tumor cells, whereas micrometastases were cancer cells that were implanted, extravasated, proliferated, and had stromal reactions, making micrometastasis a histochemical diagnosis.[24] Authors of the TNM-8 guideline write that the presence of ITCs in lymph nodes or in distant sites still suggest an N0 or M0 classification, except in malignant skin melanomas and Merkel cell carcinomas, where ITCs in a lymph node are classified as N1a or N2a.[1]

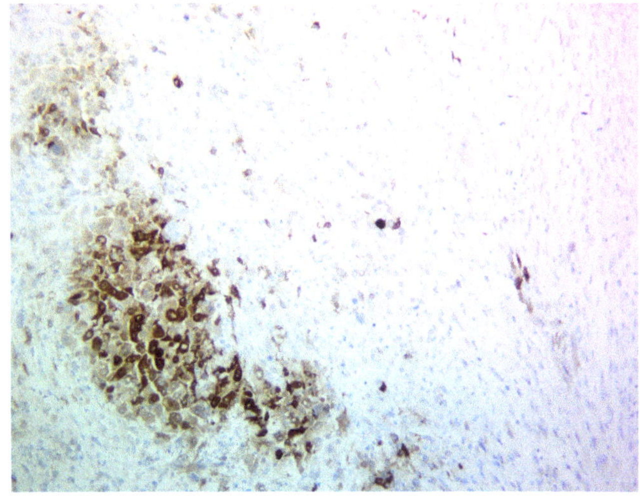

Figure 1: Mesothelioma

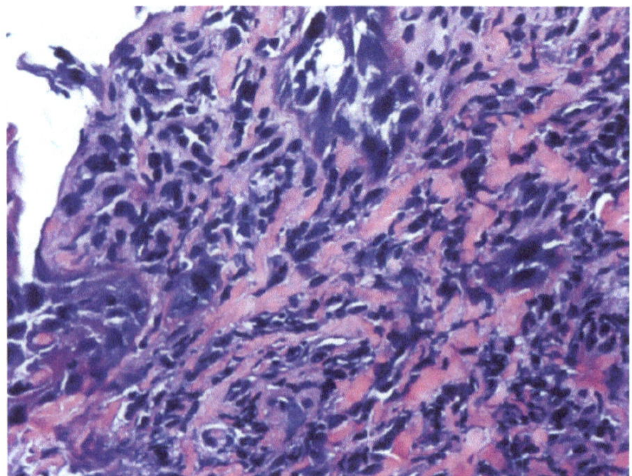

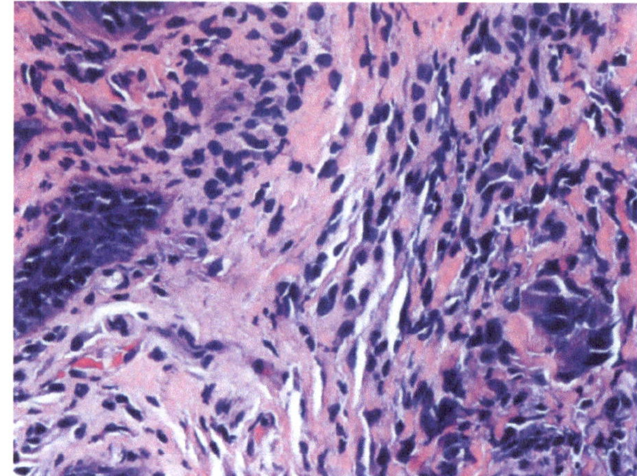

Figure 2 and 3: Isolated tumor cells from a squamous cell carcinoma of the tongue

Oropharyngeal Tumors: Presence of p16

Separate sites of the head and neck have separate classifications. Tumors with overexpression of p16 are now a part of oropharyngeal cancer classification, and it is continuing to become an important marker when forming an assessment and plan. However, classifications of p16 as driver mutations toward carcinoma remains a topic of investigation.

In addition to tobacco and alcohol, human papillomavirus (HPV) serves as an important risk factor for oropharyngeal cancers. The incidence and survival of oropharyngeal cancers in the United States population has been increasing since 1984, which can be attributed to HPV infections.[9] Fortunately, HPV-positive head and neck squamous cell cancers (HNSCC) appear to have a more favorable prognosis when compared to HPV-negative HNSCCs.[10,11]

High-risk HPV types have E6 and E7 genes which encode oncoproteins that interfere with the activity of cellular tumor suppressor proteins, p53 and RB respectively. The p16 protein is a cyclin-dependent kinase inhibitor and is thought to serve as a tumor suppressor gene.[12] High-risk HPV strains with E6 and E7 genes overexpress p16 via underexpression of p16 regulators (Figure 4).[13,14] Therefore, immunostaining for p16 may indirectly identify high-risk HPV infection in HNSCCs.[13,14] Since HPV-positive HNSCCs both overexpress p16 and have better prognosis, p16-positive head and neck cancers also indicates better prognosis. It should be noted that not all p16-positive cancers are HPV-positive, and these p16-positive HPV-negative cancers have a worse prognosis than p16-positive HPV-positive ones.[15]

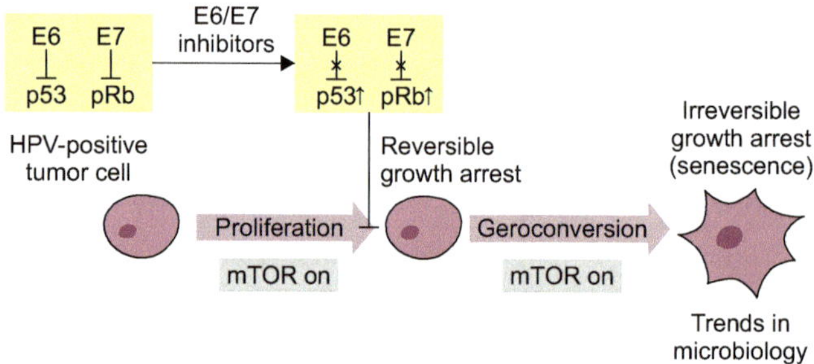

Figure 4: Pathogenesis of high-risk HPV strains containing E6 and E7 genes

Including p16 in TNM-8 outside of the context of HPV appears to have some good prognostic value. When comparing p16-positive and p16-negative oropharyngeal carcinomas, p16-positive cancers overall are more well-defined, exophytic, less ulcerated, less necrotic, and have less aggressive radiologic findings, which all indicate better prognosis.[30] Furthermore, p16-negative cancers are more frequently staged higher at III and IV when compared to p16-positive ones, and p16-positive smokers have higher staging and worse prognosis than p16-positive nonsmokers.[30] This suggests that smoking status is linked to prognosis and may need to be studied more in the future to determine if it should be included into TNM-9. As for treatment, chemotherapy and radiotherapy are efficacious therapeutic options for p16-positive HNSCC.[31,32]

TNM-8 is an improved system because it is a more informative classification for oropharyngeal cancers with better information on potential prognosis and it helps guide therapy. However, TNM-8 does not address nuances such as the presence or absence of HPV infection and the heterogeneity of high-risk HPV strains. Different high-risk HPV strains may be associated with a poorer prognosis, as seen with a worsened prognosis when comparing HPV16 and HPV33.[16] Therefore, HPV-DNA testing should be additionally performed with p16 immunostaining to ensure a proper assessment and decision for therapy.[15,17,18]

Table 2. Comparison of HNSCC markers (p16 protein, HPV status, HPV strain, and smoking status) and their associated prognosis.

HNSCC Marker	Prognosis
p16 presence	p16(+) has better prognosis than p16(–)[30]
p16 (+), HPV status	HPV(+) has better prognosis than HPV (–)[15]
HPV strain	HPV-16 has better prognosis than HPV-33[16]
p16 (+), smoking status	Non-smokers have better prognosis than smokers[30]

For both HPV-positive and -negative HNSCCs, a combination or individual use of surgery, radiation, and chemotherapy are traditional treatments, where surgery proves very effective for small primary cancers with no nodal involvement.[25] Tumors with a T stage ≥3 could be treated using chemoradiotherapy as a definitive non-surgical option, if needed.[25] Treatment of metastatic and recurrent HNSCCs with anti-PD-1 antibodies such as pembrolizumab and nivolumab is currently approved and effective for p16-negative and HPV-negative cancers, but it is ambiguous whether it is effective for metastatic or recurrent p16-positive and HPV-positive cancers.[15,33] HPV-positive HNSCCs do not express PD-1 exclusively or primarily, which may explain sub-optimal responses when using these therapies in HPV-positive carcinomas.[15]

TNM-8 has been updated and includes notable modifications for head and neck cancers. Of note, until the publication of TNM-8, the prognosis of patients within certain risk groups was based on the size of the tumor. To better classify staging of unique patients, the TNM-8 recognizes the need to categorize prognoses of almost-uniform tumors, but drastically different biological and clinical behaviors, independently. Further, important changes were seen within tumor and lymph node involvement classifications for oronasopharyngeal cancer. Finally, clinical and pathological stages for neck disease, and new HPV-16-positive HNSCC classifications have been introduced.[4]

Nasopharyngeal Tumors

With the new TNM-8 criteria, N3a and N3b were combined to just N3 to describe lower neck metastasis >6 cm in diameter.[19] Improved imaging and better detection of occult malignancies combined with improvements in radiotherapy allow for more accurate descriptions of these head and neck cancers in combination with the changes made to the T category.[19] The updates to the TNM classifications with clinical N3a and N3b stemmed from questions to the necessity of whether describing the difference of one or more nodes >6 cm with or without extra-nodal extension was helpful in predicting prognosis or guiding treatment.

Changes were seen in the T and N categories, however T1 remains unchanged.

Unknown Primary Cervical Lymph Nodes

Metastatic cervical cancers of unknown primary (MCCUP) are clinically very common, making up approximately 3-5% of all head and neck squamous cell carcinomas (HNSCCs).[21] Additionally, since a large proportion of cancers drain into cervical lymph nodes, being able to provide a more precise evaluation of cancers should improve the prognosis of patients with MCCUP. Thus, the importance of molecular diagnoses will weigh over a clinical observational diagnosis.

Papillary and Follicular Thyroid Tumors

The definition of T3 was updated for papillary, follicular, and medullary carcinomas.

T3a indicates a tumor >4 cm in the greatest dimension, limited to the thyroid. T3b indicates a tumor of any size with gross extrathyroidal extension which invades infrahyoid muscles.[1]

Additionally, the age for a poor prognosis has changed from 45-years to 55-years-old.[1] Changing the patient age for TNM staging has been shown to improve predictive ability.[20] TNM-8 reduces the staging of 41% of patients, providing a more accurate prediction of survival.[20] Therefore, the improvements seen in TNM-8 have improved patient care.

Esophagus and Gastric Tumors

Esophageal cancers have no changes in T, N, and M definitions. For these cancers, classification and staging uses the Esophageal Cancer TNM and Stage. Other cancers within this area use the Stomach Cancer TNM and Stage, even with involvement of the esophagogastric junction.

TNM-8 has redefined the gastroesophageal junction. Esophageal cancers are defined as cancers located at the center of the gastroesophageal junction, within the first two centimeters of the proximal stomach.[26]

Colon, Appendix, Rectum, and Anal Tumors

TNM-8 defines tumor deposits including the presence of venous invasion (V1, V2), lymphatic invasion (L1), or perineural invasion (Pn1) for colon, rectum, and appendiceal cancers. TNM-8 staging of appendiceal tumors excluded intraepithelial carcinoma from Tis[22] - low-grade appendiceal mucinous neoplasms (LAMN).

Anal Cancer Carcinoma is also modified within TNM-8. The N2 and N3 categories were abolished within the N category. In TNM-7, N2 was defined as metastasis to the unilateral internal iliac node with or without metastasis to the inguinal lymph node. N3 was defined as metastasis to the perirectal node as well as the inguinal lymph nodes with or without involvement of the bilateral internal iliac nodes and with or without involvement of the inguinal lymph nodes.[23] Tumors of perianal skin that are within 5 cm of the anal margin are also considered anal cancer carcinomas.[22] Originally in TNM-7, the anal verge was the boundary between the squamous mucosa and perianal skin.[23] Therefore, a tumor within the skin or distal to the mucosa is considered a perianal cancer.[23]

Liver

In TNM-8, the definitions of tumor and lymph node involvement have been updated within areas including (1) gastrointestinal-neuroendocrine tumors, (2) perihilar, intrahepatic, and distal extrahepatic bile duct tumors, (3) Ampulla of Vater tumors, and (4) gallbladder tumors. Within TNM-8, the definition for a primary tumor has changed for T1, which is now divided into T1a where the tumor is solitary and ≤2 cm, and T1b where the tumor is solitary and >2 cm without vascular invasion.[1] T2 is now defined as a solitary tumor >2 cm with vascular invasion, or multiple tumors with no single tumor being >5 cm.[1] Finally, T3a is now T3, and T3b has become T4, with T4 being a tumor containing a major portal vein or hepatic vein branch.[1]

Breast

The TNM panel felt that the tumor staging system should continue to be founded upon anatomic factors to maintain global relevancy. However, TNM-8 expands on the previous anatomical-based classifications of breast cancer by offering the flexibility to incorporate these biological factors into the staging system. These biomarkers include tumor grade, estrogen and progesterone receptor expression, and human epidermal growth factor 2 (HER2) expression, all of which were recently recognized to have great prognostic ability.[27,28,29]

Prognostic Factor Grids

TNM-8 also offers prognostic factor grids for each of the cancers discussed.[22]

Table 3. TNM-8 Prognostic Factor Grids for the Most Common Cancers in General Surgery

	Factor Impacting Prognosis		
	Tumor	Host	Environment
Papillary and Follicular Thyroid	Essential: T category - extension into extra-thyroid region. M category - Thyroglobulin post treatment.	Age	Any residual disease
Medullary	Essential: pre- and post-op calcitonin	Age	Amount of total resection
Stomach	Essential: the HER2 status within the T, N, and M categories.		Any residual disease
Biliary Tract	Essential: if tumor is resectable	Status of ECOG	Any residual disease
Soft Tissue	Essential: whether the size of the tumor is < or >5 cm. The location of the tumor anatomically. The type of histology for the tumor. How deeply the tumor has invaded. Mitotic rate of the tumor for GIST.		
Colon and rectum	Essential: T, N, and M categories with M category denoting circumferential margin around the rectal cancer	Age	Screening program
Breast	Essential: margin of surgical resection. Whether the tumor has vascular or lymphatic invasion. Histological grading of the ER HER2 receptor.	Status of menopause and age	Previous exposure to radiation toward the mediastinum or chest

Overview and Summary

With every iteration of the TNM classification system, there are advancements in the predictive capabilities across the malignancies described in the system. Providing accurate information on the progression of a malignancy is essential for planning the aggressiveness of treatment. The TNM system itself provides a standardized method of communicating cancer across specialties and physicians, and with this standardization, there is more opportunity for discourse amongst treatment options at every level of cancer progression. This standardization based on the predictive capabilities of the TNMs will push forward the treatment of these malignancies and procure changes in their classification. The staging and definitions of each TNM classification system for a malignancy will constantly change over time to reflect a more scientifically predictive system for each cancer outcome; however, this change over time will only push the capabilities of the TNM classification system forward.

REFERENCES

1. Brierley J, Gospodarowicz MK, Wittekind C. *TNM Classification of Malignant Tumours*. Chichester, West Sussex, UK: John Wiley & Sons, Inc.; 2017.
2. Reid TD, Sanyaolu LN, Chan D, Williams GT, Lewis WG. Relative prognostic value of TNM7 vs TNM6 in staging oesophageal cancer. *Br J Cancer*. 2011;105(6):842-846. doi:10.1038/bjc.2011.320.
3. TNM8: Changes from TNM7. Share and Discover Knowledge on SlideShare. https://www.slideshare.net/MauricioLema/tnm8-changes-from-tnm7. Published 2017.
4. Denaro N, Russi EG, Merlano MC. Pros and Cons of the New Edition of TNM Classification of Head and Neck Squamous Cell Carcinoma. *Oncology*. 2018;95(4):202-210. doi:10.1159/000490415.
5. Prat J; FIGO Committee on Gynecologic Oncology. Staging classification for cancer of the ovary, fallopian tube, and peritoneum. Int J Gynaecol Obstet. 2014 Jan;124(1):1-5. doi: 10.1016/j.ijgo.2013.10.001. Epub 2013 Oct 22. PMID: 24219974.
6. Cheson BD, Fisher RI, Barrington SF, et al. Recommendations for initial evaluation, staging, and response assessment of Hodgkin and non-Hodgkin lymphoma: the Lugano classification. J Clin Oncol. 2014;32: 3059-3068.
7. Feng SH, Yang ST. The new 8th TNM staging system of lung cancer and its potential imaging interpretation pitfalls and limitations with CT image demonstrations. *Diagn Interv Radiol*. 2019;25(4):270-279. doi:10.5152/dir.2019.18458.
8. Egevad L, Cheville J, Evans AJ, et al. Pathology Imagebase-a reference image database for standardization of pathology. *Histopathology*. 2017;71(5):677-685. doi:10.1111/his.13313.
9. Chaturvedi AK, Engels EA, Pfeiffer RM, et al. Human papillomavirus and rising oropharyngeal cancer incidence in the United States. J Clin Oncol. 2011;29(32):4294-4301. doi:10.1200/JCO.2011.36.4596.
10. Sedghizadeh PP, Billington WD, Paxton D, et al. Is p16-positive oropharyngeal squamous cell carcinoma associated with favorable prognosis? A systematic review and meta-analysis. Oral Oncol. 2016;54:15-27. doi:10.1016/j.oraloncology.2016.01.002.
11. Gillison ML, Koch WM, Capone RB, et al. Evidence for a causal association between human papillomavirus and a subset of head and neck cancers. J Natl Cancer Inst. 2000;92(9):709-720. doi:10.1093/jnci/92.9.709.
12. Serrano M. The tumor suppressor protein p16INK4a. Exp Cell Res. 1997;237(1):7-13. doi:10.1006/excr.1997.3824.
13. Augustin JG, Lepine C, Morini A, et al. HPV Detection in Head and Neck Squamous Cell Carcinomas: What Is the Issue?. Front Oncol. 2020;10:1751. Published 2020 Sep 15. doi:10.3389/fonc.2020.01751.
14. McLaughlin-Drubin ME, Crum CP, Münger K. Human papillomavirus E7 oncoprotein induces KDM6A and KDM6B histone demethylase expression and causes epigenetic reprogramming. Proc Natl Acad Sci U S A. 2011;108(5):2130-2135. doi:10.1073/pnas.1009933108.
15. Nauta IH, Rietbergen MM, van Bokhoven AAJD, et al. Evaluation of the eighth TNM classification on p16-positive oropharyngeal squamous cell carcinomas in the Netherlands and the importance of additional HPV DNA testing. Ann Oncol. 2018;29(5):1273-1279. doi:10.1093/annonc/mdy060.
16. Chatfield-Reed K, Gui S, O'Neill WQ, Teknos TN, Pan Q. HPV33+ HNSCC is associated with poor prognosis and has unique genomic and immunologic landscapes. Oral Oncol. 2020;100:104488. doi:10.1016/j.oraloncology.2019.104488.
17. Sharma SJ, Wagner S, Reder HSF, et al. The 8th edition AJCC/UICC TNM staging for p16-positive oropharyngeal carcinoma: is there space for improvement?. Eur Arch Otorhinolaryngol. 2018;275(12):3087-3091. doi:10.1007/s00405-018-5156-4.
18. Hammarstedt L, Holzhauser S, Zupancic M, et al. The value of p16 and HPV DNA in non-tonsillar, non-base

of tongue oropharyngeal cancer. Acta Otolaryngol. 2021;141(1):89-94. doi:10.1080/00016489.2020.1813906.

19. Huang SH, O'Sullivan B. Overview of the 8th Edition TNM Classification for Head and Neck Cancer. Curr Treat Options Oncol. 2017;18(7):40. doi:10.1007/s11864-017-0484-y.
20. Sapuppo G, Tavarelli M, Pellegriti G. The new AJCC/TNM Staging System (VIII ed.) in papillary thyroid cancer: clinical and molecular impact on overall and recurrence free survival. Ann Transl Med. 2020 Jul;8(13):838. doi: 10.21037/atm.2020.03.80. PMID: 32793683; PMCID: PMC7396237.
21. Ota I, Kitahara T. Cancer of unknown primary in the head and neck: Diagnosis and treatment. *Auris Nasus Larynx*. 2021;48(1):23-31. doi:10.1016/j.anl.2020.08.014.
22. Shida D, Kanemitsu Y, Hamaguchi T, Shimada Y. Introducing the eighth edition of the tumor-node-metastasis classification as relevant to colorectal cancer, anal cancer and appendiceal cancer: a comparison study with the seventh edition of the tumor-node-metastasis and the Japanese Classification of Colorectal, Appendiceal, and Anal Carcinoma. *Jpn J Clin Oncol*. 2019;49(4):321-328. doi:10.1093/jjco/hyy198.
22. Edge SB, Byrd DR, Compton CC, Fritz AG, Greene FL, Trotti A, editors. AJCC cancer staging manual (7th ed). New York, NY: Springer; 2010.
23. Hermanek P, Hutter RV, Sobin LH, Wittekind C. Classification of isolated tumor cells and micrometastasis. *Cancer*. 1999;86(12):2668-2673. doi:10.1002/(sici)1097-0142(19991215)86:12<2668::aid-cncr11>3.0.co;2-r.
24. Johnson DE, Burtness B, Leemans CR, Lui VWY, Bauman JE, Grandis JR. Head and neck squamous cell carcinoma. Nat Rev Dis Primers. 2020;6(1):92. Published 2020 Nov 26. doi:10.1038/s41572-020-00224-3.
25. Marano L, D'Ignazio A, Cammillini F, Angotti R, Messina M, Marrelli D, Roviello F. Comparison between 7th and 8th edition of AJCC TNM staging system for gastric cancer: old problems and new perspectives. Transl Gastroenterol Hepatol. 2019 Apr 3;4:22. doi: 10.21037/tgh.2019.03.09. PMID: 31143843; PMCID: PMC6509428.
26. Giuliano AE, Connolly JL, Edge SB, Mittendorf EA, Rugo HS, Solin LJ, Weaver DL, Winchester DJ, Hortobagyi GN. Breast Cancer-Major changes in the American Joint Committee on Cancer eighth edition cancer staging manual. CA Cancer J Clin. 2017 Jul 8;67(4):290-303. doi: 10.3322/caac.21393. Epub 2017 Mar 14. Erratum in: CA Cancer J Clin. 2017 Jul 8;67(4):345. PMID: 28294295.
27. Kalli S, Semine A, Cohen S, Naber SP, Makim SS, Bahl M. American Joint Committee on Cancer's Staging System for Breast Cancer, Eighth Edition: What the Radiologist Needs to Know. Radiographics. 2018 Nov-Dec;38(7):1921-1933. doi: 10.1148/rg.2018180056. Epub 2018 Sep 28. PMID: 30265613.
28. Chavez-MacGregor M, Mittendorf EA, Clarke CA, Lichtensztajn DY, Hunt KK, Giordano SH. Incorporating Tumor Characteristics to the American Joint Committee on Cancer Breast Cancer Staging System. Oncologist. 2017 Nov;22(11):1292-1300. doi: 10.1634/theoncologist.2017-0116. Epub 2017 Jun 7. PMID: 28592619; PMCID: PMC5679819.
29. Trinh JM, Thomas J, Salleron J, Henrot P. Differences in clinical and imaging characteristics between p16-positive non-smokers and p16-positive smokers or p16-negative patients in oropharyngeal carcinoma. Sci Rep. 2021;11(1):3314. Published 2021 Feb 8. doi:10.1038/s41598-021-82999-3.
30. Spanos WC, Nowicki P, Lee DW, et al. Immune response during therapy with cisplatin or radiation for human papillomavirus-related head and neck cancer. Arch Otolaryngol Head Neck Surg. 2009;135(11):1137-1146. doi:10.1001/archoto.2009.159.
31. Chen AM, Felix C, Wang PC, et al. Reduced-dose radiotherapy for human papillomavirus-associated squamous-cell carcinoma of the oropharynx: a single-arm, phase 2 study. Lancet Oncol. 2017;18(6):803-811. doi:10.1016/S1470-2045(17)30246-2.
32. Clancy K, Hamill CS, O'Neill WQ, et al. Impact of p16 Status and Anatomical Site in Anti-PD-1 Immunotherapy-Treated Recurrent/Metastatic Head and Neck Squamous Cell Carcinoma Patients. Cancers (Basel). 2021;13(19):4861. Published 2021 Sep 28. doi:10.3390/cancers13194861.

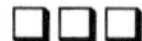